EPILEPSY

PART I

HANDBOOK OF CLINICAL NEUROLOGY

Series Editors

MICHAEL J. AMINOFF, FRANÇOIS BOLLER, AND DICK F. SWAAB

VOLUME 107

ELSEVIER

EDINBURGH LONDON NEW YORK OXFORD PHILADELPHIA
ST LOUIS SYDNEY TORONTO 2012

EPILEPSY

PART I

Series Editors

MICHAEL J. AMINOFF, FRANÇOIS BOLLER, AND DICK F. SWAAB

Volume Editors

HERMANN STEFAN AND WILLIAM H. THEODORE

VOLUME 107

3rd Series

ELSEVIER

EDINBURGH LONDON NEW YORK OXFORD PHILADELPHIA
ST LOUIS SYDNEY TORONTO 2012

ELSEVIER B.V
Radarweg 29, 1043 NX, Amsterdam, The Netherlands

ISBN: 9780444528988

British Library Cataloguing in Publication Data
A catalogue record for this book is available from the British Library

Library of Congress Cataloging in Publication Data
A catalog record for this book is available from the Library of Congress

Notice

Knowledge and best practice in this field are constantly changing. As new research and experience broaden our understanding, changes in research methods, professional practices, or medical treatment may become necessary.

Practitioners and researchers must always rely on their own experience and knowledge in evaluating and using any information, methods, compounds, or experiments described herein. In using such information or methods they should be mindful of their own safety and the safety of others, including parties for whom they have a professional responsibility.

With respect to any drug or pharmaceutical products identified, readers are advised to check the most current information provided (i) on procedures featured or (ii) by the manufacturer of each product to be administered, to verify the recommended dose or formula, the method and duration of administration, and contraindications. It is the responsibility of practitioners, relying on their own experience and knowledge of their patients, to make diagnoses, to determine dosages and the best treatment for each individual patient, and to take all appropriate safety precautions.

To the fullest extent of the law, neither the Publisher nor the contributors or editors, assume any liability for any injury and/or damage to persons or property as a matter of products liability, negligence or otherwise, or from any use or operation of any methods, products, instructions, or ideas contained in the material herein.

The Publisher

Printed and bound by CPI Group (UK) Ltd, Croydon, CR0 4YY

Transferred to digital print 2013

Commissioning Editor: Michael Houston
Development Editor: Michael Parkinson
Project Manager: Annie Victor
Designer: Alan Studholme

The Publisher's policy is to use **paper manufactured from sustainable forests**

Handbook of Clinical Neurology 3rd Series

Available titles

Vol. 79, The human hypothalamus: basic and clinical aspects, Part I, D.F. Swaab, ed. ISBN 9780444513571
Vol. 80, The human hypothalamus: basic and clinical aspects, Part II, D.F. Swaab, ed. ISBN 9780444514905
Vol. 81, Pain, F. Cervero and T.S. Jensen, eds. ISBN 9780444519016
Vol. 82, Motor neurone disorders and related diseases, A.A. Eisen and P.J. Shaw, eds. ISBN 9780444518941
Vol. 83, Parkinson's disease and related disorders, Part I, W.C. Koller and E. Melamed, eds. ISBN 9780444519009
Vol. 84, Parkinson's disease and related disorders, Part II, W.C. Koller and E. Melamed, eds. ISBN 9780444528933
Vol. 85, HIV/AIDS and the nervous system, P. Portegies and J. Berger, eds. ISBN 9780444520104
Vol. 86, Myopathies, F.L. Mastaglia and D. Hilton Jones, eds. ISBN 9780444518996
Vol. 87, Malformations of the nervous system, H.B. Sarnat and P. Curatolo, eds. ISBN 9780444518965
Vol. 88, Neuropsychology and behavioural neurology, G. Goldenberg and B.C. Miller, eds. ISBN 9780444518972
Vol. 89, Dementias, C. Duyckaerts and I. Litvan, eds. ISBN 9780444518989
Vol. 90, Disorders of consciousness, G.B. Young and E.F.M. Wijdicks, eds. ISBN 9780444518958
Vol. 91, Neuromuscular junction disorders, A.G. Engel, ed. ISBN 9780444520081
Vol. 92, Stroke – Part I: Basic and epidemiological aspects, M. Fisher, ed. ISBN 9780444520036
Vol. 93, Stroke – Part II: Clinical manifestations and pathogenesis, M. Fisher, ed. ISBN 9780444520043
Vol. 94, Stroke – Part III: Investigations and management, M. Fisher, ed. ISBN 9780444520050
Vol. 95, History of neurology, S. Finger, F. Boller, and K.L. Tyler, eds. ISBN 9780444520081
Vol. 96, Bacterial infections of the central nervous system, K.L. Roos and A.R. Tunkel, eds. ISBN 9780444520159
Vol. 97, Headache, G. Nappi and M.A. Moskowitz, eds. ISBN 9780444521392
Vol. 98, Sleep disorders, Part I, P. Montagna and S. Chokroverty, eds. ISBN 9780444520067
Vol. 99, Sleep disorders, Part II, P. Montagna and S. Chokroverty, eds. ISBN 9780444520074
Vol. 100, Hyperkinetic movement disorders, W.J. Weiner and E. Tolosa, eds. ISBN 9780444520142
Vol. 101, Muscular dystrophies, A. Amato and R.C. Griggs, eds. ISBN 9780080450315
Vol. 102, Neuro-ophthalmology, C. Kennard and R.J. Leigh, eds. ISBN 9780444529039
Vol. 103, Ataxic disorders, S.H. Subramony and A. Durr, eds. ISBN 9780444518927
Vol. 104, Neuro-oncology, Part I, W. Grisold and R. Sofietti, eds. ISBN 9780444521385
Vol. 105, Neuro-oncology, Part II, W. Grisold and R. Sofietti, eds. ISBN 9780444535023
Vol. 106, Neurobiology of psychiatric disorders, T.E. Schlaepfer and C.B. Nemeroff, eds. ISBN 9780444520029

Foreword

"My friend had it. My mommy told me to stay away from her because I could get it. I'm glad I don't have it."

The response of this fourth-grader to the question "What is epilepsy?" illustrates the paradoxical position of the condition within the field of neurology. On the one hand, epilepsy undoubtedly carries a stigma. This is less profound than in the past, particularly in industrialized countries, but it remains a reality of life for many patients who have experienced seizures. On the other hand, epilepsy is one of the most potentially treatable neurological conditions, especially since the introduction of phenytoin into our armamentarium, thanks to the pioneering work of Merritt and Putman in 1938. Much progress has taken place in the recent past that brings renewed optimism for the future of patients with epilepsy. We are pleased to introduce the present two volumes dedicated to epilepsy, with their emphasis on the most recent developments in the field. There is a new focus on the pathogenesis of the disease and on experimental models, including animal models. New neurophysiological and imaging techniques are presented. Fresh and considerable attention is given to clinical aspects of the various forms of epilepsy. Finally there is extensive coverage of the management of epilepsy and of new therapeutic strategies, including brain stimulation and other innovative techniques.

The two volumes have been edited by Hermann Stefan and William H. Theodore. As series editors, we reviewed all of the chapters in the volumes and made suggestions for improvement, but we are delighted that the volume editors and chapter authors produced such scholarly and comprehensive accounts of the different aspects of epilepsy. Hence we hope that the two volumes will appeal to clinicians and neuroscientists alike. The very significant advances presented in the two volumes lead to new insights that demand critical appraisal. Our goal is to provide basic researchers with the foundations for new approaches to the study of these disorders, and clinicians with a state-of-the-art reference that summarizes the clinical features and management of the many neurological manifestations of epilepsy. In addition to the print form, the *Handbook* series is now available electronically on Elsevier's ScienceDirect site. This should make it even more accessible to readers and should facilitate searches for specific information.

We are grateful to the volume editors and to the numerous authors who contributed their time and expertise to summarize developments in their field and helped put together these outstanding volumes. As always, we are grateful also to the team at Elsevier and in particular to Mr. Michael Parkinson, Ms. Susan Jansons, and Mr. Michael Houston, for their unfailing and expert assistance in the development and production of these two volumes.

Michael J. Aminoff
François Boller
Dick F. Swaab

Preface

The *Handbook of Clinical Neurology* has a long and distinguished history. It was an honour to be asked to edit the new volumes on epilepsy, and a challenge we can never be certain we have met.

Study of the epilepsies has been complicated by the fleeting nature of individual seizures, rarely observed by physicians who, until the advent of video-EEG, had to rely on the descriptions of patients or other observers. Moreover, seizures vary widely in their clinical manifestations and are not always recognized, even by patients themselves. They can be confused with a wide range of nonepileptic events. Epilepsy is not a single pathophysiological entity, but may be due to a bewilderingly complex array of neurological and systemic disorders, demanding differing diagnostic and treatment strategies.

Epilepsy was recognized as a brain disorder very early in recorded medical history. The writer of the Hippocratic treatise "On the Sacred Disease" regarded epilepsy as no more divine or sacred than any other illness, attributing seizures to excess accumulation of phlegm in hepatic vein branches reaching the brain, cutting off air circulation. Unfortunately, later classical and medieval writers tended to ignore Hippocrates and resurrected earlier "pathophysiological" concepts. Attribution of epilepsy to supernatural origin is still common, and patients thought guilty of ritual transgression are sometimes judged to deserve their suffering. Even in the developed world, prejudice still creates barriers to education, employment, and marriage, as well as medical care itself, as patients and their families may be unwilling to reveal the illness. An association with psychiatric illness in the 19th and early 20th centuries may have helped to reinforce prejudice by association with another stigmatized patient group. In the 1927 edition of Cecil's *Textbook of Medicine*, the "frank epileptic" is described as a "constitutional psychopath of the most disagreeable sort." Ironically, while the divergence between neurology and psychiatry later in the 20th century helped to free epilepsy from the taint of mental illness, it may have led to underappreciation of the importance of comorbidities, particularly depression and anxiety, now increasingly recognized but still undertreated.

Epilepsy is attracting increasing attention as a worldwide disease, and the Global Campaign sponsored jointly by the World Health Organization, the International League Against Epilepsy (ILAE), and the International Bureau for Epilepsy, has drawn attention to the "treatment gap" (as many as 90% of patients may receive no treatment in some developing regions), and has sponsored demonstration projects to show the value of coordinated epilepsy ascertainment and treatment programs. International travel and migration have brought major causes of epilepsy such as cysticercosis to the entire world.

Concepts of successful treatment are evolving, with recognition that good quality of life for people with epilepsy depends on freedom from both seizures and treatment side-effects. Earlier screening to diagnose and localize focal epilepsies, and a lower surgical threshold in children, are thought by many investigators to improve the chance of avoiding the psychosocial problems suffered by patients with uncontrolled seizures extending through adolescence and into adult life. The ILAE has recently published a new rubric for drug treatment outcome that incorporates these developments.

Great progress has been made in the diagnosis and treatment of epilepsy over the past 50 years. Techniques of evaluation, including video-EEG monitoring, structural and functional neuroimaging, genetic testing, invasive EEG recording, and magnetoencephalography, have paralleled a burgeoning variety of antiepileptic drugs, improved surgical techniques, and brain stimulation approaches. Nevertheless, a substantial proportion of patients continue to have seizures. Moreover, old concepts of adequate seizure control have given way to the realization that good quality of life depends on complete seizure freedom, as well as minimal antiepileptic drug toxicity. In addition, new data suggest that patients do not recognize up to 60% of their seizures, with implications for a wide range of comorbidities including sudden unexplained death. Despite dramatically improved understanding of pathophysiological mechanisms, based on animal models and clinical studies, and a wide range of "new" antiepileptic drugs, a "cure" for epilepsy seems as far away as ever.

One reason may be that drug development is still based on models that may lead to a plethora of "me too" compounds; agents with presumably novel mechanisms, however, are no more effective for seizure control than phenytoin or phenobarbital, although they may have fewer – or at least different – side-effects. New attention is being given to examining relatively neglected aspects of epilepsy pathophysiology, such as inflammation, and underlying causes, such as viruses. It is possible that future antiepileptogenic, in contrast to antiseizure, treatments may emerge. In addition, several new treatment approaches involving brain stimulation are under investigation.

Epilepsy therapeutics shares obstacles to drug development with other brain disorders. Costs and failure rates for clinical trials are higher, and perceived markets less profitable. Future therapeutic advances may depend on public–private partnerships, involvement of "third-party" payers such as insurance companies, or other innovative funding models. Cost pressures are driving practice in other arenas, including the vexed issue of generic drugs, and potential substitution of suppliers without warning to physicians or patients. The true extent and impact of this issue is uncertain.

A positive trend is the increasing recognition of epilepsy as a distinct subspecialty of neurology, and the development of fellowships for additional postresidency training. Specialized comprehensive epilepsy centers are becoming more common, and the general neurology community is recognizing their importance in the care of patients with refractory seizures.

We hope that these two volumes will provide a manageable overview of current basic and clinical aspects of epilepsy for neurologists in active clinical practice, as well as for academic investigators and students. We would like to thank all the contributors, and the general editors, Drs Michael Aminoff, François Boller, and Dick Swaab, as well as Mr. Michael Parkinson of Elsevier, for their support and encouragement.

Hermann Stefan
William H. Theodore

Contributors

B. Abou-Khalil
Epilepsy Division, Department of Neurology, Vanderbilt University Medical Center, Nashville, TN, USA

R. Badawy
Department of Neurology, Austin Health, Heidelberg; Department of Medicine, University of Melbourne, Melbourne; and Brain Research Institute, Florey Neuroscience Institutes, Heidelberg West, Victoria, Australia

S. Balosso
Laboratory of Experimental Neurology, Department of Neuroscience, Mario Negri Institute for Pharmacological Research, Milan, Italy

S. Bauer
Interdisciplinary Epilepsy Center, Department of Neurology, UKGM Marburg, Philipps University, Marburg, Germany

A.T. Berg
Epilepsy Center, Children's Memorial Hospital, Chicago, IL, USA

M.M. Berl
Center for Neuroscience, Children's National Medical Center, Washington, DC, USA

E.H. Bertram
F.E. Dreifuss Comprehensive Epilepsy Program, Department of Neurology, University of Virginia, Charlottesville, VA, USA

H.T. Chugani
Departments of Pediatrics and Neurology, School of Medicine, Wayne State University, Children's Hospital of Michigan, Detroit, MI, USA

A. Coppola
Saul R. Korey Department of Neurology, Dominick P. Purpura Department of Neuroscience, and Department of Pediatrics, Albert Einstein College of Medicine and Montefiore Medical Center, Bronx, NY, USA, and Epilepsy Center, Department of Neurology, Federico II University, Naples, Italy

J.H. Cross
Neurosciences Unit, UCL Institute of Child Health, Great Ormond Street Hospital for Children and National Centre for Young People with Epilepsy, London, UK

O. Devinsky
Comprehensive Epilepsy Center, Institute of Neurology and Neurosurgery at St. Barnabas, Livingston, NJ, and Comprehensive Epilepsy Center, NYU Langone School of Medicine, New York, NY, USA

A. Dörfler
Department of Neuroradiology, University Hospital of Erlangen, Friedrich Alexander University Erlangen-Nürnberg, Erlangen, Germany

O. Dulac
Department of Pediatric Neurology, APHP Necker-Enfants Malades, UMR663, Paris, France

B.A. Engelsen
Epilepsy Unit, Institute of Clinical Medicine, University of Bergen, and Department of Neurology, Haukeland University Hospital, Bergen, Norway

W.D. Gaillard
Center for Neuroscience, Children's National Medical Center, Washington, DC, and Clinical Epilepsy Section, National Institute of Neurological Disease and Stroke, National Institutes of Health, Bethesda, MD, USA

A. Gil-Nagel
Epilepsy Program, Department of Neurology, Hospital Ruber Internacional, Madrid, Spain

J. Gotman
Brain Imaging Center, Montreal Neurological Institute, McGill University, Montreal, Quebec, Canada

J.A. Gorter
Center for NeuroScience, Swammerdam Institute for Life Sciences, University of Amsterdam, Amsterdam, The Netherlands

R. Guerrini
Department of Neuroscience, Pediatric Neurology Unit and Laboratories, Children's Hospital A. Meyer, University of Florence, Florence, Italy

P. Halász
Department of Neurology, National Institute of Neuroscience, Budapest, Hungary

H.M. Hamer
Epilepsy Center, Department of Neurology, University Hospital Erlangen, Erlangen, Germany

T. Hammen
Neurological Clinic, University Hospital, Erlangen, Germany

W.A. Hauser
Department of Neurology, College of Physicians and Surgeons, and Mailman School of Public Health, Columbia University, New York, NY, USA

C. Helmstaedter
Department of Epileptology, University Clinic of Epileptology, Bonn, Germany

D.C. Hesdorffer
Gertrude H. Sergievsky Center, Department of Epidemiology, Columbia University, New York, NY, USA

E. Hirsch
Department of Neurology, University Hospitals of Strasbourg, Strasbourg, France

G.L. Holmes
Department of Neurology, Dartmouth Medical School, Lebanon, NH, USA

R. Kälviäinen
Department of Neurology, Kuopio Epilepsy Center, Kuopio University Hospital, Kuopio, Finland

A.M. Kanner
Department of Neurological Sciences, Rush Medical College at Rush University, Chicago, IL, USA

A. Kao
Division of Neurophysiology, Epilepsy, and Critical Care, Center for Neuroscience and Behavioral Medicine, Children's National Medical Center, Washington, DC, USA

M. Koepp
Department of Clinical and Experimental Epilepsy, UCL Institute of Neurology, London, UK

A. Kumar
Departments of Pediatrics and Neurology, School of Medicine, Wayne State University, Children's Hospital of Michigan, Detroit, MI, USA

R. Kuzniecky
NYU Epilepsy Center, Department of Neurology, New York University School of Medicine, New York, NY, USA

G.D. Jackson
Department of Neurology, Austin Health, Heidelberg; Department of Medicine, University of Melbourne, Melbourne; and Brain Research Institute, Florey Neuroscience Institutes, Heidelberg West, Victoria, Australia

T. Loddenkemper
Pediatric Neurology Center, Department of Neurology, Cleveland Clinic, Cleveland, OH, USA, and Division of Epilepsy and Clinical Neurophysiology, Children's Hospital Boston, Boston, MA, USA

F.H. Lopes Da Silva
Center for NeuroScience, Swammerdam Institute for Life Sciences, University of Amsterdam, Amsterdam, The Netherlands

K. Lukasiuk
Department of Molecular and Cellular Neurobiology, The Nencki Institute of Experimental Biology, Polish Academy of Sciences, Warsaw, Poland

M.D.M. Milh
Department of Pediatric Neurology, APHM La Timone, INMED, Marseilles, France

S.L. Moshé
Saul R. Korey Department of Neurology, Dominick P. Purpura Department of Neuroscience, and Department of Pediatrics, Albert Einstein College of Medicine and Montefiore Medical Center, Bronx, NY, USA

B. Mostacci
IRCCS Istituto delle Scienze Neurologiche, University of Bologna, Bologna, Italy

N. Nakasato
Department of Neurosurgery, Kohnan Hospital and Tohoku University, Sendai, Japan

A. Neligan
Department of Clinical and Experimental Epilepsy, UCL Institute of Neurology, London, UK

T.J. O'Brien
Department of Medicine, University of Melbourne, Melbourne, Victoria, Australia

A.C. Papanicolaou
Department of Pediatrics, University of Tennessee, Memphis, TN, USA

J.M. Pellock
Division of Child Neurology, Department of Neurology, Virginia Commonwealth University, Richmond, VA, USA

A. Pitkänen
A.I. Virtanen Institute for Molecular Sciences, University of Eastern Finland, and Department of Neurology, Kuopio University Hospital, Kuopio, Finland

J.J. Poza
Department of Neurology, Hospital Donostia, San Sebastián, Spain

P.M. Rao
Division of Child Neurology, Center for Neuroscience and Behavioral Medicine, Children's National Medical Center, Washington, DC, USA

T. Ravizza
Laboratory of Experimental Neurology, Department of Neuroscience, Mario Negri Institute for Pharmacological Research, Milan, Italy

J.W. Sander
SEIN—Epilepsy Institute in the Netherlands Foundation, Heemstede, The Netherlands

P.A. Schwartzkroin
Department of Neurological Surgery, University of California–Davis, Davis, CA, USA

F. Semah
Department of Nuclear Medicine, University Hospital of Lille, Lille, France

E.L. So
Department of Neurology, Mayo Clinic, Rochester, MN, USA

H. Stefan
Epilepsy Center, Neurology Clinic, Erlangen University Hospital, Erlangen, Germany

O.K. Steinlein
Institute of Human Genetics, School of Medicine, Ludwig-Maximilians University of Munich, Munich, Germany

W.H. Theodore
Clinical Epilepsy Section, National Institute of Neurological Disease and Stroke, National Institutes of Health, Bethesda, MD, USA

M. Thom
Institute of Neurology, National Hospital for Neurology and Neurosurgery, University College London, London, UK

P. Tinuper
IRCCS Istituto delle Scienze Neurologiche, University of Bologna, Bologna, Italy

A. Vezzani
Laboratory of Experimental Neurology, Department of Neuroscience, Mario Negri Institute for Pharmacological Research, Milan, Italy

W.J. Wadman
Center for NeuroScience, Swammerdam Institute for Life Sciences, University of Amsterdam, Amsterdam, The Netherlands

P. Widdess-Walsh
Comprehensive Epilepsy Center, Institute of Neurology and Neurosurgery at St. Barnabas, Livingston, NJ, and NYU Langone School of Medicine, New York, NY, USA

J.-A. Witt
Department of Epileptology, University Clinic of Epileptology, Bonn, Germany

P. Wolf
Danish Epilepsy Center Filadelfia, Department of Clinical Neurophysiology, Dianalund, Denmark

E. Wyllie
Pediatric Neurology Center, Department of Neurology, Cleveland Clinic, Cleveland, OH, USA

Contents of Part I

Contents of Part II

Section 1

Basic mechanisms

Handbook of Clinical Neurology, Vol. 107 (3rd series)
Epilepsy, Part I
H. Stefan and W.H. Theodore, Editors

Chapter 1

Molecular basis of acquired epileptogenesis

KATARZYNA LUKASIUK [1]* AND ASLA PITKÄNEN [2]

[1]*Department of Molecular and Cellular Neurobiology, The Nencki Institute of Experimental Biology, Polish Academy of Sciences, Warsaw, Poland*

[2]*A.I. Virtanen Institute for Molecular Sciences, University of Eastern Finland and Department of Neurology, Kuopio University Hospital, Kuopio, Finland*

INTRODUCTION

Epilepsy is one of the most common neurological diseases, affecting approximately 1% of the population (Porter, 1993). In the majority of cases, the cause of epilepsy is not identified. In about 30% of cases when the etiology of epilepsy is known, the most common causes are stroke (9.3%), trauma (8.8%), alcohol (5.8%), neurodegenerative diseases (4%), and infection (2.2%) (Banerjee and Hauser, 2008). In acquired epilepsies, the initial brain-damaging insult leads to cellular and molecular alterations that eventually culminate in spontaneous recurrent seizures (epilepsy). The latency period between the initial insult and the appearance of spontaneous seizures is called epileptogenesis. During epileptogenesis a number of molecular and cellular changes occur, including neurodegeneration, neurogenesis, axonal sprouting, axonal injury, glial cell activation, invasion of peripheral inflammatory cells, vascular damage and angiogenesis, changes in the extracellular matrix, and alterations in the molecular structure of cellular components, such as ligand and receptor-gated ion channels (for review, see Pitkanen and Lukasiuk, 2009). Epileptogenesis can take months or even years, and epilepsy typically persists for the rest of the person's life (Pitkanen and Sutula, 2002).

Many previous studies have shown that antiepileptic drugs (AEDs) that have been designed to prevent or alleviate the symptoms of the disease, that is seizures, have no beneficial effects on epileptogenesis (Temkin, 2009). To identify a roadmap for antiepileptogenesis, an understanding of the molecular events occurring during epileptogenesis and epilepsy is critical. For this purpose, the recent developments in molecular biology and bioinformatics have provided us with useful tools to address the challenge. One of the quickly expanding fields in epilepsy research is transcriptomics, which applies large-scale transcriptome profiling methods such as SAGE (serial analysis of gene expression) or microarrays in tissue analysis. Data from these studies have provided information about gene expression and the regulation of gene expression at the level of whole transcriptome (set of whole expressed mRNAs) (Diaz, 2009). These data show changes in the expression of several hundreds of genes during epileptogenesis or epilepsy (for review, see Lukasiuk et al., 2006). The next challenge is to translate these data into meaningful information about the molecular pathways critical for the development of epilepsy, and to translate this knowledge into therapies that favorably modify the epileptogenic process.

For this review we have summarized information available in the literature regarding genes changing expression level during status epilepticus (SE)-induced epileptogenesis and epilepsy, where most of the epileptogenesis related data come from. Separate gene lists were created for: (i) early effect of SE (up to 24 h), (ii) epileptogenesis, and (iii) epilepsy, including human data. Lists contain genes detected with *in situ* hybridization, polymerase chain reaction (PCR), northern blot, or other traditional methods used for evaluating gene expression, as well as genes detected with microarrays and validated with other methods, or genes detected by at least two independent microarray experiments. Subsequently, gene lists were subjected to bioinformatics analysis to detect the most common functional groups of genes. DAVID® software (http://david.abcc.ncifcrf.gov; Dennis et al., 2003; Huang et al., 2009) was used to detect GO terms (Gene Ontology terms) (http://www.geneontology.org) and KEGG pathways (Kyoto Encyclopedia of Genes

*Correspondence to: Dr. Katarzyna Lukasiuk, The Nencki Institute of Experimental Biology, Polish Academy of Sciences, 3 Pasteur Street, 02-093 Warsaw, Poland. Tel: +48 22 5892 434, Fax: +48 22 8225342, E-mail: k.lukasiuk@nencki.gov.pl

Table 1.1

Kyoto Encyclopedia of Genes and Genomes (KEGG) pathways (http://www.kegg.com/kegg/pathway.html) overrepresented in lists of genes regulated during status epilepticus, epileptogenesis, or epilepsy

Acute (up to 24 h) effect of SE	Epileptogenesis	Epilepsy
Neuroactive ligand–receptor interaction	Complement and coagulation cascades	Long-term potentiation
Complement and coagulation cascades	Neuroactive ligand–receptor interaction	Neuroactive ligand–receptor interaction
Alzheimer's disease	Alzheimer's disease	Calcium signaling pathway
Long-term potentiation	Long-term potentiation	

Gene lists were constructed on the basis of extensive literature search including genes present in at least two different microarray data sets. The conditions included are acute effect of status epilepticus (SE), epileptogenesis, or epilepsy. To detect overrepresented metabolic pathways, the genes were mapped to KEGG pathways using DAVID® software (Dennis et al., 2003; Huang et al., 2009). Only KEGG pathways with $p < 0.05$ with Bonferroni correction are presented. Genes belonging to the pathways are presented in Figures 1.1–1.4.

and Genomes Pathways Database http://www.kegg.com/kegg/pathway.html) (Kanehisa and Goto, 2000) to detect pathways that were significantly enriched in different published gene lists. Data are summarized in Table 1.1 (KEGG pathways) and Table 1.2 (GO terms). These analyses allow us to make some conclusions and generalizations about the most prevalent phenomena occurring during epileptogenesis and epilepsy, and can be used to create hypotheses regarding molecular mechanisms of the disease process.

WHICH GENES ARE ALTERED AT DIFFERENT PHASES OF EPILEPTIC PROCESS AND WHAT IS THEIR FUNCTION?

A summary of molecular changes is provided in Table 1.1 (KEGG pathways) and Table 1.2 (GO terms). We will focus on the two most prominent groups of genes that were found to be altered in both analyses, and give more details about the results in Figures 1.1–1.4.

Synaptic transmission and ion transport

Three of the metabolic pathways detected in our KEGG pathways analysis are related to synaptic function and plasticity, indicating the particular importance of these pathways in the pathogenesis of epilepsy (see Table 1.1). These pathways are: neuroactive ligand–receptor interaction (Fig. 1.1), long-term potentiation (Fig. 1.2), and calcium signaling (Fig. 1.3). These pathways substantially overlap with one another, and contain genes involved in synaptic transmission such as neurotransmitter receptors, ion channels, receptors for neuromodulators as well as molecules responsible for intracellular signaling involved in information processing of external stimuli. To identify individual genes, see the legends to Figures 1.1–1.3. The data obtained from KEGG pathways has many similarities to that revealed by analysis of GO terms in Gene Ontology database.

Analysis of the GO terms describing the biological functions indicated a clear pattern of gene expression in all three conditions studied, that is, acute SE, epileptogenesis, and epilepsy (see Table 1.2). In line with data from KEGG analysis, the two most overrepresented GO terms were synaptic transmission and ion transport. Gene sets represented by these two GO terms overlap substantially. Several remaining GO terms, such as ion transport, metal ion transport, monovalent, divalent and trivalent inorganic cation transport, and cation transport, are, in fact, fractions of ion transport GO term.

What are the individual genes behind these two GO terms? Genes altered by SE, epileptogenesis, or epilepsy within ion transport GO term contain neurotransmitter receptors, as well as calcium, potassium, and sodium channels, neuromodulators, and ion homeostasis regulators. The synaptic transmission GO term contains similar genes supplemented with others influencing neuromodulators of synaptic plasticity (prodynorphin, tumor necrosis factor, corticotropin-releasing hormone), structural proteins (Homer, synaptotagmin), or enzymes (nitric oxide synthase, glutamate decarboxylase, palmitoyl-protein thioesterase).

Obviously, alterations in the expression of genes coding neurotransmitters, neuromodulators, and their receptors will influence the electrophysiological properties of neurons and/or glia, and will therefore result in changes in network excitability, potentially leading to seizure expression. In fact, many such changes have been described. For example, changes in mRNA expression for selected $GABA_A$ receptor subunits have been reported during epileptogenesis induced by kainic acid (Nishimura et al., 2005), pilocarpine, or electrically induced status epilepticus (Nishimura et al., 2005), as well as after kindling (Clark et al., 1994). As γ-aminobutyric acid type A ($GABA_A$) receptor properties depend on subunit composition (von Blankenfeld et al., 1990; Luddens and Wisden, 1991), altered expression of its receptor subunits will result in functional abnormalities. Changes in expression of mRNAs encoding metabotropic $GABA_B$ receptors have been observed during epileptogenesis resulting from SE

Table 1.2

Biological process GO terms overrepresented in lists of genes regulated by status epilepticus, during epileptogenesis, or in epilepsy

Acute (up to 24 h) effect of epileptogenic stimulus	Epileptogenesis	Epilepsy
Synaptic transmission	Ion transport	Synaptic transmission
Ion transport	Synaptic transmission	Ion transport
Inflammatory response	Inflammatory response	Metal ion transport
Apoptosis/programmed cell death	Acute inflammatory response	Divalent and trivalent inorganic cation transport
Metal ion transport	Complement activation	Cation transport
Cell development	Metal ion transport	Regulation of neurotransmitter levels
Acute inflammatory response	Humoral immune response mediated by circulating immunoglobulin	Glutamate signaling pathway
Cation transport	Adaptive immune response	Memory
Complement activation	Activation of immune response	Cell development
Glutamate signaling pathway	Cation transport	
Adaptive immune response	B cell-mediated immunity	
Cell surface receptor-linked signal transductionx	Leukocyte-mediated immunity	
Humoral immune response	Lymphocyte-mediated immunity	
Activation of immune response	Proteolysis	
Leukocyte-mediated immunity	Regulation of cell proliferation	
Blood circulation	Glutamate signaling pathway	
B cell-mediated immunity	Blood circulation	
Cellular ion homeostasis	Cell development	
	Monovalent inorganic cation transport	
	Divalent and trivalent inorganic cation transport	

Gene lists were constructed on the basis of extensive literature search, including genes that are present in at least two microarray data sets. Then, gene lists with altered expression level after status epilepticus, during epileptogenesis, or epilepsy were analyzed using DAVID® (Dennis et al., 2003; Huang et al., 2009) to detect biological process GO terms overrepresented in comparison to whole genome. Only GO terms with $p < 0.05$ with Bonferroni correction are presented. In each column, the GO terms are presented in order of increasing p value (the most significant one is first).

induced with kainic acid (Furtinger et al., 2003) or electrical stimulation (Nishimura et al., 2005).

Glutamate, the major excitatory neurotransmitter in the brain, acts on ionotropic (AMPA (α-amino-3-hydroxy-5-methyl-4-isoxazolepropionic acid), kainate, and NMDA (*N*-methyl-D-aspartate) receptors) and metabotropic receptors (Dingledine et al., 1999). Alterations in expression of several glutamate-gated receptors have been described. Expression of subunits of AMPA receptors can be affected by kindling (Kamphuis et al., 1994) or seizures induced by an electrolytic hilar lesion (Gold et al., 1996). Interestingly, the effect on various splice variants can be differentiated (Lason et al., 1998). Alterations in the expression of subunits of kainate receptors were observed during epileptogenesis induced by kainic acid-induced SE (Ullal et al., 2005), and hippocampal or amygdala kindling (Kamphuis et al., 1995). In addition, expression of NMDA receptor 1 (NMDAR1) can be influenced by different kindling stimuli (Lason et al., 1998). There is much less information about the expression of metabotropic glutamate receptors (mGluR) in epilepsy, but kindling has been shown to induce a transient decrease in mGluR5 and an increase in mGluR1 (Akbar et al., 1996). Increase in the mGluR1 subunit was also observed following SE after intraperitoneal kainate injection (Blumcke et al., 2000).

Finally, expression of genes coding for potassium channels (Su et al., 2008), sodium channels (Aronica et al., 2001; Ellerkmann et al., 2003), calcium channels (Vigues et al., 1999), and hyperpolarization-activated cyclic nucleotide-gated cation channels (Hendriksen et al., 1997) can be regulated during epileptogenesis.

As already mentioned, not only ion channels and receptors but also other molecules, such as peptide neurotransmitters, growth factors, and other

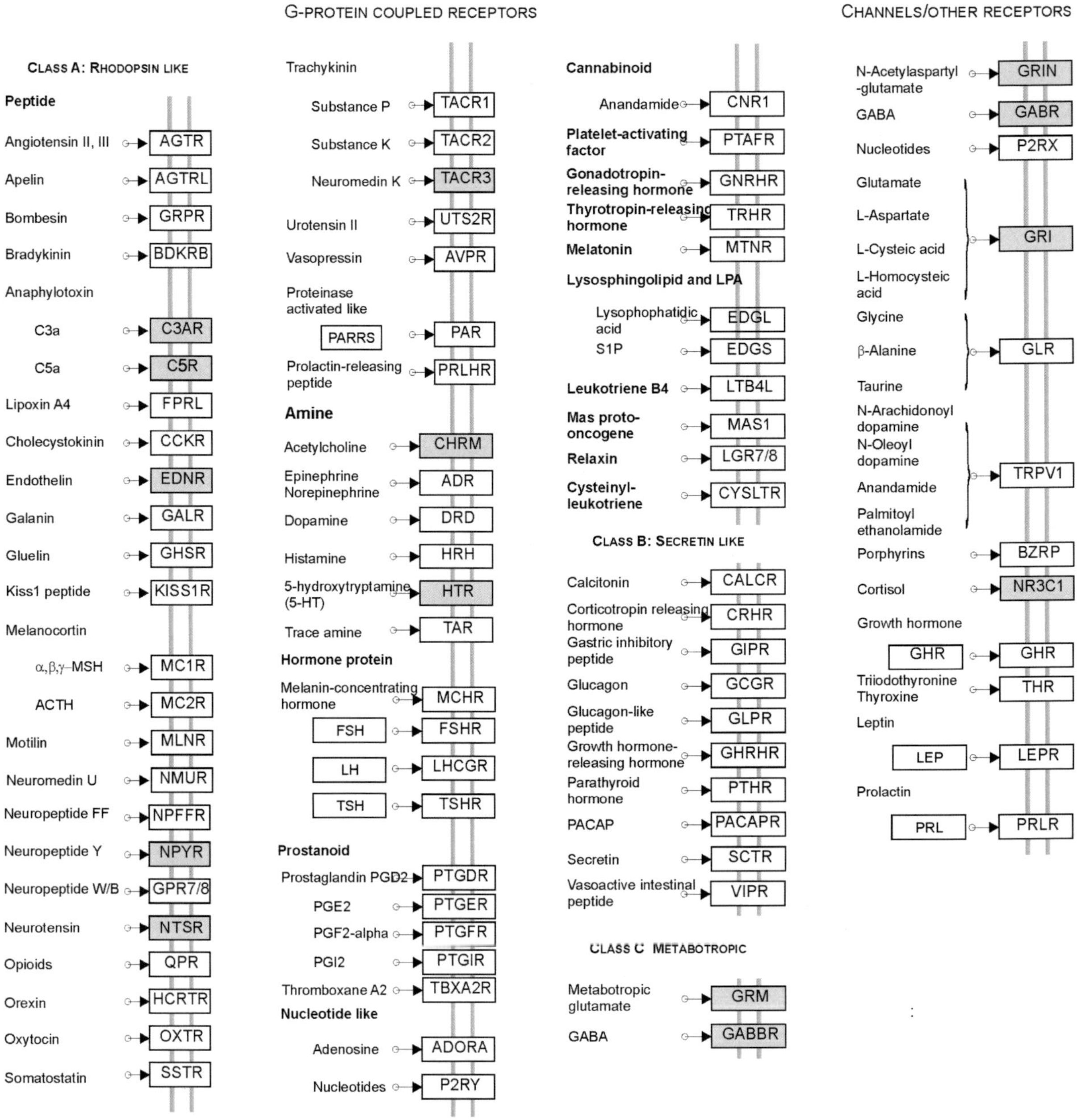

Fig. 1.1. Neuroactive ligand–receptor interaction pathway in epileptogenesis and epilepsy, as predefined by KEGG (Kyoto Encyclopedia of Genes and Genomes; http://www.kegg.com/kegg/pathway/hsa/hsa04080.html) (Kanehisa and Goto, 2000). This pathway summarizes all membrane receptors that can influence neuronal excitability. These receptors are represented by rectangles with name of the receptor protein inside. The ligands are listed on the left side and connected by arrows to rectangles symbolizing their receptors. Receptors that are regulated by epileptogenesis or epilepsy on the level of gene expression are shaded in gray. These genes code for the following receptors: C3AR, complement component 3a receptor; C5R, complement component 5 receptor; CHRM1, cholinergic receptor, muscarinic 1; EDNR, endothelin receptor; GABBR, γ-aminobutyric acid (GABA) B receptor; GABR, γ-aminobutyric acid (GABA) receptor; GRI, glutamate receptor, ionotropic; GRIN, glutamate receptor, ionotropic, *N*-methyl-D-aspartate; GRM, glutamate receptor, metabotropic; HTR1A, 5-hydroxytryptamine (serotonin) receptor 1A; NPYR, neuropeptide Y receptor; NR3C1, glucocorticoid receptor; NTSR2, neurotensin receptor 2; TACR3, tachykinin receptor 3. (Adapted from Kanehisa M, Goto S (2000). KEGG: Kyoto Encyclopedia of Genes and Genomes. Nucleic Acids Res 28: 27–30.)

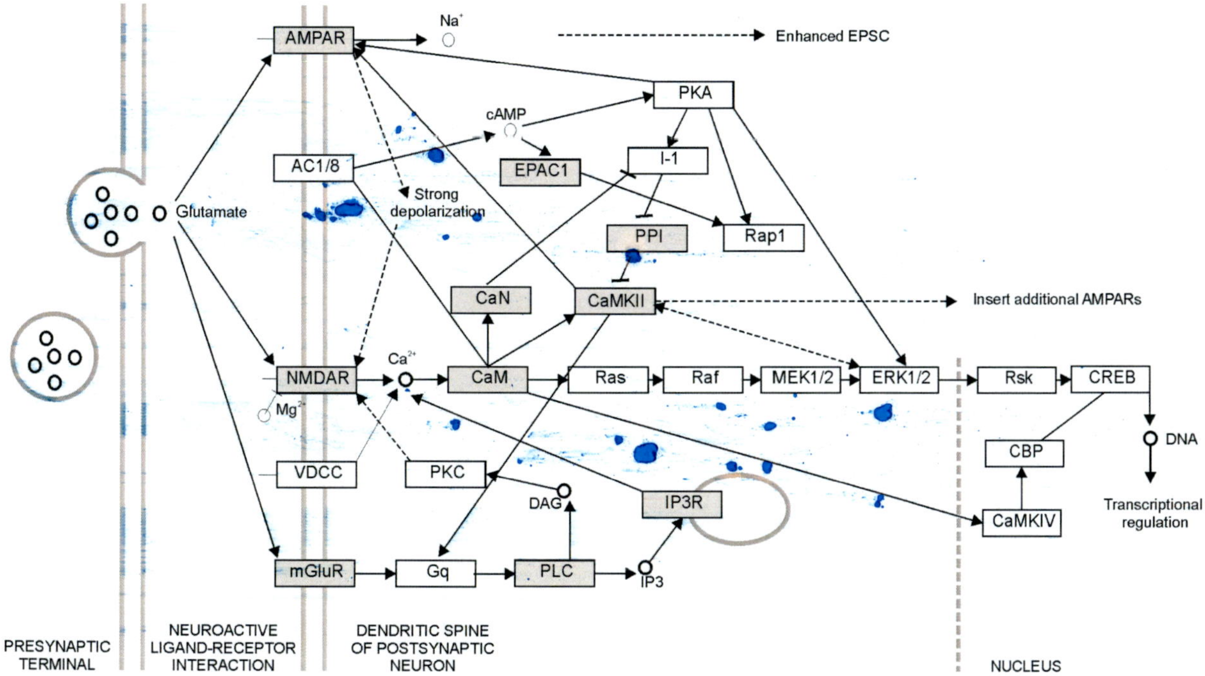

Fig. 1.2. Long-term potentiation (LTP) pathway in epileptogenesis and epilepsy, as predefined by KEGG (Kyoto Encyclopedia of Genes and Genomes; http://www.kegg.com/kegg/pathway/hsa/hsa04720.html) (Kanehisa and Goto, 2000). This pathway summarizes proteins involved in the development and modulation of LTP. Proteins are presented as rectangles with protein names inside. Arrows indicate direct (solid arrows) or indirect (dotted arrows) interactions between proteins. Proteins regulated by epileptogenesis or epilepsy on the level of gene expression are shaded in gray and include: AMPAR, glutamate receptor, ionotropic; AMPA (R), CaM, protein phosphatase 3, regulatory subunit (receptor); CaMKII, calcium/calmodulin-dependent protein kinase (CaM kinase) II; CaN, calcium-binding protein P22; EPAC1, Rap guanine nucleotide exchange factor (GEF); IP3R, inositol 1,4,5-triphosphate receptor; mGluR, glutamate receptor, metabotropic; NMDAR, glutamate receptor, ionotropic, *N*-methyl-D-aspartate; PLC, phospholipase C, beta; PP1, protein phosphatase 1 regulatory subunit. EPSC, excitatory postsynaptic current. (Adapted from Kanehisa M, Goto S (2000). KEGG: Kyoto Encyclopedia of Genes and Genomes. Nucleic Acids Res 28: 27–30.)

neuromodulators, can influence neuronal excitability (Baraban, 2004; Giorgi et al., 2004; Vezzani and Sperk, 2004; Koyama and Ikegaya, 2005; Tchekalarova and Georgiev, 2005). For example, neuropeptide Y (NPY) and its receptor have a significant role in regulating seizure activity (Gariboldi et al., 1998; Vezzani et al., 1999). Marked increases of NPY and NPY receptor mRNA have been observed following kindling (Moneta and Hollt, 1990; Kopp et al., 1999). Expression of other neuroactive peptides such as oxytocin, vasopressin or corticotropin-releasing factor can be affected by kindling as well (Greenwood et al., 1994a, b, 1997). In addition, neurotropins can influence neuronal network excitability and their expression, but little information regarding their expression in epileptogenesis is available. Expression of brain-derived neurotropic factor (BDNF) and fibroblast growth factor (FGF) can, however, be regulated by amygdala kindling (Bregola et al., 2000).

All the above-described alterations will influence synaptic function, having pronounced effects on neuronal excitability and possibly leading to functional abnormalities.

Immune function

Projecting the lists of genes changing expression level during epileptogenesis on KEGG pathways revealed overrepresentation of genes involved in complement activation cascade (see Table 1.1, Fig. 1.4). These include complement components and complement receptors, as well as regulators of complement and the coagulation cascade. Increased expression of complement factors in experimental and human temporal lobe epilepsy has been described (Aronica et al., 2007). It has been hypothesized that complement activation could contribute to a sustained inflammation and, by these means, destabilize neuronal networks involved in seizure activity (Aronica et al., 2007). Plasminogen activators may be involved in the complement activation pathway, but they can be involved also in other biological functions. It has been shown that urokinase-type plasminogen activator (uPA) is overexpressed in epileptogenesis and epilepsy, and can influence disease development by regulation of neurodegeneration and neurogenesis (Lahtinen et al., 2006, 2010; Iyer et al., 2010). Increased expression of

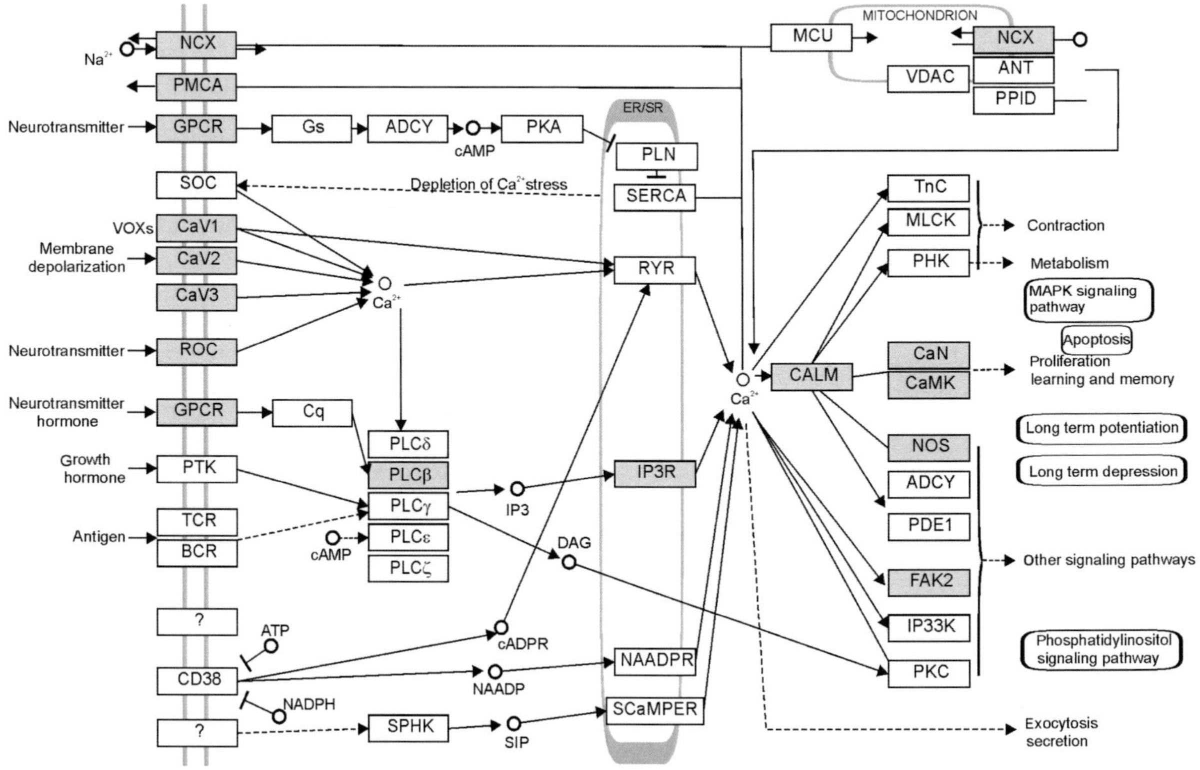

Fig. 1.3. Calcium signaling pathway in epileptogenesis and epilepsy, as predefined by KEGG (Kyoto Encyclopedia of Genes and Genomes; http://www.kegg.com/kegg/pathway/hsa/hsa04020.html) (Kanehisa and Goto, 2000). This pathway contains protein involved in regulation of intracellular calcium levels as well as proteins whose activity is regulated by calcium. Interactions between proteins, ions, cofactors, and other elements of the network are symbolized by arrows (direct interactions, solid arrows; indirect interactions, dotted arrows). Proteins regulated by epileptogenesis or epilepsy on the level of gene expression are shaded in gray and include: CALM, calmodulin; CaMK, calcium/calmodulin-dependent protein kinase; CaN, protein phosphatase 3; CaV1, calcium channel, voltage-dependent, L type; CaV2, calcium channel, voltage-dependent, P/Q type; CaV3, calcium channel, voltage-dependent, T type; FAK2, protein tyrosine kinase 2 beta; GPCR, cholinergic receptor, muscarinic 1; GPCR, cysteinyl leukotriene receptor 1; IP3R, inositol 1,4,5-triphosphate receptor; NCX, solute carrier family 8 (sodium/calcium exchanger); NCX, solute carrier family 8 (sodium/calcium exchanger); NOS, nitric oxide synthase 1; PLCβ, phospholipase C, beta; PMCA, Ca^{2+} transporting ATPase, plasma membrane; ROC; cholinergic receptor, nicotinic. (Adapted from Kanehisa M, Goto S (2000). KEGG: Kyoto Encyclopedia of Genes and Genomes. Nucleic Acids Res 28: 27–30.)

another plasminogen activator, tissue plasminogen activator (tPA), has been observed in epileptic brain (Iyer et al., 2010). Interestingly, both tPA and its inhibitor neuroserpin can regulate synaptic and seizure activity (Yepes and Lawrence, 2004; Pawlak et al., 2005).

The analysis of Gene Ontology confirmed overrepresentation of genes involved in the complement cascade among genes regulated by epileptogenesis and extended these data by additional functional groups related to immune function (see Table 1.2). Also in this analysis, the significant presence of GO terms related to immune function was observed in acute response to SE and epileptogenesis, but not in epilepsy. These GO terms include: inflammatory response, acute inflammatory response, adaptive immune response, humoral immune response, complement activation, leukocyte-mediated immunity, B cell-mediated immunity, and lymphocyte-mediated immunity. This indicates the pronounced role of mechanisms related to immune functions in epileptogenesis.

Early studies on the involvement of elements of immune system such as interleukins in epilepsy revealed the role of immune response in regulation of neuronal excitability (Shandra et al., 2002; Vezzani et al., 2002; Dube et al., 2005; Ravizza et al., 2008; Vezzani et al., 2008a; Rodgers et al., 2009). However, only recently has this topic received more attention, owing to technical developments in transcriptome profiling. Numerous studies on gene expression indicate that genes coding for proteins whose function has traditionally been linked to the immune system constitute the most prominent group of genes changing their expression level during epileptogenesis (Gorter et al., 2006; Lukasiuk et al., 2006; Aronica et al., 2008; Cacheaux et al., 2009). Much less is known about the function of protein

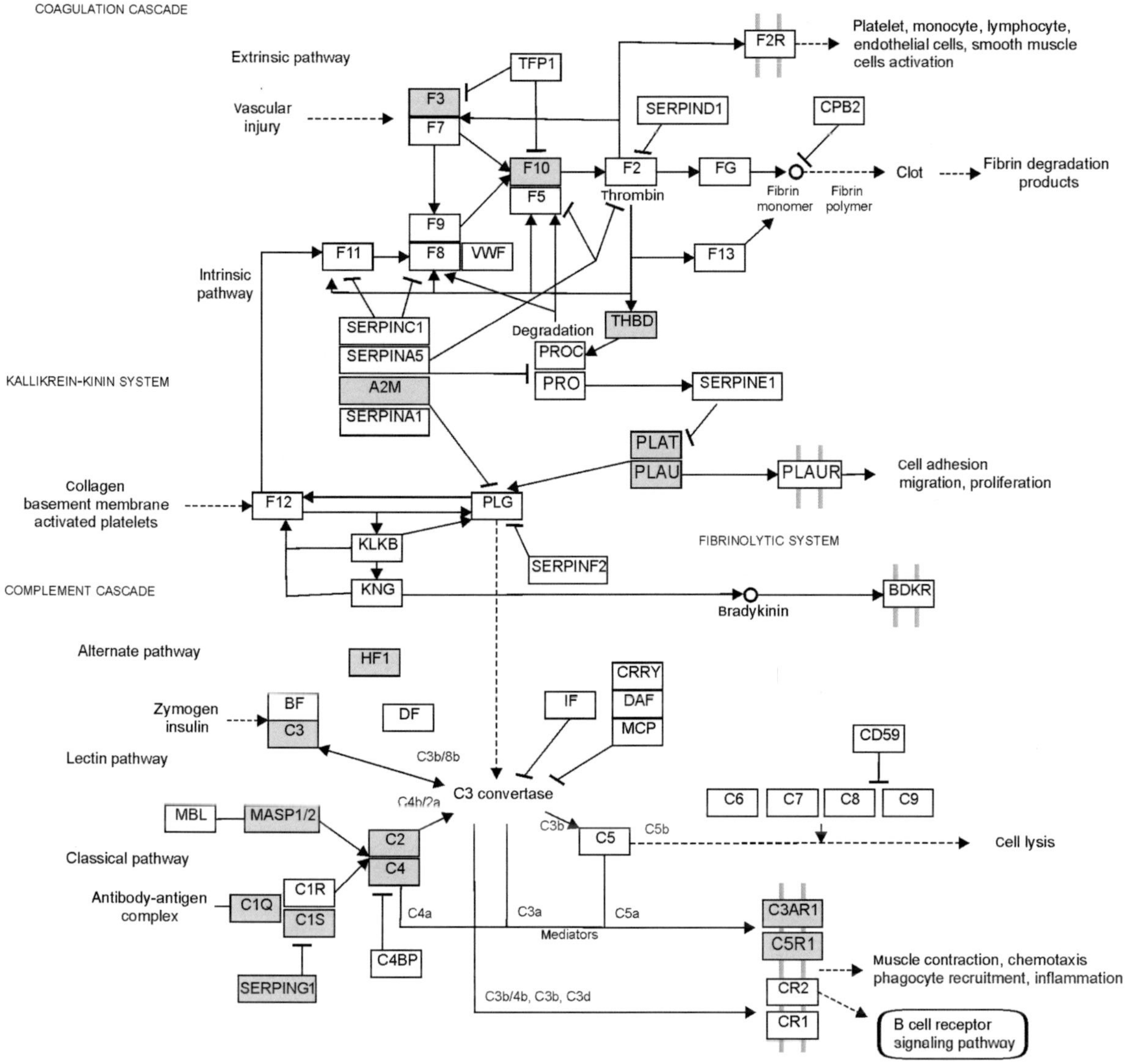

Fig. 1.4. Complement and coagulation cascades pathway in epileptogenesis and epilepsy, as predefined by KEGG (Kyoto Encyclopedia of Genes and Genomes; http://www.kegg.com/kegg/pathway/hsa/hsa04020.html) (Kanehisa and Goto, 2000). This pathway summarizes extracellularly located events of complement activation, coagulation cascade, kallikrein–kinin system, and fibrinolytic system. The membrane receptors, i.e., targets of these cascades, are also presented (membrane is symbolized by wide dark gray vertical double-lines). Proteins belonging to this metabolic pathway are symbolized by rectangles with their names inside. Interactions between elements of the network are symbolized by arrows (direct interactions, solid arrows; indirect interactions, dotted arrows). Proteins involved in complement activation and coagulation cascade that are regulated by epileptogenesis or epilepsy on the level of gene expression are shaded in gray and include: A2M, α_2-macroglobulin; C1Q, complement C1q subcomponent; C1S, complement component 1, S subcomponent; C2, complement component 2; C3, complement component 3; C3AR1, complement component 3a receptor 1; C4, complement component 4; C5R1, complement component 5 receptor 1; F10, coagulation factor X; F3, coagulation factor III (thromboplastin, tissue factor); HF1, complement factor H; MASP1/2, mannan-binding lectin serine protease 2; PLAT, tissue plasminogen activator; PLAU, urokinase plasminogen activator; SERPING1, serpin peptidase inhibitor, clade G (C1 inhibitor); THBD, thrombomodulin. (Adapted from Kanehisa M, Goto S (2000). KEGG: Kyoto Encyclopedia of Genes and Genomes. Nucleic Acids Res 28: 27–30.)

products of these genes in epilepsy. However, the pathogenetic mechanisms of some of them have already been studied. For example, interleukin (IL)-1, IL-6, and tumor necrosis factor (TNF) and their receptors have been shown to be upregulated in experimental models. More data have been gathered on IL-1β, which has been shown to have proconvulsant activity, possibly by means of functional interactions with neurotransmitters such as glutamate and GABA (Vezzani et al., 2008b). As many cytokines and chemokines are produced by glial cells, the increase in their expression can be recognized in terms of changes in communication between glia and neurons that lead to increased neuronal excitability (Vezzani et al., 2008b). Moreover, activation of peripheral immune response and lymphocyte extravasation may play a role under certain conditions in the generation of increased neuronal excitability, and even provide a therapeutic target for intervention of SE associated with infectious diseases (Fabene et al., 2008).

CONCLUSION

Analysis of changes in gene expression during epileptogenesis indicates that synaptic plasticity and transmission (represented by receptors, ion channels, and neuromodulators) and the immune response are the most prominent mechanisms affected by epileptogenesis. Importantly, some promising experimental data are already available indicating that modulation of these systems can have beneficial effects on epileptogenesis. For example, a duotherapy with BDNF and FGF-2 alleviated the severity of epilepsy in a rat pilocarpine model (Paradiso et al., 2009; Wong, 2010). In another recent study it was shown that prevention of adhesion of peripheral leukocytes to endothelial cells reduced leukocyte extravasation, and consequently, by suppressing the inflammatory response, reduced epileptogenesis (Fabene et al., 2008; Paradiso et al., 2009; Wong, 2010). Further analysis of the function of epileptogenesis-related genes revealed by bioinformatics can be expected to provide a roadmap to reveal more novel targets for tackling epileptogenesis.

ACKNOWLEDGMENTS

This study was supported by the Academy of Finland, the Sigrid Juselius Foundation, and the Polish Ministry of Science and Education (grant 3/0-PBZ-MNiI-2/1/2005).

REFERENCES

Akbar MT, Rattray M, Powell JF et al. (1996). Altered expression of group I metabotropic glutamate receptors in the hippocampus of amygdala-kindled rats. Brain Res Mol Brain Res 43: 105–116.

Aronica E, Yankaya B, Troost D et al. (2001). Induction of neonatal sodium channel II and III alpha-isoform mRNAs in neurons and microglia after status epilepticus in the rat hippocampus. Eur J Neurosci 13: 1261–1266.

Aronica E, Boer K, van Vliet EA et al. (2007). Complement activation in experimental and human temporal lobe epilepsy. Neurobiol Dis 26: 497–511.

Aronica E, Boer K, Becker A et al. (2008). Gene expression profile analysis of epilepsy-associated gangliogliomas. Neuroscience 151: 272–292.

Banerjee PN, Hauser WA (2008). Incidence and prevalence. In: JJ Engel, TA Pedley (Eds.), Epilepsy: A Comprehensive Textbook. Wolters Kluwer/Lippincott Williams & Wilkins, Baltimore, pp. 45–57.

Baraban SC (2004). Neuropeptide Y and epilepsy: recent progress, prospects and controversies. Neuropeptides 38: 261–265.

Blumcke I, Becker AJ, Klein C et al. (2000). Temporal lobe epilepsy associated up-regulation of metabotropic glutamate receptors: correlated changes in mGluR1 mRNA and protein expression in experimental animals and human patients. J Neuropathol Exp Neurol 59: 1–10.

Bregola G, Frigati L, Zucchini S et al. (2000). Different patterns of induction of fibroblast growth factor-2 and brain-derived neurotrophic factor messenger RNAs during kindling epileptogenesis, and development of a herpes simplex vector for fibroblast growth factor-2 gene transfer *in vivo*. Epilepsia 41: S122–S126.

Cacheaux LP, Ivens S, David Y et al. (2009). Transcriptome profiling reveals TGF-beta signaling involvement in epileptogenesis. J Neurosci 29: 8927–8935.

Clark M, Massenburg GS, Weiss SR et al. (1994). Analysis of the hippocampal GABAA receptor system in kindled rats by autoradiographic and in situ hybridization techniques: contingent tolerance to carbamazepine. Brain Res Mol Brain Res 26: 309–319.

Dennis G, Jr, Sherman BT, Hosack DA et al. (2003). DAVID: Database for Annotation, Visualization, and Integrated Discovery. Genome Biol 4: P3.

Diaz E (2009). From microarrays to mechanisms of brain development and function. Biochem Biophys Res Commun 385: 129–131.

Dingledine R, Borges K, Bowie D et al. (1999). The glutamate receptor ion channels. Pharmacol Rev 51: 7–61.

Dube C, Vezzani A, Behrens M et al. (2005). Interleukin-1beta contributes to the generation of experimental febrile seizures. Ann Neurol 57: 152–155.

Ellerkmann RK, Remy S, Chen J et al. (2003). Molecular and functional changes in voltage-dependent Na(+) channels following pilocarpine-induced status epilepticus in rat dentate granule cells. Neuroscience 119: 323–333.

Fabene PF, Navarro Mora G, Martinello M et al. (2008). A role for leukocyte–endothelial adhesion mechanisms in epilepsy. Nat Med 14: 1377–1383.

Furtinger S, Bettler B, Sperk G (2003). Altered expression of $GABA_B$ receptors in the hippocampus after kainic-acid induced seizures in rats. Brain Res Mol Brain Res 113: 107–115.

Gariboldi M, Conti M, Cavaleri D et al. (1998). Anticonvulsant properties of BIBP3226, a non-peptide selective antagonist at neuropeptide Y Y1 receptors. Eur J Neurosci 10: 757–759.

Giorgi FS, Pizzanelli C, Biagioni F et al. (2004). The role of norepinephrine in epilepsy: from the bench to the bedside. Neurosci Biobehav Rev 28: 507–524.

Gold SJ, Hennegriff M, Lynch G et al. (1996). Relative concentrations and seizure-induced changes in mRNAs encoding three AMPA receptor subunits in hippocampus and cortex. J Comp Neurol 365: 541–555.

Gorter JA, van Vliet EA, Aronica E et al. (2006). Potential new antiepileptogenic targets indicated by microarray analysis in a rat model for temporal lobe epilepsy. J Neurosci 26: 11083–11110.

Greenwood RS, Abdou A, Meeker RB et al. (1994a). Vasopressin mRNA changes during kindling: the effects of kindling site and stage. Brain Res Mol Brain Res 26: 286–292.

Greenwood RS, Meeker RB, Abdou A et al. (1994b). Kindled seizures induce a long-term increase in vasopressin mRNA. Brain Res Mol Brain Res 24: 20–26.

Greenwood RS, Fan Z, Meeker R (1997). Persistent elevation of corticotrophin releasing factor and vasopressin but not oxytocin mRNA in the rat after kindled seizures. Neurosci Lett 224: 66–70.

Hendriksen H, Kamphuis W, Lopes da Silva FH (1997). Changes in voltage-dependent calcium channel alpha1-subunit mRNA levels in the kindling model of epileptogenesis. Brain Res Mol Brain Res 50: 257–266.

Huang da W, Sherman BT, Lempicki RA (2009). Systematic and integrative analysis of large gene lists using DAVID bioinformatics resources. Nat Protoc 4: 44–57.

Iyer AM, Zurolo E, Boer K et al. (2010). Tissue plasminogen activator and urokinase plasminogen activator in human epileptogenic pathologies. Neuroscience 167: 929–945.

Kamphuis W, De Rijk TC, Talamini LM et al. (1994). Rat hippocampal kindling induces changes in the glutamate receptor mRNA expression patterns in dentate granule neurons. Eur J Neurosci 6: 1119–1127.

Kamphuis W, Hendriksen H, Diegenbach PC et al. (1995). N-methyl-D-aspartate and kainate receptor gene expression in hippocampal pyramidal and granular neurons in the kindling model of epileptogenesis. Neuroscience 67: 551–559.

Kanehisa M, Goto S (2000). KEGG: Kyoto Encyclopedia of Genes and Genomes. Nucleic Acids Res 28: 27–30.

Kopp J, Nanobashvili A, Kokaia Z et al. (1999). Differential regulation of mRNAs for neuropeptide Y and its receptor subtypes in widespread areas of the rat limbic system during kindling epileptogenesis. Brain Res Mol Brain Res 72: 17–29.

Koyama R, Ikegaya Y (2005). To BDNF or not to BDNF: that is the epileptic hippocampus. Neuroscientist 11: 282–287.

Lahtinen L, Lukasiuk K, Pitkanen A (2006). Increased expression and activity of urokinase-type plasminogen activator during epileptogenesis. Eur J Neurosci 24: 1935–1945.

Lahtinen L, Ndode-Ekane XE, Barinka F et al. (2010). Urokinase-type plasminogen activator regulates neurodegeneration and neurogenesis but not vascular changes in the mouse hippocampus after status epilepticus. Neurobiol Dis 37: 692–703.

Lason W, Turchan J, Przewlocka B et al. (1998). Effects of pentylenetetrazol kindling on glutamate receptor genes expression in the rat hippocampus. Brain Res 785: 355–358.

Luddens H, Wisden W (1991). Function and pharmacology of multiple GABAA receptor subunits. Trends Pharmacol Sci 12: 49–51.

Lukasiuk K, Dabrowski M, Adach A et al. (2006). Epileptogenesis-related genes revisited. Prog Brain Res 158: 223–241.

Moneta ME, Hollt V (1990). Perforant path kindling induces differential alterations in the mRNA levels coding for prodynorphin and proenkephalin in the rat hippocampus. Neurosci Lett 110: 273–278.

Nishimura T, Schwarzer C, Gasser E et al. (2005). Altered expression of GABA(A) and GABA(B) receptor subunit mRNAs in the hippocampus after kindling and electrically induced status epilepticus. Neuroscience 134: 691–704.

Paradiso B, Marconi P, Zucchini S et al. (2009). Localized delivery of fibroblast growth factor-2 and brain-derived neurotrophic factor reduces spontaneous seizures in an epilepsy model. Proc Natl Acad Sci U S A 106: 7191–7196.

Pawlak R, Rao BS, Melchor JP et al. (2005). Tissue plasminogen activator and plasminogen mediate stress-induced decline of neuronal and cognitive functions in the mouse hippocampus. Proc Natl Acad Sci U S A 102: 18201–18206.

Pitkanen A, Lukasiuk K (2009). Molecular and cellular basis of epileptogenesis in symptomatic epilepsy. Epilepsy Behav 14: 16–25.

Pitkanen A, Sutula TP (2002). Is epilepsy a progressive disorder? Prospects for new therapeutic approaches in temporal-lobe epilepsy. Lancet Neurol 1: 173–181.

Porter RJ (1993). Classification of epileptic seizures and epileptic syndromes. In: J Laidlaw, A Richens, D Chadwick (Eds.), A Textbook of Epilepsy. Churchill Livingstone, New York, pp. 1–22.

Ravizza T, Gagliardi B, Noe F et al. (2008). Innate and adaptive immunity during epileptogenesis and spontaneous seizures: evidence from experimental models and human temporal lobe epilepsy. Neurobiol Dis 29: 142–160.

Rodgers KM, Hutchinson MR, Northcutt A et al. (2009). The cortical innate immune response increases local neuronal excitability leading to seizures. Brain 132: 2478–2486.

Shandra AA, Godlevsky LS, Vastyanov RS et al. (2002). The role of TNF-alpha in amygdala kindled rats. Neurosci Res 42: 147–153.

Su T, Cong WD, Long YS et al. (2008). Altered expression of voltage-gated potassium channel 4.2 and voltage-gated potassium channel 4-interacting protein, and changes in intracellular calcium levels following lithium–pilocarpine-induced status epilepticus. Neuroscience 157: 566–576.

Tchekalarova J, Georgiev V (2005). Angiotensin peptides modulatory system: how is it implicated in the control of seizure susceptibility? Life Sci 76: 955–970.

Temkin NR (2009). Preventing and treating posttraumatic seizures: the human experience. Epilepsia 50: 10–13.

Ullal G, Fahnestock M, Racine R (2005). Time-dependent effect of kainate-induced seizures on glutamate receptor GluR5, GluR6, and GluR7 mRNA and protein expression in rat hippocampus. Epilepsia 46: 616–623.

Vezzani A, Sperk G (2004). Overexpression of NPY and Y2 receptors in epileptic brain tissue: an endogenous neuroprotective mechanism in temporal lobe epilepsy? Neuropeptides 38: 245–252.

Vezzani A, Sperk G, Colmers WF (1999). Neuropeptide Y: emerging evidence for a functional role in seizure modulation. Trends Neurosci 22: 25–30.

Vezzani A, Moneta D, Richichi C et al. (2002). Functional role of inflammatory cytokines and antiinflammatory molecules in seizures and epileptogenesis. Epilepsia 43: 30–35.

Vezzani A, Balosso S, Ravizza T (2008a). The role of cytokines in the pathophysiology of epilepsy. Brain Behav Immun 22: 797–803.

Vezzani A, Ravizza T, Balosso S et al. (2008b). Glia as a source of cytokines: implications for neuronal excitability and survival. Epilepsia 49: 24–32.

Vigues S, Gastaldi M, Chabret C et al. (1999). Regulation of calcium channel alpha(1A) subunit splice variant mRNAs in kainate-induced temporal lobe epilepsy. Neurobiol Dis 6: 288–301.

von Blankenfeld G, Ymer S, Pritchett DB et al. (1990). Differential benzodiazepine pharmacology of mammalian recombinant GABAA receptors. Neurosci Lett 115: 269–273.

Wong M (2010). Mammalian target of rapamycin (mTOR) inhibition as a potential antiepileptogenic therapy: From tuberous sclerosis to common acquired epilepsies. Epilepsia 51: 27–36.

Yepes M, Lawrence DA (2004). Tissue-type plasminogen activator and neuroserpin: a well-balanced act in the nervous system? Trends Cardiovasc Med 14: 173–180.

Handbook of Clinical Neurology, Vol. 107 (3rd series)
Epilepsy, Part I
H. Stefan and W.H. Theodore, Editors

Chapter 2

Cellular bases of focal and generalized epilepsies

PHILIP A. SCHWARTZKROIN*
Department of Neurological Surgery, University of California-Davis, Davis, CA, USA

INTRODUCTION

Epilepsy – spontaneous recurrent seizure discharge – comes in many different forms. A given type of epilepsy is determined, at least in part, by the seizure type(s) that constitutes the clinical manifestation of that epilepsy in a given individual. Understanding the cellular bases of the epilepsies, therefore, requires that one gain insight into these different seizure manifestations. Seizure activity is characterized, at the cellular level, by two primary features: (1) the imbalance between excitatory and inhibitory influences that causes abnormal (usually hyperexcitable) neuronal discharge; and (2) hypersynchrony of neuronal activity (Fig. 2.1). That is, during a seizure, neurons (at least in some parts of the brain) discharge in an unusually hypersynchronous manner, often at a much higher rate than is normally seen in that population of cells. What cellular features give rise to these pathophysiologies?

To understand the cellular bases of the epilepsies – to identify those cellular features that differentiate normal brain from epileptic brain – one must first have some sense of normal brain function, and identify the processes that maintain "normal" activity. One can then begin to characterize those differences associated with epileptic tissue. Cellular discharge patterns reflect a set of neuronal properties that are generally determined by the genetic makeup of the animal, but that can be modulated by environmental inputs. These properties can be, in a somewhat simplistic way, summarized as follows:

1. Intrinsic cellular mechanisms – as determined by the complement and distribution of channels over the cell's membrane, as well as molecules that constitute intracellular signaling pathways peculiar to that cell type.
2. Synaptic activities and interactions (both chemical and electrical) – as determined by a host of molecules that contribute to neurotransmission systems.
3. Influences of the extracellular environment – consisting of glia, extracellular space, the vascular system, and various chemicals and hormones that circulate between neurons.

This chapter will review key details of these cellular properties (Fig. 2.2), and explore how abnormalities or alterations in these properties lead to abnormal electrical discharge behaviors that we typically label "seizure" activity. It is important to note at the beginning of this discussion that, although such insights into seizure mechanisms are essential for an understanding of the epilepsies, they are not sufficient – for they often do not explain differences across seizure types or across individuals, nor do they adequately explain the bases for differences in response to treatments. Current insights into such cellular features also rarely help us understand the underlying bases for periodic, paroxysmal, and usually unpredictable discharge that defines epileptic seizures. Indeed, as complex as are the cellular mechanisms now associated with seizure occurrence, we remain woefully ignorant about such issues as how/why an individual with epilepsy may appear neurologically "normal" most of the time (i.e., between seizures). Discussion of these important features of the epileptic brain is beyond the scope of this chapter.

Finally, an understanding of the underlying bases of seizures, or even of changes that result in the sudden eruption of seizure activity in the epileptic patient, does not necessarily offer a cellular explanation for the *development* of the seizure state in a given individual. The mechanistic bases of "epileptogenesis" (the processes by which an apparently normal brain becomes an epileptic brain) are only now receiving significant attention in the laboratory – and studies suggest that the

*Correspondence to: Philip A. Schwartzkroin, Ph.D., Department of Neurological Surgery, University of California, Davis, School of Medicine Neuroscience Building, Room 612G, 1515 Newton Court, Davis, CA 95618, USA. E-mail: paschwartzkroin@ucdavis.edu

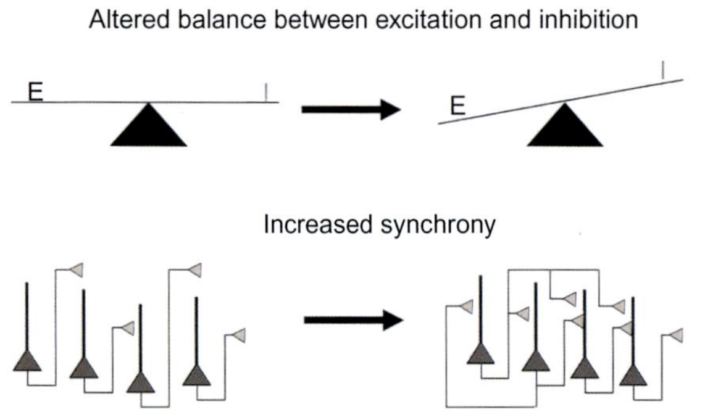

Fig. 2.1. *Top:* Diagram illustrating the delicate balance between excitatory (E) and inhibitory (I) influences that determine the level of neuronal discharge. In most (but not all) epilepsies, there is a disruption of the normal equilibrium such that excitation outweighs inhibition. *Bottom:* Perhaps more critical, seizures reflect the synchronous discharge of populations of neurons that normally do not discharge together.

cellular mechanisms of epileptogenesis may only partially overlap with those that we have identified as key to seizure discharge.

INTRINSIC PROPERTIES OF NEURONS

Excitatory projection cells

Most epilepsies involve the discharge of cortical – neocortical and/or hippocampal – pyramidal cells; absence epilepsies also involve thalamic neurons (McCormick and Contreras, 2001). In each brain region, excitatory projection cells are primarily responsible for sending signals out of the local brain region in which their cell bodies are located. These cells, then, are critical for the transmission of information (be it normal physiological information, or pathological epileptiform "information") to other brain regions. All these cell types – pyramidal cells in neocortex and hippocampus, and thalamocortical projection cells – have been well studied with respect to epileptiform discharge. In neocortex and hippocampus, pyramidal cells have been categorized into distinct types; in these regions, at least one pyramidal cell type has an intrinsic propensity for burst discharge (i.e., brief periods of electrical discharge during which action potentials are "fired" at short interspike intervals) that has led investigators to label them "initiator" or "pacemaker" cells for epileptiform activity (Fig. 2.3A). In neocortex, these "intrinsic bursters" are found in the deep layers (layer V); they are distinguished from "regular firing" pyramidal cells of more superficial layers (Prince and Connors, 1984). In the hippocampus, the CA3 pyramidal cells tend to discharge in burst patterns (even in the normal brain), and have been implicated as initiators of hippocampal epileptiform discharge – as distinguished from the more regularly firing CA1 pyramidal cells (Wong et al., 1986). Interestingly, these functionally different pyramidal cells can also be distinguished morphologically.

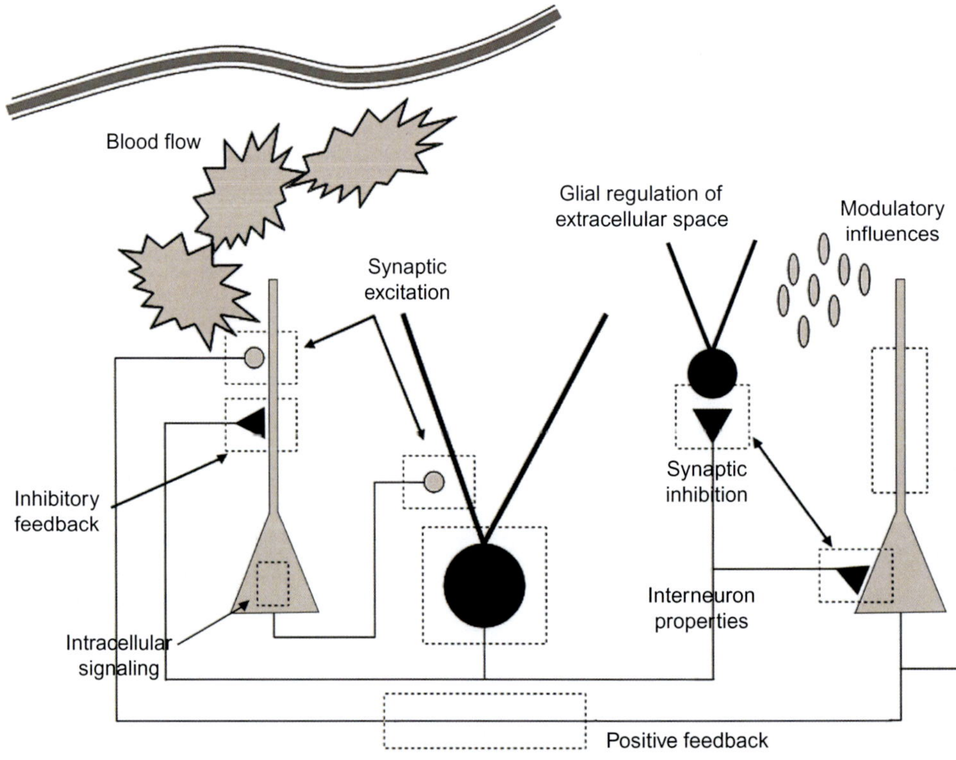

Fig. 2.2. Diagrammatic representation of the various influences that affect neuronal excitability, all of which need to be considered when trying to understand the basic mechanisms underlying seizures and epilepsies.

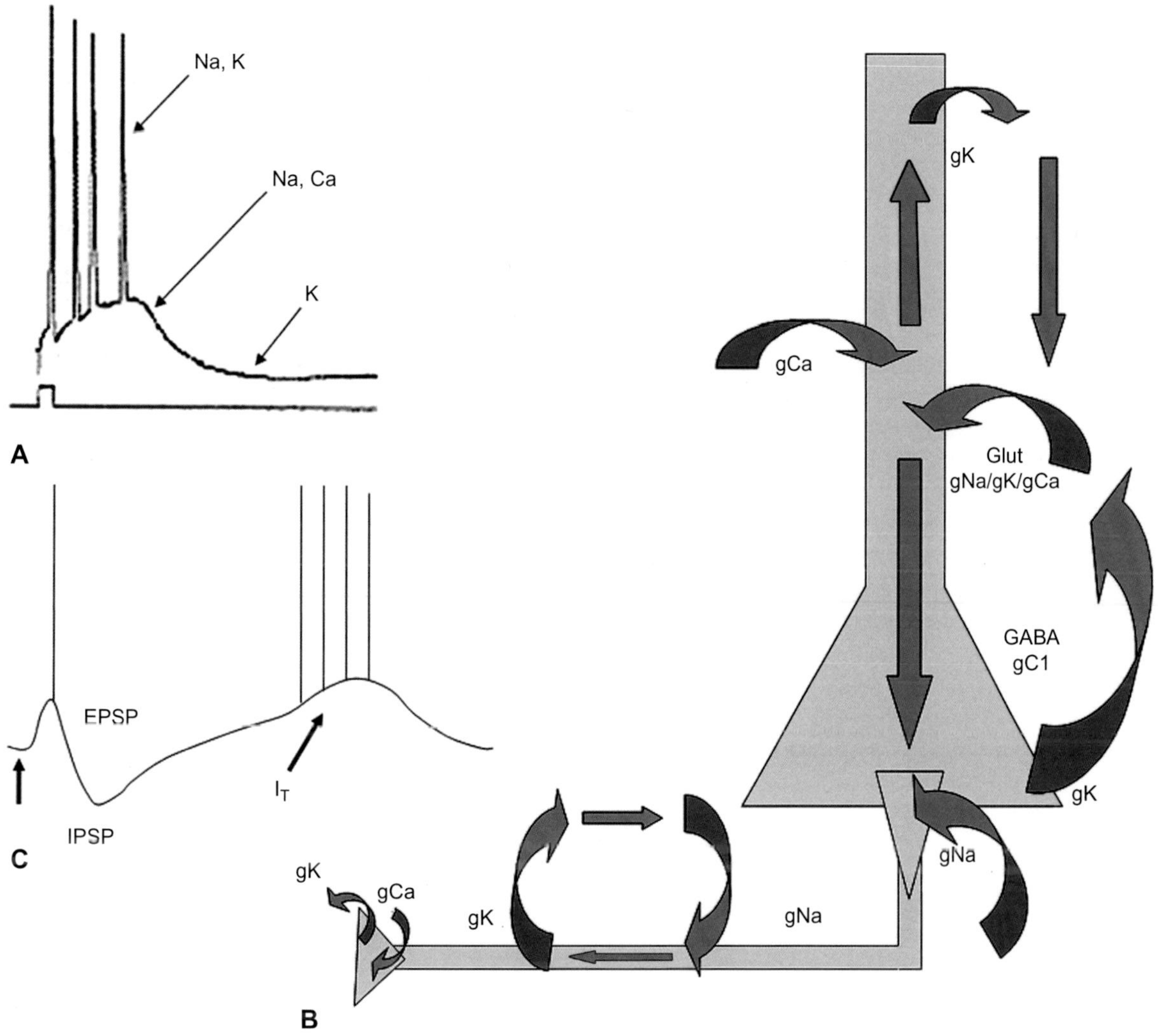

Fig. 2.3. (**A**) Burst discharge from a hippocampal pyramidal cell. Multiple action potentials are generated in response to a relatively short/low-amplitude depolarization. Membrane depolarization, due to current carried through voltage-gated sodium and calcium channels, triggers action potentials (reflecting the influx of sodium and efflux of potassium ions). Membrane repolarization is due primarily to potassium ion movement out of the neuron. (**B**) Illustration of some of the numerous intrinsic neuronal currents – in the dendrites, somata, initial segment, axon, and terminal – that determine membrane depolarizations and hyperpolarizations. GABA, γ-aminobutyric acid; Glut, glutamate. (**C**) Illustration of a neuronal discharge pattern typical of thalamic neurons, involving synaptic drives (excitatory and inhibitory postsynaptic potentials; EPSPs and IPSPs) and a voltage-gated calcium current. The latter transient (or "T") current (I_T) is mostly inactivated at cell resting potential, but is "de-inactivated" by synaptic hyperpolarization; subsequent calcium influx through these channels then depolarizes the neuron and triggers "rebound" discharge.

In neocortex, the intrinsic bursters have larger somata and more extensive dendritic arborizations compared with the regular-spiking pyramidal cells. Similarly, in hippocampus, the CA3 pyramidal cells are larger, with thicker and bushier dendrites than the regular-spiking CA1 cells.

The distinct discharge properties of these pyramidal cells, as seen in normal "baseline" activity and particularly with respect to the cells' tendency to "burst" (as a possible basis for the initiation of epileptiform discharge), is determined by a set of voltage-gated channels that are differentially expressed in these populations of projections cells. Although all neurons exhibit the well-studied sodium and potassium channels in their axons that support action potential transmission (as described by Hodgkin and Huxley), it is clear that there is a myriad of other voltage-gated channel types that determine the kinetics of soma-dendritic depolarization, the threshold for action potential initiation at the initial segment, and the release of neurotransmitter at the neuron's axon terminal (Fig. 2.3B) (Traub et al., 1991; Kager et al., 2007). For example, in the mature hippocampal CA1 neuron, dendritic depolarization (as evoked, for example, by excitatory transmitter release at dendritic synapses) is mediated not only by sodium influx but also by voltage-dependent opening of dendritic calcium channels (Beck et al., 1998; Magee et al., 1998). As the membrane depolarizes, various potassium channels open to help repolarize the membrane potential. The types of potassium channel that open (the various currents mediated via potassium channels) determine the speed at which membrane repolarization takes place, as well as the duration of the hyperpolarization. These hyperpolarizing currents prevent repetitive action potential discharge evoked by persistent membrane depolarization and/or determine the rhythm (inter-event intervals) of cell discharge (Johnston et al., 2000; Yuan and Chen, 2006). For example, some cells fire in a "regular" pattern, with an interspike interval (between each action potential) that decreases as the depolarization becomes stronger. Contrast this behavior of the hippocampal CA1 neuron with the neighboring CA3 pyramidal cell, which is endowed with a relatively high density of soma-dendritic voltage-gated calcium channels. When these CA3 cells are depolarized, the calcium channels open – and stay open much longer than the sodium channels that dominate the membrane depolarization of CA1 cells. As a result of this prolonged calcium-mediated depolarization, the CA3 neuron tends to generate multiple action potentials with short interspike intervals (i.e., a burst), even in response to relatively minimal depolarization (Fig. 2.3A) (Traub et al., 1991). That is, the opening of calcium channels acts as an amplification mechanism. Similar depolarizations, which can initiate burst discharge, are also found in some neocortical pyramidal cells. Researchers have found that these calcium-mediated events are triggered not only by the depolarizing effects of excitatory synaptic events, but also by the pressure of a slowly inactivating ("persistent") sodium current, mediated by sodium channels that stay open longer than the typical quickly inactivating sodium channel (Stafstrom et al., 1985; Stafstrom, 2007).

In many burst-generating cells, the action potential burst is followed by a long and deep hyperpolarization that is the result (at least in part) of activation of a calcium-dependent potassium conductance (Fernandez de Sevilla et al., 2006). Thus, in these cells, there is a "cellular analog" of the interictal burst discharge as expressed in the EEG – the EEG "spike" being a reflection of neuronal depolarization and action potential burst discharge, and the "wave" reflecting the neuronal hyperpolarization. One can view this set of cellular processes as "self-regulating", i.e., calcium and sodium influx mediating excitation (action potential bursts), but then almost immediately giving rise to a hyperpolarizing current that curtails the discharge. It is easy to imagine that changes in the nature of this coupling could give rise to abnormal discharge patterns. And indeed, experimental manipulations in which a component of the system is blocked (or potentiated) give rise to aberrant discharge patterns, some of which are similar to those seen in the epileptic brain (e.g., Perreault and Avoli, 1991).

In the thalamocortical projection cell, a different voltage-gated current tends to dominate the pattern of the cell's discharge. In these cells, synaptically mediated cell depolarization is followed by a powerful synaptic hyperpolarization (more of that below). This hyperpolarization "de-inactivates" a low threshold calcium conductance, leading to the so-called "T (transient) current" (Huguenard and Prince, 1992). That is, as the hyperpolarization resolves, an influx of calcium (through the gradually opening calcium channels) leads to membrane depolarization and action potential discharge ("rebound excitation") (Fig. 2.3C). This interplay of depolarization and hyperpolarization underlies the spike–wave EEG pattern seen during sleep spindles; dysregulation of the underlying mechanisms gives rise to the familiar spike–wave sequences of absence epilepsies (McCormick and Contreras, 2001).

As should be clear from the paragraphs above, the intrinsic properties of each neuron – the voltage-gated ion conductances – interact critically with those influences that depolarize (or hyperpolarize) the membrane potential. The most obvious of these influences are the synaptic inputs, excitatory and inhibitory. The channels giving rise to these voltage-gated intrinsic conductances are localized at specific subcellular sites so as best to take advantage of, or control, the effects of synaptic inputs. Thus, in neurons such as the pyramidal projection cell, where excitatory synaptic inputs terminate primarily on dendritic targets (especially dendritic spines), voltage-gated calcium channels tend to be localized in nearby dendritic membrane (Obermair et al., 2004) and are powerfully affected by synaptically mediated polarization changes that may appear rather small when recorded at the level of the cell body (Fig. 2.4). Similarly, various hyperpolarizing potassium channels have distinct dendro-somatic distributions (Johnston et al., 2000; Vacher et al., 2008), so as to shunt depolarizing currents and reduce the likelihood that a synaptically mediated depolarization will be sufficiently large – at the level of the initial segment – to induce cell discharge. The converse is also true: some types of synapse are localized strategically so as to control the excitability that results from the opening of intrinsic (i.e., voltage-gated) ion channels. For example, in addition to the high density of voltage-gated sodium channels at the initial segment, there are also powerful inhibitory synapses that reduce the likelihood of action potential discharge (Inda et al., 2006). At the nodes of Ranvier and at the terminal boutons, depolarizing and hyperpolarizing conductances interact in an intricately balanced dance to control

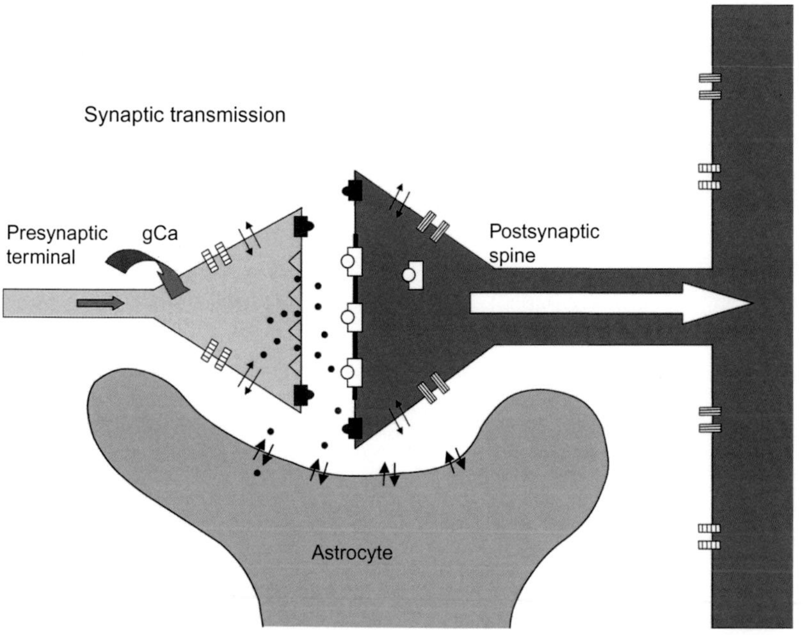

Fig. 2.4. Illustration of the various components contributing to synaptic transmission, including both synaptic and extrasynaptic receptors, pumps and transporters (on both presynaptic and postsynaptic elements), voltage-gated channels, and glial uptake of ions and transmitter. gCa, calcium conductance.

discharge and depolarization, with sodium channels and potassium channels in partnership at the nodes, and with calcium channels and potassium channels interacting at the terminal (see Fig. 2.3B). Small changes in the nature of any of these conductances, or in their precise subcellular localization, can lead to disruption of the normal balance and result in too little – or too much – excitation. Some mutant mice (and presumably some epileptic patients), with gene disruptions that lead to epileptiform activities, exhibit this loss of balance between excitatory and inhibitory voltage-gated channels (Smart et al., 1998; Burgess and Noebels, 1999).

The complexity of these systems – the large numbers of different voltage-gated channels, their precise subcellular localization, and their interaction with external synaptic drives – is orchestrated genetically. And the genetically determined expression of mRNAs for the proteins that make up specific channels is developmentally regulated (e.g., Fry, 2006). Because gene expression changes during brain development, the specific ionic properties of a given cell change during the course of maturation. These developmental changes can be seen in something as obvious as the nature of the voltage-dependent sodium channel, the changing composition of which causes changes in the kinetics of sodium flux across the membrane, the inactivation properties of the channel, and thus the ability of the cell to fire repetitively at high rates (Picken Bahrey and Moody, 2003); these developmental changes also affect the way in which these channels interact with various antiepileptic drugs (e.g., with phenytoin or carbamazepine, which target the sodium channel), and thus determine the efficacy of a given drug at different developmental stages. Cell discharge properties are also affected developmentally by the changing capabilities of the Na,K-ATPase, the molecular "pump" that moves sodium out of the cell and potassium into the cell in order to establish the resting membrane potential (and the driving force for ion flux when channels open). Another major developmental shift occurs in the expression of different chloride transporter molecules that establish the internal concentration of chloride, and thus determine the inhibitory efficacy of opening chloride channels (Payne et al., 2003; Dzhala et al., 2005) (see below). Cell properties characteristic of the adult central nervous system (CNS) may be expressed quite differently in the immature brain. Therefore, it should not be surprising that the types of pathological activity that arise from altered neuronal properties in the adult brain can be quite different in the immature CNS. As suggested above, it is important to consider these developmentally changing properties of neurons as one focuses on the unique features of seizure discharge in the immature brain, and the age-specific efficacy of antiepileptic drugs.

Finally, as we consider how these channels determine the nature of a given cell's discharge pattern in normal and in epileptic brain, it is important to factor in the "plasticity" of these systems. Although these channels have long been considered to be "hard-wired" features of a neuron, it is becoming increasingly clear that the level of channel expression, as well as the localization of various channel subunits, are in fact changeable – i.e., "plastic" (e.g., Jung et al., 2007; Catterall and Few, 2008). Normal shifts in neuronal activity may cause subtle changes in these channels; more dramatic changes in activity, as occur during seizures, may lead to significant alterations in intrinsic properties. These shifts sometimes appear to be "homeostatic" (i.e., the cell's effort to maintain normal balance). However, the changes also may give rise to a molecular "feedback" cascade that exacerbates tendencies toward hyperexcitability and seizure discharge.

Inhibitory local circuit interneurons

Interneurons are, by definition, cells that influence activity within a limited, localized brain region. That is, their axons ramify within the general area in which the cell body is embedded, influencing the activities of nearby cells. While projection cells provide the excitatory drive underlying brain discharge, interneurons generally provide the "brakes." And by applying the brakes in a very precise and selective manner, a relatively small number of interneurons sculpt the patterns of projection cell discharge.

Modern research has identified a rich complexity of different interneuron types (Freund and Buzsaki, 1996; Markram et al., 2004; Blatow et al., 2005; Houser, 2007). In the hippocampus and neocortex (those regions so key to epileptic discharge), these interneurons release γ-aminobutyric acid (GABA) as their primary inhibitory neurotransmitter. Compromises in the integrity of GABAergic transmission have been implicated in seizure disorders. Different interneuron types have been characterized on the basis of:

1. *Action potential discharge frequency and pattern.* For example, some interneurons appear to maintain a resting potential very close to the action potential threshold, and thus may discharge tonically, even with only minimal external input; such cells may fire at high tonic discharge frequencies when excited (typically by projection cells). Other interneurons maintain a much more negative resting potential and are relatively difficult to activate.
2. *Targets.* Each interneuron population has a characteristic target pattern for their axons/terminals. Some interneurons synapse specifically on, for example, the axon hillock of projection cells ("axo-axonic" interneurons), others provide a dense plexus of synapses surrounding pyramidal cell bodies ("basket cells"), and still others target dendrites of pyramidal cells, often in a pattern overlapping the excitatory inputs of specific afferent pathways. Activation of these interneurons provides precise patterns of projection cell inhibition. Importantly, some interneurons preferentially target other interneurons (i.e., not projection cells), thus giving rise to the phenomenon of "disinhibition."
3. *Inputs.* Each interneuron subtype has a characteristic somatic location and dendritic branching pattern that determines, at least in part, which inputs will make contact with (and excite) that cell. Afferent inputs from other brain regions, recurrent excitatory input from projection cells within the local region of the interneuron, and inputs from other interneurons will all be integrated to determine the cell's discharge level.
4. *Colocalized neurotransmitter.* In addition to the major inhibitory neurotransmitter, GABA, many interneurons synthesize and release other (usually peptide) neurotransmitters. Corelease (with GABA) of peptides such as neuropeptide Y or somatostatin is thought to occur particularly during high-frequency discharge of the parent interneuron, i.e., under just those conditions that are characteristic of epileptic discharge. These peptides exert specific influences separate from the inhibitory effects of GABA.
5. *Vulnerability to damage.* Different interneuron cell types appear to have dramatically different sensitivities to excitotoxic damage. This sensitivity is determined, at least in part, by the patterns and densities of excitatory inputs to the cell, characteristics that are likely a key determinant of excitability that develops during, and as a result of, seizure discharge. Different interneuron subpopulations also exhibit variable expression of calcium-binding proteins (e.g., parvalbumin, calbindin); these proteins may protect the cells from the destructive effects of the increases in intracellular calcium concentration that occur with high levels of discharge. Because of these differences across interneuron subtypes, and the fact that different brain regions are populated by different subpopulations of interneurons, different brain structures tend to show different patterns of interneuron depletion associated with various insults (including seizures). For example, in the hippocampus, somatostatin-containing interneurons appear to be selectively lost as a result of ischemia, status epilepticus, and/or chronic seizure activity. In turn, interneuron loss may lead to further hyperexcitability, as there may be a loss of inhibitory control as interneurons die.

As described above for the projection cells, different discharge patterns in interneurons are determined not only by the patterns (and locations) of synaptic inputs, but also by the patterns of voltage-gated channels that are involved in action potential generation, resting potential determination, etc. Such channels underlie currents that determine action potential duration (for example, some interneurons have extremely brief action potentials compared with those of projection cells), spike after-hyperpolarizations (some interneurons are easily recognized electrophysiologically by their profound after-hyperpolarization profile), interspike interval (determining the frequency of action potential firing), tendency to burst, spike-firing adaptation, etc.

Although it is likely that the properties of interneurons, like those of projection cells, are regulated developmentally, much less is known about how interneuron properties change with maturation. We do know, however, that (at least for cortical structures) the developmental migrational patterns of interneurons is quite different from that of pyramidal cells (Anderson et al., 1999), a difference that must be factored into discussions about developmental abnormalities associated with epileptic discharge. Cortical pyramidal cells arise in the subventricular zone and migrate in a generally "vertical" progression into their mature cortical stations, with cell type-specific features appearing as part of this process. Interneurons, in contrast, migrate into immature cortical regions from the median eminence, along a generally horizontal pathway. How their properties change along this rather complex migratory pathway, how the different interneuron subtypes find their appropriate locations within the cortical architecture, and how they establish functional inhibitory contacts with projection cells are all critical questions if we are to understand how these cells establish appropriate circuitry control. Aberrations in these developmental processes may give rise to abnormal discharge activities in cortex (Jones and Baraban, 2007).

As discussed above, the expression and location of the channels and other intrinsic interneuron features are now known to be "plastic," even in the adult brain. These interneuron features may be influenced by metabolic events, by activity levels, by circulating hormones, and by many other factors. Given the great variety of interneurons in cortical structures, the complexity of their input and output systems, and the potential for such plasticity, it is difficult to determine *a priori* the effects of activity (or loss of activity) in a given interneuron population. What does seem clear, however, is that loss of interneuron populations and/or loss of the inhibitory effects of GABA *can* have potent epileptiform consequences. Indeed, perhaps the most enduring hypothesis to explain epileptic activity revolves around loss of GABAergic interneurons.

SYNAPTIC PROPERTIES OF NEURONS

As discussed above, the epileptic state is often defined in terms of an imbalance between excitatory and inhibitory influences. In a simplistic way, this general concept has been translated into a discussion about enhanced synaptic excitation (E) (e.g., as reflected in the "power" of glutamatergic synapses) and/or reduced synaptic inhibition (I) (as determined by GABAergic synaptic power) (see Fig. 2.1). Although there are certainly other synaptic influences at play, these synapses provide the basic excitatory and inhibitory drives. Changes in glutamatergic and GABAergic synapses, and modulation of their influences by other inputs, largely determine the E–I balance.

In most discussions of synaptic properties of cortical structures, the focus is squarely on the chemical synapses associated with glutamate and GABA neurotransmission. Electrotonic neurotransmission has been somewhat neglected, since electronic transmission (via gap junctions) has been thought to be relatively rare in mammalian brain. Traditionally, electrical synapses have been considered to be nonplastic, and useful primarily for fast synchronization of limited neuronal populations (or for glial synchronization and for cell-to-cell transmission of small intracellular molecules). Such networks are, so the story goes, of questionable value in cortical structures in which synaptic modification is central to adaptive function. Recent research has again reminded us about the potential importance of electrical synapses, both in normal activities and in modulating seizure-like activities (e.g., Carlen et al., 2000; Connors and Long, 2004). Electrotonic synapses, particularly among interneurons, appear to be critical in mediating synchronous activities that in turn determine cortical outputs; high-frequency oscillatory activities (e.g., fast ripples) that appear in epileptic cortex may be generated via such connectivity (Traub et al., 2002). The role of gap junctions in linking cells in the glial syncytium will be addressed briefly below in the discussion of glia in modulating neuronal excitability.

Excitatory circuits

We typically associate excitatory synaptic effects with the transmission of information from one region of the brain to another. Indeed, such "feedforward" excitation of cortical neurons (e.g., afferent input into the neocortex from the thalamus or from other cortical regions, or afferent excitation of hippocampal neurons) constitutes important relay circuits, not only for seizure propagation but also for information transfer in the normal brain. At least as important, and until relatively recently somewhat neglected, are excitatory *feedback* circuits, whereby excitatory (projection) cells within a given area provide excitatory synaptic input (via axon collaterals) to neighboring neurons (Fig. 2.5A). Such feedback excitation is a critical feature of, for

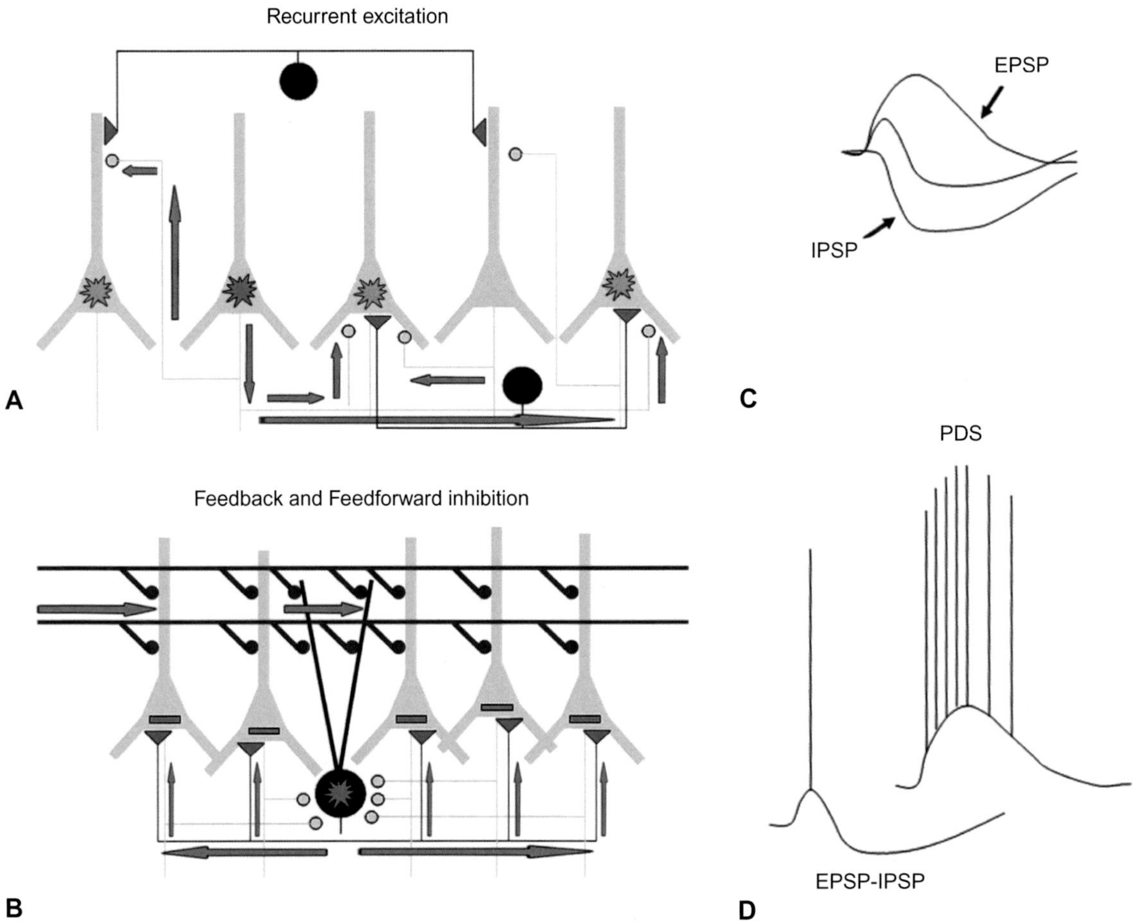

Fig. 2.5. (**A**) Diagrammatic representation of recurrent excitatory circuitry, involving excitatory connections among projection neurons. (**B**) Representation of feedforward and feedback inhibitory circuits. In the former, afferent input directly excites inhibitory interneurons, which then make synaptic contact onto projection cells. In the latter, afferents first synapse on projection cells, which then excite interneurons, which in turn provide inhibition to abort further discharge of the projection cell. (**C**) Illustration of the interplay between excitatory and inhibitory synaptic drive (EPSP and IPSP), which summate to produce the typical EPSP–IPSP sequence seen in most synaptically activated projection cells. (**D**) Normally, the EPSP triggers at most a single action potential, as the depolarization is rapidly offset by synaptic inhibition. However, when inhibition is compromised, the EPSP leads to a more prolonged depolarization that can trigger multiple action potentials, in the form of a burst discharge (or paroxysmal depolarization shift; PDS).

example, the CA3 region of hippocampus, where the CA3 pyramidal cell axon collaterals make numerous synaptic contacts onto other CA3 pyramidal cells (or even onto the parent CA3 neuron, via "autapses") (Christian and Dudek, 1988). Circuitry models of learning/memory have identified the CA3 excitatory feedback circuit as critical to normal learning-related synaptic plasticity (Hasselmo et al., 1995). And importantly, it is this region of hippocampus that appears to be the "pacemaker" for "interictal" epileptiform discharge, a role also dependent on this feedback excitatory interaction (Miles and Wong, 1987). Interestingly, in the epileptic hippocampus, the excitatory dentate granule cells, which in normal brain do not excite one another, develop excitatory recurrent collaterals of their axon system ("mossy fiber sprouting"); elaboration of this aberrant positive feedback loop appears to be highly correlated with the development of epileptic activity in hippocampus (Sutula and Dudek, 2007).

Glutamate as an excitatory agent

At the vast majority of excitatory chemical synapses in the adult mammalian forebrain, the excitatory neurotransmitter is glutamate. Glutamate is released into the synaptic cleft from synaptic vesicles, in a calcium-dependent manner. In most cases, these glutamatergic synapses consist of an axon terminal (presynaptic elements) making contact with a dendritic specialization on the target neuron. In cases where the postsynaptic neuron is an excitatory cell, the synapse most often involves a contact onto a dendritic spine; in some cases, however, when the postsynaptic cell has no spines (as is the case for "aspiny interneurons"), these contacts are directly onto dendritic shafts. Although ubiquitous and consistently excitatory, glutamate may have varied effects on its target, depending on the type of postsynaptic receptor. Ionotropic glutamate receptors (receptors that are directly associated with ion channels) come in two major varieties. The first of these, the *N*-methyl-D-aspartate (NMDA) receptors, have received considerable attention, as activation of these receptors, and subsequent opening of the channel, allows not only sodium into the cell (causing depolarization), but also calcium (Dingledine, 1983). The calcium serves as an intracellular signaling molecule, and has been implicated in a number of important cell functions, including synaptic plasticity (e.g., long-term potentiation and depression) (Malenka, 1991). The NMDA receptors have also been implicated in many of the pathologies associated with excitotoxicity, where enhanced influx of calcium triggers significant neurodegenerative changes, and can lead to aberrant gene expression. Indeed, specific blockade of NMDA channels has been shown to be neuroprotective as well as antiepileptic (Lipton, 2007). Unfortunately, interfering with this neurotransmission pathway also has – not surprisingly – significant negative cognitive side-effects; for this reason, early interest in NMDA blockade as an antiepileptic therapy has not been pursued.

Non-NMDA glutamatergic ionotropic receptor subtypes come in various forms, and are generally thought to provide the basic fast glutamatergic activation we see at excitatory synapses. Although not involved directly in triggering synaptic plasticity (as are the NMDA receptors), these non-NMDA receptor/channel molecules provide the structural basis for long-term plastic changes (Kullmann et al., 2000), moving into and out of the membrane as instructed by intracellular messenger molecules (such as calcium) (Malinow, 2003). Further, as NMDA channels open only when the membrane is depolarized (to expel the magnesium ion from the channel pore), the non-NMDA glutamatergic receptors provide the necessary membrane depolarization to make NMDA channels functional. NMDA and non-NMDA receptors often are found near each other at postsynaptic sites, where one can easily and quickly influence the function of the other.

Finally, there is a large and complex set of metabotropic glutamate receptors, i.e., receptors that are not directly associated with an ion pore, but the activation of which is mediated by intracellular signaling molecules to produce slow and prolonged changes in cellular excitability. There is growing evidence that such metabotropic glutamate receptors may be importantly involved in epileptogenic changes (Merlin, 2002, 2008; Wong et al., 2004).

Developmental and activity-dependent changes in synaptic excitation

Although the glutamatergic excitatory system is challengingly complex in the normal adult CNS, its function is complicated further by the fact that there are important maturation-dependent changes in its function. There are, for example, different sets of receptors in the immature cortex and hippocampus, including non-NMDA receptors that, because of the unique immature subunit composition of the receptor, admit calcium into the cell. In normal brain, these immature receptors are replaced over a critical period of development. But their function in the immature brain contributes to the excitability (and vulnerability) patterns of immature cortex. Further, there is growing evidence that pathological activity (e.g., seizures) may cause (and/or reflect) a "reversion" of normal mature channels to an immature state (Sanchez et al., 2001), and thus lead to functional changes in the excitatory glutamatergic system.

Other developmentally regulated changes in excitation revolve around the normally inhibitory GABAergic system (below). Indeed, in the immature cortex, GABA action on $GABA_A$ receptors can lead to chloride efflux from the neuron, with subsequent membrane depolarization and enhanced excitability (Rheims et al., 2008). This seemingly paradoxical effect is the result of the relatively slow maturational development of KCC2 chloride transporters that move chloride out of the neuron; thus, in the immature neuron, intracellular chloride concentration is relatively high compared with extracellular levels, and GABA-mediated opening of chloride channels leads to chloride efflux (and membrane depolarization). Developmental studies have suggested that this GABA-mediated depolarization plays an important trophic function in immature cortex (Owens and Kriegstein, 2002; Wang and Kriegstein, 2009). It clearly also contributes to the enhanced excitability of immature cortical tissues.

Local inhibitory circuits

The excitatory cortical circuitries are relatively simple compared with the potential complexity of local inhibitory interaction. Because there are so many different types of inhibitory cell (interneurons), and because there is potential for different patterns of synaptic interactions with different target cells, interneurons are ideally suited to provide the fine-tuning that characterizes normal cortical function. This circuitry, by the same token, represents the "weak link" in the control of excitatory–inhibitory balance. Even a relatively small reduction in inhibitory efficacy (e.g., on the order of 10–15%) can result in rather dramatic hyperexcitability (Chagnac-Amitai and Connors, 1989).

As is the case for excitatory circuits, inhibition comes in both feedforward and feedback varieties. Afferent excitation of inhibitory interneurons leads in a relatively direct way to inhibit projection cells within the region; indeed, the same afferents often excite both the projection (pyramidal) cells and the inhibitory interneurons (Fig. 2.5B). Initial afferent excitation of the pyramidal cells is followed almost immediately by interneuron-mediated inhibition, so that depolarization of the pyramidal cells is normally very brief (curtailed by powerful inhibition). This effect is accentuated by recurrent inhibitory pathways, whereby excited projection cells within a given region excite (via recurrent collaterals) local inhibitory interneurons, which in turn curtail the activity of the projection cells (Fig. 2.5C). Under normal conditions, pyramidal cell discharge is under powerful inhibitory control. If, however, there is a change in inhibitory efficacy, excitation is released and epileptiform hyperexcitability may be seen (Fig. 2.5D).

GABA as an inhibitory agent

The primary inhibitory neurotransmitter in the mammalian forebrain is γ-aminobutyric acid (GABA). It is released by inhibitory interneurons, and its effects are mediated by both ionotropic ($GABA_A$) and metabotropic ($GABA_B$) receptors. The basic function of $GABA_A$ receptors is to open a chloride-permeable channel; chloride efflux through that channel usually hyperpolarizes (inhibits) the postsynaptic neurons (except as above). The effect of GABA at those postsynaptic $GABA_A$ receptors is highly modulated, however, depending on the exact composition of the pentameric $GABA_A$ receptor (Olsen and Sieghart, 2008). The receptor/channel function is modulated by such diverse molecules/ions as barbiturates, benzodiazepines, and zinc (Gibbs et al., 2000; Harrison, 2007), which bind to specific sites on receptor subunits. This structure-dependent modulation results in importantly diverse (and plastic) receptor/channel function.

In addition to the fast/phasic GABA-mediated inhibition associated with GABA release and activation of $GABA_A$ receptors at synaptic sites, recent research has identified a tonic inhibition – also mediated by $GABA_A$ receptors that are located at "peri- or extra-synaptic" sites. These receptors, with unique subunit composition (typically containing a δ subunit rather than a γ subunit), appear to set inhibitory "tone" within a cortical circuit (Scimemi et al., 2005; Glykys and Mody, 2006). As such, modulation of these receptors can be critical in altering the thresholds for neuronal firing, and for determining thresholds for epileptiform activities.

Although the $GABA_A$ receptor is typically found on postsynaptic elements at the inhibitory synapse, $GABA_B$ receptors are often associated with both postsynaptic and presynaptic elements (e.g., synaptic terminals), and are thought to be important in modulating neurotransmitter release (Misgeld et al., 2007). When such receptors are on GABAergic neurons, their activation can hyperpolarize the neuron (soma or terminal elements), reduce GABA release, and thus somewhat paradoxically result in disinhibition (i.e., inhibition of inhibition). $GABA_B$ receptors are also found postsynaptically, where they play a role analogous to the metabotropic glutamate receptors (i.e., slow modulation of postsynaptic cell excitability via internal signaling pathways) (Avoli et al., 2004).

Plasticity mediated by changes in GABAergic function

Although there is little evidence of long-term synaptic potentiation or depression (LTP or LTD) mediated directly at GABA synapses, GABA-mediated inhibition is highly sensitive to a variety of agents and effects. For example, the efficacy of GABA-mediated inhibition appears to decrease dramatically with repetitive activation of the synapse (Kaplan et al., 2003). Thus, under conditions in which synaptic plasticity is associated with increased excitation, changes in the properties of GABAergic synapses (reduced GABA release from presynaptic neurons, altered response of receptors to prolonged presence of GABA) have been shown to reduce inhibition. This property may be of particular importance for seizure-related states in which high levels of activity – perhaps produced by an initial but transient reduction in inhibition – lead to a more prolonged excitatory state due to a chronic loss of inhibitory efficacy. Activity-dependent (or injury-dependent) alterations in $GABA_A$ receptor subunit composition may also lead to altered GABA inhibition, either increased or reduced (Raol et al., 2006). Indeed, high levels of activity may even lead to expression of GABA in terminals of nominally glutamatergic neurons, a phenomenon described for the granule cell mossy fiber terminals (Gutierrez, 2003). In this case, activity appears to lead to a homeostatic mechanism that increases inhibition in the overexcited dentate system.

It is important to note, also, that GABA-mediated inhibition is tied closely to glutamate function, as GABA is ordinarily synthesized from glutamate (via glutamic acid decarboxylase; GAD) in the terminals of inhibitory neurons. Glutamate uptake by astrocytes, conversion of glutamate to glutamine, transport of glutamine from glia to neurons, and the resynthesis of glutamate form a critical glutamine–glutamate cycle, the integrity of which has important consequences for GABA synthesis and adequate levels of inhibition (Liang et al., 2006).

MODULATION OF NEURONAL EXCITABILITY

Although the basic level of excitability of neural tissue is set by the intrinsic properties of the participating neurons and by the primary synaptic interaction among them, that excitability is modulated powerfully by a host of variables; influences of these factors may have profound consequences for the epileptogenicity of the tissue (Fig. 2.6). Some (but certainly not all) of the important players involved in these modulatory interactions are discussed briefly below.

Astrocytes

Astrocytes are now recognized as full partners with neurons in determining brain function. Studies have confirmed their critical roles not only in brain metabolic function, but also in controlling ionic and neurotransmitter levels that are central to neuronal function. Among those functions most obviously relevant to excitability and epileptogenicity are regulation of extracellular potassium concentration and glutamate uptake.

REGULATION OF EXTRACELLULAR POTASSIUM CONCENTRATION

Glia have long been recognized for their ability to take up potassium from the extracellular space. Indeed, the glia act almost like potassium indicators, as their membrane potential depolarizes in direct response to release of potassium from neurons. As neurons release potassium during excitatory activity (e.g., action potential generation), and as increasing extracellular potassium concentration in turn contributes to neuronal excitation, potassium uptake by glia is important for interrupting this potentially positive feedback system. Potassium uptake is a consequence of activation of the Na,K-ATPase (the "pump") on both neurons and glia, as well as of glial Na/K/Cl cotransport (Leis et al., 2005). In addition, glia (or at least some subpopulation of glia) are endowed with a voltage-dependent channel mechanism (inward rectifiers) for potassium uptake, and constitute a potassium "buffering" system (Sontheimer, 1994). This system appears to be designed for potassium uptake (into astrocytes) in regions of high extracellular concentration, with subsequent redistribution of the ion through the glial syncytium (large populations of glial cells linked via gap junctions), to be released in other brain regions of lower potassium concentration (but see Wallraff et al., 2006).

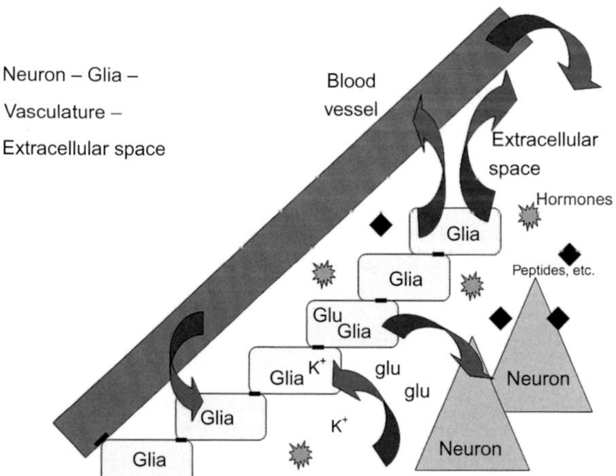

Fig. 2.6. Diagrammatic illustration of the various non-neuronal elements that contribute to excitability and its control. Astrocytes connected via gap junctions form a syncytium; they are critical in maintaining the extracellular environment. The glia are also in contact with the vasculature (their endfeet helping to form the blood–brain barrier), and are endowed with potent uptake mechanisms for regulating extracellular potassium ions and glutamate. Neuronal excitability is also affected by circulating hormones, as well as by neuromodulatory substances (peptides, neurotrophic factors, etc.) released locally by neurons and glia.

GLUTAMATE UPTAKE

Astrocytes are also critical in the process of glutamate uptake (i.e., the process of removing synaptically released glutamate from the extracellular space). Endowed with highly efficient glutamate transporter molecules, astrocytic processes typically envelope synaptic junctions so that they can rapidly remove glutamate to prevent continued/renewed excitation of neurons (Volterra and Steinhauser, 2004; Rose et al., 2009). Under some conditions (high levels of activity, such as during seizures), this transport process may run in the reverse direction, resulting in glial release of glutamate into the extracellular space – a process that would then presumably further excite nearby neurons (Haydon and Carmignoto, 2006; Malarkey and Parpura, 2008). Interestingly, astrocytes have also recently been shown to have a subset of glutamate receptors on their membranes; action of extracellular glutamate at these metabotropic receptors has been hypothesized to control, for example, neurotropin release and calcium signaling important in regulating vascular properties (D'Antoni et al., 2008; Jean et al., 2008). Indeed, when these astrocytic metabotropic glutamate receptors are activated, one can see (using calcium imaging techniques) the spread of calcium "waves" through the glial network. This widespread increase in intracellular calcium concentration, mediated via the gap junctions that connect astrocytes into a broad network of cells, provides a mechanism whereby glia may help to generalize and/or spread responses to local perturbations. Given these critical roles of astrocytes in regulating excitability, alterations in astrocyte properties in tissue from epileptic brain are of obvious significance (Bordey et al., 2001; Binder and Steinhauser, 2006).

Ionic changes

Neuronal (and glial) activity depends largely on the movement of ions across their membranes, with the extracellular concentrations of these ions in dynamic flux. Changes in the intracellular/extracellular ionic balance lead to an ongoing modulation of the excitability of neuronal elements. The relative extracellular concentrations of sodium, chloride, and potassium will affect neural excitability because of the influences of this balance on the drive to move ions into or out of the cell, and thus alter the likelihood of action potential discharge. In addition, these ionic fluxes may alter excitability by associated changes in water movement. Imbalance in intracellular versus extracellular osmolarity are associated with movement of water into, or out of, the cell through specialized channels called aquaporins (Manley et al., 2004; Nagelhus et al., 2004; Hsu et al., 2007). Subsequent swelling (or shrinkage) of neuronal volume, and concomitant shrinkage (or expansion) of the extracellular space (ECS), can have direct effects on neuronal excitability (Haglund and Hochman, 2005), mediated by several different mechanisms. For example, "ephaptic" effects of cell swelling and associated shrinkage of the ECS have been demonstrated in a number of experimental studies (e.g., Dudek et al., 1998). Current movement through the higher resistance ECS (narrower spaces = higher resistance) generates larger voltage changes, which in turn may help to depolarize neurons. This ephaptic effect has been shown to "recruit" neurons into an actively discharging population, and thus serves as a mechanism for synchronizing neurons within such a population.

Ion flux also involves the movement of H^+ ions, and leads to changes in intracellular and extracellular pH. It is now clear that even subtle changes in pH directly affect neuronal excitability, at least in part because the function of NMDA glutamate channels (and gap junction channels) is pH-sensitive. Acidification of the extracellular space reduces neuronal excitability, and alkalinization enhances neuronal firing (Somjen, 1984; Ransom, 2000; Obara et al., 2008). Interestingly, high levels of activity lead to acidification of the extracellular space, providing an intrinsic feedback mechanism for controlling discharge (i.e., reducing excitability). Small pH changes are a normal component of brain activity, and regulation of extracellular pH is one of the critical functions of astrocytes.

Neuropeptides and other neurotransmitters

Although glutamate and GABA undoubtedly function as the major neurochemical agents in the mammalian forebrain, the synaptic excitation and inhibition evoked by these neurotransmitters are modulated by a host of other chemical agents, including agents that are synaptically released and cause rapid – or slow – postsynaptic changes. Among the "classical" neurotransmitter modulatory agents are acetylcholine and a variety of catecholamines (norepinephrine, serotonin, and dopamine). These transmitter agents are typically released by afferents originating in subcortical nuclei (often in the brainstem) or from cortically localized interneurons. In addition, modern research has identified a set of peptide molecules that are also released from neurons – often only when neurons fire at high frequency – to modulate the excitability of postsynaptic elements. These "neuropeptides" include molecules such as neuropeptide Y (NPY), somatostatin, galanin, and cholecystokinin (CCK) (Mazarati, 2004; Sperk et al., 2007; Tallent, 2007). This category of modulators also includes various opioid chemicals and endocannabinoids (Simonato and Romualdi, 1996; Alger, 2004; Katona and Freund, 2008). These agents are typically released from subpopulations of interneurons; indeed, identification of interneuron subpopulations is often based on their colocalization (along with GABA) of such neuromodulatory substances.

A complete description of the action of these agents is beyond the scope of this chapter. However, a brief summary of the best studied of these modulators is useful. Acetylcholine (ACh) has been widely studied at the neuromuscular junction, where it mediates a fast excitatory effect via nicotinic receptors. However, in the forebrain, ACh is released primarily from afferents from the medial forebrain (septum, diagonal band of Broca, basal forebrain nuclei) and has been generally associated with a slower, muscarinic depolarization of cortical neurons (Gulledge and Kawaguchi, 2007). In normal brain, ACh release is importantly involved in generation of theta rhythm, acting to excite interneurons (which then inhibit excitatory projection cells) (Reich et al., 2005; Bandyopadhyay et al., 2006) and/or modulate a potassium current (the m-current) on pyramidal cells. Cholinergic input to cortex and hippocampus has been implicated in learning/memory processes (Hasselmo, 2006). Disruption of cholinergic tone (i.e., loss of ACh-containing neurons) can lead to pathology (e.g., in Alzheimer's disease), including changes in brain excitability (Mufson et al., 2003). Cholinergic muscarinic agents such as pilocarpine, injected systemically, can induce intense and prolonged hyperexcitability (status epilepticus).

The role of catecholaminergic drugs has been explored primarily within the context of psychiatric disorders (Howes and Kapur, 2009; Sara, 2009), but there is a significant literature on their effects on brain epileptogenicity (Jobe, 2003; Giorgi et al., 2004; Kanner, 2007). In general, the monoamines – serotonin and dopamine – appear to have inhibitory effects on their postsynaptic targets. Norepinephrine (NE), however, has complex and multiple effects, depending on the nature of the receptor with which it interacts. Although many studies have shown that NE has a net inhibitory effect (i.e., loss of NE leads to increased excitability, as seen in the epileptic phenotype of a knockout mouse in which the NE-synthesizing enzyme, dopamine β-hydroxylase, is deleted; Weinshenker and Szot, 2002), activation of some NE receptor subtypes clearly excites the postsynaptic neuron. Thus, as is the case for ACh, it is impossible to predict change of cortical excitability associated with disruption of the NE system without having detailed knowledge about which cells, and which receptors, are affected by the disruption (Gulyas et al., 1999; Kruglikov and Rudy, 2008).

Like NE, most of the neuropeptide agents have been shown to have primarily inhibitory effects. Because they are released primarily by specific subpopulations of interneurons, their influence can be exquisitely localized. However, recent studies have shown that treatments that increase release of these neuropeptides within specific brain regions (e.g., through transplantation of peptide-releasing neurons, or through neuronal transfection with genetic material leading to overproduction of, for example, NPY or galanin) (Mazarati et al., 2000; Noe et al., 2008; Riban et al., 2009) can cause a general antiepileptic effect. This influence presumably is due to the powerful influence of these agents on key excitatory elements in cortex or hippocampus. Unlike NPY or somatostatin or galanin, opioid peptides often appear to have a net excitatory effect. Yet, they too produce primarily inhibition on their postsynaptic targets. As those targets are predominantly inhibitory interneurons, the opioid effect is thought to be "disinhibitory." Other modulatory molecules (neurotrophic factors, adenosine, etc.) that are released from neurons (and glia) provide intrinsic antiepileptic protection, and upregulation of these chemicals (e.g., via grafts engineered to release these agents), appear to have real potential as novel antiepileptic therapies (Rao et al., 2007; Boison, 2009).

Circulating agents

In contrast to the modulatory agents described above, which are released from presynaptic cells to influence the excitability of rather specific postsynaptic targets, there is another type of modulatory agent that is released into the circulatory system. Such agents, in the form of hormones, may provide slowly acting modulation of neuronal excitability, often as a part of a feedback loop whereby changes in brain activity (e.g., in the hypothalamus) increase, or decrease, the release of these hormones. For example, the hypothalamic–pituitary–adrenal (HPA) axis not only provides signals for the release of steroid hormones (glucocorticoids and mineralocorticoids, as well as sex hormones), but is also regulated by the effects of these molecules at the CNS level. Of particular significance with respect to seizure discharge are the effects of stress hormones, which have profound effects on neuronal viability, and act on specific neuronal receptors to cause changes in cell discharge (Joels, 2009). Another reflection of hormonal modulation of brain excitability can be seen in the catemenial epilepsies (Penovich and Helmers, 2008), which appear to result from large swings in the release of estrogen- and progesterone-like molecules; these steroid hormones, and their metabolites, have excitatory and inhibitory effects (respectively) on central neurons, and also may trigger neuronal signaling mechanisms that result in various forms of neuronal plasticity (Smith and Woolley, 2004; Foy et al., 2008). The sex steroid molecules have also been implicated in neuroprotection (Suzuki et al., 2006; Veliskova, 2006). Although these hormones are, by definition, produced and released into the circulatory system at some distance from the brain, some steroid-like molecules appear to be manufactured within the brain itself. Such "neurosteroids" act on specific receptors (both membrane and nuclear) and regulate neuronal function; there is considerable interest in the application of these molecules in antiepileptic treatment (Reddy and Rogawski, 2009).

Similarly, another category of modulatory molecules that are made and released within the brain can have important (and still poorly explored) effects on neuronal integrity and excitability. These molecules include neurotrophic agents such as brain-derived neurotrophic factor (BDNF), which has been shown to have direct excitatory effects on subpopulations of neurons (e.g., in the CA3 region of hippocampus), can induce long-term synaptic potentiation-like effects, and appears to be critical for kindling-like plasticity as well as for neuronal repair and growth (Binder and Scharfman, 2004; He et al., 2004). In the hippocampus, these tropic agents are localized to mossy fiber terminals (Danzer and McNamara, 2004), and are released to act at specific receptors, triggering complex intracellular signaling pathways (Paradiso et al., 2009).

Finally, immune system-related molecules – often associated with inflammatory reactions to infection or injury – are now known to have various effects on neuronal excitability as well as on cell viability. Cytokine release from astrocytes (as well as from microglia) represent the brain's immediate protective response to foreign substances (or to the products of cell damage), and may also increase tissue excitability and thus contribute to seizure activity. There is now considerable interest in, and analysis of, immune-related molecules as they relate to changes in the epileptic brain (Vezzani et al., 2008).

PATHOLOGICAL PROCESSES

Developmental abnormalities

Many (perhaps most) epilepsies can be thought of as pediatric disorders, in the sense that the initiating factor(s) appears early in brain development. In some cases, genetic mutations lead to epilepsies that are seen early in the life of the child, but have little or no gross cellular manifestations. Understanding of these disorders begins, therefore, at the genetic/molecular level; insights into the abnormal production or localization of specific proteins (e.g., channels or receptors) can then be pursued within the context of altered brain excitability. Another set of genetic disorders gives rise to aberrations in molecular signaling, which in turn alters the physical processes of brain development, resulting in morphologically and/or histologically identifiable abnormalities in brain structure that are highly associated with seizure activity. These structural abnormalities may be rather subtle, for example focal cortical dysplasia consisting of relatively small numbers of heterotopic and/or morphologically aberrant neurons (Eriksson et al., 2005; Blumcke, 2009), or they may be quite dramatic, e.g., shrunken cortex as in the various lissencephalies (Schwartzkroin and Walsh, 2000). Although there is often an intuitively attractive "explanation" for the underlying basis of epilepsies with genetic/molecular abnormalities of channels or receptors, it is rarely obvious how the more overt structural changes lead to epileptiform discharges. In general, the epileptogenic bases of these developmental "lesions" can be viewed as arising from one or more of the following pathologies:

- *Formation of aberrant neurons or glia* – i.e., cells that have hyperexcitable intrinsic properties, which then act as "pacemaker" cells that drive surrounding tissue into seizure activity. Although some developmental abnormalities do present with such aberrant neurons (e.g., the "balloon cells" of focal cortical dysplasia and tuberous sclerosis), there is currently little evidence that such cells are major epileptogenic factors. In contrast, relatively normal-appearing pyramidal cells have been shown to have abnormal complements of channels or receptors that might be viewed as "epileptic" (Cepeda et al., 2003). Not to be ignored, aberrant ("reactive") astrocytes may also contribute to hyperexcitability, as a result of abnormal function resulting from alterations in their channels, receptors, coupling mechanisms, or transporter molecules (Bordey et al., 2001; Wong et al., 2003; Binder and Steinhauser, 2006).
- *Loss of interneurons resulting in reduced inhibition.* Interneuron generation and migration into cortical structures follows a program quite different from that of the resident pyramidal cells. Several of the disorders of cortical development are associated with specific aberrations that affect interneuron migration and/or differentiation and/or survival, with the functional consequence of too little inhibitory control of the excitatory cortical circuitry (Friocourt et al., 2007; Gant et al., 2009).
- *Reduced or enhanced production of cortical pyramidal neurons (and/or glia).* This type of process leads to abnormal circuits, often with excitatory cells synapsing directly on other excitatory cells to form aberrant networks (Haas et al., 2002).
- *Heterotopic localization of young neurons* – results not only in abnormal cortical structure, but also in epileptogenic circuits due to aberrant synaptic patterns with incoming afferents or other local neurons (Scharfman et al., 2003).

Some developmental brain abnormalities consist of more than one of the above conditions, or a given primary cellular condition may give rise, over the course of development, to other types of abnormality that affect cortical function. As indicated above, the precise epileptogenic mechanism is rarely obvious. Particularly in order to understand appropriate points of therapeutic intervention, it is necessary to explore each condition to assess the developmental epileptogenic processes. Such studies are now being carried out using a variety of animal models in which appropriate genetic alterations are induced, and/or parallel structural lesions are experimentally generated.

Trauma-induced changes

Although we now recognize that many epilepsies have aberrant genetic bases, that recognition is relatively recent. Indeed, for years, it was thought that most epilepsies – the "acquired" epilepsies – reflected some form of traumatic brain injury (TBI). Developmental epilepsies, including those with structural phenotypes, were thought to result from early, sometimes *in utero*, insults. Clearly, trauma-induced changes, in the absence of any "epilepsy genes," can lead to epileptic conditions. The underlying mechanisms of such epilepsies depend heavily on the type of insult, the timing of the insult, the location of the insult (if focal), and any underlying genetic predispositions. Thus, identification of mechanisms of trauma-induced epilepsies is difficult and complex. Again, however, the contributing factors are likely to include one of more of the following:

1. Specific loss of inhibitory interneuron (selective vulnerability of subclasses of interneurons)

2. General excitotoxicity, with loss of sensitive neuronal populations (including both inhibitory and excitatory neurons)
3. Cell damage (but not death), resulting in cell populations with aberrant discharge features (e.g., altered expression of channels or receptors)
4. Reorganization of circuits
5. Alteration of channel/receptor patterns on neurons and glia.

These types of change have been implicated as epileptogenic factors that can influence brain function following various types of insult and injury, from TBI (automobile accidents, wartime injuries) to brain infections to stroke (Lowenstein, 2009). Several of the above features can be – indeed, are likely to be – present concomitantly, making it difficult to determine the initial (initiating?) or salient (with respect to epilepsy) brain change associated with the trauma. For example, in animal models of TBI, status epilepticus, and ischemia (stroke), investigators have found: massive release of glutamate that leads to excitotoxic damage and cell death in focal brain regions; early loss of sensitive neuronal populations, which most often include subpopulations of inhibitory interneurons; progressive large-scale loss of principal neurons; and synaptic reorganization involving the formation of new (and usually aberrant) synaptic relationships (Dudek and Shao, 2002; Prince et al., 2009). Altered properties of surviving neurons have also been reported in many of these models. In most cases, it is unclear which changes are "primary" and which changes (e.g., circuitry reorganization) are subsequent to earlier primary events (e.g., altered patterns of synaptic input or different levels of neuronal activity). The fact that all of these features have been observed in human tissue samples seems to confirm the clinical significance of such findings in animal models.

Despite the consistency of these pathologies, the determination of which change constitutes the *epileptogenic* factor remains controversial. Perhaps the most influential current hypothesis views neuronal injury – and particularly cell death – as the precipitating event, and the reorganizational consequence as the key to epileptogenesis. However, epileptogenicity has been demonstrated under conditions of little obvious synaptic reorganization, making it unclear what abnormalities should be targeted in attempts at therapy. Further, the possibility that initial (and ongoing) abnormal activities help to maintain and expand the epileptic zone remains of significant concern, with many investigators still studying the potential of "seizures begetting seizures" (Ben-Ari, 2006).

In the following paragraphs, I have tried to provide a couple of clinically relevant examples of epilepsies in which some of the pathological changes mentioned above have been identified. I have chosen one example of focal epilepsy – temporal lobe epilepsy (TLE) – and one example of generalized epilepsy – generalized epilepsy with febrile seizures plus (GEFS+). These are epilepsy syndromes about which considerable information, clinical and laboratory, has been generated, leading to a perception that we understand the mechanisms fairly well. Although it is clear that we have identified many potential epilepsy-related features of these syndromes, it is important to recognize that the *causal* relationships (with respect to the epilepsy) remain complex and often puzzling.

Example of focal epilepsy – temporal lobe epilepsy

TLE is the most common of the drug-resistant epilepsies among the adult population. It has not only been the focus of extensive pharmacological and clinical investigation, but also the target of surgical intervention, which is often successful. Because TLE is generally considered to be focal (i.e., associated with a discrete regional abnormality that constitutes the initiation zone for seizure genesis), it lends itself well to experimental model investigation. Indeed, the vast majority of our animal models have focused on the hippocampus and related temporal lobe structures. These studies have revealed a number of interesting features that help to explain both the focal nature of this disorder and its relatively high frequency. In particular, hippocampal pyramidal cells (or at least some subpopulations, such as the CA3 cells) have been shown to have "pacemaker"-like potential – the tendency to discharge in bursts of action potentials that provide potent input to their targets, especially when that discharge is synchronized across a significant cell population. Further, these cells are synaptically connected (i.e., they excite one another), giving rise to a positive feedback loop. The potential for high levels of excitation is normally kept in check by powerful interneuronal inhibitory mechanisms. However, some subpopulations of interneurons are particularly vulnerable to excitotoxic injury (as are some hippocampal principal cells, the CA1 pyramidal cells, and the mossy cells). Under conditions of excitotoxic insult (e.g., status epilepticus or TBI), sensitive cell populations die, leading to dramatic circuitry reorganization (e.g., mossy fiber sprouting) that exacerbates the excitatory feedback characteristics of the hippocampus (Fig. 2.7). The cell injury/death process may be intensified by inflammatory reactions to the initial injury (reactive astrocytes, microglial proliferation), with release of cytokines which themselves appear to have excitatory actions on neurons. In addition, some conditions that lead to brain injury

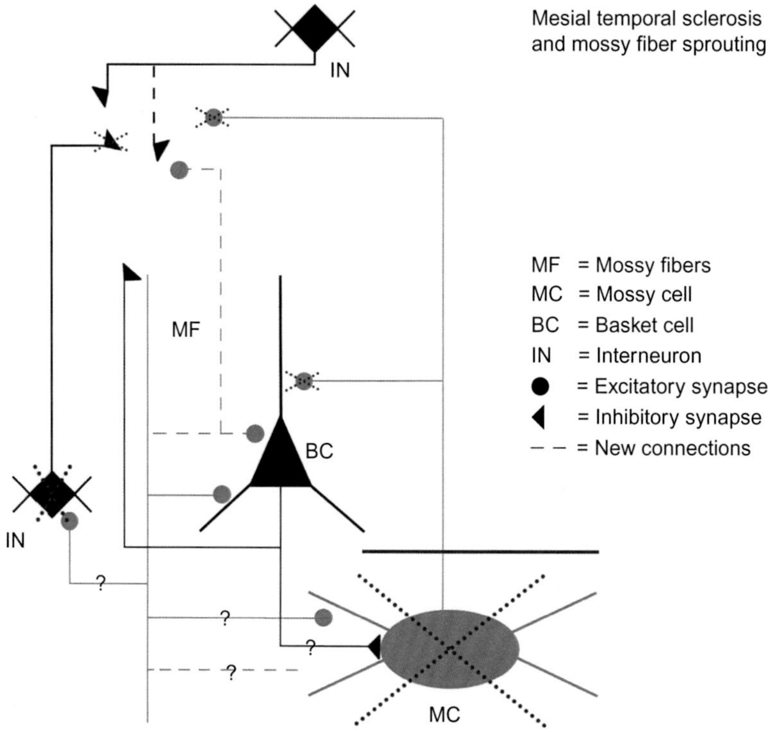

Fig. 2.7. Illustration of processes that are thought to occur in the genesis of temporal lobe epilepsy with hippocampal sclerosis. Excitotoxic influences cause degeneration of sensitive neuronal populations (e.g., excitatory mossy cells and subpopulations of inhibitory interneurons). Subsequent reorganization of hippocampal circuitry includes the formation of aberrant recurrent excitatory connections among granule cells (mossy fiber sprouting).

also tend to enhance neurogenesis, presumably to replace lost/damaged elements in the brain. Neurogenesis is relatively restricted within the brain, but one of the major sites of neurogenesis is the hippocampal dentate region. Newborn cells migrate within the dentate gyrus, and those that survive must establish new connections with the already-resident neurons. Aberrant migration and/or abnormal connectivity has been suggested to be a key element in some forms of TLE.

There is much compelling evidence for the epileptogenic nature of these sclerosis-associated and/or neurogenic pathologies in TLE. However, there is a significant population of clinical TLE cases in which no such processes are evident (e.g., no significant neuronal death, no obvious sprouting/circuitry reorganization, no aberrantly localized neurons). How might one explain these cases? Animal studies, particularly using the kindling model, have shed light on potential underlying mechanisms that appear to depend on relatively normal "plasticity" processes. Among these mechanisms is long-term potentiation of synaptic efficacy. Indeed, increased excitatory effects at already established synapses have been shown to be activity-dependent, reinforcing the concept that "seizures beget seizures", i.e., brief and/or acute increases in neuronal discharge can "kindle" seizure activity in otherwise normal brain regions. Kindling-like plasticity has been shown to involve changes in gene expression, altered channel/receptor number and/or subtype, subtle changes in axon/terminal connectivity (i.e., sprouting), and loss of inhibitory interneurons – sufficiently subtle changes to go undetected with current methods of analysis. Further, TLE tissue is increasingly associated with subtle forms of dysplasia (e.g., altered lamination patterns, heterotopic neurons, etc.) (Smart et al., 1998), suggesting an underlying disturbance in brain development or some early pathological process that affected small populations of neurons. Finally, a number of studies have suggested that the glia in TLE tissue may be aberrant in function (e.g., abnormal glutamate transport), with consequent effects on neuronal output.

Although clinical and basic laboratory studies have generally assumed that TLE is a result of focal abnormalities, it is important to recognize that even focal seizure initiation is likely to reflect potential abnormalities in broad neuronal networks. For example, it is increasingly clear that some gene mutations can promote, contribute to, or even cause a TLE-like syndrome. Recent clinical studies have identified a TLE associated with mutation of the *LGI1* gene, and laboratory research has characterized TLE-like epilepsies in gene knockout mice (Ottman et al., 2004). Although such gene abnormalities presumably are found in every cell (throughout the brain), the cell-type and region-specific expression of some genes may give rise to an apparently focal/partial brain excitability. Further, while focal temporal lobe abnormality can lead to local discharge, it is primarily when that discharge spreads, and involves other brain regions, that it becomes a significant clinical problem. Widespread brain circuitry is inevitably involved in the restriction and/or propagation of temporal lobe seizures; when efficient inhibitory control mechanisms break down in brain regions outside the temporal lobe (e.g., in the thalamus), focal hyperexcitability becomes widespread seizure activity.

Example of generalized epilepsy – generalized epilepsy with febrile seizures plus (GEFS+)

In contrast to partial/focal epilepsies such as TLE, there is a large set of so-called "idiopathic" epilepsies that represent a large proportion of the epilepsies in early development and childhood. These epilepsies are characterized by the apparently simultaneous onset of electrical abnormality (seizures) across broad regions of the brain, and so have been labeled "generalized." As obvious cell death or other tissue pathology is often absent (thus the term "idiopathic"), these epilepsies are typically associated with genetic abnormalities. Increasingly, investigators have identified gene mutations as a cause of these epilepsies, and in some cases mutations in a single gene have been shown to be responsible for the seizure condition (Burgess, 2005). One such case is the GEFS+ syndrome, a seizure condition that appears in childhood and is characterized by febrile generalized seizures in combination with afebrile seizure types (e.g., atonic or myoclonic seizures) (Scheffer et al., 2005). Early characterization of this syndrome identified mutations in the β subunit of the voltage-gated sodium channel; subsequently, other mutations (α subunit of the sodium channel, γ2 subunit of the $GABA_A$ receptor) were identified that gave rise to a similar clinical phenotype. Severe myoclonic epilepsy of infancy (SMEI), Dravet syndrome, has been shown to arise due to sodium channel α-subunit mutations (Scheffer et al., 2009). That loss of function mutations of a sodium channel subunit could lead to a seizure phenotype has been somewhat of a puzzle, because such a mutation would, intuitively, be expected to lead to *decreased* neuronal excitability. Recently, this apparent paradox has been "solved" by the demonstration that the channel subunit in question in SMEI is preferentially expressed in interneurons, and thus results in reduced activity in the inhibitory system (Yu et al., 2006; Yamakawa, 2009).

This "discovery" is important not only in understanding GEFS+ and Dravet syndrome, but also in the more general interpretation of gene-based epilepsies. The loss of a functional gene, or even the malfunction (or loss) of a specific cell population, does not necessarily provide insight into the underlying basis of a widespread seizure phenomenon. It is not sufficient simply to identify the gene mutation, or even to demonstrate the effect of the mutation on the function of the associated protein. One must also understand the pattern of gene expression, and the role of the expressing cells within large brain networks.

For example, past studies have elucidated the circuitry thought to be involved in generalized seizure generation, particularly the 3/sec spike–wave discharge (e.g., characteristic of absence seizures) (McCormick and Contreras, 2001). A network involving cortical pyramidal cell excitatory output to the thalamus and associated reticular nucleus (nRT), the powerful inhibitory effects of nRT neurons on thalamic relay cells, and the positive feedback of thalamic relay neurons to the cortex, have all been shown to be involved in generating a regular pattern of inhibition and excitation that is synchronized across large areas of the brain. A key feature of this circuit seems to be the enhancement of nRT-mediated inhibition onto the thalamic neurons, as reflected in powerful bursts of action potentials in the nRT neurons. What is clear from the animal models in which such circuits have been functionally dissected is that mutations in several different genes, including those that code for calcium channel subunits and $GABA_B$ receptor subunits, can give rise to this abnormal generalized electrical pattern.

Remarkably, in GEFS+, the phenotype may include many different seizure types. One characteristic of GEFS+ is the involvement of febrile seizures, a condition that extends beyond the occasional episode of febrile seizure seen commonly in young children. In animal models of febrile seizures, investigators have identified alterations in the genes encoding hyperpolarizing activated cyclic nucleotide-gated channels (HCN channels) (Dube et al., 2009). It remains unclear whether these alterations should be interpreted as cause or effect of seizure activity. Certainly, this gene plasticity is only part of the febrile seizures story, as hyperthermia is also associated with inflammatory reactivity (expression, for example, of the cytokine interleukin-1β) as well as endocannabinoid signaling (Bartfai et al., 2007). Interestingly, HCN plasticity – not only changes in the subunit interactions, but also the subcellular localization of these channels – has been also demonstrated in other forms of epilepsy, suggesting that channel plasticity (not just channel pathology) may be an important contributor to seizure activity (Chen et al., 2003).

CONCLUDING COMMENT

The underlying cellular bases of seizures, both partial and generalized, are complex. Even in those cases where a single gene mutation "causes" the epilepsy, the cascade of mechanisms that lead to seizure activity inevitably involves many different processes. For the most part, the cellular mechanisms associated with seizure activity are variations on a "normal" theme. Thus, an understanding of seizure mechanisms must start with a detailed view of normal brain function.

ACKNOWLEDGMENTS

The author is grateful to Ms. Laurie Beninsig for her help in preparing this manuscript.

References

Alger BE (2004). Endocannabinoids and their implications for epilepsy. Epilepsy Curr 4: 169–173.

Anderson S, Mione M, Yun K et al. (1999). Differential origins of neocortical projection and local circuit neurons: role of Dlx genes in neocortical interneuronogenesis. Cereb Cortex 9: 646–654.

Avoli M, Benini R, de Guzman P et al. (2004). GABA(B) receptor activation and limbic network ictogenesis. Neuropharmacology 46: 43–51.

Bandyopadhyay S, Sutor B, Hablitz JJ (2006). Endogenous acetylcholine enhances synchronized interneuron activity in rat neocortex. J Neurophysiol 95: 1908–1916.

Bartfai T, Sanchez-Alavez M, Andell-Jonsson S et al. (2007). Interleukin-1 system in CNS stress: seizures, fever, and neurotrauma. Ann N Y Acad Sci 1113: 173–177.

Beck H, Steffens R, Elger CE et al. (1998). Voltage-dependent Ca^{2+} currents in epilepsy. Epilepsy Res 32: 321–332.

Ben-Ari Y (2006). Seizures beget seizures: the quest for GABA as a key player. Crit Rev Neurobiol 18: 135–144.

Binder DK, Scharfman HE (2004). Brain-derived neurotrophic factor. Growth Factors 22: 123–131.

Binder DK, Steinhauser C (2006). Functional changes in astroglial cells in epilepsy. Glia 54: 358–368.

Blatow M, Caputi A, Monyer H (2005). Molecular diversity of neocortical GABAergic interneurons. J Physiol 562: 99–105.

Blumcke I (2009). Neuropathology of focal epilepsies: a critical review. Epilepsy Behav 15: 34–39.

Boison D (2009). Adenosine augmentation therapies (AATs) for epilepsy: prospect of cell and gene therapies. Epilepsy Res 85: 131–141.

Bordey A, Lyons SA, Hablitz JJ et al. (2001). Electrophysiological characteristics of reactive astrocytes in experimental cortical dysplasia. J Neurophysiol 85: 1719–1731.

Burgess DL (2005). Neonatal epilepsy syndromes and DEFS+: mechanistic considerations. Epilepsia 46: 51–58.

Burgess DL, Noebels JL (1999). Single gene defects in mice: the role of voltage-dependent calcium channels in absence models. Epilepsy Res 36: 11–122.

Carlen PL, Skinner F, Zhang L et al. (2000). The role of gap junctions in seizures. Brain Res Rev 32: 235–241.

Catterall WA, Few AP (2008). Calcium channel regulation and presynaptic plasticity. Neuron 59: 882–901.

Cepeda C, Hurst RS, Flores-Hernandez J et al. (2003). Morphological and electrophysiological characterization of abnormal cell types in pediatric cortical dysplasia. J Neurosci Res 15: 472–486.

Chagnac-Amitai Y, Connors BW (1989). Synchronized excitation and inhibition driven by intrinsically bursting neurons in neocortex. J Neurosci 62: 1149–1162.

Chen K, Ratzliff A, Hilgenberg L et al. (2003). Long-term plasticity of endocannabinoid signaling induced by developmental febrile seizures. Neuron 39: 599–611.

Christian EP, Dudek FE (1988). Characteristics of local excitatory circuits studied with glutamate microapplication in the CA3 area of rat hippocampal slices. J Neurophysiol 59: 90–109.

Connors BW, Long MA (2004). Electrical synapses in the mammalian brain. Annu Rev Neurosci 27: 393–418.

D'Antoni S, Berretta A, Bonaccorso CM et al. (2008). Metabotropic glutamate receptors in glial cells. Neurochem Res 33: 2436–2443.

Danzer SC, McNamara JO (2004). Localization of brain-derived neurotrophic factor to distinct terminals of mossy fiber axons implies regulation of both excitation and feed-forward inhibition of CA3 pyramidal cells. J Neurosci 24: 11346–11355.

Dingledine R (1983). Excitatory amino acids: modes of action on hippocampal pyramidal cells. Fed Proc 42: 2881–2885.

Dube CM, Brewster AL, Baram TZ (2009). Febrile seizures: mechanisms and relationship to epilepsy. Brain Dev 31: 366–371.

Dudek FE, Shao LR (2002). Synaptic reorganization in an experimental model of posttraumatic epilepsy. Epilepsy Curr 2: 198–199.

Dudek FE, Yasumura T, Rash JE (1998). 'Non-synaptic' mechanisms in seizures and epileptogenesis. Cell Biol Int 22: 793–805.

Dzhala VI, Talos DM, Sdrulla DA et al. (2005). NKCC1 transporter facilitates seizures in the developing brain. Nat Med 11: 1205–1213.

Eriksson SH, Malmgren K, Nordborg C (2005). Microdysgenesis in epilepsy. Acta Neurol Scand 111: 279–290.

Fernandez de Sevilla D, Garduno J, Galvan E et al. (2006). Calcium-activated afterhyperpolarizations regulate synchronization and timing of epileptiform bursts in hippocampal neurons. J Neurophysiol 96: 3028–3041.

Foy MR, Baudry M, Diaz Brinton R et al. (2008). Estrogen and hippocampal plasticity in rodents models. J Alzheimers Dis 15: 589–603.

Freund TF, Buzsaki G (1996). Interneurons of the hippocampus. Hippocampus 6: 347–470.

Friocourt G, Liu JS, Antypa M et al. (2007). Both doublecortin and doublecortin-like kinase play a role in cortical interneuron migration. J Neurosci 27: 3875–3883.

Fry M (2006). Developmental expression of Na^{+} currents in mouse Purkinje neurons. Eur J Neurosci 24: 2557–2566.

Gant JC, Thibault O, Blalock EM et al. (2009). Decreased number of interneurons and increased seizures in neuropilin-2 deficient mice: implications for autism and epilepsy. Epilepsia 50: 629–645.

Gibbs JW, 3rd, Zhang YF, Shumate MD et al. (2000). Regionally selective blockade of GABAergic inhibition by zinc in the thalamocortical system: functional significance. J Neurophysiol 83: 1510–1521.

Giorgi FS, Pizzanelli C, Biagioni F et al. (2004). The role of norepinephrine in epilepsy: from the bench to the bedside. Neurosci Biobehav Rev 28: 507–524.

Glykys J, Mody I (2006). Hippocampal network hyperactivity after selective reduction of tonic inhibition in GABA(A) receptor alpha5 subunit-deficient mice. J Neurophysiol 95: 2796–2807.

Gulledge AT, Kawaguchi Y (2007). Phasic cholinergic signaling in the hippocampus: functional homology with the neocortex? Hippocampus 17: 327–332.

Gulyas AI, Acsady L, Freund TF (1999). Structural basis of the cholinergic and serotonergic modulation of GABAergic neurons in the hippocampus. Neurochem Int 34: 359–372.

Gutierrez R (2003). The GABAergic phenotype of the "glutamatergic" granule cells of the dentate gyrus. Prog Neurobiol 71: 337–358.

Haas CA, Dudeck O, Kirsch M et al. (2002). Role for reelin in the development of granule cell dispersion in temporal lobe epilepsy. J Neurosci 22: 5797–5802.

Haglund MM, Hochman DW (2005). Furosemide and mannitol suppression of epileptic activity in the human brain. J Neurophysiol 94: 907–918.

Harrison NL (2007). Mechanisms of sleep induction by GABA(A) receptor agonists. J Clin Psychiatry 68: 6–12.

Hasselmo ME (2006). The role of acetylcholine in learning and memory. Curr Opin Neurobiol 16: 710–715.

Hasselmo ME, Schnell E, Barkai E (1995). Dynamics of learning and recall at excitatory recurrent synapses and cholinergic modulation in rat hippocampal region CA3. J Neurosci 15: 5249–5262.

Haydon PG, Carmignoto G (2006). Astrocyte control of synaptic transmission and neurovascular coupling. Physiol Rev 86: 1009–1031.

He XP, Kotloski R, Nef S et al. (2004). Conditional deletion of the TrkB but not BDNF prevents epileptogenesis in the kindling model. Neuron 43: 31–42.

Houser CR (2007). Interneurons of the dentate gyrus: an overview of cell types, terminal fields and neurochemical identity. Prog Brain Res 163: 217–232.

Howes OK, Kapur S (2009). The dopamine hypothesis of schizophrenia: version III – the final common pathway. Schizophr Bull 35: 549–562.

Hsu MS, Lee DJ, Binder DK (2007). Potential role of the glial water channel aquaporin-4 in epilepsy. Neuron Glia Biol 3: 287–297.

Huguenard JR, Prince DA (1992). A novel T-type current underlies prolonged Ca(2+)-dependent burst firing in GABAergic neurons of rat thalamic reticular nucleus. J Neurosci 12: 3804–3817.

Inda MC, DeFelipe J, Munoz A (2006). Voltage-gated ion channels in the axon initial segment of human cortical pyramidal cells and their relationship with chandelier cells. Proc Natl Acad Sci U S A 103: 2920–2925.

Jean YY, Lercher LD, Dreyfus CF (2008). Glutamate elicits release of BDNF from basal forebrain astrocytes in a process dependent on metabotropic receptors and the PLC pathway. Neuron Glia Biol 4: 35–42.

Jobe PC (2003). Common pathogenic mechanisms between depression and epilepsy: an experimental perspective. Epilepsy Behav 4: 14–24.

Joels M (2009). Stress, the hippocampus, and epilepsy. Epilepsia 50: 586–597.

Johnston D, Hoffman DA, Magee JC et al. (2000). Dendritic potassium channels in hippocampal neurons. J Physiol 525: 75–81.

Jones DL, Baraban SC (2007). Characterization of inhibitory circuits in the malformed hippocampus of Lis1 mutant mice. J Neurophysiol 98: 2737–2746.

Jung S, Jones TD, Lugo JN Jr et al. (2007). Progressive dendritic HCN channelopathy during epileptogenesis in the rat pilocarpine model of epilepsy. J Neurosci 27: 13012–13021.

Kager H, Wadman WJ, Somjen GG (2007). Seizure-like afterdischarges simulated in a model neuron. J Comput Neurosci 22: 105–128.

Kanner AM (2007). Epilepsy and mood disorders. Epilepsia 48: 20–22.

Kaplan MP, Wilcox KS, Dichter MA (2003). Differences in multiple forms of short-term plasticity between excitatory and inhibitory hippocampal neurons in culture. Synapse 50: 41–52.

Katona I, Freund TF (2008). Endocannabinoid signaling as a synaptic circuit breaker in neurological disease. Nat Med 14: 923–930.

Kruglikov I, Rudy B (2008). Persomatic GABA release and thalamocortical integration onto neocortical excitatory cells are regulated by neuromodulators. Neuron 58: 911–924.

Kullmann DM, Asztely F, Walker MC (2000). The role of mammalian ionotropic receptors in synaptic plasticity: LTP, LTD and epilepsy. Cell Mol Life Sci 57: 1551–1561.

Leis JA, Bekar LK, Walz W (2005). Potassium homeostasis in the ischemic brain. Glia 50: 407–416.

Liang SL, Carlson GC, Coulter DA (2006). Dynamic regulation of synaptic GABA release by the glutamate–glutamine cycle in hippocampal area CA1. J Neurosci 26: 8537–8548.

Lipton SA (2007). Pathologically activated therapeutics for neuroprotection. Nat Rev Neurosci 8: 803–808.

Lowenstein DH (2009). Epilepsy after head injury: an overview. Epilepsia 50: 4–9.

Magee J, Hoffman D, Colbert C et al. (1998). Electrical and calcium signaling in dendrites of hippocampal pyramidal cells. Annu Rev Physiol 60: 327–346.

Malarkey EB, Parpura V (2008). Mechanisms of glutamate release from astrocytes. Neurochem Int 52: 142–154.

Malenka RC (1991). The role of postsynaptic calcium in the induction of long-term potentiation. Mol Neurobiol 5: 289–295.

Malinow R (2003). AMPA receptor trafficking and long-term potentiation. Philos Trans R Soc Lond B Biol Sci 358: 707–714.

Manley GT, Binder DK, Papadopoulos MC et al. (2004). New insights into water transport and edema in the central nervous system from phenotype analysis of aquaporin-4 null mice. Neuroscience 129: 983–991.

Markram H, Toledo-Rodriguez M, Wang Y et al. (2004). Interneurons of the neocortical inhibitory system. Nat Rev Neurosci 5: 793–807.

Mazarati AM (2004). Galanin and galanin receptors in epilepsy. Neuropeptides 38: 331–343.

Mazarati AM, Hohmann JG, Bacon A et al. (2000). Modulation of hippocampal excitability and seizures by galanin. J Neurosci 20: 6276–6281.

McCormick DA, Contreras D (2001). On the cellular and network bases of epileptic seizures. Annu Rev Physiol 63: 815–846.

Merlin LR (2002). Differential roles for mGluR1 and mGluR5 in the persistent prolongation of epileptiform bursts. J Neurophysiol 87: 621–625.

Merlin LR (2008). The ups and downs of hippocampal metabotropic glutamate receptors: ramifications for epileptogenesis and cognitive impairment following status epilepticus. Epilepsy Curr 8: 43–45.

Miles R, Wong RK (1987). Inhibitory control of local excitatory circuits in the guinea-pig hippocampus. J Physiol 388: 611–629.

Misgeld U, Drew G, Yanovsky Y (2007). Presynaptic modulation of GABA release in the basal ganglia. Prog Brain Res 160: 245–259.

Mufson EJ, Ginsberg SD, Ikonomovic MD et al. (2003). Human cholinergic basal forebrain: chemoanatomy and neurologic dysfunction. J Chem Neuroanat 26: 233–242.

Nagelhus EA, Mathiisen TM, Ottersen OP (2004). Aquaporin-4 in the central nervous system: cellular and subcellular distribution and coexpression with KIR4.1. Neuroscience 129: 905–913.

Noe F, Pool AH, Nissinen J et al. (2008). Neuropeptide Y gene therapy decreases chronic spontaneous seizures in a rat model of temporal lobe epilepsy. Brain 131: 1506–1515.

Obara M, Szeliga M, Albrecht J (2008). Regulation of pH in the mammalian central nervous system under normal and pathological conditions: facts and hypotheses. Neurochem Int 52: 905–919.

Obermair GJ, Szabo Z, Bourinet E et al. (2004). Differential targeting of the L-type Ca^{2+} channel alpha 1 C (Cav1.2) to synaptic and extrasynaptic compartments in hippocampal neurons. Eur J Neurosci 19: 2109–2122.

Olsen RW, Sieghart W (2008). Subtypes of gamma-aminobutyric acid (A) receptors: classification on the basis of subunit composition, pharmacology, and function. Update. Pharmacol Rev 60: 243–260.

Ottman R, Winawer MR, Kalachikov S et al. (2004). LGI1 mutations in autosomal dominant partial epilepsy with auditory features. Neurology 62: 1120–1126.

Owens DF, Kriegstein AR (2002). Is there more to GABA than synaptic inhibition? Nat Rev Neurosci 3: 715–727.

Paradiso B, Marconi P, Zucchini S et al. (2009). Localized delivery of fibroblast growth factor-2 and brain-derived neurotrophic factor reduces spontaneous seizures in an epilepsy model. Proc Natl Acad Sci U S A 106: 7191–7196.

Payne JA, Rivera C, Viopio J et al. (2003). Cation–chloride co-transporters in neuronal communication, development and trauma. Trends Neurosci 26: 199–206.

Penovich PE, Helmers S (2008). Catamenial epilepsy. Int Rev Neurobiol 83: 79–90.

Perreault P, Avoli M (1991). Physiology and pharmacology of epileptiform activity induced by 4-aminopyridine in rat hippocampal slices. J Neurophysiol 65: 771–785.

Picken Bahrey HL, Moody WJ (2003). Early development of voltage-gated ion currents and firing properties in neurons of the mouse cerebral cortex. J Neurophysiol 89: 1761–1773.

Prince DA, Connors BW (1984). Mechanisms of epileptogenesis in cortical structures. Ann Neurol 16: S59–S64.

Prince DA, Parada I, Scalise K et al. (2009). Epilepsy following cortical injury: cellular and molecular mechanisms as targets for potential prophylaxis. Epilepsia 50: 30–40.

Ransom BR (2000). Glial modulation of neural excitability mediated by extracellular pH: a hypothesis revisited. Prog Brain Res 125: 217–228.

Rao MS, Hattiangady B, Rai KS et al. (2007). Strategies for promoting anti-seizure effects of hippocampal fetal cells grated into the hippocampus of rats exhibiting chronic temporal lobe epilepsy. Neurobiol Dis 27: 117–132.

Raol YH, Zhang G, Lund IV et al. (2006). Increased GABA (A)-receptor alpha1-subunit expression in hippocampal dentate gyrus after early life status epilepticus. Epilepsia 47: 1665–1673.

Reddy DS, Rogawski MA (2009). Neurosteroid replacement therapy for catamenial epilepsy. Neurotherapeutics 6: 392–401.

Reich CG, Karson MA, Karnup SV et al. (2005). Regulation of IPSP theta rhythm by muscarinic receptors and endocannabinoids in hippocampus. J Neurophysiol 94: 4290–4299.

Rheims S, Minlebaev M, Ivanov A et al. (2008). Excitatory GABA in rodent developing neocortex *in vitro*. J Neurophysiol 100: 609–619.

Riban V, Fitzsimons HL, During MJ (2009). Gene therapy in epilepsy. Epilepsia 20: 24–32.

Rose EM, Koo JC, Antflick JE et al. (2009). Glutamate transporter coupling to Na, K-ATPase. J Neurosci 29: 8143–8155.

Sanchez RM, Koh S, Rio C et al. (2001). Decreased glutamate receptor 2 expression and enhanced epileptogenesis in immature rat hippocampus after prenatal hypoxia-induced seizures. J Neurosci 21: 8154–8163.

Sara SJ (2009). The locus coeruleus and noradrenergic modulation of cognition. Nat Rev Neurosci 10: 211–223.

Scharfman HE, Sollas AE, Berger RE et al. (2003). Perforant path activation of ectopic granule cells that are born after pilocarpine-induced seizures. Neuroscience 121: 1017–1029.

Scheffer IE, Harkin LA, Dibbens LM et al. (2005). Neonatal epilepsy syndromes and generalized epilepsy with febrile seizures plus (GEFS+). Epilepsia 46: 41–47.

Scheffer IE, Zhang YH, Jansen FE et al. (2009). Dravet syndrome or genetic (generalized) epilepsy with febrile seizures plus? Brain Dev 31: 394–400.

Schwartzkroin PA, Walsh CA (2000). Cortical malformations and epilepsy. Ment Retard Dev Disabil Res Rev 6: 268–280.

Scimemi A, Semyanov A, Sperk G et al. (2005). Multiple and plastic receptors mediate tonic GABA(A)receptor currents in the hippocampus. J Neurosci 25: 10016–10024.

Simonato M, Romualdi P (1996). Dynorphin and epilepsy. Prog Neurobiol 50: 557–583.

Smart SL, Lopantsev V, Zhang CL et al. (1998). Deletion of the Kv1.1 potassium channel causes epilepsy in mice. Neuron 20: 809–819.

Smith SS, Woolley CS (2004). Cellular and molecular effects of steroid hormones on CNS excitability. Cleve Clin J Med 71: 4–10.

Somjen GG (1984). Acidification of interstitial fluid in hippocampal formation caused by seizures and spreading depression. Brain Res 311: 186–188.

Sontheimer H (1994). Voltage-dependent ion channels in glial cells. Glia 11: 156–172.

Sperk G, Hamilton T, Colmers WF (2007). Neuropeptide Y in the dentate gyrus. Prog Brain Res 163: 285–297.

Stafstrom CE (2007). Persistent sodium current and its role in epilepsy. Epilepsy Curr 7: 15–22.

Stafstrom CE, Schwindt PC, Chubb MC et al. (1985). Properties of persistent sodium conductance and calcium conductance of layer V neurons from cat sensorimotor cortex in vitro. J Neurophysiol 53: 153–170.

Sutula TP, Dudek FE (2007). Unmasking recurrent excitation generated by mossy fiber sprouting in the epileptic dentate gyrus: an emergent property of a complex system. Prog Brain Res 163: 541–563.

Suzuki S, Brown CM, Wise PM (2006). Mechanisms of neuroprotection by estrogen. Endocrine 29: 209–215.

Tallent MK (2007). Somatostatin in the dentate gyrus. Prog Brain Res 163: 265–284.

Traub RD, Wong RK, Miles R et al. (1991). A model of a CA3 hippocampal pyramidal neuron incorporating voltage-clamp data on intrinsic conductances. J Neurophysiol 66: 635–650.

Traub RD, Draguhn A, Whittington MA et al. (2002). Axonal gap junctions between principal neurons: a novel source of network oscillations, and perhaps epileptogenesis. Rev Neurosci 13: 1–30.

Vacher H, Mohapatra DP, Trimmer JS (2008). Localization and targeting of voltage-dependent ion channels in mammalian central neurons. Physiol Rev 88: 1407–1447.

Veliskova J (2006). The role of estrogens in seizures and epilepsy: the bad guys or the good guys? Neuroscience 138: 837–844.

Vezzani A, Balosso S, Ravizza T (2008). The role of cytokines in the pathophysiology of epilepsy. Brain Behav Immun 22: 797–803.

Volterra A, Steinhauser C (2004). Glial modulation of synaptic transmission in the hippocampus. Glia 47: 249–257.

Wallraff A, Kohling R, Heinemann U et al. (2006). The impact of astrocytic gap junctional coupling on potassium buffering in the hippocampus. J Neurosci 26: 5438–5447.

Wang DD, Kriegstein AR (2009). Defining the role of GABA in cortical development. J Physiol 587: 1873–1879.

Weinshenker D, Szot P (2002). The role of catecholamines in seizure susceptibility: new results using genetically engineered mice. Pharmacol Ther 94: 213–233.

Wong RK, Traub RD, Miles R (1986). Cellular basis of neuronal synchrony in epilepsy. Adv Neurol 44: 583–592.

Wong M, Ess KC, Uhlmann EJ et al. (2003). Impaired glial glutamate transport in a mouse tuberous sclerosis epilepsy model. Ann Neurol 54: 251–256.

Wong RK, Chuang SC, Bianchi R (2004). Plasticity mechanisms underlying mGluR-induced epileptogenesis. Adv Exp Med Biol 548: 69–75.

Yamakawa K (2009). Molecular basis of severe myoclonic epilepsy in infancy. Brain Dev 31: 401–404.

Yu FH, Mantegrazza M, Westenbroek RE et al. (2006). Reduced sodium current in GABAergic interneurons in a mouse model of severe myoclonic epilepsy in infancy. Nat Neurosci 9: 1142–1149.

Yuan LL, Chen X (2006). Diversity of potassium channels in neuronal dendrites. Prog Neurobiol 78: 374–389.

Handbook of Clinical Neurology, Vol. 107 (3rd series)
Epilepsy, Part I
H. Stefan and W.H. Theodore, Editors

Chapter 3

Epilepsy as a dynamic disease of neuronal networks

FERNANDO H. LOPES DA SILVA*, JAN A. GORTER, AND WYTSE J. WADMAN
Center for NeuroScience, Swammerdam Institute for Life Sciences, University of Amsterdam, Amsterdam, The Netherlands

INTRODUCTION

The brain consists of a multitude of neuronal networks interconnected by short- and long-range connections. From some descriptions of the brain, particularly those studies based on imaging techniques, one may get the impression that what counts is the existence of *brain areas* to which functions are ascribed, that are often described in rather specific terms. This perspective has yielded insight into how the brain works but has submerged the complementary approach, according to which brain functions are the result of the activity of interconnected *neuronal networks* that may engage several cortical and subcortical systems. These general considerations are relevant in the context of this chapter because epilepsy is a dynamic disease of such neuronal networks. This means that epilepsy is characterized by qualitative changes in the dynamic state of neuronal networks.

These networks can function in a normal state in which information processing takes place normally, but can also jump to another state where these same networks display abnormal oscillations, disturbing the normal functioning of the brain. The latter constitute what is generally called epileptiform paroxysmal activity or ictal activity, as reflected on the electroencephalogram (EEG).

Indeed, epileptic subjects display (long) periods of normal behavior and EEG activity, sometimes presenting short-lived epileptiform events (spikes, sharp waves, fast ripples) that are not associated with overt behavioral manifestations, although these periods are occasionally interrupted by episodes characterized by paroxysmal EEG activity and abnormal behavior, i.e., by seizures (ictal activity). This can be illustrated most typically with respect to absence (nonconvulsive) seizures, which are characterized by brief episodes of loss of consciousness without much abnormal movement and relatively long periods of normal EEG and behavior.

This implies that, in order to understand how epileptic seizures occur, it is necessary to take into account that the brain of epileptic subjects can function in two very distinct modes. A main question is how transitions occur in the dynamics of the neuronal networks of the brain of these subjects whereby a jump from the normal to the epileptic state takes place, and is followed by a return to the normal state. This kind of behavior, however, does not occur only in brain systems; it is found in many other physical systems – generally termed nonlinear complex systems – and has been the object of intense mathematical analysis.

According to the terminology of the theory of complex systems, this kind of behavior represents a bifurcation in a bistable system. We hypothesized that some types of epileptic transition represent bifurcations occurring in a bistable system. Bistable systems feature two stable operational states that exist simultaneously for the same set of system parameters. One of these states is the normal, interictal state, and the other is the epileptic or ictal state of the network. We can assume that transitions between states are relatively fast with respect to the time spent by the system in these states; thus, the current state is always well defined. Transitions between the two states may occur due to an external stimulus, for example in cases of reflex epilepsy, or from the influence of random fluctuations of inputs and/or of changes of certain network parameters.

It should be noted that the parameters that control the dynamic behavior of neuronal networks extend from membrane phenomena, such as ion channel kinetics, to processes of neurotransmission (chemical and electrical, presynaptic and postsynaptic), and may encompass

*Correspondence to: F.H. Lopes da Silva, M.D., Ph.D., Emeritus Professor, Swammerdam Institute for Life Sciences, Center of NeuroSciences, Kamer C3-269, Science Park 904, 1098 XH Amsterdam, The Netherlands. Tel: +(31)020-5257622, Fax: +(31) 020 5257675, E-mail: F.H.LopesdaSilva@uva.nl

several timescales, including long-term plastic properties involving the collective behavior of neuronal populations.

Epileptic phenomena can emerge in many different systems in the brain. There are, however, two systems that appear particularly prone to display epileptic behaviors, albeit of different kinds:

- the thalamocortical system, which plays an important role in absence epilepsy
- the mesial temporal system, in which the hippocampal formation occupies a central position and is responsible for the mesial temporal lobe epileptic syndrome.

Interestingly these two systems show a remarkable degree of plasticity and are associated with the transition between wakefulness and sleep in the case of the thalamocortical system, and with the formation, consolidation, and retrieval of memories in the case of the hippocampus and associated structures. This means that these systems are very changeable, and may undergo frequent transitions of dynamic state. Nonetheless, in the normal brain such dynamic changes are kept under well-controlled limits owing to the parameters that maintain the stability of the neuronal networks. In the brain of epileptic subjects, however, these parameters are disturbed so that the threshold for transitions that go beyond the controlled limits is much lower. This is the essential difference between the dynamics of a normal and an epileptic brain.

In the following sections we consider the main aspects of how the stability of neuronal networks may be maintained and disturbed in epilepsy; how transitions between normal and epileptic behavior may occur in thalamocortical networks; how transitions between normal and epileptic behavior may occur in neuronal networks of the hippocampal system; and how neuronal networks involved in epileptic behavior may be identified and analyzed in the clinic. We end with a short conclusion, in which some conceptual models are presented.

HOW MAY THE STABILITY OF NEURONAL NETWORKS BE MAINTAINED AND DISTURBED IN EPILEPSY?

Neuronal networks display many forms of plasticity, the most obvious ones occurring during development and aging, where substantial changes can take place in a network. The more subtle forms of plasticity constitute the basis of the formation of memory traces and are best exemplified by the phenomena of long-term potentiation (LTP) and depression (LTD), two mechanisms that specifically enhance and decrease synaptic strength, respectively.

If LTP were to accumulate progressively, however, the stability of a neuronal network would be put at risk, with the possible consequence that epileptic activity would develop. This is indeed what may happen in the case of electrical kindling (Maru et al., 1982; Kamphuis et al., 1988), where daily use of an electrical tetanic stimulation capable of inducing LTP over a period of weeks leads to an epileptic focus. Conversely, a depression of synaptic activity can affect brain functioning, and has to be counteracted to redress efficient synaptic transmission such that brain functions may be recovered.

Thus neuronal networks possess mechanisms that promote their stabilization, i.e., *homeostatic mechanisms of regulation of neuronal excitability*. Epileptic behavior may result from a disruption of such homeostatic mechanisms and it is appropriate to discuss those homeostatic processes briefly here.

What kind of mechanism can mediate homeostatic regulation of neuronal excitability?

Homeostatic regulation of neuronal excitability can be attained in two fundamentally different ways: (1) by regulation of synaptic strength, or (2) by regulation of ion channels that translate changes of membrane potential into a pattern of action potential firing. There is ample evidence that both mechanisms exist and that they are not mutually exclusive.

According to Turrigiano et al. (1998) homeostatic synaptic scaling is a form of synaptic plasticity that adjusts the strength of the complete set of a neuron's excitatory synapses up or down to stabilize firing under conditions of changing input. One can envisage that a neuronal network possesses a set of homeostatic mechanisms that operate over different temporal and spatial scales (Turrigiano, 2008). Their existence has been demonstrated both *in vitro* and *in vivo*, in neocortical as well as in hippocampal pyramidal neurons (Lissin et al., 1998; O'Brien et al., 1998; Turrigiano et al., 1998; Thiagarajan et al., 2005).

The second important mechanism is the regulation of membrane excitability by changes in ion conductances. This was shown by van Welie et al. (2006) in hippocampal CA1 pyramidal neurons, who found an increase in the amplitude of the hyperpolarization-activated cation current I_h after a strong bombardment of glutamatergic synaptic activity. This modulation of I_h is specific for AMPA (2-amino-3-(5-methyl-3-oxo-1,2- oxazol-4-yl)propanoic acid) receptor activity, depends on a rise of intracellular calcium ($[Ca^{2+}]_i$), and most likely involves signalling pathways downstream to $[Ca^{2+}]_i$. Along the same line, the investigations of Fan et al. (2005) showed that hippocampal LTP is accompanied by a decrease in cellular excitability mediated by an increase in HCN1 (hyperpolarization-activated cyclic nucleotide-gated) channels that carry I_h, which results in a decrease in overall excitability and an increase of resting membrane conductance. Indeed, these authors demonstrated that increased I_h can speed the decay rate of excitatory postsynaptic potentials (EPSPs) and reduce EPSP efficacy to initiate action potential firing (Fan et al., 2005). The opposite change in synaptic strength, LTD, induced by 3-Hz synaptic stimulation, downregulates I_h via activation of group 1 metabotropic glutamate receptors (mGluRs) and subsequent stimulation of protein kinase C (Brager and Johnston, 2007). These findings, taken together, justify the proposal that modulation of I_h behaves as a homeostatic and bidirectional mechanism that assures the stability of the neuronal network, under conditions where synaptic plastic changes (LTP or LTD) take place.

The modulation of I_h , however, is not the only process at the membrane level contributing to the homeostatic control of neuronal excitability. Van Welie et al. (2006) showed in hippocampal slices that the reduction of background activity results within a short timeframe (a few minutes) in an upregulation of the excitability of CA1 pyramidal neurons. The responsible mechanism is a *reduction* in K^+ current, mediated by Kv2.1, that is the soma-dendritic sustained or delayed rectifier voltage-gated potassium conductance. This results in a shift in the input–output gain relationship in the direction of lowering the threshold for the generation of action potentials. Interestingly, an opposite phenomenon has also been reported, namely that glutamate stimulation causing an increase in synaptic activity results in increased K^+ conductance in cultured rat hippocampal neurons, and thus in a hyperpolarizing shift (Misonou et al., 2004) and decreased excitability. The latter authors in a series of experiments showed that the glutamate-induced hyperpolarizing shifts in K-channel gating are mediated by a pathway involving the activation of ionotropic glutamate receptors, increased $[Ca^{2+}]_i$, and the activation of calcineurin. It should be noted that still other types of ion channel, including Ca^{2+}-dependent K^+ channels (Carr et al., 2003), and voltage-dependent Na^+ channels (Brager and Johnston, 2007), have also been proposed as possibly mediating changes in excitability associated with homeostatic plasticity.

We should emphasize that the findings of van Welie et al. (2006) are complementary to those of Misonou et al. (2004), revealing that the modulation of this K^+ conductance can *increase* or *decrease* neuronal threshold within a relatively short timescale, depending on whether the neuronal activity state is *enhanced* respectively *depressed*.

Besides these mechanisms at the level of ion conductance, modifications of synaptic transmission, either presynaptic or postsynaptic, can also contribute significantly to the processes underlying neuronal homeostasis. The nature of these mechanisms is a matter of debate. A possible mechanism of synaptic upscaling is the postsynaptic accumulation of glutamate AMPA and/or *N*-methyl-D-aspartate (NMDA) receptors (O'Brien et al., 1998; Watt et al., 2000; Wierenga et al., 2006; Gainey et al., 2009). We cannot enter here into a discussion of the experimental evidence for different mechanisms, but it should be noted that several studies have suggested that synaptic homeostatic scaling involves changes in synaptic delivery, turnover, or tethering of AMPA receptors in the synaptic membrane, especially the glutamate receptor GluR2 subunit. Gainey et al., (2009) showed that the molecular process by which the expression of AMPA receptors can be enhanced in LTP is different from the process underlying synaptic upscaling; the former involves a pathway that depends on the subunit GluR1, whereas the latter depends on the GluR2 subunit. This suggests that synaptic scaling may take place while LTP may be left unimpaired.

Further, the mechanisms responsible for "scaling down" and "scaling up" synaptic strength may be different (for a detailed discussion, see the review of Turrigiano, 2008). Several molecular mechanisms have been proposed to account for the process by which a neuron "senses" deviations in synaptic strength, taking it away from the desired setpoint, and subsequently triggers the *signaling pathway* that restores the homeostatic equilibrium.

Three main processes have been put forward as candidate signaling pathways for synaptic scaling: (1) brain-derived nerve growth factor (BDNF) (Rutherford et al., 1998); (2) tumor necrosis factor α (TNFα) (Stellwagen and Malenka, 2006); and (3) intracellular Ca^{2+}. The fact that the administration of BDNF can prevent the upscaling of synaptic strength *in vitro* suggests a role of BDNF as a possible signaling molecule, but it is not yet clear how it may act *in vivo*. The cytokine TNFα, once released from glial cells, can upscale synaptic strength in neurons where it was previously decreased by tetrodotoxin (TTX). TNFα can increase AMPA receptor surface expression in hippocampal neurons, thus strengthening excitatory synapse, while it can elicit endocytosis of γ-aminobutyric acid type A ($GABA_A$) receptors (Stellwagen and Malenka, 2006). However, there are some reservations regarding the role of TNFα in this process, as its action is rather slow, and it is not clear whether it can also reduce the strength of synapses that were previously enhanced. Nonetheless, the results obtained by the computational study of Savin et al. (2009) suggest that this factor may be relevant in epileptogenesis, where the speed of the process is not a critical factor. Regarding the role of Ca^{2+}, there is ample experimental evidence that the intracellular Ca^{2+} concentration modulates synaptic strength (Thiagarajan et al., 2005; Ibata et al., 2008; de Jong and Verhage, 2009). Turrigiano (2008) put forward the interesting concept that "synaptic scaling does not act to stabilize mean firing rate, but instead acts to stabilize somatic calcium".

It should be emphasized that synaptic scaling may involve both presynaptic and postsynaptic processes. Wierenga et al. (2006) showed in neuronal cultures that there is a shift in the scaling mechanism after TTX application from a predominantly postsynaptic response at early stages (< 14 DIV, days *in vitro*), to a combined presynaptic and postsynaptic response at later stages (> 18 DIV).

What is the role of disturbance of cellular homeostatic processes (ionic or synaptic) in promoting changes to the stability of neuronal networks, leading to epileptogenesis?

A review of the literature does not allow a clear answer to this question, although it may be hypothesized that disturbances in these processes can contribute to the emergence of abnormal dynamics manifest as epileptic seizures. Nonetheless, it is interesting briefly to review here three experimental observations, supported by computational modeling, that are relevant in this context.

The first is the experiment carried out by Houweling et al. (2005), who used as an experimental model of posttraumatic epilepsy the chronically isolated neocortex, where deafferentation results in a chronic blockade of activity. Indeed a few days of pharmacologically induced blockade of activity in cortical cell cultures leads to increases in the amplitude of miniature excitatory postsynaptic currents (mEPSCs) and evoked EPSCs in pyramidal cells (Turrigiano et al., 1998; Watt et al., 2000). Houweling et al. (2005) constructed a computer model of this process in order to investigate the effect of homeostatic upregulation of excitatory synapses on network stability. They found that burst discharges emerged in their computer simulations resembling the epileptiform discharges recorded in chronically isolated neocortex. This suggests that the molecular mechanisms responsible for homeostatic upregulation, described above (Watt et al., 2000; Wierenga et al., 2006; Gainey et al., 2009) may underlie postdeafferentation epileptogenesis. The most critical parameter that emerged from this study was the upregulation of excitatory synapses between pyramidal cells mediated by AMPA receptors, either with or without a concurrent downregulation of inhibitory synapses and/or upregulation of intrinsic excitability. These observations led to the speculation that this homeostatic upregulation may be a target to counteract posttraumatic epileptogenesis.

The second observation relates to the role of neuron–glia interaction in homeostatic ion regulation, particularly under conditions where extensive neuronal activity induces ion accumulation, osmotic changes, and cell swelling (for reviews see Somjen, 2002, 2004). The computational studies of Kager et al. (2007) and Somjen et al. (2008) demonstrated that even relative simple cellular models of neuron–glia interaction can reproduce quite realistic epileptic seizures. However, they also show that the mere complexity of the neuron–glia system makes it difficult to attribute the instabilities to specific parameters. However, even mild deregulations of excitatory input suffice to initiate the process of seizure generation.

The third observation concerns the role of TNFα in mediating homeostatic synaptic scaling in response to a state of depression of neuronal activity. Savin et al. (2009) showed in a computational model of neuron–glia interaction that under normal conditions TNFα can redress neuronal excitability, but following overexpression of TNFα by glia the network develops seizure-like activity patterns. This may account for the fact that brain inflammation increases the risk of seizure. In line with this finding in the microarray study of gene expression in the rat after status epilepticus (SE) (Gorter et al., 2006), TNFα showed upregulation both at 1 day and 1 week after SE in CA3 and entorhinal cortex, and even in the chronic stage (3 months after SE) in CA3, although less pronounced. In this way the balance between excitation and inhibition in the neuronal network of CA3 would be heavily disturbed, resulting in epileptic seizure activity.

HOW MAY TRANSITIONS BETWEEN NORMAL AND EPILEPTIC BEHAVIOR OCCUR IN THALAMOCORTICAL NETWORKS?

The typical form of epilepsy that is associated with disturbances of the dynamics of thalamocortical networks is characterized by absence seizures. Absence seizures are paroxysmal losses of consciousness that start and end abruptly, and are accompanied by bilaterally synchronous spike and wave discharges (SWDs) that can be recorded on the EEG.

The functional integrity of both cortex and thalamus is required for generation of SWDs, as suggested by lesion studies (Vergnes and Marescaux, 1992; Meeren et al., 2009).

This pathological condition is determined by an abnormal set of parameters of the neuronal elements involved that likely have a genetic origin but may also depend on developmental factors. The genetic abnormalities responsible for this epileptic phenotype in humans are not yet clear (Crunelli and Leresche, 2002). The development of animal models of absence seizures – the Wag/Rij rat (van Luijtelaar and Coenen, 1986; Coenen and van Luijtelaar, 2003) and the generalized absence epilepsy rat from Strasbourg (GAERS; Marescaux et al., 1992; Danober et al., 1998) – and, more recently, the construction of computational models have contributed to a better understanding of basic neuronal mechanisms of this type of epilepsy. It is likely that the mechanisms underlying SWDs are related to those responsible for the oscillations occurring in superficial sleep, the so-called sleep spindles (Steriade et al., 1993; Avoli et al., 2001; McCormick and Contreras, 2001). The latter, however, are phenomena that occur under normal conditions, whereas SWDs appear only in patients with epilepsy.

Therefore, *three main questions* have to be put forward:

1. How can the same basic neuronal network cause sleep spindles and, in certain cases, also SWDs?
2. What makes the neuronal network switch its behavior from a state characterized by normal oscillations and normal behavior to another state characterized by SWD and absences?
3. What are the roles of the thalamus and the cortex in the generation of SWDs?

Experimental studies in animal models have yielded interesting findings (reviewed in McCormick, 2002; Destexhe and Sejnowski, 2003), but these are still fragmentary and answers to these questions remain limited. In order to integrate, in a comprehensive way, diverse experimental findings, computational models constitute useful tools.

A number of such models of thalamic and thalamocortical networks have been developed (e.g., Wang et al., 1995; Lytton et al., 1996; Destexhe et al., 1998, 1999). Some of the model studies, however, show only how a given set of parameters of these neuronal networks may account for the generation of SWDs, and do not address specifically the most essential issue of this type of epileptic activity: namely, that a given thalamocortical network can display both normal and epileptic activity, without making adjustments of parameters. In order to overcome this limitation, we explored a new type of computational model. In these models, populations of interacting neurons integrating neuronal and network properties are simulated. This model approach is based on theoretical (Wilson and Cowan, 1972) and experimental (Freeman, 1975, 1979) principles, and provides the possibility of investigating network dynamics at the macroscopic level, i.e., at the level where electrical brain signals such as local field potentials or EEG signals are recorded.

How can the same basic neuronal network cause spindle oscillations and, occasionally, also SWDs?

The models developed by our group (Suffczynski et al., 2004, 2005, 2006, 2008; Kalitzin et al., 2011; Koppert et al., 2011) give answers to this question, as they show that the same neuronal network can exhibit two qualitatively different types of behavior, as seen in experimental animals (WAG/Rij and GAERS) and in patients with absence epilepsy. Namely, the output signal may display a waxing and waning oscillation of relatively low amplitude typical of sleep spindles, having a spectrum with a peak at approximately 11 Hz in the "normal state" or a high-amplitude "seizure-like" oscillation (SWD) at a frequency of around 9 Hz in the "abnormal state." We refer to the former behavior as "normal ongoing" activity and to the latter as "paroxysmal" activity. This means that the thalamocortical network displays bistable dynamics, as represented symbolically in Figure 3.1.

Spindle activity in the model is generated by the cyclical interaction between the thalamocortical relay (TC) and reticular neuronal (RE) populations. Inhibitory postsynaptic potentials (IPSPs) of RE origin facilitate the generation of rebound low-threshold calcium spikes (I_T calcium current) in the TC population, which in turn activates GABAergic RE neurons. The dominant frequency (approximately 11 Hz) of this rhythmic activity is determined largely by the time course of both AMPA and $GABA_A$ postsynaptic currents and membrane time constants, and by other factors such as the kinetics of low-threshold calcium spikes (I_T), synaptic coupling constants, and sensory (noise) input level. The thalamic-generated spindle activity induces activity at the same frequency in the cortical populations.

$GABA_B$ receptor-mediated IPSPs may contribute to the sudden transition of the model's behavior from "normal ongoing" activity to "seizure-like" 9-Hz large-amplitude oscillations (SWDs). The frequency and amplitude of paroxysmal oscillations depend on the relative contribution of $GABA_A$ and $GABA_B$ components.

Thus, in reply to question (1), it is necessary to determine which are the most critical parameters with respect to the regulation of the threshold level above which SWDs occur.

Critical parameters of the thalamocortical network

In order to make estimates of these critical parameters, we investigated the sensitivity of the network dynamics to the variation of a number of parameters using the model (Suffczynski et al., 2006); as the model has a large number of parameters, we choose those most

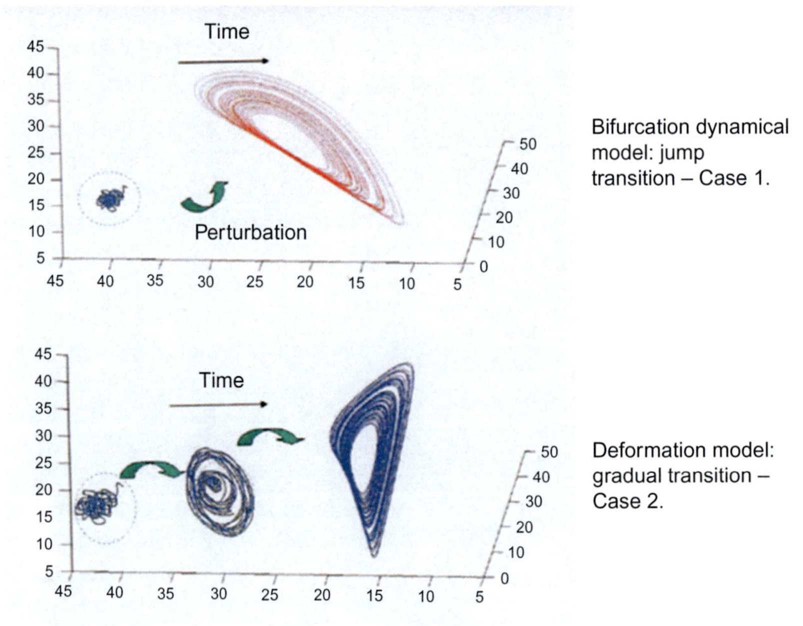

Fig. 3.1. Symbolic representation of the evolution in time of two models of transition between interictal and seizure states in a two-dimensional view of state space. The axes represent time and two state variables: neuronal network excitatory and inhibitory activity (numerical scales are arbitrary values). *Top:* Case 1 or *bifurcation model*: the dynamics of the neuronal network display a bifurcation from the interictal ("normal") state attractor to the ictal attractor that corresponds to large-amplitude spike-and-wave oscillations, as the result of a randomly occurring perturbation. *Bottom:* Case 2 or *deformation model*: the dynamics of the neuronal network evolve through a series of states (here only one intermediary state is indicated for simplicity) corresponding to a sequence of attractors due to a progressive deformation of network parameters, from an interictal state ("normal") attractor until an ictal attractor is reached. Seizures may not be anticipated in Case 1, but forecasting of seizure occurrence may be possible in Case 2 if appropriate tools can be applied to detect the intermediary dynamic states. (Adapted from Lopes da Silva, 2008. © Wiley.)

likely to be relevant, taking into consideration the following pathophysiological experimental data: $GABA_A$ in the cortex (Spreafico et al., 1993; Luhmann et al., 1995), I_T current in RE cells (Tsakiridou et al., 1995), burst firing in TC cells (Coulter et al., 1989; Leresche et al., 1998), and $GABA_A$ inhibition between RE cells (Huguenard and Prince, 1994). Furthermore, the influence of neuromodulatory inputs originating from brainstem mesencephalic cholinergic neurons was also investigated, as these inputs play an important role in the control of the level of vigilance and sleep. Indeed, acetylcholine released by cholinergic pathways affects the main cellular elements of the thalamocortical network, by decreasing the potassium conductance in the TC cells that brings about depolarization of the TC population, while increasing potassium conductance in the RE neurons and thereby inducing hyperpolarization of the RE population (McCormick and Prince, 1986).

The parameter sensitivity study in the model allowed a number of conclusions to be drawn regarding the parameters most likely to be critical in enhancing the probability of transition to the SWD state. The following appeared to be the most relevant in this respect: (i) a reduction of cortical $GABA_A$ inhibition and of intra-RE $GABA_A$ inhibition; (ii) an increase in $GABA_B$ conductance; (iii) increased burst firing in RE or TC populations; (iv) an increase in the slope of the function relating membrane potential and firing rate in the population of cortical interneurons; and (v) the level of the cholinergic input. Clearly there are several parameters that may be critical, either alone or in various combinations. Below, we review the experimental evidence with respect to the parameters that emerged as being most critical from the model sensitivity study.

Sensitivity to the cortical $GABA_A$ inhibition (i) is consistent with experimental data showing that one of the primary abnormalities underlying absence seizures in GAERS rats is an impairment of $GABA_A$-mediated transmission in the neocortex (Spreafico et al., 1993). Similarly, the cortical hyperexcitability in WAG/Rij rats was demonstrated to be due to decreased GABA-mediated inhibition (Luhmann et al., 1995). Injection of $GABA_A$ antagonists such as penicillin or bicuculline to the cortex produced SWDs in the cat (Gloor et al., 1979; Steriade and Contreras, 1998). Powerful control of cortical excitability by intracortical $GABA_A$ inhibition was also demonstrated *in vivo* and in another modeling study by Contreras et al. (1997).

The activation of $GABA_B$ inhibition in thalamic relay nuclei (ii) is essential for paroxysmal discharges in animal models of absence epilepsy (Hosford et al., 1992; Liu et al., 1992; Snead, 1992; Puigcerver et al., 1996; Smith and Fisher, 1996; Vergnes et al., 1997; Bowery et al., 1999), although it was not confirmed in all studies (Staak and Pape, 2001). In the model, the beginning of a paroxysmal epoch was detected when $GABA_B$ conductance in the TC cells was relatively large, and the end of a paroxysmal epoch was detected when $GABA_B$ conductance decreased again.

An increase of burst firing in RE or TC populations (iii) is compatible with the experimental findings in epileptic GAERS rats (Tsakiridou et al., 1995), which showed that the underlying low-threshold (I_T) calcium conductance in RE nucleus neurons is increased in comparison with that in nonepileptic controls. An increase of I_T current is detectable prior to the time of first SWD appearance (Tsakiridou et al., 1995). In the same strain of epileptic rats, a pharmacological reduction of burst firing in the RE nucleus, attributed to a decrease in the I_T calcium current and consequent decrease in the calcium-dependent potassium current, resulted in a decrement of paroxysmal discharge duration (Avanzini et al., 1992). Thomas and Grisar (2000) put forward an interesting hypothesis that the increased synchrony of the thalamic network, due to an increase of I_T current conductance in the RE neurons, may be related to a phase-shift in the activity of TC and RE neurons rather than to an increase in the amplitude of I_T in RE cells, as the latter was unaffected by I_T conductance changes. We also found in our model that an increase of I_T current in the RE population changes the phase relation between TC and RE neurons, increasing the network synchrony as indicated by the enhancement of the peak in the power spectrum of the thalamic signals.

The critical dependence of paroxysmal activity on the slope of the function relating membrane potential and firing rate in the population of cortical interneurons (iv) may indicate that the distribution of firing thresholds in this neuronal population is narrower than under normal conditions; in this way, this population can be more easily synchronized. It may be conceived that the slope parameter is related to the strength of gap–junctional connections within a population of interneurons. In this context it may be of interest to note that Velazquez and Carlen (2000) proposed that hyperventilation, which reduces blood carbon dioxide levels and causes alkalosis, may enhance gap–junctional communication and neural synchrony. Histological data indicate that gap junctions in the neocortex are specifically formed among inhibitory cells; in addition, they play a role in the communication between glial cells. It is known that during SWD glial cells swell (Amzica and Nekelmann, 1999), facilitating intercellular ephaptic transmission, which can facilitate the spreading of the discharge activity through gap junctions throughout the glial syncytium. In the light of these observations, the modeling results showing that an increase in the slope parameter has a powerful effect on paroxysmal activity may be related to an increase of electrotonic coupling.

The model results are also in agreement with the experimental observations in the WAG/Rij rats (v), that the SW seizures predominantly occur during drowsiness and light non-rapid eye movement (non-REM) sleep (Coenen and van Luijtelaar, 2003), where sleep spindles are prevalent. In the model, we found that a decrease in cholinergic activation from the brainstem, which underlies mainly the transition from the waking state to sleep (McCormick and Bal, 1997), facilitates the generation of paroxysmal activity. The latter result is also in line with the behavioral observation that paroxysmal discharges in GAERS occur primarily when attention and activity are reduced (Snead et al., 1999), and with the antiburst action of cholinergic thalamic input as proposed by Buzsáki et al. (1990).

The relevance of the network parameters that critically make the network prone to a transition to the epileptic state may be validated by investigating the effects of pharmacological agents in the model.

The most selective antiabsence drug, ethosuximide, is believed to exert its antiepileptic effect by antagonizing the burst firing in TC neurons, either by decreasing the I_T current (Coulter et al., 1989) or by acting on the noninactivating Na^+ current and on a Ca^{2+}-activated K^+ current in thalamic cells (Leresche et al., 1998).

The effect of benzodiazepines, such as clonazepam, is related to specific cellular targets mainly within the thalamic networks. RE and TC neurons do not have the same kind of $GABA_A$ receptor; those of the former have molecular subunits with binding sites for benzodiazepines, in contrast to the latter (Browne et al., 2001). Thus, these antiabsence drugs are likely to enhance $GABA_A$-mediated inhibition within the RE nucleus (Huguenard and Prince, 1994) but not in TC cells, and in this way they may attenuate GABA-mediated inhibition of the RE to TC neurons and thus prevent absence seizures. This hypothesis is confirmed by our model, as an increase in inhibitory strength between RE cells leads to a decrease of RE output and antagonizes paroxysmal activity. These modeling results are also in agreement with an experimental study showing that suppression of $GABA_A$ inhibition in the RE nucleus of GAERS led to an increased duration of SW activity (Aker et al., 2002). Additionally, antiabsence action of clonazepam may include also augmentation of $GABA_A$

currents in rat cortical neurons (Oh et al., 1995), which, as discussed above, is also consistent with the results of the model.

What makes the neuronal network switch its behavior from a state characterized by normal oscillations and normal behavior to another state characterized by SWD and absence seizures?

With respect to the second question, as formulated above, the model provided useful insight and led to predictions that could be tested in practice. The model revealed that transitions occur when random fluctuations in cortical and sensory (noise) inputs occur and peaks of these fluctuations take place above a certain level. Thus, the transition to SWDs in the model depends on a random process, i.e., the onset of paroxysms occurs randomly over time with particular probabilities.

Accordingly, the distribution of the duration of paroxysmal and normal epochs can be predicted to be exponential. In the model the histograms of durations of paroxysmal epochs and of the intervals between the occurrence of bursts of SWDs detected during 24 h of simulated time could be optimally fitted with exponential functions. The same applies to experimental results obtained in rat and human (Suffczynski et al., 2005) but only under certain circumstances. We noted that the distribution of durations of bursts of SWDs could differ from an exponential distribution suggesting that the probability of paroxysmal processes ending can change in the course of a paroxysmal epoch, due to the action of some use-dependent processes; the model study of Koppert et al. (2011) showed that such a process may be activation of the I_h current which, as discussed above, may act as a homeostatic mechanism resulting in a decrease in overall excitability, and thus in the reduction of seizure duration.

What are the roles of the thalamus and cortex in the generation of SWDs?

This third question, concerning the roles of the thalamus and the cortex in the initiation of SWDs, has a long history in neurophysiology since Jasper and Kershman (1941) analyzed the EEGs of patients with "petit mal" absence seizures, and proposed that the SWDs had a subcortical origin, because they could not find evidence for a cortical origin with the techniques available at that time. They concluded that this putative subcortical pacemaker should project to both hemispheres simultaneously, as SWDs appeared to be generalized over the whole head. This interpretation was reinforced by the discovery by Morison and Dempsey in 1941 of a thalamocortical projection system originating in the intralaminar nuclei of the thalamus. Later, Penfield and Jasper (1954) introduced the term "centrencephalic integrating system" for the putative diffuse neural system projecting to both hemispheres, which was assumed to be responsible for the control of the level of consciousness. This constitutes the "centrencephalic theory of absence seizures." In contrast, Bancaud (1969), Niedermeyer (1972), and Lüders et al. (1984) argued, based particularly on intracerebal recordings, that the cortex probably had also a role in the onset of SWDs. The search for mechanisms initiating SWDs in animal models of epilepsy was further elaborated by Gloor et al. (1990), who proposed that a "corticoreticular mechanism" was involved in the generation of SWDs, or, in other words, Gloor formulated the "corticoreticular theory of absence seizures." Gloor interpreted experimental data obtained using the "feline generalized penicillin model" (FGPE) as indicating that both the cortex and the reticular system of thalamus, and also the brainstem, play an essential role in the genesis of SWDs. This experimental model consisted of the intramuscular injection of penicillin in the cat, which was able to induce generalized, bilaterally synchronous, SWDs in the cortex. This FGPE model was considered a model for human primary absence epilepsy. The question as to whether the epileptic discharges were the result of abnormal responses of the cortex or abnormal volleys from the thalamus was answered partially by an experiment in which diffuse application of penicillin on the cortex was also able to produce SWDs, whereas an injection of penicillin in the thalamus failed to do so. Avoli and Gloor (1982) investigated in bilaterally and unilaterally decorticated cats whether or not the thalamus plays a primary role in the production of SWDs in the FGPE model. These authors found that an intramuscular dose of penicillin sufficient to induce FGPE in intact cats failed to elicit thalamic SWDs in the decorticated thalamus. They concluded that the development of generalized SWDs in FGPE depends primarily on a change in cortical excitability, and that thalamic SWDs in intact animals following penicillin appear to be imposed upon the thalamus by the cortex. Subsequently, Gloor et al. (1990) proposed that the crucial factor responsible for the SWDs was a diffuse increase in the excitability of the cortex. In this hyperexcitable state of the cortex, local neurons would respond to afferent thalamocortical volleys by producing SWDs instead of spindles, and thus the presence of both thalamus and cortex would be important for the typical cortical SWDs to develop, whereas the bilateral synchrony of the SWDs would depend on commissural connections. More recently our group carried out an extensive electrophysiological study of WAG/Rij rats with the objective of clarifying how SWDs occur and how these spread throughout the brain (Meeren et al., 2002).

Field potentials were simultaneously recorded from multiple cortical and thalamic sites. The corticocortical, intrathalamic, and corticothalamic interrelationships between local field potentials were quantified by means of the method of nonlinear association analysis developed by Pijn et al. (1989). This method yields a direct measure of the strength of association between signals recorded from different electrodes, regardless of whether the relationship is linear (estimated by the r^2 coefficient) or nonlinear (estimated by the h^2 coefficient), and also an estimate of the corresponding time delay. This analysis revealed that SWDs had an onset in a defined site of the somatosensory cortex, namely in a network that receives sensory inputs from the perioral region (nose, upper lip and vibrissae) of the body (Fig. 3.2). SWDs recorded at other cortical sites consistently lagged behind those recorded from this onset site with an average "propagation velocity" over the cortex of about 1.4 m/s. The analysis of corticothalamic relationships yielded very interesting results. First, the leading cortical sites started to display SWDs earlier than other cortical sites; similarly, sites of the ventroposteromedial thalamic nucleus (VPM), which are functionally related to the same region of the somatosensory cortex, also displayed SWDs earlier than other thalamic sites. Second, cortical SWDs could sometimes occur without concomitant thalamic SWDs, whereas the reverse was not observed. Third, we compared the results obtained using r^2 and h^2,

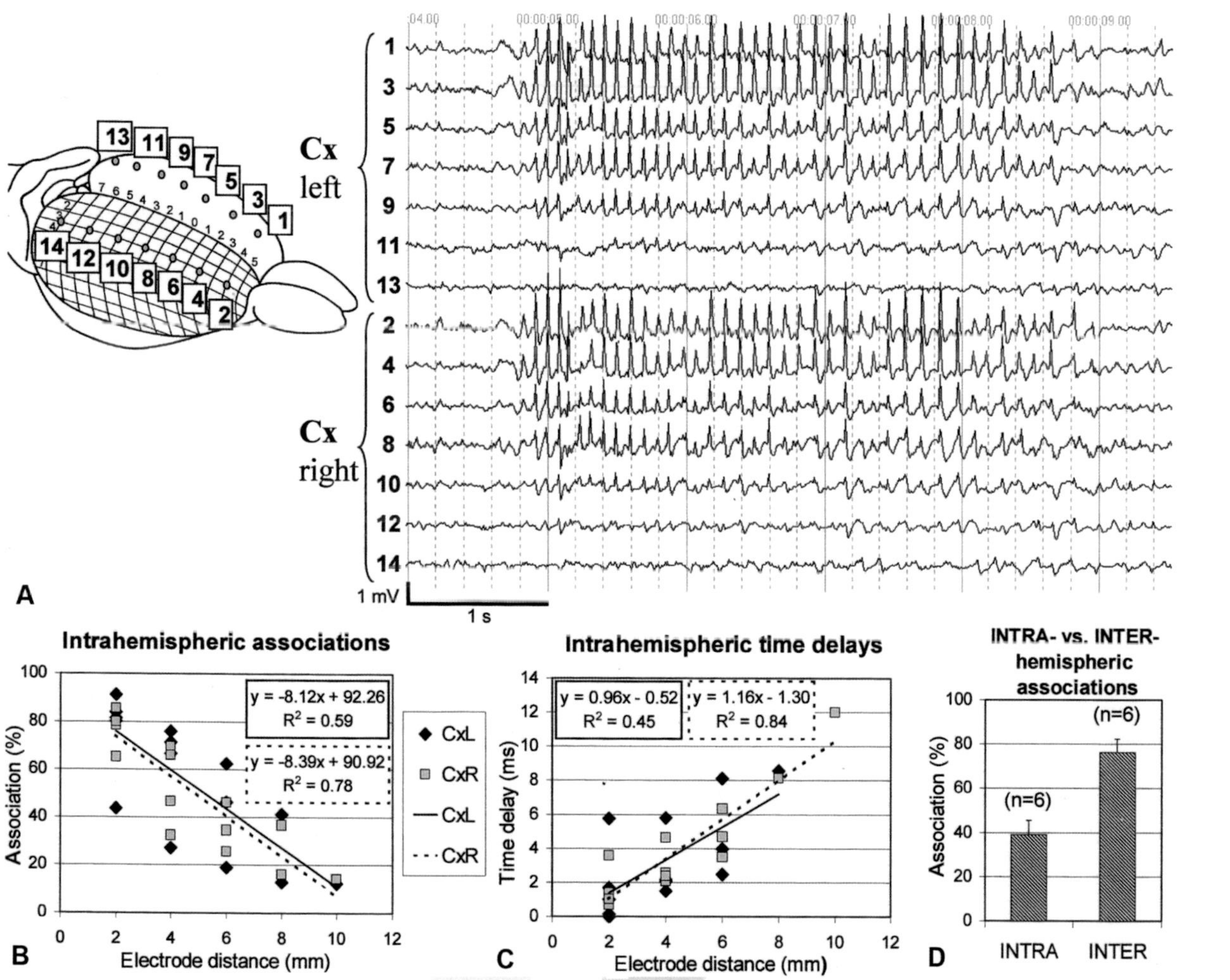

Fig. 3.2. (**A**) Distribution over the cortex of spike and wave discharges recorded from the rat genetic absence model WAG/Rij. The associations between the electrocorticographic (ECoG) signals recorded from different sites were estimated using the nonlinear association index h^2. (**B**) Intrahemispheric associations. (**C**) Intrahemispheric time delays. (**D**) Histogram showing the intra- versus inter-hemispheric associations (average of 6 rats). Note the decrease in association strength with distance from the reference site in the perioral area of the somatosensory cortex (**B**), the increase in time delay (**C**) reflecting a propagation velocity of about 1.4 m/s; the histograms in (**D**) show that interhemispheric associations between symmetrical sites are systematically larger than intrahemispheric associations, regardless of distance. (Adapted from Meeren et al., 2002. © Society for Neuroscience.)

which gives the possibility of estimating the degree of nonlinearity of the relationship between two signals. For the corticocortical and intrathalamic relationships, h^2 was similar or only marginally larger than r^2, indicating that these relationships can be described as approximately linear. For the corticothalamic relations, however, large differences were found most often between r^2 and h^2, with the latter being larger. This indicates that the corticothalamic relationships have strong nonlinear characteristics.

Fourth, the most important result in the light of this discussion, however, was the finding that during the early part of a SWD burst, namely during the initial period of about 500 ms of a SWD burst, the variability in corticothalamic time delays was very low, and the cortical sites consistently led the thalamus by about 8 ms (Fig. 3.3). This means that, at the onset of a burst of SWD, the cortical sites are leading and the thalamus follows this lead. In the course of the evolution of a SWD burst, however, these time relations may become variable and the direction of the time delay may even be inverted. This indicates that during sustainment of a SWD burst, cortex and thalamus form a unified network with strong re-entrant components, and that the SWD oscillation may be considered an emergent property of the whole complex network.

Therefore, to detect the onset of SWDs it is necessary to analyze the very early beginning of a burst.

The cortical driver of SWDs

The finding of a cortical network that is responsible for the onset of SWDs in rats with absence epilepsy led to a number of further studies:

- cortical electrophysiological studies at the intracellular level (Pinault, 2003; Polack et al., 2007)
- pharmacological studies to test the "cortical onset site" interpretation (Manning et al., 2004; Gurbanova et al., 2006)
- molecular studies at the level of ion channels and receptor subunits to test whether the SWD onset site presents specific abnormalities at the molecular level (Klein et al., 2004; Blumenfeld et al., 2008).

All of the above studies yielded results supporting the notion that there is indeed a cortical driver of SWDs in the somatosensory cortex in the rat genetic models.

- human and imaging studies to test whether the rat findings can be generalized to patients with absence epilepsy and to complement the findings obtained electrophysiologically with functional magnetic resonance imaging (fMRI) methods.

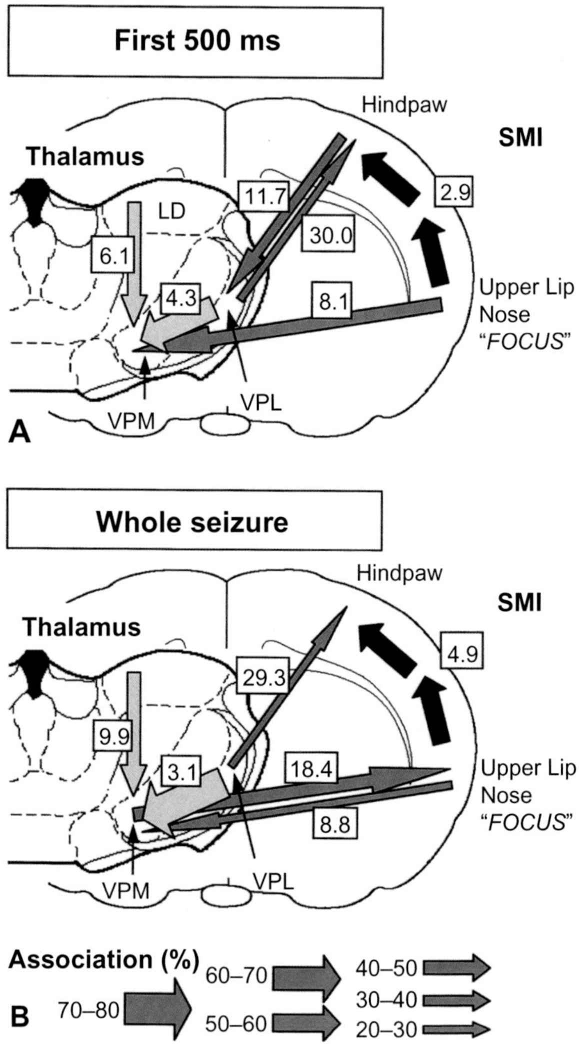

Fig. 3.3. Thalamocortical neuronal network. Dynamics of the interactions between thalamus and cortex during spike-and-wave discharges (SWDs). (**A**) During the first 500 ms the driver of SWDs is in the perioral area of the somatosensory cortex; the activity spreads from there to the rest of the cortex and to the thalamus. (**B**) Analysis of the whole seizure shows much more complex relationships and it is not possible to detect a clear driver. The value of the associations (as %) is indicated by the width of the arrows; the corresponding time delays (in milliseconds) are indicated in the boxes on the sides of the arrows. VPL, ventroposterolateral nucleus; VPM, ventroposteromedial thalamic nucleus. (Adapted from Meeren et al., 2002. © Society for Neuroscience.)

We refer to the last in more detail, as these studies are specifically relevant to the human case.

Holmes et al. (2004) recorded absence seizures in five patients by means of 256-channel dense-array scalp EEG recordings. They analyzed SWDs using source analysis methods and found that the onset of seizures was localized to discrete areas of the dorsofrontal or orbital frontal lobe. In particular, the spike component was highly localized over the frontopolar regions of orbital frontal cortex. In addition to frontopolar sources, other sources were also localized in the anterior cingulate gyrus, which has an important role in the maintenance of arousal. These findings demonstrate that, as in the rat, absence seizures are not "generalized" from the onset but have a cortical onset site. Tucker et al. (2007) made similar recordings in patients with absences and noted that neither the onset nor the spread of these seizures was generalized. Based on the finding of specific involvement of the frontal cortex, they proposed the hypothesis that absence seizures are associated with pathology in a circuit comprising the ventromedial frontal cortex, rostral thalamic reticular nucleus, and limbic nuclei of the thalamus. This network would be disrupted in absences. Using magnetoencephalography (MEG) recordings, Westmijse et al. (2009) found the onset of SWDs in human absence epilepsy at frontal and parietal sites.

The issue of the sequence of brain areas of the thalamocortical network involved in SWD was also analyzed in seven patients with idiopathic generalized epilepsy (IGE) using fMRI (Vaudano et al., 2009) and dynamic causal modeling (DCM). These authors tested three possible dynamic models that differed in the region where SWDs would have the onset: thalamus (model A), ventromedial prefrontal cortex (model B), and precuneus (model C). Model C (SWDs as autonomous input to precuneus) appeared to fit the data the best in five patients, and model A prevailed in two. The authors concluded that activity in the precuneus gates SWDs in the thalamo-(fronto) cortical network. The involvement of precuneus is interesting, considering its role in the control of awareness. These results, however, pose a problem: if the dynamics of the onset and propagation of SWDs in humans follow the same pattern as in the rat genetic models, the possibility of finding the onset area is limited to the very first 500 ms. This time resolution cannot be achieved with the hemodynamic signals. Therefore, studies based on the latter can indicate grossly which brain regions are involved in the propagation of SWDs and are recruited into this abnormal pattern of activity, but not the area of onset.

This limitation of fMRI with respect to the question of determining the onset of SWDs is also illustrated by the interesting study of David et al. (2008) in GAERS. They used both electrophysiological (using intracerebral electrodes) and fMRI methods to investigate the onset and development of SWDs in these animals and asked precisely the question whether fMRI allows the identification of SWD neural drivers. Furthermore, they analyzed fMRI time series directly using DCM, which relates synaptic activity in a lumped model of the cortical population to hemodynamic signals (David and Friston, 2003), and Granger causality in order to estimate where in the brain the driver of SWD might be localized. The estimates based on fMRI signals indicated that the somatosensory (barrel field SIBF) cortex was most likely the driver of SWDs, but did not allow the determination of time delays. Electrophysiologically, however, this study showed that the averaged SWD in the cortical barrel field SIBF preceded by 5.5 and 10 ms those measured in the thalamus and striatum, respectively. This average sequence of activation confirms previous findings in both GAERS and WAG/Rij rats. Mishra et al. (2011) also recorded electrophysiological and fMRI (9.4 Tesla) signals during SWDs in rats displaying absence seizures (WAG/Rij rats). They found that during these discharges the somatosensory cortex and the thalamus showed increased BOLD (blood oxygen dependent) signal and cerebral blood volume (CBV) as well as cerebral blood flow (CBF), associated with an increase in local field potential and multiunit activity, but no time relations between cortex and thalamus were analyzed.

HOW MAY TRANSITIONS BETWEEN NORMAL AND EPILEPTIC BEHAVIOR OCCUR IN NEURONAL NETWORKS OF THE HIPPOCAMPAL SYSTEM?

Temporal lobe epilepsy, in general, is characterized by the occurrence of complex partial seizures, and is the most common form of medically refractory epilepsy. This makes these patients very often candidates for the surgical removal of the epileptogenic zone. A system that shows a remarkable tendency to exhibit epileptic seizures is the mesial temporal lobe, where the hippocampal formation occupies a prominent position. The fact that the brain of these patients is usually investigated in great detail before surgery, in order to determine whether, or not, an estimate of the epileptogenic zone might be obtained, has yielded an appreciable amount of data regarding the pathophysiology of these syndromes. Many electrophysiological, imaging, and even biochemical and molecular studies have been carried out which have enriched our knowledge about the neuronal networks involved in mesial temporal lobe epilepsy (MTLE). In addition, a long series of experimental studies in animal models of MTLE has led to new insights into the cellular and network processes that may account for epileptic seizures, providing good models of the human pathological condition. Furthermore, computational models have been developed with the aim of making comprehensive integration of experimental data and formulating hypotheses that may be tested in experimental or clinical situations.

These studies led to the concept that the epileptogenic zone in MTLE is "multistructural" (Bragin et al., 2000; Bartolomei et al., 2004). Indeed, in many cases several structures of the mesial temporal lobe are involved at the initiation of seizures, mainly the hippocampus, subiculum, entorhinal cortex, and amygdala. In this way, the notion of a well-circumscribed focus within a specific structure is not applicable. On the contrary, one should formulate the hypothesis that the abnormality responsible for the epileptic seizures is a property of a complex network involving different structures.

Contrary to absence seizures, where the cortical driver does not show conspicuous macroscopic abnormalities, the MTLE syndrome displays characteristic neuropathological changes that are clearly seen on histological examination of brain tissue of patients, and that in many cases are also evident on MRI.

A hallmark of MTLE is the extensive loss of neurons of the hippocampal hilar region, without comparable cell loss of granule cells in the dentate gyrus (Margerison and Corsellis, 1966; de Lanerolle et al., 1989; Sloviter, 1991a, b), and considerable gliosis, which is termed endfolium sclerosis. In addition there is remarkable sprouting of mossy fibers into the granule cell layer of the dentate gyrus associated with synaptic reorganization. The sprouted mossy fibers may form recurrent excitatory collaterals on the granule cell dendrites in the inner molecular layer (Golarai and Sutula, 1996; Wuarin and Dudek, 1996; Lynch and Sutula, 2000).

These pathological changes can be reproduced in animal models, namely in post-SE in the rat (Gorter et al., 2001). SE may be induced in a variety of ways: by repeated high-frequency electrical stimulation according to the method devised by Lothman et al. (1989); by injection of several drugs such as kainate (Ben-Ari and Cossart, 2000), either locally (Cavalheiro et al., 1982) or systemically (Hellier et al., 1998); or by pilocarpine (Turski et al., 1983).

A general feature of the post-SE evolution of epileptic seizures is that spontaneous seizures do not start immediately in the rat but take a week or more to appear, depending on the paradigm used to induce SE. Thus there exists a *latent period* between the initial precipitating event and the occurrence of spontaneous seizures. This indicates that the epileptogenic process involves the development of structural and functional changes in and around the damaged area before seizures may emerge. It is assumed that a similar process occurs also in humans, although the "latent period" is much longer than in the rat and may last for years. Indeed, studies of MTLE in humans support the hypothesis that hippocampal sclerosis is an acquired pathology in which most of the neuronal loss occurs with the initial precipitating insult, which is most commonly a complex febrile seizure. After a latent period, spontaneous seizures occur that commonly show a progressive evolution. We may state that during this latent period a *deformation of parameters* that are critical with respect to the stability of these neuronal networks takes place.

A basic question is how these structural changes create the conditions that change the dynamic state of the underlying neuronal networks such that spontaneous seizures may occur. As in the case of absence seizures discussed above, we have to emphasize here that the same hippocampal network can generate both normal activity and occasionally partial complex seizures; the latter can propagate throughout the brain and produce dramatic transient behavioral abnormalities.

How can neuronal networks of the mesial temporal lobe cause normal behavior and occasionally also epileptic seizures?

In the case of limbic seizures, characteristic of MTLE, there is a set of cellular/molecular changes that render certain parameters controlling the stability of the networks extremely vulnerable to the influence of endogenous and/or exogenous factors. We should note, however, that most of the time these networks display normal oscillations – such as theta or gamma rhythmic activities – typical of the interictal state, but occasionally can display epileptic seizure activity – the ictal state. If we represent these two states in a theoretical space as two attractors, we may state that the distance between the two attractors (normal interictal activity and ictal seizure) becomes relatively small during the process of epileptogenesis, owing to the changes that occur in the network, as represented symbolically in Figure 3.1. Under perfect normal conditions this distance would be so large that the probability of the dynamic state changing from one to the other attractor would be extremely small (Lopes da Silva et al., 2003). Only the application of a strong electric shock to the head might trigger such a transition in a normal brain. However, because of modifications of the control parameters of the neuronal networks in MTLE, this distance becomes gradually smaller due to changes in some critical unstable parameters in such a way that a transition to a seizure eventually takes place. Thus we may state that these parameters suffer a deformation in the course of time. This means that, in principle, it should be possible to detect the dynamic changes that precede the transition to a seizure, and thus that seizures might be anticipated. We discuss whether this may be possible to realize in practice briefly below.

What are the critical parameters responsible for the change in network dynamics leading to MTLE seizures?

The MTLE syndrome does not result from abnormal neuronal activity in a highly circumscribed focal area; rather, it involves a tightly connected neuronal network that includes several structures of the limbic brain (Bertram et al., 1998; Bartolomei et al., 2001). There exists a relationship between the number of brain structures with epileptogenic characteristics and the duration of the epileptic condition in patients with MTLE (Bartolomei et al., 2008). The core of this network is created by the hippocampal formation and directly associated structures such as the entorhinal cortex (EC).

In the process of epileptogenicity of MTLE, the hippocampus plays a central role. Thus, we will start by focusing on the processes that take place at the level of the hippocampus and then consider its interconnections with the EC. Recently developed computational models (Wendling et al., 2002, 2005) give us some clues regarding critical parameters that control the dynamics of these neuronal networks.

These models are based on a simplified cellular organization of the hippocampus, and include:

- recurrent excitatory connections from pyramidal cells to pyramidal cells (Thomson and Radpour, 1991; Whittington et al., 1997)
- two types of $GABA_A$ synaptic response in CA1 pyramidal neurons: a fast one that is perisomatic, and a slow one that is located at the dendrites; the first one, $GABA_A$,fast, is a rapidly activated and decaying IPSC mediated by somatic synapses, and the second, $GABA_A$,slow, is a slowly rising and decaying IPSC mediated by dendritic synapses (Miles et al., 1996)
- stimulation of two main classes of interneuron: basket cells (B) and interneurons of the stratum lacunosum-moleculare (LM), respectively called, for simplicity, $GABA_A$,fast interneurons and $GABA_A$,slow interneurons, responsible for the two types of IPSC (Banks et al., 1998), as indicated above
- both classes of interneuron interact: $GABA_A$,slow interneurons inhibit not only pyramidal cells but also $GABA_A$,fast interneurons (Banks et al., 2000).

These elements of the neuronal network are presented schematically in Figure 3.4.

In the modeled network, three parameters emerge as the most significant ones in this respect: the levels of excitation (EXC), of slow dendritic inhibition (SDI), and of fast somatic inhibition (FSI). Parameter EXC represents the average amplitude of EPSPs at the synapses between pyramidal neurons and interneurons, as well as among pyramidal cells themselves; parameter SDI represents the average amplitude of IPSPs with slow kinetics at the synapses formed by LM interneurons (somatostatin-immunoreactive) on the dendrites of pyramidal cells and other interneurons (B, basket cells); parameter FSI represents the average amplitude of postsynaptic potentials with fast kinetics at the synapses formed by B interneurons (parvalbumin-immunoreactive) on pyramidal cells.

What makes the neuronal network switch its behavior from a state characterized by normal oscillations and normal behavior to a state characterized by epileptiform activity and seizures?

Using the model described above in forward mode, Wendling et al. (2002) were able to reproduce EEG signals, and the corresponding power spectra, very similar to those observed during successive periods: the interictal period, the period just before the onset of a seizure (pre-onset), the period at seizure onset, and the period during the seizure (ictal period). The major change in power spectra occurs at seizure onset, which is characterized by the appearance of EEG signals with low amplitude mainly in the frequency band from 15 to about 40 Hz; this is followed during the ictal phase by a transition to narrow-band large-amplitude signals ranging from 3 to 10 Hz. Most interesting, Wendling et al. (2005) later tested the model, in inverse mode, based on real EEG signals recorded intracerebrally from five patients with typical MTLE seizures. Applying an evolutionary algorithm, these authors were able to estimate values of the three critical parameters (EXC, SDI, FSI) corresponding to the real EEG signals and their evolution along the different periods leading to the ictal phase. These analyses revealed the parameter changes that make the neuronal network switch from the interictal phase characterized by normal oscillations to an abnormal state where epileptiform oscillations occur.

In the model this switch is realized by the following evolution of the three critical parameters, as follows: (i) *parameter EXC* increases during the transition between the interictal and the preonset and onset phases, and stays large during the transition to the ictal phase; (ii) *parameter SDI* increases from the interictal period to the period just before the onset (following the increase in EXC), but decreases markedly at the onset (the phase characterized by fast oscillations in the EEG) and increases again at the transition between onset and ictal periods; (iii) *parameter FSI* is stable or increases in the preonset period, but decreases markedly during the transition from onset to ictal.

The evolution of these critical parameters can be translated into the following (patho)physiological processes: at the onset of a seizure there is a breakdown of SDI (i.e., of slow GABA inhibition), which provokes disinhibition of fast GABAergic interneurons (basket cell, B interneurons), with the appearance of EEG fast oscillations; the subsequent EEG slowing could be due

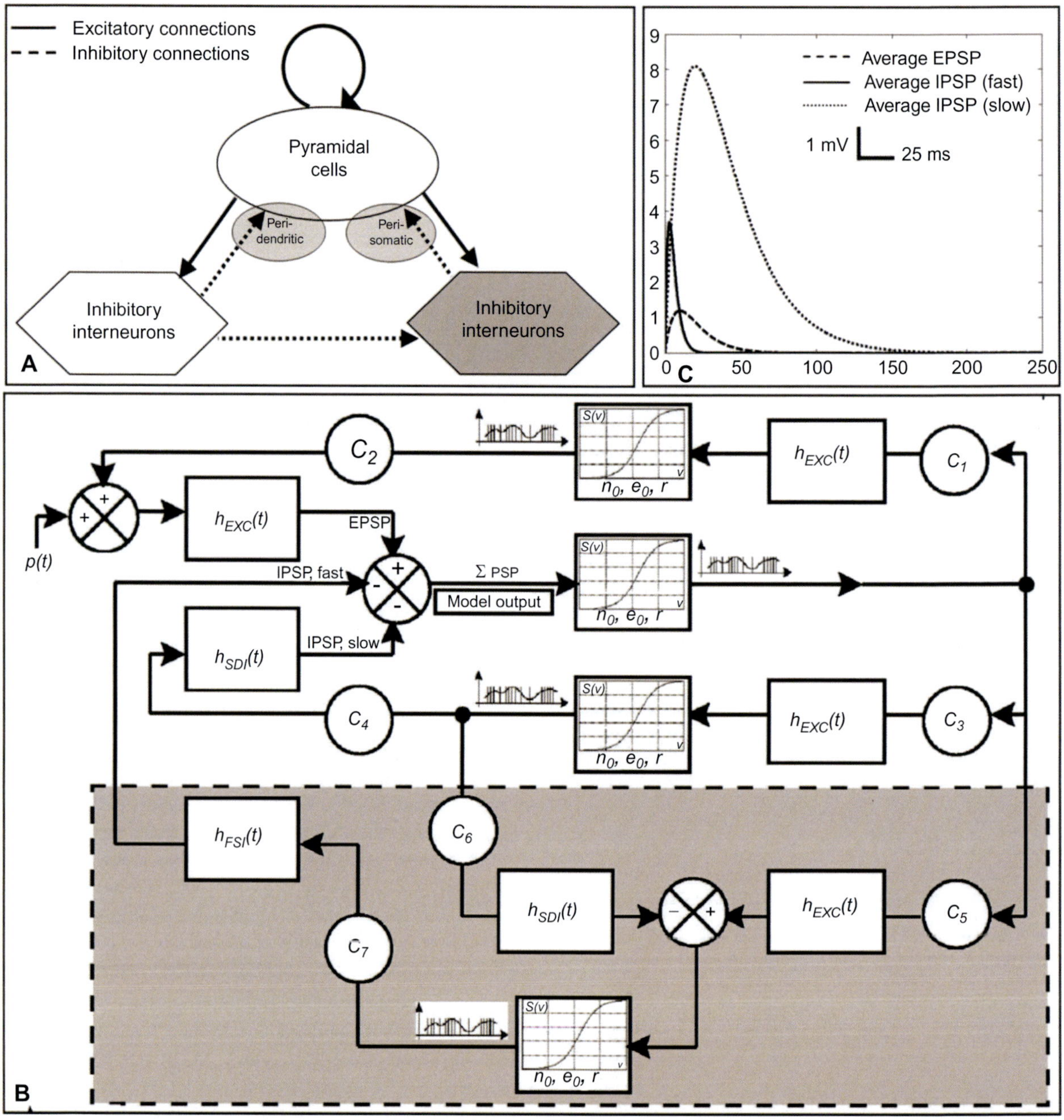

Fig. 3.4. Neuronal network of the hippocampus involved in mesial temporal lobe epilepsy (MTLE). Neural mass model based on the cellular organization of the hippocampus. (**A**) A population of principal cells (pyramidal cells) project to and receive feedback from other local interneurons. Input to interneurons is excitatory (AMPA receptor-mediated). Feedback to pyramidal cells is either excitatory (recurrent excitation) or inhibitory: dendritic synapses with slow kinetics, $GABA_A$, slow (slow dendritic, SD); somatic synapses, grey rectangle; with faster kinetics, $GABA_A$,fast (fast somatic, FS). In addition, "slow interneurons" project to "fast ones". (**C**) Time courses of the corresponding excitatory postsynaptic potentials (EPSPs) and inhibitory postsynaptic potentials (fast and slow IPSPs). (**B**) Corresponding block diagram representation. In each subset, the average pulse density of afferent action potentials is changed into an average inhibitory or excitatory postsynaptic membrane potential using a linear dynamic transfer function of impulse response $h_{EXC}(t)$, $h_{SDI}(t)$, and $h_{FSI}(t)$, while this potential is converted into an average pulse density of potentials fired by the neurons by way of a static nonlinear function (asymmetrical sigmoid curve, $S(v)$). The subset of somatic-projecting interneurons (grey rectangle) receives input from both subsets of pyramidal and dendritic interneurons. One of the model outputs represents the summated average of postsynaptic potentials on pyramidal cells; this reflects an EEG signal. (Adapted from Wendling et al., 2005.)

to a process of exhaustion of this fast inhibition according to Wendling's model (2005).

It should be noted that these conclusions are based on a computational model, and are not necessarily unique. Nonetheless, the fact that these results have already been tested in a number of real cases, namely using EEG recordings obtained by way of intracerebral electrodes in patients with MTLE, provides the assurance that these conclusions are plausible, even though they may not be unique. Therefore, it is important to examine next how these changes in the network parameters may be accounted for by physiological/molecular changes in real neuronal elements.

Starting with the increase of EXC: this may reflect the enhancement of EPSPs in CA1 subarea as has been seen in experimental models of MTLE. In an experimental investigation in the kainate post-SE rat, Wu and Leung (2003) reported that 2–4 months after SE when usually the animals have spontaneous seizures, the basal and distal apical EPSPs were enhanced in CA1 following stimulation of CA3 or of the input from the Entorhinal Cortex (EC). In addition, in experimental models of focal epilepsy enhanced and/or prolonged EPSPs were found (Bernard et al., 2001; Gorter et al., 2002), as well as in slices from human hippocampus (Schwartzkroin, 1994), showing that epileptic seizures susceptibility is associated with this increase in excitability. Huberfeld et al. (2011) examined this process in tissue slices from human subjects with MTLE, where seizure-like discharges were induced in the subiculum by alkalinization or low Mg^{2+}. These authors concluded that in these patients the subiculum is involved in the generation of seizures and that the latter are an "emergent glutamatergic population activity."

Regarding the inhibitory parameters (SDI and FSI), it should be noted that just before the onset of a seizure the SDI increases; this may simply be a reaction to the increase of EXC, as was described by Khalilov et al. (2003) in the intact hippocampus preparation kept *in vitro*. From a dynamic point of view this would act as a compensatory homeostatic mechanism to avoid the excessive excitation leading to an unstable network. An important aspect of the transition to a seizure, however, is that this increase of SDI is not sustained, and is promptly followed by a decrease at seizure onset as the fast oscillations appear in the EEG. How can this be accounted for? A possibility is that in the abnormal hippocampus the SDI is too "labile" to be able to compensate for the excessive excitatory activity. An important feature of the inhibitory circuits of the hippocampus is that the slow GABAergic interneurons, responsible for SDI, inhibit the fast GABAergic interneurons responsible for FSI (Banks et al., 2000). If the former break down, the latter are disinhibited; this would be reflected in the occurrence of fast oscillations at the onset of a seizure. As this process evolves, the FSI gradually decreases in these epileptic animals and the fast oscillations and the dynamics become dominated by large-amplitude, slower oscillations characteristic of the full-blown seizure.

In this context it is interesting to note that Cossart et al. (2001) showed a decrease in dendritic inhibition (corresponding to parameter SDI) but not in somatic inhibition (FSI) in experimental epilepsy. The loss of dendritic inhibition may enhance the tendency for dendritic spiking, as found experimentally (Wu and Leung, 2003). Other local cellular changes may also contribute to the enhancement of dendritic excitability in CA1, such as changes in calcium channel density (Bernstein et al., 1999), enhancement of Na^+ and Ca^{2+} currents (Vreugdenhil and Wadman, 1994; Faas et al., 1996), and a decrease in A-current (Castro et al., 2001). These processes can increase seizure susceptibility in the CA1 subarea, as the entorhinal inputs bypass the dentate gyrus, where inhibitory processes may even be enhanced (Buckmaster and Dudek, 1997). Interestingly, Wu and Leung (2003) point out that enhancement of the activity in the pathways from the EC to CA1 will reinforce the re-entrant multisynaptic circuit: CA1 – subiculum – EC – medial perforant path – CA1 (Kloosterman et al., 2004). In addition, we may speculate that enhanced activity in this re-entrant circuit may constitute the anatomical and physiological substrate for reverberation to occur, i.e., persistent activity in these loops in the absence of external input. Indeed, it has been suggested that in the subcortically denervated hippocampus of the freely moving rat, removal of tonic inhibitory influences allows reverberation of information in the entorhinal–hippocampal–entorhinal cortex circuitry (Buzsáki et al., 1989). It has not yet been established experimentally, however, whether this kind of reverberation is an important mechanism making these rats more susceptible to the occurrence of epileptic seizures.

In short, two main mechanisms appear to be responsible for the transition from the interictal to the ictal state: (a) enhancement of parameter EXC, and (b) the lability or instability of GABAergic processes.

We consider first the former (a). Taking into consideration that the main excitatory input of the hippocampus arises from the EC, it is appropriate to examine what happens in the EC in this rat post-SE experimental model and also in patients with MTLE. In patients with MTLE, the superficial part of the rostral EC presents marked cell loss, which is particularly noticeable in layer III (Du et al., 1993) and can be detected with MRI (Bernasconi et al., 1999; Jutila et al., 2001). This characteristic cell loss in layer III of the EC has been reproduced in several rat post-SE models of MTLE (Du et al., 1995; Gorter et al., 2001; van Vliet et al., 2004) and is confined mostly to the medial portion of the entorhinal cortex (medial entorhinal area, MEA). It has been suggested that within the MEA, the deep cortical layers are responsible primarily for the onset of epileptiform activity (Iijima et al., 1996; Dickson and Alonso, 1997; Lopantsev and Avoli, 1998), although this was based on investigations carried in slice preparations *in vitro*. In an *in vivo* study of post-SE rats elicited by kainate with spontaneous seizures (Tolner et al., 2005), however, we found no evidence for this role of deep layers of the EC. On the contrary, we found diminished control of the activity of the interneurons in superficial layers (II and III), due to the absence of excitatory input from MEA-III principal neurons on inhibitory interneurons, as the number of the former is diminished substantially. This would lead to a decrease of the inhibitory drive on pyramidal cells of the superficial layers. It is likely, although not directly proven, that this may cause the threshold for excitation of layer II neurons to be lowered, which could facilitate the occurrence of oscillations and lead to enhancement of the excitatory input from these superficial EC layers to the hippocampal formation. In this way, enhancement of the critical parameter EXC, the excitatory drive, of the model described above would be accounted for. As in the case of the hippocampus, computer models of the EC may also shed new light on the processes underlying seizure susceptibility in this structure.

Regarding the second mechanism (b), there is experimental evidence that the $GABA_A$ receptors behave deficiently in epileptic tissue. It was shown by Palma et al. (2007) in surgically removed brain tissue from patients with MTLE that the ionic current elicited by stimulation of $GABA_A$ receptors presents a strong rundown (an effect enhanced by zinc) in comparison with that of control tissue. This was also found in cortical neurons of rats with spontaneous epileptic seizures after the administration of pilocarpine. The authors concluded that the rundown of $GABA_A$ receptors is a hallmark of MTLE and may favor the development of seizures.

Later the same group (Mazzuferi et al., 2010) carried out an investigation at the molecular level to determine the cause of this "rundown" phenomenon; they reported a relative increase in the $\alpha4$ subunit, relative to $\alpha1$-containing $GABA_A$ receptors, occurring at the same time as the increased rundown appears in pilocarpine-treated epileptic rats. According to these authors, this could represent the switch leading to the occurrence of spontaneous seizures. Other studies at the molecular level in the post-SE rat model of MTLE (Gorter et al., 2006) also revealed changes of the expression of genes involved in GABAergic transmission that could contribute to instability of the neuronal networks. A particularly consistent finding was that the genes encoding the subunits $\alpha5$ (CA3) and delta (EC) were downregulated. Both subunits are present in extrasynaptic receptors that control tonic inhibition (Houser and Esclapez, 2003; Dibbens et al., 2004; Peng et al., 2004; Glykys and Mody, 2006). Further, it has been shown in clinical studies that the GABA-$\alpha5$ subunit is also downregulated in humans (de Lanerolle and Lee, 2005; Arion et al., 2006; Ozbas-Gerceker et al., 2006). In addition, the expression of chloride (Cl^-) transporters (NKCC1 and KCC2), which regulate the intracellular chloride concentration and thus the nature of the Cl^- ionic flux associated with GABA synapses, has been shown to be altered in a number of developmental lesions, including focal cortical dysplasia, hemimegalencephaly, and ganglioglioma in patients with medically intractable epilepsy, where NKCC1 was highly expressed while KCC2 was reduced. This pattern is suggestive of what is found in immature cortex, and may cause depolarizing GABAergic synaptic responses that will destabilize the neuronal networks. The existence of GABAergic depolarizing responses was reported in the subiculum of slices from patients with temporal lobe epilepsy in neurons downstream of the sclerotic CA1 region (Cohen et al., 2002). Ionic mechanisms causing depolarizing GABAergic events were also investigated by Lamsa and Kaila (1997). In the search for proepileptic changes in slices from mice that had received a focal kainate injection into one hippocampus, Le Duigou et al. (2008) also found a depolarized reversal potential for GABAergic events and a depolarized resting potential in CA1 pyramidal neurons. This study led to another interesting conclusion in the light of the present discussion, namely that both depolarizing GABAergic responses and an independent increase in cellular excitability are needed for the initiation of epileptic seizures.

Labyt et al. (2007) constructed a model of the EC neuronal networks including the following elements: (i) subpopulations of neurons (pyramidal cells, stellate cells) and interneurons that are encountered in deep and superficial layers of the EC; and (ii) a set of intralayer and interlayer interaction links between these subpopulations (see Fig. 3.4) by means of glutamatergic excitatory synapses and GABAergic synapses of three kinds: $GABA_A$ with slow and fast kinetics, and $GABA_B$; in addition, glycinergic synapses (Keck and White, 2009) were also included. The transfer function between membrane potential and firing rate is represented by a nonlinear sigmoid function with a given steepness, which incorporates a threshold and saturation level (maximal firing rate). The model receives a random input that represents the synaptic afferents coming from surrounding and distant neuronal populations; the output is constituted by the sum of postsynaptic potentials of the pyramidal cell subpopulations. The data included in the model were inferred from experimental data obtained from recording of electrical activities in guinea-pig brains maintained *in vitro* by perfusion (de Curtis et al., 1991). Epileptiform discharges were induced by arterial applications of the $GABA_A$ receptor antagonist, bicuculline, diluted in the perfusion solution. The model can display different types of EEG-like signal, including fast discharges corresponding to the pattern seen during seizure onset in real conditions. Epileptic activities start to appear when the value of $GABA_B$ inhibition decreases below a given threshold. Different kinds of spike burst (spikes mixed to fast activity, polyspikes) may appear depending on the value of $GABA_A$ fast inhibition. Without entering here into details of the model study (but see Labyt et al., 2007), the critical parameters leading to model instability (i.e., to the onset of epileptiform discharges) were mainly a decrease in $GABA_A$ slow and $GABA_B$ receptor-mediated inhibition.

Considering that the condition leading to MTLE syndrome is characterized by changes in the parameters controlling the stability of limbic neuronal networks distributed over different brain structures, where the EC and the hippocampal formation form the central core, it is important to know how seizure activity *propagates* within and beyond this network. This issue was considered in an investigation by Bartolomei et al. (2004) of patients with MTLE, where intracerebral electrodes were placed in different areas of the hippocampus, EC, and amygdala, as well as some other areas such as the frontal, parietal, and other temporal lobe areas (temporobasal, insular cortex). Interactions between the EEG signals recorded from these areas were estimated using a nonlinear association index (h^2; Lopes da Silva et al., 1989; Pijn et al., 1989) combined with a "direction index" that indicates the direction of signal flow (Wendling et al., 2001; Bartolomei et al., 2004). Three 10-s periods were analyzed using analysis windows of 4 s – periods before (BRD), during (DRD), and after (ARD) the EEG rapid discharge that occurs at seizure onset – as well as a control period far away from the seizure (Fig. 3.5). The onset of all seizures was found at electrode sites within the mesial temporal lobe. EEG changes at the transition to the characteristic seizure rapid tonic discharge could be preceded by a period of large-amplitude, low-frequency spiking (Spencer et al., 1992; Velasco et al., 2000), or not. The hippocampus, but not the amygdala, was involved in most of the couplings, and the EC was the leading structure in some situations, as specified below. Above, we indicated that two types of evolution of seizure activity can be distinguished in patients with MTLE. We may raise the question of whether these two types may correspond to different processes, concerning onset and propagation routes. Bartolomei et al. (2004) concluded that this may be very well the case. Indeed, in cases where the rapid tonic discharge was preceded by large-amplitude, low-frequency spiking, the latter appeared to originate in the hippocampus and not in the EC; the involvement of the latter during the subsequent seizure phase indicates that the seizure propagates from the hippocampus to the EC, from where it may be distributed to many cortical areas. In contrast, those cases where no spiking was observed in the period before rapid discharge (BRD), a marked synchrony between EC, hippocampus, and amygdala was found, with the first leading, suggesting that the rapid discharge started in the EC. We have to make a critical remark regarding these conclusions, as the analysis window used in this study was relatively long (4 s); if these flows are as quick as those encountered in the case of the propagation of SWDs in the rat with absence seizures (Meeren et al., 2002), it is possible that this window may have been too long to catch very quick propagation flows of seizure activity.

Are there EEG markers of hyperexcitability of limbic neuronal networks in epileptic conditions?

In the last decade, specific bursts of oscillations, the so-called fast ripples (FRs), were described in hippocampal recordings from rats with post-SE spontaneous seizures, and also in the hippocampus of patients with MTLE (Bragin et al., 1999a, b, c; Jacobs et al., 2008). Previously, ripples at a lower frequency, consisting of bursts of oscillations at 100–200 Hz were described in normal brain (Buzsáki et al., 1992).The FRs consist of oscillations at frequencies above 200 Hz, primarily near the seizure onset region. This discovery led to the hypothesis that FRs reflect a state of high excitability of the underlying networks and are generated by synchronous discharges of pyramidal neurons. The interpretation is that these FRs result from the activity of clusters of interconnected neurons capable of sustaining synchrony of discharges, surrounded by a strong inhibitory ring; if feedback inhibition is surpassed, the formation of similar clusters in target areas may occur, and these clusters may become synchronized, ultimately leading to seizures (Bragin et al., 2002).

It is therefore important to know what is the relationship between the occurrence of FRs and the propensity for the occurrence of spontaneous seizures. Initially, FRs were recorded using microelectrodes and it was even doubted whether these oscillations could be detected using macroelectrodes, as they appeared to be localized within small volumes of brain tissue. Nonetheless, Jirsch et al. (2006) showed that FRs can be recorded from human focal epileptic brain using depth

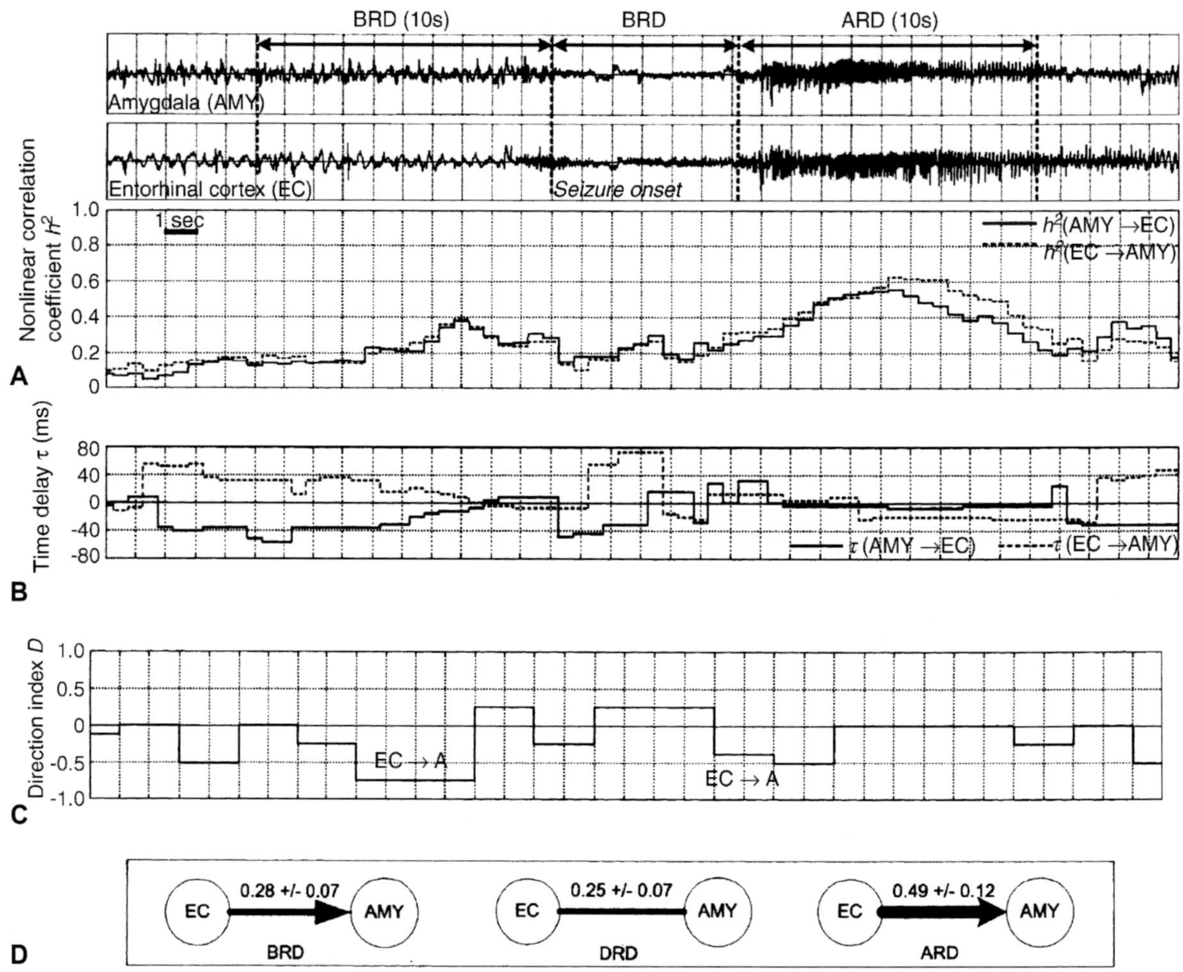

Fig. 3.5. Analysis of the dynamics of a seizure in a patient with mesial temporal lobe epilepsy (MTLE) recorded from the entorhinal cortex (EC) and amygdala (AMY). On each pair of signals, nonlinear regression analysis is used to calculate: (**A**) the nonlinear correlation coefficient h^2 and (**B**) the time delay τ from upper signal to lower (solid line, AMY to EC) and vice versa (dotted line, EC to AMY). (**C**) Asymmetry information (difference between h^2 coefficients) and time delays are used jointly to calculate the direction index D, which characterizes the direction of coupling. When greater than 0.5 (respectively lower than -0.5), D indicates a coupling from upper to lower signal (respectively lower to upper signal). (**D**) Values of h^2 are averaged over given periods (BRD, before rapid discharge; DRD, during rapid discharge; ARD, after rapid discharge), and information is represented as a graph in which line thickness is proportional to the average h^2 value and in which the arrow indicates coupling direction, when significant. Standard deviation of coefficient h^2 is also provided. Note the increase in the association index before the occurrence of the "rapid discharge" (BRD), followed by a decrease during the "rapid discharge" (DRD), with the EC leading during part of the time, and large increase during the large-amplitude seizure oscillations where the latter appear to be synchronous (time delay is approximately zero). (Adapted from Bartolomei et al., 2004. © Elsevier.)

macroelectrodes, and concluded that these "macro FRs" reflect the partial synchronization of local oscillations, an interpretation comparable to that made for FRs recorded with microelectrodes. Jacobs et al. (2009) evaluated whether the occurrence of FRs (250–500 Hz) showed any association with the preictal period, in seven patients with MTLE. Total rates of FRs were significantly higher in the seizure onset zone than outside, but the rates did not change in a systematic way in the preictal period. Thus, it appears that the occurrence and rate of FRs are not clearly associated with the evolution of preictal to ictal EEG periods; FRs, however, are likely relevant markers of the epileptogenic onset zone. Another line of research focused on studying the dynamics of a large number of single neurons recorded simultaneously using multichannel microelectrode arrays in epileptic patients (Truccolo et al., 2011). Although to date only a few patients have been studied using this technique, the authors found that many neurons changed their firing pattern activity significantly as the seizure approached. These patterns differed from those observed in periods remote from the seizure, but were somewhat heterogeneous among cortical patches. These authors suggested that using this kind of multichannel unit recording "it may be possible to obtain predictive information from individual neuronal activity without necessarily localizing what has been traditionally considered the seizure focus" (Truccolo et al., 2011, p. 640). Clearly this suggestion has to be tested in much larger data sets.

An alternative way to determine the excitability state of hippocampal networks is to apply in the interictal period a stimulation protocol by means of which the state of the neuronal networks is perturbed, and to record their subsequent reactions. This may reveal relevant features of the network's excitability state (Suffczynski et al., 2008). In our group, we used intermittent electrical pulse stimulation (frequency range 10–20 Hz) applied through the same indwelling electrodes that are used for presurgical evaluation in patients with MTLE, and calculated a quantitative measure of spectral phase demodulation, the relative phase clustering index (rPCI), of the EEG signals evoked by the stimuli. In the interictal periods, high values of rPCI were found at the sites close to the seizure onset zone; furthermore, the values of rPCI increased as the time to the next seizure decreased. A first proof-of-principle clinical study indicated that, applying this methodology, the probabilistic forecasting of impeding seizures may be possible (Kalitzin et al., 2002, 2005, 2010).

HOW MAY NEURONAL NETWORKS INVOLVED IN EPILEPTIC BEHAVIOR BE IDENTIFIED AND ANALYZED IN A CLINICAL SETTING?

The identification of a neuronal network responsible for the onset of an epileptic seizure implies an appropriate *sampling in brain space*. In many cases this is difficult to realize in practice. Be as it may, the brain areas likely to be involved have to be estimated based on high-density EEG or MEG recordings, ideally complemented by magnetic resonance images of associated brain lesions (hippocampal sclerosis) or malformations (dysplasias). Assuming that an appropriate set of recordings is available, it is necessary to analyze the data using quantitative methods to estimate the degree of association between the recordings. The question is to determine which EEG signals recorded during a seizure are significantly associated with one another, and which are the time relations between the different signals, i.e., which are leading and which are lagging, and what are the corresponding time delays. Ultimately one wishes to estimate causal relations within the set of EEG signals that belong to the epileptogenic network. One important aspect of seizure activity is that during the course of a seizure the EEG signals may change considerably, i.e. the signals show strong *nonstationarity*. This implies that an analysis method has to take this essential feature into account and that any analysis must be carried out in successive epochs, which should be short enough to avoid nonstationary segments but long enough to obtain the desired level of accuracy. These epochs should partially overlap in order to obtain smooth estimates of the association indices. Two experimental examples provide clear evidence for the presence of nonstationarity in EEG signals recorded during seizures. One is the study of Meeren et al. (2002), which showed, using the nonlinear association index h^2 computed within successive epochs of 0.5-s duration with 50% overlap, that during absence seizures in the WAG/Rij genetic rat model the time delays between cortical and thalamic signals are consistent only in the first 500-ms epoch at seizure onset, but may change considerably in the course of the seizure. Another example is the study of Boucetta et al. (2008) in a cortically generated Lennox–Gastaut-type seizure in cat, which showed, using cross-correlation analysis on successive 1-s long epochs with 0.5-s overlap, that several patterns of synchronization could be observed between signals recorded from different sites: synchronous, either in phase or with phase shift, or showing phase shift transitions, and even showing nonsynchronous periods. This implies that analysis of seizures that use epochs longer than about 1 s may yield ambiguous results, because there may be mixing signals with different degrees of association and a variety of time relations. Such data should be considered with great caution. Indeed, the degree of synchrony at the onset and during a seizure may change appreciably; Netoff and Schiff (2002), in an experimental model of seizures using microelectrode recordings, observed a decrease in neuronal synchronization at fast timescales, whereas synchronization was increased with respect to brief burst-firing events at slow timescales, and as seizures stopped; Wendling et al. (2003), in EEG signals recorded with intracerebral electrodes in patients suffering from partial epilepsy, found evidence for "decorrelation" at seizure onset as very fast (mainly within the 60–90-Hz band) oscillations of low amplitude are present in the EEG, followed by an abnormally high degree of synchronization as the seizure develops.

A classical method for determining time delays between EEG signals during epileptic seizures consists of calculating coherence and the corresponding phase functions as proposed by Brazier (1972). The interpretation of phase shifts in terms of time delays can be concluded with certainty only when the coherence is sufficiently large (Gotman and Levtova, 1996), and when there is a linear relationship between phase and frequency within a certain frequency band (for a discussion of methodological aspects, see Lopes da Silva, 2006).

A fundamental problem with these methods of analysis, however, is that very often the relations between EEG signals cannot be considered linear, so that the use of coherence is not justified, as referred to above in relation to thalamocortical SWDs. Alternative methods have been developed over recent decades. One is computation of the average amount of mutual information (AAMI), in the sense of Gelfand and Yaglom (1959), between pairs of EEG signals as a function of the delay time introduced between both signals. AAMI was used for localization of epileptic networks in animals having a kindled epileptogenic focus (Mars and Lopes da Silva, 1983), allowing the spread pattern of these seizures to be estimated. The same method was also applied to human seizures (Mars et al., 1985). The algorithms based on AAMI, however, proved to be rather cumbersome to apply in practice. This led to the creation of a new method of *nonlinear regression analysis, the h^2 method,* by Pijn et al. (1989) (Lopes da Silva et al., 1989; Kalitzin et al., 2007). This consists of calculating a general coefficient of nonlinear fit between pairs of signals. Application of this nonlinear regression coefficient to EEG signals recorded during seizures in animals (Fernandes de Lima et al., 1990) revealed that a large number of EEG signals recorded from different brain sites belonging to an epileptogenic network present clear nonlinear relations. The same applies to EEG signals recorded from intracranial electrodes in patients (Pijn and Lopes da Silva, 1993; Bartolomei et al., 2004), in rats with absence-like seizures (Meeren et al., 2002), and in the study of the propagation dynamics of seizure activity in the hippocampal–parahippocampal region of the isolated guinea-pig brain (Uva and de Curtis, 2005). Thus, this method offers perspectives for the characterization of an epileptogenic network, based on a set of simultaneously recorded EEG signals. In addition to the estimation of h^2, a derived quantity was proposed by Guye et al. (2006) that gives information about the causality of the association, called the direction index, D. This quantity takes into account both the estimated time delay (Δt) between signals x and y, and the asymmetrical nature of the nonlinear correlation coefficient, h^2. A further refinement of the nonlinear association analysis is the so-called *"partialization"* of the association measure between two signals. Indeed, in cases where a nonlinear association index, h^2, between two signals may be caused by a third one, acting as a common source, the influence of the third one can be removed and the association of the residual signals may be calculated to determine whether the association between them is caused by the common influence of the third signal or not. More recently, Kalitzin et al. (2007) presented a general definition of the nonlinear association index, h^2, demonstrating rigorously that this index measures the best dynamic range of any nonlinear map between signals.

Another method that is currently used, particularly in the field of fMRI, is the estimation of Granger causality (Roebroeck et al., 2005; David et al., 2008). This approach is based on the assumption that an observed time series $x(n)$ causes another time series $y(n)$, if knowledge of the past of $x(n)$ significantly improves the prediction of $y(n)$. This relationship is not reciprocal, i.e., $x(n)$ may cause $y(n)$ without $y(n)$ necessarily causing $x(n)$. It is beyond the scope of this chapter to discuss this and a variety of other methods to estimate synchronization between EEG signals that have been proposed to study functional connectivity in the brain, because most applications have not, as yet, addressed directly the analysis of signals recorded *during* seizures. A recent development, however, consists of applying the "small world" graphical approach to estimate measures of clustering within a set of EEG signals. Ponten et al. (2007) analyzed intracerebral recordings of patients with MTLE during interictal, before, during, and after rapid discharges (in which the last two periods were ictal) and postictal. They calculated the synchronization matrix of this set of signals and constructed abstract network representations (graphs), which were characterized by a clustering coefficient C (measure of local connectedness) and a shortest path length L (measure of overall network integration). They found that, during seizures, the neuronal network moved in the direction of a more ordered configuration (higher C combined with a slightly, but significantly, higher L) compared with the more randomly organized interictal network. Similar analyses (Kramer et al., 2010) revealed an interesting feature of seizures, namely that at the macroscopic spatial scale epileptic seizures should not be considered as reflecting simply hypersynchrony but rather as a product of neuronal network reorganization.

It should be noted that these analyses were based on relatively long EEG epochs, of the order of many seconds (Ponten et al., 2007; van Dellen et al., 2010), which does not take into account the nonstationary nature of these signals; consequently these analyses may not be sensitive enough to reveal phenomena occurring at the timescale that is essential to catch the speed at which seizure activity develops and propagates, particularly in the initial second or fraction of a second.

Confronted with so many methods of analysis, the choice of a specific method to apply in patients may be difficult for clinical neurophysiologists and neurologists. Therefore, it is important to have critical comparative studies of the performance of different methods applied under similar circumstances. In a recent study, Wendling et al. (2009a, b) dealt with this question and assessed functional brain connectivity based on signals recorded from different brain areas during partial complex epileptic seizures, namely linear and nonlinear regression, phase synchronization, and generalized synchronization, using a model-based methodology. This comparison revealed that there was no "ideal" method, i.e., none of the methods performed better than the others in all situations studied. Nevertheless, it should be emphasized that *regression methods (linear or nonlinear)* showed sensitivity to the coupling parameter in all tested models with average or good performances.

Finally, an interesting concept that was proposed with the aim of identifying brain areas that may belong to an epileptogenic neuronal network is the notion of "epileptogenicity," put forward by Bartolomei et al. (2008). These authors introduced a measure, the "epileptogenicity index" (EI), that is based on the relative power of EEG rapid (beta + gamma) oscillations with respect to low-frequency components (theta + alpha) and on the time delay between the moment defined as "seizure onset" and the appearance of the rapid discharges, recorded by means of intracerebral recordings from multiple electrodes. In 17 patients with MTLE, large EI values were found for signals recorded from mesial structures. Interestingly, a significant correlation was found between the duration of the epileptic clinical condition and the number of structures disclosing large EIs. This suggests that MTLE is a slowly evolving process, involving gradually more areas of the temporal lobe as a patient becomes older.

In summary, it is advisable first to apply linear *and* nonlinear regression methods in order to characterize functional brain connectivity at seizure onset and during seizure development, before using more sophisticated methods that require specific assumptions about the underlying model of relationship. In addition, it is recommended to use time–frequency methods employing different frequency sub-bands and relatively short, sliding time windows, in order to determine functional coupling in ("frequency locking") between EEG/MEG signals recorded from different sites, within a fine timescale. In this context it should be noted that the choice of frequency bands may be critical.

CONCLUSION: GENERAL CONCEPTS AND MODELS

In conclusion, we have presented some general concepts with respect to the dynamic properties of neuronal networks that are relevant to understand how transitions between brain normal state and seizure states take place. In the introduction, we put forward the concept that epilepsy is a *dynamic disease* of neuronal networks, and emphasized that a main question in epileptology is how such transitions (i.e., bifurcations) occur. In addition to the intrinsic theoretical interest of this issue, which can be evidenced by means of computer models of neuronal networks in epilepsy (Lytton, 2008), it has also practical implications in the clinic, because an insight into this process may help to develop procedures with the aim of anticipating and, eventually, controlling the occurrence of seizures. While discussing basic neurobiological mechanisms above, we stressed that neuronal networks possess mechanisms that promote their stabilization, i.e., homeostatic processes of regulation of neuronal excitability, and that epileptic conditions may result from a disruption of such homeostatic processes. Indeed, a critical parameter in this context is the upregulation of excitatory synapses, either with, or without, a concurrent downregulation of inhibitory synapses and/or upregulation of intrinsic excitability at the level of ionic membrane mechanisms. A deficit or deregulation of such processes can lead to abnormal dynamics of the involved neuronal networks, which may become manifest as epileptic seizures.

Accordingly, seizures may be preceded by a state of enhanced excitability, at least in some forms of epilepsy. This is the case in mesial temporal lobe epilepsy (MTLE). This conclusion is supported by the computational model studies of Wendling et al. (2002, 2005), as described above. Nonetheless, in some other forms of epilepsy, namely in absence epilepsy, transition to seizure can result from random fluctuations in cortical and sensory (noise) inputs, and thus may not be preceded by a specific enhanced excitability state that may be detectable; in such cases, these seizures are not predictable. This conclusion has also been evidenced by the model studies of Suffczynski et al. (2004, 2005, 2008).

Thus, we may state that there are two major processes by means of which transitions to seizures can occur, as shown in Fig. 3.1:

- as a consequence of random fluctuations in inputs to specific neuronal networks that have steady-state abnormal parameters, such that the threshold for these transitions is much lower than in normal brains
- as a consequence of progressive deformation of parameters responsible for maintaining homeostatic control of the excitability state of neuronal networks, which results in an abnormal dynamic state of enhanced excitability preceding a seizure.

Finally, an important practical question is whether it may be possible to detect these changes in excitability before a seizure becomes manifest, i.e., whether it may be possible to anticipate this kind of seizure. In a nutshell, we propose three possible ways by which such changes might be detected: (i) by analyzing spontaneous EEG signals, which has been attempted extensively but with little success until now, as reviewed by Mormann et al. (2007) and

Andrzejak et al. (2009); (ii) by means of recording fast ripples, although the rate of these does not appear to be associated with the evolution of preictal to ictal EEG periods, even though these FRs are likely relevant markers of the epileptogenic onset zone, as discussed above; and (iii) by recording the neural activity evoked by electrical stimuli applied via intracerebral electrodes to probe the excitability state of the neuronal networks involved in seizure generation (Kalitzin et al., 2005, 2010).

Assuming that, in a neuronal network with multiattractor dynamic states, transition from a normal dynamic state to a seizure state is caused by a *deformation* of critical parameters, responsible for maintaining the dynamic state of the neuronal networks within the normal working range (homeostatic condition), the probabilistic forecasting of impeding seizures may be possible, particularly using an active stimulation paradigm (Kalitzin et al., 2005, 2010). In this way, characteristic features of the excitability state of the neuronal networks may be detected as, for example, by means of the phase-clustering index. Furthermore, if these features are detected early, transitions into seizures might be blocked by an adequate counterstimulation (Kalitzin et al., 2010; Osorio and Frei, 2010).

References

Aker RG, Ozkara C, Dervent A et al. (2002). Enhancement of spike and wave discharges by microinjection of bicuculline into the reticular nucleus of rats with absence epilepsy. Neurosci Lett 322: 71–74.

Andrzejak RG, Chicharro D, Elger CE et al. (2009). Seizure prediction: any better than chance? Clin Neurophysiol 120: 1465–1478.

Arion D, Sabatini M, Unger T et al. (2006). Correlation of transcriptome profile with electrical activity in temporal lobe epilepsy. Neurobiol Dis 22: 374–387.

Avanzini G, de Curtis M, Marescaux C et al. (1992). Role of the thalamic reticular nucleus in the generation of rhythmic thalamo-cortical activities subserving spike and waves. J Neural Transm Suppl 35: 85–95.

Avoli M, Gloor P (1982). Role of the thalamus in generalized penicillin epilepsy: observations on decorticated cats. Exp Neurol 77: 386–402.

Avoli M, Rogawski MA, Avanzini G (2001). Generalized epileptic disorders: an update. Epilepsia 42: 445–457.

Bancaud J (1969). Physiopathogenesis of generalized epilepsies of organic nature (stereoencephalographic study). In: H Gastaut, HH Jasper, J Bancaud et al. (Eds.), The Physiopathogenesis of the Epilepsies. Charles C Thomas, Springfield, IL, pp. 158–185.

Banks MI, Li TB, Pearce RA (1998). The synaptic basis of GABA-A, slow. J Neurosci 18: 1305–1317.

Banks MI, White JA, Pearce RA (2000). Interactions between distinct GABA(A) circuits in hippocampus. Neuron 25: 449–457.

Bartolomei F, Wendling F, Bellanger JJ et al. (2001). Neural networks involving the medial temporal structures in temporal lobe epilepsy. Clin Neurophysiol 112: 1746–1760.

Bartolomei F, Wendling F, Régis J et al. (2004). Pre-ictal synchronicity in limbic networks of mesial temporal lobe epilepsy. Epilepsy Res 61: 89–104.

Bartolomei F, Chauvel P, Wendling F (2008). Epileptogenicity of brain structures in human temporal lobe epilepsy: a quantified study from intracerebral EEG. Brain 131: 1818–1830.

Ben-Ari Y, Cossart R (2000). Kainate, a double agent that generates seizures: two decades of progress. Trends Neurosci 23: 580–587.

Bernard C, Marsden DP, Wheal HV (2001). Changes in neuronal excitability and synaptic function in a chronic model of temporal lobe epilepsy. Neuroscience 103: 17–26.

Bernasconi N, Bernasconi A, Andermann F et al. (1999). Entorhinal cortex in temporal lobe epilepsy: a quantitative MRI study. Neurology 52: 1870–1876.

Bernstein GM, Mendonça A, Wadia J et al. (1999). Kindling induces a long-term enhancement in the density of N-type calcium channels in the rat hippocampus. Neuroscience 94: 1083–1095.

Bertram EH, Zhang DX, Mangan P et al. (1998). Functional anatomy of limbic epilepsy: a proposal for central synchronization of a diffusely hyperexcitable network. Epilepsy Res 32: 194–205.

Blumenfeld H, Klein JP, Schridde U et al. (2008). Early treatment suppresses the development of spike–wave epilepsy in a rat model. Epilepsia 49: 400–409.

Boucetta S, Chauvette S, Bazhenov M et al. (2008). Focal generation of paroxysmal fast runs during electrographic seizures. Epilepsia 49: 1925–1940.

Bowery NG, Parry K, Boehrer A et al. (1999). Pertussis toxin decreases absence seizures and GABA(B) receptor binding in thalamus of a genetically prone rat (GAERS). Neuropharmacology 38: 1691–1697.

Brager DH, Johnston D (2007). Plasticity of intrinsic excitability during long-term depression is mediated through mGluR-dependent changes in I(h) in hippocampal CA1 pyramidal neurons. J Neurosci 27: 13926–13937.

Bragin A, Engel J Jr, Wilson CL et al. (1999a). Electrophysiologic analysis of a chronic seizure model after unilateral hippocampal KA injection. Epilepsia 40: 1210–1221.

Bragin A, Engel J Jr, Wilson CL et al. (1999b). High-frequency oscillations in human brain. Hippocampus 9: 137–142.

Bragin A, Engel J Jr, Wilson CL et al. (1999c). Hippocampal and entorhinal cortex high-frequency oscillations (100–500 Hz) in human epileptic brain and in kainic acid-treated rats with chronic seizures. Epilepsia 40: 127–137.

Bragin A, Wilson CL, Engel J Jr. (2000). Chronic epileptogenesis requires development of a network of pathologically interconnected neuron clusters: a hypothesis. Epilepsia 41: S144–S152.

Bragin A, Mody I, Wilson CL et al. (2002). Local generation of fast ripples in epileptic brain. J Neurosci 22: 2012–2021.

Brazier MAB (1972). Spread of seizure discharges in epilepsy: anatomical and electrophysiological considerations. Exp Neurol 36: 263–272.

Browne SH, Kang J, Akk G et al. (2001). Kinetic and pharmacological properties of GABA(A) receptors in single thalamic neurons and GABA(A) subunit expression. J Neurophysiol 86: 2312–2322.

Buckmaster PS, Dudek FE (1997). Neuron loss, granule cell axon reorganization, and functional changes in the dentate gyrus of epileptic kainate-treated rats. J Comp Neurol 385: 385–404.

Buzsáki G, Ponomareff GL, Bayardo F et al. (1989). Neuronal activity in the subcortically denervated hippocampus: a chronic model for epilepsy. Neuroscience 28: 527–538.

Buzsáki G, Smith A, Berger S et al. (1990). Petit mal epilepsy and parkinsonian tremor: hypothesis of a common pacemaker. Neuroscience 36: 1–14.

Buzsáki G, Horváth Z, Urioste R et al. (1992). High-frequency network oscillation in the hippocampus. Science 256: 1025–1027.

Carr DB, Day M, Cantrell AR et al. (2003). Transmitter modulation of slow, activity-dependent alterations in sodium channel availability endows neurons with a novel form of cellular plasticity. Neuron 39: 793–806.

Castro PA, Cooper EC, Lowenstein DH et al. (2001). Hippocampal heterotopia lack functional Kv4.2 potassium channels in the methylazoxymethanol model of cortical malformations and epilepsy. J Neurosci 21: 6626–6634.

Cavalheiro EA, Riche DA, Le Gal La Salle G (1982). Long-term effects of intrahippocampal kainic acid injection in rats: a method for inducing spontaneous recurrent seizures. Electroencephalogr Clin Neurophysiol 53: 581–589.

Coenen AM, Van Luijtelaar EL (2003). Genetic animal models for absence epilepsy: a review of the WAG/Rij strain of rats. Behav Genet 33: 635–655.

Cohen I, Navarro V, Clemenceau S et al. (2002). On the origin of interictal activity in human temporal lobe epilepsy in vitro. Science 298: 1418–1421.

Contreras D, Dürmüller N, Steriade M (1997). Plateau potentials in cat neocortical association cells in vivo: synaptic control of dendritic excitability. Eur J Neurosci 9: 2588–2595.

Cossart R, Dinocourt C, Hirsch JC et al. (2001). Dendritic but not somatic GABAergic inhibition is decreased in experimental epilepsy. Nat Neurosci 4: 52–62.

Coulter DA, Huguenard JR, Prince DA (1989). Calcium currents in rat thalamocortical relay neurones: kinetic properties of the transient, low-threshold current. J Physiol 414: 587–604.

Crunelli V, Leresche N (2002). Childhood absence epilepsy: genes, channels, neurons and networks. Nat Rev Neurosci 3: 371–382.

Danober L, Deransart C, Depaulis A et al. (1998). Pathophysiological mechanisms of genetic absence epilepsy in the rat. Prog Neurobiol 55: 27–57.

David O, Friston KJ (2003). A neural mass model for MEG/EEG: coupling and neuronal dynamics. Neuroimage 20: 1743–1755.

David O, Guillemain I, Saillet S et al. (2008). Identifying neural drivers with functional MRI: an electrophysiological validation. PLoS Biol 6: e315.

de Curtis M, Paré D, Llinas RR (1991). The electrophysiology of the olfactory hippocampal circuit in the isolated and perfused adult mammalian brain in vitro. Hippocampus 1: 341–354.

de Jong AP, Verhage M (2009). Presynaptic signal transduction pathways that modulate synaptic transmission. Curr Opin Neurobiol 19: 245–253.

de Lanerolle NC, Lee TS (2005). New facets of the neuropathology and molecular profile of human temporal lobe epilepsy. Epilepsy Behav 7: 190–203.

de Lanerolle NC, Kim JH, Robbins RJ et al. (1989). Hippocampal interneuron loss and plasticity in human temporal lobe epilepsy. Brain Res 495: 387–395.

Destexhe A, Sejnowski TJ (2003). Interactions between membrane conductances underlying thalamocortical slow-wave oscillations. Physiol Rev 83: 1401–1453.

Destexhe A, Contreras D, Steriade M (1998). Mechanisms underlying the synchronizing action of corticothalamic feedback through inhibition of thalamic relay cells. J Neurophysiol 79: 999–1016.

Destexhe A, McCormick DA, Sejnowski TJ (1999). Thalamic and thalamocortical mechanisms underlying 3 Hz spike-and-wave discharges. Prog Brain Res 121: 289–307.

Dibbens LM, Feng HJ, Richards MC et al. (2004). GABRD encoding a protein for extra- or perisynaptic GABAA receptors is a susceptibility locus for generalized epilepsies. Hum Mol Genet 13: 1315–1319.

Dickson CT, Alonso A (1997). Muscarinic induction of synchronous population activity in the entorhinal cortex. J Neurosci 17: 6729–6744.

Du F, Whetsell WO, Jr., Abou-Khalil B et al. (1993). Preferential neuronal loss in layer III of the entorhinal cortex in patients with temporal lobe epilepsy. Epilepsy Res 16: 223–233.

Du F, Eid T, Lothman EW et al. (1995). Preferential neuronal loss in layer III of the medial entorhinal cortex in rat models of temporal lobe epilepsy. J Neurosci 15: 6301–6313.

Faas GC, Vreugdenhil M, Wadman WJ (1996). Calcium currents in pyramidal CA1 neurons in vitro after kindling epileptogenesis in the hippocampus of the rat. Neuroscience 75: 57–67.

Fan Y, Fricker D, Brager DH et al. (2005). Activity-dependent decrease of excitability in rat hippocampal neurons through increases in I(h). Nat Neurosci 8: 1542–1551.

Fernandes de Lima VM, Pijn JPM, Filipe CN et al. (1990). The role of hippocampal commissures in the interhemispheric transfer of epileptiform after-discharges in the rat: a study using linear and nonlinear regression analysis. Electroencephalogr Clin Neurophysiol 76: 520–540.

Freeman WJ (1975). Mass Action in the Nervous System. Academic Press, New York.

Freeman WJ (1979). Nonlinear dynamics of paleocortex manifested in the olfactory EEG. Biol Cybern 35: 21–37.

Gainey MA, Hurvitz-Wolff JR, Lambo ME et al. (2009). Synaptic scaling requires the GluR2 subunit of the AMPA receptor. J Neurosci 29: 6479–6489.

Gelfand IM, Yaglom AM (1959). Calculation of the amount of information about a random function contained in another such function. Usp Mat Nauk 12: 3–52. (English translation in American Mathematical Society Translations, Providence, R.I. Series 2, vol. 12).

Gloor P, Pellegrini A, Kostopoulos GK (1979). Effects of changes in cortical excitability upon the epileptic bursts in generalized penicillin epilepsy of the cat. Electroencephalogr Clin Neurophysiol 46: 274–289.

Gloor P, Avoli M, Kostopoulos G (1990). Thalamocortical relationships in generalized epilepsy with bilaterally synchronous spike-and-wave discharge. In: M Avoli, P Gloor, G Kostopoulos et al. (Eds.), Generalized Epilepsy: Neurobiological Approaches. Birkhäuser, Boston, MA, pp. 190–212.

Glykys J, Mody I (2006). Hippocampal network hyperactivity after selective reduction of tonic inhibition in GABA A receptor alpha5 subunit deficient mice. J Neurophysiol 95: 2796–2807.

Golarai G, Sutula TP (1996). Functional alterations in the dentate gyrus after induction of long-term potentiation, kindling, and mossy fiber sprouting. J Neurophysiol 75: 343–353.

Gorter JA, van Vliet EA, Aronica E et al. (2001). Progression of spontaneous seizures after status epilepticus is associated with mossy fibre sprouting and extensive bilateral loss of hilar parvalbumin and somatostatin-immunoreactive neurons. Eur J Neurosci 13: 657–669.

Gorter JA, van Vliet EA, Aronica E et al. (2002). Long-lasting increased excitability differs in dentate gyrus vs. CA1 in freely moving chronic epileptic rats after electrically induced status epilepticus. Hippocampus 12: 311–324.

Gorter JA, van Vliet EA, Aronica E et al. (2006). Potential new antiepileptogenic targets indicated by microarray analysis in a rat model for temporal lobe epilepsy. J Neurosci 26: 11083–11110.

Gotman J, Levtova V (1996). Amygdala–hippocampus relationships in temporal lobe seizures: a phase-coherence study. Epilepsy Res 25: 51–57.

Gurbanova AA, Aker R, Berkman K et al. (2006). Effect of systemic and intracortical administration of phenytoin in two genetic models of absence epilepsy. Br J Pharmacol 148: 1076–1082.

Guye M, Régis J, Tamura M et al. (2006). The role of corticothalamic coupling in human temporal lobe epilepsy. Brain 129: 1917–1928.

Hellier JL, Patrylo PR, Buckmaster PS et al. (1998). Recurrent spontaneous motor seizures after repeated low-dose systemic treatment with kainate: assessment of a rat model of temporal lobe epilepsy. Epilepsy Res 31: 73–84.

Holmes MD, Brown M, Tucker DM (2004). Are "generalized" seizures truly generalized? Evidence of localized mesial frontal and frontopolar discharges in absence. Epilepsia 45: 1568–1579.

Hosford DA, Clark S, Cao Z et al. (1992). The role of GABAB receptor activation in absence seizures of lethargic (lh/lh) mice. Science 257: 398–401.

Houser CR, Esclapez M (2003). Downregulation of the alpha5 subunit of the GABA(A) receptor in the pilocarpine model of temporal lobe epilepsy. Hippocampus 13: 633–645.

Houweling AR, Bazhenov M, Timofeev I et al. (2005). Homeostatic synaptic plasticity can explain post-traumatic epileptogenesis in chronically isolated neocortex. Cereb Cortex 15: 834–845.

Huberfeld G, Menendez de la Prida L, Pallud J et al. (2011). Glutamatergic pre-ictal discharges emerge at the transition to seizure in human epilepsy. Nat Neurosci 14: 627–634.

Huguenard JR, Prince DA (1994). Intrathalamic rhythmicity studied in vitro: nominal T-current modulation causes robust antioscillatory effects. J Neurosci 14: 5485–5502.

Ibata K, Sun Q, Turrigiano GG (2008). Rapid synaptic scaling induced by changes in postsynaptic firing. Neuron 57: 819–826.

Iijima T, Witter MP, Ichikawa M et al. (1996). Entorhinal–hippocampal interactions revealed by real-time imaging. Science 272: 1176–1179.

Jacobs J, LeVan P, Chander R et al. (2008). Interictal high-frequency oscillations (80–500 Hz) are an indicator of seizure onset areas independent of spikes in the human epileptic brain. Epilepsia 49: 1893–1907.

Jacobs J, Zelmann R, Jirsch J et al. (2009). High frequency oscillations (80–500 Hz) in the preictal period in patients with focal seizures. Epilepsia 50: 1780–1792.

Jasper HH, Kershman J (1941). Electroencephalographic classification of the epilepsies. Arch Neurol Psychiatry 45: 903–943.

Jirsch JD, Urrestarazu E, LeVan P et al. (2006). High-frequency oscillations during human focal seizures. Brain 129: 1593–1608.

Jutila L, Ylinen A, Partanen K et al. (2001). MR volumetry of the entorhinal, perirhinal, and temporopolar cortices in drug-refractory temporal lobe epilepsy. AJNR Am J Neuroradiol 22: 1490–1501.

Kager H, Wadman WJ, Somjen GG (2007). Seizure-like afterdischarges simulated in a model neuron. J Comput Neurosci 22: 105–128.

Kalitzin S, Parra J, Velis DN et al. (2002). Enhancement of phase clustering in the EEG/MEG gamma frequency band anticipates transitions to paroxysmal epileptiform activity in epileptic patients with known visual sensitivity. IEEE Trans Biomed Eng 49: 1279–1286.

Kalitzin S, Velis D, Suffczynski P et al. (2005). Electrical brain-stimulation paradigm for estimating the seizure onset site and the time to ictal transition in temporal lobe epilepsy. Clin Neurophysiol 116: 718–728.

Kalitzin SN, Parra J, Velis D et al. (2007). Quantification of unidirectional nonlinear associations between multidimensional signals. IEEE Trans Biomed Eng 54: 454–461.

Kalitzin SN, Velis DN, Lopes da Silva FH (2010). Stimulation-based anticipation and control of state transitions in the epileptic brain. Epilepsy Behav 17: 310–323.

Kalitzin S, Koppert M, Petkov G et al. (2011). Computational model prospective on the observation of proictal states in epileptic neuronal systems. Epilepsy Behav 22: S102–S109.

Kamphuis W, Lopes da Silva FH, Wadman WJ (1988). Changes in local evoked potentials in the rat hippocampus (CA1) during kindling epileptogenesis. Brain Res 440: 205–215.

Keck T, White JA (2009). Glycinergic inhibition in the hippocampus. Rev Neurosci 20: 13–22.

Khalilov I, Holmes GL, Ben-Ari Y (2003). In vitro formation of a secondary epileptogenic mirror focus by interhippocampal propagation of seizures. Nat Neurosci 6: 1079–1085.

Klein JP, Khera DS, Nersesyan H et al. (2004). Dysregulation of sodium channel expression in cortical neurons in a rodent model of absence epilepsy. Brain Res 1000: 102–109.

Kloosterman F, van Haeften T, Lopes da Silva FH (2004). Two reentrant pathways in the hippocampal–entorhinal system. Hippocampus 14: 1026–1039.

Koppert MM, Kalitzin S, Lopes da Silva FH et al. (2011). Plasticity-modulated seizure dynamics for seizure termination in realistic neuronal models. J Neural Eng 8: 046027.

Kramer MA, Eden UT, Kolaczyk ED et al. (2010). Coalescence and fragmentation of cortical networks during focal seizures. J Neurosci 30: 10076–10085.

Labyt E, Frogerais P, Uva L et al. (2007). Modeling of entorhinal cortex and simulation of epileptic activity: insights into the role of inhibition-related parameters. IEEE Trans Inf Technol Biomed 11: 450–461.

Lamsa K, Kaila K (1997). Ionic mechanisms of spontaneous GABAergic events in rat hippocampal slices exposed to 4-aminopyridine. J Neurophysiol 78: 2582–2591.

Le Duigou C, Bouilleret V, Miles R (2008). Epileptiform activities in slices of hippocampus from mice after intra-hippocampal injection of kainic acid. J Physiol 586: 4891–4904.

Leresche N, Parri HR, Erdemli G et al. (1998). On the action of the anti-absence drug ethosuximide in the rat and cat thalamus. J Neurosci 18: 4842–4853.

Lissin DV, Gomperts SN, Carroll RC et al. (1998). Activity differentially regulates the surface expression of synaptic AMPA and NMDA glutamate receptors. Proc Natl Acad Sci U S A 95: 7097–7102.

Liu Z, Vergnes M, Depaulis A et al. (1992). Involvement of intrathalamic $GABA_B$ neurotransmission in the control of absence seizures in the rat. Neuroscience 48: 87–93.

Lopantsev V, Avoli M (1998). Laminar organization of epileptiform discharges in the rat entorhinal cortex in vitro. J Physiol 509: 785–796.

Lopes da Silva FH (2006). Event-related neural activities: what about phase? Prog Brain Res 159: 3–17.

Lopes da Silva FH (2008). Epilepsy as a disease of the dynamics of neuronal networks – models and predictions. In: B Schelter, J Timmer, A Schulze-Bonhage (Eds.), Seizure Prediction in Epilepsy: From Basic Mechanisms to Clinical Applications. Wiley, Weinheim, pp. 97–108.

Lopes da Silva F, Pijn JP, Boeijinga P (1989). Interdependence of EEG signals: linear vs. nonlinear associations and the significance of time delays and phase shifts. Brain Topogr 2: 9–18.

Lopes da Silva F, Blanes W, Kalitzin SN et al. (2003). Epilepsies as dynamical diseases of brain systems: basic models of the transition between normal and epileptic activity. Epilepsia 44: 72–83.

Lothman EW, Bertram EH, Bekenstein JW et al. (1989). Self-sustaining limbic status epilepticus induced by 'continuous' hippocampal stimulation: electrographic and behavioral characteristics. Epilepsy Res 3: 107–119.

Lüders H, Lesser RP, Dinner DS et al. (1984). Generalized epilepsies: a review. Cleve Clin Q 51: 205–226.

Luhmann HJ, Mittmann T, van Luijtelaar G et al. (1995). Impairment of intracortical GABAergic inhibition in a rat model of absence epilepsy. Epilepsy Res 22: 43–51.

Lynch M, Sutula T (2000). Recurrent excitatory connectivity in the dentate gyrus of kindled and kainic acid-treated rats. J Neurophysiol 83: 693–704.

Lytton WW (2008). Computer modeling of epilepsy. Nat Rev Neurosci 9: 626–637.

Lytton WW, Destexhe A, Sejnowski TJ (1996). Control of slow oscillations in the thalamocortical neuron: a computer model. Neuroscience 70: 673–684.

Manning JP, Richards DA, Leresche N et al. (2004). Cortical-area specific block of genetically determined absence seizures by ethosuximide. Neuroscience 123: 5–9.

Marescaux C, Vergnes M, Depaulis A (1992). Genetic absence epilepsy in rats from Strasbourg – a review. J Neural Transm Suppl 35: 37–69.

Margerison JH, Corsellis JA (1966). Epilepsy and the temporal lobes. A clinical, electroencephalographic and neuropathological study of the brain in epilepsy, with particular reference to the temporal lobes. Brain 89: 499–530.

Mars NJI, Lopes da Silva FH (1983). Propagation of seizure activity in kindled dogs. Electroencephalogr Clin Neurophysiol 56: 194–209.

Mars NJI, Thompson PM, Wilkus RJ (1985). The spread of epileptic seizures activity in humans. Epilepsia 26: 85–94.

Maru E, Tatsuno J, Okamoto J et al. (1982). Development and reduction of synaptic potentiation induced by perforant path kindling. Exp Neurol 78: 409–424.

Mazzuferi M, Palma E, Martinello K et al. (2010). Enhancement of GABA(A)-current run-down in the hippocampus occurs at the first spontaneous seizure in a model of temporal lobe epilepsy. Proc Natl Acad Sci U S A 107: 3180–3185.

McCormick DA (2002). Cortical and subcortical generators of normal and abnormal rhythmicity. Int Rev Neurobiol 49: 99–114.

McCormick DA, Bal T (1997). Sleep and arousal: thalamocortical mechanisms. Annu Rev Neurosci 20: 185–215.

McCormick DA, Contreras D (2001). On the cellular and network bases of epileptic seizures. Annu Rev Physiol 63: 815–846.

McCormick DA, Prince DA (1986). Acetylcholine induces burst firing in thalamic reticular neurones by activating a potassium conductance. Nature 319: 402–405.

Meeren HK, Pijn JP, Van Luijtelaar EL et al. (2002). Cortical focus drives widespread corticothalamic networks during spontaneous absence seizures in rats. J Neurosci 22: 1480–1495.

Meeren HK, Veening JG, Möderscheim TA et al. (2009). Thalamic lesions in a genetic rat model of absence epilepsy: dissociation between spike–wave discharges and sleep spindles. Exp Neurol 217: 25–37.

Miles R, Tóth K, Gulyás AI et al. (1996). Differences between somatic and dendritic inhibition in the hippocampus. Neuron 16: 815–823.

Mishra AM, Ellens DJ, Schridde U et al. (2011). Where fMRI and Electrophysiology Agree to Disagree: Corticothalamic and Striatal Activity Patterns in the WAG/Rij Rat. J Neurosci 31: 15053–15064.

Misonou H, Mohapatra DP, Park EW et al. (2004). Regulation of ion channel localization and phosphorylation by neuronal activity. Nat Neurosci 7: 711–718.

Morison RS, Dempsey EW (1941). A study of thalamocortical relations. Am J Physiol 135: 281–292.

Mormann F, Andrzejak RG, Elger CE et al. (2007). Seizure prediction: the long and winding road. Brain 130: 314–333.

Netoff TI, Schiff SJ (2002). Decreased neuronal synchronization during experimental seizures. J Neurosci 22: 7297–7307.

Niedermeyer E (1972). The Generalized Epilepsies: A Clinical Electroencephalographical Study. Charles C Thomas, Springfield, IL.

O'Brien RJ, Kamboj S, Ehlers MD et al. (1998). Activity-dependent modulation of synaptic AMPA receptor accumulation. Neuron 21: 1067–1078.

Oh KS, Lee CJ, Gibbs JW et al. (1995). Postnatal development of $GABA_A$ receptor function in somatosensory thalamus and cortex: whole-cell voltage-clamp recordings in acutely isolated rat neurons. J Neurosci 15: 1341–1351.

Osorio I, Frei M (2010). Feasibility of automated warning in subjects with localization-related epilepsies. Epilepsy Behav 19: 602–607.

Ozbas-Gerceker F, Redeker S, Boer K et al. (2006). Serial analysis of gene expression in the hippocampus of patients with mesial temporal lobe epilepsy. Neuroscience 138: 457–474.

Palma E, Roseti C, Maiolino F et al. (2007). GABA(A)-current rundown of temporal lobe epilepsy is associated with repetitive activation of GABA(A) "phasic" receptors. Proc Natl Acad Sci USA 104: 20944–20948.

Penfield WG, Jasper HH (1954). Epilepsy and the Functional Anatomy of the Human Brain. Little Brown & Co, Boston, MA.

Peng Z, Huang CS, Stell BM et al. (2004). Altered expression of the delta subunit of the GABA-A receptor in a mouse model of temporal lobe epilepsy. J Neurosci 24: 8629–8639.

Pijn JP, Lopes da Silva FH (1993). Propagation of electrical activity: nonlinear associations and time delays between EEG signals. In: S Zschocke, EJ Speckmann (Eds.), Basic Mechanisms of the EEG. Birkhauser, Boston, pp. 41–61.

Pijn JPM, Vijn PCM, Lopes da Silva FH et al. (1989). The use of signal-analysis for the localization of an epileptogenic focus: a new approach. Adv Epileptol 17: 272–276.

Pinault D (2003). Cellular interactions in the rat somatosensory thalamocortical system during normal and epileptic 5–9 Hz oscillations. J Physiol 552: 881–905.

Polack PO, Guillemain I, Hu E et al. (2007). Deep layer somatosensory cortical neurons initiate spike-and-wave discharges in a genetic model of absence seizures. J Neurosci 27: 6590–6599.

Ponten SC, Bartolomei F, Stam CJ (2007). Small-world networks and epilepsy: graph theoretical analysis of intracerebrally recorded mesial temporal lobe seizures. Clin Neurophysiol 118: 918–927.

Puigcerver A, van Luijtelaar EL, Drinkenburg WH et al. (1996). Effects of the $GABA_B$ antagonist CGP 35348 on sleep–wake states, behaviour, and spike–wave discharges in old rats. Brain Res Bull 40: 157–162.

Roebroeck A, Formisano E, Goebel R (2005). Mapping directed influence over the brain using Granger causality and fMRI. Neuroimage 25: 230–242.

Rutherford LC, Nelson SB, Turrigiano GG (1998). BDNF has opposite effects on the quantal amplitude of pyramidal neuron and interneuron excitatory synapses. Neuron 21: 521–530.

Savin C, Triesch J, Meyer-Hermann M (2009). Epileptogenesis due to glia-mediated synaptic scaling. J R Soc Interface 6: 655–668.

Schwartzkroin PA (1994). Cellular electrophysiology of human epilepsy. Epilepsy Res 17: 185–192.

Sloviter RS (1991a). Feedforward and feedback inhibition of hippocampal principal cell activity evoked by perforant path stimulation: GABA-mediated mechanisms that regulate excitability in vivo. Hippocampus 1: 31–40.

Sloviter RS (1991b). Permanently altered hippocampal structure, excitability, and inhibition after experimental status epilepticus in the rat: the "dormant basket cell" hypothesis and its possible relevance to temporal lobe epilepsy. Hippocampus 1: 41–66.

Smith KA, Fisher RS (1996). The selective $GABA_B$ antagonist CGP-35348 blocks spike–wave bursts in the cholesterol synthesis rat absence epilepsy model. Brain Res 729: 147–150.

Snead OC 3rd (1992). Evidence for $GABA_B$-mediated mechanisms in experimental generalized absence seizures. Eur J Pharmacol 213: 343–349.

Snead OC 3rd Depaulis A, Vergnes M et al. (1999). Jasper's basic mechanisms of the epilepsies. Adv Neurol 79: 253–279.

Somjen GG (2002). Ion regulation in the brain: implications for pathophysiology. Neuroscientist 8: 254–267.

Somjen GG (2004). Ions in the Brain: Normal Function, Seizures, and Stroke. Oxford University Press, New York.

Somjen GG, Kager H, Wadman WJ (2008). Computer simulations of neuron–glia interactions mediated by ion flux. J Comput Neurosci 25: 349–365.

Spencer SS, Guimaraes P, Katz A et al. (1992). Morphological patterns of seizures recorded intracranially. Epilepsia 33: 537–545.

Spreafico R, Mennini T, Danober L et al. (1993). $GABA_A$ receptor impairment in the genetic absence epilepsy rats from Strasbourg (GAERS): an immunocytochemical and receptor binding autoradiographic study. Epilepsy Res 15: 229–238.

Staak R, Pape HC (2001). Contribution of GABA(A) and GABA(B) receptors to thalamic neuronal activity during spontaneous absence seizures in rats. J Neurosci 21: 1378–1384.

Stellwagen D, Malenka RC (2006). Synaptic scaling mediated by glial TNF-alpha. Nature 440: 1054–1059.

Steriade M, Contreras D (1998). Spike–wave complexes and fast components of cortically generated seizures. I. Role of neocortex and thalamus. J Neurophysiol 80: 1439–1455.

Steriade M, McCormick DA, Sejnowski TJ (1993). Thalamocortical oscillations in the sleeping and aroused brain. Science 262: 679–685.

Suffczynski P, Kalitzin S, Lopes Da Silva FH (2004). Dynamics of non-convulsive epileptic phenomena modeled by a bistable neuronal network. Neuroscience 126: 467–484.

Suffczynski P, Lopes da Silva F, Parra J et al. (2005). Epileptic transitions: model predictions and experimental validation. J Clin Neurophysiol 22: 288–299.

Suffczynski P, Lopes da Silva FH, Parra J et al. (2006). Dynamics of epileptic phenomena determined from statistics of ictal transitions. IEEE Trans Biomed Eng 53: 524–532.

Suffczynski P, Kalitzin S, da Silva FL et al. (2008). Active paradigms of seizure anticipation: computer model evidence for necessity of stimulation. Phys Rev E Stat Nonlin Soft Matter Phys 78: 051917.

Thiagarajan TC, Lindskog M, Tsien RW (2005). Adaptation to synaptic inactivity in hippocampal neurons. Neuron 47: 725–737.

Thomas E, Grisar T (2000). Increased synchrony with increase of a low-threshold calcium conductance in a model thalamic network: a phase-shift mechanism. Neural Comput 12: 1553–1571.

Thomson AM, Radpour S (1991). Excitatory connections between CA1 pyramidal cells revealed by spike triggered averaging in slices of rat hippocampus are partially NMDA receptor mediated. Eur J Neurosci 3: 587–601.

Tolner EA, Kloosterman F, Kalitzin SN et al. (2005). Physiological changes in chronic epileptic rats are prominent in superficial layers of the medial entorhinal area. Epilepsia 46: 72–81.

Truccolo W, Donoghue JA, Hochberg LR et al. (2011). Single-neuron dynamics in human focal epilepsy. Nat Neurosci 14: 635–641.

Tsakiridou E, Bertollini L, de Curtis M et al. (1995). Selective increase in T-type calcium conductance of reticular thalamic neurons in a rat model of absence epilepsy. J Neurosci 15: 3110–3117.

Tucker DM, Brown M, Luu P et al. (2007). Discharges in ventromedial frontal cortex during absence spells. Epilepsy Behav 11: 546–557.

Turrigiano GG (2008). The self-tuning neuron: synaptic scaling of excitatory synapses. Cell 135: 422–435.

Turrigiano GG, Leslie KR, Desai NS et al. (1998). Activity-dependent scaling of quantal amplitude in neocortical neurons. Nature 391: 892–896.

Turski WA, Czuczwar SJ, Kleinrok Z et al. (1983). Cholinomimetics produce seizures and brain damage in rats. Experientia 39: 1408–1411.

Uva L, de Curtis M (2005). Polysynaptic olfactory pathway to the ipsi- and contralateral entorhinal cortex mediated via the hippocampus. Neuroscience 130: 249–258.

van Dellen E, Douw L, Baayen JC et al. (2010). Long-term effects of temporal lobe epilepsy on local neural networks: a graph theoretical analysis of corticography recordings. PLoS One 4: e8081.

van Luijtelaar EL, Coenen AM (1986). Two types of electrocortical paroxysms in an inbred strain of rats. Neurosci Lett 70: 393–397.

van Vliet EA, Aronica E, Tolner EA et al. (2004). Progression of temporal lobe epilepsy in the rat is associated with immunocytochemical changes in inhibitory interneurons in specific regions of the hippocampal formation. Exp Neurol 187: 367–379.

van Welie I, van Hooft JA, Wadman WJ (2006). Background activity regulates excitability of rat hippocampal CA1 pyramidal neurons by adaptation of a K^+ conductance. J Neurophysiol 95: 2007–2012.

Vaudano AE, Laufs H, Kiebel SJ et al. (2009). Causal hierarchy within the thalamo-cortical network in spike and wave discharges. PLoS One 4: e6475.

Velasco AL, Wilson CL, Babb TL et al. (2000). Functional and anatomic correlates of two frequently observed temporal lobe seizure-onset patterns. Neural Plast 7: 49–63.

Velazquez JLP, Carlen PL (2000). Gap junctions, synchrony and seizures. Trends Neurosci 23: 68–74.

Vergnes M, Marescaux C (1992). Cortical and thalamic lesions in rats with genetic absence epilepsy. J Neural Transm Suppl 35: 71–83.

Vergnes M, Boehrer A, Simler S et al. (1997). Opposite effects of $GABA_B$ receptor antagonists on absences and convulsive seizures. Eur J Pharmacol 332: 245–255.

Vreugdenhil M, Wadman WJ (1994). Kindling-induced long-lasting enhancement of calcium current in hippocampal CA1 area of the rat: relation to calcium-dependent inactivation. Neuroscience 59: 105–114.

Wang X-J, Golomb D, Rinzel J (1995). Emergent spindle oscillations and intermittent burst firing in a thalamic model: specific neuronal parameters. Proc Natl Acad Sci U S A 92: 5577–5581.

Watt AJ, van Rossum MCW, MacLeod KM et al. (2000). Activity coregulates quantal AMPA and NMDA currents at neocortical synapses. Neuron 26: 659–670.

Wendling F, Bartolomei F, Bellanger JJ et al. (2001). Interpretation of interdependencies in epileptic signals using a macroscopic physiological model of the EEG. Clin Neurophysiol 112: 1201–1218.

Wendling F, Bartolomei F, Bellanger JJ et al. (2002). Epileptic fast activity can be explained by a model of impaired GABAergic dendritic inhibition. Eur J Neurosci 15: 1499–1508.

Wendling F, Bartolomei F, Bellanger JJ et al. (2003). Epileptic fast intracerebral EEG activity: evidence for spatial decorrelation at seizure onset. Brain 126: 1449–1459.

Wendling F, Hernandez A, Bellanger JJ et al. (2005). Interictal to ictal transition in human temporal lobe epilepsy: insights from a computational model of intracerebral EEG. J Clin Neurophysiol 22: 343–356.

Wendling F (2005). Neurocomputational models in the study of epileptic phenomena. J Clin Neurophysiol 22: 285–287.

Wendling F, Ansari-Asl K, Bartolomei F et al. (2009a). From EEG signals to brain connectivity: a model-based evaluation of interdependence measures. J Neurosci Methods 183: 9–18.

Wendling F, Bartolomei F, Senhadji L (2009b). Spatial analysis of intracerebral electroencephalographic signals in the time and frequency domain: identification of epileptogenic networks in partial epilepsy. Philos Transact A Math Phys Eng Sci 367: 297–316.

Westmijse I, Ossenblok P, Gunning B et al. (2009). Onset and propagation of spike and slow wave discharges in human absence epilepsy: a MEG study. Epilepsia 50: 2538–2548.

Whittington MA, Traub RD, Faulkner HJ et al. (1997). Recurrent excitatory postsynaptic potentials induced by synchronized fast cortical oscillations. Proc Natl Acad Sci U S A 94: 12198–12203.

Wierenga CJ, Walsh MF, Turrigiano GG (2006). Temporal regulation of the expression locus of homeostatic plasticity. J Neurophysiol 96: 2127–2133.

Wilson HR, Cowan JD (1972). Excitatory and inhibitory interactions in localized populations of model neurons. Biophys J 12: 1–24.

Wu K, Leung LS (2003). Increased dendritic excitability in hippocampal CA1 in vivo in the kainic acid model of temporal lobe epilepsy: a study using current source density analysis. Neuroscience 116: 599–616.

Wuarin JP, Dudek FE (1996). Electrographic seizures and new recurrent excitatory circuits in the dentate gyrus of hippocampal slices from kainate-treated epileptic rats. J Neurosci 16: 4438–4448.

Handbook of Clinical Neurology, Vol. 107 (3rd series)
Epilepsy, Part I
H. Stefan and W.H. Theodore, Editors

Chapter 4

Animal models

ANTONIETTA COPPOLA[1,2] AND SOLOMON L. MOSHÉ[1*]

[1]*Saul R. Korey Department of Neurology, Dominick P. Purpura Department of Neuroscience and Department of Pediatrics, Albert Einstein College of Medicine and Montefiore Medical Center, Bronx, NY, USA*

[2]*Epilepsy Center, Department of Neurology, Federico II University, Naples, Italy*

INTRODUCTION

Why model?

Epilepsy is an unresolved problem with an enormous burden on its victims and on society. Epilepsy is an episodic disorder that imposes a substantial burden on individuals and society as a whole. The economic, social, and personal costs of this disorder are due largely to uncontrolled seizures but also to the underlying disease (Begley et al., 2000; Strzelczyk et al., 2008). Patients with epilepsy have decreased lifespan (Yuen et al., 2007; Sillanpaa and Shinnar, 2010). The treatments themselves may be associated with significant morbidity; the behavioral disturbances may be exaggerated by the stigma associated with epilepsy. Long-term educational/social outcomes are often unsatisfactory and not always related to seizure control or remission.

The epilepsies present unique challenges in their diversity and unmatched complexity. Research regarding the pathophysiology, diagnosis, treatment, and prevention of epilepsy is needed. Ideally, research on human epilepsy should use humans, but it is obvious that this approach is not always possible. Despite a tremendous increase in the opportunities for noninvasive research on the human brain provided by epidemiological studies, modern neuroimaging and electrophysiological techniques, randomized clinical trials, and growing access to direct investigations in the setting of epilepsy surgery, animal models of epilepsy are still essential to epilepsy research.

What to model

The International League Against Epilepsy defines an epileptic seizure as the occurrence of signs and or symptoms due to abnormal excessive and/or synchronous, usually self-limited neuronal activity in the brain (Blume et al., 2001; Fisher et al., 2005). The most accepted definition of epilepsy is of a disorder associated with at least two unprovoked seizures separated by 24 hours. Epilepsy is a chronic disorder characterized by an enduring predisposition to generate epileptic seizures associated with the neurobiological, cognitive, psychosocial, and social consequences.

In animal models, the majority of the seizures are provoked. They are elicited by different means, such as administration of convulsant drugs, electrical stimulation, and other insults (i.e., head trauma). The models can be acute, semi-chronic, and chronic. Acute models consist of provoked seizures. They permit the investigation of the fundamental neuronal basis of ictogenesis, propagation, and seizure termination. These models can be used easily to screen antiepileptic drugs. In chronic models, spontaneous seizures are not correlated to any induced stimuli (i.e., GAERS – Genetic Absence Epilepsy Rat from Strasbourg); in other chronic models spontaneous seizures appear long after the initial epileptogenic event has occurred. In the chronic models, the presence of epilepsy is associated with permanent epileptogenic/epileptic disturbances. They allow the neuroscientists to investigate progressive epileptogenesis and the subsequent enduring state with interictal/ictal/postictal abnormalities. They are also useful to study the consequences and comorbidities of epilepsy and to develop effective treatments and eventually cures.

*Correspondence to: Solomon L. Moshé, M.D., Charles Frost Chair of Neurosurgery and Neurology, Vice-Chairman, Department of Neurology, Director Pediatric Neurology & Clinical Neurophysiology, Albert Einstein College of Medicine, 1410 Pelham Parkway South, K316, Bronx, NY 10461, USA. Tel: +1-718-430-2447, Fax: +1-718-430-8899, E-mail: solomon.moshe@einstein.yu.edu

An interesting "inbetween" model is kindling. Kindling is often considered to be a semi-chronic model of epilepsy, with features between those of acute and chronic models. Indeed, in kindling, provoked seizures occur initially after repetitive trivial stimuli with increasing severity. Eventually, long after the kindling state has been reached, spontaneous seizures occur (Goddard et al., 1969). Spontaneous seizures following kindling readily occur in developing animals (Haas et al., 1990; Shouse et al., 1990). Indeed, in all chronic models investigators need to address age- and sex-specific features of ictogenesis and of epileptic state.

How to model

It has often been said that the best model of a cat is another cat, and preferably the same cat. This is a description of imitative models, which attempt to come as close as possible to the human condition studied. Thus, the models of epilepsy should have two basic characteristics. First, the models should be *realistic*, by closely mimicking the clinical entity of interest in terms of behavioral and electrographic seizures. Second, they should be *reproducible* across various laboratories. Imitative models are particularly useful for therapeutic studies.

Models can also be reductionist; to study pathophysiology, for example, there is often no point in closely mimicking a human condition that may be too complex. On the contrary, it is advantageous to isolate one of its features and reduce it to its simplest components in order to be able to understand its molecular mechanisms. Often the model is built upon a specific research question that targets other criteria (age of onset, etiology, consequences, and pharmacological response). Indeed, for example, methylazoxymethanol (MAM)-induced heterotopias mimic some of the features of epilepsy syndromes associated with cortical dysplasia (Jurgen Wenzel et al., 2000) and thus may be useful in studying developmental dysplastic lesions often associated with early-onset epilepsy. These animals, however, do not have (or rarely have) spontaneous seizures and, thus, are inappropriate for assessing treatment possibilities. In contrast, the pilocarpine model reproduces the spontaneous limbic seizures pattern and neuropathological features of human mesial temporal lobe epilepsy (MTLE).

Ideally an animal model should be under the control of the scientist, meaning that the scientist should be able to control or even better predict when the seizures are happening and thus be able to interfere with them. Obviously this is not always the case, as it is not the case in humans.

There are *in silico* (Estrada and Pena, 2000), *in vitro*, and *in vivo* models of seizures and epilepsy. *In vitro* models can utilize acutely dissociated neurons, cell culture, organotypical slices, and organotypic cultures. *In vivo* models involve alive animals, and seizures or epilepsy are induced by chemical or physical (stimulation and lesion) means, or they are genetic models. Data from both approaches are often complementary.

IN VITRO MODELS

Acutely dissociated single neurons can be obtained from many different animal species and even from humans (from surgical specimens). The procedure includes microdissection of brain slices to isolate a specific brain region and cell population followed by an enzyme treatment to facilitate cell dissociation. These cells remain sufficiently intact to generate many types of cellular activity, including action potentials, voltage-gated currents, and currents associated with activation of specific receptor-transmitted systems. The advantage of such preparations is that different stages of neuron development or different pathological conditions can be studied by harvesting cells from animals of different ages or from brains with existing pathology. The limit of these preparations is that acutely dissociated cells remain viable for recording for minutes to hours, and when the functionality is only partially preserved results are distorted. Furthermore the absence of synaptic connectivity is a limit that does not allow for the study of interactions between cells.

Dissociated cell cultures usually consist of neurons cocultured with glial cells in a relatively enriched medium. These neurons can be prepared from any mammalian species and are harvested to a different density according to the experiment. They have contributed to the study of the mechanisms of action of different antiepileptic drugs (AEDs). However, they have some drawbacks. First, these cells are produced somewhat artificially and usually there is a significant variability among laboratories. Cultured neurons may not express some proteins that are expressed by neurons in intact brain. In addition, dissociated cells form a two-dimensional network that cannot be considered as representative of the complex network of neurons in the intact brain.

Acute organotypic slices preserve the synaptic activity and the network feature of the neuronal tissue. Acute brain slices consist of 200–600-μm thin sections of living brain tissue that can be obtained from any living animal with a complex brain. Those preparations partially preserve interarea connectivity, but inevitably they have undergone a period of ischemia and some projections have been cut. As there is a limitation in oxygen diffusion and glucose supply, solutions with 95% oxygen and high glucose content are typically used to maintain the slices, and this approach results in superficial cells being exposed to high oxygen tension and glucose levels, whereas cells in the center have a low oxygen tension and less glucose.

Organotypic cultures consist of slices of embryonic tissue harvested in a controlled condition. They have several of the intrinsic properties of the tissue from which they are derived, including aspects of connectivity. The advantages over dissociated cultures and acute slices are that organotypic slices possess a limited extracellular space and contain many of the neuron types present in the comparable area *in vivo*, they are not acutely damaged, and as they are thinner they do not require high oxygenation and glucose for maintenance. Finally, they can be placed back in the incubator after a series of seizures, allowing for exploration of the long-term effect. However, the preparations are usually made from very immature animals and then studied after 7–30 days *in vitro*; the exact analogy to the brain development of the animals is not known. In addition, as the preparations are more or less deafferented, abnormal connectivity may develop. Because some of this abnormal connectivity mimics aberrant connectivity in epileptic brain, organotypic slice cultures may provide insights pertaining to the chronically epileptic tissue, where abnormal connectivity is one of the hallmarks of tissue reorganization.

IN VIVO ANIMAL MODELS

Animals used to create models

Different animals have been used to model epileptic seizure and epilepsy. They include invertebrates such as worms (*Caenorhabditis elegans*), fruitflies (*Drosophila melanogaster*), vertebrates from simpler organisms such as zebrafish (*Danio serio*), and tadpoles, as well as more complex organisms such as chickens, cats, dogs, and primates.

Currently rodents (rats and mice) are the most commonly used animals because they are easily handled, have a high reproductive rate, require simple facilities and small space to live, and overall costs are low.

Worms

C. elegans is a transparent nematode whose nervous system consists of 302 neurons. All major hallmarks of mammalian neuronal function are conserved, including ion channels, axon guidance cues, receptors, transporters, synaptic components, and neurotransmitters (Williams et al., 2004). This worm has been used to study lissencephaly, a cortical malformation often associated with epilepsy. As the central nervous system is extremely complex, the genetic analysis in a simple organism like this nematode may provide a rapid and complementary means to discern the role of the gene *LIS1*, mutation of which is responsible for the disease. In fact, these worms have been found to have convulsions in the presence of a γ-aminobutyric acid type A ($GABA_A$) agonist (Weimer et al., 2003; Williams et al., 2004).

Fruitflies

Fruitflies are widely used in the field of neurobiology and have been explored as animal models of seizures or epilepsy as well (Baraban, 2007).

D. melanogaster has related sequences with 75% of all human disease genes (Bier, 2005), and these genes can be manipulated. Thus, a large number of seizure-sensitive mutants, for instance the temperature-sensitive paralytic seizure (hERG), slowpoke (BK) (Titus et al., 1997; Ganetzky, 2000), and seizure-suppressor mutants, have been developed to study new AED strategies. The identification of the $top1^{js}$ mutation (a seizure-suppressor gene) has led to consideration of a class of DNA topoisomerase I inhibitors as potentially effective AEDs. Indeed, these drugs have been found to be effective at ameliorating some seizure phenotypes in the *Drosophila* model (Song and Tanouye, 2008).

Zebrafish

Zebrafish (*D. Serio*) are freshwater teleosts. They have the important features of being small and lower in the phylogenetically vertebrates scale, with a relatively short life cycle. They also give birth to hundreds of offspring and they develop *ex utero* in a transparent egg. Even though the maturational stage of this fish is not clearly comparable to higher order vertebrates, genes that have been identified as controlling development in zebrafish (*hedgehog*, *cadherin*, *notch*, *Wnt*) often have similar roles in higher vertebrates. Studies in zebrafish offer a unique combination of genetic manipulation, close homology with higher vertebrates, and accessible experimental methodologies such as optical imaging, behavioral analysis, and electrophysiological recording, and zebrafish may be a good candidate to develop animal models of epilepsy (Baraban et al., 2005). Several commonly used convulsants, such as picrotoxin, pentylenetetrazole (PTZ), pilocarpine, and kainic acid (KA) have been used to induce seizures in larval zebrafish.

It is likely that the potential mechanisms of action in zebrafish are similar to those reported for higher vertebrates, because glutamate, GABA, and acetylcholinergic receptors are highly conserved across species. In fact, freely swimming zebrafish exposed to PTZ (as a bath application) show increased swimming activity (stage 1), whirlpool-like behavior (stage 2), and brief head-to-tail clonic movements leading to a loss of posture (stage 3). Zebrafish brain lacks the highly ordered laminar cortical structures of higher-order vertebrates, and the larva are so small that chronic electroencephalographic (EEG) recording in freely moving fish is impossible. However, by immobilizing the zebrafish on a low melting point agar block, it is possible to place microelectrodes in the central brain structures and to record changes in accessible structures such as the tectum. The recorded activity consists of population bursts with an abrupt onset, primarily monophasic, brief duration discharge that precedes convulsive activity, monitored electromyographically in fish-tail muscle and never observed in fish exposed to normal bath (Berghmans et al., 2007). Zebrafish have also been used for drug screening. AEDs previously demonstrated to suppress PTZ-induced seizures in rodents (benzodiazepines or valproic acid; VPA) also suppress PTZ-induced epileptiform discharge in a concentration-dependent manner in zebrafish. An inherent limitation is the difficulty in controlling the amount of drug being delivered, as it is administered as a bath application. This model is considered more robust than *Drosophila*-based models because zebrafish are vertebrates and thus phylogenetically closer to humans. Furthermore, because larval zebrafish possess far fewer neurons and synaptic circuits than immature rodents (but exhibit similar types of complex epileptiform discharge), analysis of cellular mechanisms in this model could be a fruitful experimental strategy to identify the basic elements required for generation of epileptic seizures.

Tadpoles

The albino *Xenopus laevis* tadpole is a transparent vertebrate used extensively for *in vivo* imaging of neuronal growth and synaptogenesis (Cantallops et al., 2000; Haas et al., 2006; Sanchez et al., 2006). This animal can be immobilized by immersion in agar, leading to a reversible paralysis. Tadpoles have been used recently to study *in vivo* electrophysiology, seizure discharges, and seizure-induced effects on neuronal development (with *in vivo* calcium imaging) within the intact unanesthetized brain (Hewapathirane et al., 2008).

Mongolian gerbils

Epilepsy is common in Mongolian gerbils, and seizure-sensitive strains have been bred. Gerbils usually begin to have seizures after 1 month of age. Seizure susceptibility and severity increases with age, reaching a permanent plateau at approximately 6 months (Loscher and Frey, 1984). Environmental factors such as housing with other epileptic animals can worsen the seizures, and various relatively mild external stressors (handling, air blowing, exposure to a novel environment) can trigger seizures (Thiessen et al., 1968). The latter allows the scientist to control the timing of the seizures.

Behaviorally, the seizures range from brief immobility to severe, generalized, tonic–clonic convulsions followed by wild running. After each seizure the animals usually experience a refractory period. The EEG recorded from neocortex and dentate gyrus shows electrographic spikes followed by a postictal depression. It is still debated whether the onset is in the hippocampus or the cortex.

Notwithstanding the number of seizures, chronically epileptic gerbils do not display hilar neuronal loss or granule cell reorganization, suggesting that not all seizures may lead to hippocampal sclerosis.

The efficacy of currently available AEDs has been tested and compared with that in other rodent models. Gerbils are more sensitive to the anticonvulsant effects of drugs that enhance GABA and dopamine, and less sensitive to drugs that block excitatory amino acid neurotransmission or increase serotonin levels (Loscher, 1985).

The pathophysiology of the epileptic disorder is still unknown. It may be species-specific as, for example, gerbils are unique among small animals in developing ischemic lesions after only unilateral carotid ligation because they lack the circle of Willis. Interestingly, the induction and extent of the stroke is not related to seizure propensity (Donadio et al., 1982). Genetic factors seem to be important, but the seizure susceptibility does not show a simple mendelian inheritance (Thiessen et al., 1968).

Because the seizures do not appear until after the animals are more than 1 month old, studies can be performed before the onset of seizures. Many of the abnormalities (frontal reduced glutamic acid decarboxylase (GAD) activity, fewer $GABA_A$ receptors in the substantia nigra pars reticulata) reported for pre-epileptic gerbils involve GABAergic synaptic transmission, consistent with the unusually high anticonvulsant potency of GABA mimetic drugs in controlling these seizures (Asano and Mizutani, 1980; Loscher, 1987).

The value of gerbils as a model of human epilepsy is high, as these animals experience spontaneous seizures and can also have timely induced seizures triggered by handling. The progressive age-dependent development of seizure susceptibility in gerbils resembles human absence or myoclonic epilepsy in childhood, which at a later age often proceeds to generalized tonic–clonic seizures (Loscher, 1987). Their seizures could be classified as reflex seizures, but spontaneous seizures have also been observed, though rarely. Perhaps the seizures can be classified as complex reflex epilepsy or genetic epilepsy, based on inheritance patterns, age dependence, and lack of a structural brain lesion.

Chicken

Another animal model with a genetic predisposition to seizures is the Fayoumi strain of chickens (Fepi). This chicken carries a recessive autosomal gene mutation in which homozygotes are afflicted with photogenic and audiogenic reflex epilepsy. Seizures consist of stimulus-locked motor symptoms followed by generalized self-sustained convulsions (Batini et al., 2004). The use of these animals is limited nowadays. Recently, Scorza and coworkers used a chicken model, *Gallus gallus*, to study sudden unexpected death in epilepsy (SUDEP). In these animals, death occurs in close association with a tonic–clonic seizure (Scorza et al., 2009).

Cats and dogs

Cats and kittens have been used successfully to induce kindling (Racine, 1978) and to induce generalized epilepsy. Shouse and colleagues have described such seizures in cats and kittens, including sleep-related aspects (Shouse et al., 2004). Amygdala kindling was performed in weaned, prepubertal kittens between 2.5 and 6.5 months of age and in 1-year-old adults (female kittens reach puberty at 7–9 months and male kittens at around 1 year). Electrical kindling is performed 1–2 weeks after surgery, using a protocol of one stimulation per day in adult cats, and multiple stimulations per day in kittens. Young kittens require only about 14 afterdischarges (ADs) to the first generalized tonic–clonic seizure, whereas adults require at least 24 ADs. The behavioral manifestations consist of unilateral then bilateral eye, nose, and/or cheek twitches (stage 1–2), lip smacking or chewing, salivation and head clonus, body rotating to the contralateral side of the kindling (stage 3), circling (stage 4), jumping or rocking (stage 5), and violent generalized tonic–clonic seizures (stage 6). Kittens may also display apparently generalized tonic–clonic seizures or ipsilateral eye blinking during stage 3. Young kittens are more likely than older kittens and adults to develop spontaneous seizures, defined by seizures occurring 1 hour after an evoked seizure (Shouse et al., 1990).

Feline generalized penicillin epilepsy represents an experimental model of generalized spike-and-wave discharges (SWDs) occurring during clinical absence attacks (Avoli, 1995). Intramuscular administration of penicillin to the cat consistently produces generalized, bilateral, synchronous SWDs associated with blinking, myoclonus, and staring. These are sensitive to antiabsence drugs (Fisher and Prince, 1977).

Dogs have been used in kindling too (Racine, 1978). More recently, epileptic dogs with different types of spontaneous recurrent seizure have been used as animal model of intractable/drug-resistant epilepsy (Loscher, 1997).

Monkeys

Monkeys are phylogenetically the closest animal to humans, but obviously their use as animal model is limited by ethical concerns, costs, and the need for large facilities. Different strains of monkey have been used to induce seizures, including the *Papio papio* baboon, pig-tailed macaques (Jurgen Wenzel et al., 2000), the rhesus monkey and *Macaca mullata*. *P. papio* is a nonhuman primate that shows naturally occurring photosensitive epilepsy very similar to that observed in some humans with epilepsy (Killam et al., 1966). Intermittent light stimulation induces bilateral and synchronous eye, facial, and limb myoclonic twitches, which are associated with paroxysmal discharges (bursts of polyspikes and waves predominantly in the frontal cortex) (Menini and Silva-Barrat, 1990). If the seizure progresses, loud vocalization with maximal opening of the mouth occurs just before the rhythmic EEG discharges are displaced by an electrodecremental interval consisting of low-amplitude fast activity and a generalized tonic convulsion (Fischer-Williams et al., 1968). Interictal spikes are characteristic of the epileptic *P. papio* and may give rise to spontaneous seizures. The high prevalence of epileptic *P. papio* in Senegal, Africa, with their susceptibility to light-induced and spontaneous seizures, plus the absence of known morphological defects, supports the concept that there is a genetic determinant for this disorder (Loscher, 1984). Another approach used in rhesus monkeys involves an alumina gel injection into sensorimotor cortex (Lockard, 1980) or temporal lobe (Ribak et al., 1998). Injections in the sensorimotor cortex lead to the development of a chronic model that follows a time course similar to that seen in posttraumatic epilepsy in humans. Spontaneous focal seizures begin 4–8 weeks following application of the alumina gel. The area bordered by the injection often shows a disruption in the laminar pattern with a significant loss of neurons and reactive gliosis. The neuronal loss involves mainly GABAergic neurons. There is also evidence of decreased GABA receptor binding, GABA concentration, and GAD activity at the epileptic focus. This model has many similarities with the human condition. The alumina injection provides a localized focus and a well-known interval before the beginning of the seizures that can allow for the study of interictal anatomical changes.

Injection of aluminum into hippocampus, entorhinal and perirhinal cortices, and the amygdala creates a model of temporal lobe epilepsy (Ribak et al., 1998). Seizures begin 12–14 days after the injection. They are classified as focal and secondary generalized seizures. Seizures start with blank stares followed by head turning. Other symptoms can include sniffing of the fingers, followed by an arrest of movements with a motionless stare for up to a minute. As the seizure progresses, vocalization, drooling, orofacial automatisms, chewing motions, and head turning appear. Sometimes a tonic–clonic jacksonian march can be observed. The EEG pattern consists of ictal and interictal epileptiform abnormalities limited to the mesial inferior temporal lobe on the ipsilateral side of the injection site. Neuronal loss is visible at the injection site. Reactive gliosis and mossy fiber sprouting are observed in the molecular layer of the dentate gyrus.

This model provides useful information about the pathophysiological mechanisms related to temporal lobe epilepsy in humans, because its features are very close to those of human temporal lobe epilepsy, including behavior and some aspects of pathology.

Classification

As discussed, the *in vivo* models can be separated into models of acute seizure and models of chronic epilepsy that are associated with permanent epileptogenic disturbances. Some of the currently available models of acute seizure are considered to be correlates of human epileptic seizures as described in the International Classification of Epileptic Seizures from the Commission on Classification and Terminology of the International League Against Epilepsy (1981). Thus, there are models of focal-onset seizures and models of generalized-onset seizures (Table 4.1) based on the organization proposed by Berg et al. (2010). It is worth noting that the 1981 classification differentiated between simple and complex partial (focal seizures). However, as the presumed simple types depend on the person orally identifying the symptoms, it is impossible to create such models in animals.

Most chronic models are designed to study partial epilepsies, especially of temporal lobe origin (Wieser, 2004). Nevertheless there are several models used to study other epilepsies or syndromes. The term syndrome is often used for a group of clinical entities, consistently identified based on the combination of clinical/behavioral and EEG features (Berg et al., 2010). Table 4.2 shows the chronic models arranged by the age of onset (Berg et al., 2010).

Table 4.1

Available models of specific epilepsy seizure types according to the recently proposed organization of Berg et al. (2010)

Seizure type	Model	Reference (reviewed in)
Focal onset		
	Electrical and chemical kindling	Goddard et al., 1969; McNamara and Wada, 1997
	Tetanus toxin, intracerebrally	Mellanby et al., 1977
	KA, intrahippocampally or i.p.	Nadler, 1981
	Pilocarpine, i.p.	Cavalheiro, 1995
	Electrical stimulation	Fisher et al., 2005
Generalized onset		
Absence seizures	THIP, i.p.	Fariello and Golden, 1987
	GHB, i.p.	Snead, 1992
	PTZ, i.p., s.c., i.v. (low doses)	Snead, 1992
	Penicillin, i.m.	Avoli, 1995
	AY-9944 sc (inhibitor of cholesterol synthesis)	Cortez et al., 2001
Tonic or clonic	PTZ, s.c., i.p., i.v. (high doses)	Mody et al., 1997
(or a combination) seizures	Bicuculline, i.p.	Fisher, 1989
	Flurothyl, by inhalation	Mody, 1997
	Picrotoxin, s.c., i.p., i.v.	Fisher, 1989
	KA, i.p.	Mody, 1997
	AMPA or NMDA, intracerebrally	Fisher, 1989
	Pilocarpine, i.p.	Fisher, 1989
	Electroshock	Fisher, 1989
	Alcohol withdrawal	Becker et al., 1997
	Alumina gel injection in monkeys	Lockard, 1980
Myoclonic seizures	Maximal electroshock seizures (MES)	Fisher, 1989

AMPA, 2-amino-3-(5-methyl-3-oxo-1,2- oxazol-4-yl) propanoic acid; GHB, γ-hydroxybutyric acid; i.m., intramuscularly; i.p., intraperitoneally; i.v., intravenously; KA, kainic acid; NMDA, *N*-methyl-D-aspartate; PTZ, pentylenetetrazole; s.c., subcutaneously; THIP, 4,5,6,7-tetrahydroxyisoxazole [4,5-c]pyridine-3-ol.

Table 4.2

Models of chronic epilepsy arranged according to the recently proposed organization of Berg et al. (2010)

Epilepsy	Model	Species
Neonatal period		
Familial neonatal seizures	*KCNQ2* knockout	Mouse
Early infantile epileptic encephalopathy	*STXBP1* knockout	Mouse
Pyridoxine-dependent epilepsy	*TNAP*-deficient mice	Mouse
	BALBc	
Infancy		
West syndrome	TTX, intrahippocampally	Rat
	Multiple hit (see below)	
	CRH, i.p. or intracerebrally	
	NMDA, i.p.	
	ARX plus 7	
	Triplet ARX expansion	
Severe myoclonic epilepsy of infancy (Dravet syndrome)	*SCN1a* knockout	Mouse
Childhood		
Absence epilepsies	Genetic models: GAERS,	Rat
	WAG/Rij, DBA(R43Q)	Mouse
Adolescence–Adult		
Progressive myoclonic epilepsy (Unverricht–Lundborg's disease)	Cystatin B deficiency	Mouse
Progressive myoclonic epilepsy (Lafora's disease)		Beagle
Less specific age relationship		
Epilepsy with specific triggers	GEPR (audiogenic seizures)	Rat
	DBA/2 (audiogenic seizures)	Mouse
	Photosensitive epilepsy	Baboon
	Photogenic and audiogenic	Chicken
	Hot water	Rat
Distinctive constellation		
Temporal lobe epilepsy	KA	Rat
	Pilocarpine	
	Kindling	
Rasmussen encephalitis	Anti-GluR3 antibodies	Rabbit
Epilepsia partialis continua	GABA withdrawal	Baboon
	Tetanus toxin	Cat
Epilepsies attributed and organized by structural–metabolic causes		
Epilepsy associated with cortical malformations: heterotopias (subcortical band)	*Tish* mutation	Rat
Tuberous sclerosis complex	*Tsc1* knockout	Mouse
Epilepsy associated with Krabbe disease	Twitcher	Mouse
Post-traumatic seizures	Lateral fluid-percussion injury	Rat
Epilepsy due to drug abuse	Ethanol withdrawal	Mouse
	Cocaine-induced	Rat
		Mouse
		Rabbit
Hypoxia related	Global hypoxia	Rat
Angelman syndrome	GABA receptor β3 knockout	Mouse
Epilepsies of unknown cause (conditions with epileptic seizures that are traditionally not diagnosed as a form of epilepsy *per se*)		
Febrile seizures	Hyperthermia-induced	Rat
		Mouse?

ARX, Aristaless related homeobox; CRH, corticotropin-releasing hormone; GABA, γ-aminobutyric acid; GAERS, genetic absence epilepsy rat from Strasbourg; GEPR, genetically epilepsy-prone rat; GluR, glutamate receptor; KA, kainic acid; NMDA, *N*-methyl-D-aspartate; TTX, tetrodotoxin.

DETERMINATION OF SEIZURE SUSCEPTIBILITY

To determine differences in seizure susceptibility several measurements have been developed. One approach is to determine the minimum stimulus intensity that is required to induce an electrographic discharge (AD threshold). Another parameter is the minimum stimulus required to induce a behavioral seizure; there are various levels at which this measurement can be applied – determination of the development of generalized clonic seizures versus the development of chronic seizures. Another parameter includes the latency to the onset to the first behavioral seizure and subsequent seizures, as has frequently been done in the flurothyl model (Veliskova, 2006). Other parameters include seizure duration for a particular seizure type within the animal model. This indicates the duration of the behavior versus the electrographic seizure, with seizure severity determined by a scoring system according to several scales (Tables 4.3–4.5).

The careful description of the behavior characterizing a rat or a mouse seizure is extremely important; this behavior is different in adult and immature animals. In fact, particular seizure behaviors occur as a function of age, appearing or disappearing during development, depending on the maturity of the networks involved. Several of the "seizure" events may be an exacerbation of normal behavior seen in various age groups. For example, excessive scratching can be a sign of initial seizure in 2-week-old pups subjected to KA-induced seizures (Veliskova, 2006).

Behavioral seizures

Before assessing a critical behavior it is important to recognize a normal behavior. In developing rats up to postnatal day (PN) 12, occasional jerking and short-lasting head and body tremor may occur. In older rats, normal behaviors are exploration, sniffing, rearing, washing, and resting, usually in a dark corner.

It is also important to take into account all the conditions that can influence the behavior: light–dark cycle (rats are nocturnal animals), number of rats within a cage, stress (handling, separation from the dam), temperature (very young rats cannot control their body temperature), sex and hormonal changes, and strain differences.

The expression of an epileptic seizure depends on many factors. The phenotype is correlated to the site in the brain where the seizure originates. It is influenced by other variables such as age, sex, and strain. As a general rule, it is very important that any "seizure-like" behavior first be confirmed and correlated with electrographic discharges.

Behavioral arrest and staring. In adult animals, behavioral arrest and episodes of staring can be seen in both focal and absence seizures. One cannot differentiate whether it is focal or generalized without an EEG record.

Automatisms. Automatisms are repetitive movements that originally may have served a purpose. Automatisms are characteristic of limbic seizures. Depending on the drug, automatisms can be presented as excessive washing, water licking, sniffing, rearing, scratching, circling, or wet dog shakes (WDS).

Table 4.3

Scoring system for focal seizures with secondary generalization

Seizure stage	Adult rats: amygdala kindling (Racine et al., 1973; Pinel and Rovner, 1978)	Developing rats: kindling (Haas et al., 1990)	KA-/pilocarpine-induced seizures
0	–	Behavioral arrest	–
1	Mouth and facial movement	Mouth clonus	Staring with mouth clonus
?	Head nodding	Head bobbing	Automatisms (WDS, scratching)
3	Contralateral forelimb clonus	Unilateral forelimb clonus	Unilateral forelimb clonus
3.5	–	Alternating forelimb clonus	–
4	Symmetrical forelimb clonus with rearing	Bilateral forelimb clonus	Bilateral forelimb clonus
5	Rearing and falling	Bilateral forelimb clonus (with rearing and falling after 10 days of age)	Bilateral forelimb clonus with rearing and falling
6	Wild running, jumping, rolling, and vocalization. Loss of righting reflex	Wild running, jumping, rolling, and vocalization	Tonic–clonic seizures
7	Tonic posturing	Tonus	

KA, kainic acid; WDS, wet dog shakes.

Table 4.4

Scoring system for primary generalized seizures with forebrain origin (Pohl and Mares, 1987; Veliskova et al., 1990)

Seizure stage	Behavioral expression
0	No changes in behavior
0.5	Abnormal behavior (sniffing, extensive washing, orientation)
1	Isolated myoclonic jerks
2	Atypical (unilateral or incomplete) clonic seizures
3	Fully developed bilateral forelimb clonus
3.5	Forelimb clonus with a tonic component and twist of body
4	Tonic–clonic seizure with suppressed tonic phase; only clonus of all limbs. Loss of righting reflex
5	Fully developed tonic–clonic seizure

Table 4.5

Scoring system for generalized tonic–clonic seizures originating in the brainstem: audiogenic seizures (Jobe et al., 1973)

Seizure stage	Behavioral expression
0	No response
1	Wild running only
2	Two running phases separated by a refractory period; generalized clonus involving forelimbs, hindlimbs, pinnae, and/or vibrissae
3	Same as (2), but only one running phase and no refractory period
4	Two running phases separated by a refractory period; tonic flexion of neck, trunk, and forelimbs with clonus of hindlimbs
5	Same as (4), but only one running phase and no refractory period
6	Two running phases separated by a refractory period; convulsive endpoint similar to (4), except that hindlimbs are in partial tonic extension (i.e., tonic extension of thighs and legs with clonus of feet)
7	Same as (6), but only one running phase and no refractory period
8	Two running phases separated by a refractory period; convulsive endpoint similar to (4), except that hindlimbs are in complete tonic extension
9	Same as (8), but only one running phase and no refractory period

Myoclonic twitches. These are usually whole-body twitches that, if very frequent, can lead to occurrence of tonic–clonic seizures.

Wild running and barrel rotation. Wild running can be an early epileptic manifestation seen in amygdala kindling and audiogenic seizures. Barrel rotation is another epileptic manifestation that can be seen in hypoglycemic seizures (Velisek, 2008).

Clonic seizures. These are presumed to be of forebrain origin. Clonic seizures involve rhythmic movements of forelimbs often accompanied by facial clonus and lasting for seconds to tens of seconds. The forelimb clonus can be unilateral or bilateral with or without rearing or Straub tail (Veliskova, 2006). Clonic seizures can be elicited in all ages, but during the first two postnatal weeks clonic seizures in most models progress rapidly to tonic–clonic seizures.

Tonic–clonic seizures. Tonic–clonic seizures are generalized seizures consisting of tonic flexion and extension of forelimb, hindlimb, or both – longlasting clonus of all limbs with the animal unable to stand (Veliskova, 2006).

The origin of tonic seizures is not known; some investigators believe it to be in the brainstem structures (Browning, 1985). In most models, tonic–clonic seizures represent the spread of paroxysmal activity from the forebrain to the brainstem (Browning, 1985). However, few models show seizures with a primary origin in the brainstem structure, such as in maximal electroshock stimulation (MES) or in genetically prone animals such as genetically epilepsy-prone rats (GEPRs) (Ludvig and Moshé, 1989).

During early life, tonic–clonic seizures are readily elicited by most convulsants, but variability of the phases can be observed depending on the seizure model. In most models, tonic–clonic seizures can start with swimming-like movements. Rearing depends on the developmental stage of the rodent and is rarely seen before 15 days of age. The tonic phase consists of tonic flexion and extension of forelimbs and flexion of hindlimbs of variable duration. There may be periods of gasping and opisthotonus (de Feo et al., 1985; Velisek et al., 1992).

Spasms. Spasms consist of seizures of short duration characterized by abrupt flexion or extension (see Scantlebury et al., 2010). A particular type of flexion spasm is emprosthotonus, which is triggered by *N*-methyl-D-aspartate (NMDA) or homocysteic acid (Mares and Velisek, 1992; Mares et al., 1997). Emprosthotonus is observed only in rats younger than 25 days of age (Mares and Velisek, 1992).

MODELS

Electrical stimulation-induced models of seizure

Seizures induced by electrical stimulation can be divided into those elicited by stimulation of the whole brain (electroshock seizures) and those induced by local stimulation of a defined brain structure (epileptic ADs).

The advantage of these procedures is that the agent provoking the seizures acts only during application of the current and does not remain in the body, in contrast to drugs, thus the epileptic activity is no longer influenced by the agent. However, electrical stimuli are not specific as they can act on both neuronal and non-neuronal elements.

Electroshock seizures

Two methods are commonly used to induce electroshock seizures: stimulation with an alternating current of 60 or 50 Hz (according to the local current) frequency and low-frequency stimulation (6 Hz). Two types of seizure can be induced in relation to the localization of the stimulating electrodes and intensity of the stimulation current: (1) minimal clonic seizures involving muscles of head and forelimbs and (2) maximal seizures with tonic–clonic seizures.

Minimal clonic seizures are generated in the forebrain using threshold and slightly suprathreshold stimulation with corneal electrodes. They probably represent a model of myoclonic seizures (Loscher and Schmidt, 1988). Minimal threshold electroshock seizures consist of clonic movements of the head and the forelimb muscles with preservation of the righting reflex.

MES are generalized seizures characterized by tonic flexion followed by tonic extension and clonus accompanied by loss of posture (Browning and Nelson, 1985). They are considered to be of brainstem origin. MES can be induced with corneal, auricular, or transcranial stimulations with a similar procedure. Classically the MES test is performed with 0.2-second series of alternating current with a frequency of 60 Hz and an intensity of 50 mA for mice and 150 mA for rats. To assess the efficacy of an intervention, the occurrence and latency to onset of tonic hindlimb extension is taken as the criterion. The auricular stimulation can evoke the seizure even at the threshold current, whereas with the other procedures the seizures occur at suprathreshold current. The endpoint is tonic extension of hindlimbs extended 180° at the plane of the body. These seizures are followed by a period of refractoriness to the same stimulus.

There are no consistent data on EEG during MES because the high intensity of the stimulation current and the violent movements during the tonic–clonic phase mask the EEG. Morphological studies have not found any significant neuropathological changes after a single MES (Meldrum, 1986).

The advantage of this test is the ease of its performance, even though a reliable stimulator is needed. The disadvantage is that animals are used only once. It represents a convenient screening tool and is used routinely to screen potential AEDs.

Local electrical stimulation

In this model electrical stimuli are delivered to a specific structure. This paradigm can be used to determine the threshold intensities of electrical current necessary for elicitation of ADs. The AD is defined as a discharge of neuronal potentials after termination of the initiating stimulus. The AD threshold (ADT) is considered the lowest stimulus intensity that is able to induce an AD (Dyer et al., 1979).

Neocortical and limbic structures (hippocampus, amygdala, and entorhinal cortex) are the sites that are used most frequently. Electrodes can be placed epidurally or into the cerebral cortex via a stereotaxic apparatus. The recovery period, before the stimulations begin, depends on the age of the animal (Moshé, 1981). Different frequencies (high or low) of stimulation can be used similarly to the electroshock model, and the duration of stimulation series is in inverse relation to frequency. When stimuli are applied with the same intensity but with short interstimulus intervals (not leading to kindling), status epilepticus occurs.

The monitoring requires an EEG apparatus, and the evaluation focuses on the presence or absence of ADs (5 seconds at least), their pattern, and accompanying behavioral phenomena.

ADs may be of different types and duration in relation to the stimulated structure; cortical or thalamic low-frequency stimulation elicits brief spike-and-wave rhythm, whereas limbic ADs are characterized by longer trains of fast spikes, large delta waves, or sharp theta waves. Immediately after the end of ASDs, postictal depression may occur preventing the elicitation of subsequent seizures. Depression is followed by potentiation; thus, if stimulation is repeated with long intervals, kindling may be induced (Dyer et al., 1979).

Kindling

Kindling is the progressive development of seizures in response to a previously subconvulsant stimulus administered in a repeated and intermittent fashion (Goddard et al., 1969). Traditionally kindling has been performed using brief, low-intensity trains of electrical stimulation (electrical kindling), but kindling can also be obtained using chemicals (chemical kindling). Kindling is an epilepsy model of focal seizures with secondary generalization (McIntyre, 1970).

Electrical kindling in adult rats

Localized, intracranial, repetitive, low-intensity, usually electrical, stimulations lead to the development of focal ADs, behavioral automatisms, and, eventually, generalized motor convulsions. This gradual alteration in brain function and expression, once induced, is permanent (Goddard et al., 1969). Different animals have been used for the kindling studies, but here we will focus our attention to rats.

Electrical kindling requires that the animals are surgically implanted with electrodes. After the electrodes have been implanted, rats are allowed to recover for several days depending on their age. The interval is the shortest in younger animals. The most common sites used for induction of kindling include the amygdala, perforant path, dorsal hippocampus, olfactory bulb, and perirhinal cortex. Thus, electrical kindling is used most commonly as a model of temporal lobe or "limbic" epilepsy.

The stimulus usually consists of 60-Hz current delivered for 1–2 seconds, although other stimulus paradigms have been also employed. The first step is to determine the AD threshold, which is the stimulus intensity that will trigger an AD that outlasts the stimulus itself for 2 seconds or longer. Then, on all subsequent stimulus applications, the stimulus intensity is presented at that threshold value or suprathreshold intensity. According to Racine's protocol (Racine, 1972), the procedure begins with a low intensity, such as 10 μA. If this stimulus does not trigger an AD, the intensity is doubled for the next trial until an AD is triggered. Once the AD is triggered, the next step is to use a stimulus intensity halfway between the intensity that triggered the AD and the immediate previous value that did not.

Another parameter is the interstimulus interval (ISI), which can considerably influence the speed of epileptogenesis. In adults, the most used interval is 24 hours because it is practical and, with this interval, kindling can be achieved with the fewest stimuli (Mares et al., 1997). Longer intervals (e.g., weekly) are impractical. Shorter intervals may require more stimulations. The genetic makeup can influence the choice of ISI in an adult. In fact, some rats are more naturally seizure prone (fast kindlers) and kindle at shorter ISIs, and there are naturally seizure-resistant rats (slow kindlers) that will not kindle at that intensity ((Elmer et al., 1998).

During kindling the severity of the induced seizures is determined by the Racine scale and is based on amygdala kindling (see Table 4.3). Other sites may show different patterns (Racine et al., 1977; McIntyre et al., 1999). For example, frontal kindling presents with a short clonic–tonic–clonic seizure. The perirhinal cortex is the quickest to kindle among the structures in the forebrain, and the seizure behavior does not follow the Racine scale; indeed, the first seizure triggered from the perirhinal area is usually a convulsive stage 3–5 response. A peculiarity of hippocampal kindling is the early appearance of WDS; once they disappear, kindling ensues (Ludvig and Moshé, 1988).

The kindling phenomenon includes two important aspects: kindling transfer and kindling antagonism. Once a stage 5 seizure has been reached with a kindling protocol, the kindling of a second site usually proceeds at a much faster rate than if kindling of the first site had been omitted. This phenomenon is called positive transfer and occurs throughout the forebrain between structures in both the ipsilateral and contralateral hemispheres (McIntyre, 1970).

However, if two sites are kindled at the same time, one site usually progressively kindles at a normal rate while seizures from the other site are suppressed. This phenomenon is called "kindling antagonism", and appears to make use of natural inhibitory mechanisms recruited by the seizure activity from the more dominant site (Applegate et al., 1986).

Various anticonvulsant drugs have been tested for their effect on kindling. Diazepam has been found to be much more effective in blocking amygdala-kindled convulsions than cortex-kindled convulsions (Racine et al., 1973). Conversely, procaine hydrochloride and diphenylhydantoin are much more effective at blocking seizures triggered by cortical stimulation. Phenobarbital is effective in the suppression of amygdala (Wise and Chinerman, 1974) and hippocampal (Albertson et al., 1976) seizure responses.

The occurrence of neuropathological damage after kindling has been debated. Although kindling does not seem to result in significant neuronal loss, there is a kindling-induced reorganization of neuronal circuitry, as new connections are presumably being formed. Sutula et al. (1988) have shown sprouting in kindled brains depicted by a change in pattern of Timm staining of the mossy fiber of the inner molecular layer of the dentate gyrus.

Kindling is a model that is very easy to induce once the animal has been prepared surgically. In addition, it is not associated with a life-threatening physical insult – in fact, the mortality rate is practically zero. It offers also the advantage that it is easily replicated.

Electrical kindling in developing rats

Kindling of immature rats has been considered a reliable method of assessing seizure susceptibility in the developing brain. Once induced, it persists into adulthood. Kindling was the first model to document the increased seizure susceptibility of the immature brain (Moshé,

1981). Kindling is a useful model to study the consequences of repetitive seizures in the developing brain and persistence of any seizure-induced deficit. Thus, this model has been used to assess the efficacy and effects of drugs on the developing brain. Drugs can be tested for altering either the sensitivity to kindling (in this case they are injected the day before the stimulus is applied) or the establishment of the kindling state (in this case the drug is administered once the rat is fully kindled). The first protocol of amygdala kindling in infantile pups was published by Moshé and colleagues in 1981. The surgical procedure is similar to adult protocol but, because the head of the pups grows rapidly, the recovery period is shorter than for adults. Usually 1-week-old rats recover for 1 day (Baram et al., 1993) and 2-week-old animals for 2 days. Moshé used an ISI of 1 hour and 60-Hz alternating current stimulations. Later, this group also tried with shorter intervals such as 15 minutes and were still able to obtain kindling phenomenon within 1 day (Moshé, 1981; Moshé et al., 1981; Moshé and Albala, 1983).

The severity of kindling can be measured using the Haas scale (see Table 4.3) (Haas et al., 1990).

Postnatal day (PN) 7–9 kindled rats rarely develop bilateral clonic seizures or rearing, and progress from unilateral clonic seizures to tonic seizures (Baram et al., 1998). PN15–17 pups are also more prone to develop recurrent kindled seizures (Moshé and Albala, 1983). This may occur because of the absence of postictal refractoriness (Moshé and Albala, 1983).

A peculiar feature of kindling in young animals is that they do not develop kindling antagonism; thus, if alternating stimuli are delivered to two sites, kindling is accelerated in both sites (Haas et al., 1990). This observation suggests that in rat pups the available circuits that can contain the expression of seizures are not mature and thus not able to suppress multiple foci. One of these circuits appears to involve the substantia nigra pars reticulata and its output systems (Moshé, 1987).

In young rats, kindling of the limbic structures appears to lead to persistent alterations in the brain. Kindled PN15–18 rats can be rekindled faster during adulthood whether the stimulation is done at the ipsilateral or the contralateral amygdala (Moshé and Albala, 1983). However, those rats do not show any significant cell loss at the CA3 or CA1 hippocampus, nor any mossy fiber sprouting, demonstrating that the permanent kindling phenomenon occurs without any underlined histological modifications. Deoxyglucose uptake is increased in rhinencephalic structures, but not in basal ganglia or neocortex in PN15–16 rats that have reached stage 6 and 7 seizure (Ackermann et al., 1989).

Among the drugs that have been tested for their efficacy in kindling so far, diazepam (Albertson et al., 1982) and gabapentin (Lado et al., 2001) are able to modify kindled seizures in immature rats, whereas adrenocorticotropic hormone (ACTH) is able to inhibit the development of the kindling state but has no effect if administered once the kindling state is already established (Holmes and Weber, 1986). Holmes and Weber (1984) also studied the effect of progesterone; they observed no effect on kindling in the adult animal, whereas in the immature animal progesterone markedly inhibited kindling, preventing generalization of seizures.

Chemical kindling

Chemical kindling can be induced by direct intracerebral administration of low doses of excitatory agents or, more routinely, by repeated systemic administration of convulsant agents at subthreshold concentrations. The most common form of chemical kindling is systemic (intravenous, intraperitoneal, or subcutaneous) administration, with injections at intervals of 24–72 hours (Ono et al., 1990).

When the drug is administered intracerebrally, the injection site is the amygdala or the hippocampus, through a permanently implanted cannula at a slow rate to avoid damage (Ono et al., 1990).

As with electrical kindling, rats chemically kindled require many fewer stimulations to reach generalized seizures when subsequently challenged in a standard electrical kindling paradigm (Cain et al., 1986).

This model closely mimics focal seizures with secondary generalization (Bradford, 1995). However, when PTZ is used to induce kindling, there may be more cortical involvement, and thus this is considered to be a close model of primary generalized epilepsy (Ono et al., 1990).

In a typical chemical kindling experiment, animals are injected on an intermittent schedule with a proconvulsant drug at a subthreshold concentration; they are then recorded for behavioral manifestations.

With chemical kindling it is possible to study the severity of seizure responses, frequency, latency of onset and duration of the behavior, and finally the number of drug treatments required to induce a convulsive response.

The most common drug used to induce chemical kindling is PTZ, which can produce the kindling phenomenon even when administered every 2–3 days. Using PTZ, the seizures originate in the forebrain and a state of fully generalized convulsions and even status epilepticus can be reached (Mason and Cooper, 1972; Corda et al., 1991). Chemical kindling can also be used in association with other drugs that can slow (antiepileptic) or accelerate (proconvulsant, e.g., pesticides) the rate of kindling development. To avoid the effects of drug accumulation, the drug should be administered at intervals that allow their washout. With this paradigm there is a degree of neuronal cell loss in the dentate hilum and synaptic reorganization of the mossy fibers into the inner molecular layer in kindled animals (Cavazos et al., 2004).

The advantage of chemical kindling is that it does not require the implantation of chronic indwelling electrodes, as an EEG is not screened, which can be also a limitation. Chemical kindling has not been studied extensively in developing animals.

Single drug application

Chemical models can use different methods of administration:

- systemic injection of convulsant substances – GABA-related substances (PTZ, bicuculline, picrotoxin), excitatory amino acid-related substances (KA, NMDA), or cholinergic substances (pilocarpine)
- inhalation of convulsant agents (flurothyl)
- topical application of various agents, namely metals, convulsant drugs, antibiotics, and tetanus toxin.

GABA-related substances

This group of drugs is probably that used most commonly to produce acute seizures. It includes $GABA_A$ receptor antagonists, chloride channel blockers, inhibitors of GABA synthesis, convulsant benzodiazepines, and drugs with prevailing or suspected effects on the $GABA_A$ receptor, including flurothyl (Velisek, 2006). Usually the seizures do not produce neuropathological changes unless status is induced.

All of these drugs induce different phenomena, usually occurring in the following sequence: freezing behavior, myoclonic twitches, clonic seizures, and tonic–clonic seizures. With EEG monitoring, four different patterns may appear – not all of them occurring with every drug (Velisek, 2006):

1. Isolated spikes, usually associated with myoclonic jerks. In developing animals, slow and sharp waves appear instead of spikes.
2. Spindles of spike-and-wave activity associated with freezing.
3. Decrescendo spike-and-wave activity associated with clonic seizures. This pattern also depends on the drug; dissociation of this EEG pattern from behavioral seizures is frequent.
4. Polyspikes or polyspike and slow waves associated with the start of tonic–clonic seizures.

PTZ

Originally used as a cardiostimulant, PTZ has significant convulsant potency in mice, rats, monkeys, and humans. The most common administration route is intraperitoneal, but PTZ can be also administered subcutaneously or intravenously because it dissolves freely in saline or water.

PTZ induces all four behavioral phenomena – freezing, myoclonic twitches, clonic seizures, and tonic–clonic seizures – although the occurrence of freezing and clonic seizures is limited during the first two postnatal weeks in the rat. Graded doses of PTZ in adult rats will induce specific seizures. Thus, low doses can be titrated to induce only freezing with underlying EEG spindles, somewhat higher doses for kindling, even higher doses for clonic seizures, and doses above 100 mg/kg for tonic–clonic seizures.

Repeated low doses of PTZ administered intraperitoneally may be used to induce status epilepticus (SE) in immature rats (Nehlig and Pereira de Vasconcelos, 1996).

PTZ-induced clonic seizures represent a routine test for screening anticonvulsants, as ethosuximide (ETX), clonazepam, and valproic acid (VPA) suppress EEG spindles (Brabcova et al., 1993) and tonic–clonic seizures (Mares et al., 1981).

Bicuculline

Bicuculline acts as a competitive antagonist at the GABA-binding site of the $GABA_A$ receptor. This model can be used for screening for AEDs as classical anticonvulsant drugs, and especially $GABA_A$ receptor-acting drugs, are effective in this model.

Bicuculline is usually administered intraperitoneally because of the low pH. In fact, the final solution with bicuculline is obtained using a weak acid (0.1-N hydrochloric acid) as a solvent and a weak base (0.1-N sodium hydroxide) for careful titration to the resulting pH of 5.6 (Velisek and Mares, 1995). Bicuculline can also be administered intravenously, especially in adult rats where higher doses are usually required if used intraperitoneally because of a first-pass effect. Usual doses for intraperitoneal injection are 2–4 mg/kg for developing rats and 6–8 mg/kg for prepubertal and adult rats (Veliskova et al., 1990). If administered intraperitoneally, 2 mg/kg is sufficient for adult rats. Seizures occur after 20 minutes, producing all behavioral phenomena, with the only exception that clonic seizures begin to occur during the second postnatal week.

Myoclonic jerks are rare in 7-day-old compared with adult animals.

Picrotoxin

Picrotoxin blocks the $GABA_A$ receptor/chloride channel. As for PTZ and bicuculline, this model is useful for screening of putative AEDs. Picrotoxin can be administered subcutaneously, intraperitoneally, or intravenously, because it dissolves readily in saline. Seizures occur within 30–40 minutes, showing all behavioral phenomena. Thus, the seizures develop at a slower pace than PTZ- and bicuculline-induced seizures.

It should be noted that the incidence of clonic seizures is relatively low in PN7 rats and increases to nearly 100% after PN18. In pups, clonic seizures are often unilateral (Veliskova and Velisek, 1992).

Excitatory amino acid-related substances

KA

KA is the most popular neurotoxin used to produce SE and the consequent neuropathological changes (Sperk, 1994). It is an agonist for the KA subtype of ionotropic glutamate receptor, which is highly concentrated in the hippocampus, especially in the CA3 region, also in the amygdala, perirhinal and entorhinal cortex (Miller et al., 1990). As these areas are affected preferentially following systemic administration, KA is considered a valuable model of focal seizures with complex symptomatology and secondary generalization from the limbic focus (Ben-Ari, 1985), as well as a model of epileptogenesis after SE (Cavalheiro et al., 1982).

KA can be dissolved in normal saline; however, the resulting pH is acidic, so the intraperitoneal route of administration is widely preferred. Nevertheless, KA exerts a potent convulsive action when applied systematically into the cerebral fluid or locally into limbic brain areas (Nadler et al., 1980). The dosage depends both on the maturational state of the animal and on the strain (Sperk, 1994). In general, lower doses are used in immature animals.

When administered systemically, seizures usually occur within the first 60 minutes. KA produces hypoactivity for about 20–30 minutes (Ben-Ari et al., 1981). After that there is variability in the behavior depending on the age of the rats. During the first 2 weeks they show profuse scratching. The following week they start to present with WDS, which increases with aging. Two-week-old rats develop bilateral motor manifestations much more quickly than adult rats, but the seizures can be asymmetrical. Rearing is seldom seen (Albala et al., 1984). When administered locally, depending on the dose, KA can induce mild limbic seizures, full-blown limbic motor seizures, or a longlasting SE (Nadler, 1980, Nadler et al., 1981). EEG includes spikes, spike-and-wave and polyspike-and-wave activity. Electrographic seizures may last for many hours after the behavioral seizures have stopped (Giorgi et al., 2005).

Metabolic studies in adult rats have revealed an increase in 2-deoxyglucose (2-DG) uptake in the hippocampal formation, lateral septum (Ben-Ari et al., 1981), and substantia nigra pars reticulata (Albala et al., 1984) during the early stages of KA seizures, where there is a decrease in the neocortex, forebrain, mesencephalon, and brainstem. In immature rats (PN15–18), 2-DG uptake is increased in hippocampus and lateral septum, deep cortical layers, and ventromedial thalamic nuclei, but not in substantia nigra pars reticulata (Albala et al., 1984).

Neuropathology is also age-specific, being represented by only minimal nonspecific changes in limbic structures in younger animals (Albala et al., 1984), whereas in adults there is significant cell loss after KA administration in the hippocampus associated with synaptic remodeling (Sperber et al., 1999b).

Even though KA administration is one of the most common methods used to induce seizures in animal models, some limitations should be considered: the doses required may be quite specific for the strain, and the location and extent of KA seizure-induced damage is different among the different strains (Brandt et al., 2003).

NMDA

NMDA is a prototype agonist at the NMDA subtype of the ionotropic glutamate receptor, expressed mostly in the hippocampal CA1, dentate gyrus, and striatum.

NMDA dissolves in normal saline but its blood–brain barrier permeability is very poor, so it usually provokes seizures when administered intracerebrally at a dose of 2–10 nmol (Ishimoto et al., 2000), or at much higher doses (> 100 mg/kg) when administered systemically. Seizures occur within 15–45 minutes, depending on the dose. As this model is associated with very low survival rates, administration of the NMDA receptor antagonist ketamine (50 mg/kg intraperitoneally) after 15–30 min of seizure duration is used to increase the survival rate.

The first symptom is increased locomotor activity including wild running. The rats then develop automatisms, which usually start with tail flicking. Biting is also a common manifestation. Interestingly, in rats younger than 3 weeks of age, NMDA induces a special seizure pattern consisting of hyperflexion of the head, body, and tail while the rat is lying on its side (emprosthotonic seizures) (Mares and Velisek, 1992). These seizures are usually pharmacoresistant and lead to long-term learning impairments (Velisek and Mares, 1995); thus, they are considered an equivalent of infantile spasms, although with some reservations. NMDA induces tonic–clonic seizures throughout development, and clonus regularly precedes tonus, which is indicative of imminent death (Mares and Velisek, 1992).The EEG pattern is characterized by long suppression that usually corresponds to hyperactivity or tonic–clonic seizures, followed by slow waves. The EEG pattern is chaotic between motor seizures.

When administered intracerebrally in adult rats, NMDA produces severe neuronal damage (McDonald et al., 1998) . No damage is found in young rats when NMDA is injected systemically (Kabova et al., 1999).

Acetylcholine-related substances

Pilocarpine

Pilocarpine is an acetylcholine agonist acting on muscarinic receptors, which are found mainly in the hippocampus, striatum, and cortex. This model has been useful for testing drugs for focal seizures. When administered alone, pilocarpine has significant peripheral effects. Therefore, when pilocarpine is used with a systemic injection of high doses (300–400 mg/kg), a muscarinic antagonist is also injected subcutaneously. Otherwise, to decrease the dosage and subsequent effect, pretreatment with lithium chloride is injected 24 hours before a pilocarpine dose of 30–60 mg/kg (Turski et al., 1989).

Pilocarpine-induced seizures consist of automatisms, WDS, clonic seizures, and SE. Starting from PN3, the EEG correlate consists of spikes that start from the hippocampus and spread to the cortex (Cavalheiro et al., 1987).

In this model seizure-induced damage appears to be age-specific. Neuropathology is more extensive in adults, less so in P15 and begins in earnest at PN21. In the adults, the hippocampus is the structure predominantly damaged (Turski et al., 1989). In immature animals at PN12–21, some damage can be found in the hippocampus, thalamus, olfactory cortex, septum, and neocortex (Cavalheiro et al., 1987). In the younger animals (PN12), neuronal damage is found in thalamic nuclei (Kubova et al., 2001).

Inhalation of convulsant substances

Flurothyl

Drugs with easy evaporation at room temperature are used as inhalant substances to provoke seizures.

Flurothyl (*bis*-2,2,2-trifluoroethyl ether) has an uncertain mechanism of action that may involve different systems ($GABA_A$ receptors, sodium channels, cholinergic system) (Woodbury, 1980). Seizures have been described in various animals including mice, rats, gerbils, and humans. Flurothyl is usually delivered by means of a microinfusion pump at a constant rate. When flurothyl evaporates, it forms convulsant fumes. The latency to seizure onset depends both on the amount of flurothyl and also on the environmental conditions (barometric pressure, air humidity). In this model, mortality is usually low.

The behavioral features of the seizures are age-specific (Sperber and Moshé, 1988). During development, flurothyl induces agitation followed by exploratory activity. During the first postnatal week, swimming movements occur followed by tonus.

Clonic seizures develop after PN10. Beginning from this age, rats usually experience several myoclonic twitches followed by a clonic seizure, which can evolve into a tonic–clonic seizure with loss of posture. After PN20 the tonic–clonic seizure is usually preceded by several separated clonic seizures. Flurothyl-induced seizures appear to be more violent than seizures induced by injection of a GABA-related agent. The EEG shows rhythmic discharges. Individual spikes can be also recorded, and in young animals also sharp waves. The correlation with myoclonic twitches is not tight for young animals (Sperber et al., 1999a).

Flurothyl can induce a motionless stare with accompanying EEG spindles. This can be considered a model of typical absence seizures. Clonic seizures can be considered a model of generalized clonic seizures, and tonic–clonic a model of generalized tonic–clonic seizures (Engel, 2001).

Metabolic studies using 2-DG in adult rats demonstrate complex involvement of basal ganglia structures, including the substantia nigra pars reticulata. In immature rats mild seizures induce decreases in 2-DG uptake, whereas severe seizures produce increases in the brainstem and decreases in the cortex. There is no activation of the substantia nigra pars reticulata (Veliskova et al., 2005). C-fos immunoreactivity after flurothyl seizures was found throughout the cortex, but only in the deep neocortical layer in PN10 rats (Jensen et al., 1993).

The limitation of this model is the need for special equipment (airtight glass cylinder, fume hood to eliminate excessive fumes of the convulsant). Flurothyl is also expensive.

Topical (focal) application of substances

This approach can produce acute or chronic seizure foci in a brain area, usually the cortex. Drugs can also be injected in the ventricles in very small amounts. However, in this case it is difficult to determine the actual focus as many regions can be affected almost simultaneously. Many substances have been used for this purpose, such as metals, antibiotics, tetanus toxin, and convulsant drugs.

Metals

The models utilizing metals are expensive and require intensive labor. Among the metals, alumina cream is a very potent convulsant, but its effect is limited to monkeys and rabbits. In this model, the latency to the expression of seizures is long, as seizures appear after several months but can last for several years.

A major advantage is that these seizures occur spontaneously. However, their detection requires video-EEG monitoring, which is expensive and labor-intensive.

Antibiotics

Focally administered epileptogenic antibiotics produce a model of focal seizures with initial symptoms depending on the exact localization (Engel, 2001). Among the antibiotics, penicillin produces an epileptogenic effect in different species including rats and cats (Noebels and Pedley, 1977). Cephalosporins have also substantial epileptogenic potency when applied focally. It should be emphasized that the first identification of neurons displaying the paroxysmal depolarizing shift, the hallmark of epileptic neurons in the epileptic focus (Matsumoto and Ajmonemarsan, 1964), was in the penicillin model.

Tetanus toxin

Tetanus toxin was first described as a means to induce experimental seizures by Roux and Borrell in 1989. Tetanus toxin is a zinc-dependent protease that cleaves synaptobrevin (Schiavo et al., 1992) and hence blocks synaptic release. Tetanus toxins can induce seizures in any vertebrate species, but have been utilized mostly in mice and rats (Mellanby et al., 1977). Different approaches have been used: hippocampal injections that model focal seizures (temporal lobe seizures), and intracortical injections, which model focal neocortical epilepsy, secondary generalized seizures, and epilepsia partialis continua.

With the intrahippocampal injection, up to 30 seizures, each lasting for 2 minutes, occur per day (Jefferys et al., 1995). They usually consist of behavioral arrest, vibrissae twitching, followed by forelimb myoclonus, and ultimately rearing and falling (stage 5 in the Racine scale). Monitoring reveals partial seizures with bilateral manifestations when induced in dorsal hippocampus (Mellanby et al., 1977). Electrographic seizures recorded from the hippocampus start either with a sudden prolonged burst of activity or with short bursts at 2–3 Hz, developing into faster burst discharges at about 20 Hz and then slowing to a bilaterally synchronous 9–16-Hz activity, which is often a prelude to secondary generalization. The seizure often ends with a 2–5-Hz discharge (Finnerty and Jefferys, 2000). These seizures usually remit after 6–8 weeks, but none of the rats returns to normal – they always show impairments of learning and memory (George and Mellanby, 1982). From an anatomical point of view there is a reduction of synaptic responses and changes in several intrinsic neuronal properties (Vreugdenhil et al., 2002). There is mossy fiber sprouting in the dentate gyrus (Mitchell et al., 1996) and CA1 pyramidal cell axons into the stratum radiatum (Vreugdenhil et al., 2002). This model has been used to study the effect of AEDs and in fact responds to different AEDs (carbamazepine, lamotrigine).

In pups, the behavior is different. During the first week of life, seizures occur frequently, typically about one per hour. They can last from a few seconds to a few minutes and are often associated with WDS and wild running. After the first week the generalized seizures remit, but interictal spiking continues. Once adult, these rats can show rare spontaneous seizures (Lee et al., 1995). A high proportion of rats will remain epileptic permanently.

When tetanus toxin is administered intracortically, the seizure depends on the specific site of injection and on the amount of toxin. Injection into sensory cortex provokes frequent interictal spikes, motor seizures, and occasional generalized seizures (Brener et al., 1991). These seizures appear a few days after the injection, but last for at least 7 months. When the toxin is injected in the motor cortex, focal motor seizures, epilepsia partialis continua, and occasional secondary generalization occur (Nilsen et al., 2005). These seizures are associated with a burst of fast EEG activity (>20 Hz), evolving into rhythmic spiking at 1–2 Hz with higher (15 Hz) frequencies intermixed. In this model, monitoring is of essential importance because the number of observed motor seizures underestimates the number of electrographic seizures. With the intracortical injection there is no sprouting within the hippocampus. This model is considered to be a model of epilepsia partialis continua. It is resistant to the systemic administration of high doses of phenytoin or diazepam, mimicking the drug resistance typical of this condition (Nilsen et al., 2005).

Overall, the application of tetanus toxin results in a robust model, but careful attention should be paid because of the powerful toxic implication of this drug to the experimenters. In addition, tetanus toxin can be destroyed by bacterial contamination, so it is important to create an aseptic environment and refrigeration is essential.

Other acquired focal models

In this section, we discuss other focally acquired models, including models of abnormal cortical development (cortical freeze lesion, MAM, *in utero* irradiation), hypoxia-induced seizures, complex febrile seizures, seizures associated with hemorrhage–iron deposition, and post-traumatic epilepsy (lateral fluid–percussion brain injury).

Models of abnormal cortical development

Neuronal migration disorders are structural malformations resulting from early developmental disturbances or genetic defects in the process of migration of new neurons to their final region. These disorders are often associated with pharmacoresistant epilepsy (Guerrini et al., 2003). Different models have been developed to study these disorders, such as the cortical freeze lesion model, the MAM model, and the *in utero* irradiation model. Two spontaneous mutants, the *Flathead* and the *Tish*, showing abnormal cortical development have been reported in the literature (Lee et al., 1997; Sarkisian et al., 1999).

The cortical freeze lesion model

Dvorak and Feit first described the cortical freeze lesion in newborn rodents as a model of human neuronal migration disorders such as polymicrogyria, focal heterotopia, cortical dysplasia, and schizencephaly (Dvorak and Feit, 1977).

The neocortical freeze lesion model has been used in various strains of newborn rat. The result is strictly dependent on the age of the animal. When the lesion is induced from PN1 to PN4, cortical dysplasia (three- or four-layered cerebral cortex), microgyria, and heterotopia in layer I can be obtained. In adult rodents the cortical freeze lesion has been used as a model of traumatic brain injury or brain edema (Stoffel et al., 2001).

The procedure described by Dvorak and Feit (1977) consists of anesthesia by hypothermia, surgical exposure of the cortical area of interest, and induction of three contiguous freeze lesions by liquid nitrogen delivered by a copper rod. According to this protocol, a four-layered microgyrus lesion is obtained when the procedure is carried out in newborn rats (less than 24 hours after birth). Other freeze lesions have been described, including layer I and white matter heterotopia, laminar necrosis, and porencephaly (Ferrer et al., 1993). Using larger freezing probes and freezing times, it is possible to obtain a cortical cleft resembling human schizencephaly.

Spontaneous seizures have not yet been described in cortical freeze lesion models. However, young freeze-lesioned rats have a significant lower threshold temperature, shorter latency to seizure onset, and a longer duration compared with control animals when exposed to hyperthermia-induced seizures. These seizures begin with jaw myoclonus, followed by hindlimb clonus and generalized convulsions, and are terminated with a period of posthyperthermia depression (Scantlebury et al., 2004). Epileptiform synaptic responses have been demonstrated using electrical stimulation of different afferent inputs. This activity originates from a focal hyperexcitable region around the lesion and not from the microgyrus itself (Jacobs et al., 1996). The architecture of this area appears normal but there is upregulation of binding to AMPA (2-amino-3-(5-methyl-3-oxo-1,2- oxazol-4-yl)propanoic acid) and KA receptors, and downregulation of $GABA_A$ receptors.

Even though this model does not show spontaneous seizures, it is considered useful to study the pathophysiology of malformations due to abnormal cortical development. It is a very reproducible model with a low mortality rate. Limitations are the strict dependence of the lesion on the age of the animal and the possibility that the pup may be neglected by the mother after the lesion has been induced.

MAM model

Compounds that inhibit DNA synthesis (5-azacytidine, methyl-mercury, nitrosoureas, and carmustine) can lead to neuronal cellular ablation and thus to cerebral malformations when used during embryonic development (Hallas and Das, 1978; Taylor and Jones, 1979; Rodier, 1990; Benardete and Kriegstein, 2002). Among these, MAM is the only one that has been used widely to induce developmental brain dysfunction in rodents. MAM is an alkylating agent found naturally in a palm-like plant belonging to the *Cycas* genus of the Cycads that is found in tropical areas all over the world. It shows a high selectivity for neuronal precursors undergoing their final mitotic division at the time of administration. It does not affect gestational parameters and has no teratogenic effects on other organs in the offspring (Cattabeni and Luca, 1997).

When administered intraperitoneally to pregnant rats, MAM is rapidly converted to methyl-diazonium, which is able to pass the placenta and also the blood–brain barrier and damage DNA by methylating the O^6 or N^7 position of guanine. MAM selectively affects actively dividing neuroepithelial cells during the S phase, whereas postmitotic neurons or neuroblasts in the G0 phase are spared. This killing effect lasts for a period of 2–24 hours, with maximal activity at 12 hours after administration.

The lesion caused by MAM depends on the day the drug has been delivered. MAM administration on embryonic day (E) 14 results in a reduction of the thickness of all cortical layers, whereas MAM treatment on E15 or E16 results in the selective ablation of layers II–IV and sparing of layers V–VI (Tamaru et al., 1988; de Feo et al., 1995). Paredes et al. (2006) demonstrated that in

MAM-exposed rats the abnormal cell clusters (heterotopia) first appear postnatally in the hippocampus (PN1–2) and that their appearance is preceded by a distinct sequence of perturbations in neocortical development: (1) disruption of the radial glial scaffolding with premature astroglial differentiation; and (2) thickening of the marginal zone with redistribution of Cajal–Retzius neurons to deeper layers.

Double MAM administration on embryonic day E15 (with a 12-hour interval) resulted in severe cortical hypoplasia and layering abnormalities, with a clear rostrocaudal and mediolateral gradient. In addition there were conspicuous cerebral heterotopias (Colacitti et al., 1998). Thus, MAM-treated rats can be considered a useful model for human brain dysgeneses, such as periventricular nodular heterotopias (PNH).

Rats subjected to MAM administration do not develop spontaneous seizures. However, they do have a decreased seizure threshold to flurothyl *in vivo* (Baraban and Schwartzkroin, 1996), PTZ (Chevassus-Au-Louis et al., 1998), KA (Germano and Sperber, 1997), and kindling (Chevassus-Au-Louis et al., 1998). In addition, *in vitro* studies with intracellular recordings have shown evidence of hyperexcitability in both the subcortical and the intracortical heterotopias. These neurons show excessive and longlasting repetitive bursts of action potentials in response to low-amplitude depolarizing current pulses, until reaching longlasting trains of high-frequency action potentials outlasting the duration of the pulses (Colacitti et al., 1999).

In utero irradiation

The *in utero* irradiation model has been developed as an attempt to model human cortical dysplasia. It uses pregnant rats with known insemination dates that can be irradiated with a different radiation source (McGrath et al., 1956). The pups are born at term. The result is very sensitive on the timing of the irradiation. Irradiation at E12 produces a thin cortex with an almost normal lamination. Irradiation at E16 generates the most severe dysplasia with a markedly thinned cortex and heterotopic gray matter. By E17, only neurons and interneurons from the intermediate plate (II, III, and IV) are affected from the radiation because the others have already reached the cortical plate (Cowen and Geller, 1960).

Irradiated brains are microcephalic and the cortex thickness is one-third that of the control cortex (Marin-Padilla et al., 2003). The effect of the irradiation is not uniform. The dorsomedial cortex is most severely affected, showing complete loss of lamination. Small and large neurons are sparse in the cortical mantle, and pyramidal cells show an abnormal orientation. Interneurons (parvalbumin and calbindin-positive cells) are reduced by about 50% compared with control tissue (Roper, 1998). Unlike the human cortical dysplasias, irradiated brains do not reproduce balloon cells and giant neurons are rare.

Irradiated animals appear normal, being able to feed and live a long life. However, they typically exhibit behavioral deficits (increased reactivity to novel stimuli, impaired maze learning, and abnormalities of locomotion) that vary depending on the time of exposure. The incidence of seizures is not clear. Kellinghaus and coworkers reported seizures in 3 of 5 rats exposed to 175 cGy on E17. The semiology of these seizures consisted of staring, behavioral arrest, facial twitching, WDS, loss of postural reflexes, and asymmetrical forelimb and hindlimb clonus (Kellinghaus et al., 2004); the seizure onset was localized to the hippocampus, with eventual secondary generalization. Others have not reproduced these results.

This is an easy model to study. However, the primary limitation is that it does not reproduce balloon cells and giant neurons of Taylor's type or type cortical dysplasia. It more closely models sporadic acquired cortical dysplasia.

Flathead mutant rat

The *flathead* rat is a spontaneous mutant from a colony of Wistar rats discovered in 1995 in Connecticut. The mutation responsible for this phenotype is in the citron kinase gene (*CitK*) (Sarkisian et al., 2002). Homozygous mutants display generalized seizures with regular intervals from the first trough the second week after birth, resting tremor, severe ataxia, dystonia, atonia, and astatic episodes (Sarkisian et al., 1999). They show microcephaly, neuronal and glial cytomegalic cells, and GABAergic interneuron loss similar to that in human dysplasia (Roberts et al., 2000). The rats usually die within the third week of life. The *flathead* is a completely penetrant autosomal recessive mutation; thus 25% of the offspring from heterozygous rats show the mutant phenotype. This model is a valuable resource for exploring cellular changes associated with seizures progression because seizures occur regularly, with early onset, and the phenotype is very different from that of heterozygous and normal littermates.

Tish mutant rat

The *Tish* rat is a spontaneous mutant from a colony of Sprague-Dawley rats. As in the *flathead*, *Tish* is a completely penetrant autosomal recessive mutation, but it is not lethal (Lee et al., 1997). The rats show well-developed bilateral subcortical band heterotopias and spontaneous seizures from 1–6 months of age. The mutation responsible for this phenotype has not yet been identified. Its identification could be useful to help the study of human double cortex cases that are not caused by the X-linked *DCX* or *LIS1* mutations (Pilz et al., 1998; D'Agostino et al., 2002).

Hypoxia-induced seizures

Neonatal seizures occurring during hypoxic encephalopathy are usually prolonged and refractory to conventional AED therapy. A rodent model of perinatal seizures induced by hypoxia has been developed by Jensen and coworkers (1991) using Long-Evans rats at PN9–12.

The model consists of a 15-minute exposure to graded global hypoxia in an airtight chamber using nitrogen. During the procedure, strict control of the body temperature is maintained with a heating pad. Seizures appear after 3–7 minutes and only during an age window (PN10–12). These episodes consist of brief tonic–clonic seizures, which become progressively longer. These episodes can occur up to 4 days after the hypoxia has been induced. The EEG shows fast spike activity that starts at a low amplitude. Interestingly, younger and older rats have diminished EEG activity and an isoelectric EEG in adulthood (PN50). Cell loss and gliosis are not evident after hypoxia-induced seizures.

Rats that have experienced hypoxia-induced seizures at PN10 show a long term increase in susceptibility to seizures induced by PTZ, flurothyl, and KA (Jensen et al., 1992).

These seizures are blocked by systemic administration of an AMPA receptor antagonist (NBQX) given before hypoxia is induced (Jensen et al., 1995). Topiramate is also effective in reducing the number of seizures when given as a pretreatment. Both NBQX and topiramate pretreatment are able to protect against permanent changes in flurothyl threshold in adulthood (Koh and Jensen, 2001). In contrast, NMDA receptor antagonists (MK801), GABA receptor agonists (lorazepam), and phenytoin do not prevent these hypoxia-related epileptogenic effects and are not able to block these seizures (Jensen et al., 1995).

This model is easy to develop and the mortality rate is extremely low if hyperthermia is avoided (Jensen et al., 1991).

Complex febrile seizures model

This model uses PN7–14 rat pups. The induction of seizures is obtained with hyperthermia as fever is very difficult to induce in young pups. The aim of the procedure is to increase the brain temperature by 2°C/minute until seizure onset. Using this protocol the latency to seizure onset is usually 2–4 minutes. The hyperthermia is maintained for 30 minutes unless the rat's temperature is above 41.5°C (Dubé et al., 2000). In this case the pup is moved to a cool metal surface to prevent excessive heating (Olson et al., 1984; Baram et al., 1997).

After the experiment, pups are submerged for 1 second in water at room temperature, then hydrated orally and transferred to a cool surface until their core temperature reaches 32–34°C.

The seizures start with sudden arrest of the running (freezing) followed by oral automatisms (chewing, biting) and often forelimb clonic movements. Later, tonic body flexion can be seen. The EEG shows spike trains in hippocampus and amygdala that coincide with the immobility and oral automatisms, although there is no change (or just flattening) in cortical EEG activity. The ictal EEG activity consist of trains of spikes and spike–waves with progressively increasing amplitude in hippocampal and amygdala leads, with variable progression to the cortex (Dubé et al., 2004). There is evidence for the occurrence of spontaneous seizures (epilepsy) in a subgroup of the rats that had sustained experimental febrile seizures.

Spontaneous recurrent seizures have been reported to occur in adulthood in about 35% of the rats and interictal spiking was recorded in about 88% of the rats (Dubé et al., 2010). Lesioned rats with hyperthermic seizures also showed an impaired performance on the Morris water maze when compared with naive control rats, suggesting mild deficits in learning and memory (Scantlebury et al., 2005). In this model seizures are not followed by acute (Toth et al., 1998) or long-term neuronal death in the hippocampus (Bender et al., 2003), although transient neuronal injury is detectable over 2 weeks in hippocampus, amygdala, and perirhinal cortex (Toth et al., 1998). These seizures can provoke only transient neuronal injury in limbic structures (Dubé et al., 2010). Inflammation contributes to increased neuronal excitability and seizures, as the temperature necessary to induce febrile seizures is reduced after intracerebroventricular administration of interleukin-1β to rat pups (Dubé et al., 2010).

According to Baram et al. (1997), this model is very reproducible because 99% of the rats develop prolonged seizures. They emphasize that attention should be paid to controlling the temperature of the animals. To avoid direct hyperthermic injury and agonal, terminal seizures, temperatures should be carefully controlled and maintained at 40–42°C. Specifically, temperatures higher than 43 °C may lead to direct injury.

Post-traumatic epilepsy

Hemorrhage–iron deposition and lateral fluid percussion brain injury

Traumatic brain injuries are known to cause 20% of all symptomatic epilepsies (Hauser and Annegers, 1991).

There have been many attempts to model post-traumatic epilepsy (PTE). The subpial application of ferrous or ferric chloride into the rat or cat sensorimotor cortex (Willmore et al., 1978) was based on the observation that hemosiderin deposits are associated with high risk of PTE. This model consists of injection of ferric chloride into rat amygdala, which causes the development of and gradual increase in spike discharges. Epileptiform activity is recorded from the ipsilateral amygdala within 5–10 minutes after the injection. In the following days isolated spikes can be recorded, also arising from the contralateral hippocampus, while epileptiform discharges usually arise from the ispilateral hippocampus.

By the fifth day after injection, 92% of the animals will develop spontaneous seizures represented by limb clonus, rearing, and limb clonus (stage 4 or 5 on the Racine scale). Histopathological analysis shows mossy fiber sprouting and cell loss in both hippocampi. A genetic and molecular study has shown that 30 days after the injection, the production of a glutamate transporter (GLAST) is downregulated in both hippocampi. This can lead to an impaired ability to remove synaptic glutamate, facilitating the epileptic process. On the other hand, GABA transporters, particularly GAT3, are upregulated, suggesting a compensatory response (Ueda and Willmore, 2000).

The lateral fluid percussion brain injury (FPI) is currently the most widely used animal model for human traumatic brain injury because so far it is the only model that leads to spontaneous seizures (Thompson et al., 2005). It reproduces several characteristics of closed head injury in humans (head contusion, blood–brain barrier disruption, altered cerebral metabolism and flow, hematomas and hemorrhages, axonal injury, progressive neuronal loss, altered electrical activity, and behavioral abnormalities) (Thompson et al., 2005).

The procedure was first described by McIntosh et al. in 1989. It consists of a traumatic brain injury produced in an anesthetized rat with a fluid percussion device on a specified area of the brain. With this procedure, a 33% mortality rate is observed. Brief acute clonic seizures occur immediately after induction of the injury in 30% of rats. At the 42-week follow-up, 50% of the animals developed epilepsy. The ictal pattern recorded from the ventral ipsilateral hippocampus is characterized by repetitive, rhythmic, polymorphic spike-and-wave or polyspike–slow wave complexes. Interictal activity consists of spike–wave paroxysmal discharges in the hippocampus ipsilateral to the trauma. Seizures are approximately 1 minute long, with a seizure frequency of about 0.3 seizures per day. The frequency has a tendency to increase with time. Analysis of thionin-stained sections reveals substantial neuronal loss in both hemispheres. There is also mossy fiber sprouting in the septal hippocampus ipsilateral to the trauma.

The limitations of this model consist of the high mortality rate and the long follow-up needed to detect the seizures (6–12 months).

Recently, Sankar and coworkers applied this model to developing rats to demonstrate that, following a traumatic brain injury, the central nervous system may experience a period of protection. They used PN19 rats subjected to a severe lateral fluid percussion injury followed by pilocarpine-induced SE. The injury produced a temporary state of neuroprotection from seizure-induced cell death in the developing rat; no long-term protection from altered hippocampal circuit rearrangements, enhanced excitability, or later convulsive seizures were found (Gurkoff et al., 2009).

SYNDROMES OR ENCEPHALOPATHIES (NOT GENETICALLY INDUCED)

Pharmacological models of generalized absence seizures in rodents

Absence epilepsy is an epilepsy syndrome with generalized nonconvulsive seizures characterized by a brief unresponsiveness and cessation of activity, which may be accompanied by automatisms or moderate tonic or clonic components affecting the limbs, eyeballs, or eyelids (Panayiotopoulos, 1999).

Typical absence seizures are associated with bilateral, synchronous, 3 cycles/second spike-and-wave discharges on the EEG that are presumed to start and end abruptly. These abnormalities are generalized, synchronous, and symmetrical. The background activity is normal (Commission on Classification and Terminology of the International League Against Epilepsy, 1981). They are usually well controlled by specific AEDs and, apart from the absences, patients do not present any other neurological abnormality.

Atypical absence seizures may have heterogeneous EEG patterns including spike and slow-wave complexes, fast activity, or other paroxysmal activity. These abnormalities are bilateral, but often asymmetrical and irregular. The background is usually abnormal (Commission on Classification and Terminology of the International League Against Epilepsy, 1981). The prognosis of the patients suffering from atypical absences seizures is usually poor.

Models displaying electrical, behavioral, and pharmacological characteristics of absence seizures have been developed in rodents, cats, and primates by injection of different compounds. Experimental generalized absence seizure models should meet some criteria: EEG and behavior similar to the human condition, reproducibility and predictability, quantifiable, involvement of thalamocortical mechanisms, and appropriate pharmacology (seizures exacerbated by GABAergic agents and blocked by $GABA_B$ receptor antagonists) (Cortez and Snead, 2006).

Acute models of typical absence epilepsy have been obtained using PTZ (Marescaux et al., 1984), penicillin (Avoli, 1995), 4,5,6,7-tetrahydroxyisoxazole [4,5-c]pyridine-3-ol (THIP) (Fariello and Golden, 1987), and γ-butyrolactone (GBL) (Snead, 1988). All of these models are self-limiting and resolve within a defined period of administration of the respective drugs. Neither cell loss nor reactive gliosis has been reported for any of these models.

Chronic animal models of typical absence epilepsy include the Genetic Absence Epilepsy Rat from Strasbourg (GAERS) (Marescaux et al., 1984) and the WAG/Rij (Wistar Albino Glaxo Strain bred in Rijswijk, the Netherlands) (Coenen and Van Luijtelaar, 1987).

There are also chronic models that are considered to be models of atypical absence epilepsy, the AY9944 and MAM (Cortez et al., 2001; Serbanescu et al., 2004). In these models, seizures persist long after administration of the compound.

THIP, GHB, PTZ, and penicillin models

THIP is a GABA agonist that, when administered intraperitoneally, induces bilaterally synchronous SWDs in rats lasting for 7–9 seconds (Fariello and Golden, 1987). These abnormalities correspond to immobility and vibrissal twitching. This model differs from the others here described because valproic acid (VPA) exacerbates these episodes (Vergnes et al., 1985).

GHB (γ-hydroxybutyric acid) is a GABA metabolite that occurs naturally in the mammalian brain. When administered intraperitoneally it can induce generalized seizures. GBL (γ-butyrolactone) is the prodrug of GHB and is biologically inactive in the brain. However, an active lactonase in the serum and liver convert GBL to GHB. Thus, when GBL is administered intraperitoneally to rats it results in the rapid onset of bilaterally synchronous SWDs in rats that correlate with an almost immediate appearance of GHB in the brain. If GHB is administered intraperitoneally, the EEG discharges do not occur until 20 minutes after its administration, corresponding with the peak of GHB levels in the brain. When GHB is injected into the thalamus, brief bursts of SWDs appear, whereas if GBL is injected there is no effect (Snead, 1991). In rats, the behavior of seizures consists of complete arrest with facial myoclonus and vibrissae twitching. When GHB is administered to prepubescent monkeys, they present with immobility, head drops, staring, papillary dilation, eyelid fluttering, rhythmic eye movements, and stereotypical automatisms (Snead, 1978).

PTZ is the most commonly used $GABA_A$ receptor antagonist to induce absence-like seizures with low doses, even though all the $GABA_A$ receptor antagonists are capable of inducing them. Low doses of PTZ induce absence seizures that meet all the criteria for absence seizure models, while clonic seizures appear when the dosage is increased (Marescaux et al., 1984).

Penicillin has been used to induce absence in cats (Fisher and Prince, 1977; Kostopoulos, 2000). In fact, when administered intramuscularly penicillin produces generalized, bilaterally synchronous, SWD discharges associated with blinking, myoclonus, and staring. These abnormalities are sensitive to most of the AEDs commonly used to treat absence seizures, and are exacerbated by photic stimulation (Avoli, 1980) and GABAergic agonists (Fariello and Golden, 1987). When penicillin is administered to rats, the occurrence of SWDs is not always reproduced.

Chronic models of typical absence epilepsy

Genetic models of absence epilepsy in rats

Two models of spontaneous occurrence of SWDs evocative of absence seizures in untreated rats have been described so far: the GAERS and the WAG/Rij.

The GAERS strain was selected from Wistar colonies that displayed spontaneous SWDs on routine cortical EEG. Breeding then selected pairs for three or four generations, and a strain with 100% of rats displaying SWDs was produced (Vergnes et al., 1982). It is important to note that in old age 100% of Wistar rats show SWDs activity that is not distinguishable from the GAERS activity, suggesting that aging is associated with aggravation of SWDs. At the same time, it was discovered serendipitously in Nijmegen that the already fully inbred WAG/Rij strain of rats showed SWDs in their cortical EEG (van Luijtelaar and Coenen, 1986).

In both WAG/Rij and GAERS, SWDs start and end abruptly on a normal cortical desynchronized EEG background. In adult animals the frequency of these complexes varies in a range of 7–11 cycles/second (c/s) (Drinkenburg et al., 1993). In GAERS, SWDs can last from 25 to 60 seconds and absences occur about every minute (Vergnes et al., 1982). These complexes are detected when the GAERS are around 60–80 days old and 100% of the rats show the complexes by the age of 3 months. In WAG/Rij they last less, about 5 seconds and the maximum number of complexes is during the dark period of their 24-hour light/dark cycle. Some WAG/Rij animals (60%) also show localized SWDs recorded bilaterally at the occipital and parietal cortex (Midzianovskaia et al., 2001). In WAG/Rij, the SWD complexes are detectable at around 3 months of age, and at 6 months 100% of the rats show the complexes.

In both strains the SWDs are always concomitant with behavioral immobility and sometimes rhythmic twitching of the vibrissae and facial muscles. This is accompanied by diminished neck muscle tone. At the end of the SWDs the animal resumes its behavior and the muscle tone of the neck is restored (van Luijtelaar and Coenen, 1986). Beyond the epileptic episodes these rats show a normal behavior, including feeding, exploration, social interaction, and learning.

No gross morphological modification has been observed in either model, although an increase in glial fibrillary acidic protein (GFAP) expression has been reported in the cortex and thalamus of both adult and young GAERS, suggesting that reactive astrocytes are already present before the onset of absences (Dutuit et al., 2000).

In both models SWDs are suppressed by ETX, trimethadione, VPA, and benzodiazepines, and worsened by carbamazepine and phenytoin, as in the human condition (Micheletti et al., 1985).

Even though these two models share many features with the human absence syndrome, several discrepancies exist. First, the frequency in the humans is 3 c/s, whereas in these animals it is between 7 and 11 c/s. This could be species-dependent, as this frequency has never been observed in rodents (Snead, 1978). Further, SWDs in GAERS and WAG/Rij occur when brain maturation has finished and last throughout the life of the animals, whereas in humans they occur during development and tend to disappear once development is completed.

Recently another model of absences has been described by Tan et al. (2007). Based on a mutation found in an Australian family affected by childhood absence epilepsy, a knock-in mouse for the $GABA_A$ receptor γ2 subunit point mutation (R43Q) has been constructed. The homozygous mice die before the age of 18 days. Heterozygous mice demonstrate behavioral arrest associated with 6–7-Hz SWDs. These appear with an abrupt onset at PN20, corresponding to human childhood. These EEG abnormalities are suppressed by ETX, which is also a peculiar finding in childhood absence epilepsy syndrome. Thus, this model can be considered as a model of childhood absence epilepsy. These mice are also sensitive to PTZ, a $GABA_A$ receptor blocker.

Interestingly, Reid et al. (2011) recently demonstrated that an insulin-mediated reduction in blood glucose levels was sufficient to double the occurrence of SWDs in two absence models: the DBA(R43Q) model and the SWD-prone DBA/2 J mouse strain. Conversely, injection of glucose was able to reverse the impact of insulin on SWDs in the DBA(R43Q) model. These findings suggest that low blood glucose levels can precipitate SWD in genetically predisposed animal models and should be considered as a potential environmental risk factor in patients with absence epilepsy (Reid et al., 2011).

Chronic models of atypical absence epilepsy

The AY-9944 and the MAM–AY model

AY-9944 is a compound able to inhibit the reduction of 7-dehydrocholesterol to cholesterol (Willmore et al., 2009). When administered subcutaneously every 6 days to rat pups at PN 2, 6, 8, 14, and 20, AY-9944 leads to absence-like seizures that persist into adulthood. The seizures begin to appear at PN21 (Cortez et al., 2001), and are also associated with an abnormal cognitive outcome. The onset and offset of these seizures is gradual and the animals maintain their ability to move purposefully, as occurs in children with atypical absences.

Antiabsence drugs such as VPA and ETX reduce the frequency of the seizures, whereas phenytoin and GABA agonists exacerbate them (Cortez et al., 2001).

The MAM–AY model is also known as the double-hit model, as atypical recurrent absence seizures occur after the two compounds are administered to pups (Serbanescu et al., 2004). The antimitotic agent MAM is administered on gestation day (G), leading to a neuronal migration disorder similar to cortical dysplasia. The pups are then injected with AY-9944 as described above. The rats show spontaneous, recurrent, atypical absence seizures characterized by bilaterally synchronous slow SWDs with a frequency of 4–6 Hz. The seizures are refractory to ETX and VPA, thus creating a model of refractory atypical absence seizures as might occur in children with brain dysgenesis (Serbanescu et al., 2004).

Animal models of infantile spasm

Infantile spasm or West syndrome is an early childhood encephalopathy usually characterized by a triad: infantile spasms, arrest of psychomotor development, and hypsarrhythmia on EEG. The syndrome usually begins in the first year of life, commonly between 3 and 10 months of age, and can have different etiologies (Dulac et al., 2002). Unfortunately, most AEDs are ineffective, although the spasms may respond to ACTH and vigabatrin (Vigevano and Cilio, 1997; Willmore et al., 2009). The outcome is usually poor because of the progression to other types of seizure and abnormal cognitive and neurological development (Riikonen, 2001). The pathophysiology is still unknown and the absence of an animal model to study this peculiar syndrome has been a limiting factor for years. Several promising animal models have been described recently (Stafstrom, 2009). They include genetic models, such as Down syndrome, the Aristaless-related homeobox (*ARX*) mutation, the triplet repeat expansion of the *ARX* gene model, and acquired models such as those induced with toxins (tetrodotoxin (TTX) model and multiple-hit models) or with stress hormones (corticotropin-releasing hormone (CRH) model), or by blockade of neuronal activity (NMDA model following *in utero* treatment with betamethasone).

Down syndrome model – Ts65Dn mouse

Infantile spasms occur in up to 10% of children with Down syndrome (Stafstrom and Konkol, 1994). The Ts65Dn mouse is a model overexpressing $GABA_B$ receptors and exhibiting spontaneous SWDs on EEG (Galdzicki and Siarey, 2003; Rachidi and Lopes, 2008). In this model the administration of baclofen or GBL causes clusters of extensor spasms observed when the animal is suspended. The spasms decrease with ACTH, VPA, ETX, and vigabatrin (Cortez et al., 2009). This model suggests the involvement of the $GABA_B$ receptors in the genesis of the infantile spasms, at least in Down syndrome. Seizures do not occur spontaneously or chronically.

Aristaless-related homeobox (*ARX*) mutation model

The X-linked Aristaless-related homeobox (*ARX*) gene is one of the family homeobox genes that encodes for a transcription factor involved in development of the nervous system. Mutations of this gene can be associated with different phenotypes including mental retardation, epilepsy, and specifically infantile spasms (Hirose and Mitsudome, 2003). *ARX* knockout mice show a deficient proliferation and migration of the GABAergic interneurons that may be responsible for the epilepsy phenotype (Kitamura et al., 2002). A conditional deletion of *ARX* from inhibitory interneurons of the cortex constitutes a new model exhibiting a variety of seizure types during development. These rats show first limbic seizures in the early (limited) recordings and then spasm-like episodes (in adulthood) (Marsh et al., 2009). The EEG shows interictal spikes and an ictal electrodecremental response. The importance of this model is that the phenotype is obtained with a mutation of a known infantile spasm gene and the *ARX* knockout mouse has the advantage of being closely related to human *ARX* mutations. Although X-linked, with males showing a more severe phenotype, female carriers also exhibit seizures and cognitive changes. Thus, this model is also appropriate for studying sex differences in susceptibility to epilepsy. It is still not clear whether the cognitive and behavioral abnormalities observed in *ARX*-deficient mice are the result of the seizures or the mutation.

Triplet repeat expansion of the *ARX* gene model of infantile spasm

Price and colleagues have recently generated a nonlethal genetic mouse model of infantile spasm engineered by targeted expansion of the first polyalanine tract in the X-linked *Arx* gene, Arx(GCG). This polyalanine tract expansion is the mutation most commonly associated with West syndrome and mental retardation in human patients with infantile spasm (Poirier et al., 2008). Null mutation of the *Arx* gene impairs GABA and cholinergic interneuronal migration but results in a neonatal lethal phenotype, whereas the newly generated mice do have metabolic abnormalities leading to early lethality. Wild-type pups display spontaneous brief focal myoclonic twitches and generalized startles. The mutants also display twitches and startles, and in addition they exhibit sustained spasm-like movements so strong as to cause the pup to flip or fall over. Regarding the EEG, different patterns have been described. In pups younger than 21 days, there is a high-voltage slow-wave transient followed by attenuation of the background EEG amplitude and a transient increase of higher frequency activity. This corresponds to a brief myoclonic jerk involving the head and body at the onset of the attenuation event. Other patterns include high-amplitude multifocal cortical spikes and sharp waves, high-voltage slow waves associated with a spike occurring independently over both hemispheres. There is no obvious motor behavior linked to these discharges.

Mice older than 3.5 weeks show spontaneous electrographic seizures characterized by generalized attenuation of the background activity and low-voltage fast activity, followed by generalized high-frequency and high-amplitude spike and polyspike activity. This activity corresponds to versive movements of the head and or trunk, clonic movements, and grooming suggestive of limbic seizures (Price et al., 2009).

The neurobehavioral profile of *Arx* mutants includes lowered anxiety, impaired associative learning, and abnormal social interaction (Price et al., 2009).

Neuropathology includes laminar decreases of Arx^+ cortical interneurons and a selective reduction of interneurons expressing calbindin, but not parvalbumin or calretinin, in neocortical layers and hippocampus, indicating that specific classes of synaptic inhibition are missing from the adult forebrain, and providing a basis for the seizures and cognitive disorder (Price et al., 2009).

Corticotropin-releasing hormone (CRH) model

Based on the knowledge that ACTH can be effective in infantile spasms, it has been hypothesized that stress plays a role in increasing brain excitability and provoking infantile spasms. As stress results in release of CRH, Baram and colleagues have injected this hormone in rats, intraperitoneally or intracerebroventricularly, during the second week of life. These rats showed severe seizures, that phenotypically were limbic seizures rather than infantile spasms (Baram and Schultz, 1995). Acute ACTH administration does not stop these seizures (Baram and Schultz, 1991). Ictal EEG for CRH seizures can be either an electrodecremental response or rhythmic sharp activity, whereas the interictal EEG is like hypsarrhythmia (Baram and Schultz, 1991). Excess CRH, as initiated by multiple stressors, results in seizures and dendritic and neuronal structural abnormalities, as well as long-term cognitive, learning, and memory deficit. Because this model does not involve damage to the brain, any cognitive deficits may be a result of the seizures themselves.

NMDA model after *in utero* treatment with betamethasone

Intraperitoneal administration of the glutamate receptor agonist NMDA to rat pups between PN12 and PN18 causes hyperflexion and tonic spasms of the entire body, with loss of the righting reflex. This type of seizure is termed emprosthotonus (Mares and Velisek, 1992; Kubova et al., 2001). Recently, a modification to this model was proposed, consisting of the administration of betamethasone on gestational day 15, mimicking a stressor for the hypothalamic–pituitary–adrenal (HPA) axis (Velisek et al., 2010). This treatment is meant to sensitize the brain to postnatal exposure to NMDA (Welberg et al., 2001; Velisek et al., 2007, 2010; Chachua et al., 2011). The prenatally exposed rats are then injected with NMDA, beginning on PN15, and following a short latency period exhibit tail twisting and then flexor spasms. ACTH is able to modify the latency of these seizures when given before the administration of NMDA (Velisek et al., 2010). The limitations of this model are the absence of spontaneous seizures and the fact that seizures do not occur without NMDA administration.

Tetrodotoxin (TTX) model

Intrahippocampal infusion of the sodium channel blocker, TTX, from PN10 to PN12, causes recurrent seizures in rat pups, consisting of brief spasm-like seizures (Galvan et al., 2000, 2003). These seizures are associated with fast activity on EEG. When TTX is injected for 28 days with an osmotic micropump, one-third of the pups at about PN21 develop flexor or extensor spasms, singly or in cluster. The interictal EEG pattern shows high-voltage, chaotic waves and multispikes, especially during non-rapid eye movement (non-REM) sleep. The ictal EEG includes a generalized slow wave, followed by an electrodecremental response, low-voltage fast activity. These ictal and interictal features closely resemble the EEG pattern of human infantile spasms. These EEG abnormalities persist following pump removal. After disappearance of the spasms, limbic seizures appear.

Multiple-hit model

Based on the hypothesis that infantile spasms result from an interaction between cortical, subcortical, and brainstem pathologies (Lado and Moshé, 2002), a multiple-hit model of symptomatic infantile spasms has been developed (Scantlebury et al., 2010). This model consists of the injection of three drugs: on PN3, doxorubicin is injected into the cerebral ventricles and lipopolysaccharide is injected in the right cerebral cortex. Doxorubicin is an anthracycline chemotherapeutic agent that creates neuronal damage through oxidative stress (Chen et al., 2007). Lipopolysaccharide is a toxin released by Gram-negative bacteria that is able to damage white matter and activate inflammatory cells (Wang et al., 2006). Then, on PN5, *p*-chlorophenylalanine is administered intraperitoneally to reduce the serotonin level by blocking its synthetic enzyme, tryptophan hydroxylase (Sharma et al., 2000). This is based on the knowledge that serotonin is able to lessen brain excitability (Trindade-Filho et al., 2008). Animals treated with these three drugs develop clusters of flexor or extensor spasms from PN4 to PN12. In both epidural and depth recordings, electrodecremental patterns are correlated to each spasm episode. Spike and sharp-wave discharges and/or fast rhythmic activities can also be associated with the spasms (73% of electrographic correlates). Interictally, frequent spikes or complexes of high-amplitude spike and slow-wave discharges are observed only in PN7–13 pups. Other seizures may emerge after PN9 that resemble limbic seizures.

$ACTH_{1-24}$ at a dose of 1.25 units per kg per day (Cosyntropin® depot at a dose of 0.0125 mg per kg per day) intraperitoneally is not effective in treating the spasms. Vigabatrin transiently suppresses spasms at PN5 (Scantlebury et al., 2010).

These rats also exhibit neurodevelopmental deficits such as memory and learning impairment, and socialization deficits, including decreased exploration, indifference to other rats, and excessive grooming. These features have been related to autism spectrum disorder, which is often found in patients suffering from infantile spasms (Tuchman et al., 2009).

A limitation of the model is the significant mortality rate (up to 30%; A.S. Galanopoulou, personal communication), although the literature reports that 5–30% of children with infantile spasms die and that 50% of these deaths are disease-related. Furthermore, mortality is greater in symptomatic cases (Dulac and Jallon, 1997).

Rasmussen encephalitis

Rasmussen encephalitis (RE) is a neurological condition characterized by refractory epilepsy that usually begins in the first decade of life leading to progressive degeneration of one cerebral hemisphere. The progressively worsening unilateral seizures are accompanied by progressive atrophy of the hemisphere and hemispheric neurological symptoms.

The etiology and pathogenesis of RE are incompletely understood. However, a humoral autoimmune mechanism has been found to contribute to the pathogenesis. This has been demonstrated with the immunization of rabbits with the glutamate receptor subunit GluR3, resulting in epileptic seizures, with neurological deficit and similar histopathology of the cortex (Rogers et al., 1994). Accordingly a subset of patients with RE were found to have circulating anti-GluR3 immunoglobulin (Ig) G. Importantly, in some patients seizure severity and frequency are reduced following plasmapheresis of IgG-selective immunoadsorption, in parallel with reduction of GluR3 antibody titers (Rogers et al., 1994; Andrews and McNamara, 1996; Antozzi et al., 1998).

This model has been developed with repeated subcutaneous injection of a GluR3 protein linked to a glutathione-*S*-transferase (GST) in White New Zealand male rabbits (He et al., 1998). Two weeks after the second immunization, 2 of 5 injected animals developed motor incoordination while ambulating and epileptic seizures (repetitive tonic or clonic movements of all four extremities). Subsequently the animals developed persistent obtundation and failure to thrive with weight loss. Immunization of rabbits with other GluR (1, 2, 5, or 6) and *N*-acetylcholine receptor subunits did not induce this disorder.

Histopathological examination revealed multifocal inflammatory abnormalities consisting of microglial nodules and perivascular lymphocytic cuffing, principally in cerebral cortex with lymphocytic infiltration of the meninges. In contrast to the human pathology, these occurred bilaterally (He et al., 1998). Interestingly anti-GluR3 IgG-stained cortical neurons were present in the two ill rabbits but not in healthy GluR3-immunized rabbits, suggesting that GluR3 antibodies gained access to GluR3 *in vivo* in the ill, but not in the healthy GluR3-immunized rabbits.

A limitation of this model is the cost of purchasing and maintaining rabbits, which is much greater than that for mice and rats.

GENETIC MODELS

Many research approaches are available to build a genetic model of epilepsy. The earliest models were obtained with spontaneous mutations in mice. These models were usually due to monogenic mutations, which alone were able to produce an epileptic phenotype (Noebels, 2006). Later, scientists produced engineered genetic models, trying to reproduce a phenotype or genotype of a human epileptic condition. One of the most common approaches is to inactivate a given gene in the mouse germline by homologous recombination in embryonic stem cells. This procedure is called *knockout* (Noebels, 2006). With this approach the scientist is able to observe whether the resulting phenotype presents with epilepsy. Another approach is to model exactly a human mutation known to cause epilepsy. For example, a sequence of a gene that is present in epileptic patients but not in unaffected controls is identified. It is possible to create a model in which the candidate mutated gene is inserted by homologous recombination into the same molecular context in the orthologous mouse gene. This method is called *knockin* (Noebels, 2006). This has the advantage of better reflecting the human condition than the complete obliteration of gene expression. Practically, this method is also more convenient when the knockout approach produces a lethal phenotype.

In some cases the investigator may wish to study a phenotype of the epilepsy without caring about the genotype. In this case, the approach would be to produce a *transgenic model* that serves to overexpress a protein and can be useful to produce the desired phenotype (Noebels, 2006). With this approach it is also possible to express the protein ectopically and to choose when to express the protein, turning expression on and off by adding appropriate chemicals (e.g., doxycycline) to the animal's drinking water.

Knockout models

Gene knockout strategies are also known as gene replacement. This approach can be used to study either gain of function or loss of function phenotypes. This technique was developed beginning in the late 1980s by Capecchi (1989a, b). It is based on the concept that a piece of DNA, when introduced into a nucleus, is able to find its matching sequence in the host genome and "trade places" through a mechanism called homologous recombination. In this way the investigator can replace a specific target gene with a completely inactive copy or a mutated version of the piece, and study the resulting phenotype. Once a genomic target has been identified, a gene replacement transcript is constructed and transfected into embryonic stem cells by electroporation or lipofection. Following selection, the genomic DNA of the cells is tested by polymerase chain reaction (PCR) to verify that the correct homologous recombination has occurred. Correctly targeted embryonic stem cells are microinjected into normal donor mouse blastocysts, where they mix with the population of normal embryonic stem cells that constitute the inner stem mass of the early embryo. The injected blastocysts are then implanted into surrogate females, and the subsequent procedure is similar to that of the transgene approach.

Gene knockout models are much more expensive than standard transgene procedure because of the extensive embryonic stem cell culturing and analysis. Other limitations are the possibility of incomplete inactivation, and disruption of overlapping or adjacent genes.

Transgenic models

We usually refers to homologous recombination as the process of introducing exogenous DNA into a specific position in the genome of a recipient animal, and to transgenesis as the introduction of DNA into a random position (Noebels, 2006).

Usually, a transgene consists of the same element as the endogenous gene, a promoter, a region of transcribed sequences that encode a protein, and a poly(A) additional signal. The protein-coding segment usually consists of an intronless cDNA fragment. It is constructed by standard recombinant DNA techniques in a plasmid, and amplified by growth in *Escherichia coli*. The vector is then removed and the transgene is injected into one of the two pronuclei of a newly fertilized zygote from a female donor mouse. The insertion site into the genome is believed to be random. The injected embryos are then implanted into a surrogate female. The pups born from this mouse are the F0 generation. They may or may not carry the mutation and PCR analysis is necessary to genotype the genomic DNA of the pups to determine whether the procedure has been successful and the gene expressed or not. Another approach to create a transgenic mouse is to use a retrovirus. Theoretically, any gene can be transfected, depending on the availability of the promoter.

There are many limitations to using transgenic approaches. The expression can result in the death of the transgenic animals. Occasionally the animals can be born as a "chimeric" form for the transgene and carry it in some cells but not others. Insertion of the transgene in the genome can produce an unintended loss of function if it interrupts or disturbs the expression of an endogenous gene. The phenotype can also vary as a result of differences in the level or site of transgene expression. Also, multiple insertion can occur and the expression may not be inhibited. Transgenes can be inserted into the Y chromosome and thus expressed only by males. Lastly, when the transgene is expressed in a heterozygous manner, it can become unstable during rearrangements (Noebels, 2006).

Genetic models of epileptic syndromes

Genetic models of reflex seizures in rats

Some epilepsy syndromes are known as reflex epilepsy because seizures are objectively and consistently demonstrated to be evoked by a specific afferent stimulus (light flashes, listening to music, or hearing sounds) or by activity (thinking, reading, playing chess, eating) of the patient (Blume et al., 2001). Scientists have obtained animals with seizure predisposition and expression by breeding individual animals. In this section we focus our attention on genetic models of reflex seizures in rats.

Among rats models, the genetically epilepsy-prone rat (GEPR) is a model susceptible to seizure for different stimuli. A 100% epilepsy-relevant trait has been obtained via inbreeding of naturally occurring epilepsy occasionally seen in Sprague-Dawley rats (Mishra et al., 1988, 1989). Two independently derived strains have been developed: the moderate GEPR-3 and the severe GEPR-9. Three types of seizure predisposition are exhibited by GEPRs. First, seizures can be triggered by endogenous and exogenous stimuli that do not cause seizures in normal animals. Both strains are sensitive to sound and hyperthermia, and some GEPRs also show seizures in response to handling and postural changes. GEPRs also present with infrequent spontaneous seizures that cannot easily be correlated to a stimulus. Second, they show exaggerated seizure responsiveness to stimuli that also cause seizures in nonepileptic animals. Third, they have an abnormally low threshold to many convulsant drugs such as aminophylline (De Sarro and De Sarro, 1991), to electroshock (Browning et al., 1990), to flurothyl (Franck et al., 1989), to hyperbaric conditions (Millan et al., 1991), to PTZ (Browning et al., 1990), and to barbiturate withdrawal (Bourn and Garrett, 1983). They also have an accelerated rate of limbic kindling, representing another aspect of seizure predisposition in GEPRs (Coffey et al., 1996). Both GEPR-3 and GEPR-9 are highly susceptible to sound-induced generalized tonic–clonic seizures. The genetic background is characterized by a complex interaction between multiple genes, with incomplete penetrance and variable expressivity of these factors (Kurtz et al., 2001).

A generalized tonic–clonic seizure in GEPR-9 is characterized by the sudden onset of massive myoclonus coupled with initial high-amplitude polyspikes and waves. This is followed by a sudden marked electrodecremental interval in the EEG with tonic rigidity of all muscles. High-amplitude spike–wave complexes with partial reduction and recurrence of tonus then appear, followed by progressive displacement of tonus with clonus of increasing amplitude. A postictal reduction of EEG amplitude with muscular flaccidity is the final event (Jobe et al., 1995; Moraes et al., 2005).

A sound stimulus is able to produce a brainstem seizure (running fit) in both strains (Ludvig and Moshé, 1989). The seizure is almost the same, except that in GEPR-3 a 10–20-second running episode precedes the seizure, which is also less severe than that in GEPR-9.

Spontaneous seizures occur more frequently in GEPR-9 than in GEPR-3.

The major drawback of this model is that it is not commercially available and is in danger of disappearing (Kiesmann et al., 1988).

Over the years, other models of genetic reflex seizure have been described, such as a strain of Wistar rat that was inbred in Strasbourg (Kiesmann et al., 1988), the DBA/2 mouse (see Schreiber and Graham, 1976), and the EL mouse (see Seyfried et al., 1999). The first is a model of rats that present with susceptibility to audiogenic seizures characterized by one or two wild running fits followed by tonic dorsiflexion with open mouth and then a catatonic state. The corresponding cortical EEG was flat for 1–2 seconds, followed by slow, regular, low-amplitude discharges. When these rats were exposed to 40 daily 90-second auditory stimuli, a kindling state was developed with the seizures propagating from the brainstem to forebrain structures. The wild running became disorganized by myoclonic jerks of the limbs and body. In some animals, the tonic extension disappeared and a myoclonic seizure developed progressively, with facial and forelimb clonus, and rearing and falling. In others, the tonic phase was followed by a generalized clonic phase. The EEG during the myoclonic and tonic–clonic seizures showed high-amplitude rhythmic spikes, polyspikes, and spike–waves (Kiesmann et al., 1988).

Benign familial neonatal epilepsy (BFNE)

Benign familial neonatal convulsion is an autosomal dominant epilepsy. Recently, two voltage-dependent potassium channel genes, *KCNQ2* and *KCNQ3*, have been identified by positional cloning as being responsible for BFNE. Watanabe et al. (2000) disrupted the mouse *KCNQ2* gene using a gene targeting strategy. Homozygous pups ($KCNQ2^{-/-}$) died within a few hours of birth from pulmonary atelectasis. Heterozygous mice had decreased expression of *KCNQ2* and showed hypersensitivity to develop seizures when treated with epileptogenic agents such as pentylenetetrazole (Watanabe et al., 2000).

Early infantile encephalopathy with suppression burst (EIEE) – Ohtahara syndrome

Early infantile epileptic encephalopathy with suppression burst (EIEE), also known as Ohtahara syndrome, is one of the most severe and earliest forms of epilepsy. Recently, Saitsu et al. (2008) found a *de novo* 2.0-Mb microdeletion at 9q33.3–q34.11 in a girl with EIEE. Mutational analysis of candidate genes mapped to the deletion revealed that four unrelated individuals with EIEE had heterozygous missense mutations in the gene encoding syntaxin binding protein 1 (*STXBP1*) (Saitsu et al., 2008). More recently, a *de novo* mutation in *STXBP1* has been identified in individuals with mental retardation and nonsyndromic epilepsy (Hamdan et al., 2009).

STXBP1 (also known as MUNC18-1) is an evolutionally conserved neuronal protein expressed throughout the brain. It regulates cell polarization as well as focal secretion at synapses (Verhage et al., 2000). Abolishing *munc18-1* expression in mice by homologous recombination results in complete loss of neurotransmitter secretion from synaptic vesicles throughout development in mice, although seizures have never been described (Verhage et al., 2000).

Severe myoclonic epilepsy in infancy (SMEI) – Dravet syndrome

Heterozygous loss-of-function mutations in voltage-gated sodium channels cause severe myoclonic epilepsy in infancy (SMEI). A knockout mouse for *SCN1A*, the gene encoding for this channel, has been developed by Catterall's group (Yu et al., 2006). Homozygous $Scn1a^{-/-}$ mice developed ataxia and seizures beginning on PN9 and died on PN15. Heterozygous $Scn1a^{+/-}$ mice had spontaneous seizures at around PN21–27, and sporadic deaths beginning after PN21. Seizures began with stereotypical behaviors such as myoclonic jerks and hindlimb flexion, progressed to forelimb clonus and head bobbing, and ended with relaxed muscle tone. The seizure duration was typically 20 seconds (Yu et al., 2006). This model seems to be very promising for the development of new therapeutic strategies to cure Dravet syndrome.

The tuberous sclerosis model – *TSC1* knockout mouse

Tuberous sclerosis complex (TSC) is one of the most common causes of epilepsy. This disease is caused by mutation of the *TSC1* (tuberin) or *TSC2* (hamartin) gene and is characterized by tumors or hamartomas in multiple organs including the brain. The neurological involvement accounts for intractable seizures, autism, and mental retardation (Crino et al., 2006). Because mice homozygous for *Tsc1* or *Tsc2* targeted mutations die by mid embryogenesis, it is not possible to study the consequence of tuberin or hamartin loss postnatally. To circumvent this problem, Uhlmann et al. (2002) generated mice with astrocyte-specific inactivation of *Tsc1*. Although these mice are phenotypically normal at birth, they begin to die by 3 months of age. However, from approximately 2 months of age they show behavioral seizures consisting of brief periods of tonic stiffening of the trunk or extremities without loss of posture, followed by rhythmic bouncing of the head and trunk with forearm clonus. Occasionally, there are other seizures characterized by behavioral arrest, wild running, or severe tonic posturing with loss of upright posture. Electrographically, most seizures appeared to have a simultaneous onset in both hemispheres. These mice usually have an abnormal interictal EEG background showing a burst-suppression pattern with frequent spikes. Histopathology demonstrates an overall increase in size of the brain, increased GFAP-immunoreactive cells, enlarged hippocampi, and aberrant pyramidal neurons (Uhlmann et al., 2002).

Wong and coworkers recently assessed the efficacy of rapamycin, a compound able to inhibit the mTOR (mammalian target of rapamycin) pathway, in curing epilepsy in this model. They found that early treatment with rapamycin prevented the development of epilepsy and premature death observed in vehicle-treated mice. Late treatment with rapamycin suppressed seizures and prolonged survival in mutated mice that had already developed epilepsy. Correspondingly, rapamycin inhibited the abnormal activation of the mTOR pathway, astrogliosis, and neuronal disorganization, and increased brain size in mutated mice (Zeng et al., 2008).

Progressive myoclonus epilepsy type 1

The progressive myoclonus epilepsies (PMEs) are diseases characterized by tonic–clonic seizures, myoclonic seizures, and progressive neurological dysfunction, including dementia and ataxia (Berkovic et al., 1986). The five major PME types are myoclonic epilepsy and ragged-red fiber disease, Unverricht–Lundborg disease (EPM1), neuronal ceroid lipofuscinosis, sialidosis, and Lafora disease.

EPM1 is an autosomal recessive inherited disorder due to a mutation in a gene that encodes for a protein, cystatin B (CstB), a cysteine protease inhibitor. The onset of symptoms is around 6–15 years of age, and the disorder is characterized by myoclonic and tonic–clonic seizures. In 1998, Pennacchio et al. developed a mouse model of EPM1 by knocking out the cystatin B gene. *Cstb*-deficient mice are developmentally normal and fertile, but develop myoclonic seizures during sleep and mild signs of ataxia at 6 months of age that worsen as the animal ages. This ataxic phenotype is associated with widespread granule cell loss in the cerebellum (Pennacchio et al., 1998). The phenotype resulting from the loss of *Cstb* provides parallels to the human disease resulting from the same genetic lesion. However, there are some differences. The mutant mice do not develop tonic–clonic seizures, show no photosensitivity, display seizures with myoclonus only during sleep, and the spike–wave complexes reported in patients have not been observed in the mutant model. Whether these differences indicate additional contributing factors in humans, or reflect the differences between human and mouse biology, brain development, or a background strain effect, remains to be investigated (Pennacchio et al., 1998).

SUMMARY

Epilepsy accounts for a significant portion of the disease burden worldwide. Research in this field is fundamental and mandatory. Animal models have played, and still play, a substantial role in understanding the pathophysiology and treatment of human epilepsies. A large number and variety of approaches are available, and they have been applied to many animals. In this chapter the *in vitro* and *in vivo* animal models are discussed, with major emphasis on the *in vivo* studies. Models have used phylogenetically different animals – from worms to monkeys. Our attention has been dedicated mainly to rodents.

In clinical practice, developmental aspects of epilepsy often differ from those in adults. Animal models have often helped to clarify these differences. In this chapter, developmental aspects have been emphasized.

Electrical stimulation and chemical-induced models of seizures have been described first, as they represent the oldest and most common models. Among these models, kindling raised great interest, especially for the study of the epileptogenesis. Acquired focal models mimic seizures and occasionally epilepsies secondary to abnormal cortical development, hypoxia, trauma, and hemorrhage.

Better knowledge of epileptic syndromes will help to create new animal models. To date, absence epilepsy is one of the most common and (often) benign forms of epilepsy. There are several models, including acute pharmacological models (PTZ, penicillin, THIP, GBL) and chronic models (GAERS, WAG/Rij). Although atypical absence seizures are less benign, thus needing more investigation, only two models are so far available (AY-9944, MAM–AY). Infantile spasms are an early childhood encephalopathy that is usually associated with a poor outcome. The investigation of this syndrome in animal models is recent and fascinating. Different approaches have been used including genetic (Down syndrome, *ARX* mutation) and acquired (multiple hit, TTX, CRH, betamethasone–NMDA) models.

An entire section has been dedicated to genetic models, from the older models obtained with spontaneous mutations (GEPRs) to the new engineered knockout, knockin, and transgenic models. Some of these models have been created based on recently recognized pathogenesis such as benign familial neonatal epilepsy, early infantile encephalopathy with suppression bursts, severe myoclonic epilepsy of infancy, the tuberous sclerosis model, and the progressive myoclonic epilepsy.

The contribution of animal models to epilepsy research is unquestionable. The development of further strategies is necessary to find novel strategies to cure epileptic patients, and optimistically to allow scientists first and clinicians subsequently to prevent epilepsy and its consequences.

ACKNOWLEDGMENTS

This work was supported by grants NS-20253, NS-43209, NS-45911, and NS-058303 from the National Institute of Neurologic Diseases and Stroke, and grants from Parents Against Childhood Epilepsy, Rett Syndrome Research Foundation, and the Heffer Family Medical Foundation.

REFERENCES

Ackermann RF, Moshé SL, Albala BJ (1989). Restriction of enhanced [2-14 C]deoxyglucose utilization to rhinencephalic structures in immature amygdala-kindled rats. Exp Neurol 104: 73–81.

Albala BJ, Moshé SL, Okada R (1984). Kainic-acid-induced seizures: a developmental study. Brain Res 315: 139–148.

Albertson TE, Stark LG, Peterson SL et al. (1976). The effects of phenobarbital and SC-13504 on the "kindled" seizures of rats. Proc West Pharmacol Soc 19: 204–208.

Albertson TE, Bowyer JF, Paule MG (1982). Modification of the anticonvulsant efficacy of diazepam by Ro-15-1788 in the kindled amygdaloid seizure model. Life Sci 31: 1597–1601.

Andrews PI, McNamara JO (1996). Rasmussen's encephalitis: an autoimmune disorder? Curr Opin Neurobiol 6: 673–678.

Antozzi C, Granata T, Aurisano N et al. (1998). Long-term selective IgG immuno-adsorption improves Rasmussen's encephalitis. Neurology 51: 302–305.

Applegate CD, Burchfiel JL, Konkol RJ (1986). Kindling antagonism: effects of norepinephrine depletion on kindled seizure suppression after concurrent, alternate stimulation in rats. Exp Neurol 94: 379–390.

Asano T, Mizutani A (1980). Brain benzodiazepine receptors and their rapid changes after seizures in the Mongolian gerbil. Jpn J Pharmacol 30: 783–788.

Avoli M (1980). Electroencephalographic and pathophysiologic features of rat parenteral penicillin epilepsy. Exp Neurol 69: 373–382.

Avoli M (1995). Feline generalized penicillin epilepsy. Ital J Neurol Sci 16: 79–82.

Baraban SC (2007). Emerging epilepsy models: insights from mice, flies, worms and fish. Curr Opin Neurol 20: 164–168.

Baraban SC, Schwartzkroin PA (1996). Flurothyl seizure susceptibility in rats following prenatal methylazoxymethanol treatment. Epilepsy Res 23: 189–194.

Baraban SC, Taylor MR, Castro PA et al. (2005). Pentylenetetrazole induced changes in zebrafish behavior, neural activity and c-fos expression. Neuroscience 131: 759–768.

Baram TZ, Schultz L (1991). Corticotropin-releasing hormone is a rapid and potent convulsant in the infant rat. Brain Res Dev Brain Res 61: 97–101.

Baram TZ, Schultz L (1995). ACTH does not control neonatal seizures induced by administration of exogenous corticotropin-releasing hormone. Epilepsia 36: 174–178.

Baram TZ, Hirsch E, Schultz L (1993). Short-interval amygdala kindling in neonatal rats. Brain Res Dev Brain Res 73: 79–83.

Baram TZ, Gerth A, Schultz L (1997). Febrile seizures: an appropriate-aged model suitable for long-term studies. Brain Res Dev Brain Res 98: 265–270.

Baram TZ, Hirsch E, Schultz L (1998). Short interval electrical amygdala kindling in infant rats: the paradigm and its application to the study of age-specific convulsants. In: ME Corcoran, SL Moshé (Eds.), Kindling 5. Vol. 48. Plenum Press, New York, pp. 35–44.

Batini C, Teillet MA, Naquet R (2004). An avian model of genetic reflex epilepsy. Arch Ital Biol 142: 297–312.

Becker HC, Diaz-Granados JL, Weathersby RT (1997). Repeated ethanol withdrawal experience increases the severity and duration of subsequent withdrawal seizures in mice. Alcohol 14: 319–326.

Begley CE, Famulari M, Annegers JF et al. (2000). The cost of epilepsy in the United States: an estimate from population-based clinical and survey data. Epilepsia 41: 342–351.

Benardete EA, Kriegstein AR (2002). Increased excitability and decreased sensitivity to GABA in an animal model of dysplastic cortex. Epilepsia 43: 970–982.

Ben-Ari Y (1985). Limbic seizure and brain damage produced by kainic acid: mechanisms and relevance to human temporal lobe epilepsy. Neuroscience 14: 375–403.

Ben-Ari Y, Tremblay E, Riche D et al. (1981). Electrographic, clinical and pathological alterations following systemic administration of kainic acid, bicuculline or pentetrazole: metabolic mapping using the deoxyglucose method with special reference to the pathology of epilepsy. Neuroscience 6: 1361–1391.

Bender RA, Dubé C, Gonzalez-Vega R et al. (2003). Mossy fiber plasticity and enhanced hippocampal excitability, without hippocampal cell loss or altered neurogenesis, in an animal model of prolonged febrile seizures. Hippocampus 13: 399–412.

Berg AT, Berkovic SF, Brodie MJ et al. (2010). Revised terminology and concepts for organization of seizures and epilepsies: report of the ILAE Commission on Classification and Terminology, 2005–2009. Epilepsia 51: 676–685.

Berghmans S, Hunt J, Roach A et al. (2007). Zebrafish offer the potential for a primary screen to identify a wide variety of potential anticonvulsants. Epilepsy Res 75: 18–28.

Berkovic SF, Andermann F, Carpenter S et al. (1986). Progressive myoclonus epilepsies: specific causes and diagnosis. N Engl J Med 315: 296–305.

Bier E (2005). *Drosophila*, the golden bug, emerges as a tool for human genetics. Nat Rev Genet 6: 9–23.

Blume WT, Lüders HO, Mizrahi E et al. (2001). Glossary of descriptive terminology for ictal semiology: report of the ILAE task force on classification and terminology. Epilepsia 42: 1212–1218.

Bourn WM, Garrett RL (1983). Increased susceptibility of audiogenic rats to barbital withdrawal convulsions. Pharmacol Biochem Behav 19: 839–841.

Brabcova R, Kubova H, Velisek L et al. (1993). Effects of a benzodiazepine, bretazenil (Ro 16-6028), on rhythmic metrazol EEG activity: comparison with standard anticonvulsants. Epilepsia 34: 1135–1140.

Bradford HF (1995). Glutamate, GABA and epilepsy. Prog Neurobiol 47: 477–511.

Brandt C, Potschka H, Loscher W et al. (2003). N-methyl-D-aspartate receptor blockade after status epilepticus protects against limbic brain damage but not against epilepsy in the kainate model of temporal lobe epilepsy. Neuroscience 118: 727–740.

Brener K, Amitai Y, Jefferys JG et al. (1991). Chronic epileptic foci in neocortex: in vivo and in vitro effects of tetanus toxin. Eur J Neurosci 3: 47–54.

Browning RA (1985). Role of the brain-stem reticular formation in tonic–clonic seizures: lesion and pharmacological studies. Fed Proc 44: 2425–2431.

Browning RA, Nelson DK (1985). Variation in threshold and pattern of electroshock-induced seizures in rats depending on site of stimulation. Life Sci 37: 2205–2211.

Browning RA, Wang C, Lanker ML et al. (1990). Electroshock- and pentylenetetrazol-induced seizures in genetically epilepsy-prone rats (GEPRs): differences in threshold and pattern. Epilepsy Res 6: 1–11.

Cain DP, Plant J, Rouleau S et al. (1986). Failure to kindle seizures after repeated intracerebral administration of arginine vasopressin. Life Sci 38: 985–989.

Cantallops I, Haas K, Cline HT (2000). Postsynaptic CPG15 promotes synaptic maturation and presynaptic axon arbor elaboration in vivo. Nat Neurosci 3: 1004–1011.

Capecchi MR (1989a). Altering the genome by homologous recombination. Science 244: 1288–1292.

Capecchi MR (1989b). The new mouse genetics: altering the genome by gene targeting. Trends Genet 5: 70–76.

Cattabeni F, Di Luca M (1997). Developmental models of brain dysfunctions induced by targeted cellular ablations with methylazoxymethanol. Physiol Rev 77: 199–215.

Cavalheiro EA (1995). The pilocarpine model of epilepsy. Ital J Neurol Sci 16: 33–37.

Cavalheiro EA, Riche DA, Le Gal La Salle G (1982). Long-term effects of intrahippocampal kainic acid injection in rats: a method for inducing spontaneous recurrent seizures. Electroencephalogr Clin Neurophysiol 53: 581–589.

Cavalheiro EA, Silva DF, Turski WA et al. (1987). The susceptibility of rats to pilocarpine-induced seizures is age-dependent. Brain Res 465: 43–58.

Cavazos JE, Jones SM, Cross DJ (2004). Sprouting and synaptic reorganization in the subiculum and CA1 region of the hippocampus in acute and chronic models of partial-onset epilepsy. Neuroscience 126: 677–688.

Chachua T, Yum MS, Velíšková J et al. (2011). Validation of the rat model of cryptogenic infantile spasms. Epilepsia 52: 1666–1677.

Chen Y, Jungsuwadee P, Vore M et al. (2007). Collateral damage in cancer chemotherapy: oxidative stress in nontargeted tissues. Mol Interv 7: 147–156.

Chevassus-Au-Louis N, Rafiki A, Jorquera I et al. (1998). Neocortex in the hippocampus: an anatomical and functional study of CA1 heterotopias after prenatal treatment with methylazoxymethanol in rats. J Comp Neurol 394: 520–536.

Coenen AM, Van Luijtelaar EL (1987). The WAG/Rij rat model for absence epilepsy: age and sex factors. Epilepsy Res 1: 297–301.

Coffey LL, Reith ME, Chen NH et al. (1996). Amygdala kindling of forebrain seizures and the occurrence of brainstem seizures in genetically epilepsy-prone rats. Epilepsia 37: 188–197.

Colacitti C, Sancini G, Franceschetti S et al. (1998). Altered connections between neocortical and heterotopic areas in methylazoxymethanol-treated rat. Epilepsy Res 32: 49–62.

Colacitti C, Sancini G, DeBiasi S et al. (1999). Prenatal methylazoxymethanol treatment in rats produces brain abnormalities with morphological similarities to human developmental brain dysgeneses. J Neuropathol Exp Neurol 58: 92–106.

Commission on Classification and Terminology of the International League Against Epilepsy (1981). Proposal for revised clinical and electroencephalographic classification of epileptic seizures. Epilepsia 22: 489–501.

Corda MG, Orlandi M, Lecca D et al. (1991). Pentylenetetrazol-induced kindling in rats: effect of GABA function inhibitors. Pharmacol Biochem Behav 40: 329–333.

Cortez MA, Snead PC (2006). Pharmacologic models of generalized absence seizures in rodents. In: A Pitkänen, PA Schwartzkroin, SL Moshé (Eds.), Models of Seizures and Epilepsy. Elsevier Academic Press, Burlington, MA, pp. 111–126.

Cortez MA, McKerlie C, Snead OC, 3rd (2001). A model of atypical absence seizures: EEG, pharmacology, and developmental characterization. Neurology 56: 341–349.

Cortez MA, Shen L, Wu Y et al. (2009). Infantile spasms and Down syndrome: a new animal model. Pediatr Res 65: 499–503.

Cowen D, Geller LM (1960). Long-term pathological effects of prenatal x-irradiation on the central nervous system of the rat. J Neuropathol Exp Neurol 19: 488–527.

Crino PB, Nathanson KL, Henske EP (2006). The tuberous sclerosis complex. N Engl J Med 355: 1345–1356.

D'Agostino MD, Bernasconi A, Das S et al. (2002). Subcortical band heterotopia (SBH) in males: clinical, imaging and genetic findings in comparison with females. Brain 125: 2507–2522.

de Feo MR, Mecarelli O, Ricci GF (1985). Bicuculline- and allylglycine-induced epilepsy in developing rats. Exp Neurol 90: 411–421.

de Feo MR, Mecarelli O, Ricci GF (1995). Seizure susceptibility in immature rats with micrencephaly induced by prenatal exposure to methylazoxymethanol acetate. Pharmacol Res 31: 109–114.

De Sarro A, De Sarro GB (1991). Responsiveness of genetically epilepsy-prone rats to aminophylline-induced seizures and interactions with quinolones. Neuropharmacology 30: 169–176.

Donadio MF, Kozlowski PB, Kaplan H et al. (1982). Brain vasculature and induced ischemia in seizure-prone and non-seizure-prone gerbils. Brain Res 234: 263–273.

Drinkenburg WH, van Luijtelaar EL, van Schaijk WJ et al. (1993). Aberrant transients in the EEG of epileptic rats: a spectral analytical approach. Physiol Behav 54: 779–783.

Dubé C, Chen K, Eghbal-Ahmadi M et al. (2000). Prolonged febrile seizures in the immature rat model enhance hippocampal excitability long term. Ann Neurol 47: 336–344.

Dubé C, Chen K, Eghbal-Ahmadi M et al. (2004). Serial MRI after experimental febrile seizures: altered T2 signal without neuronal death. Ann Neurol 56: 709–714.

Dubé CM, Ravizza T, Hamamura M et al. (2010). Epileptogenesis provoked by prolonged experimental febrile seizures: mechanisms and biomarkers. J Neurosci 30: 7484–7494.

Dulac O, Jallon P (1997). Patterns of care for patients with epilepsy in France. Neurology 48: S30–S32.

Dulac O, Soufflet C, Chiron C et al. (2002). What is West syndrome? Int Rev Neurobiol 49: 1–22.

Dutuit M, Didier-Bazes M, Vergnes M et al. (2000). Specific alteration in the expression of glial fibrillary acidic protein, glutamate dehydrogenase, and glutamine synthetase in rats with genetic absence epilepsy. Glia 32: 15–24.

Dvorak K, Feit J (1977). Migration of neuroblasts through partial necrosis of the cerebral cortex in newborn rats–contribution to the problems of morphological development and developmental period of cerebral microgyria. Histological and autoradiographical study. Acta Neuropathol (Berl) 38: 203–212.

Dyer RS, Swartzwelder HS, Eccles CU et al. (1979). Hippocampal afterdischarges and their post-ictal sequelae in rats: a potential tool for assessment of CNS neurotoxicity. Neurobehav Toxicol 1: 5–19.

Elmer E, Kokaia M, Kokaia Z et al. (1998). Epileptogenesis induced by rapidly recurring seizures in genetically fast- but not slow-kindling rats. Brain Res 789: 111–117.

Engel J Jr (2001) A proposed diagnostic scheme for people with epileptic seizures and with epilepsy: report of the ILAE Task Force on Classification and Terminology. Epilepsia 42: 796–803.

Estrada E, Peña A (2000). In silico studies for the rational discovery of anticonvulsant compounds. Bioorg Med Chem 8: 2755–2770.

Fariello RG, Golden GT (1987). The THIP-induced model of bilateral synchronous spike and wave in rodents. Neuropharmacology 26: 161–165.

Ferrer I, Alcantara S, Catala I et al. (1993). Experimentally induced laminar necrosis, status verrucosus, focal cortical dysplasia reminiscent of microgyria, and porencephaly in the rat. Exp Brain Res 94: 261–269.

Finnerty GT, Jefferys JG (2000). 9–16 Hz oscillation precedes secondary generalization of seizures in the rat tetanus toxin model of epilepsy. J Neurophysiol 83: 2217–2226.

Fischer-Williams M, Poncet M, Riche DM et al. (1968). Light-induced epilepsy in the baboon, *Papio papio*: cortical and depth recordings. Electroencephalogr Clin Neurophysiol 25: 557–569.

Fisher RS (1989). Animal models of the epilepsies. Brain Res Brain Res Rev 14: 245–278.

Fisher RS, Prince DA (1977). Spike–wave rhythms in cat cortex induced by parenteral penicillin. II. Cellular features. Electroencephalogr Clin Neurophysiol 42: 625–639.

Fisher RS, van Emde Boas W, Blume W et al. (2005). Epileptic seizures and epilepsy: definitions proposed by the International League Against Epilepsy (ILAE) and the International Bureau for Epilepsy (IBE). Epilepsia 46: 470–472.

Franck JE, Ginter KL, Schwartzkroin PA (1989). Developing genetically epilepsy-prone rats have an abnormal seizure response to flurothyl. Epilepsia 30: 1–6.

Galdzicki Z, Siarey RJ (2003). Understanding mental retardation in Down's syndrome using trisomy 16 mouse models. Genes Brain Behav 2: 167–178.

Galvan CD, Hrachovy RA, Smith KL et al. (2000). Blockade of neuronal activity during hippocampal development produces a chronic focal epilepsy in the rat. J Neurosci 20: 2904–2916.

Galvan CD, Hrachovy RA, Smith KL et al. (2003). Postsynaptic contributions to hippocampal network hyperexcitability induced by chronic activity blockade in vivo. Eur J Neurosci 18: 1861–1872.

Ganetzky B (2000). Genetic analysis of ion channel dysfunction in *Drosophila*. Kidney Int 57: 766–771.

George G, Mellanby J (1982). Memory deficits in an experimental hippocampal epileptiform syndrome in rats. Exp Neurol 75: 678–689.

Germano IM, Sperber EF (1997). Increased seizure susceptibility in adult rats with neuronal migration disorders. Brain Res 777: 219–222.

Giorgi FS, Malhotra S, Hasson H et al. (2005). Effects of status epilepticus early in life on susceptibility to ischemic injury in adulthood. Epilepsia 46: 490–498.

Goddard GV, McIntyre DC, Leech CK (1969). A permanent change in brain function resulting from daily electrical stimulation. Exp Neurol 25: 295–330.

Guerrini R, Sicca F, Parmeggiani L (2003). Epilepsy and malformations of the cerebral cortex. Epileptic Disord 5: S9–S26.

Gurkoff GG, Giza CC, Shin D et al. (2009). Acute neuroprotection to pilocarpine-induced seizures is not sustained after traumatic brain injury in the developing rat. Neuroscience 164: 862–876.

Haas KZ, Sperber EF, Moshé SL (1990). Kindling in developing animals: expression of severe seizures and enhanced development of bilateral foci. Brain Res Dev Brain Res 56: 275–280.

Haas K, Li J, Cline HT (2006). AMPA receptors regulate experience-dependent dendritic arbor growth in vivo. Proc Natl Acad Sci U S A 103: 12127–12131.

Hallas BH, Das GD (1978). N-ethyl-N-nitrosourea-induced teratogenesis of brain in the rat. A cellular and cytoarchitectural analysis of the neocortex. J Neurol Sci 39: 111–122.

Hamdan FF, Piton A, Gauthier J et al. (2009). De novo STXBP1 mutations in mental retardation and nonsyndromic epilepsy. Ann Neurol 65: 748–753.

Hauser WA, Annegers JF (1991). Risk factors for epilepsy. Epilepsy Res Suppl 4: 45–52.

He XP, Patel M, Whitney KD et al. (1998). Glutamate receptor GluR3 antibodies and death of cortical cells. Neuron 20: 153–163.

Hewapathirane DS, Dunfield D, Yen W et al. (2008). In vivo imaging of seizure activity in a novel developmental seizure model. Exp Neurol 211: 480–488.

Hirose S, Mitsudome A (2003). X-linked mental retardation and epilepsy: pathogenetic significance of ARX mutations. Brain Dev 25: 161–165.

Holmes GL, Weber DA (1984). The effect of progesterone on kindling: a developmental study. Brain Res 318: 45–53.

Holmes GL, Weber DA (1986). Effects of ACTH on seizure susceptibility in the developing brain. Ann Neurol 20: 82–88.

Ishimoto T, Omori N, Mutoh F et al. (2000). Convulsive seizures induced by N-methyl-D-aspartate microinjection into the mesencephalic reticular formation in rats. Brain Res 881: 152–158.

Jacobs KM, Gutnick MJ, Prince DA (1996). Hyperexcitability in a model of cortical maldevelopment. Cereb Cortex 6: 514–523.

Jefferys JG, Borck C, Mellanby J (1995). Chronic focal epilepsy induced by intracerebral tetanus toxin. Ital J Neurol Sci 16: 27–32.

Jensen FE, Applegate CD, Holtzman D et al. (1991). Epileptogenic effect of hypoxia in the immature rodent brain. Ann Neurol 29: 629–637.

Jensen FE, Holmes GL, Lombroso CT et al. (1992). Age-dependent changes in long-term seizure susceptibility and behavior after hypoxia in rats. Epilepsia 33: 971–980.

Jensen FE, Firkusny IR, Mower GD (1993). Differences in c-fos immunoreactivity due to age and mode of seizure induction. Brain Res Mol Brain Res 17: 185–193.

Jensen FE, Blume H, Alvarado S et al. (1995). NBQX blocks acute and late epileptogenic effects of perinatal hypoxia. Epilepsia 36: 966–972.

Jobe PC, Picchioni AL, Chin L (1973). Role of brain norepinephrine in audiogenic seizure in the rat. J Pharmacol Exp Ther 184: 1–10.

Jobe PC, Mishra PK, Adams-Curtis LE et al. (1995). The genetically epilepsy-prone rat (GEPR). Ital J Neurol Sci 16: 91–99.

Jurgen Wenzel H, Born DE, Dubach MF et al. (2000). Morphological plasticity in an infant monkey model of temporal lobe epilepsy. Epilepsia 41: S70–S75.

Kabova R, Liptakova S, Slamberova R et al. (1999). Age-specific N-methyl-D-aspartate-induced seizures: perspectives for the West syndrome model. Epilepsia 40: 1357–1369.

Kellinghaus C, Kunieda T, Ying Z et al. (2004). Severity of histopathologic abnormalities and in vivo epileptogenicity in the in utero radiation model of rats is dose dependent. Epilepsia 45: 583–591.

Kiesmann M, Marescaux C, Vergnes M et al. (1988). Audiogenic seizures in Wistar rats before and after repeated auditory stimuli: clinical, pharmacological, and electroencephalographic studies. J Neural Transm 72: 235–244.

Killam KF, Killam EK, Naquet R (1966). Study of responses evoked by intermittent light stimulation in monkeys presenting paroxysmal responses to this type of stimulation. Rev Neurol (Paris) 115: 422–423.

Kitamura K, Yanazawa M, Sugiyama N et al. (2002). Mutation of ARX causes abnormal development of forebrain and testes in mice and X-linked lissencephaly with abnormal genitalia in humans. Nat Genet 32: 359–369.

Koh S, Jensen FE (2001). Topiramate blocks perinatal hypoxia-induced seizures in rat pups. Ann Neurol 50: 366–372.

Kostopoulos GK (2000). Spike-and-wave discharges of absence seizures as a transformation of sleep spindles: the continuing development of a hypothesis. Clin Neurophysiol 111: S27–S38.

Kubova H, Druga R, Lukasiuk K et al. (2001). Status epilepticus causes necrotic damage in the mediodorsal nucleus of the thalamus in immature rats. J Neurosci 21: 3593–3599.

Kurtz BS, Lehman J, Garlick P et al. (2001). Penetrance and expressivity of genes involved in the development of epilepsy in the genetically epilepsy-prone rat (GEPR). J Neurogenet 15: 233–244.

Lado FA, Moshé SL (2002). Role of subcortical structures in the pathogenesis of infantile spasms: what are possible subcortical mediators? Int Rev Neurobiol 49: 115–140.

Lado FA, Sperber EF, Moshé SL (2001). Anticonvulsant efficacy of gabapentin on kindling in the immature brain. Epilepsia 42: 458–463.

Lee CL, Hrachovy RA, Smith KL et al. (1995). Tetanus toxin-induced seizures in infant rats and their effects on hippocampal excitability in adulthood. Brain Res 677: 97–109.

Lee KS, Schottler F, Collins JL et al. (1997). A genetic animal model of human neocortical heterotopia associated with seizures. J Neurosci 17: 6236–6242.

Lockard JS (1980). A primate model of clinical epilepsy: mechanisms of action through quantification of therapeutic effects. In: JS Lockard, AA Ward (Eds.), Epilepsy: A Window to Brain Mechanisms. Raven Press, New York, pp. 11–49.

Loscher W (1984). Genetic animal models of epilepsy as a unique resource for the evaluation of anticonvulsant drugs. A review. Methods Find Exp Clin Pharmacol 6: 531–547.

Loscher W (1985). Influence of pharmacological manipulation of inhibitory and excitatory neurotransmitter systems on seizure behavior in the Mongolian gerbil. J Pharmacol Exp Ther 233: 204–213.

Loscher W (1987). Hippocampal glutamate decarboxylase activity is not altered in gerbils with high seizure susceptibility. Biochem Pharmacol 36: 979–982.

Loscher W (1997). Animal models of intractable epilepsy. Prog Neurobiol 53: 239–258.

Loscher W, Frey HH (1984). Evaluation of anticonvulsant drugs in gerbils with reflex epilepsy. Arzneimittelforschung 34: 1484–1488.

Loscher W, Schmidt D (1988). Which animal models should be used in the search for new antiepileptic drugs? A proposal based on experimental and clinical considerations. Epilepsy Res 2: 145–181.

Ludvig N, Moshé SL (1988). Deep prepiriform cortex lesion and development of amygdala kindling. Epilepsia 29: 401–403.

Ludvig N, Moshé SL (1989). Different behavioral and electrographic effects of acoustic stimulation and dibutyryl cyclic AMP injection into the inferior colliculus in normal and in genetically epilepsy-prone rats. Epilepsy Res 3: 185–190.

Mares P, Velisek L (1992). N-methyl-D-aspartate (NMDA)-induced seizures in developing rats. Brain Res Dev Brain Res 65: 185–189.

Mares P, Maresova D, Schickerova R (1981). Effect of antiepileptic drugs on metrazol convulsions during ontogenesis in the rat. Physiol Bohemoslov 30: 113–121.

Mares P, Folbergrova J, Langmeier M et al. (1997). Convulsant action of D, L-homocysteic acid and its stereoisomers in immature rats. Epilepsia 38: 767–776.

Marescaux C, Micheletti G, Vergnes M et al. (1984). A model of chronic spontaneous petit mal-like seizures in the rat: comparison with pentylenetetrazol-induced seizures. Epilepsia 25: 326–331.

Marin-Padilla M, Tsai RJ, King MA et al. (2003). Altered corticogenesis and neuronal morphology in irradiation-induced cortical dysplasia: a Golgi–Cox study. J Neuropathol Exp Neurol 62: 1129–1143.

Marsh E, Fulp C, Gomez E et al. (2009). Targeted loss of Arx results in a developmental epilepsy mouse model and recapitulates the human phenotype in heterozygous females. Brain 132: 1563–1576.

Mason CR, Cooper RM (1972). A permanent change in convulsive threshold in normal and brain-damaged rats with repeated small doses of pentylenetetrazol. Epilepsia 13: 663–674.

Matsumoto H, Ajmonemarsan C (1964). Cellular mechanisms in experimental epileptic seizures. Science 144: 193–194.

McDonald JW, Shapiro SM, Silverstein FS et al. (1998). Role of glutamate receptor-mediated excitotoxicity in bilirubin-induced brain injury in the Gunn rat model. Exp Neurol 150: 21–29.

McGrath JJ, Riggs HE, Schwarz HP (1956). Malformation of the adult brain (albino rat) resulting from prenatal irradiation. J Neuropathol Exp Neurol 15: 432–446.

McIntosh TK, Vink R, Noble L et al. (1989). Traumatic brain injury in the rat: characterization of a lateral fluid-percussion model. Neuroscience 28: 233–244.

McIntyre DC (1970). Differential amnestic effect of cortical vs. amygdaloid elicited convulsions in rats. Physiol Behav 5: 747–753.

McIntyre DC, Kelly ME, Dufresne C (1999). FAST and SLOW amygdala kindling rat strains: comparison of amygdala, hippocampal, piriform and perirhinal cortex kindling. Epilepsy Res 35: 197–209.

McNamara JO, Wada JA (1997). Kindling model. In: J Engel, T Pedley (Eds.), Epilepsy: A Comprehensive Textbook. Lippincott-Raven, Philadelphia, pp. 419–425.

Meldrum BS (1986). Neuropathological consequences of chemically and electrically induced seizures. Ann N Y Acad Sci 462: 186–193.

Mellanby J, George G, Robinson A et al. (1977). Epileptiform syndrome in rats produced by injecting tetanus toxin into the hippocampus. J Neurol Neurosurg Psychiatry 40: 404–414.

Menini C, Silva-Barrat C (1990). Value of the monkey *Papio papio* for the study of epilepsy. Pathol Biol (Paris) 38: 205–213.

Micheletti G, Vergnes M, Marescaux C et al. (1985). Antiepileptic drug evaluation in a new animal model: spontaneous petit mal epilepsy in the rat. Arzneimittelforschung 35: 483–485.

Midzianovskaia IS, Kuznetsova GD, Coenen AM et al. (2001). Electrophysiological and pharmacological characteristics of two types of spike–wave discharges in WAG/Rij rats. Brain Res 911: 62–70.

Millan MH, Wardley-Smith B, Durmuller N et al. (1991). The high pressure neurological syndrome in genetically epilepsy prone rats: protective effect of 2-amino-7-phosphono heptanoate. Exp Neurol 112: 317–320.

Miller LP, Johnson AE, Gelhard RE et al. (1990). The ontogeny of excitatory amino acid receptors in the rat forebrain – II. Kainic acid receptors. Neuroscience 35: 45–51.

Mishra PK, Dailey JW, Reigel CE et al. (1988). Brain norepinephrine and convulsions in the genetically epilepsy-prone rat: sex-dependent responses to Ro 4-1284 treatment. Life Sci 42: 1131–1137.

Mishra PK, Dailey JW, Reigel CE et al. (1989). Audiogenic convulsions in moderate seizure genetically epilepsy-prone rats (GEPR-3s). Epilepsy Res 3: 191–198.

Mitchell J, Gatherer M, Sundstrom LE (1996). Aberrant Timm-stained fibres in the dentate gyrus following tetanus toxin-induced seizures in the rat. Neuropathol Appl Neurobiol 22: 129–135.

Mody I, Schwartzkroin PA (1997). Acute seizure models (intact animals). In: J Engel, T Pedley (Eds.), Epilepsy: A Comprehensive Textbook. Lippincott-Raven, Philadelphia, pp. 397–404.

Moraes MF, Mishra PK, Jobe PC et al. (2005). An electrographic analysis of the synchronous discharge patterns of GEPR-9s generalized seizures. Brain Res 1046: 1–9.

Moshé SL (1981). The effects of age on the kindling phenomenon. Dev Psychobiol 14: 75–81.

Moshé SL (1987). Epileptogenesis and the immature brain. Epilepsia 28: S3–S15.

Moshé SL, Albala BJ (1983). Maturational changes in postictal refractoriness and seizure susceptibility in developing rats. Ann Neurol 13: 552–557.

Moshé SL, Sharpless NS, Kaplan J (1981). Kindling in developing rats: variability of afterdischarge thresholds with age. Brain Res 211: 190–195.

Nadler JV (1981). Minireview. Kainic acid as a tool for the study of temporal lobe epilepsy. Life Sci 29: 2031–2042.

Nadler JV, Perry BW, Gentry C et al. (1980). Degeneration of hippocampal CA3 pyramidal cells induced by intraventricular kainic acid. J Comp Neurol 192: 333–359.

Nehlig A, Pereira de Vasconcelos A (1996). The model of pentylenetetrazol-induced status epilepticus in the immature rat: short- and long-term effects. Epilepsy Res 26: 93–103.

Nilsen KE, Walker MC, Cock HR (2005). Characterization of the tetanus toxin model of refractory focal neocortical epilepsy in the rat. Epilepsia 46: 179–187.

Noebels JL (2006). Spontaneous epileptic mutation in the mouse. In: A Pitkänen, PA Schwartzkroin, SL Moshé (Eds.), Models of Seizures and Epilepsy. Elsevier Academic Press, Burlington, MA, pp. 223–232.

Noebels JL, Pedley TA (1977). Anatomic localization of topically applied [^{14}C]penicillin during experimental focal epilepsy in cat neocortex. Brain Res 125: 293–303.

Olson JE, Scher MS, Holtzman D (1984). Effects of anticonvulsants on hyperthermia-induced seizures in the rat pup. Epilepsia 25: 96–99.

Ono J, Vieth RF, Walson PD (1990). Electrocorticographical observation of seizures induced by pentylenetetrazol (PTZ) injection in rats. Funct Neurol 5: 345–352.

Panayiotopoulos CP (1999). Typical absence seizures and their treatment. Arch Dis Child 81: 351–355.

Paredes M, Pleasure SJ, Baraban SC (2006). Embryonic and early postnatal abnormalities contributing to the development of hippocampal malformations in a rodent model of dysplasia. J Comp Neurol 495: 133–148.

Pennacchio LA, Bouley DM, Higgins KM et al. (1998). Progressive ataxia, myoclonic epilepsy and cerebellar apoptosis in cystatin B-deficient mice. Nat Genet 20: 251–258.

Pilz DT, Matsumoto N, Minnerath S et al. (1998). LIS1 and XLIS (DCX) mutations cause most classical lissencephaly, but different patterns of malformation. Hum Mol Genet 7: 2029–2037.

Pinel JP, Rovner LI (1978). Experimental epileptogenesis: kindling-induced epilepsy in rats. Exp Neurol 58: 190–202.

Pohl M, Mares P (1987). Effects of flunarizine on metrazol-induced seizures in developing rats. Epilepsy Res 1: 302–305.

Poirier K, Eisermann M, Caubel I et al. (2008). Combination of infantile spasms, non-epileptic seizures and complex movement disorder: a new case of ARX-related epilepsy. Epilepsy Res 80: 224–228.

Price MG, Yoo JW, Burgess DL et al. (2009). A triplet repeat expansion genetic mouse model of infantile spasms syndrome, Arx(GCG)10 + 7, with interneuronopathy, spasms in infancy, persistent seizures, and adult cognitive and behavioral impairment. J Neurosci 29: 8752–8763.

Rachidi M, Lopes C (2008). Mental retardation and associated neurological dysfunctions in Down syndrome: a consequence of dysregulation in critical chromosome 21 genes and associated molecular pathways. Eur J Paediatr Neurol 12: 168–182.

Racine RJ (1972). Modification of seizure activity by electrical stimulation. II. Motor seizure. Electroencephalogr Clin Neurophysiol 32: 281–294.

Racine R (1978). Kindling: the first decade. Neurosurgery 3: 234–252.

Racine RJ, Burnham WM, Gartner JG et al. (1973). Rates of motor seizure development in rats subjected to electrical brain stimulation: strain and inter-stimulation interval effects. Electroencephalogr Clin Neurophysiol 35: 553–556.

Racine R, Rose PA, Burnham WM (1977). Afterdischarge thresholds and kindling rates in dorsal and ventral hippocampus and dentate gyrus. Can J Neurol Sci 4: 273–278.

Reid CA, Kim TH, Berkovic SF et al. (2011). Low blood glucose precipitates spike-and-wave activity in genetically predisposed animals. Epilepsia 52: 115–120.

Ribak CE, Seress L, Weber P et al. (1998). Alumina gel injections into the temporal lobe of rhesus monkeys cause complex partial seizures and morphological changes found in human temporal lobe epilepsy. J Comp Neurol 401: 266–290.

Riikonen R (2001). Long-term outcome of patients with West syndrome. Brain Dev 23: 683–687.

Roberts MR, Bittman K, Li WW et al. (2000). The flathead mutation causes CNS-specific developmental abnormalities and apoptosis. J Neurosci 20: 2295–2306.

Rodier PM (1990). Developmental neurotoxicology. Toxicol Pathol 18: 89–95.

Rogers SW, Andrews PI, Gahring LC et al. (1994). Autoantibodies to glutamate receptor GluR3 in Rasmussen's encephalitis. Science 265: 648–651.

Roper SN (1998). In utero irradiation of rats as a model of human cerebrocortical dysgenesis: a review. Epilepsy Res 32: 63–74.

Roux E, Borrell A (1989). Tétanos cérébral et innunité contre le tétanos. Annal de l''institut Pasteur 4: 126–138.

Saitsu H, Kato M, Mizuguchi T et al. (2008). De novo mutations in the gene encoding STXBP1 (MUNC18-1) cause early infantile epileptic encephalopathy. Nat Genet 40: 782–788.

Sanchez AL, Matthews BJ, Meynard MM et al. (2006). BDNF increases synapse density in dendrites of developing tectal neurons in vivo. Development 133: 2477–2486.

Sarkisian MR, Rattan S, D'Mello SR et al. (1999). Characterization of seizures in the flathead rat: a new genetic model of epilepsy in early postnatal development. Epilepsia 40: 394–400.

Sarkisian MR, Li W, Di Cunto F et al. (2002). Citron-kinase, a protein essential to cytokinesis in neuronal progenitors, is deleted in the flathead mutant rat. J Neurosci 22: RC217.

Scantlebury MH, Ouellet PL, Psarropoulou C et al. (2004). Freeze lesion-induced focal cortical dysplasia predisposes to atypical hyperthermic seizures in the immature rat. Epilepsia 45: 592–600.

Scantlebury MH, Gibbs SA, Foadjo B et al. (2005). Febrile seizures in the predisposed brain: a new model of temporal lobe epilepsy. Ann Neurol 58: 41–49.

Scantlebury MH, Galanopoulou AS, Chudomelova L et al. (2010). A model of symptomatic infantile spasms syndrome. Neurobiol Dis 37: 604–612.

Schiavo G, Poulain B, Rossetto O et al. (1992). Tetanus toxin is a zinc protein and its inhibition of neurotransmitter release and protease activity depend on zinc. EMBO J 11: 3577–3583.

Schreiber RA, Graham JM Jr (1976). Audiogenic priming in DBA/2 J and C57BL/6 J mice: interactions among age, prime-to-test interval and index of seizure. Dev Psychobiol 9: 57–66.

Scorza FA, de Albuquerque R, Arida RM et al. (2009). Could sudden death syndrome (SDS) in chickens (*Gallus gallus*) be a valid animal model for sudden unexpected death in epilepsy (SUDEP)? Med Hypotheses 73: 67–69.

Serbanescu I, Cortez MA, McKerlie C et al. (2004). Refractory atypical absence seizures in rat: a two hit model. Epilepsy Res 62: 53–63.

Sharma HS, Winkler T, Stalberg E et al. (2000). p-Chlorophenylalanine, an inhibitor of serotonin synthesis reduces blood–brain barrier permeability, cerebral blood flow, edema formation and cell injury following trauma to the rat brain. Acta Neurochir Suppl 76: 91–95.

Shouse MN, King A, Langer J et al. (1990). The ontogeny of feline temporal lobe epilepsy: kindling a spontaneous seizure disorder in kittens. Brain Res 525: 215–224.

Shouse MN, Scordato JC, Farber PR (2004). Sleep and arousal mechanisms in experimental epilepsy: epileptic components of NREM and antiepileptic components of REM sleep. Ment Retard Dev Disabil Res Rev 10: 117–121.

Sillanpaa M, Shinnar S (2010). Long-term mortality in childhood-onset epilepsy. N Engl J Med 363: 2522–2529.

Snead OC, 3rd (1978). Gamma hydroxybutyrate in the monkey. I. Electroencephalographic, behavioral, and pharmacokinetic studies. Neurology 28: 636–642.

Snead OC, 3rd (1988). gamma-Hydroxybutyrate model of generalized absence seizures: further characterization and comparison with other absence models. Epilepsia 29: 361–368.

Snead OC, 3rd (1991). The gamma-hydroxybutyrate model of absence seizures: correlation of regional brain levels of gamma-hydroxybutyric acid and gamma-butyrolactone with spike wave discharges. Neuropharmacology 30: 161–167.

Snead OC, 3rd (1992). Pharmacological models of generalized absence seizures in rodents. J Neural Transm Suppl 35: 7–19.

Song J, Tanouye MA (2008). From bench to drug: human seizure modeling using *Drosophila*. Prog Neurobiol 84: 182–191.

Sperber EF, Moshé SL (1988). Age-related differences in seizure susceptibility to flurothyl. Brain Res 467: 295–297.

Sperber EF, Haas KZ, Romero MT et al. (1999a). Flurothyl status epilepticus in developing rats: behavioral, electrographic, histological and electrophysiological studies. Brain Res Dev Brain Res 116: 59–68.

Sperber EF, Veliskova J, Germano IM et al. (1999b). Age-dependent vulnerability to seizures. Adv Neurol 79: 161–169.

Sperk G (1994). Kainic acid seizures in the rat. Prog Neurobiol 42: 1–32.

Stafstrom CE (2009). Infantile spasms: a critical review of emerging animal models. Epilepsy Curr 9: 75–81.

Stafstrom CE, Konkol RJ (1994). Infantile spasms in children with Down syndrome. Dev Med Child Neurol 36: 576–585.

Stoffel M, Rinecker M, Plesnila N et al. (2001). Role of nitric oxide in the secondary expansion of a cortical brain lesion from cold injury. J Neurotrauma 18: 425–434.

Strzelczyk A, Reese JP, Dodel R et al. (2008). Cost of epilepsy: a systematic review. Pharmacoeconomics 26: 463–476.

Sutula T, He XX, Cavazos J et al. (1988). Synaptic reorganization in the hippocampus induced by abnormal functional activity. Science 239: 1147–1150.

Tamaru M, Hirata Y, Nagayoshi M et al. (1988). Brain changes in rats induced by prenatal injection of methylazoxymethanol. Teratology 37: 149–157.

Tan HO, Reid CA, Single FN et al. (2007). Reduced cortical inhibition in a mouse model of familial childhood absence epilepsy. Proc Natl Acad Sci U S A 104: 17536–17541.

Taylor SM, Jones PA (1979). Multiple new phenotypes induced in 10 T1/2 and 3 T3 cells treated with 5-azacytidine. Cell 17: 771–779.

Thiessen DD, Friend HC, Lindzey G (1968). Androgen control of territorial marking in the Mongolian gerbil. Science 160: 432–434.

Thompson HJ, Lifshitz J, Marklund N et al. (2005). Lateral fluid percussion brain injury: a 15-year review and evaluation. J Neurotrauma 22: 42–75.

Titus SA, Warmke JW, Ganetzky B (1997). The *Drosophila* erg K^+ channel polypeptide is encoded by the seizure locus. J Neurosci 17: 875–881.

Toth Z, Yan XX, Haftoglou S et al. (1998). Seizure-induced neuronal injury: vulnerability to febrile seizures in an immature rat model. J Neurosci 18: 4285–4294.

Trindade-Filho EM, de Castro-Neto EF, de Carvalho RA et al. (2008). Serotonin depletion effects on the pilocarpine model of epilepsy. Epilepsy Res 82: 194–199.

Tuchman R, Moshé SL, Rapin I (2009). Convulsing toward the pathophysiology of autism. Brain Dev 31: 95–103.

Turski L, Ikonomidou C, Turski WA et al. (1989). Review: cholinergic mechanisms and epileptogenesis. The seizures induced by pilocarpine: a novel experimental model of intractable epilepsy. Synapse 3: 154–171.

Ueda Y, Willmore LJ (2000). Hippocampal gamma-aminobutyric acid transporter alterations following focal epileptogenesis induced in rat amygdala. Brain Res Bull 52: 357–361.

Uhlmann EJ, Wong M, Baldwin RL et al. (2002). Astrocyte-specific TSC1 conditional knockout mice exhibit abnormal neuronal organization and seizures. Ann Neurol 52: 285–296.

van Luijtelaar EL, Coenen AM (1986). Two types of electrocortical paroxysms in an inbred strain of rats. Neurosci Lett 70: 393–397.

Velisek L (2006). Models of chemically-induced acute seizures. In: A Pitkänen, PA Schwartzkroin, SL Moshé (Eds.), Models of Seizures and Epilepsy. Elsevier Academic Press, Burlington, MA, pp. 127–152.

Velisek L (2008). Age, sex, and hormonal status can be additional variables in prenatal dexamethasone exposure. Neurosci Res 61: 333–334.

Velisek L, Mares P (1995). Age-dependent anticonvulsant action of clonazepam in the N-methyl-D-aspartate model of seizures. Pharmacol Biochem Behav 52: 291–296.

Velisek L, Kubova H, Pohl M et al. (1992). Pentylenetetrazol-induced seizures in rats: an ontogenetic study. Naunyn Schmiedebergs Arch Pharmacol 346: 588–591.

Velisek L, Jehle K, Asche S et al. (2007). Model of infantile spasms induced by N-methyl-D-aspartic acid in prenatally impaired brain. Ann Neurol 61: 109–119.

Velisek L, Chachua T, Yum MS et al. (2010). Model of cryptogenic infantile spasms after prenatal corticosteroid priming. Epilepsia 51: 145–149.

Veliskova J (2006). Behavioral characterization of seizures in rats. In: A Pitkänen, PA Schwartzkroin, SL Moshé (Eds.), Models of Seizures and Epilepsy. Elsevier Academic Press, Burlington, MA, pp. 601–611.

Veliskova J, Velisek LS (1992). Picrotoxin-induced tonic–clonic seizures and lethality are decreased by MK-801 in developing rats. Pharmacol Biochem Behav 43: 291–295.

Veliskova J, Velisek L, Mares P et al. (1990). Ketamine suppresses both bicuculline- and picrotoxin-induced generalized tonic-clonic seizures during ontogenesis. Pharmacol Biochem Behav 37: 667–674.

Veliskova J, Miller AM, Nunes ML et al. (2005). Regional neural activity within the substantia nigra during peri-ictal flurothyl generalized seizure stages. Neurobiol Dis 20: 752–759.

Vergnes M, Marescaux C, Micheletti G et al. (1982). Spontaneous paroxysmal electroclinical patterns in rat: a model of generalized non-convulsive epilepsy. Neurosci Lett 33: 97–101.

Vergnes M, Vergnes M, Marescaux C et al. (1985). Blockade of "antiabsence" activity of sodium valproate by THIP in rats with petit mal-like seizures. Comparison with ethosuximide. J Neural Transm 63: 133–141.

Verhage M, Maia AS, Plomp JJ et al. (2000). Synaptic assembly of the brain in the absence of neurotransmitter secretion. Science 287: 864–869.

Vigevano F, Cilio MR (1997). Vigabatrin versus ACTH as first-line treatment for infantile spasms: a randomized, prospective study. Epilepsia 38: 1270–1274.

Vreugdenhil M, Hack SP, Draguhn A et al. (2002). Tetanus toxin induces long-term changes in excitation and inhibition in the rat hippocampal CA1 area. Neuroscience 114: 983–994.

Wang X, Rousset CI, Hagberg H et al. (2006). Lipopolysaccharide-induced inflammation and perinatal brain injury. Semin Fetal Neonatal Med 11: 343–353.

Watanabe H, Nagata E, Kosakai A et al. (2000). Disruption of the epilepsy *KCNQ2* gene results in neural hyperexcitability. J Neurochem 75: 28–33.

Weimer RM, Richmond JE, Davis WS et al. (2003). Defects in synaptic vesicle docking in unc-18 mutants. Nat Neurosci 6: 1023–1030.

Welberg LA, Seckl JR, Holmes MC (2001). Prenatal glucocorticoid programming of brain corticosteroid receptors and corticotrophin-releasing hormone: possible implications for behaviour. Neuroscience 104: 71–79.

Wieser HG (2004). ILAE Commission Report. Mesial temporal lobe epilepsy with hippocampal sclerosis. Epilepsia 45: 695–714.

Williams SN, Locke CJ, Braden AL et al. (2004). Epileptic-like convulsions associated with LIS-1 in the cytoskeletal control of neurotransmitter signaling in *Caenorhabditis elegans*. Hum Mol Genet 13: 2043–2059.

Willmore LJ, Sypert GW, Munson JV et al. (1978). Chronic focal epileptiform discharges induced by injection of iron into rat and cat cortex. Science 200: 1501–1503.

Willmore LJ, Abelson MB, Ben-Menachem E et al. (2009). Vigabatrin: 2008 update. Epilepsia 50: 163–173.

Wise RA, Chinerman J (1974). Effects of diazepam and phenobarbital on electrically-induced amygdaloid seizures and seizure development. Exp Neurol 45: 355–363.

Woodbury DM (1980). Convulsant drugs: mechanisms of action. Adv Neurol 27: 249–303.

Yu FH, Mantegazza M, Westenbroek RE et al. (2006). Reduced sodium current in GABAergic interneurons in a mouse model of severe myoclonic epilepsy in infancy. Nat Neurosci 9: 1142–1149.

Yuen AW, Thompson PJ, Flugel D et al. (2007). Mortality and morbidity rates are increased in people with epilepsy: is stress part of the equation? Epilepsy Behav 10: 1–7.

Zeng LH, Xu L, Gutmann DH et al. (2008). Rapamycin prevents epilepsy in a mouse model of tuberous sclerosis complex. Ann Neurol 63: 444–453.

Handbook of Clinical Neurology, Vol. 107 (3rd series)
Epilepsy, Part I
H. Stefan and W.H. Theodore, Editors

Chapter 5

Classification of epilepsies and seizures: historical perspective and future directions

ANNE T. BERG[1]* AND J. HELEN CROSS[2]

[1]*Epilepsy Center, Children's Memorial Hospital, Chicago, IL, USA*

[2]*Neurosciences Unit, UCL Institute of Child Health, Great Ormond Street Hospital for Children and National Centre for Young People with Epilepsy, London, UK*

INTRODUCTION

The classifications of seizures and epilepsies, as we know them, had their roots in two proposals circulated by Henri Gastaut and published in 1969 (Gastaut, 1969a, b). The proposals (one for seizures, one for epilepsies) were formally accepted and published in 1970 (Merlis, 1970). The seizure classification was revised in 1981. An interim revision for epilepsies was made in 1985 and then again in 1989. The 1981 and 1989 reports were, until recently, the official classifications of the International League Against Epilepsy (ILAE) and widely regarded around the world as the authoritative statements for "classification."

Between 1970 and 1981 for seizures (Commission on Classification and Terminology of the ILAE, 1981) and in 1989 for epilepsies (Commission on Classification and Terminology of the ILAE, 1989), some minor changes occurred in terminology. For example, primary and secondary were replaced with idiopathic and symptomatic. Cryptogenic was introduced and intended to mean "presumed symptomatic." Different elements were introduced as seizure and epilepsy types. Some additional documents were published that addressed some peripheral, although still important, issues, but these did not offer any changes to the actual classifications (Blume et al., 2001; Engel, 2001, 2006; Fisher et al., 2005). The 2001 report, really a proposal for a diagnostic scheme, did attempt to make a break with the old approach by proposing a five-axis system for classifying epilepsy and seizures (Engel, 2001). It also acknowledged the need for flexibility. Although the specific approach proposed in the document was never formally accepted as a new classification, it did pave the way for the changes that came later. For the most part, the concepts on which the original classifications had been based remained unchanged until recently.

The purpose of the original classifications was a laudable one: to provide a common terminology to facilitate research and progress in epilepsy. This provided a shared language to discuss shared concepts prevalent at the time. Originally, the classification efforts were focused primarily on clinical issues, largely treatment, and research into causes and mechanisms was not the dominant purpose, certainly not as it is today. Over the past 50 years, roughly the same timeframe covered since the early efforts in classification, the world of epilepsy – in fact, of all biology and medicine – has changed considerably. The human genome was sequenced (Venter et al., 2001). Genetic technologies took off with the development of the polymerase chain reaction (PCR), followed by array technology, high-speed optical techniques, and so forth. Concepts and discoveries in genomics have reduced earlier ideas about gene–disease correspondence to an almost quaint state. For example, errors in the same gene can lead to different disorders. Errors in *SLC2A1*, which codes for glucose transporter 1 (GLUT1), can lead to a form of exercise-induced dystonia (Suls et al., 2008), but can also cause epilepsies of varying severity, often treatable with the ketogenic diet (Klepper and Leiendecker, 2007). *SCN1A* errors, which are found in roughly 80% of patients with Dravet syndrome, are associated with a broader range of epilepsy phenotypes (Harkin et al., 2007) and are also implicated in a form of hemiplegic migraine (Vahedi et al., 2009). Discoveries about alternate splicing, the

*Correspondence to: Anne T. Berg, Ph.D., Epilepsy Center, Children's Memorial Hospital, 2300 Children's Plaza, Box #29, Chicago, IL 60614, USA. Tel: 1-773-883-6159, Fax: 1-773-868-8904, E-mail: atberg@childrensmemorial.org

regulatory role of conserved genetic elements, the role of intronic DNA, and so forth, keep challenging us to expand our understanding of the amazing but dauntingly complex mechanisms involved in the regulation of cell growth, motility, proliferation, and function (Feero et al., 2010; Hayden, 2010). Neuroimaging has evolved from pneumoencephalography to computed tomography (CT) to magnetic resonance imaging (MRI) to high-strength MRI, diffusion tensor imaging (DTI), positron emission tomography (PET), single-photon emission CT (SPECT), tractology, and functional MRI with blood-oxygen-level-dependent contrast (fMRI-BOLD), and the list seems to grow every year (Madan and Grant, 2009; Jackson et al., 2010). Simple scalp electroencephalography (EEG) has been augmented by simultaneous video recording, and digital technology allows far more detailed and sophisticated analysis of the EEG tracing; magnetoencephalography (MEG), EEG source imaging (Stefan et al., 2009; Sakurai et al., 2010; Vulliemoz et al., 2010) and transcranial magnetic stimulation (TMS) (Badawy et al., 2009; Kimiskidis, 2009) are giving us glimpses into brain function that could only be imagined when the classifications were first put forward. These technologies and new ones continue to improve our ability to study the brain in a clinical setting. In the process of providing us with this ever-expanding understanding of the brain and its disorders, they have also given us new terminology and an entirely new and growing set of concepts with which to communicate and organize our knowledge.

The 1989 and 1981 documents rested on ideas that were prevalent when the original classifications were first introduced, and have remained largely unchanged since that time. The old terminology and concepts do not readily accommodate; in fact, they almost actively repel the new concepts and information developed from basic and clinical science research, and which are gradually being translated into improvements in patient care. In addition, the old classification's terminology and concepts were not accepted by many who complained that they were too complicated and too difficult. One is forced to learn a tortuous series of exceptions: West syndrome is a "generalized" epilepsy but is frequently found secondary to focal pathology and may itself present with focal seizures and focal EEG abnormalities. Lennox–Gastaut syndrome is a "generalized" epilepsy, often accompanied by "complex partial" seizures (the latter a term that has now been discarded). Benign rolandic epilepsy is "idiopathic," meaning presumed genetic, yet there is no evidence that the epilepsy itself (the electroclinical syndrome with seizures) aggregates in families. Dravet syndrome, clearly a genetic form of epilepsy, is not welcomed into the fold of idiopathic. These are just a few of the more obvious contradictions that require apologies and hand-waving to explain.

Another perceived but very real concern was that, although many of the "electroclinical" syndromes clearly have an objective and clinically valuable basis, there has been too much hair-splitting (Panayiotopoulos, 2008), rarely of any clinical value, and often in the search for self-named syndromes (Panayiotopoulos, 2007). This has detracted considerably from the validity of the entire classification effort.

Changing the old approach to classification has proven to be an extraordinarily difficult task, not the least because there has been such obstinate opposition to modernizing this outdated and increasingly irrelevant system. This opposition occasionally rises to a fevered pitch in which no coherent arguments are proffered, merely assertions that the classification of the epilepsies must be kept simple for physicians. Interestingly, no such arguments are made for biochemistry or molecular cell biology, or any other areas that physicians are expected to study.

In 2010, the ILAE Commission on Classification and Terminology presented a series of recommendations for changes in classification terminology and concepts (Berg et al., 2010). Ultimately, the Commission was only partially successful in updating classification in epilepsy. In considering what was accomplished and what remains to be done, it is helpful to review how the word "classification" has been used with respect to epilepsy. Classification, at least in the English language, is used to refer to categories or, perhaps more properly, diagnoses that might be made (e.g., West syndrome or childhood absence epilepsy, CAE). No changes were made to those diagnoses that reflected well-recognized electroclinical syndromes. The term is sometimes used to refer to the process by which entities come to be recognized as syndromes. This will be discussed later. Finally, and perhaps most usefully, classification refers to the system and terminology by which we organize information. The Tree of Life and the periodic table of the elements are examples of such classifications. It is classification in this last sense that was addressed by the Commission and which succeeded in breaking with old traditions and bad habits with respect to some key concepts and the language used to describe them. This should pave the way in the future to develop a new, useful classification that is not weighed down by outmoded concepts and terminology. The following provides a summary of what has not been changed, as well as the main changes and the implications of those changes. Of note, at this time, there is no final classification and there should not be one until we, as a field and not just a small committee of self-appointed experts, have reached a consensus on how best to build such a classification. Furthermore, there will be no "final" version until we have learned all there is to know about the epilepsies.

GENERALIZED VERSUS FOCAL: A NONDICHOTOMY?

Seizures

The standard uses of the terms generalized versus focal for seizures are not entirely straightforward; however, they do have some descriptive relevance for the manifestations of seizures. Consequently, they were retained but specifically redefined. In particular, focal was defined, or more accurately reconceptualized, as referring to seizures that arose within a network limited to one hemisphere. The activity may later spread and involve the other hemisphere. Generalized, by contrast, was reconceptualized as referring to seizures that began within and rapidly engaged bilaterally distributed networks. This change to the concept of generalized represents a paradigmatic breakthrough in that it allows that generalized seizures may arise from focal lesions. This is seen in epileptic spasms, which are frequently due to focal pathology. The response of intractable atonic seizures to callosotomy provides another example. Atonic seizures are considered to be generalized seizures (including in the new seizure classification). Disruption of the bilateral pathways that these seizure rapidly engage can modify their expression to one of a unilateral event. In fact, this may apply to a greater or lesser extent to virtually any type of seizure and may simply be a matter of degree and speed. In the end, Hughlings Jackson summarized the situation best when he wrote about focal discharging lesions leading to both focal ("epileptiform seizures") and generalized seizures ("ordinary epilepsy") (York and Steinberg, 2009).

The concept of networks is an exciting one in the neurosciences and especially in epilepsy (Spencer, 2002). Eventually, and perhaps very soon, the field will have the tools to study them objectively as hypotheses. Until then, however, they must be recognized as concepts and should not become the center of heated debates, nor should they be relied upon as solid explanations until such time as networks and their functions can be measured and studied objectively.

In terms of the specific seizure types recognized (i.e., the classification of generalized seizures), what resulted was admittedly arbitrary but at least represented a consensus. Table 5.1 presents the seizure types. The placement of eyelid myoclonia with absence and not with myoclonic seizures created concern from the start. What is perhaps most important is that eyelid myoclonia representing an epileptic seizure be recognized. Interestingly, there were strong and divided opinions concerning how best to characterize epileptic spasms. Consequently, this seizure type was simply left in its own category as unknown. In the end, that holds true to a certain extent of any seizure type.

Table 5.1

"Classification" of epileptic seizures (Berg et al., 2010)

Type of seizure	Subtype/Comment
Generalized seizures	
Tonic–clonic	These components may occur in any order and combination
Absence	Typical (as occurring in the setting of CAE, JAE, or JME)
	Atypical (as occurring in the setting of LGS, Dravet, etc.)
	Absence with special features
	Myoclonic absence
	Eyelid myoclonia
Myoclonic	Myoclonic
	Myoclonic atonic
	Myoclonic tonic
Clonic	
Tonic	
Atonic	
Focal seizures	No specific subtypes recognized; however, these may be described according to their semiological features*
Unknown as to whether focal, generalized, or depending on context	Epileptic spasms

*Descriptive features include but are not limited to: focal motor (and by more specific motor components), auras, dyscognitive, hemiconvulsion, evolving to a generalized convulsion (with tonic, clonic, or both components).

CAE, childhood absence epilepsy; JAE, juvenile absence epilepsy; JME, juvenile myoclonic epilepsy; LGS, Lennox–Gastaut syndrome.

The terms simple partial, complex partial, and secondarily generalized were not always used consistently and tended to encompass highly heterogeneous seizure phenomena. In fact, the 2001 report recommended that the terms simple and complex partial be dropped, although no replacements were recommended at the time. In the 2010 Classification report, it was noted that, for focal seizures, there was no evidence based on any understanding of mechanisms that allowed division of focal seizures into defensible categories. Consequently, no specific classification of focal seizure was offered as there was no rational basis on which to create one. Instead, an interim solution was simply to describe the seizure semiology in accurate terms with reference to the Glossary of Ictal Semiology (Blume et al., 2001). In fact, the 2001 and 2006 Task Force reports had proposed a "classification" based largely on ictal semiology

(Engel, 2001, 2006). The 2010 report built on this idea but emphasized that these terms be considered descriptors and not necessarily identifiers of unique seizure types. Hemiconvulsions, which never clearly fit into the old classification approach, would be labeled as hemiconvulsions, and so forth. For seizures in which impairment of cognition is the most apparent predominant feature, the term dyscognitive has been recommended. Although some would prefer to eschew an apparent neologism, in fact words such as dyslexia, dystonia, and dysplasia are routinely accepted and used. The term dyscognitive reasonably conveys the notion of impaired cognition. The term dialeptic was not received with great enthusiasm, but may eventually find its place in the lexicon. Finally, the expression secondarily generalized has been widely misapplied and overapplied to mean that there may be motor manifestations on both sides of the body. Evolution to a generalized tonic–clonic seizure is a distinct clinical event. Although specific terms have not yet been recommended for this event, it should be specifically identified and separated from events in which there may be bilateral manifestations but not a generalized convulsion. Clear characterization of the actual motor or other components may provide some insight into mechanisms that are currently obscured by the simple–complex partial dichotomy. For example, a seizure involving focal clonic activity could simply be described as "focal clonic." Focal epileptic spasms, often not recognized and likely called simple partial seizures by some, may have very specific implications for treatment.

In retrospect, there is some irony in the elevation of a "generalized myoclonic seizure" to reflect a classification of seizure type, whereas a focal myoclonic event is merely a description of semiology. For example, we do not know whether the "generalized myoclonic" seizures seen in juvenile myoclonic epilepsy (JME) are the same entity as seen in Dravet syndrome or Lennox–Gastaut syndrome. This is an area where much still needs to be done.

Epilepsies

Traditionally, epilepsies (the underlying disorders) have been referred to as generalized or focal. Other terms that have been replaced by focal include partial and localization-related. Although these terms are also ingrained in our vocabulary for describing epilepsy, they are inaccurate, misleading, and inconsistently applied. For example, Dravet syndrome is a diffuse genetic channelopathy. It presents with focal and generalized seizures and was classified in the 1989 classification not as a generalized epilepsy but as one with both generalized and focal features. West and Lennox–Gastaut syndromes, both of which often present with focal features and may arise from focal lesions, were classified as generalized epilepsies.

The use of these terms in this way provided little, if any, insight into the nature or process of the underlying disorder, and required constant explanation and apologies for the resulting inconsistencies and confusions. In fact, new investigative techniques (MEG/electron spectroscopic imaging (ESI)) are quickly challenging the simplistic notion of generalized, even in those epilepsies traditionally called "idiopathic generalized" (van Luijtelaar and Sitnikova, 2006; Stefan et al., 2009; Sakurai et al., 2010). Furthermore, the implications of this change for clinical practice and patient care may, at times, be profound. The use of surgical treatment of epilepsy has increased, particularly in children. Generalized was often interpreted as implying nonsurgical. In fact, "generalized" appearing disorders can often, upon careful evaluation, be successfully treated surgically with resective procedures (Jonas et al., 2005; Chugani et al., 2010; Lee et al., 2010). The interpretation, particularly by nonepilepsy specialists, of generalized seizures or EEG abnormalities as a contraindication for surgery can result in delay or even complete failure to refer for specialty evaluation. At the other extreme, just because a focal functional abnormality can be identified does not mean that the area should be resected. There have unfortunately been cases of children with Dravet syndrome who were operated on because their physicians did not understand that the focal features did not signal focal pathology that should be resected but were a consequence of a diffuse genetic disorder. These are extreme cases; however, the basic principle likely applies to virtually any form of epilepsy and becomes especially critical once a patient's seizures are seen to be drug-resistant.

TERMS AND CONCEPTS FOR GROUPING ETIOLOGY

The terms in the 1989 classification for grouped etiology – idiopathic, cryptogenic, and symptomatic – were poorly defined, based on presumptions, and had taken on connotations regarding treatability and long-term outcome that interfered with clear communication, treatment and management, and rational attempts to organize our knowledge concerning these diagnoses. They were replaced and new concepts were defined.

Instead of idiopathic "presumed genetic," the label genetic was chosen and explicitly defined to mean that the epilepsy, as best as understood, is the direct result of one or more known genetic defects (established through well-designed and replicated studies) or that the genetic contributions can be inferred, based upon evidence from appropriately designed family studies showing that the epilepsy is indeed transmitted within families. Seizures are the core symptom of the disorder. This, of course, requires knowledge of the mechanism by which the genetic defect occurs – something we often do not fully know. This will be revisited and likely revised in the near future as molecular discoveries challenge this notion. The concept also rests on the impression that there are generally no other symptoms associated with, or at least preceding, the epilepsy.

The idea that one can have epilepsy alone with no other consequences has been dismantled in recent years. It is now abundantly clear that all epilepsies, including those that were once called "benign" and "idiopathic" epilepsies, cosegregate with a range of psychiatric, behavioral, and cognitive disorders. This has become a rich area for research and is providing new insights into brain function, not just epilepsy. Ample evidence points to the likelihood of some common mechanisms that may contribute both to various forms of epilepsy and to specific cognitive and psychiatric disorders (Kanner, 2003, 2008). Although the notion of "just epilepsy" has been discarded, many of these associated other disorders which are seen more frequently in people with epilepsy may result from shared or related underlying mechanisms and not the intermediate cause of epilepsy. Thus, a direct genetic effect is not precluded by the presence of these other disorders.

Symptomatic was defined as "secondary to a known or presumed disorder of the brain." This seems tautological, as all epilepsy is symptomatic of something that affects the brain. In its place, a somewhat unwieldy but more direct phrase, "structural–metabolic," was recommended. The accompanying concept is that the epilepsy is due to the effects of a structural lesion or metabolic disorder of the brain, although other factors, such as immunological, should be included as well. There is a separate identifiable or discernible disorder, and the patient would generally have another diagnosis in addition to the epilepsy. The nature of that disorder may be highly varied and may come from either or both acquired or genetic sources.

In many cases, distinguishing a genetic epilepsy from a structural metabolic epilepsy will require knowledge of the actual mechanism, which is not always available. This distinction is really only temporary until such time as we are able reliably to identify and characterize those underlying mechanisms.

Finally, cryptogenic had been defined as unknown but presumed symptomatic. This is an unfathomable obfuscation, especially today in light of the progress being made in the genetic basis of seizures and epilepsies, in neuroimaging, and in our understanding of the role of various metabolic errors that may be associated with epilepsy. Autosomal dominant nocturnal frontal lobe epilepsy (ADNFLE) and Dravet syndrome are prime examples. The first is due to a mutation in *CHRNA4* or *CHRNB2*, which respectively code for the α4 and β2 subunits of the neuronal nicotinic acetylcholine receptor (nAChR) (Steinlein et al., 1995, 1997; Hoda et al., 2008). The second is the closest we have to a genetic epilepsy disease, in that mutations in a single gene, *SCN1A*, which codes for the α1 subunit of the voltage-gated neuronal sodium channel, account for roughly 80% of all cases of the disorder (Harkin et al., 2007). On the other hand, advances in neuroimaging are demonstrating lesions that previously went undetected (Lerner et al., 2009). To replace cryptogenic, the term "of unknown cause" was recommended to reflect true uncertainty when the cause is not yet identified.

In rejecting the term cryptogenic and replacing it with unknown cause, the Commission also encouraged plain language and direct communication between physician and patient, as well as a greater degree of intellectual honesty than did the previous terminology.

In time, all of these terms will be replaced as we develop a more refined understanding of the "causes" of different forms of epilepsy. For example, instead of "genetic" epilepsies, perhaps we will eventually talk about channelopathies as one group of genetic causes of epilepsy. Until that time, these terms allow a break with a past terminology that did little to reflect our growing knowledge, and they should serve as a valuable intermediate step toward classifying according to a specific underlying cause and mechanism. The terms encourage a focus on the underlying cause of the epilepsy which has tremendous implications for patient care including genetic testing, genetic counseling, the use of high-quality imaging, consideration of alternative therapies such as the ketogenic diet, and referral for surgical evaluation.

New and abandoned terms and concepts

Catastrophic and benign

Certain terms were considered to be problematic when discussing epilepsy. "Catastrophic," often used in reference to some of the worst forms of epilepsy occurring in infancy and early childhood, was thought to be too emotionally charged and not a helpful way to present a diagnosis to parents. In fairness, it was never part of the ILAE lexicon. At the same time and more controversial, it was also recommended that the term "benign" not be used to characterize epilepsy or that certain epilepsies be identified as "benign" epilepsies. In referring to a form of epilepsy, benign was defined at the Monreale Workshop (Capovilla et al., 2009) as meaning the epilepsy reliably disappeared (resolved) in time; there were no sequelae with respect to development and cognition, quality of life and fulfilment of expectations; it could be readily identified at initial presentation and thus could be predictive of outcome; and treatment was not always necessary. The reason for abandoning it was due to the considerable burden of cognitive, behavioral, and psychiatric comorbidities as well as the risk of sudden unexplained death in epilepsy (SUDEP), which may accompany any form of epilepsy. Many of the consequences that accompany epilepsy can present significant challenges in the educational setting, for employment, and for general social functioning even, it would seem, in people with well-controlled seizures.

The terms benign and idiopathic were used for anticipatory guidance. Although they were misleading or abstruse, the purposes for which they were used were of value but could be better served with clear, plain language. Alternative language was considered. In particular, rather than either benign or idiopathic, if the concept to be conveyed is that the epilepsy will most likely resolve in time, self-limited would be an appropriate term. The term was already used in reference to seizures that terminated on their own (Engel, 2006), and its use with respect to electroclinical syndromes would be very consistent with that for seizure duration. If the concept to be conveyed is that the epilepsy is likely to be highly responsive to pharmacological therapy, one could refer to it as being pharmacoresponsive or easily treated. Such a simple, unadorned approach would do much for improving patients' understanding of their disorder, while still leaving room to discuss potential cognitive and psychiatric concerns as well as SUDEP.

A few changes to the names of some syndromes were made, including changing seizures to epilepsy and partial to focal epilepsy in syndromes such as "migrating partial seizures," which was renamed "epilepsy with migrating focal seizures." Removing the modifier "benign" from such electroclinical syndromes as "benign epilepsy with central-temporal spikes," however, has not occurred at this point in time.

Epileptic encephalopathy

The term of epileptic encephalopathy is not new (Dulac, 2001). It has been defined explicitly to mean that the epileptic activity itself contributes to behavioral and cognitive disorders above and beyond any compromise that could be attributed to the underlying lesion or condition itself. Originally, the concept and term arose from the observation that a group of disorders with onset in infancy and early childhood appeared to be associated with a failure to develop and even a loss of developmental milestones. These included West, Lennox–Gastaut, Dravet, and Doose syndromes. Ultimately, children fail to develop normally and can be left with varying degrees of intellectual disability and behavioral disorders. Inherent in the term as it was applied to the very young was the notion that the epileptic activity or other electrographic abnormalities directly interfered with normal developmental events during critical times in neurodevelopment. This could, if severe and persistent, result in permanent derailment of development and lasting intellectual and behavioral disability. The concept, however, has been expanded. It is recognized as applying to any form of epilepsy, not just those previously called "epileptic encephalopathies," and it may occur at any age. A recent study had demonstrated the encephalopathic effect of seizure in adult rats (Lin et al., 2009). Studies in humans have demonstrated that changes in brain activity can be detected up to a day before and a day after a seizure (Badawy et al., 2009). Following a seizure, decreased excitation occurs. One could speculate that, if this occurs in cognitively eloquent cortex, it may be a basis for some of the cognitive difficulties seen in patients with frequent seizures. Permanent losses in cognitive function in adults over time (Hermann et al., 2006) and changes in brain anatomy (Berhardt et al., 2009) may also occur. These and other sources of evidence amply demonstrate the potential for the persistent and cumulative effects of seizures on the brain and cognition.

ABANDONING THE RIGID STRUCTURE OF THE 1989 CLASSIFICATION

The 1989 classification of the epilepsies, both the terminology and the structure, imposed a rigid and ultimately artificial organization and way of thinking that hobbled our ability to represent biologically relevant and clinically useful information about different forms of epilepsy. The value of a classification of epilepsies should be in its ability to improve patient care by allowing meaningful translation of relevant basic and clinical research discoveries into clinical practice. This can in part be accomplished by presenting and organizing information regarding key features that are relevant to clinical practice. At this time, pieces that might eventually contribute to such a classification are becoming apparent. For example, GLUT1 deficiency syndrome is now recognized as a highly treatable encephalopathy (Klepper and Leiendecker, 2007; Leen et al., 2010). The increasing ability to recognize milder forms of GLUT1 deficiency has important diagnostic and therapeutic implications (Roulet-Perez et al., 2008; Suls et al., 2009). The recent discovery of not only the gene but the mechanisms behind DEND (developmental delay, epilepsy, and neonatal diabetes) also has very specific and useful treatment implications (Koster et al., 2008a, b). The new evidence regarding mTOR (mammalian target of rapamycin) and epileptogenicity may translate into specific therapeutic options in time, perhaps soon (Wong, 2010), and evidence regarding abnormalities in glutamate receptors in tuberous sclerosis may contribute to prevention of the epileptogenicity of cortical tubers (Talos et al., 2008). For the most part, however, we are still just on the threshold of being able to translate such scientific discoveries into clinical practice. Rather than fabricating an incomplete, inaccurate, and inadequate classification, the Commission held back. In place of a "classification," a simple justifiable organization based on well-established information, and not presumptions and assertions, was recommended. To do this, the diagnostic specificity of different entities previously contained in the classification of epilepsies was considered and ranked.

Diseases and syndromes

The terms disease and syndrome have defined meanings in medicine; however, they are not used consistently, for example Alzheimer disease and Rett syndrome. Although the concept of disease may well apply to some currently recognized forms of epilepsy, the Commission held back from insisting on its use for specific entities. The term syndrome, however, has clearly been much overused to the point that it is frequently meaningless. An electroclinical syndrome was intended to refer to a distinct disorder characterized by a cluster of signs and symptoms including age at onset, specific electrographic signatures, specific seizure types, certain antecedents (or lack thereof), imaging findings, nocturnal patterns and triggers for seizure occurrence, and other features. To the extent that patients who share an electroclinical syndrome are homogeneous, they tend to share similar if not the same underlying causes and mechanisms, and also may be treated in a fairly uniform manner. For example, most physicians who understand electroclinical syndromes if faced with 10 patients with CAE would provide similar information to the patient and family and tend to initiate the same treatments. Faced with 10 patients with West syndrome, those same physicians would all provide similar information to the parents and select from among a limited number of first treatment options (Wheless et al., 2005, 2007). The information given to families and the treatments initiated for children would be vastly different depending on the specific syndrome, CAE or West syndrome. In this sense, "syndrome" is highly meaningful. Distinctive electroclinical syndromes can also become the target for genetic investigations and have yielded some valuable findings. ADNFLE (*CHRNA4* and *CHRNB2*) (Hoda et al., 2008), Dravet (*SCN1A*) (Claes et al., 2001; Sugawara et al., 2002), epilepsy in females with mental retardation (EFMR) (*PCDH19*) (Dibbens et al., 2008), and Ohtahara syndrome (*STXBP1*) (Saitsu et al., 2008) are just some examples. Once the term "syndrome" was applied to "garden variety" epilepsy, for example "cryptogenic parietal lobe epilepsy," which is an incomplete description at best, it lost its utility.

Consequently, an explicit change in the approach to thinking about epilepsy entailed resurrecting the concept of electroclinical syndrome and encouraging a more selective and informative use of the term with the recognition that some "syndromes" would be better characterized as diseases. The 1989 classification organized electroclinical syndromes and other forms of epilepsy together into a system that was neither natural nor especially relevant. Rather than impose any specific system of classification, these syndromes should be organized in a manner that best suits the purpose for which they are being organized. For example, from a diagnostic viewpoint, organization by age at onset has some clear clinical utility. Organization can be by any feature that reflects useful understanding or improves understanding of these disorders.

Of note, there has traditionally been a cluster of syndrome known as the "idiopathic generalized epilepsies" (IGE). Although the recognition of some commonalities among these syndromes is helpful in genetic investigations, in fact, for choice of therapy there are some striking differences. For example, the first drug of choice for CAE would not be the same as for juvenile myoclonic epilepsy. Myoclonic atonic epilepsy (MAE or Doose syndrome) appears to be a genetic epilepsy but was included under the "generalized cryptogenic or symptomatic" heading in the 1989 classification. A 2001 taskforce report suggested it should be incorporated into the idiopathic generalized epilepsies (Engel, 2001). Whether inclusion of MAE within the same cluster as CAE, juvenile absence epilepsy (JAE), and JME is biologically (genetically) relevant is not clear. Such an affiliation would do little to improve one's ability to treat this particular disorder. Just being able to recognize the syndrome and knowing the appropriate approaches to treatment is likely of greatest clinical utility, not artificially grouping it or imbuing it with certain qualities by association.

Distinctive constellations

A small group of highly distinctive epilepsies that do not have the same genetic–developmental cohesiveness as the traditional electroclinical syndromes must also be recognized. Chief among these are mesial temporal lobe epilepsy with hippocampal sclerosis, Rasmussen encephalitis, and gelastic seizures with hypothalamic hamartoma. Whether these are ultimately called "electroclinical" syndromes or not is unimportant. They can be identified based on distinctive characteristics and they have very specific implications for specific surgical therapies. In time, these may be referred to as surgical epilepsy syndromes.

A caveat must be placed, however, on the notion that mesial temporal lobe epilepsy is necessarily a surgical syndrome as the natural history of this disorder is complicated and does not necessarily involve refractory seizures (Berg, 2008).

Nonsyndromic epilepsies

Apart from the electroclinical syndromes and epilepsy diseases, what remains is the majority of epilepsies that do not fit clearly into any of the recognized electroclinical syndromes or clear patterns. In the past, the classification partitioned most of these into groups for localization-related symptomatic and localization-related cryptogenic, although some remained as unclassified generalized epilepsies. These were further subdivided according to the lobe from which the seizures were thought to originate (frontal, temporal, parietal, occipital) as well as generalized symptomatic or cryptogenic (many of which were already specific electroclinical syndromes) and generalized symptomatic (some of which were specific syndromes). Instead, these nonsyndromic epilepsies might most usefully continue to be organized first based upon whether or not a specific underlying structural–metabolic cause can be identified.

Nonsyndromic epilepsy associated with structural–metabolic lesions

The somewhat unwieldy term applied to this group for now is structural–metabolic epilepsy. The term structural–metabolic is not exclusive to nonsyndromic epilepsy and can be used to refer to the underlying cause of electroclinical syndromes in which a recognized structural insult or metabolic condition is responsible for the epilepsy. The purpose of recognizing this group, however, is that these are epilepsies that do not fit a clear electroclinical pattern but for which there are specific recognized, associated causes. Consequently, until we have reason to think otherwise, we might consider organizing them according to cause, for example by malformations of cortical development, gliomas, vascular accidents, respiratory chain defects, and so forth. Within or across such groups and depending on the purpose, further subdivisions might be made following meaningful classification schemes. For example, one well-regarded classification scheme for malformations of cortical development has been available for several years (Barkovich et al., 2005). The focus on underlying cause highlights meaningful information about a patient's epilepsy and treatment. It also emphasizes the importance of identifying a specific cause, many of which may have specific implications for treatment, including surgical. This is something the emphasis on lobe or apparent onset did not do. Understanding the mechanisms through which the causes act may bring certain, apparently distinct, causes together, for example disorders that involve dysregulation of mTOR (tuberous sclerosis complex, focal cortical dysplasia (FCD), trauma; (Wong, 2010). In this regard, note that the segregation of electroclinical syndromes from these nonsyndromic epilepsies does not preclude reorganizing all epilepsies according to, say, underlying cause. In this way, some forms of West syndrome, Lennox–Gastaut syndrome, and nonsyndromic epilepsy characterized by focal seizures might be grouped together as being secondary to tuberous sclerosis or secondary to focal cortical dysplasia.

Within the nonsyndromic epilepsies with structural–metabolic causes, age at onset of epilepsy may help to reveal relevant clinical patterns. A combination of age at onset and underlying cause may be particularly helpful. For example, one study found different patterns in terms of age at onset and location of lesion as a function of type I versus type II focal cortical dysplasia (Lerner et al., 2009). This has relevance to surgical evaluation as well as to understanding underlying mechanisms that produced the lesions in the first place.

Nonsyndromic epilepsies of unknown cause

The last group of epilepsies is the most difficult as they have no obvious features for organizing them, at least none that, as currently understood, could improve understanding of cause, improve selection of pharmacological treatment, or inform prognosis (anticipatory guidance). The previous approach of classifying based on lobe of the brain did none of this based on any current understanding. Even for the purposes of surgery, it provided only very crude information. In the future, identification of specific networks with different neurochemical profiles may change this; however, as we currently understand it, the use of lobe is unhelpful in nonsyndromic epilepsy. This is the group of epilepsies previously "presumed symptomatic" from which genetic syndromes such as ADNFLE have been found. It is also the group in which advanced imaging protocols have revealed subtle lesions. For now, careful phenotyping of all features (including diurnal pattern of occurrence, triggers, specific semiological features, and specific EEG characteristics) might, in the proper context, result in recognition of clinically relevant patterns not previously appreciated and which might improve clinical care if identified.

In the end, rather than having a classification or organization of epilepsies that implies certain relationships, the proposed organization of epilepsy diagnoses does no such thing (Table 5.2). Instead, it simply lays out epilepsy diagnoses based on what is known about the epilepsy and strives to avoid presumptions, assumptions, and assertions.

Table 5.2

Pragmatic organization of epilepsies: electroclinical syndromes, arranged by typical age range of onset (Berg et al., 2010)

Typical age at onset	Syndrome
Neonatal period	Benign familial neonatal epilepsy (BFNE)
	Early myoclonic encephalopathy (EME)
	Ohtahara syndrome
Infancy	Epilepsy of infancy with migrating partial seizures
	West syndrome
	Myoclonic epilepsy in infancy (MEI)
	Benign infantile epilepsy
	Benign familial infantile epilepsy
	Dravet syndrome
	Myoclonic encephalopathy in nonprogressive disorders
Childhood	Epilepsy in females with mental retardation (EFMR)*
	Febrile seizures plus (FS+) (can start in infancy)
	Panayiotopoulos syndrome
	Epilepsy with myoclonic atonic (previously astatic) seizures
	Benign epilepsy with centrotemporal spikes (BECTS)
	Autosomal-dominant nocturnal frontal lobe epilepsy (ADNFLE)
	Late-onset childhood occipital epilepsy (Gastaut type)
	Epilepsy with myoclonic absences
	Lennox–Gastaut syndrome
	Epileptic encephalopathy with continuous spike-and-wave during sleep (CSWS)
	Landau–Kleffner syndrome (LKS)
	Childhood absence epilepsy (CAE)
Adolescence–adulthood	Juvenile absence epilepsy (JAE)
	Juvenile myoclonic epilepsy (JME)
	Epilepsy with generalized tonic/clonic seizures alone
	Autosomal dominant partial epilepsy with auditory features (ADPEAF)
	Other familial temporal lobe epilepsies
Less specific age relationship	Familial focal epilepsy with variable foci (childhood to adulthood)
	Reflex epilepsies
	Progressive myoclonus epilepsies (PME)
Distinctive constellations	These do not have the genetic–developmental characteristics of the electroclinical syndromes above but may, in the future, be incorporated into that group or left separately as surgical syndromes
	Mesial temporal lobe epilepsy with hippocampal sclerosis (MTLE with HS)
	Rasmussen syndrome
	Gelastic seizures with hypothalamic hamartoma
Nonsyndromic structural–metabolic epilepsies	Epilepsies attributed to and organized by structural–metabolic causes
	Malformations of cortical development
	Hemimegalencephaly
	Lissencephaly
	Pachygyria
	Polymicrogyria
	Heterotopias
	Focal cortical dysplasia, types I and II
	Other
	Neurocutaneous syndromes
	Tuberous sclerosis complex
	Sturge–Weber
	Neurofibromatosis
	Metabolic
	GLUT1 deficiency*
	Neonatal diabetes, *KCNG11* mutation*
	Mitochondrial respiratory chain deficiencies*

Continued

Table 5.2

Continued

Typical age at onset	Syndrome
	Pyruvate dehydrogenase deficiency
	Isolated sulphite oxidase/molybdenum cofactor deficiency
	Guanadinoacetate methyltransferase (GAMT) deficiency
	Neuronal ceroid lipofuscinosis
	Tumors
	Infections
	Trauma
	Perinatal insults
	Postneonatal strokes
Nonsyndromic epilepsies of unknown cause	No single feature or group of features is currently known to provide helpful information for treatment, management, and prediction of prognosis for these undifferentiated epilepsies
	Conditions with epileptic seizures that are traditionally not diagnosed as a form of epilepsy *per se*
	Benign neonatal seizures (BNS)
	Febrile seizures (FS)

*Not previously recognized in International League Against Epilepsy documents. EFMR fits the notion of a syndrome. Neonatal diabetes secondary to *KCNG11* mutation is likely best characterized as a disease causing the developmental delay, epilepsy, and neonatal diabetes syndrome (DEND). Glucose transporter type 1 (GLUT1) deficiency is associated with a spectrum of clinical phenotypes. Again, whether this is best characterized as a disease or syndrome has not been determined, but the phenomenon should be recognized. Likewise, mitochondrial respiratory chain defects are increasingly recognized as a cause of early-onset epilepsy.

The process of classification

The final area of concern for classification is one that has caused considerable controversy in the past. Expert opinion, often accompanied by a certain amount of emotionalism and even vitriol, was the primary, in fact only, criterion for determining whether or not to allow a new entity into the august list of syndrome types. For those not among the cognoscenti of classification, the process was often viewed as arcane and its results arbitrary. Although that is not entirely fair, there is some truth to that characterization none the less. As previously reviewed (Berg and Blackstone, 2003, 2006), evolutionary biology went through a similar phase. One evolutionary biologist was famously paraphrased upon being asked, "What is a species?": "A species is whatever an expert says it is." Evolutionary biology has become the exemplar of scientific classification. It has given us molecular phylogeny, which is the backbone of bioinformatics, a key tool in molecular medicine. Epilepsy has much to learn from studying how evolutionary biology evolved from an expert opinion and assertion dominated field to a scientific endeavor explicitly involved in hypothesis testing.

As it is, the ILAE, perhaps in part because of its slowness to make any useful contributions to developing a transparent and rigorous process for identifying new epilepsy entities and distinguishing amongst syndromes, has largely become irrelevant to that process. Instead, the peer-reviewed scientific literature, driven largely by genomics and in part by neuroimaging, has taken this over. For example, the "syndrome" of EFMR was described in 2008 (Scheffer et al., 2008) and now, in 2012, there is a genetic test that can be ordered to assist in confirming its diagnosis. Developmental delay, epilepsy, and neonatal diabetes (DEND), a rare but treatable encephalopathy condition, is widely recognized. Neither appears in any ILAE document. They do not need to be condoned by the ILAE in order for their clinical importance to be recognized and for genetic testing to be made available. For that matter, GLUT1 deficiency does not appear in the ILAE lists either, yet is considered perhaps one of the most treatable forms of developmental encephalopathy associated with epilepsy (Klepper and Leiendecker, 2007). In fact, many of the very early-onset disorders, particularly those with inborn errors of metabolism, do not need to pass through the stage of being recognized as syndromes, and the concept of disease will increasingly take the place of syndrome. This is likely the way in which "classification" will and should proceed.

Pragmatic approach to epilepsy

A useful classification should highlight key information needed in patient care and should help organize information in a useful manner. In the absence of such a classification, the following pragmatic approach is suggested, particularly for the nonepilepsy specialist. It rests largely on diagnostic strategies and recommendations that have been developed over the past several years from several professional societies, and also on epidemiological data showing that, especially in children, there are a limited number of diagnoses that account for the vast majority of patients whose epilepsies fit criteria for specific electroclinical syndromes in the general population (Callenbach et al., 1998; Berg et al., 1999; Jallon et al., 2001).

1. In general, any child with the onset of epilepsy under age 2 years should be evaluated by a pediatric epilepsy specialist as this is the age group in which some of the most serious encephalopathic conditions arise. Although this specific recommendation has not been made by any panel in the USA, it is consistent with the NICE guidelines in the UK (National Institute for Clinical Excellence, 2004), which recommend evaluation at a tertiary center of all children with onset of epilepsy under age 2 years. In this group, neuroimaging with MRI and, in the absence of structural abnormalities, further investigation of genetic and metabolic disorders is imperative.
2. Determine whether a patient has one of the more common and easily recognized and easily treated electroclinical syndromes. Four syndromes, benign epilepsy with centrotemporal spikes (BECTS), CAE, JAE, and JME, are highly distinctive and with a little training are readily recognizable. Together, they account for 20–30% of all epilepsy occurring in children and adolescents. There is generally good agreement about initial treatment approaches for these four syndromes (Wheless et al., 2005, 2007), and they are usually highly amenable to treatment. Very few adult patients have recognized electroclinical syndromes, and the concept is not currently of as great utility as in children and adolescents.
3. Patients of any age who have generalized features and whose form of epilepsy cannot be diagnosed as CAE, JAE, or JME should probably be evaluated by a specialist. This is especially true in children where syndromes such as MAE and Lennox–Gastaut syndrome may occur, but in adults as well in whom rare but serious progressive disorders such as the progressive myoclonus epilepsies may arise.
4. Any patient who at onset has a deficit of unexplained origin, or who develops a new neurological, including cognitive, deficit during the course of his epilepsy should be fully evaluated to determine the cause.
5. For individuals not clearly meeting criteria for one of the more tractable epilepsy syndromes (BECTS, CAE, JAE, JME), and whose presentation has not already raised concern regarding a specialty evaluation, available diagnostic resources should be used to determine whether there is a structural brain lesion that itself may become the focus of treatment or which may influence treatment decisions in the future. MRI is the imaging modality preferred for epilepsy and is recommended in any patient, especially in children, not clearly conforming to one of a handful of syndromes already identified as highly treatable (Hirtz et al., 2000; National Institute for Clinical Excellence, 2004; Gaillard et al., 2009).
6. Over time, any individual, child or adult, whose seizures fail to come under full control after appropriate treatment with informative trials of two antiepileptic drugs should be considered to have drug-resistant epilepsy (Kwan et al., 2010).
7. Patients of any age who meet basic criteria for drug-resistant epilepsy should be referred for specialty evaluation at a center that is able to investigate the underlying cause and offer a range of therapies including nonpharmacological and surgical (National Association of Epilepsy Centers, 2001; Cross et al., 2006).

This straightforward, pragmatic approach is not supported by the 1989 Classification of the Epilepsies, which itself is of limited clinical value for treating and managing patients. Although some will lament the “loss” of the 1989 Classification, it is, in the end, no great loss but a step forward toward integrating clinical epilepsy into the neurosciences. The final chapter has not been written and likely will not be for a good long while. The temporary new approach does, at least, provide a rational and meaningful framework for organizing information relative to patient care and remains flexible for future approaches for incorporating new information as it develops. That alone is a tremendous advance over the system that was in place for the last half century.

References

Badawy R, Macdonell R, Jackson G et al. (2009). The periictal state: cortical excitability changes within 24 h of a seizure. Brain 132: 1013–1021.

Barkovich AJ, Kuzniecky RI, Jackson GD et al. (2005). A developmental and genetic classification for malformations of cortical development. Neurology 65: 1873–1887.

Berg AT (2008). The natural history of mesial temporal lobe epilepsy. Current Opin Neurol 21: 173–178.

Berg AT, Blackstone NW (2003). Of cabbages and kings: perspectives on classification from the field of systematics. Epilepsia 44: 8–12.

Berg AT, Blackstone NW (2006). Concepts in classification and their relevance to epilepsy. Epilepsy Res 70: 11–19.

Berg AT, Levy SR, Testa FM et al. (1999). Classification of childhood epilepsy syndromes in newly diagnosed epilepsy: interrater agreement and reasons for disagreement. Epilepsia 40: 439–444.

Berg AT, Berkovic SF, Brodie MJ et al. (2010). Revised terminology and concepts for organization of seizures and epilepsies: report of the ILAE Commission on Classification and Terminology, 2005–2009. Epilepsia 51: 676–685.

Berhardt BC, Worsley KJ, Kim H et al. (2009). Longitudinal and cross sectional analysis of atrophy in pharmacoresistant temporal lobe epilepsy. Neurology 72: 1747–1754.

Blume WT, Luders HO, Mizrahi E et al. (2001). Glossary of descriptive terminology for ictal semiology. International League Against Epilepsy. Epilepsia 42: 1212–1218.

Callenbach PM, Geerts AT, Arts WF et al. (1998). Familial occurrence of epilepsy in children with newly diagnosed multiple seizures: Dutch Study of Epilepsy in Childhood. Epilepsia 39: 331–336.

Capovilla G, Berg AT, Cross JH et al. (2009). Conceptual dichotomies in classifying epilepsies: partial versus generalized and idiopathic versus symptomatic (April 18–20th, 2008, Monreale, Italy). Epilepsia (Epub ahead of print).

Chugani HT, Asano E, Sood S (2010). Infantile spasms: who are the ideal surgical candidates? Epilepsia 51: 94–96.

Claes L, Del-Favero J, Ceulemans B et al. (2001). *De novo* mutations in the sodium-channel gene *SCN1A* cause severe myoclonic epilepsy of infancy. Am J Hum Genet 68: 1327–1332.

Commission on Classification and Terminology of the International League Against Epilepsy (1981). Proposal for revised clinical and electrographic classification of epileptic seizures. Epilepsia 22: 489–501.

Commission on Classification and Terminology of the International League Against Epilepsy (1989). Proposal for revised classification of epilepsies and epileptic syndromes. Epilepsia 30: 389–399.

Cross JH, Jaykar P, Nordli D et al. (2006). Proposed criteria for referral and evaluation of children for epilepsy surgery: recommendations of the Subcommission for Pediatric Epilepsy Surgery. Epilepsia 47: 953–959.

Dibbens LM, Tarpey PS, Hynes K et al. (2008). X-linked protocadherin 19 mutations cause female-limited epilepsy and cognitive impairment. Nat Genet 40: 776–781.

Dulac O (2001). Epileptic encephalopathy. Epilepsia 42: 23–26.

Engel J (2001). A proposed diagnostic scheme for people with epileptic seizures and with epilepsy: report of the ILAE Task Force on Classification and Terminology. Epilepsia 42: 796–803.

Engel J (2006). Report of the ILAE Classification Core Group. Epilepsia 47: 1558–1568.

Feero WG, Guttmacher AE, Collins FS (2010). Genomic medicine – an updated primer. N Engl J Med 362: 2001–2011.

Fisher RS, Boas WVE, Blume W et al. (2005). Epileptic seizures and epilepsy: definitions proposed by the International League Against Epilepsy (ILAE) and the International Bureau for Epilepsy (IBE). Epilepsia 46: 470–472.

Gaillard WD, Chiron C, Cross JH et al. (2009). Guidelines for imaging infants and children with recent-onset epilepsy. Epilepsia 50: 2147–2153.

Gastaut H (1969a). Clinical and electroencephalographical classification of epileptic seizures. Epilepsia 10: S2–S13.

Gastaut H (1969b). Classification of the epilepsies. Proposal for an international classification. Epilepsia 10: S14–S21.

Harkin LA, McMahon JM, Iona X et al. (2007). The spectrum of *SCN1A*-related infantile epileptic encephalopathies. Brain 130: 843–852.

Hayden EC (2010). Life is complicated. Nature 464: 664–669.

Hermann BP, Seidenberg M, Dow C et al. (2006). Cognitive prognosis in chronic temporal lobe epilepsy. Ann Neurol 60: 80–87.

Hirtz D, Ashwal S, Berg AT et al. (2000). Evaluating a first nonfebrile seizure in children: an evidence-based practice parameter. Neurology 55: 616–623.

Hoda J-C, Gu W, Friedli M et al. (2008). Human nocturnal frontal lobe epilepsy: pharmacogenomic profiles of pathogenic nicotinic acetylcholine receptor B-subunit mutations outside the ion channel pore. Mol Pharmacol 74: 379–391.

Jackson GD, Calamante F, Tournier J-D et al. (2010). New anatomic MRI techniques. Epilepsia 51: 80–82.

Jallon P, Loiseau P, Loiseau J (2001). Newly diagnosed unprovoked epileptic seizures: presentation at diagnosis in CAROLE study. Epilepsia 42: 464–475.

Jonas R, Asarnow RF, LoPresti C et al. (2005). Surgery for symptomatic infant-onset epileptic encephalopathy with and without infantile spasms. Neurology 64: 746–750.

Kanner AM (2003). Depression in epilepsy: prevalence, clinical semiology, pathogenic mechanisms, and treatment. Biol Psychiatry 54: 388–398.

Kanner AM (2008). Depression in epilepsy: a complex relation with unexpected consequences. Curr Opin Neurol 21: 190–194.

Kimiskidis VK (2009). Transcranial magnetic stimulation for drug-resistant epilepsies: rational and clinical experience. Eur Neurol 63: 205–210.

Klepper J, Leiendecker B (2007). GLUT1 deficiency syndrome – 2007 update. Dev Med Child Neurol 49: 707–716.

Koster JC, Cadario F, Peruzzi C et al. (2008a). The G53D mutation in Kir6.2 (*KCNJ11*) is associated with neonatal diabetes and motor dysfunction in adulthood that is improved with sulfonylurea therapy. J Clin Endocrinol Metab 93: 1054–1061.

Koster JC, Kurtara HT, Enkvetchakul D et al. (2008b). DEND mutation in Kir6.2 (*KCNJ11*) reveals a flexible *N*-terminal region critical for ATP-sensing of the KATP channel. Biophys J 95: 4689–4697.

Kwan P, Arzimanoglou A, Berg AT et al. (2010). Definition of drug resistant epilepsy: consensus proposal by the *ad hoc* Task Force of the ILAE Commission on Therapeutic Strategies. Epilepsia 51: 1069–1077.

Lee YJ, Kang H-C, Lee JS et al. (2010). Resective pediatric epilepsy surgery in Lennox–Gastaut syndrome. Pediatrics 125: e58–e66.

Leen WG, Klepper J, Verbeek MM et al. (2010). Glucose transporter-1 deficiency syndrome: the expanding clinical and genetic spectrum of a treatable disorder. Brain 133: 655–670.

Lerner JT, Salamon N, Hauptman JS et al. (2009). Assessment and surgical outcomes for mild type I and severe type II cortical dysplasia: a critical review and the UCLA experience. Epilepsia 50: 1310–1335.

Lin H, Holmes GL, Kubie JL et al. (2009). Recurrent seizures induce a reversible impairment in a spatial hidden goal task. Hippocampus 19: 817–827.

Madan N, Grant PE (2009). New directions in clinical imaging of cortical dysplasias. Epilepsia 50: 9–18.

Merlis JK (1970). Proposal for an international classification of the epilepsies. Epilepsia 11: 114–119.

National Association of Epilepsy Centers (2001). Guidelines for essential services, personnel, and facilities in specialized epilepsy centers in the United States. Epilepsia 42: 804–814.

National Institute for Clinical Excellence (2004). The Epilepsies: Diagnosis and Management of the Epilepsies in Children and Young People in Primary and Secondary Care. Clinical Guideline 20. NICE, London.

Panayiotopoulos CP (2007). The birth and evolution of the concept of Panayiotopoulos syndrome. Epilepsia 48: 1041–1043.

Panayiotopoulos CP (2008). Typical absence seizures and related epileptic syndromes: assessment of current state and directions for future research. Epilepsia 49: 2131–2139.

Roulet-Perez E, Ballhausen D, Bonafé L et al. (2008). Glut-1 deficiency syndrome masquerading as idiopathic generalized epilepsy. Epilepsia 49: 1955–1958.

Saitsu H, Kato M, Mizuguchi T et al. (2008). *De novo* mutations in the gene encoding *STXBP1* (*MUNC18-1*) cause early infantile epileptic encephalopathy. Nat Genet 40: 782–788.

Sakurai K, Takeda Y, Tanaka N et al. (2010). Generalized spike–wave discharges involve a default mode network in patients with juvenile absence epilepsy: a MEG study. Epilepsy Res 89: 176–184.

Scheffer IE, Turner SJ, Dibbens LM et al. (2008). Epilepsy and mental retardation limited to females: an underrecognized disorder. Brain 131: 918–927.

Spencer SS (2002). Neural networks in human epilepsy: evidence of and implications for treatment. Epilepsia 43: 219–227.

Stefan H, Paulini-Ruf A, Hopfengärtner R et al. (2009). Network characteristics of idiopathic generalized epilepsies in combined MEG/EEG. Epilepsy Res 85: 187–198.

Steinlein OK, Mulley JC, Propping P et al. (1995). A missense mutation in the neuronal nicotinic acetylcholine receptor alpha 4 subunit is associated with autosomal dominant nocturnal frontal lobe epilepsy. Nat Genet 11: 201–203.

Steinlein OK, Magnusson A, Stoodt J et al. (1997). An insertion mutation of the *CHRNA4* gene in a family with autosomal dominant nocturnal frontal lobe epilepsy. Hum Mol Genet 6: 943–947.

Sugawara T, Mazaki-Miyazaki E, Fukushima K et al. (2002). Frequent mutations of *SCN1A* in severe myoclonic epilepsy in infancy. Neurology 58: 1122–1124.

Suls A, Dedeken P, Goffin K et al. (2008). Paroxysmal exercise-induced dyskinesia and epilepsy is due to mutations in *SLC2A1*, encoding the glucose transporter GLUT1. Brain 131: 1831–1844.

Suls A, Mullen SA, Weber YG et al. (2009). Early-onset absence epilepsy caused by mutations in the glucose transporter GLUT1. Ann Neurol 66: 415–419.

Talos DM, Kwiatkowski DJ, Cordero K et al. (2008). Cell-specific alterations of glutamate receptor expression in tuberous sclerosis complex cortical tubers. Ann Neurol 63: 454–465.

Vahedi K, Depienne C, Le Fort D et al. (2009). Elicited repetitive daily blindness: a new phenotype associated with hemiplegic migraine and *SCN1A* mutations. Neurology 72: 1178–1183.

van Luijtelaar G, Sitnikova E (2006). Global and focal aspects of absence epilepsy: the contribution of genetic models. Neurosci Biobehav Rev 30: 983–1003.

Venter JC, Adams MD, Myers EW et al. (2001). The sequence of the human genome. Science 291: 1304–1351.

Vulliemoz S, Lemieux L, Daunizeau J et al. (2010). The combination of EEG source imaging and EEG-correlated functional MRI to map epileptic networks. Epilepsia 51: 491–505.

Wheless JW, Clarke DF, Carpenter D (2005). Treatment of pediatric epilepsy: expert opinion, 2005. J Child Neurol 20: S1–S56.

Wheless JW, Clarke DF, Arzimanoglou A et al. (2007). Treatment of pediatric epilepsy: European expert opinion, 2007. Epileptic Disord 9: 353–412.

Wong M (2010). Mammalian target of rapamycin (mTOR) inhibition as a potential antiepileptogenic therapy: from tuberous sclerosis to common acquired epilepsies. Epilepsia 51: 27–36.

York GK, Steinberg DA (2009). Hughlings Jackson's suggestion for the treatment of epilepsy. Neurology 73: 1155–1158.

Handbook of Clinical Neurology, Vol. 107 (3rd series)
Epilepsy, Part I
H. Stefan and W.H. Theodore, Editors

Chapter 6

The epidemiology of the epilepsies

AIDAN NELIGAN[1], WILLARD A. HAUSER[2], AND JOSEMIR W. SANDER[1,3]*

[1]*Department of Clinical and Experimental Epilepsy, UCL Institute of Neurology, London, UK*

[2]*Department of Neurology, College of Physicians and Surgeons, and Mailman School of Public Health, Columbia University, New York, NY, USA*

[3]*SEIN – Epilepsy Institute in the Netherlands Foundation, Heemstede, The Netherlands*

INTRODUCTION

Epilepsy is the commonest neurological condition affecting people of all ages, races, and social classes. Worldwide it is estimated that over 50 million people have epilepsy, of whom three-quarters live in resource-poor countries with little or no access to medical services and treatment (Meinardi et al., 2001; Ngugi et al., 2010).

Epidemiology is the study of health determinants, and the distribution and natural history of disease in populations. Epidemiological studies can be descriptive, analytical, or experimental. Descriptive epidemiology deals with the distribution and vital statistics (incidence and prevalence) of a condition in a population, without regard to causation, and usually involves observational studies. Analytical epidemiology tests hypotheses, for example examining risk factors for a disease, often using cohort and case–control studies. Experimental epidemiology consists of studies in which relevant risk factors are controlled. Epidemiological studies in epilepsy are mostly descriptive or analytical (Sander, 2003).

Until the 1960s, epidemiological studies in epilepsy were carried out in tertiary referral centers; this suggested that epilepsy was a chronic, progressive, incurable condition with little chance of remission (Sander, 2003).

Methodological differences, lack of standardized classification, problems with case ascertainment and diagnostic accuracy, as well as the heterogeneous nature of epilepsy, result in disparity in study findings.

Diagnostic accuracy is a particular problem in epilepsy as seizures are a symptom of diverse underlying cerebral etiologies and may not have permanent physical manifestations (Sander, 2003). The diagnosis of epilepsy is dependent on the chance recording of an event, the availability of a detailed eye-witness account (which may be misleading; Rugg-Gunn et al., 2001), and the expertise and experience of the diagnosing specialist, with opinions differing in ambiguous cases (van Donselaar et al., 1989; Stroink et al., 2004). Consequently a definitive diagnosis is often made only after an extended period of follow-up (Hauser and Kurland, 1975; Sander et al., 1990) Moreover, 20–30% of those attending tertiary referral centers with refractory epilepsy do not have epilepsy (Smith et al., 1999); the most common differential diagnoses are dissociative seizures and syncope. Neurologists are better at diagnosing epilepsy than nonspecialists (misdiagnosis rate 5.6% versus 18.9%) (Leach et al., 2005), but at least 5% of diagnoses may be wrong.

People with epilepsy may not seek medical attention, through either ignorance or lack of awareness of the symptoms. Some absence and complex partial seizures may be recognized only in retrospect following a convulsion (Hauser et al., 1990). One study found that only 20% of patients with seizures suspected the diagnosis prior to consultation (Hopkins and Scambler, 1977). A community study using a door-to-door survey found that one-quarter of people with seizures had not sought medical attention (Zielinski, 1974a).

Fear of stigmatization may also cause concealment. This may be a particular problem in certain communities; in one study, the low prevalence rate was interpreted as being the result of concealment (Rocca et al., 2001). In another study, 10% of those with a confirmed diagnosis of epilepsy denied having seizures (Beran et al., 1985).

*Correspondence to: J.W. Sander, Department of Clinical Experimental Epilepsy, UCL Institute of Neurology, Queen Square, London WC1N 3BG, UK. E-mail: l.sander@ucl.ac.uk

Thus, epidemiological studies of epilepsy should be community-based, prospective (to identify risk factors), and independent of existing medical records (or supplemented by use of door-to-door surveys, questionnaires, or interview) to allow as complete as possible case ascertainment.

DEFINITIONS

To allow meaningful comparisons, the same definition of epilepsy and a standardized classification of seizures need to be applied across all studies. The International League Against Epilepsy (ILAE) (Commission on Epidemiology and Prognosis of the ILAE, 1993) provides guidelines for epidemiological studies in epilepsy. Epilepsy is defined as a condition characterized by recurrent (two or more) seizures that are unprovoked by any identifiable cause. Febrile seizures and neonatal seizures are excluded. A single seizure is defined as one seizure or as multiple seizures occurring within a 24-hour period. A person with active epilepsy is defined as someone with known epilepsy who has had at least one unprovoked seizure in the previous 5 years irrespective of treatment status, whereas a person with prevalent epilepsy in remission is defined as someone with known epilepsy who has had no seizures in 5 years or more regardless of treatment.

Epidemiological studies in epilepsy are typically divided into studies from resource-poor and developed countries, because of differences in etiologies and medical services; this division is somewhat arbitrary.

INCIDENCE STUDIES

Incidence is defined as the number of new cases of epilepsy or seizures in a well-defined population during a specified time period (usually 1 year) and is normally expressed as the number of cases per 100 000 people in the population per year. Incidence studies are important for identifying risk factors as well as for providing information on prognosis. Most incidence studies have been conducted in developed countries and are retrospective, although some recent studies have been population-based prospective studies as recommended by the Commission on Epidemiology and Prognosis of the ILAE (1997).

Incidence studies of first epileptic seizures

A new-onset seizure can be unprovoked or provoked (acute symptomatic seizure; ASS). The latter occur within close temporal proximity of an acute cerebral or systemic insult and are considered distinct from epilepsy because they tend to recur only with a recurrence of the precipitant. The prognosis is also different. The likelihood of further seizures is less and mortality is greater when compared with that of individuals with unprovoked seizures (Hesdorffer et al., 1998, 2009) The annual incidence of ASS was 20 per 100 000 in one study (Forsgren et al., 1996a) and 35 per 100 000 in another (Hauser et al., 1993).

Although many people presenting with seizures have a history of prior events, up to half present with a single unprovoked seizure (Sander et al., 1990; Adelow et al., 2009). Most studies combine the incidence rates for all newly diagnosed unprovoked seizures (single seizures and newly diagnosed epilepsy), but this is usually higher than the incidence of epilepsy in a population followed over a long period of time, as not all people with a single seizure develop epilepsy. This was demonstrated in one study over a 50-year period. The incidence of a first unprovoked seizure or newly diagnosed epilepsy was 61 per 100 000 person-years and the incidence of newly diagnosed epilepsy alone was 44 per 100 000 person-years (Hauser et al., 1993). Overall the incidence of first single unprovoked seizure or newly diagnosed epilepsy is probably between 50 and 70 per 100 000 per year in industrialized countries (Table 6.1), but may be much higher in developing countries.

Incidence of epilepsy in more developed countries

Incidence studies have been conducted in European countries and the USA with remarkable consistency across different countries (Table 6.2). In general, the incidence of epilepsy in the Western world is around 50 (range 40–70) per 100 000 per year (Sander, 2003). A systematic review of incidence studies identified 40 studies (9 prospective and 7 from resource-poor countries). The median annual incidence of epilepsy was 47.4 per 100 000 and that of unprovoked seizures was 56 per 100 000. When the analysis was limited to studies of the highest quality, the median annual incidence of both decreased slightly (Kotsopoulos et al., 2002).

Annual incidence rates of epilepsy in Europe were shown to range from 43 to 47 per 100 000 person-years (Forsgren et al., 2005a). Two more recent studies provided annual incidences of 33.3 (Iceland) (Olafsson et al., 2005) and 68.8 (Denmark) (Christensen et al., 2007b) per 100 000.

Incidence of epilepsy in resource-poor countries

There are fewer incidence studies from resource-poor countries (Table 6.3). In the systematic review, the seven studies from the developing world had a median annual incidence of 68.7 per 100 000, compared with 43.4 per 100 000 for more industrialized countries

Table 6.1

Incidence of first epileptic seizure (per 100 000)

Reference	Country	Population size	Total	Provoked	Unprovoked	Single	Study design
Loiseau et al., 1990	France	1 128 164	71.3	29.0	42.3	18.3	Prospective
Hauser et al., 1993	USA	2 003 357	100	35.0	61.0	NA	Retrospective
Forsgren et al., 1996a	Sweden	101 583	76.0	20.0	56.0	NA	Prospective (adults ≥ 17 years)
Jallon et al., 1997	Switzerland	384 657	70.8	25.2	45.6	NA	Prospective
Jallon et al., 1999	Martinique	383 596	80.5	16.4	64.1	NA	Prospective
MacDonald et al., 2000a	UK	100 230	NA	NA	57.0	11.0	Prospective
Olafsson et al., 2005	Iceland	272 512	NA	NA	56.8	23.5	Prospective
Benn et al., 2008	USA	270 677	NA	NA	40.3	16.4	Prospective
Adelöw et al., 2009	Sweden	998 500	NA	NA	33.9	14.4	Prospective

NA, not available.

Table 6.2

Prospective population-based incidence studies

Reference	Country	No. of cases	Age-adjusted incidence rate per 100 000	Comments
Hauser et al., 1993	USA	880	44	Comprehensive medical review; 1935–1984
Sidenvall et al., 1993	Sweden	61	73	Age 0–15 years; 20 months
Forsgren et al., 1996a	Sweden	160	56	Population register; SS included; age > 16 years
Olafsson et al., 1996	Iceland	42	47	Medical record; review (1993)
Zarrelli et al., 1999	USA	157	52.3	Comprehensive medical review; 1980–1984
Annegers et al., 1999	USA	197 78 (SS)	35.5 50.9 (SS)	HMO population; age 0–64 years; 1988–1994
Beilmann et al., 1999	Estonia	216	45	Age 1 month to 19 years; 1995–1997
Oün et al., 2003	Estonia	81	35.4	Database review (1994–1997); age ≥20 years
Olafsson et al., 2005	Iceland	294 207 (SS)	32.4 22.8 (SS)	Nationwide surveillance system; 1995–1999
Christensen et al., 2007b	Denmark	88 616	68.8	Database review; 1977–2002; all ages
Adelow et al., 2009	Sweden	585 430 (SS)	33.9*	Incidence registry; 2001–2004; all ages

*All first unprovoked seizures.
SS, single seizure.

Table 6.3

Incidence studies in resource-poor countries

Reference	Country	No. of cases	Age-adjusted incidence rate per 100 000	Comments
Li et al., 1985	China	16	35	Wide confidence intervals
Placencia et al., 1992	Ecuador	137	122–190	Wide geographical variation
Lavados et al., 1992	Chile	102	113	
Rwiza et al., 1992	Tanzania	122	55	Crude incidence 73.3 per 100 000
Tekle-Haimanot et al., 1997	Ethiopia	139	49	Crude incidence 64 per 100 000
Kaiser et al., 1998	Uganda	80	156	Crude incidence 215 per 100 000
Mani et al., 1998	India	32	49.3	
Sawhney et al., 1999	India	34	60.0	
Wang et al., 2002	China	16	28.8	Door-to-door survey in 5 rural provinces
Tuan et al., 2010	Vietnam	19/21	44.8	Door-to-door surveys (×2) in rural area

(Kotsopoulos et al., 2002). Incidence rates from South America are among the highest reported; a well-designed study reported incidence between 122 and 190 per 100 000 per year in Ecuador (Placencia et al., 1992). Age-adjusted annual incidence rates from Chile (113 per 100 000) (Lavados et al., 1992) and Honduras (92.7 per 100 000) (Medina et al., 2005) were similarly high. Incidence in India (Mani et al., 1998; Sawhney et al., 1999) was similar to that in developed countries, while that in China was lower (Li et al., 1985; Wang et al., 2002); both Chinese studies were small. In Africa, there is wide geographical variation in incidence; the incidence reported in Uganda (Kaiser et al., 1998) is twice that of Tanzania (Rwiza et al., 1992) and Ethiopia (Tekle-Haimanot et al., 1997), which have an age-adjusted incidence similar to that of Western countries. Such variations may be largely explained by infestations; a Ugandan study (Kaiser et al., 1998) reported that the age-adjusted incidence was 232 per 100 000 person-years in an onchocerciasis endemic area and 77 per 100 000 person-years in a nonendemic area. Other factors such as poor sanitation and poor health services may also contribute.

Cumulative incidence

The cumulative incidence of epilepsy is the proportion of a fixed population that develops epilepsy in a certain time. An early study found the cumulative incidence of unprovoked seizures was 2.4% by age 80 years (Juul-Jensen and Foldspang, 1983). Later studies have found higher rates. In a US study the cumulative incidence was 1.2% by age 24, 3% by age 75, and 4.4% by age 85 years (Hauser et al., 1993). Almost identical figures were found in Sweden (Forsgren et al., 1996a) and in Iceland (Olafsson et al., 1996). In contrast, in Martinique (Jallon et al., 1999) the cumulative incidence was 2.2% by age 15, 4.5% by age 50, and 7.2% by age 75 years. A similarly high figure was found recently in Denmark, where approximately 2% were diagnosed with epilepsy by age 25 years (Christensen et al., 2007b). In summary, almost 1 in 15 people will experience an unprovoked seizure at some stage.

Gender

Most incidence studies report that epilepsy is more common in males than in females, in both developing and more developed countries (Lavados et al., 1992; Hauser et al., 1993; Olafsson et al., 1996; Christensen et al., 2007b); this difference is rarely statistically significant (Jallon et al., 1999). In the systematic review of incidence studies, the median annual incidence of epilepsy was 50.7 per 100 000 for males and 46.2 per 100 000 for females, with slightly higher rates for unprovoked seizures (Kotsopoulos et al., 2002). Some incidence studies have reported a female predominance (Placencia et al., 1992; Cockerell et al., 1995).

Age-specific incidence

Studies in developed countries consistently show a bimodal distribution. There is a very high incidence in infancy and early childhood, with a relative decrease in adolescence. Incidence is at its lowest in young adults and steadily increases after the age of 50 years, with the greatest increase seen in those over age 80. The incidence of epilepsy is now higher in elderly people than in children (Everitt and Sander, 1998). The Iceland study (Olafsson et al., 2005) found an incidence of 130.2 per 100 000 person-years in infants and 110.5 per 100 000 person-years in those aged over 65 years. The highest incidence of 168.5 per 100 000 person-years was in those aged between 75 and 84 years.

There is evidence to suggest that there are age-specific differences in incidence between men and women, particularly in the elderly. In one study (Forsgren et al., 1996a), the incidence increased sharply in men between the ages of 60 and 69 and peaked at age 70–79 years. In contrast, the sharp increase occurred later in women, peaking in those aged 80 years and above.

The temporal changes in incidence of epilepsy in Finland between 1986 and 2002 were examined using a nationwide database. The total incidence decreased significantly from 71.6 to 52.9 per 100 000 person-years during that interval. The incidence decreased in children and adults but increased in the elderly, particularly in women (Sillanpaa et al., 2006). In the Rochester studies (Hauser and Kurland, 1975; Hauser et al., 1993) there was no significant change in total annual incidence over a 50-year period, although the incidence of epilepsy decreased by 40% in children aged less than 10 years over that interval whereas the incidence of epilepsy in the elderly almost doubled. A study from Denmark investigating the incidence of epilepsy between 1995 and 2002 (Christensen et al., 2007b) found that, although the overall incidence rates remained constant, the incidence increased for those aged more than 60 years (particularly for those aged above 80) while decreasing in children (particularly in infants). It has been suggested that this increase in the elderly is due to improved survival following cerebrovascular accidents (Annegers et al., 1995; Hallstrom et al., 2002) despite the incidence of cerebrovascular accidents falling dramatically over the same time period (Muntner et al., 2002).

The pediatric population has the highest incidence in studies from Africa. In sub-Saharan Africa (Preux and Druet-Cabanac, 2005), more than three-quarters of those with incident epilepsy were under 20 years old, with low incidence rates in the elderly. This may be due to the lower life expectancy in sub-Saharan countries, in addition to the increased mortality rate associated with epilepsy and its underlying causes. In South American studies, incidence rates were higher in the pediatric population than in Western countries, but the incidence rates were also increased in the elderly (Placencia et al., 1992; Medina et al., 2005). Studies from Asia show similar age-specific incidence patterns to those in Western countries.

Socioeconomic factors and ethnicity

A study of the incidence of epilepsy (including febrile and neonatal seizures) in childhood reported annual incidence of 136 per 100 000 for African American males and 99 per 100 000 for African American females, compared with 63 per 100 000 for Caucasian males and 60 per 100 000 for Caucasian females. The study also demonstrated an excess of epilepsy in children (of either ethnicity) living in lower socioeconomic areas (Shamansky and Glaser, 1979). Later studies limited to unprovoked seizures have failed to replicate such findings. No significant differences in ethnicity-specific incidence rates were found in a study of an Health Maintenance Organization (HMO) population (Annegers et al., 1999), while the annual incidence among Hispanics (36.5 per 100 000) was similar to that of non-Hispanic whites (39.4 per 100 000) and non-Hispanic blacks (37.6 per 100 000) in a study of incidence in a low-income community in New York. Lower income was associated with a higher incidence of epilepsy (Benn et al., 2008). A strong association between socioeconomic deprivation and the age-adjusted incidence of epilepsy was demonstrated in London, where the age-adjusted incidence of epilepsy in the most deprived fifth of the population was 2.3 times that of the least deprived fifth (Heaney et al., 2002). No overall differences in incidence were found when South Asian children in Bradford were compared with white children. Children with seizures from both communities were significantly more likely to come from deprived areas (Hamdy et al., 2007).

Seizure types

Epileptic seizures are classified into seizure types based on clinical description and EEG findings according to the ILAE guidelines (Commission on Classification and Terminology of the ILAE, 1981). While many studies have noted a majority of people with generalized seizures (Li et al., 1985; Rwiza et al., 1992; Jallon et al., 1999), it is likely that in many cases partial seizures with secondary generalization have been misclassified as generalized seizures. Partial seizures predominate in studies from the UK (59%) (Sander et al., 1990), the USA (57%) (Hauser et al., 1993), Sweden (68%) (Forsgren et al., 1996a, and France (46%) (Jallon et al., 2001). A systematic review (Kotsopoulos et al., 2002) found that partial seizures occurred in 55% of patients. In one study, age-specific incidences of generalized and partial seizures were compared; generalized seizures were more common in the first 5 years of life, the incidence was similar for both between the ages of 6 and 24 years, and partial seizures were twice as common as generalized onset seizures in adults aged over 24 years (Hauser et al., 1993). In a community-based study of newly diagnosed epilepsy in children, 55% had partial seizures (Berg et al., 1999).

Incidence of epileptic syndromes

Epilepsy syndromes are classified according to the ILAE classification (Commission on Classification and Terminology of the ILAE, 1989), which is based on age, clinical semiology, and electrophysiological findings. Epilepsy is defined as idiopathic (assumed genetic), cryptogenic (assumed symptomatic), and remote symptomatic. Many cases in epidemiological studies, however, are unclassifiable according to the current classification (Everitt and Sander, 1999). In one study, only 34% of 564 cases of definite epilepsy were classifiable into ILAE diagnostic categories, with many rare syndromes not represented (Manford et al., 1992b). Localization-related epilepsies are the most frequent form of epilepsy in studies such as the EPIMART study (Jallon et al., 1999), where 47% had localization-related epilepsy and 34% had generalized epilepsy. In the Rochester study (Zarrelli et al., 1999), 18% lacked clear focal or generalized features; this has been a feature in other studies (Manford et al., 1992a; Forsgren et al., 1996a) Other studies limited to children have achieved a higher rate of specific classification (Berg et al., 1999). It is clear that the syndrome classification is better suited to classifying childhood-onset epilepsy. In prospective follow-up studies the relative distributions of the epilepsy syndromes will change over time; in one study limited to children (Shinnar et al., 1999) the proportion of undetermined cases decreased from 26% to 18%.

In a study from Iceland (Olafsson et al., 2005), the following incidence rates for the epileptic syndromes were calculated: juvenile myoclonic epilepsy (0.7 per 100 000), childhood absence epilepsy (0.8 per 100 000), benign rolandic epilepsy (2.8 per 100 000), West syndrome (0.007 per 100 000), Landau–Kleffner syndrome (0.2 per 100 000), benign familial infantile convulsions (0.3 per 100 000), primary reading epilepsy and benign occipital epilepsy (0.2 per 100 000 each) (Table 6.4).

Table 6.4

Incidence of epileptic syndromes (per 100 000 person-years)

Type of epilepsy	South-West France (Loiseau et al., 1990)	Rochester, USA (Zarrelli et al., 1999)	Iceland (Olafssson et al., 2005)
Localization-related epilepsies			
Total	15.3	34.9	18.6
Idiopathic partial epilepsies	1.7	0.2	1.6
Symptomatic partial epilepsies	13.6	17.2	8.4
Cryptogenic partial epilepsies	–	17.5	8.6
Generalized epilepsies			
Total	7.2	7.7	3.9
Idiopathic	6.1	3.7	3.1
Cryptogenic or symptomatic	1.1	1.7	0.7
Symptomatic	–	2.3	0.1
Epilepsies with both generalized and focal features	–	1.7	0.8
Epilepsies without unequivocal focal or generalized features	1.9	8.0	8.5
Isolated unprovoked seizures	18.3	–	22.8

PREVALENCE

Prevalence is defined as the number of people with a disease in a defined population as a proportion of the total population and is usually expressed as the number of cases per 1000 population. Point prevalence is the number of existing cases in the population at a particular point in time, whereas period prevalence is the prevalence over a particular interval (usually 1 year). Information about a disease's prevalence is important for service provision and planning. Prevalence studies use cross-sectional studies, so are fairly quick and easy to perform, and much less expensive than cohort studies. Consequently there is a far greater number of prevalence studies. Most of these were carried out using door-to-door surveys with standardized validated screening questionnaires; this is considered the gold standard methodology.

Prevalence in developed countries

Prevalence studies in developed countries have reported the prevalence for active epilepsy to be between 4 and 10 per 1000 (Sander, 2003); most studies report a prevalence of active epilepsy of 4–7 per 1000 (Forsgren, 1992; Sidenvall et al., 1996; Olafsson and Hauser, 1999). The lowest prevalence reported was 1.5 per 1000 in Japan (Sato, 1964), although more recent studies have estimated prevalence rates of active epilepsy more in concordance with other Western countries (Oka et al., 2006). A systematic review (Forsgren et al., 2005a) found that the range of prevalence in Europe was 3.3–7.8 per 1000 with a median prevalence of active epilepsy of 5.2 per 1000. European studies with the lowest reported prevalence were from Italy: 3.3 per 1000 in Sicily (Rocca et al., 2001) and 3.0 per 1000 in the Aeolian Islands (Gallitto et al., 2005), although the authors of both studies suggested that the low reported prevalence rates might have resulted from concealment. In the Rochester study the prevalence of active epilepsy, at 10-year intervals over 50 years, ranged from 2.7 to 6.8 per 1000 (Hauser et al., 1991).

Prevalence of epilepsy in resource-poor countries

The median prevalence in Africa or Latin America is significantly higher than that reported in Western countries, whereas the reported prevalence in Asia is broadly similar to that in Western countries (Table 6.5).

In Latin America, prevalence studies from 12 countries reported a median lifetime prevalence of 17.8 (range 6–44.3) per 1000 and a median prevalence of active epilepsy of 12.4 (range 5.1–57) per 1000 (Burneo et al., 2005). There is, however, significant heterogeneity between different countries and even between different regions within the same country. The highest prevalence reported, based upon a small number of cases, was from rural Panama (prevalence of active epilepsy 57 per 1000; Gracia et al., 1990) compared with a previously reported prevalence of 22 per 1000 in Panama city (Gracia et al., 1988). This contrasts with a prevalence of active epilepsy of 5.1 per 1000 in Rio de Janeiro (Gomes et al., 2002). Although methodological differences cause difficulties in comparing prevalence between countries or even between studies performed in the same country, marked differences in prevalence have been reported between

Table 6.5

Selected prevalence studies in resource-poor countries

Reference	Country	Prevalence per 1000 population	No. of cases
Placencia et al., 1992	Ecuador	6.7–8.0	575
Aziz et al., 1997	Pakistan (P)/Turkey (T)	9.98 (P) 7.0 (T)	24 130 (P) 11 497 (T)
Nicoletti et al., 1999	Bolivia	12.3 11.1 active epilepsy	124
Sridharan and Murthy, 1999	India	5.35	3207
Wang et al., 2003	China	7.0 4.6 active epilepsy	387
Burneo et al., 2005	Latin America (1974–2002)	17.8 (6–43.2)*	Pooled analysis of 32 prevalence studies
Medina et al., 2005	Rural Honduras	23.3 15.4 active epilepsy	151
Preux and Druet-Cabanac, 2005	Sub-Saharan Africa (1986–2004)	15.0 (5.2–70.0)	Pooled analysis of 26 door-to-door surveys in 15 countries, all but 3 rural populations
Ndoye et al., 2005	Senegal	14.2	64
Dent et al., 2005	Tanzania	7.4 active epilepsy	42
Almu et al., 2006	Ethiopia	29.5	82
Velez and Eslava-Cobos, 2006	Columbia	11.3 (9.2–13.8) 10.1 (8.1–12.4)	92
Mac et al., 2007	Asia (1985–2006)	6.0 (1.5–14.0)	Pooled analysis of 20 studies from 12 countries
Edwards et al., 2008	Kenya	4.5 active epilepsy	466
Tuan et al., 2008	Vietnam	4.4 active epilepsy	206

*Values in parentheses represent the range of different prevalence rates of epilepsy in 32 studies from Latin America.

rural and urban areas (15.4 compared with 9.1 per 1000 in Ecuador) (Placencia et al., 1992).

Twelve countries in Asia have an estimated median lifetime prevalence of 6 (range 1.5–14) per 1000 (Mac et al., 2007). A meta-analysis of 20 prevalence studies in India estimated the overall age-adjusted prevalence as 5.6 per 1000, with nonsignificantly higher prevalence in urban areas (Sridharan and Murthy, 1999). Three studies from China reported an age-adjusted point prevalence of 4.4 per 1000 in six cities (Li et al., 1985), 3.6 per 1000 in a rural province (Huang et al., 2002), and a prevalence of 4.6 per 1000 for active epilepsy and lifetime prevalence rate of 7 per 1000 (Wang et al., 2003). A recent study from rural Tibet estimated a lifetime prevalence of 2.5 per 1000 (Zhao et al., 2008), emphasizing the geographical variation in prevalence in China. A comparative study of prevalence in urban and rural populations in Pakistan and Turkey used identical methodology. The overall prevalence was 9.98 per 1000 in Pakistan and 7.0 per 1000 in Turkey, but the prevalence was twice as high in rural areas than in urban areas in both countries (Aziz et al., 1997).

Prevalence studies in Africa demonstrate significant variation between countries and even within the same country. A systematic review estimated a median prevalence of 15 (range 5.2–70.0) per 1000 in sub-Saharan Africa (Preux and Druet-Cabanac, 2005). Many of the included studies were small with variable methodology, with the inherent risk of overestimation or underestimation of the true prevalence. The study from the Cameroon (point prevalence 70 per 1000) was based on a population of only 500 (Nkwi and Ndonko, 1989). The five studies with populations of greater than 15 000 displayed greater concordance, with prevalence ranging from 5.3 to 12.5 per 1000 (Preux and Druet-Cabanac, 2005). The largest study, in a rural population of over

150 000 in Kenya, estimated the prevalence of active epilepsy as 4.5 (95% confidence interval (CI) 4.1 to 4.9) per 1000 (Edwards et al., 2008).

Gender

As with incidence studies, most prevalence studies demonstrate a slight predominance of males that is rarely significant. A few studies have, however, shown a female predominance (Ndoye et al., 2005). In the Rochester study (Hauser et al., 1991) the prevalence was higher in males in each successive decade, except the last. Although most studies report an overall predominance of males, this may shift between different age groups.

Prevalence and ethnicity

True differences in prevalence are difficult to assess owing to the confounding of socioeconomic factors, which may themselves be causative or a consequence of epilepsy. In a study examining racial differences, the age-adjusted prevalence was higher in African American people than in Caucasian people, with the prevalence of active epilepsy 10.0 per 1000 in African American males and 6.9 per 1000 in African American females, compared with 6.7 per 1000 in Caucasian males and 4.0 per 1000 in Caucasian females (Haerer et al., 1986). The prevalence of epilepsy in South Asian people in Bradford was half that of the rest of the population, which may reflect different cultural perceptions, selective immigration, and fear of stigmatization (Wright et al., 2000).

A higher prevalence in Hispanics (active epilepsy 6.3 per 1000) compared with non-Hispanics (4.1 per 1000) was found in a US study of self-reported epilepsy. African American people had a lower prevalence of active epilepsy but higher lifetime prevalence rates than Caucasian people (Kelvin et al., 2007).

Prevalence and socioeconomic factors

Social deprivation appears to be causal for, and a consequence of, epilepsy. Unemployment, a commonly used substrate for social deprivation, has been found to be high (46%) in people with epilepsy (59% in those with active epilepsy), compared with 19% in an age- and sex-matched control population (Elwes et al., 1991). In a Welsh study, a strong correlation between social deprivation and prevalence of epilepsy was found ($r = 0.75$), which persisted when patients with an underlying psychiatric illness or learning disability were excluded ($r = 0.70$). Moreover, this strong correlation was evident in the youngest age group (less than 20 years) when indicators of social deprivation such as unemployment would have minimal effect (Morgan et al., 2000).

Lower socioeconomic status was found to be associated with an increased risk of epilepsy in adults but not children in Iceland. Low education was associated with a higher risk (odds ratio (OR) 2.29, 95% CI 1.21 to 4.34), whereas home ownership was associated with a decreased risk (OR 0.69, 95% CI 0.43 to 0.92) in adults (Hesdorffer et al., 2005).

One study (Abib et al., 2007) examined factors associated with epilepsy in young children in a socially deprived area in Brazil. The overall prevalence of seizures was high (45.2 per 1000), with the risk significantly associated with poor housing (OR 3.0, 95% CI 1.4 to 7.1) and lack of tap water (OR 2.5, 95% CI 1.0 to 5.8) on multivariable analysis.

Age-specific prevalence

In European studies, the median prevalence per 1000 people was 5.5 (95% CI 3.5 to 9.3) for those aged 0–19 years, 5.4 (95% CI 3.3 to 8.6) for those aged 20–59 years, and 4.7 (95% CI 3.0 to 7.3) in people more than 60 years (Forsgren et al., 2005a). Case ascertainment in the elderly can be problematic, with epilepsy frequently misdiagnosed; thus, the true prevalence of epilepsy has frequently been underestimated. In one study, there was a tendency for the prevalence to be highest in the elderly (aged above 75 years), with the most dramatic change of prevalence over time seen in this age group (1.9 per 1000 in 1940, increasing to 14.8 per 1000 in 1980) (Hauser et al., 1991). In another study (Olafsson and Hauser, 1999), the prevalence of epilepsy increased with age, with the highest prevalence reported in those aged 85 years or more (9.4 per 1000).

The impression that the prevalence of epilepsy increases with age is supported by the findings of a study that looked at the prevalence of epilepsy in those aged over 55 years. The prevalence of active epilepsy increased from 0.7 per 1000 in those aged 55–64 years to 1.2 per 1000 in those aged 85–94 years (De La Court et al., 1996).

Studies from resource-poor countries tend to show a high prevalence in adolescents and young adults, with much lower prevalences in the elderly (Edwards et al., 2008). This may be related to the high frequency of infections in the young and the lower life expectancy in such countries.

Seizure type

Most studies in the Western world show a predominance of partial seizures over generalized seizures (more than 60% of all active epilepsy cases in Rochester; Hauser et al., 1991). The difference seems most marked in the elderly, as shown in the Rotterdam study (73% partial seizures in all those aged above 55 years) (De La Court et al., 1996).

In contrast, many studies from the developing world have found more people with generalized seizures

(80.5% in Pakistan and 65.4% in Turkey) (Aziz et al., 1997). The use of EEG with clinical data may allow the reclassification of some cases clinically diagnosed as generalized seizures to partial seizures with secondary generalization (Nicoletti et al., 1999). One-third of cases were clinically diagnosed with partial seizures, but with the addition of electroclinical data the proportion with partial seizures increased to 53%.

RISK FACTORS FOR EPILEPSY

The etiology of any chronic condition is best determined by use of population-based studies of newly diagnosed cases. Prevalence studies of active epilepsy will miss cases at both ends of the severity spectrum (severe cases with causes associated with increased mortality and more benign cases with early remission). Epilepsy is divided into different categories according to causation: remote symptomatic, progressive symptomatic, idiopathic (presumed genetic), and cryptogenic or unknown.

In population-based studies the epilepsy is most frequently cryptogenic or idiopathic, 44.5% (Oün et al., 2003) to 67% (Olafsson et al., 2005), with the proportion of other causes increasing with age. The number of cases classified as cryptogenic has remained broadly similar over the past 20 years despite significant improvements in neuroimaging. An American study (Benn et al., 2008) defined 55% of cases as idiopathic/cryptogenic, similar to 61% reported in a UK study (Sander et al., 1990) almost 20 years earlier. Etiologies tend to be age-specific, with cerebral palsy, congenital brain damage, and learning disability predominating in the young, whereas tumors, neurodegenerative disorders, and cerebrovascular disease dominate in the elderly.

PROGNOSIS

For patients with seizures, the prognosis is the risk of further seizures after a single unprovoked seizure, or the likelihood of achieving seizure freedom after a pattern of recurring seizures has been established (Sander, 1993). Various aspects of the prognosis of epilepsy can be considered: the likelihood of recurrence following a single seizure; the impact of early versus late treatment; the probability of relapse after prolonged remission, following epilepsy surgery, or following antiepileptic medication withdrawal; and the morbidity and mortality associated with epilepsy.

Recurrence after a single seizure

Prospective population studies of single seizures are difficult as many seizures go unrecognized or are unwitnessed and patients may not present to medical attention unless the seizure is convulsive. The overall risk of recurrence following a single seizure has been reported as 27–71%. A meta-analysis found that the average risk of seizure recurrence was 40% in prospective studies and 52% in retrospective studies (Berg and Shinnar, 1991). The time interval between the seizure and inclusion in the follow-up influences recurrence; a patient who has a recurrence soon after the index seizure may be classified as having epilepsy, artificially lowering the estimated recurrence rate following a single seizure (Hopkins et al., 1988). The risk of subsequent seizures decreases with time, with up to 80% of recurrences occurring within 2 years of the initial seizure. Reported recurrence rates are 36% in prospective studies and 47% in retrospective at 2 years (Berg and Shinnar, 1991). In a UK study, the National General Practice Study of Epilepsy (NGPSE), 67% of those with a single seizure had a recurrence within 12 months and 78% within 36 months (Hart et al., 1990).

In a prospective study of 407 children with a first unprovoked seizure, 45% had a second seizure (median time to recurrence 6.2 months). The cumulative risk of a second seizure was 29% (1 year), 37% (2 years), and 46% (10 years) (Shinnar et al., 2000). In a study of epilepsy in childhood (Stroink et al., 1998), 156 children, none of whom received treatment, were followed up from the time of a first unprovoked seizure; 54% had a recurrence within 2 years. Similarly, another study (Lindsten et al., 2001b) found a recurrence rate of 58% at 750 days in 107 adults. No further recurrences were recorded thereafter during a median follow-up of 10.3 years, confirming the impression that the risk of seizure recurrence decreases with time.

Recurrence after a second seizure

The risk of recurrent seizures following a second seizure was investigated in a predominantly adult population (Hauser et al., 1998). In patients with a second seizure, the cumulative risk of a further seizure was 32% at 3 months, 41% at 6 months, 57% at 1 year, and 74% at 4 years. Of those who did not have a recurrence within the first 4 years of follow-up, none had a relapse in the subsequent 3 years. The majority (63%) of those with a third seizure had a further seizure, with the risk of a fourth seizure being 78% at 3 years. As with single seizures, the risk of further seizures is highest immediately after the last one. Similarly for children, the risk of a third seizure was 72% at 5 years after a second seizure (Shinnar et al., 2000).

Short- and medium-term prognosis

The prognosis of epilepsy is generally favorable, with 60–70% achieving remission (Sander, 1993). In a prospective study of children with newly diagnosed epilepsy followed from diagnosis, 74% achieved a period of remission (seizure freedom of 2 years or more), of whom 24% had a further seizure. In those who relapsed, approximately 50% occurred when antiepileptic medication was being withdrawn or had been stopped (Berg et al., 2001a). In the NGPSE after 9 years, 86% of those with definite epilepsy had achieved a remission of 3 years and 68% a remission of 5 years (Cockerell et al., 1997). In a study of 107 adults with newly diagnosed epilepsy, after 10 years the cumulative remission rates were 68% (1 year), 64% (3 years), and 58% (5 years) (Lindsten et al., 2001a).

Long-term prognosis

Few studies have investigated the long-term prognosis of people with epilepsy and most are retrospective. In the Rochester study (Annegers et al., 1979), 76% had achieved a 5-year period of remission at 20 years after diagnosis and 70% were in terminal remission. Of those in remission, 20% continued on antiepileptic medication whereas 50% had successfully discontinued medication and remained seizure-free for 5 years or more. In a cohort of children with active epilepsy, 64% were in a 3-year terminal remission after 12 years (Brorson and Wranne, 1987).

Two-thirds of 144 children with epilepsy were in terminal remission, on or off medication, after 37 years' follow-up. Early remission, occurring within the first year of treatment, occurred in 45 (31%), and the remission continued to terminal remission in 23. Remission without relapse occurred in another 72 (50%) with a mean delay of 9 years. Twenty (14%) entered remission but subsequently relapsed with further remission in a relapse-remitting pattern, whereas 27 (19%) continued with seizures from the onset (Sillanpaa and Schmidt, 2006a).

Of 102 children from the same cohort followed up for a median of 40 years, 95 (93%) had one or more periods of remission (1 year) (Sillanpaa and Schmidt, 2009), confirming an overall excellent prognosis for childhood epilepsy.

Prognostic factors

Many studies have looked at possible predictors of seizure prognosis, including age of onset, gender, etiology, seizure type, EEG patterns, number of seizures prior to treatment, and early response to treatment (Sander, 2003). In patients presenting with a first-ever seizure, neither multiple discrete seizures within 24 hours nor presentation as status epilepticus were associated with a higher risk for seizure recurrence than a single seizure (Hauser et al., 1990; Shinnar et al., 1996; Kho et al., 2006). Remote symptomatic epilepsy, the presence of a neurological birth deficit, and learning disability are consistently shown to be associated with a poorer prognosis. In one study (Brorson and Wranne, 1987), the 3-year remission rate was 89% for those with idiopathic epilepsy and normal examination, compared with only 49% for those with a neurological deficit or learning disability. The number of seizures in the first 6 months after onset is a strong determinant of the probability of subsequent remission, with 95% of those with two seizures in the first 6 months achieving a 5-year remission compared with only 24% of those with more than 10 seizures (MacDonald et al., 2000b).

A high initial seizure frequency, focal EEG slowing, and ASSs or neonatal status epilepticus are all significantly associated with an increased risk of developing refractory or intractable epilepsy in children (Berg et al., 2001b).

Seizure type is an inconsistent prognostic factor, with some studies indicating that those with partial seizures have a poorer prognosis (Annegers et al., 1979), whereas others have demonstrated a poorer prognosis for generalized onset seizures (Shafer et al., 1988). Patients with multiple seizure types, as typical in the childhood encephalopathies, appear to have a poorer prognosis (Collaborative Group for the Study of Epilepsy, 1992).

A significant reduction or complete cessation of seizures within 3 months of initiating treatment seems to be a strong predictor of subsequent remission (Camfield and Camfield, 1996; Sillanpaa et al., 1998). The probability of seizure remission decreases significantly with each successive treatment failure (Kwan and Brodie, 2000). Only 11% of patients who discontinued the first appropriate antiepileptic drug (AED) due to lack of efficacy became seizure-free on a second AED, and only 4% on a third medication or polypharmacy.

Children with clusters of seizures during treatment were more likely to have refractory epilepsy than children without clusters (42% versus 13%, $p = 0.01$) and less likely to achieve 5-year terminal remission ($p = 0.004$) (Sillanpaa and Schmidt, 2008). Children who had weekly seizures during the first year of treatment had an 8-fold increased risk of developing intractable epilepsy and twice the risk of not achieving 1-year terminal remission compared with those without weekly seizures (Sillanpaa and Schmidt, 2009).

The impact of etiology on prognosis

Patients with idiopathic generalized epilepsy appear to have a better prognosis than others. Most (82%) patients with idiopathic generalized seizures achieved 1-year seizure freedom, compared with only 35% of patients with symptomatic partial epilepsy and 45% of those with cryptogenic partial epilepsy (Semah et al., 1998).

Temporal lobe epilepsy (TLE) was associated with a poorer prognosis than extratemporal lobe epilepsy (36% versus 20% seizure-free). For patients with a single identified lesion, TLE with hippocampal sclerosis (HS) had a particularly bad prognosis (11% seizure-free) compared with other etiologies. Patients with HS and another identified pathology (dual pathology) had the worst prognosis (3% seizure-free) (Semah et al., 1998). Others found a similar prognosis in those with symptomatic and cryptogenic partial epilepsy (58% versus 56% seizure-free for at least 1 year) (Stephen et al., 2001). Comparing patients by etiology, they found that mesial TLE had the worst prognosis (42% seizure-free), compared with rates of 54% (cortical dysplasia), 55% (cerebral atrophy), 57% (cortical gliosis), 63% (cerebral infarction), and 78% (arteriovenous malformation).

The impact of medication on prognosis

In developed countries most patients start AEDs after two unprovoked seizures; prognostic studies from these countries are thus essentially those of treated epilepsy. Evidence from studies from resource-poor countries where a significant treatment gap exists suggests that many patients enter spontaneous remission without AEDs (Placencia et al., 1994); moreover, the response to AEDs in patients with chronic longstanding epilepsy is comparable to that of patients with new-onset seizures (Feksi et al., 1991; Watts, 1992; Placencia et al., 1994). This implies that the belief that epilepsy is a chronic progressive condition is false. It has been suggested that patients with epilepsy can be subdivided into prognostic groups based on their etiology and epileptic syndrome, which in turn determines their need and response to antiepileptic treatment (Sander, 1993).

Two studies have assessed the impact of medication on the risk of seizure recurrence. In the FIRST study, people with a first unprovoked (primary or secondary) generalized seizure were randomized either to immediate treatment (treated group) or to treatment only after a further seizure (untreated group). Although immediate treatment reduced the risk of early relapse, it did not affect the long-term prognosis. The 2-year remission rate was 72% in the treated group (57% in the untreated group), with rates of 84% versus 79% at 3 years and 85% versus 86% at 10 years. The comparable probabilities of attaining a 5-year remission were identical at 5 years (Leone et al., 2006).

In the MESS study (Marson et al., 2005), patients with a single seizure or early epilepsy (all types) were randomized to receive immediate or deferred treatment. Patients in the immediate treatment group had increased time to seizure recurrence, in addition to a reduced time to 2-year remission. At 5-year follow-up, however, three-quarters of both groups had achieved 3–5-year seizure freedom.

In conclusion, immediate treatment delays the early recurrence of seizures but does not affect the medium- or long-term prognosis.

Prognosis following AED withdrawal

In the largest randomized controlled trial of continued treatment versus drug withdrawal in 1013 patients in remission (2 years or more seizure-free), at 2 years after randomization 41% of those who discontinued medication had had a recurrence of seizures compared with 22% of those who stayed on medication. The rate of relapse was higher in the discontinuation group for up to 2 years of follow-up, but by 2–4 years the risk of relapse was higher in those continuing treatment (MRC AED Withdrawal Study Group, 1991). By 5 years after a relapse, 90% of those who had experienced a relapse had had a further 2-year remission period, indicating that the long-term prognosis was similar in both groups (Chadwick et al., 1996). An analysis of 14 AED withdrawal studies (Schmidt and Loscher, 2005) found that the recurrence rate following AED discontinuation ranged from 12% to 66% (mean 34%; 95% CI 27% to 43%) and reinstatement of treatment was successful in obtaining further remission in, on average, 80% (95% CI 75% to 85%) with no significant differences between age groups. A second remission may, however, take many years to achieve, while in an average of 19% (95% CI 15% to 24%) the reintroduction of medication did not control the seizures as before. Up to 23% of those discontinuing treatment developed intractable epilepsy. Risk factors for subsequent poor treatment outcome were symptomatic partial epilepsy and cognitive deficits (Schmidt and Loscher, 2005).

Ninety children who discontinued treatment following remission were followed for an average of 32 years from seizure onset (Sillanpaa and Schmidt, 2006b). Seizure relapse occurred in 33 (37%), with 36% of relapses occurring within the first year, 46% within 2 years, and 67% within 3 years. The last relapse occurred after 28 years of follow-up. Eight restarted treatment, with two achieving subsequent 5-year terminal remission with a delay of 10–19 years after restarting treatment. The other six patients did not achieve 5-year terminal remission, with two considered to have drug-resistant epilepsy. Factors associated with failure to achieve 5-year terminal remission following reinstatement of treatment were symptomatic and localization-related etiology (Sillanpaa and Schmidt, 2006b).

Despite the risk of seizure recurrence, patients may choose to discontinue treatment because of the impact of continuing AEDs on quality of life. In the Akershus study, the effect of AED withdrawal on quality of life was assessed. At 1 year, seizure recurrence had occurred in 15% of the withdrawal group compared with 7% in the no-withdrawal group (relative risk (RR) 2.46, 95% CI 0.85 to 7.08). The proportion of patients having completely normal neuropsychological findings increased from 11% to 28% in the withdrawal group, while decreasing from 11% to 9% in the no-withdrawal group. No differences in quality of life were observed between the two groups. At 41 months' follow-up, predictors of continued seizure freedom following treatment withdrawal were prior use of carbamazepine and a normal neurological examination (Lossius et al., 2008).

Prognosis following epilepsy surgery

In the only study of its type (Wiebe et al., 2001), 80 patients with temporal lobe epilepsy were randomized to either epilepsy surgery or continued medical treatment for 1 year. In the surgery group, 90% of patients had undergone surgery with 64% free from seizures impairing consciousness (42% completely seizure-free) compared with 8% (3% completely seizure-free overall) in the medical group at 1 year. Quality of life also improved in patients after surgery compared with that in patients in the medical group ($p < 0.001$).

In a recent review of controlled studies (2734 patients; all but one study nonrandomized), 44% of patients in the surgical group (mainly temporal lobe surgery) were seizure-free compared with 12% who had medical treatment only (pooled RR 4.26, 95% CI 3.03 to 5.98), and surgical patients were four times more likely to be able to discontinue medication than nonsurgical patients (RR 4.67, 95% CI 2.18 to 10.01) (Schmidt and Stavem, 2009).

In summary, in appropriately selected patients, surgery is four times as likely to render patients seizure-free as medical treatment alone.

Prognosis in those with intractable epilepsy

Studies suggest that failure to control seizures with the first or second AED implies that the probability of subsequent seizure control with further AEDs is small (Kwan and Brodie, 2000). Such a view may, however, be overly pessimistic. In a retrospective review of the effect of 265 medication changes in 155 patients with uncontrolled epilepsy of at least 5 years' duration, 16% of all patients were rendered seizure-free (12 months or more) following a drug introduction, and a further 21% had a reduction of seizure frequency of 50–99%. Overall, 28% of the cohort was rendered seizure-free by medical changes (Luciano and Shorvon, 2007).

A group of 246 patients with refractory epilepsy was followed for 3 years (Callaghan et al., 2007). Excluding 11 (4%) who became seizure-free as a result of surgery, 26 (11%) became seizure-free (6 months of terminal remission) as a result of medication change. No single AED was significantly associated with seizure freedom. Patients with mental retardation were less likely to achieve a remission. Overall, approximately 5% per year became seizure-free, highlighting that, irrespective of the number of AEDs previously tried, there is still a possibility of inducing meaningful seizure remission in this population.

The probability of seizure relapse following remission was studied retrospectively in a cohort of 186 patients with intractable epilepsy followed for median 3.8 years (Choi et al., 2008). Overall 20 patients achieved a remission of 12 months or more, with a 4% probability of remission per year. Of these, five subsequently suffered a relapse, with an estimated cumulative probability of relapse of 33% at 2 years and 44% at 3 years. No clear predictors of remission or subsequent relapse were identified.

In summary, approximately 4–5% a year of those with refractory epilepsy will achieve a remission of 12 months on medication; many will subsequently relapse.

MORTALITY

People diagnosed with epilepsy need to know whether this will have any impact on their life expectancy. It is accepted that people with epilepsy have a 2–3-fold increased risk of premature death compared with the general population. It has consistently been shown that people with neurological deficits or symptomatic seizures have a significantly increased risk of premature death, whereas the risk for those with idiopathic or cryptogenic epilepsy is broadly similar to that of the general population. Long-term population-based prospective cohort studies provide the most reliable estimates of the risk of mortality and of the way it changes over time (Neligan et al., 2010), although there are very few studies with follow-up of more than 20 years.

Methodological issues

Mortality studies in epilepsy should be community-based studies of people with incident epilepsy. Studies of people with prevalent epilepsy may underestimate the short-term mortality rate (as mortality in patients with epilepsy has consistently been shown to be highest soon after diagnosis), while simultaneously overestimating the long-term mortality rate (as patients who have gone into remission may not be included in the cohort). The risk of premature death in people with epilepsy has been studied using death certificates, hospital or institutional records, and through follow-up of community cohorts. Death certificates have been shown to be an unreliable source (Harvey et al., 1993; Bell et al., 2004). The use of hospital or institution registries may lead to selection bias of more severe cases and therefore an overestimation of the mortality risk.

The most commonly reported measure of mortality is the standardized mortality ratio (SMR), which is defined as the ratio of the observed deaths in the cohort divided by the number of expected deaths if the age–sex-specific rates are the same as those of the standard population. This measures how much more (or less) likely a person in the study population is to die during a certain period of time than someone of the same age and sex in the standard population. Comparisons of SMRs between studies are difficult because of differences of the age and sex distribution between study populations (Logroscino and Hesdorffer, 2005).

The proportionate mortality rate (PMR) is not a direct measure of mortality but gives the proportion of deaths due to one specific cause. This is influenced both by an increase of one cause of death and also by decreases in other causes.

Death after a first seizure

The SMR in patients with a newly diagnosed unprovoked seizure ranges from 2.5 to 4.1, with the highest SMRs in young children and in those with symptomatic epilepsy (Hauser and Beghi, 2008).

In the Gironde study, the SMR at 1 year after an unprovoked seizure was 4.1 (95% CI 2.5 to 6.2) (Loiseau et al., 1999). Mortality was significantly increased in patients with ASSs (SMR 10.3, 95% CI 8.3 to 12.7), remote symptomatic seizures (SMR 6.4, 95% CI 3.6 to 10.3), and progressive symptomatic seizures (SMR 19.8, 95% CI 14.0 to 27.3), but not in people with idiopathic or cryptogenic epilepsy.

In a Swedish population-based cohort study of adults, the SMR was 2.5 (95% CI 1.2 to 3.2) in people with a newly diagnosed unprovoked seizure and was markedly increased in the first 2 years after diagnosis (SMR 7.3, 95% CI 4.4 to 12.1) with a second peak at 9–11 years (SMR 5.4, 95% CI 2.7 to 11.2) (Lindsten et al., 2000). The SMR was significantly increased in patients with remote symptomatic epilepsy (SMR 3.3, 95% CI 2.4 to 4.5) but not in patients with idiopathic epilepsy. The increased risk of mortality was most pronounced in those aged less than 60 years.

In a prospective study of 407 children with a single unprovoked seizure followed for a mean of 14.2 years, it was found that treatment after a single seizure did not alter the mortality rate (Shinnar et al., 2005).

In the NGPSE cohort, 15% had acute symptomatic seizures and had an SMR of 3.0 (95% CI 2.0 to 4.3) at 11–14 years after diagnosis (Lhatoo et al., 2001).

Mortality in epilepsy

The mortality of patients with epilepsy has been studied in hospital-based cohorts (Nilsson et al., 1997; Shackleton et al., 2002; Mohanraj et al., 2006), institutionalized cohorts (White et al., 1979; Klenerman et al., 1993), and population-based cohorts (Zielinski, 1974b; Hauser et al., 1980; Olafsson et al., 1998; Loiseau et al., 1999; Lhatoo et al., 2001; Neligan et al., 2011) (Table 6.6). Reported SMRs in mortality studies from developed countries range from 1.6 to 4.1 (Forsgren et al., 2005b). Much of the variation of the risk estimation for mortality is

Table 6.6

Population studies of mortality in people with epilepsy

Reference	Country	SMR	Age group	Comments
Zielinski, 1974b	Poland	1.8	All	Retrospective prevalent cohort
Hauser et al., 1980	USA	2.3 (1.9, 2.6)	All	Historical incident cohort (Rochester)
Annegers et al., 1984	USA	2.1 (1.9, 2.5)	All	Heart disease mortality in Rochester cohort
Olafsson et al., 1998	Iceland	1.6 (1.2, 2.2)	All	Historical incident cohort
Loiseau et al., 1999	France	4.1 (2.5, 6.2)	All	Prospective, incident cohort; 1-year mortality
Lindsten et al., 2000	Sweden	2.5 (1.2, 3.2)	≥ 17 years	Prospective incident cohort with first seizure
Camfield et al., 2002	Canada	5.3 (2.3, 8.3)	< 17 years	Historical incident cohort
Ding et al., 2006	China	3.9 (3.8, 3.9)	> 2 years	Prospective incident and prevalent cohort
Neligan et al., 2011	UK	2.6 (2.2, 2.9)* 2.2 (2.0, 2.5)†	All	Prospective incident cohort (NGPSE); 1984–2009

SMR, standardized mortality rates (with 95% confidence intervals); NGPSE, National General Practice Study of Epilepsy.
*Definite epilepsy; †definite and possible epilepsy.

determined by the "source population," with community-based studies reporting SMRs between 1.3 and 3.1 whereas SMRs from institutionalized cohorts are between 1.9 and 5.1 (Shackleton et al., 2002).

In one study, the SMR for the total group after 29 years of follow-up was 2.3, with the most significant increase being in the first 10 years (Hauser et al., 1980). In another study the SMR was 2.5 after a median of 6.9 years, with the highest SMR (5.1) in the first year (Cockerell et al., 1994). The SMR further decreased to 2.1 after 11–14 years of follow-up (Lhatoo et al., 2001). The highest SMRs were estimated in patients with remote symptomatic epilepsy (SMR 3.7, 95% CI 2.9 to 4.6) and epilepsy due to a congenital neurological deficit (SMR 25, 95% CI 5.1 to 73.1). By contrast patients with idiopathic epilepsy (defined as etiology not determined) did not have a significantly increased long-term mortality rate (SMR 1.3, 95% CI 0.9 to 1.9), a finding that has been replicated in community-based studies in Iceland and France.

Overall, people with epilepsy have been found to have a reduced life expectancy, which is highest at the time of diagnosis and reduces with time. This reduction can be up to 2 years in people with idiopathic/cryptogenic epilepsy and up to 10 years in people with symptomatic epilepsy (Gaitatzis et al., 2004).

The impact of age and sex

Most studies have shown that males have a higher mortality risk than females, although no clear explanation for this has been demonstrated. Age also influences the risk. The SMR tends to be high in children, but this relates principally to the underlying cause of the epilepsy (remote symptomatic, perinatal insults) rather than to the epilepsy itself.

In a cohort of children, 75% of children who died had remote symptomatic epilepsy (Sillanpaa et al., 1998), with similarly high representations of remote symptomatic epilepsy in childhood mortality studies from Australia (Harvey et al., 1993) and Nova Scotia (Camfield et al., 2002). Decreasing SMRs are found with increasing age groups. The lowest SMRs are reported in those aged over 75 years; this relates in part to the fact that this age group has a high mortality rate (Hauser et al., 1993).

Causes of death

Causes of death in people with epilepsy can be divided into epilepsy-related and non-epilepsy-related deaths. For people with symptomatic epilepsy (both remote and progressive), the excess mortality risk relates primarily to the underlying cause of the epilepsy rather than to the epilepsy itself. In a study of 692 children with epilepsy followed up over an average of 13 years, the SMR was 5.3, with functional neurological deficit being the only independent predictor of mortality (Camfield et al., 2002). In a Dutch study of mortality in people with epilepsy followed up over 40 years, the SMR was 16 in the first 2 years, decreasing to 2.8 thereafter (Shackleton et al., 1999). After 2 years, approximately one-third of deaths were directly or indirectly attributable to epilepsy.

The importance of the underlying cause as a contributor to the mortality rate in people with epilepsy, particularly in the early years after diagnosis, was demonstrated in the Gironde study, where the causes of death after 1 year were the underlying pathology in 64%, an unrelated cause in 20%, unknown in 9%, and seizure-related in 6%. There were no reported deaths in people with idiopathic generalized epilepsy (Loiseau et al., 1999).

Common nonepileptic causes of death include pneumonia, cerebrovascular disease, malignancy, and heart disease. SMRs and PMRs are consistently raised for these causes in the population-based, and often markedly so in the first few years of follow-up. In a study investigating cause-specific mortality in over 9000 adults with epilepsy, the overall SMR was 3.6 (95% CI 3.5 to 3.7), with SMR increased for specific causes such as cancer (SMR 2.6, 95% CI 2.4 to 2.8), respiratory disease (SMR 4.0, 95% CI 3.6 to 4.5), heart and cerebrovascular disease (SMR 3.1, 95% CI 3.0 to 3.3), and accidents and poisoning (SMR 5.6, 95% CI 5.0 to 6.3) (Nilsson et al., 1997). The risk of premature death with heart disease was found to be increased in those aged 25–64 years, but not in those aged 65 years or more in a US cohort (Annegers et al., 1984). Bronchopneumonia is an important cause of death in people with epilepsy of all ages, not just the elderly, and was associated with the highest SMR (7.2) in a UK study (Cockerell et al., 1994).

The influence of intellectual disability (ID) and epilepsy on mortality was investigated in one study (Forsgren et al., 1996b). The SMR was 1.6 (95% CI 1.3 to 2.0) in people with ID alone, but 5.0 (95% CI 3.3 to 7.5) for those with ID and epilepsy.

In studies from institutions and hospitals, epilepsy-related deaths are more common. In one study, PMRs were 26% for cancer, 25% for bronchopneumonia, 24% for circulatory diseases, 12% for seizure-related deaths (other than sudden unexplained death in epilepsy; SUDEP), and 6% for SUDEP (Klenerman et al., 1993).

Epilepsy-related deaths

Deaths directly related to epilepsy include SUDEP, status epilepticus, accidents as a consequence of a seizure (including drowning), iatrogenic (drug toxicity and idiosyncratic), and suicide.

Status epilepticus

The fatality rate following status epilepticus is between 10% and 22% (Logroscino et al., 2005) (Rochester cohort 21%; DeLorenzo et al., 1996), with lower rates in Europe possibly as a result of the exclusion of deaths due to status epilepticus following anoxic encephalopathy. The primary determinant of prognosis in status epilepticus is etiology (Neligan and Shorvon, 2010), with the highest mortality rate seen in those with acute symptomatic status epilepticus, while mortality is less in those with a prior history of epilepsy (Logroscino et al., 2008). There is a suggestion that the fatality rate following status epilepticus may be decreasing (Wu et al., 2002), and is particularly low in children (Chin et al., 2006).

SUDEP

SUDEP is defined as a sudden unexpected death in an individual with epilepsy with or without evidence of a seizure where autopsy does not reveal a specific cause of death (Nashef, 1997; Lhatoo and Sander, 2002). Estimates of SUDEP rates are heavily influenced by the population under study, with much higher rates in those with severe or refractory epilepsy. Identified risk factors for SUDEP include younger age of onset, long duration of epilepsy, and refractory epilepsy (Tomson et al., 2005). In a prospective cohort study, the incidence of SUDEP was 1.21 per 1000 patient-years and accounted for 18% of all deaths. Independent risk factors identified for SUDEP were the occurrence of tonic–clonic seizures, mental retardation (IQ below 70), and treatment with more than two AEDs, after adjustment for seizure frequency (Walczak et al., 2001). The incidence of SUDEP was 0.35 per 1000 person-years in the Rochester cohort (Ficker et al., 1998), while an incidence of 1 in 295 per year was found in children with more severe epilepsy and learning difficulties (Nashef et al., 1995).

Accidents

People with epilepsy may die as a result of an accident during a seizure. The risk of injury as a result of a seizure has been estimated as 29.5 per 100 000 population per year (Kirby and Sadler, 1995). Many seizure-related injuries tend to be minor, with an increased risk related to background seizure frequency (Lawn et al., 2004), but some injuries can be fatal.

Drowning

People with epilepsy have an increased risk of drowning (15–19-fold) compared with the general population. In a meta-analysis of the risk of drowning, the overall SMR was 18.7. The SMR varied depending on the population under study, with an SMR of 5.4 in community-based incident cohorts, 18 for people with prevalent epilepsy, 25.7 for people with epilepsy and learning disability, and 96.9 for people in institutional care (Bell et al., 2008).

Suicide

People with epilepsy have been shown to be at increased risk of suicide in some studies (Zielinski, 1974b; Nilsson et al., 1997) but not in others (Hauser et al., 1980; Lhatoo et al., 2001). In a meta-analysis, the SMR for people with epilepsy and suicide was markedly increased, particularly for those with temporal lobe epilepsy (Harris and Barraclough, 1997). In a population-based control study from Denmark, 2.3% of people with epilepsy committed suicide, compared with 0.74% in the general population, corresponding to a 3-fold increased risk (risk ratio 3.17, 95% CI 2.88 to 3.50). This risk was particularly high in people with comorbid psychiatric illness and in the first 6 months after diagnosis (Christensen et al., 2007a). A more recent meta-analysis found that the overall SMR for suicide in people with epilepsy was 3.3 (95% CI 2.8 to 3.7), with highest rates in those following temporal lobe excision (SMR 13.9), following other forms of epilepsy surgery (SMR 6.4), and in people with temporal lobe epilepsy (SMR 6.4) (Bell et al., 2009a).

Mortality and seizure control

In one study, the risk of premature death persisted in patients in remission, particularly in the first 5 years following remission (Hauser et al., 1980). Most (87%) children who died during 30 years of follow-up continued to have seizures at the time of death (Sillanpaa et al., 1998). In a study of people with newly diagnosed epilepsy, the SMR for those who continued to have seizures despite treatment was 2.54 (95% CI 1.84 to 3.44), compared with 0.95 (95% CI 0.68 to 1.29) for those who had entered remission (Mohanraj et al., 2006).

The hypothesis that patients with complete seizure freedom have lower mortality rates than those who continue to have seizures was tested in a cohort of postsurgical patients. The SMR for patients with recurrent seizures following surgery was 4.7 (95% CI 2.3 to 7.9) with no recorded deaths in people in remission (Sperling et al., 2005).

Mortality in resource-poor countries

In contrast to developed countries, there are few data for epilepsy mortality in resource-poor settings. Indeed, there is only one prospective population-based mortality study of epilepsy from one such setting (Ding et al., 2006). The overall SMR was 3.9 (95% CI 3.8 to 3.9) with a higher SMR in women. The SMRs were particularly high in those aged 15–29 years, with SMRs between

23.3 and 40.2. Cause-specific PMRs were 30% for injury and stroke, 15% for cancer, 6% for myocardial infarction, and 5% for pneumonia.

Although the reported SMR in this study was just in the range reported from developed countries (1.6–4.1) (Forsgren et al., 2005b), it is likely that mortality rates and SMRs are higher in resource-poor countries. This is suggested by small studies from Martinique and Ecuador with reported SMRs of 5.7 and 6.3 respectively (Carpio et al., 2005). Further prospective population-based mortality studies from developing countries are needed to confirm this.

Antiepileptic medication and mortality

It has been suggested that antiepileptic treatment with more than two AEDs increases the risk of premature death and in particular of SUDEP (Walczak et al., 2001), although other studies have not shown an increased risk of SUDEP with any AED in monotherapy or in combination (Opeskin and Berkovic, 2003). Moreover the risk of suicide in people taking AEDs for epilepsy, although slightly increased, appears to be low (Bell et al., 2009b).

It has been reported that long-term use of AEDs is associated with an increased risk of fracture, particularly in women, with the risk increasing with the duration of treatment (Souverein et al., 2006).

Nonadherence to AED treatment is associated with a 3-fold increased risk of death (hazard ratio 3.32, 95% CI 3.11 to 3.54) after controlling for possible confounding factors. Nonadherence was also associated with an 86% increased risk of hospital admission and a 50% increased risk of emergency department attendance (Faught et al., 2008).

Cancer

SMRs and PMRs for cancer have been consistently shown to be raised in people with epilepsy, even after excluding central nervous system (CNS) neoplasms. Cancer mortality was compared between two cohorts with epilepsy, one from an institution with more severe epilepsy and the other a community-based population with milder epilepsy. The SMR for all cancers was increased in those with severe epilepsy (SMR 1.42, 95% CI 1.18 to 1.69) but not in the community-based population (SMR 0.93, 95% CI 0.84 to 1.03). The SMR for brain and CNS neoplasms was significantly increased in the group with milder epilepsy (Singh et al., 2009).

CONCLUSION

Further epidemiological studies should be prospective population-based incident cohort studies, focusing on outcome and possible temporal changes of the incidence of different epileptic syndromes in defined populations. Furthermore, research should focus on differences (real or perceived) between people of different ethnicity and social background. This may, in turn, lead to the identification of inherent risk factors in particular subpopulations for the subsequent development of epilepsy.

The overall prognosis for people with newly diagnosed epilepsy is good in terms of achieving seizure freedom, with many becoming seizure-free in the early course of the condition. The probability of obtaining seizure freedom is particularly high in those with idiopathic generalized epilepsy and normal neurological examination. For those who continue to have seizures despite multiple appropriate AED treatments, in appropriate candidates epilepsy surgery is four times more likely to render seizure freedom then continued medical treatment alone. Despite this, medical changes will result in seizure freedom for a year in 4–5% of those with seemingly intractable epilepsy.

A diagnosis of epilepsy is associated with an increased risk of premature death, particularly in the early years following diagnosis. Up to one-third of such deaths can be directly or indirectly attributable to epilepsy. This risk is decreased, but possibly not eliminated, by rendering the person completely seizure-free by treatment.

References

Abib CR, Mendoza-Sassi RA, Bech-Nappi J et al. (2007). Prevalence of seizures and associated factors in children under five living in a deprived municipality of southern Brazil. Arq Neuropsiquiatr 65: 581–586.

Adelow C, Andell E, Amark P et al. (2009). Newly diagnosed single unprovoked seizures and epilepsy in Stockholm, Sweden: first report from the Stockholm Incidence Registry of Epilepsy (SIRE). Epilepsia 50: 1094–1101.

Almu S, Tadesse Z, Cooper P et al. (2006). The prevalence of epilepsy in the Zay Society, Ethiopia – an area of high prevalence. Seizure 15: 211–213.

Annegers JF, Hauser WA, Elveback LR (1979). Remission of seizures and relapse in patients with epilepsy. Epilepsia 20: 729–737.

Annegers JF, Hauser WA, Shirts SB (1984). Heart disease mortality and morbidity in patients with epilepsy. Epilepsia 25: 699–704.

Annegers JF, Hauser WA, Lee JR et al. (1995). Secular trends and birth cohort effects in unprovoked seizures: Rochester, Minnesota 1935–1984. Epilepsia 36: 575–579.

Annegers JF, Dubinsky S, Coan SP et al. (1999). The incidence of epilepsy and unprovoked seizures in multiethnic, urban health maintenance organizations. Epilepsia 40: 502–506.

Aziz H, Guvener A, Akhtar SW et al. (1997). Comparative epidemiology of epilepsy in Pakistan and Turkey: population-based studies using identical protocols. Epilepsia 38: 716–722.

Beilmann A, Napa A, Hamarik M et al. (1999). Incidence of childhood epilepsy in Estonia. Brain Dev 21: 166–174.

Bell GS, Gaitatzis A, Johnson AL et al. (2004). Predictive value of death certification in the case ascertainment of epilepsy. J Neurol Neurosurg Psychiatry 75: 1756–1758.

Bell GS, Gaitatzis A, Bell CL et al. (2008). Drowning in people with epilepsy: how great is the risk? Neurology 71: 578–582.

Bell GS, Gaitatzis A, Bell CL et al. (2009a). Suicide in people with epilepsy: how great is the risk? Epilepsia 50: 1933–1942.

Bell GS, Mula M, Sander JW (2009b). Suicidality in people taking antiepileptic drugs: what is the evidence? CNS Drugs 23: 281–292.

Benn EK, Hauser WA, Shih T et al. (2008). Estimating the incidence of first unprovoked seizure and newly diagnosed epilepsy in the low-income urban community of northern Manhattan, New York City. Epilepsia 49: 1431–1439.

Beran RG, Michelazzi J, Hall L et al. (1985). False-negative response rate in epidemiologic studies to define prevalence ratios of epilepsy. Neuroepidemiology 4: 82–85.

Berg AT, Shinnar S (1991). The risk of seizure recurrence following a first unprovoked seizure: a quantitative review. Neurology 41: 965–972.

Berg AT, Shinnar S, Levy SR et al. (1999). Newly diagnosed epilepsy in children: presentation at diagnosis. Epilepsia 40: 445–452.

Berg AT, Shinnar S, Levy SR et al. (2001a). Two-year remission and subsequent relapse in children with newly diagnosed epilepsy. Epilepsia 42: 1553–1562.

Berg AT, Shinnar S, Levy SR et al. (2001b). Early development of intractable epilepsy in children: a prospective study. Neurology 56: 1445–1452.

Brorson LO, Wranne L (1987). Long-term prognosis in childhood epilepsy: survival and seizure prognosis. Epilepsia 28: 324–330.

Burneo JG, Tellez-Zenteno J, Wiebe S (2005). Understanding the burden of epilepsy in Latin America: a systematic review of its prevalence and incidence. Epilepsy Res 66: 63–74.

Callaghan BC, Anand K, Hesdorffer D et al. (2007). Likelihood of seizure remission in an adult population with refractory epilepsy. Ann Neurol 62: 382–389.

Camfield PR, Camfield CS (1996). Antiepileptic drug therapy: when is epilepsy truly intractable? Epilepsia 37: S60–S65.

Camfield CS, Camfield PR, Veugelers PJ (2002). Death in children with epilepsy: a population-based study. Lancet 359: 1891–1895.

Carpio A, Bharucha NE, Jallon P et al. (2005). Mortality of epilepsy in developing countries. Epilepsia 46: 28–32.

Chadwick D, Taylor J, Johnson T (1996). Outcomes after seizure recurrence in people with well-controlled epilepsy and the factors that influence it. The MRC Antiepileptic Drug Withdrawal Group. Epilepsia 37: 1043–1050.

Chin RF, Neville BG, Peckham C et al. (2006). Incidence, cause, and short-term outcome of convulsive status epilepticus in childhood: prospective population-based study. Lancet 368: 222–229.

Choi H, Heiman G, Pandis D et al. (2008). Seizure remission and relapse in adults with intractable epilepsy: a cohort study. Epilepsia 49: 1440–1445.

Christensen J, Vestergaard M, Mortensen PB et al. (2007a). Epilepsy and risk of suicide: a population-based case–control study. Lancet Neurol 6: 693–698.

Christensen J, Vestergaard M, Pedersen MG et al. (2007b). Incidence and prevalence of epilepsy in Denmark. Epilepsy Res 76: 60–65.

Cockerell OC, Johnson AL, Sander JW et al. (1994). Mortality from epilepsy: results from a prospective population-based study. Lancet 344: 918–921.

Cockerell OC, Eckle I, Goodridge DM et al. (1995). Epilepsy in a population of 6000 re-examined: secular trends in first attendance rates, prevalence, and prognosis. J Neurol Neurosurg Psychiatry 58: 570–576.

Cockerell OC, Johnson AL, Sander JW et al. (1997). Prognosis of epilepsy: a review and further analysis of the first nine years of the British National General Practice Study of Epilepsy, a prospective population-based study. Epilepsia 38: 31–46.

Collaborative Group for the Study of Epilepsy (1992). Prognosis of epilepsy in newly referred patients: a multicenter prospective study of the effects of monotherapy on the long-term course of epilepsy. Epilepsia 33: 45–51.

Commission on Classification and Terminology of the ILAE (1981). Proposal for revised clinical and electroencephalographic classification of epileptic seizures. Epilepsia 22: 489–501.

Commission on Classification and Terminology of the ILAE (1989). Proposal for revised classification of epilepsies and epileptic syndromes. Epilepsia 30: 389–399.

Commission on Epidemiology and Prognosis of the ILAE (1993). Guidelines on epidemiologic studies on epilepsy. Epilepsia 34: 592–596.

Commission on Epidemiology and Prognosis of the ILAE (1997). The epidemiology of the epilepsies: future directions. Epilepsia 38: 614–618.

De La Court A, Breteler MM, Meinardi H et al. (1996). Prevalence of epilepsy in the elderly: the Rotterdam Study. Epilepsia 37: 141–147.

DeLorenzo RJ, Hauser WA, Towne AR et al. (1996). A prospective, population-based epidemiologic study of status epilepticus in Richmond, Virginia. Neurology 46: 1029–1035.

Dent W, Helbok R, Matuja WB et al. (2005). Prevalence of active epilepsy in a rural area in South Tanzania: a door-to-door survey. Epilepsia 46: 1963–1969.

Ding D, Wang W, Wu J et al. (2006). Premature mortality in people with epilepsy in rural China: a prospective study. Lancet Neurol 5: 823–827.

Edwards T, Scott AG, Munyoki G et al. (2008). Active convulsive epilepsy in a rural district of Kenya: a study of prevalence and possible risk factors. Lancet Neurol 7: 50–56.

Elwes RD, Marshall J, Beattie A et al. (1991). Epilepsy and employment. A community based survey in an area of high unemployment. J Neurol Neurosurg Psychiatry 54: 200–203.

Everitt AD, Sander JW (1998). Incidence of epilepsy is now higher in elderly people than children. BMJ 316: 780.

Everitt AD, Sander JW (1999). Classification of the epilepsies: time for a change? A critical review of the International Classification of the Epilepsies and Epileptic Syndromes (ICEES) and its usefulness in clinical practice and epidemiological studies of epilepsy. Eur Neurol 42: 1–10.

Faught E, Duh MS, Weiner JR et al. (2008). Nonadherence to antiepileptic drugs and increased mortality: findings from the RANSOM Study. Neurology 71: 1572–1578.

Feksi AT, Kaamugisha J, Sander JW et al. (1991). Comprehensive primary health care antiepileptic drug treatment programme in rural and semi-urban Kenya. ICBERG (International Community-based Epilepsy Research Group). Lancet 337: 406–409.

Ficker DM, So EL, Shen WK et al. (1998). Population-based study of the incidence of sudden unexplained death in epilepsy. Neurology 51: 1270–1274.

Forsgren L (1992). Prevalence of epilepsy in adults in northern Sweden. Epilepsia 33: 450–458.

Forsgren L, Bucht G, Eriksson S et al. (1996a). Incidence and clinical characterization of unprovoked seizures in adults: a prospective population-based study. Epilepsia 37: 224–229.

Forsgren L, Edvinsson SO, Nystrom L et al. (1996b). Influence of epilepsy on mortality in mental retardation: an epidemiologic study. Epilepsia 37: 956–963.

Forsgren L, Beghi E, Oün A et al. (2005a). The epidemiology of epilepsy in Europe – a systematic review. Eur J Neurol 12: 245–253.

Forsgren L, Hauser WA, Olafsson E et al. (2005b). Mortality of epilepsy in developed countries: a review. Epilepsia 46: 18–27.

Gaitatzis A, Johnson AL, Chadwick DW et al. (2004). Life expectancy in people with newly diagnosed epilepsy. Brain 127: 2427–2432.

Gallitto G, Serra S, La SP et al. (2005). Prevalence and characteristics of epilepsy in the Aeolian islands. Epilepsia 46: 1828–1835.

Gomes Md Mda M, Zeitoune RG, Kropf LA et al. (2002). A house-to-house survey of epileptic seizures in an urban community of Rio de Janeiro, Brazil. Arq Neuropsiquiatr 60: 708–711.

Gracia FJ, Bayard V, Triana E et al. (1988). Prevalence of neurologic diseases in Belisario Porras municipality, District of San Miguelito, Panama, 1986. Rev Med Panama 13: 40–45.

Gracia F, de Lao SL, Castillo L et al. (1990). Epidemiology of epilepsy in Guaymi Indians from Bocas del Toro Province, Republic of Panama. Epilepsia 31: 718–723.

Haerer AF, Anderson DW, Schoenberg BS (1986). Prevalence and clinical features of epilepsy in a biracial United States population. Epilepsia 27: 66–75.

Hallstrom B, Norrving B, Lindgren A (2002). Stroke in Lund-Orup, Sweden: improved long-term survival among elderly stroke patients. Stroke 33: 1624–1629.

Hamdy NA, Ginby D, Feltbower R et al. (2007). Ethnic differences in the incidence of seizure disorders in children from Bradford, United Kingdom. Epilepsia 48: 913–916.

Harris EC, Barraclough B (1997). Suicide as an outcome for mental disorders. A meta-analysis. Br J Psychiatry 170: 205–228.

Hart YM, Sander JW, Johnson AL et al. (1990). National General Practice Study of Epilepsy: recurrence after a first seizure. Lancet 336: 1271–1274.

Harvey AS, Nolan T, Carlin JB (1993). Community-based study of mortality in children with epilepsy. Epilepsia 34: 597–603.

Hauser WA, Beghi E (2008). First seizure definitions and worldwide incidence and mortality. Epilepsia 49: 8–12.

Hauser WA, Kurland LT (1975). The epidemiology of epilepsy in Rochester, Minnesota, 1935 through 1967. Epilepsia 16: 1–66.

Hauser WA, Annegers JF, Elveback LR (1980). Mortality in patients with epilepsy. Epilepsia 21: 399–412.

Hauser WA, Rich SS, Annegers JF et al. (1990). Seizure recurrence after a 1st unprovoked seizure: an extended follow-up. Neurology 40: 1163–1170.

Hauser WA, Annegers JF, Kurland LT (1991). Prevalence of epilepsy in Rochester, Minnesota: 1940–1980. Epilepsia 32: 429–445.

Hauser WA, Annegers JF, Kurland LT (1993). Incidence of epilepsy and unprovoked seizures in Rochester, Minnesota: 1935–1984. Epilepsia 34: 453–468.

Hauser WA, Rich SS, Lee JR et al. (1998). Risk of recurrent seizures after two unprovoked seizures. N Engl J Med 338: 429–434.

Heaney DC, MacDonald BK, Everitt A et al. (2002). Socioeconomic variation in incidence of epilepsy: prospective community based study in south east England. BMJ 325: 1013–1016.

Hesdorffer DC, Logroscino G, Cascino G et al. (1998). Risk of unprovoked seizure after acute symptomatic seizure: effect of status epilepticus. Ann Neurol 44: 908–912.

Hesdorffer DC, Tian H, Anand K et al. (2005). Socioeconomic status is a risk factor for epilepsy in Icelandic adults but not in children. Epilepsia 46: 1297–1303.

Hesdorffer DC, Benn EK, Cascino GD et al. (2009). Is a first acute symptomatic seizure epilepsy? Mortality and risk for recurrent seizure. Epilepsia 50: 1102–1108.

Hopkins A, Scambler G (1977). How doctors deal with epilepsy. Lancet 1: 183–186.

Hopkins A, Garman A, Clarke C (1988). The first seizure in adult life. Value of clinical features, electroencephalography, and computerised tomographic scanning in prediction of seizure recurrence. Lancet 1: 721–726.

Huang M, Hong Z, Zeng J et al. (2002). The prevalence of epilepsy in rural Jinshan in Shanghai. Zhonghua Liu Xing Bing Xue Za Zhi 23: 345–346.

Jallon P, Goumaz M, Haenggeli C et al. (1997). Incidence of first epileptic seizures in the Canton of Geneva, Switzerland. Epilepsia 38: 547–552.

Jallon P, Smadja D, Cabre P et al. (1999). EPIMART: prospective incidence study of epileptic seizures in newly referred patients in a French Carribean island (Martinique). Epilepsia 40: 1103–1109.

Jallon P, Loiseau P, Loiseau J (2001). Newly diagnosed unprovoked epileptic seizures: presentation at diagnosis in CAROLE study. Coordination Active du Reseau Observatoire Longitudinal de l'Epilepsie. Epilepsia 42: 464–475.

Juul-Jensen P, Foldspang A (1983). Natural history of epileptic seizures. Epilepsia 24: 297–312.

Kaiser C, Asaba G, Leichsenring M et al. (1998). High incidence of epilepsy related to onchocerciasis in West Uganda. Epilepsy Res 30: 247–251.

Kelvin EA, Hesdorffer DC, Bagiella E et al. (2007). Prevalence of self-reported epilepsy in a multiracial and multiethnic community in New York City. Epilepsy Res 77: 141–150.

Kho LK, Lawn ND, Dunne JW et al. (2006). First seizure presentation: do multiple seizures within 24 hours predict recurrence? Neurology 67: 1047–1049.

Kirby S, Sadler RM (1995). Injury and death as a result of seizures. Epilepsia 36: 25–28.

Klenerman P, Sander JW, Shorvon SD (1993). Mortality in patients with epilepsy: a study of patients in long term residential care. J Neurol Neurosurg Psychiatry 56: 149–152.

Kotsopoulos IA, van Merode T, Kessels FG et al. (2002). Systematic review and meta-analysis of incidence studies of epilepsy and unprovoked seizures. Epilepsia 43: 1402–1409.

Kwan P, Brodie MJ (2000). Early identification of refractory epilepsy. N Engl J Med 342: 314–319.

Lavados J, Germain L, Morales A et al. (1992). A descriptive study of epilepsy in the district of El Salvador, Chile, 1984–1988. Acta Neurol Scand 85: 249–256.

Lawn ND, Bamlet WR, Radhakrishnan K et al. (2004). Injuries due to seizures in persons with epilepsy: a population-based study. Neurology 63: 1565–1570.

Leach JP, Lauder R, Nicolson A et al. (2005). Epilepsy in the UK: misdiagnosis, mistreatment, and undertreatment? The Wrexham Area Epilepsy Project. Seizure 14: 514–520.

Leone MA, Solari A, Beghi E (2006). Treatment of the first tonic–clonic seizure does not affect long-term remission of epilepsy. Neurology 67: 2227–2229.

Lhatoo SD, Sander JW (2002). Sudden unexpected death in epilepsy. Hong Kong Med J 8: 354–358.

Lhatoo SD, Johnson AL, Goodridge DM et al. (2001). Mortality in epilepsy in the first 11 to 14 years after diagnosis: multivariate analysis of a long-term, prospective, population-based cohort. Ann Neurol 49: 336–344.

Li SC, Schoenberg BS, Wang CC et al. (1985). Epidemiology of epilepsy in urban areas of the People's Republic of China. Epilepsia 26: 391–394.

Lindsten H, Nystrom L, Forsgren L (2000). Mortality risk in an adult cohort with a newly diagnosed unprovoked epileptic seizure: a population-based study. Epilepsia 41: 1469–1473.

Lindsten H, Stenlund H, Forsgren L (2001a). Remission of seizures in a population-based adult cohort with a newly diagnosed unprovoked epileptic seizure. Epilepsia 42: 1025–1030.

Lindsten H, Stenlund H, Forsgren L (2001b). Seizure recurrence in adults after a newly diagnosed unprovoked epileptic seizure. Acta Neurol Scand 104: 202–207.

Logroscino G, Hesdorffer DC (2005). Methodologic issues in studies of mortality following epilepsy: measures, types of studies, sources of cases, cohort effects, and competing risks. Epilepsia 46: 3–7.

Logroscino G, Hesdorffer DC, Cascino G et al. (2005). Mortality after a first episode of status epilepticus in the United States and Europe. Epilepsia 46: 46–48.

Logroscino G, Hesdorffer DC, Cascino G et al. (2008). Status epilepticus without an underlying cause and risk of death: a population-based study. Arch Neurol 65: 221–224.

Loiseau J, Loiseau P, Guyot M et al. (1990). Survey of seizure disorders in the French southwest. I. Incidence of epileptic syndromes. Epilepsia 31: 391–396.

Loiseau J, Picot MC, Loiseau P (1999). Short-term mortality after a first epileptic seizure: a population-based study. Epilepsia 40: 1388–1392.

Lossius MI, Hessen E, Mowinckel P et al. (2008). Consequences of antiepileptic drug withdrawal: a randomized, double-blind study (Akershus Study). Epilepsia 49: 455–463.

Luciano AL, Shorvon SD (2007). Results of treatment changes in patients with apparently drug-resistant chronic epilepsy. Ann Neurol 62: 375–381.

Mac TL, Tran DS, Quet F et al. (2007). Epidemiology, aetiology, and clinical management of epilepsy in Asia: a systematic review. Lancet Neurol 6: 533–543.

MacDonald BK, Cockerell OC, Sander JW et al. (2000a). The incidence and lifetime prevalence of neurological disorders in a prospective community-based study in the UK. Brain 123: 665–676.

MacDonald BK, Johnson AL, Goodridge DM et al. (2000b). Factors predicting prognosis of epilepsy after presentation with seizures. Ann Neurol 48: 833–841.

Manford M, Hart YM, Sander JW et al. (1992a). National General Practice Study of Epilepsy (NGPSE): partial seizure patterns in a general population. Neurology 42: 1911–1917.

Manford M, Hart YM, Sander JW et al. (1992b). The National General Practice Study of Epilepsy. The syndromic classification of the International League Against Epilepsy applied to epilepsy in a general population. Arch Neurol 49: 801–808.

Mani KS, Rangan G, Srinivas HV et al. (1998). The Yelandur study: a community-based approach to epilepsy in rural South India – epidemiological aspects. Seizure 7: 281–288.

Marson A, Jacoby A, Johnson A et al. (2005). Immediate versus deferred antiepileptic drug treatment for early epilepsy and single seizures: a randomised controlled trial. Lancet 365: 2007–2013.

Medina MT, Duron RM, Martinez L et al. (2005). Prevalence, incidence, and etiology of epilepsies in rural Honduras: the Salama Study. Epilepsia 46: 124–131.

Meinardi H, Scott RA, Reis R et al. (2001). The treatment gap in epilepsy: the current situation and ways forward. Epilepsia 42: 136–149.

Mohanraj R, Norrie J, Stephen LJ et al. (2006). Mortality in adults with newly diagnosed and chronic epilepsy: a retrospective comparative study. Lancet Neurol 5: 481–487.

Morgan CL, Ahmed Z, Kerr MP (2000). Social deprivation and prevalence of epilepsy and associated health usage. J Neurol Neurosurg Psychiatry 69: 13–17.

MRC AED Withdrawal Study Group (1991). Randomised study of antiepilepetic drug withdrawal in patients in remission. Lancet 337: 1175–1180.

Muntner P, Garrett E, Klag MJ et al. (2002). Trends in stroke prevalence between 1973 and 1991 in the US population 25 to 74 years of age. Stroke 33: 1209–1213.

Nashef L (1997). Sudden unexpected death in epilepsy: terminology and definitions. Epilepsia 38: 6–8.

Nashef L, Fish DR, Garner S et al. (1995). Sudden death in epilepsy: a study of incidence in a young cohort with epilepsy and learning difficulty. Epilepsia 36: 1187–1194.

Ndoye NF, Sow AD, Diop AG et al. (2005). Prevalence of epilepsy its treatment gap and knowledge, attitude and practice of its population in sub-urban Senegal an ILAE/IBE/WHO study. Seizure 14: 106–111.

Neligan A, Shorvon SD (2010). Frequency and prognosis of convulsive status epilepticus of different causes: a systematic review. Arch Neurol 67: 931–940.

Neligan A, Bell GS, Shorvon SD et al. (2010). Temporal trends in the mortality of people with epilepsy: a review. Epilepsia 51: 2241–2246.

Neligan A, Bell GS, Johnson AL et al. (2011). The long-term risk of premature mortality in people with epilepsy. Brain 134: 388–395.

Ngugi AK, Bottomley C, Kleinschmidt I et al. (2010). Estimation of the burden of active and life-time epilepsy: a meta-analytic approach. Epilepsia 51: 883–890.

Nicoletti A, Reggio A, Bartoloni A et al. (1999). Prevalence of epilepsy in rural Bolivia: a door-to-door survey. Neurology 53: 2064–2069.

Nilsson L, Tomson T, Farahmand BY et al. (1997). Cause-specific mortality in epilepsy: a cohort study of more than 9,000 patients once hospitalized for epilepsy. Epilepsia 38: 1062–1068.

Nkwi PN, Ndonko FT (1989). The epileptic among the Bamileke of Maham in the Nde Division, West Province of Cameroon. Cult Med Psychiatry 13: 437–448.

Oka E, Ohtsuka Y, Yoshinaga H et al. (2006). Prevalence of childhood epilepsy and distribution of epileptic syndromes: a population-based survey in Okayama, Japan. Epilepsia 47: 626–630.

Olafsson E, Hauser WA (1999). Prevalence of epilepsy in rural Iceland: a population-based study. Epilepsia 40: 1529–1534.

Olafsson E, Hauser WA, Ludvigsson P et al. (1996). Incidence of epilepsy in rural Iceland: a population-based study. Epilepsia 37: 951–955.

Olafsson E, Hauser WA, Gudmundsson G (1998). Long-term survival of people with unprovoked seizures: a population-based study. Epilepsia 39: 89–92.

Olafsson E, Ludvigsson P, Gudmundsson G et al. (2005). Incidence of unprovoked seizures and epilepsy in Iceland and assessment of the epilepsy syndrome classification: a prospective study. Lancet Neurol 4: 627–634.

Opeskin K, Berkovic SF (2003). Risk factors for sudden unexpected death in epilepsy: a controlled prospective study based on coroners cases. Seizure 12: 456–464.

Oün A, Haldre S, Magi M (2003). Incidence of adult epilepsy in Estonia. Acta Neurol Scand 108: 245–251.

Placencia M, Shorvon SD, Paredes V et al. (1992). Epileptic seizures in an Andean region of Ecuador. Incidence and prevalence and regional variation. Brain 115: 771–782.

Placencia M, Sander JW, Roman M et al. (1994). The characteristics of epilepsy in a largely untreated population in rural Ecuador. J Neurol Neurosurg Psychiatry 57: 320–325.

Preux PM, Druet-Cabanac M (2005). Epidemiology and aetiology of epilepsy in sub-Saharan Africa. Lancet Neurol 4: 21–31.

Rocca WA, Savettieri G, Anderson DW et al. (2001). Door-to-door prevalence survey of epilepsy in three Sicilian municipalities. Neuroepidemiology 20: 237–241.

Rugg-Gunn FJ, Harrison NA, Duncan JS (2001). Evaluation of the accuracy of seizure descriptions by the relatives of patients with epilepsy. Epilepsy Res 43: 193–199.

Rwiza HT, Kilonzo GP, Haule J et al. (1992). Prevalence and incidence of epilepsy in Ulanga, a rural Tanzanian district: a community-based study. Epilepsia 33: 1051–1056.

Sander JW (1993). Some aspects of prognosis in the epilepsies: a review. Epilepsia 34: 1007–1016.

Sander JW (2003). The epidemiology of epilepsy revisited. Curr Opin Neurol 16: 165–170.

Sander JW, Hart YM, Johnson AL et al. (1990). National General Practice Study of Epilepsy: newly diagnosed epileptic seizures in a general population. Lancet 336: 1267–1271.

Sato S (1964). The epidemiological and clinico-statistical study of epilepsy in Nigata City. Clin Neurol (Tokio) 4: 413–424.

Sawhney IM, Singh A, Kaur P et al. (1999). A case control study and one year follow-up of registered epilepsy cases in a resettlement colony of North India, a developing tropical country. J Neurol Sci 165: 31–35.

Schmidt D, Loscher W (2005). Uncontrolled epilepsy following discontinuation of antiepileptic drugs in seizure-free patients: a review of current clinical experience. Acta Neurol Scand 111: 291–300.

Schmidt D, Stavem K (2009). Long-term seizure outcome of surgery versus no surgery for drug-resistant partial epilepsy: a review of controlled studies. Epilepsia 50: 1301–1309.

Semah F, Picot MC, Adam C et al. (1998). Is the underlying cause of epilepsy a major prognostic factor for recurrence? Neurology 51: 1256–1262.

Shackleton DP, Westendorp RG, Trenite DG et al. (1999). Mortality in patients with epilepsy: 40 years of follow up in a Dutch cohort study. J Neurol Neurosurg Psychiatry 66: 636–640.

Shackleton DP, Westendorp RG, Kasteleijn-Nolst Trenite DG et al. (2002). Survival of patients with epilepsy: an estimate of the mortality risk. Epilepsia 43: 445–450.

Shafer SQ, Hauser WA, Annegers JF et al. (1988). EEG and other early predictors of epilepsy remission: a community study. Epilepsia 29: 590–600.

Shamansky SL, Glaser GH (1979). Socioeconomic characteristics of childhood seizure disorders in the New Haven area: an epidemiologic study. Epilepsia 20: 457–474.

Shinnar S, Berg AT, Moshe SL et al. (1996). The risk of seizure recurrence after a first unprovoked afebrile seizure in childhood: an extended follow-up. Pediatrics 98: 216–225.

Shinnar S, O'Dell C, Berg AT (1999). Distribution of epilepsy syndromes in a cohort of children prospectively monitored from the time of their first unprovoked seizure. Epilepsia 40: 1378–1383.

Shinnar S, Berg AT, O'Dell C et al. (2000). Predictors of multiple seizures in a cohort of children prospectively followed from the time of their first unprovoked seizure. Ann Neurol 48: 140–147.

Shinnar S, O'Dell C, Berg AT (2005). Mortality following a first unprovoked seizure in children: a prospective study. Neurology 64: 880–882.

Sidenvall R, Forsgren L, Blomquist HK et al. (1993). A community-based prospective incidence study of epileptic seizures in children. Acta Paediatr 82: 60–65.

Sidenvall R, Forsgren L, Heijbel J (1996). Prevalence and characteristics of epilepsy in children in northern Sweden. Seizure 5: 139–146.

Sillanpaa M, Schmidt D (2006a). Natural history of treated childhood-onset epilepsy: prospective, long-term population-based study. Brain 129: 617–624.

Sillanpaa M, Schmidt D (2006b). Prognosis of seizure recurrence after stopping antiepileptic drugs in seizure-free patients: a long-term population-based study of childhood-onset epilepsy. Epilepsy Behav 8: 713–719.

Sillanpaa M, Schmidt D (2008). Seizure clustering during drug treatment affects seizure outcome and mortality of childhood-onset epilepsy. Brain 131: 938–944.

Sillanpaa M, Schmidt D (2009). Early seizure frequency and aetiology predict long-term medical outcome in childhood-onset epilepsy. Brain 132: 989–998.

Sillanpaa M, Jalava M, Kaleva O et al. (1998). Long-term prognosis of seizures with onset in childhood. N Engl J Med 338: 1715–1722.

Sillanpaa M, Kalviainen R, Klaukka T et al. (2006). Temporal changes in the incidence of epilepsy in Finland: nationwide study. Epilepsy Res 71: 206–215.

Singh G, Fletcher O, Bell GS et al. (2009). Cancer mortality amongst people with epilepsy: a study of two cohorts with severe and presumed milder epilepsy. Epilepsy Res 83: 190–197.

Smith D, Defalla BA, Chadwick DW (1999). The misdiagnosis of epilepsy and the management of refractory epilepsy in a specialist clinic. QJM 92: 15–23.

Souverein PC, Webb DJ, Weil JG et al. (2006). Use of antiepileptic drugs and risk of fractures: case–control study among patients with epilepsy. Neurology 66: 1318–1324.

Sperling MR, Harris A, Nei M et al. (2005). Mortality after epilepsy surgery. Epilepsia 46: 49–53.

Sridharan R, Murthy BN (1999). Prevalence and pattern of epilepsy in India. Epilepsia 40: 631–636.

Stephen LJ, Kwan P, Brodie MJ (2001). Does the cause of localisation-related epilepsy influence the response to antiepileptic drug treatment? Epilepsia 42: 357–362.

Stroink H, Brouwer OF, Arts WF et al. (1998). The first unprovoked, untreated seizure in childhood: a hospital based study of the accuracy of the diagnosis, rate of recurrence, and long term outcome after recurrence. Dutch Study of Epilepsy in Childhood. J Neurol Neurosurg Psychiatry 64: 595–600.

Stroink H, van Donselaar CA, Geerts AT et al. (2004). Interrater agreement of the diagnosis and classification of a first seizure in childhood. The Dutch Study of Epilepsy in Childhood. J Neurol Neurosurg Psychiatry 75: 241–245.

Tekle-Haimanot R, Forsgren L, Ekstedt J (1997). Incidence of epilepsy in rural central Ethiopia. Epilepsia 38: 541–546.

Tomson T, Walczak T, Sillanpaa M et al. (2005). Sudden unexpected death in epilepsy: a review of incidence and risk factors. Epilepsia 46: 54–61.

Tuan NA, Cuong le Q, Allebeck P et al. (2008). The prevalence of epilepsy in a rural district of Vietnam: a population-based study from the EPIBAVI project. Epilepsia 49: 1634–1637.

Tuan NA, Cuong le Q, Allebeck P et al. (2010). The incidence of epilepsy in a rural district of Vietnam: a community-based epidemiologic study. Epilepsia 51: 2377–2383.

van Donselaar CA, Geerts AT, Meulstee J et al. (1989). Reliability of the diagnosis of a first seizure. Neurology 39: 267–271.

Velez A, Eslava-Cobos J (2006). Epilepsy in Colombia: epidemiologic profile and classification of epileptic seizures and syndromes. Epilepsia 47: 193–201.

Walczak TS, Leppik IE, D'Amelio M et al. (2001). Incidence and risk factors in sudden unexpected death in epilepsy: a prospective cohort study. Neurology 56: 519–525.

Wang W, Wu J, Wang D et al. (2002). Epidemiological survey on epilepsy among rural populations in five provinces in China. Zhonghua Yi Xue Za Zhi 82: 449–452.

Wang WZ, Wu JZ, Wang DS et al. (2003). The prevalence and treatment gap in epilepsy in China: an ILAE/IBE/WHO study. Neurology 60: 1544–1545.

Watts AE (1992). The natural history of untreated epilepsy in a rural community in Africa. Epilepsia 33: 464–468.

White SJ, McLean AE, Howland C (1979). Anticonvulsant drugs and cancer. A cohort study in patients with severe epilepsy. Lancet 2: 458–461.

Wiebe S, Blume WT, Girvin JP et al. (2001). A randomized, controlled trial of surgery for temporal-lobe epilepsy. N Engl J Med 345: 311–318.

Wright J, Pickard N, Whitfield A et al. (2000). A population-based study of the prevalence, clinical characteristics and effect of ethnicity in epilepsy. Seizure 9: 309–313.

Wu YW, Shek DW, Garcia PA et al. (2002). Incidence and mortality of generalized convulsive status epilepticus in California. Neurology 58: 1070–1076.

Zarrelli MM, Beghi E, Rocca WA et al. (1999). Incidence of epileptic syndromes in Rochester, Minnesota: 1980–1984. Epilepsia 40: 1708–1714.

Zhao Y, Zhang Q, Tsering T et al. (2008). Prevalence of convulsive epilepsy and health-related quality of life of the population with convulsive epilepsy in rural areas of Tibet Autonomous Region in China: an initial survey. Epilepsy Behav 12: 373–381.

Zielinski JJ (1974a). Epidemiology and Medicosocial Problems of Epilepsy in Warsaw. Final Report on Research Program no. 19-P-58325-F-01. Psychoneurological Institute, Warsaw.

Zielinski JJ (1974b). Epilepsy and mortality rate and cause of death. Epilepsia 15: 191–201.

Handbook of Clinical Neurology, Vol. 107 (3rd series)
Epilepsy, Part I
H. Stefan and W.H. Theodore, Editors

Chapter 7

Maturation of the human brain and epilepsy

GREGORY L. HOLMES[1]*, M.D. MATHIEU MILH[2], AND OLIVIER DULAC[3]

[1]*Department of Neurology, Dartmouth Medical School, Lebanon, NH, USA*

[2]*Department of Pediatric Neurology, APHM La Timone, INMED, Marseilles, France*

[3]*Department of Pediatric Neurology, APHP Necker-Enfants Malades, UMR663, Paris, France*

INTRODUCTION

Age plays a major role in virtually all aspects of epilepsy (Hauser, 1992). Children are at substantially higher risk for epilepsy than young and middle-aged adults (Hauser, 1994, 1995; Forsgren et al., 2005). In addition to the higher incidence of epilepsy in children than in adults, precipitating factors such as fever are far more likely to induce a seizure in a young child than in an adult (Hauser, 1992; Fetveit, 2008). Age is critical in the clinical and electroencephalographic (EEG) features of seizures. Disorders such as infantile spasms and Landau–Kleffner syndrome always begin in early childhood. EEG features such as hypsarrhythmia and electrical status epilepticus of sleep (ESES) are confined to childhood. Age is also a determinant for prognosis. Intellectual impairment (Huttenlocher and Hapke, 1990; Glosser et al., 1997; Bulteau et al., 2000; Bjornaes et al., 2001; Hermann et al., 2002; Cormack et al., 2007), learning disabilities (Sillanpaa, 2004; Soria et al., 2007; Fastenau et al., 2008), social outcome (Lindsay et al., 1979; Sillanpaa, 1983), and medical refractoriness (Berg et al., 1996; Casetta et al., 1999; Camfield and Camfield, 2007) all appear to be influenced by age of onset.

The reason age is such an important factor in pediatric epilepsy is that it serves as a surrogate marker for brain development. Enormous developmental changes occur in the brain. In fact, from birth to adulthood the human brain expands by a factor of 3.3. The adult brain has approximately 10 billion neurons, which on average are connected to other neurons through roughly 10 000 synapses. Infants start off with only about 10% of the synapses found in the adult brain. Hundreds of new γ-aminobutyric acid (GABA)ergic and glutamatergic synapses are established every day on a pyramidal neuron during the last third of gestation and first months of life. Along with the massive increase in connectivity and cell growth, myelination occurs throughout childhood and early adulthood. In addition to growth, the developing brain also is continuously redesigning itself through apoptosis and pruning of connections.

Understanding the morphological and physiological developmental changes provides insight into the unique features of childhood epilepsy. In this chapter, key features of brain development, as it relates to pediatric epilepsy, will be reviewed. As many key features of ontogeny are similar in the rat and human brain, this chapter will incorporate information from both animals and humans.

DEVELOPMENTAL CHANGES IN BRAIN MORPHOLOGY

Brain weight reaches adult values (about 1.45 kg) between 10 and 12 years of age. The fastest growth occurs during the first 3 years of life so that by the age of 5 years the infant's brain weighs about 90% of the adult value (Dekaban, 1978). Although the brain continues to change throughout life, changes in brain morphology during childhood and adolescence are more subtle than those in the first 4 years of life.

Synapse number peaks during infancy and then declines (Huttenlocher et al., 1982a; Huttenlocher, 1984, 1990). Huttenlocher (1979) used the phosphotungstic acid method to study the density of synaptic profiles in layer 3 of middle frontal gyrus in 21 normal human brains ranging from newborn to age 90 years. Synaptic density increased during infancy, reaching a maximum

*Correspondence to: Gregory L. Holmes, M.D., Dartmouth Medical School, One Medical Center Drive, Lebanon, New Hampshire 03756, USA. Tel: +1-603-650-7610, Fax: +1-603-650-7617, E-mail: Gregory.L.Holmes@Dartmouth.edu

at age 1–2 years, which was about 50% above the adult mean. The decline in synaptic density observed between ages 2 and 16 years was accompanied by a slight decrease in neuronal density. Synaptic density was constant throughout adult life (ages 16–72 years) with a mean of 11.05×10^8 synapses/mm^3. Similar time profiles have been found in the visual cortex (Huttenlocher et al., 1982b) and striatum (Huttenlocher and de Courten, 1987). In addition to development of synapses, there is a progressive increase in arborization of the dendrites and an increase in dendritic spines with age. The phenomenal growth of the dendritic tree and formation of synapses occurs at a time when cortical networks are developing. There is increasing evidence that neuronal network development is driven by external or endogenous stimuli such as light (Desai et al., 2002) and muscle twitches (Khazipov et al., 2004b). In addition, as will be described below, seizures can also dramatically alter brain development.

Paralleling morphological brain maturation are biochemical changes characterized by an increase in *N*-acetyl-aspartate (NAA) and creatine, and a concomitant decrease in choline, myoinositol, and lipids (Kreis et al., 1993). The choline peak includes free choline, glycerophosphorylcholine, and phosphorylcholine. It represents the high levels of substrate needed for the formation of cell membranes, with gradual reduction as soon as incorporation of lipids has taken place. NAA is considered as a neuronal marker and is also expressed in immature and mature oligodendrocytes. Therefore, NAA also reflects oligodendrocyte proliferation and differentiation (Bhakoo and Pearce, 2000). As neuronal cell density in cortex decreases with dendritic maturation, the increase in NAA with age reflects a contribution from non-neuronal origins.

Regional variations are pronounced at all ages between gray and white matter, and also within different areas of gray and white matter. Highest choline, creatine, and NAA peak intensities occur in the thalamus, followed by basal ganglia, and then other regions in preterm and term infants (Barkovich et al., 2001). This probably reflects the high cellular density in these areas and the more mature status of deep brain structures compared with white matter. Concentration of NAA is higher in gray matter than in white matter, probably because NAA is expressed in mitochondria located in the cellular soma and not in axons or oligodendrocytes. Creatine concentration is also higher in gray matter than in white matter, whereas choline levels are slightly lower in gray matter than in white matter.

DEVELOPMENTAL CHANGES IN MYELINATION

Myelination is an important developmental process that begins during the fifth fetal month with myelination of the cranial nerves, and continues throughout life. The major changes in myelination occur from 3 weeks to 1 year for all brain regions. Myelination appears to occur earliest in the posterior fossa, with the middle cerebellar peduncle identifiable by age 3 months. By the age of 1 year, all major white matter tracts including the corpus callosum, subcortical white matter, and the internal capsule are well defined. In contrast to the high rate of myelination in the first year, the changes between 1 and 2 years are more subtle, although changes in radial diffusivity on diffusion tensor imaging suggest a pruning process. The development of white matter begins from the center to the periphery and from the occipital to the frontal lobes (Gao et al., 2009).

During the first year of life, the magnetic resonance imaging (MRI) white matter signal on T2 changes from hyperintense to hypointense, and vice versa on T1 (Barkovich, 2000). Like other membranes, myelin is composed of a bilayer of lipids with several large proteins, most of which span the bilayer (including myelin basic protein and proteolipid protein). The outer lipid layers are composed mainly of cholesterol and glycolipids, whereas the inner portion of the lipid bilayer is composed mainly of phospholipids. It is thought that the high signal intensity seen on T1-weighted images with the maturation of white matter results from T1 shortening caused by the cholesterol, glycolipids, and possibly the proteins in the outer lipid layers of the membrane, whereas it is thought that the diminishing signal intensity seen on the T2-weighted images with maturation results from a decreased number of water molecules caused by development of the hydrophobic phospholipid inner layer (Svennerholm and Vanier, 1978; Svennerholm et al., 1978; Holland et al., 1986; Barkovich et al., 1988).

The changes in signal intensity in myelin with age may make interpretation of MRI scans in children with epilepsy difficult. Distinguishing leukoencephalopathies from normal age-dependent changes in myelination can be challenging. In addition, how well cortical dysplasias are seen on the MRI may be related to the degree of myelination. In some cortical dysplasias the lesion may be seen better on MRI before extensive myelination occurs (Eltze et al., 2005). However, in some cases cortical dysplasias may be more evident with increased myelination (Yoshida et al., 2008).

In addition to myelination affecting the clinical and EEG features of seizures, epilepsy and its causes may alter myelination. For example, delays in myelination have been seen in children with infantile spasms (Muroi et al., 1996; Natsume et al., 1996; Takano et al., 2007). Children with prenatally or perinatally acquired brain lesions appear to have more severe delays of myelination (Schropp et al., 1994). The mechanism by which seizures alter the rate of myelination is not known.

The myelination pattern may also have a significant role in when infantile spasms begin. Koo et al. (1993) reviewed 93 cases of infantile spasms with focal cerebral lesions confined to frontal, centrotemporoparietal, or occipital regions. The mean age of onset of infantile spasms was around 3 months in patients with occipital lesions, versus 6 months in those with centrotemporoparietal lesions, and 10 months in those with frontal lesions. It is therefore of considerable interest that myelination occurs in the occipital lobe and moves forward into the temporal, parietal, and frontal lobes. The age distribution pattern of spasm onset according to localization of cortical lesion was therefore closely correlated with that of the normal sequence of brain maturation, suggesting that myelination may be necessary for the seizures to occur.

With greater myelination of the frontal lobes there is a greater likelihood of seeing spike–wave discharges arising frontally. Lennox–Gastaut syndrome, with frontal predominantly slow spike–wave discharges, typically does not begin in the first year of life but may evolve from West syndrome as the brain myelinates more fully. Likewise, the development of epilepsy with myoclonic–astatic seizures is an age-related phenomenon, occurring in toddlers but not in infants (Doose, 1992).

BEHAVIORAL AND ELECTROENCEPHALOGRAPHIC CORRELATES OF BRAIN DEVELOPMENT

As described above, the most robust changes involve cell growth, connectivity, and myelination. These changes in brain growth are reflected in the EEG and behavioral manifestations of seizures. In very preterm infants (< 30 weeks estimated conceptional age; ECA), the EEG is discontinuous with long periods of inactivity with intermittent bursts of higher voltage slow activity. From around 30 weeks ECA, the EEG exhibits no interhemispheric synchronization and consists of poorly organized waveforms. The asymmetry and discontinuous nature of the record likely relates to the poor myelination in the cerebral hemispheres as well as the lack of developed neuronal networks. With increasing age and increasing connectivity and myelination, the EEG becomes more continuous with better interhemispheric synchronization of activity. This occurs simultaneously with development of thalamocortical connections (Minlebaev et al., 2009).

Electrographic ictal discharges in neonates are focal and may be limited to a small cortical area due to lack of myelin in the forebrain combined with limited connectivity between cortical regions. If seizures propagate, they do so very slowly. Behaviorally, the most common seizure type in infants is focal or multifocal seizures. Generalized seizures, either electrographically or behaviorally, are quite unusual in newborns.

As connectivity and myelination occur during the first year of life, thalamocortical and intrahemispheric and interhemispheric networks are organized and features such as sleep spindles and rhythmic delta and theta background patterns emerge. During the first year of life generalized seizures (partial with secondary generalization) begin to occur. Infantile spasms with generalized hypsarrhythmia rarely occur before 3 months of age, but start to occur when the cerebral hemispheres begin to myelinate.

DEVELOPMENTAL CHANGES IN THE BRAIN PHYSIOLOGY

Children during the first months of life are at particularly high risk for seizures, with the largest number of new-onset seizure disorders occurring during this time (Hauser, 1995). There is considerable evidence that the immature brain is more susceptible to seizures than the mature brain. The propensity for seizures in the immature brain has been demonstrated in a number of experimental models, including kainic acid (Tremblay et al., 1984; Khalilov et al., 2003), electrical stimulation (Moshe, 1981), hypoxia (Jensen et al., 1991), penicillin (Swann and Brady, 1984), picrotoxin (Gomez-Di Cesare et al., 1997), $GABA_B$ receptor antagonists (McLean et al., 1996), and increased extracellular potassium (Dzhala and Staley, 2003; Khazipov et al., 2004a).

The enhanced excitability of the immature brain compared with the mature brain is related to the sequential development and expression of essential signaling pathways. In the adult brain, glutamate is the primary excitatory neurotransmitter and GABA is the principal inhibitory transmitter. Synaptic transmission is mediated by glutamate, which is released from the pyramidal neurons and depolarizes and excites the target neurons via ionotropic receptors: *N*-methyl-D-aspartate (NMDA), α-amino-3-hydroxy-5-methylisoxazole-4-proprionic acid (AMPA), and kainic acid (KA). Fast inhibition is through GABA activation of GABA receptors.

Although all of the glutamate subreceptors respond to glutamate, they have individual characteristics. NMDA receptors are heteromeric with an obligate NR1 subunit. In the immature brain, the predominant NR2 subunit is the NR2B subunit (Chang et al., 2009). The NMDA receptor has characteristics of both a ligand-mediated and voltage-gated channel. The ion Mg^{2+} lies in the pore of the channel, preventing permeability of Na^+ and Ca^{2+} ions. When Mg^{2+} is released from the pore by membrane depolarization, the flow of Na^+ and Ca^{2+} ions can occur. Compared with the NR2A subunit, which is highly expressed on mature neurons, NR2B subunits have reduced Mg^{2+} sensitivity, resulting in increased excitability (Hollmann and Heinemann, 1994). Other developmentally regulated subunits (NR2C, NR2D, and NR3A) also are increased in the first two postnatal weeks (Monyer et al., 1994).

The AMPA receptor is responsible for fast excitatory neurotransmission. AMPA receptors are heteromeric and made up of four subunits, including combinations of the glutamate receptor (GluR) 1, GluR2, GluR3, or GlurR4 subunits (Hollmann and Heinemann, 1994). In the immature rodent and human brain, AMPA receptors are Ca^{2+} permeable because they lack the GluR2 subunit (Hollmann et al., 1991; Sanchez et al., 2001; Kumar et al., 2002). The enhanced Ca^{2+} permeability would result in greater excitability and increase the likelihood of seizures in the immature brain.

The development of GABAergic and glutamatergic synapses follows distinct timelines. During fetal development, GABAergic synapses develop before glutamatergic synapses (Khazipov et al., 2001). During the first few weeks of life there is enhanced excitation due to an overabundance of NMDA and AMPA receptors (McDonald et al., 1990; Miller et al., 1990). With maturation, axonal collaterals and attendant synapses regress (Swann et al., 1991).

In addition to changes in the receptors, structures that anchor the synapses to the membrane also change with age. The postsynaptic density (PSD) is a cytoskeleton specialization at neuronal synapses that comprises glutamate receptors, their molecular scaffolding molecules, cell adhesion molecules, and a diverse set of other signaling proteins. The PSD has been proposed to concentrate and organize neurotransmitter receptors to respond rapidly to neurotransmitter in the synaptic cleft. The ontogeny of PSD parallels the ontogeny of NMDA receptors, with substantial decreases in NR2B and increases in NR2A and PSD during development (Sans et al., 2000).

There are also developmental changes in the neurophysiology of the receptors. The NMDA excitatory postsynaptic currents (EPSCs) show a maturational decrease in rise time but no change in decay time, whereas AMPA EPSCs show neither rise nor decay time changes with development (Ye et al., 2005). AMPA receptors possess mature kinetics and become the dominant glutamatergic current during early brain development.

The AMPA receptor responds rapidly to glutamate with opening of the channel to allow Na^{+} to enter the cell and depolarize the membrane. This influx of Na^{+} is sufficient to allow the displacement of Mg^{2+} from the NMDA channel, and to permit Na^{+} and Ca^{2+} ions to enter the cell through the NMDA receptor. The rise in intracellular Ca^{2+} is an essential signal for memory processes; hence the NMDA receptor plays an important role in learning and plasticity.

During the early postnatal period, at a time when the immature brain is highly susceptible to seizures (Jensen and Baram, 2000; Khazipov et al., 2004a), GABA, which in the adult brain is the primary inhibitory neurotransmitter, exerts paradoxical excitatory action (Dzhala and Staley, 2003; Khazipov et al., 2004a). GABA is excitatory in the immature brain because of a larger intracellular concentration of chloride in immature neurons than mature ones (Ben-Ari et al., 1989; Ben-Ari, 2002; Ben-Ari and Holmes, 2005). The shift from a depolarizing to a hyperpolarizing chloride current occurs over an extended period depending on the age and developmental stage of the structure (Glykys et al., 2009). The shift is mediated by an active Na^{+}–K^{+}–$2Cl^{-}$ cotransporter (NKCC1) that facilitates the accumulation of chloride in neurons, and a delayed expression of a K^{+}–Cl^{-} cotransporter (KCC2) that extrudes Cl^{-} to establish adult concentrations of intracellular Cl^{-} (Dzhala et al., 2005). The depolarization by GABA of immature neurons is sufficient to generate Na^{+} action potentials and to remove the voltage-dependent Mg^{2+} blockade of NMDA channels and activate voltage-dependent Ca^{2+} channels, leading to a large influx of Ca^{2+} that in turn triggers long-term changes of synaptic efficacy. The synergistic action of GABA with NMDA and Ca^{2+} channels is unique to the developing brain and has many consequences on the impact of GABAergic synapses on the network. In addition, agents that interfere with the transport of Cl^{-} exert an antiepileptogenic action (Dzhala et al., 2005). With maturation there is increasing function of KCC2 and decreasing function of NKCC1, a transporter that brings Cl^{-} into the cell resulting in an inhibitory effect of GABA. Figure 7.1 shows in cartoon form the developmental changes in the chloride content of pyramidal cells.

The lack of an efficient time locked inhibition, the delayed maturation of postsynaptic $GABA_B$-mediated currents, and the high input resistance of immature neurons will facilitate the generation of action potentials and synchronized activities (Gaiarsa et al., 1995; McLean et al., 1996).

The imbalance of excitation over inhibition may help to explain some of the early-life epileptic syndromes. For example, encephalopathy with suppression bursts may have its onset even before birth (Ohtahara et al., 1987). The EEG shows bilateral bursts of polyspikes contrasting with very little slow-wave activity (Aicardi and Goutières, 1978). The premature activation of NMDA neurotransmission, before GABA has become inhibitory, likely plays a major role in this very hyperexcitable EEG picture (Milh et al., 2007).

In summary, the immature brain's high susceptibility for seizures can be explained by the morphological and physiological events occurring during early life. The overabundance of synaptic connections, the increased

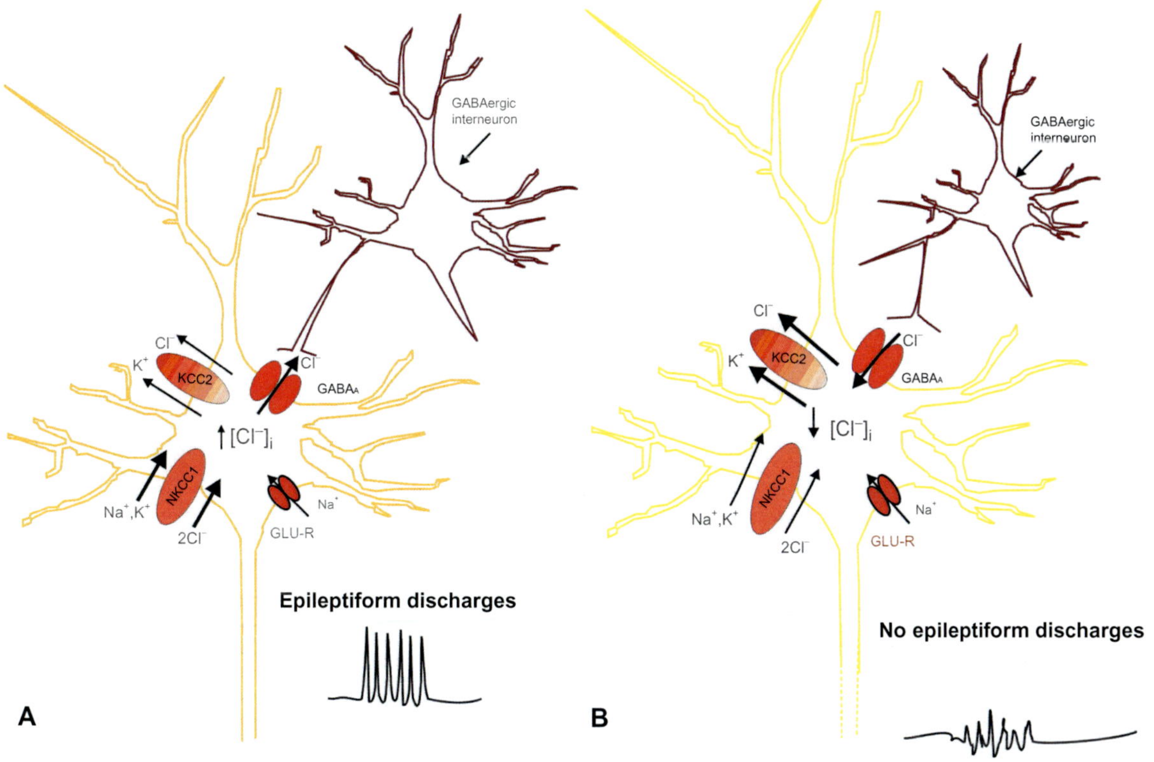

Fig. 7.1. Cartoons of (**A**) immature and (**B**) mature neurons. The immature neuron (**A**) is in a more excitable state than the mature neuron (**B**). Because the Na^+–K^+–$2Cl^-$ cotransporter (NKCC1) develops and functions sooner than the K^+–Cl^- cotransporter (KCC2) there is an increase of chloride within immature neurons compared with that in mature neurons (**A**). The increase in intracellular chloride results in a depolarized chloride equilibrium potential. When the γ-aminobutyric acid (GABA) channel is activated by GABA, there is a flow of chloride from inside the cell to outside the cell. As chloride carries a negative charge, the exodus of chloride served to depolarize the cell, making it more likely to discharge when sodium enters the cell. In the mature neuron (**B**), KCC2 is functional and balances the increase of chloride through NKCC1 with an outward flow of chloride. Because of lower intracellular chloride levels when the GABA receptor is activated, chloride enters the cell carrying a negative charge, thus resulting in hyperpolarization. GLU-R, glutamate receptor.

intracellular Cl^- resulting in a depolarizing effect of GABA, and the overexpression of AMPA and NMDA receptors with a composition that enhances excitability of neuronal networks, and the lack of developed inhibitory networks, leads to a situation were the immature brain is at high risk for seizures.

ALTERATIONS IN BRAIN DEVELOPMENT AS A CONSEQUENCE OF SEIZURES

As described above, the construction of cortical networks is associated with a sequential shift from an ensemble of immature cells with little or no organized communication devices to an active network composed of neurons endowed with thousands of active synapses. This shift is mediated by a series of processes that include intrinsic programs and extrinsic factors. It is known that seizures, like other insults, will modify these developmental processes leading to persistent deleterious sequels.

In the adult animals, prolonged or frequent seizures cause neuronal loss in hippocampal fields CA1, CA3, and the dentate hilus (Nadler, 1981; Cavazos and Sutula, 1990; Cavazos et al., 1991; Ben-Ari, 2001). Although the threshold for seizure generation is lower in immature brains than in adult brains, developing neurons are less vulnerable, in terms of neuronal damage and cell loss, than adult neurons to a wide variety of pathological insults. Compared with adult animals, young animals have far less cell loss in the hippocampus following a prolonged seizure (Albala et al., 1984; Berger et al., 1984; Holmes and Thompson, 1988; Sankar et al., 1998; Sankar et al., 2000).

Although cell loss does not occur in the young brain, early-life seizures can result in spine loss in CA3 pyramidal cells (Jiang et al., 1998) and synaptic reorganization of the axons and terminals of the mossy fibers of the dentate granule cells (Holmes et al., 1998; Huang et al., 1999, 2002; Sogawa et al., 2001). The mossy fiber sprouting differs significantly from the sprouting seen after status epilepticus in adult rats, occurring primarily in the CA3 pyramidal cell layer (de Rogalski Landrot et al., 2001) rather than the supragranular region. Recurrent seizures in developing rats can also adversely affect neurogenesis. McCabe and colleagues (2001) studied the extent of neurogenesis in the granule cell layer of the dentate gyrus over multiple time points following a series of 25 flurothyl-induced seizures administered during the first 5 days of life. Rats with neonatal seizures had a significant reduction in the number of newly formed neurons in the dentate gyrus and hilus compared with controls, with reductions in new cell formation continuing for 6 days after the final seizure.

In addition to sprouting and impaired neurogenesis, recurrent early-life seizures have been shown to result in immunohistological alterations of glutamate (Sogawa et al., 2001; Bo et al., 2004) and GABA subunit expression (Ni et al., 2004). Neonatal seizures have been associated with a decrease in GluR2 mRNA expression and protein levels (Zhang et al., 2004b), and selective reduction in the membrane pool of GluR subunits and decrease in the total amount of NMDA receptor 2A (Cornejo et al., 2007). In addition, excitatory amino acid carrier 1 (EAAC1) was reduced in rats with neonatal seizures compared with controls (Zhang et al., 2004b). Animals with alterations in glutamate receptors have been shown to have deficits in hippocampal-dependent radial arm water maze (Cornejo et al., 2007), demonstrating the relationship between neonatal seizures and memory deficits with specific alterations in glutamatergic synaptic function.

Significant alterations in GABAergic function have also been reported following neonatal seizures. Rats subjected to lithium–pilocarpine-induced seizures at postnatal day 10 show long-term $GABA_A$ receptor changes, including a 2-fold increase in α1-subunit expression (compared with lithium-injected controls) and enhanced type I benzodiazepine augmentation, the opposite to those seen after status epilepticus in adult rats (Zhang et al., 2004a). Persistent decreases in GABA amplitude in the hippocampus in rats also occur following neonatal seizures (Isaeva et al., 2006).

SUMMARY

All features of childhood epilepsy are intimately related to brain development. The clinical EEG features of seizures are closely related to developmental changes in cell growth, synapse formation, and myelination. The immature brain is highly excitable due to the depolarizing effects of GABA, overexpression of glutamatergic receptors, and lack of efficient inhibitory control. Seizures have an age-specific effect on brain development. Whereas early life seizures rarely result in cell loss, they can induce changes in synapse organization and receptor physiology.

ACKNOWLEDGMENTS

Supported by grants from the National Institutes of Health (NINDS): NS0415951 and NS056170.

References

Aicardi J, Goutières F (1978). Encéphalopathie myoclonique néonatale. Rev Electroencephalogr Neurophysiol Clin 8: 99–101.

Albala BJ, Moshé SL, Okada R (1984). Kainic-acid-induced seizures: a developmental study. Dev Brain Res 13: 139–148.

Barkovich AJ (2000). Concepts of myelin and myelination in neuroradiology. AJNR Am J Neuroradiol 21: 1099–1109.

Barkovich AJ, Kjos BO, Jackson DE, Jr et al. (1988). Normal maturation of the neonatal and infant brain: MR imaging at 1.5 T. Radiology 166: 173–180.

Barkovich AJ, Westmark KD, Bedi HS et al. (2001). Proton spectroscopy and diffusion imaging on the first day of life after perinatal asphyxia: preliminary report. AJNR Am J Neuroradiol 22: 1786–1794.

Ben-Ari Y (2001). Cell death and synaptic reorganizations produced by seizures. Epilepsia 42: 5–7.

Ben-Ari Y (2002). Excitatory actions of GABA during development: the nature of the nurture. Nat Rev Neurosci 3: 728–739.

Ben-Ari Y, Holmes GL (2005). The multiple facets of gamma-aminobutyric acid dysfunction in epilepsy. Curr Opin Neurol 18: 141–145.

Ben-Ari Y, Cherubini E, Corradetti R et al. (1989). Giant synaptic potentials in immature rat CA3 hippocampal neurones. J Physiol 416: 303–325.

Berg AT, Levy SR, Novotny EJ et al. (1996). Predictors of intractable epilepsy in childhood: a case–control study. Epilepsia 37: 24–30.

Berger ML, Tremblay E, Nitecka L et al. (1984). Maturation of kainic acid seizure–brain damage syndrome in the rat. III. Postnatal development of kainic acid binding sites in the limbic system. Neuroscience 13: 1095–1104.

Bhakoo KK, Pearce D (2000). In vitro expression of N-acetyl aspartate by oligodendrocytes: implications for proton magnetic resonance spectroscopy signal in vivo. J Neurochem 74: 254–262.

Bjornaes H, Stabell K, Henriksen O et al. (2001). The effects of refractory epilepsy on intellectual functioning in children and adults. A longitudinal study. Seizure 10: 250–259.

Bo T, Jiang Y, Cao H et al. (2004). Long-term effects of seizures in neonatal rats on spatial learning ability and N-methyl-D-aspartate receptor expression in the brain. Brain Res Dev Brain Res 152: 137–142.

Bulteau C, Jambaque I, Viguier D et al. (2000). Epileptic syndromes, cognitive assessment and school placement: a study of 251 children. Dev Med Child Neurol 42: 319–327.

Camfield P, Camfield C (2007). Long-term prognosis for symptomatic (secondarily) generalized epilepsies: a population-based study. Epilepsia 48: 1128–1132.

Casetta I, Granieri E, Monetti VC et al. (1999). Early predictors of intractability in childhood epilepsy: a community-based case–control study in Copparo, Italy. Acta Neurol Scand 99: 329–333.

Cavazos JE, Sutula TP (1990). Progressive neuronal loss induced by kindling: a possible mechanism for mossy fiber synaptic reorganization and hippocampal sclerosis. Brain Res 527: 1–6.

Cavazos JE, Golarai G, Sutula TP (1991). Mossy fiber synaptic reorganization induced by kindling: time course of development, progression, and permanence. J Neurosci 11: 2795–2803.

Chang LR, Liu JP, Zhang N et al. (2009). Different expression of NR2B and PSD-95 in rat hippocampal subregions during postnatal development. Microsc Res Tech 72: 517–524.

Cormack F, Helen CJ, Isaacs E et al. (2007). The development of intellectual abilities in pediatric temporal lobe epilepsy. Epilepsia 48: 201–204.

Cornejo BJ, Mesches MH, Coultrap S et al. (2007). A single episode of neonatal seizures permanently alters glutamatergic synapses. Ann Neurol 61: 411–426.

de Rogalski Landrot I, Minokoshi M, Silveira DC et al. (2001). Recurrent neonatal seizures: relationship of pathology to the electroencephalogram and cognition. Brain Res Dev Brain Res 129: 27–38.

Dekaban AS (1978). Changes in brain weights during the span of human life: relation of brain weights to body heights and body weights. Ann Neurol 4: 345–356.

Desai NS, Cudmore RH, Nelson SB et al. (2002). Critical periods for experience-dependent synaptic scaling in visual cortex. Nat Neurosci 5: 783–789.

Doose H (1992). Myoclonic–astatic epilepsy. Epilepsy Res Suppl 6: 163–168.

Dzhala VI, Staley KJ (2003). Transition from interictal to ictal activity in limbic networks in vitro. J Neurosci 23: 7873–7880.

Dzhala VI, Talos DM, Sdrulla DA et al. (2005). NKCC1 transporter facilitates seizures in the developing brain. Nat Med 11: 1205–1213.

Eltze CM, Chong WK, Bhate S et al. (2005). Taylor-type focal cortical dysplasia in infants: some MRI lesions almost disappear with maturation of myelination. Epilepsia 46: 1988–1992.

Fastenau PS, Jianzhao S, Dunn DW et al. (2008). Academic underachievement among children with epilepsy: proportion exceeding psychometric criteria for learning disability and associated risk factors. J Learn Disabil 41: 195–207.

Fetveit A (2008). Assessment of febrile seizures in children. Eur J Pediatr 167: 17–27.

Forsgren L, Beghi E, Oun A et al. (2005). The epidemiology of epilepsy in Europe – a systematic review. Eur J Neurol 12: 245–253.

Gaiarsa JL, Tseeb V, Ben-Ari Y (1995). Postnatal development of pre- and postsynaptic $GABA_B$-mediated inhibitions in the CA3 hippocampal region of the rat. J Neurophysiol 73: 246–255.

Gao W, Lin W, Chen Y et al. (2009). Temporal and spatial development of axonal maturation and myelination of white matter in the developing brain. AJNR Am J Neuroradiol 30: 290–296.

Glosser G, Cole LC, French JA et al. (1997). Predictors of intellectual performance in adults with intractable temporal lobe epilepsy. J Int Neuropsychol Soc 3: 252–259.

Glykys J, Dzhala VI, Kuchibhotla KV et al. (2009). Differences in cortical versus subcortical GABAergic signaling: a candidate mechanism of electroclinical uncoupling of neonatal seizures. Neuron 63: 657–672.

Gomez-Di Cesare CM, Smith KL, Rice FL et al. (1997). Axonal remodeling during postnatal maturation of CA3 hippocampal pyramidal neurons. J Comp Neurol 384: 165–180.

Hauser WA (1992). Seizure disorders: the changes with age. Epilepsia 33: S6–S14.

Hauser WA (1994). The prevalence and incidence of convulsive disorders in children. Epilepsia 35: S1–S6.

Hauser WA (1995). Epidemiology of epilepsy in children. Neurosurg Clin N Am 6: 419–429.

Hermann BP, Seidenberg M, Bell B (2002). The neurodevelopmental impact of childhood onset temporal lobe epilepsy on brain structure and function and the risk of progressive cognitive effects. Prog Brain Res 135: 429–438.

Holland BA, Haas DK, Norman D et al. (1986). MRI of normal brain maturation. AJNR Am J Neuroradiol 7: 201–208.

Hollmann M, Heinemann S (1994). Cloned glutamate receptors. Annu Rev Neurosci 17: 31–108.

Hollmann M, Hartley M, Heinemann S (1991). Ca^{2+} permeability of KA-AMPA-gated glutamate receptor channels depends on subunit composition. Science 252: 851–853.

Holmes GL, Thompson JL (1988). Effects of kainic acid on seizure susceptibility in the developing brain. Brain Res 467: 51–59.

Holmes GL, Gairsa JL, Chevassus-Au-Louis N et al. (1998). Consequences of neonatal seizures in the rat: morphological and behavioral effects. Ann Neurol 44: 845–857.

Huang L, Cilio MR, Silveira DC et al. (1999). Long-term effects of neonatal seizures: a behavioral, electrophysiological, and histological study. Brain Res Dev Brain Res 118: 99–107.

Huang LT, Yang SN, Liou CW et al. (2002). Pentylenetetrazol-induced recurrent seizures in rat pups: time course on spatial learning and long-term effects. Epilepsia 43: 567–573.

Huttenlocher PR (1979). Synaptic density in human frontal cortex – developmental changes and effects of aging. Brain Res 163: 195–205.

Huttenlocher PR (1984). Synapse elimination and plasticity in developing human cerebral cortex. Am J Ment Defic 88: 488–496.

Huttenlocher PR (1990). Morphometric study of human cerebral cortex development. Neuropsychologia 28: 517–527.

Huttenlocher PR, de Courten C (1987). The development of synapses in striate cortex of man. Hum Neurobiol 6: 1–9.

Huttenlocher PR, Hapke RJ (1990). A follow-up study of intractable seizures in childhood. Ann Neurol 28: 699–705.

Huttenlocher PR, de Courten C, Garey LJ et al. (1982a). Synaptic development in human cerebral cortex. Int J Neurol 16–17: 144–154.

Huttenlocher PR, de Courten C, Garey LJ et al. (1982b). Synaptogenesis in human visual cortex – evidence for synapse elimination during normal development. Neurosci Lett 33: 247–252.

Isaeva E, Isaev D, Khazipov R et al. (2006). Selective impairment of GABAergic synaptic transmission in the flurothyl model of neonatal seizures. Eur J Neurosci 23: 1559–1566.

Jensen FE, Baram TZ (2000). Developmental seizures induced by common early-life insults: short- and long-term effects on seizure susceptibility. Ment Retard Dev Disabil Res Rev 6: 253–257.

Jensen FE, Applegate CD, Holtzman D et al. (1991). Epileptogenic effect of hypoxia in the immature rodent brain. Ann Neurol 29: 629–637.

Jiang M, Lee CL, Smith KL et al. (1998). Spine loss and other persistent alterations of hippocampal pyramidal cell dendrites in a model of early-onset epilepsy. J Neurosci 18: 8356–8368.

Khalilov I, Holmes GL, Ben-Ari Y (2003). In vitro formation of a secondary epileptogenic mirror focus by interhippocampal propagation of seizures. Nat Neurosci 6: 1079–1085.

Khazipov R, Esclapez M, Caillard O et al. (2001). Early development of neuronal activity in the primate hippocampus in utero. J Neurosci 21: 9770–9781.

Khazipov R, Khalilov I, Tyzio R et al. (2004a). Developmental changes in GABAergic actions and seizure susceptibility in the rat hippocampus. Eur J Neurosci 19: 590–600.

Khazipov R, Sirota A, Leinekugel X et al. (2004b). Early motor activity drives spindle bursts in the developing somatosensory cortex. Nature 432: 758–761.

Koo B, Hwang PA, Logan WJ (1993). Infantile spasms: outcome and prognostic factors of cryptogenic and symptomatic group. Neurology 43: 2322–2327.

Kreis R, Ernst T, Ross BD (1993). Development of the human brain: in vivo quantification of metabolite and water content with proton magnetic resonance spectroscopy. Magn Reson Med 30: 424–437.

Kumar SS, Bacci A, Kharazia V et al. (2002). A developmental switch of AMPA receptor subunits in neocortical pyramidal neurons. J Neurosci 22: 3005–3015.

Lindsay J, Ounsted C, Richards P (1979). Long-term outcome in children with temporal lobe seizures. I: Social outcome and childhood factors. Dev Med Child Neurol 21: 285–298.

McCabe BK, Silveira DC, Cilio MR et al. (2001). Reduced neurogenesis after neonatal seizures. J Neurosci 21: 2094–2103.

McDonald JW, Johnston MV, Young AB (1990). Differential ontogenic development of three receptors comprising the NMDA receptor/channel complex in the rat hippocampus. Exp Neurol 110: 237–247.

McLean HA, Caillard O, Khazipov R et al. (1996). Spontaneous release of GABA activates $GABA_B$ receptors and controls network activity in the neonatal rat hippocampus. J Neurophysiol 76: 1036–1046.

Milh M, Becq H, Villeneuve N et al. (2007). Inhibition of glutamate transporters results in a "suppression-burst" pattern and partial seizures in the newborn rat. Epilepsia 1: 169–174.

Miller LP, Johnson AE, Gelhard RE et al. (1990). The ontogeny of excitatory amino acid receptors in the rat forebrain – II. Kainic acid receptors. Neuroscience 35: 45–51.

Minlebaev M, Ben-Ari Y, Khazipov R (2009). NMDA receptors pattern early activity in the developing barrel cortex in vivo. Cereb Cortex 19: 688–696.

Monyer H, Burnashev N, Laurie DJ et al. (1994). Developmental and regional expression in the rat brain and functional properties of four NMDA receptors. Neuron 12: 529–540.

Moshe SL (1981). The effects of age on the kindling phenomenon. Dev Psychobiol 14: 75–81.

Muroi J, Okuno T, Kuno C et al. (1996). An MRI study of the myelination pattern in West syndrome. Brain Dev 18: 179–184.

Nadler JV (1981). Kainic acid as a tool for the study of temporal lobe epilepsy. Life Sci 29: 2031–2042.

Natsume J, Watanabe K, Maeda N et al. (1996). Cortical hypometabolism and delayed myelination in West syndrome. Epilepsia 37: 1180–1184.

Ni H, Jiang YW, Bo T et al. (2004). Long-term effects of neonatal seizures on subsequent N-methyl-D-aspartate receptor-1 and gamma-aminobutyric acid receptor A-alpha1 receptor expression in hippocampus of the Wistar rat. Neurosci Lett 368: 254–257.

Ohtahara S, Ohtuska Y, Yamatogi Y et al. (1987). The early-infantile-epileptic encephalopathy with suppression-burst: developmental aspects. Brain Dev 9: 371–376.

Sanchez RM, Koh S, Rio C et al. (2001). Decreased glutamate receptor 2 expression and enhanced epileptogenesis in immature rat hippocampus after perinatal hypoxia-induced seizures. J Neurosci 21: 8154–8163.

Sankar R, Shin DH, Liu H et al. (1998). Patterns of status epilepticus-induced neuronal injury during development and long-term consequences. J Neurosci 18: 8382–8393.

Sankar R, Shin D, Mazarati AM et al. (2000). Epileptogenesis after status epilepticus reflects age- and model-dependent plasticity. Ann Neurol 48: 580–589.

Sans N, Petralia RS, Wang YX et al. (2000). A developmental change in NMDA receptor-associated proteins at hippocampal synapses. J Neurosci 20: 1260–1271.

Schropp C, Staudt M, Staudt F et al. (1994). Delayed myelination in children with West syndrome: an MRI-study. Neuropediatrics 25: 116–120.

Sillanpaa M (1983). Social functioning and seizure status of young adults with onset of epilepsy in childhood. An epidemiological 20-year follow-up study. Acta Neurol Scand Suppl 96: 1–81.

Sillanpaa M (2004). Learning disability: occurrence and long-term consequences in childhood-onset epilepsy. Epilepsy Behav 5: 937–944.

Sogawa Y, Monokoshi M, Silveira DC et al. (2001). Timing of cognitive deficits following neonatal seizures: relationship to histological changes in the hippocampus. Brain Res Dev Brain Res 131: 73–83.

Soria C, El Sabbagh S, Escolano S et al. (2007). Quality of life in children with epilepsy and cognitive impairment: a review and a pilot study. Dev Neurorehabil 10: 213–221.

Svennerholm L, Vanier MT (1978). Lipid and fatty acid composition of human cerebral myelin during development. Adv Exp Med Biol 100: 27–41.

Svennerholm L, Vanier MT, Jungbjer B (1978). Changes in fatty acid composition of human brain myelin lipids during maturation. J Neurochem 30: 1383–1390.

Swann JW, Brady RJ (1984). Penicillin-induced epileptogenesis in immature rats CA_3 hippocampal pyramidal cells. Dev Brain Res 12: 243–254.

Swann JW, Smith KL, Brady RJ (1991). Age-dependent alterations in the operations of hippocampal neural networks. Ann N Y Acad Sci 627: 264–276.

Takano T, Hayashi A, Sokoda T et al. (2007). Delayed myelination at the onset of cryptogenic West syndrome. Pediatr Neurol 37: 417–420.

Tremblay E, Nitecka L, Berger ML et al. (1984). Maturation of kainic acid seizure-brain damage syndrome in the rat. I. Clinical, electrographic and metabolic observations. Neuroscience 13: 1051–1072.

Ye GL, Yi S, Gamkrelidze G et al. (2005). AMPA and NMDA receptor-mediated currents in developing dentate gyrus granule cells. Brain Res Dev Brain Res 155: 26–32.

Yoshida F, Morioka T, Hashiguchi K et al. (2008). Appearance of focal cortical dysplasia on serial MRI after maturation of myelination. Childs Nerv Syst 24: 269–273.

Zhang G, Raol YH, Hsu FC et al. (2004a). Effects of status epilepticus on hippocampal $GABA_A$ receptors are age-dependent. Neuroscience 125: 299–303.

Zhang G, Raol YS, Hsu FC et al. (2004b). Long-term alterations in glutamate receptor and transporter expression following early-life seizures are associated with increased seizure susceptibility. J Neurochem 88: 91–101.

Handbook of Clinical Neurology, Vol. 107 (3rd series)
Epilepsy, Part I
H. Stefan and W.H. Theodore, Editors

Chapter 8

Genetics of idiopathic epilepsies

ORTRUD K. STEINLEIN*

Institute of Human Genetics, School of Medicine, Ludwig-Maximilians University of Munich, Munich, Germany

THE CONCEPT OF IDIOPATHIC EPILEPSIES

The term "idiopathic" was first used to separate the large group of epilepsies that seemed to "have no underlying cause other than a possible inherited predisposition" (Commission on Classification and Terminology of the International League Against Epilepsy, 1989) from the heterogeneous group of symptomatic epilepsies that had a known etiology such as tumor, metabolic disorder, or inborn brain malformation. The assumption about the inherited predisposition of idiopathic epilepsies has been proven correct by the progress made in molecular genetic techniques that helped to uncover many different gene defects. However, genetic predisposition can no longer be used to differentiate between idiopathic and symptomatic epilepsies because it has become obvious that many symptomatic epilepsies are genetic disorders, too. Nevertheless, the term "idiopathic epilepsy" is, mostly by tradition, still used today to describe a group of epilepsies that are characterized by a relatively benign course and the rarity with which additional neurological or other symptoms are observed in patients. It includes rare monogenic epilepsies such as familial nocturnal frontal lobe epilepsy and benign familial neonatal convulsions, as well as oligogenic and polygenic epilepsies including juvenile myoclonic epilepsy or the childhood and juvenile absence epilepsies.

THE PREDOMINANT PATHOGENETIC CONCEPT: ION CHANNEL DYSFUNCTION

Voltage- or ligand-gated ion channels are directly involved in the regulation of neuronal excitability and have therefore always been regarded as prime candidates for epileptic disorders. In particular, the excitatory channels such as glutamate receptors appeared to be the most logical choice when the progress in molecular genetics first offered the opportunity to study genes in detail. However, most researchers were surprised when the first epilepsy mutation that was detected happened to be located in a subunit of the nicotinic acetylcholine receptor, an ion channel that no-one would have put on top of the list of candidates (Steinlein et al., 1995). The epilepsy genes that followed coded for different voltage-gated channel subunits, a super-class of ion channels that more easily fits into existing pathogenetic concepts of epileptogenesis. Today, several monogenic idiopathic epilepsies are known to be channelopathies, and numerous studies have found evidence for associations between common subtypes of idiopathic epilepsy and specific ion channel genes (Table 8.1). Thus, mutations and susceptibility variants in voltage-gated and ligand-gated ion channels represent a major, although not the only, cause of idiopathic epilepsies. Ion channels have the advantage that their function can be studied in relatively simple experimental setups, and the detailed genetic and electrophysiological analyses of mutations found in different idiopathic epilepsies have already provided significant knowledge on the pathophysiological pathways leading from mutation to seizure (Avanzini et al., 2007). Several of the idiopathic epilepsies with known mutations are discussed in detail below.

Autosomal dominant nocturnal frontal lobe epilepsy

Of the rare monogenic idiopathic epilepsies, autosomal dominant nocturnal frontal lobe epilepsy (ADNFLE) is one of the best characterized at the pathophysiological and genetic level. ADNFLE shows considerable intrafamilial and interfamilial variance, both in age of onset and

*Correspondence to: Ortrud K. Steinlein, M.D., Ph.D., Head of Department, Ludwig-Maximilians University of Munich, School of Medicine, Institute of Human Genetics, Goethestrasse 29, 80336 Munich, Germany. Tel: 49/89-5160-4470, Fax: 49/89-5160-4468, E-mail: Ortrud.Steinlein@med.uni-muenchen.de

Table 8.1

Ion channel mutations in idiopathic epilepsies

Ion channel subfamilies	Subunits	Idiopathic epilepsies
Ligand-gated channels		
Nicotinic acetylcholine receptors	*CHRNA4**	Autosomal dominant nocturnal frontal lobe epilepsy
	*CHRNB2**	
	CHRNA2	
GABAergic receptors	*GABRG2*	Generalized epilepsy with febrile seizures plus
		Severe myoclonic epilepsy of childhood
	GABRA1	Childhood absence epilepsy and febrile seizures
		Autosomal dominant juvenile myoclonic epilepsy
	GABRD	Generalized epilepsy with febrile seizures plus
Voltage-gated channels		
Potassium channels	*KCNQ2**	Benign familial neonatal convulsions*
		Benign familial neonatal convulsions/myokymia syndrome
	KCNQ3	Benign familial neonatal convulsions
Sodium channels	*SCN1A**	Generalized epilepsy with febrile seizures plus
	SCN2A	
	SCN1B	
	*SCN1A**	Severe myoclonic epilepsy of childhood
	SCN2A	Benign familial neonatal-infantile convulsions

*Indicates the major genes for the respective epilepsies. Mutations in unmarked genes have been found mostly in fewer than five families.

in the severity of the clinical phenotype. The mean age of onset in ADNFLE is during adolescence or young adulthood, but a wide age range is observed even within families (between 1 and 64 years of age). Typically, clusters of brief motor seizures occur, mostly out of non-rapid eye movement (non-REM) sleep. Patients show episodes of recurrent paroxysmal awakenings associated with stereotyped movements. Seizures often start with gasps, grunts, or vocalizations followed by thrashing hyperkinetic activity or tonic stiffening of the limbs, and superimposed clonic jerking. Most seizure episodes are of 2–20 seconds in duration, but some of them might last considerably longer. In some families sleepwalking is a common feature and patients are reported to move around, talk unintelligibly, or scream for 3 minutes or more. An aura phenomenon including epigastric, sensory, or psychic symptoms often precedes the seizures. The clusters of nightly seizures often lead to poor sleep quality and cause tiredness during the daytime. Antiepileptic drugs such as carbamazepine are effective in some patients, but not in all (Scheffer et al., 1995).

ADNFLE: genes and mutations

The first ADNFLE mutation was identified in *CHRNA4,* the gene coding for the α4 subunit of the neuronal nicotinic acetylcholine receptor (nAChR). The *CHRNA4* gene represents one of the major subunits in one of the largest families of neuronal ligand-gated ion channels. nAChRs consist of five homologous or heterologous subunits that assemble around a central axis and form a cation-selective ion channel. Subsequently, two additional genes were identified to be involved in the pathogenesis of ADNFLE, *CHRNB2* and *CHRNA4*, which encode the β2 and α2 subunits of the nAChR. All but one of the known ADNFLE mutations are missense mutations that cluster within the second or, less frequently, first or third transmembrane regions (Fusco et al., 2000; Phillips et al., 2001; Aridon et al., 2006). The transmembrane regions either form the walls of the ion channel (TM2) or contribute indirectly to it (TM1, TM3). This suggests that only mutations that target the crucial functional mechanism of channel gating can cause ADNFLE.

Nonepileptic features in ADNFLE

Most known ADNFLE mutations are private, i.e., they have been detected only in a single family. However, some amino acid substitutions such as S248F and S252L were found in two or more ADNFLE families that often came from different parts of the world. This makes it likely that at least some of these mutations occurred independently in the respective families, offering the possibility to study the impact of different genetic backgrounds on ADNFLE mutations (Steinlein, 2007). In most ADNFLE families the patients are not only affected by seizures but present with additional neurological features. These might include psychiatric disorders, especially negative symptoms of schizophrenia (*CHRNA4*-776ins3), mental retardation (*CHRNA4*-S252L), or cognitive problems (*CHRNB2*-I312M) (Steinlein et al., 1997; Hirose et al., 1999; Magnusson et al., 2003; Bertrand et al., 2005). Interestingly, the pattern of nonepileptic features remained the same if unrelated families carried identical nAChR mutations, strongly suggesting that the mutations themselves rather than the genetic background or environmental factors determine the clinical phenotype. This hypothesis is supported not only by the complex and far from completely understood involvement of nAChRs in higher brain function, but also by functional studies. Expression analysis of the different ADNFLE mutations in *Xenopus* oocytes and HEK cells showed that each mutation has its individual biopharmacological profile. For example, some of the mutations increase the receptor's nicotine sensitivity, whereas others decrease it. Likewise, some of the mutated receptors can be blocked effectively by carbamazepine, whereas others are even less sensitive with respect to this antiepileptic drug than the wild type. Nevertheless, all ADNFLE mutations have in common that they increase the receptor's sensitivity to acetylcholine, most likely causing a gain-of-function effect. It is tempting to speculate that the gain-of-function effect might be responsible for the epilepsy phenotype, whereas the particular functional signatures of each mutant contribute to the associated neurological features in patients with ADNFLE (Steinlein and Bertrand, 2008).

It is still largely unknown how the mutated nAChRs are able to cause epilepsy. One plausible explanation could be that the gain-of-function effect causes presynaptically located nAChRs to overactivate inhibitory γ-aminobutyric acid (GABA)ergic interneurons. This could lead to the temporary inhibition of an unusually large number of pyramidal neurons. Once the inhibition resolves, all of these neurons are likely to produce action potentials at the same time, causing a hypersynchronization of neuronal networks that could easily escalate into a seizure (Fig. 8.1).

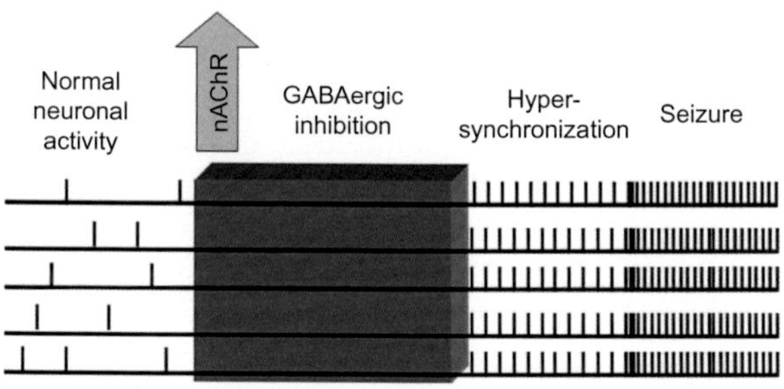

Fig. 8.1. Neuronal hypersynchronization in autosomal dominant nocturnal frontal lobe epilepsy (ADNFLE). The black box represents the phase of increased inhibition induced by gain-of-function mutations in nicotinic acetylcholine receptors (nAChRs). GABA, γ-aminobutyric acid.

Benign familial neonatal convulsions

Neonatal seizures that segregate in families were first described in 1964 (Rett and Teubel, 1964). More than three decades later, the molecular basis of benign familial neonatal convulsions (BFNC) was uncovered by the detection of the first mutations in the voltage-gated potassium channel genes *KCNQ2* and *KCNQ3* (Biervert et al., 1998; Charlier et al., 1998; Singh et al., 1998). BFNC is a rare autosomal dominantly inherited seizure disorder that starts between the first day and (at the latest) the fourth month of life. The seizures, which are generalized or multifocal, consist mostly of tonic posturing which can progress to clonic movements. They are frequently accompanied by features such as dyspnea, ocular symptoms, or autonomic signs. The course of the disorder is usually described as benign and self-limiting, and, with or without pharmacotherapy, in the majority of patients the seizures remit spontaneously within a few days or weeks. Most patients are seizure-free by the age of 6 months (Ronen et al., 1993). However, about 10–15% of the patients will experience mostly provoked seizures later in life. These "late-onset" seizures usually start in adolescence or young adulthood, an age when the brain seems to be especially vulnerable to the development of epilepsy. One explanation for these late-onset seizures might be that the mutations underlying BFNC generally lower the seizure threshold, rendering their carriers more likely to develop epilepsy in vulnerable developmental periods. Most of these seizures can be easily controlled by lifestyle changes and only rarely require long-term treatment with antiepileptic drugs. More disturbing are the recent reports that seriously question whether the condition is benign. Several BFNC families have come to attention in which developmental delay or mild retardation co-occurred with BFNC. In some families, single affected members have even presented with a disastrous course of the disorder, including epileptic encephalopathy and severe psychomotor retardation (Dedek et al., 2003; Borgatti et al., 2004; Schmitt et al., 2005). The outcome seems not to be related directly to the underlying mutation, as some of these patients inherited their mutations from a parent with a mild form of BFNC. Thus, the pathophysiological effect of BFNC mutations is likely to be modulated either by unknown genetic factors or by certain environmental influences.

Potassium channels genes and BFNC

The genes causing BFNC, *KCNQ2* (chromosome 20q13.3) and (more rarely) *KCNQ3* (chromosome 8q24), encode two highly homologous subunits that together form a heteropentameric potassium channel (Biervert et al., 1998; Charlier et al., 1998; Singh et al., 1998; Wang et al.,

1998). The channel subunits have identical structures including six transmembrane regions (TM), a voltage sensor in TM4, a loop between TM5 and TM6 that builds the ion channel pore, and a long C-terminal region that contains sequence motifs for subunit assembly. Most mutations are found in *KCNQ2*, which can be regarded as the major gene for BFNC. The mutational spectrum includes point mutations such as missense mutations, splice site aberrations, and single base-pair deletions or insertions as well as multiexon deletions. The mutations are usually private, meaning that they are not found in additional BFNC families. Expressed in the heteromeric *KCNQ2/KCNQ3* combination, most mutations do not exhibit a dominant negative effect with respect to the unmutated subunits but cause haploinsufficiency of the voltage-gated potassium channel (Biervert et al., 1998). That such a rather mild effect can nevertheless cause epilepsy is easily explained by the importance of the KCNQ2/KCNQ3 channel in brain. The heteromeric channel is thought to underlie most of the so-called M-current, which is a widely distributed K^+ current characterized by slow activation and deactivation kinetics as well as by a low activation threshold. The M-current is a powerful controller of neuronal firing and regulates the frequency with which action potentials are building. It is crucial in controlling excess neuronal excitability and in the prevention of seizures (Wang et al., 1998), which might explain why even modest reductions of the M-current are sufficient to increase seizure susceptibility in affected newborns (Watanabe et al., 2000).

BFNC–myokymia syndrome

One *KCNQ2* mutation has been identified that, at least in an experimental setup, is able to display a dominant negative effect on channel function by reducing the potassium current of the heteromeric receptor by more than 50%. The R207W missense mutation affects one of the positively charged amino acids that serve as the channel's voltage sensor. Interestingly, it causes not only BFNC but also myokymia, a spontaneous and repetitive involuntary contraction of muscle fiber groups. The mutation displays an unusual biopharmacological profile, which might help to explain the occurrence of both central and peripheral features in the affected family. Its effect on the potassium currents changes with respect to the pattern and time course of the depolarization. The dominant negative effect is observed only with short depolarization times, which are more likely found in motoneurons than in central neurons. The distinct biopharmacological characteristics that the mutation displays in reconstitution experiments might explain why R207W can cause both epilepsy and myokymia (Dedek et al., 2001).

Other early childhood idiopathic epilepsies

Two more rare autosomal dominant idiopathic epilepsies are known that typically start within the first year of life. BFNC, the earliest of the three with an age of onset (and usually also remission) within the first 4–5 months of life, is clinically and genetically distinct from the syndrome of benign familial infantile convulsions (BFIC). Children affected by BFIC usually develop their first seizure after their fourth month but before they complete their first year of life. The age of onset of the third of the early childhood epilepsies, benign familial neonatal/infantile convulsions (BFNIC), overlaps with both BFNC and BFIC. BFIC is genetically heterogeneous, and has been linked to various chromosomal loci including 1q23, 2q24, 19q, and 16p12-q12. The candidate region on chromosome 16p12-q12 overlaps with the putative loci for the infantile convulsions and choreoathetosis syndrome (ICCA), paroxysmal kinesigenic choreoathetosis (PKC), and rolandic epilepsy with paroxysmal exercise-induced dystonia and writer's cramp (EPRPDC) (Vigevano et al., 1992). In BFNIC, both neonatal and early infantile onset of the seizures may be present in the same family. In some patients, BFNIC is caused by mutations in the voltage-gated sodium channel subunit gene *SCN2A*, a gene that is also discussed as a minor gene for $GEFS^+$ below (Heron et al., 2002).

Generalized epilepsy with febrile seizures plus ($GEFS^+$)

Affecting 3–5% of children under the age of 6 years at least once, febrile seizures are the most common seizure type in humans. They are usually thought to have an oligogenic or polygenic background, but rare families with monogenic inheritance of febrile seizures have been identified and used tentatively to assign several putative gene loci to different genomic regions (*FEB1–FEB11*). In the syndrome named "generalized epilepsy with febrile seizures plus" ($GEFS^+$), febrile seizures not only affect an above-average number of family members but also often persist beyond the age of 6 years. $GEFS^+$ families also show a high incidence of different types of afebrile seizure, including generalized tonic–clonic seizures, absence seizures, atonic or myoclonic seizures, and, more rarely, also partial seizures (Scheffer and Berkovic, 1997). Owing to the variability of the seizure phenotype, the mode of inheritance underlying $GEFS^+$ is not always easy to determine. In some families the seizure susceptibility seems to follow an autosomal dominant inheritance pattern with high penetrance, while in most families the underlying genetic trait is more likely to be oligogenic, a major gene effect or a combination of both. The ion channel genes that have been implicated in $GEFS^+$ include the voltage-gated sodium channel genes *SCN1B*, *SCN1A*, and *SCN2A* as well as the GABAergic receptor subunit *GABRG2* (Wallace et al., 1998). However, the mutation detection rate in $GEFS^+$ remains very low, which would be in accordance with a mostly complex genetic background. Most mutations are found in the *SCN1A* gene, which codes for one of the major, pore-forming α subunits of the voltage-gated sodium channel. The subunit is composed of four domains each containing six transmembrane domains. $GEFS^+$ mutations are mostly missense mutations that are distributed over the whole length of the gene (Escayg et al., 2000).

Dravet syndrome (severe myoclonic epilepsy of infancy)

Mutations in the *SCN1A* gene also cause an epileptic encephalopathy termed Dravet syndrome or severe myoclonic epilepsy of infancy (SMEI). Phenotypically, the syndrome overlaps with the syndromes of borderline SMEI (SMEB) or intractable childhood epilepsy with generalized tonic–clonic seizures (ICEGTC) (Claes et al., 2003). In SMEI, febrile seizures usually occur around the age of 6 months in formerly normally developed children. During the second year various afebrile seizure types can occur, including absence, myoclonic, and partial seizures. The seizures are therapy-resistant and developmental delay becomes obvious, resulting in profound mental and motoric retardation. Nearly all patients are sporadic, resulting from *de novo* mutations in the *SCN1A* gene. The mutations are either truncating or missense mutations located in functionally critical parts of the gene. The differences in functional severity of the respective mutations probably explain why SMEI and $GEFS^+$ are allelic disorders with different clinical severity and outcomes (Rhodes et al., 2004).

NON-ION CHANNEL GENES IN IDIOPATHIC EPILEPSY

Autosomal dominant lateral lobe epilepsy

In 2002, mutations in the first non-ion channel gene were identified in an idiopathic epilepsy, demonstrating that ion channels are an important but obviously not the only pathogenetic mechanism underlying this group of epilepsies. The *LGI1* gene (leucine-rich glioma inactivated gene 1) was found to be mutated in autosomal dominant partial epilepsy with auditory features, also named autosomal dominant lateral temporal lobe epilepsy (ADLTLE) (Kalachikov et al., 2002). ADLTLE is a rare focal epilepsy syndrome characterized by recurrent unprovoked seizures with mainly acoustic and sometimes also visual hallucinations (Winawer et al., 2000). In some families the seizures start with a brief sensory aphasia triggered by unexpected environmental sounds or noises. The patients experience a brief period in which they have difficulties in speaking or understanding spoken language (Gu et al., 2002a). The *LGI1* gene on chromosome 10q24 was originally identified because it was disrupted by a reciprocal chromosome translocation in a glioma cell line. It is still a matter of debate whether *LGI1* indeed has a role in tumorigenesis, as has been hypothesized based on its reduced expression in malignant brain tumors, or whether it serves only as an unrelated marker for the decreased content of neuronal cells in gliomas. On the other hand, its role in epilepsy has been verified by several independent reports.

The mutational spectrum in ADLTLE includes both missense and truncating mutations that are distributed over the whole length of the *LGI1* gene. Its protein is characterized by a leucine-rich repeat motif (LRR) in its N-terminal end and seven so-called epilepsy-associated repeats (EARs) in the C-terminal half. The LRR motif shows high homology with comparable motifs in Slit and other proteins that are involved in protein–protein interaction or receptor function (Gu et al., 2002b; Staub et al., 2002). It has been shown that two different isoforms of LGI1 protein are expressed in brain. The longer isoform is secreted and has been shown to interact on the cell surface specifically with ADAM22, a transmembrane protein that can cause hypomyelinization of peripheral nerves and fatal epilepsy in the mouse model (Sagane et al., 2005). The EARs in LGI1 interact with the ectodomain of ADAM22 in a ligand–receptor manner, a mechanism that might point to a general pathomechanism in epileptogenesis. The ADAM22 protein interacts with stargazin, a transmembrane α-amino-3-hydroxy-5-methyl-4-isoxazolepropionic acid (AMPA) receptor regulatory protein. It has therefore been hypothesized that the LGI1/ADAM22–protein complex influences glutamatergic transmission, which would mean that ADLTLE mutations could interfere directly with the most important excitatory transmitter system in the brain (Fukata et al., 2006). The putative role of EARs in epilepsy is also underlined by the observation that this sequence motif is also present in the *MASS1/VLGR1/USH2C* gene, which causes seizures phenotype in mice and is mutated in a single family with febrile seizures (Skradski et al., 2001; Nakayama et al., 2002).

Familial juvenile myoclonic epilepsy

Juvenile myoclonic epilepsy (JME) is one of the most common idiopathic epilepsies. Clinically it is characterized by 15–30-Hz multispikes that can be recorded during myoclonic and tonic–clonic convulsions but are also found in clinically asymptomatic family members.

In most families JME runs as an oligogenic trait, with moderate recurrence risks. A few families have been identified in which a rare monogenic form of JME is present. In these families mutations in a gene of unknown function, *EFHC1* (EF-hand domain containing 1), segregate with the epilepsy phenotype (Suzuki et al., 2004; Medina et al., 2008). The same gene has also been found to be mutated in other types of idiopathic epilepsy, including rare cases of juvenile absence epilepsy and unclassified generalized idiopathic epilepsy (Stogmann et al., 2006).

References

Aridon P, Marini C, Di Resta C et al. (2006). Increased sensitivity of the neuronal nicotinic receptor alpha 2 subunit causes familial epilepsy with nocturnal wandering and ictal fear. Am J Hum Genet 7: 342–350.

Avanzini G, Franceschetti S, Mantegazza M (2007). Epileptogenic channelopathies: experimental models of human pathologies. Epilepsia 48: 51–64.

Bertrand D, Elmslie F, Hughes E et al. (2005). The CHRNB2 mutation I312M is associated with epilepsy and distinct memory deficits. Neurobiol Dis 20: 799–804.

Biervert C, Schroeder BC, Kubisch C et al. (1998). A potassium channel mutation in neonatal human epilepsy. Science 279: 403–406.

Borgatti R, Zucca C, Cavallini A et al. (2004). A novel mutation in KCNQ2 associated with BFNC, drug resistant epilepsy, and mental retardation. Neurology 63: 57–65.

Charlier C, Singh NA, Ryan SG et al. (1998). A pore mutation in a novel KQT-like potassium channel gene in an idiopathic epilepsy family. Nat Genet 18: 53–55.

Claes L, Ceulemans B, Audenaert D et al. (2003). De novo SCN1A mutations are a major cause of severe myoclonic epilepsy of infancy. Hum Mutat 21: 615–621.

Commission on Classification and Terminology of the International League Against Epilepsy (1989). Proposal for revised classification of epilepsies and epileptic syndromes. Epilepsia 30: 389–399.

Dedek K, Kunath B, Kananura C et al. (2001). Myokymia and neonatal epilepsy caused by a mutation in the voltage sensor of the KCNQ2 K^+ channel. Proc Natl Acad Sci U S A 98: 12272–12277.

Dedek K, Fusco L, Teloy N et al. (2003). Neonatal convulsions and epileptic encephalopathy in an Italian family with a missense mutation in the fifth transmembrane region of KCNQ2. Epilepsy Res 54: 21–27.

Escayg A, MacDonald BT, Meisler MH et al. (2000). Mutations of SCN1A, encoding a neuronal sodium channel, in two families with GEFS + 2. Nat Genet 24: 343–345.

Fukata Y, Adesnik H, Iwanaga T et al. (2006). Epilepsy-related ligand/receptor complex LGI1 and ADAM22 regulate synaptic transmission. Science 313: 1792–1795.

Fusco MD, Becchetti A, Patrignani A et al. (2000). The nicotinic receptor beta2 subunit is mutant in nocturnal frontal lobe epilepsy. Nat Genet 26: 275–276.

Gu W, Brodtkorb E, Steinlein OK (2002a). LGI1 is mutated in familial temporal lobe epilepsy characterized by aphasic seizures. Ann Neurol 52: 364–367.

Gu W, Wevers A, Schröder H et al. (2002b). The LGI1 gene involved in lateral temporal lobe epilepsy belongs to a new subfamily of leucine-rich repeat proteins. FEBS Lett 519: 71–76.

Heron SE, Crossland KM, Andermann E et al. (2002). Sodium-channel defects in benign familial neonatal–infantile seizures. Lancet 360: 851–852.

Hirose S, Iwata H, Akiyoshi H et al. (1999). A novel mutation of CHRNA4 responsible for autosomal dominant nocturnal frontal lobe epilepsy. Neurology 53: 1749–1753.

Kalachikov S, Evgrafov O, Ross B et al. (2002). Mutations in LGI1 cause autosomal-dominant partial epilepsy with auditory features. Nat Genet 30: 335–341.

Magnusson A, Stordal E, Brodtkorb E et al. (2003). Schizophrenia, psychotic illness and other psychiatric symptoms in families with autosomal dominant nocturnal frontal lobe epilepsy. Psychiatr Genet 13: 91–95.

Medina MT, Suzuki T, Alonso ME et al. (2008). Novel mutations in Myoclonin1/EFHC1 in sporadic and familial juvenile myoclonic epilepsy. Neurology 70: 2137–2144.

Nakayama J, Fu YH, Clark AM et al. (2002). A nonsense mutation of the MASS1 gene in a family with febrile and afebrile seizures. Ann Neurol 52: 654–657.

Phillips HA, Favre I, Kirkpatrick M et al. (2001). CHRNB2 is the second acetylcholine receptor subunit associated with autosomal dominant nocturnal frontal lobe epilepsy. Am J Hum Genet 68: 225–231.

Rett A, Teubel R (1964). Neugeborenen Krampfe im Rahmen einer epileptisch belasten Familie. Wien Klin Wochenschr 76: 609–613.

Rhodes TH, Lossin C, Vanoye CG et al. (2004). Noninactivating voltage-gated sodium channels in severe myoclonic epilepsy of infancy. Proc Natl Acad Sci U S A 101: 11147–11152.

Ronen GM, Rosales TO, Connolly M et al. (1993). Seizure characteristics in chromosome 20 benign familial neonatal convulsions. Neurology 43: 1355–1360.

Sagane K, Hayakawa K, Kai J (2005). Ataxia and peripheral nerve hypomyelination in ADAM22-deficient mice. BMC Neurosci 6: 33.

Scheffer IE, Berkovic SF (1997). Generalized epilepsy with febrile seizures plus. A genetic disorder with heterogeneous clinical phenotypes. Brain 120: 479–490.

Scheffer IE, Bhatia KP, Lopes-Cendes I et al. (1995). Autosomal dominant nocturnal frontal lobe epilepsy: a distinctive clinical disorder. Brain 118: 61–73.

Schmitt B, Wohlrab G, Sander T et al. (2005). Neonatal seizures with tonic clonic sequences and poor developmental outcome. Epilepsy Res 65: 161–168.

Singh NA, Charlier C, Stauffer D et al. (1998). A novel potassium channel gene, KCNQ2, is mutated in an inherited epilepsy of newborns. Nat Genet 18: 25–29.

Skradski SL, Clark AM, Jiang H et al. (2001). A novel gene causing a mendelian audiogenic mouse epilepsy. Neuron 31: 537–544.

Staub E, Perez-Tur J, Siebert R et al. (2002). The novel EPTP repeat defines a superfamily of proteins implicated in epileptic disorders. Trends Biochem Sci 27: 441–444.

Steinlein OK (2007). Genetic disorders caused by mutated acetylcholine receptors. Life Sci 80: 2186–2190.

Steinlein OK, Bertrand D (2008). Neuronal nicotinic acetylcholine receptors: from the genetic analysis to neurological disease. Biochem Pharmacol 76: 1175–1183.

Steinlein O, Mulley JC, Propping P et al. (1995). A missense mutation in the neuronal nicotinic acetylcholine receptor alpha 4 subunit is associated with autosomal dominant nocturnal frontal lobe epilepsy. Nat Genet 11: 201–203.

Steinlein OK, Magnusson A, Stoodt J et al. (1997). An insertion mutation of the CHRNA4 gene in a family with autosomal dominant nocturnal frontal lobe epilepsy. Hum Mol Genet 6: 943–947.

Stogmann E, Lichtner P, Baumgartner C et al. (2006). Idiopathic generalized epilepsy phenotypes associated with different EFHC1 mutations. Neurology 67: 2029–2031.

Suzuki T, Delgado-Escueta AV, Aguan K et al. (2004). Mutations in EFHC1 cause juvenile myoclonic epilepsy. Nat Genet 36: 842–849.

Vigevano F, Fusco L, Di Capua M et al. (1992). Benign infantile familial convulsions. Eur J Pediatr 151: 608–612.

Wallace RH, Wang DW, Singh R et al. (1998). Febrile seizures and generalized epilepsy associated with a mutation in the Na^+-channel beta1 subunit gene SCN1B. Nat Genet 19: 366–370.

Wang HS, Oan Z, Shi W et al. (1998). KCNQ2 and KCNQ3 potassium channel subunits: molecular correlates of the M-channel. Science 282: 1890–1893.

Watanabe H, Nagata E, Kosakai A et al. (2000). Disruption of the epilepsy KCNQ2 gene results in neural hyperexcitability. J Neurochem 75: 28–33.

Winawer MR, Ottman R, Hauser WA et al. (2000). Autosomal dominant partial epilepsy with auditory features: defining the phenotype. Neurology 54: 2173–2176.

Handbook of Clinical Neurology, Vol. 107 (3rd series)
Epilepsy, Part I
H. Stefan and W.H. Theodore, Editors

Chapter 9

The genetics of focal epilepsies

JUAN JOSÉ POZA*
Department of Neurology, Hospital Donostia, San Sebastián, Spain

INTRODUCTION

From a genetic point of view, epilepsies can be classified into three large groups.

1. *Monogenic epilepsies* are produced by the mutation of a gene that usually codes for a protein related to a neurotransmitter receptor or an ion channel. The mutation involves an important structural change in the protein that leads to a loss or gain in function that is sufficiently powerful to generate a change in the potential of the neuronal membrane, increasing its excitability.
2. *Oligogenic epilepsies* are caused by the mutation of a small number of genes, two or three at most. Patients who are carriers of mutations in all of these genes may develop the relevant phenotype, whereas someone with only one of the mutations will not develop the disease.
3. *Polygenic epilepsies* are those occasioned by a broad group of genes related to neuronal excitability. This genetic modification takes the form of a polymorphism, that is to say, alleles of the gene with differing degrees of efficacy in performing their function, but without being clearly deficient. Each individual has a collection of genes that make their neurons more or less excitable, and neuronal excitability is distributed in the population according to a Gaussian curve. Individuals at one extreme of that spectrum, those with the most excitable neurons, are most predisposed to develop epilepsy, especially if a brain injury occurs such as through trauma, tumor, or cerebrovascular disease.

The interest of geneticists has been centered primarily on the monogenic epilepsies, which are the easiest to study, and it is to these that the greater part of this chapter is dedicated. However, it should not be forgotten that these forms represent only a small proportion of epilepsies, and that the majority are of polygenic origin. What is more, even in monogenic epilepsies, other genes involved in neuronal excitability also influence phenotypic expression, so that not everyone who bears the mutation develops the epileptic syndrome. As with many other genetically based diseases, the penetrance (percentage of people with the mutation who actually develop the disease) for monogenic epilepsies is high, but it is not complete, and within a single family one can find individual carriers of the same mutation with very different clinical expressions.

AUTOSOMAL DOMINANT NOCTURNAL FRONTAL LOBE EPILEPSY

In 1994, autosomal dominant nocturnal frontal lobe epilepsy (ADNFLE) was described, and characterized by nocturnal motor seizures, usually during phase II nonrapid eye movement (NREM) sleep, that appear in clusters (average of eight seizures per night), are of short duration (usually less than 1 minute), are fundamentally motor-based (dystonic, tonic, or hyperkinetic), and are frequently preceded by an aura that may be tactile (local or generalized paresthesia), sensorial (auditory hallucinations, vertigo), psychic (fear, *déjà vu*), or autonomic (tachycardia, difficulty breathing), and are transmitted in an autosomal dominant pattern beginning in childhood or adolescence (Scheffer et al., 1994, 1995a). Its presentation during sleep, the complexity of its motor component (with shouts, groans, or moans, pedaling movements, disordered violent movements of the limbs, rhythmic movement of the pelvis, or dystonic postures), while retaining consciousness and with frequently normal EEG monitoring, have often caused patients to be diagnosed with

*Correspondence to: Dr. Juan José Poza, Servicio de Neurología, Hospital Donostia, P/Dr. Beguiristain S/N, Apdo correos 477, 20080 San Sebastián, Spain. E-mail: JUANJOSE.POZAALDEA@osakidetza.net

nocturnal paroxystic dystonia (Lugaresi et al., 1986), parasomnias, or psychiatric disorders (Godbout et al., 1985). More recently, a large number of families of different national origin (Anglo-Saxon, French-Canadian, Norwegian, French, Italian, Spanish, and Japanese) have been described, confirming the worldwide distribution of the syndrome (Berkovic et al., 1995; Oldani et al., 1998; Peraita et al., 1998; Ito et al., 2000). In just one centre in Italy, 28 families have been identified, indicating that the condition is more common than was previously thought.

Polysomnographic and video monitoring is crucial for the diagnosis of this disorder, although it is not unusual for even a critical EEG to fail to show a clear epileptic pattern; the most commonly found pattern is that of slow or spiked waves which are not necessarily focal. Notable interfamilial and intrafamilial variety can exist in the clinical picture, with regard to age of onset, severity, frequency of seizures, and response to treatment. Patients with the most severe forms of the disease may have generalized daytime tonic/clonic seizures and even repeated status epilepticus seizures, often precipitated by lack of sleep or by stress. Neurological examination is normal, although a thorough neuropsychological evaluation may show mild frontal dysfunction (Bertrand et al., 2005). A tendency to present schizophrenic or psychotic symptoms has been described (Picard et al., 2000; Magnusson et al., 2003). Carbamazepine is the drug of choice, although some 20–30% of patients are refractory to it (Picard et al., 1999). Valproic acid is usually ineffective for this type of epilepsy. An improvement in control of seizures has been reported with the use of tobacco or nicotine patches (Brodtkorb and Picard, 2006).

A linkage has been found to chromosome 20q13.3 (Phillips et al., 1995) and various gene mutations in the gene coding the α4 subunit of the cholinergic receptor, nicotinic, α4 (*CHRNA4*) in families of different national origin (Steinlein et al., 1995, 1997; Saénz et al., 1999). A second locus has been identified on chromosome 15q24, in a region where various genes that code for the synthesis of different subunits of the cholinergic neurone receptor (α3, α5, and β4) are found, although the causative gene for this locus has not yet been identified (Phillips et al., 1998). In 2000, another locus was identified in chromosome 1 (Gambardella et al., 2000), and a second gene related to the disease was cloned that codes for the β2 subunit of the CHRNB2 nicotinic receptor (De Fusco et al., 2000). From a clinical point of view, families with this mutation are indistinguishable from those with mutations of the *CHRNA4* gene (McLellan et al., 2003). Finally, one Italian family with a mutation of the α2 subunit of the CHRNA2 nicotinic receptor situated on chromosome 8 (Aridon et al., 2006) was described as presenting nocturnal epileptic seizures that included feelings of fear, tongue movements, and sleepwalking.

The effect of all these mutations in the subunits of the cholinergic receptors mentioned is that of increasing the sensitivity of the acetylcholine (ACh) receptor and even its usually inactive metabolites, such as choline (Phillips et al., 2001; Bertrand et al., 2002; Matsushima et al., 2002; Raggenbass and Bertrand, 2002). Carbamazepine reverses this effect, but this does not occur with valproic acid, which explains the differing sensitivity of ADNFLE to these two antiepileptic drugs, and indicates rational treatment strategies for epileptic syndromes for which the molecular basis is still being determined (Picard and Chauvel, 1999). The varied composition of nicotinic receptors, comprised of varying proportions of different subunits in distinct regions of the cerebral cortex, could explain the focal nature of these seizures. Finally, the progressive reduction in the number of cholinergic receptors in the frontal lobe, which occurs physiologically, could explain the favorable evolution and tendency for the number of seizures to diminish with age in ADNFLE (Gotti et al., 1997).

However, ADNFLE appears to be very heterogeneous from a genetic point of view, given that nearly 90% of these families do not show mutations of the indicated genes (Duga et al., 2002). In some families, a relationship with the known nicotinic receptors (Bonati et al., 2002) has been ruled out, and other mechanisms related to the disorder have been sought. To this end, two Italian families have been identified in which changes have been found in the gene promoter located on chromosome 8 (Combi et al., 2005) that codes for corticotropin-releasing hormone (CRH). The functional result of the changes is variable, in some cases resulting in increased gene expression, and in other cases in reduced expression. In addition, one of these changes has been found in unaffected individuals, so the pathogenetic role of the changes and their involvement in the appearance of ADNFLE remains to be confirmed.

FAMILIAL TEMPORAL LOBE EPILEPSY

Familial temporal lobe epilepsy is clinically and genetically heterogeneous (Cendes et al., 1998). To date, two very clinically different temporal epileptic syndromes with mendelian inheritance have been described; the seizures originate in the temporal lobe, but in the lateral or neocortical area in one syndrome and in the mesial area in the other.

Autosomal dominant lateral temporal lobe epilepsy (ADLTE), *or* autosomal dominant partial epilepsy with auditory features (ADPEAF)

This is an autosomal dominant disorder with penetrance that varies by family, but on average reaches 67% (Rosanof and Ottman, 2008). It includes simple partial visual seizures (simple images) or auditory seizures (buzzing, machinery noises), often with secondary generalization, that frequently appear during the first hours of sleep. Seizures are few and respond well to antiepileptic drugs, although they generally reappear upon discontinuing medication. There is not usually any postictal stupor, although patients often report headache following the seizure. The EEG between seizures is typically normal, although temporo-occipital epileptic activity may be detected, usually unilaterally (left). Neuroimaging is normal (Ottman et al., 1995; Poza et al., 1999). Other families present aphasic seizures (Gu et al., 2002), sometimes induced by auditory stimuli, generally language (Brodtkorb et al., 2005a). In some patients, a subtle change in left cortical auditory evoked potential has been reported, which suggests a change in language processing in this disorder (Brodtkorb et al., 2005b).

In some families of differing national origins, mutations have been found in the *LGI1* gene located on chromosome 10q (Kalachikov et al., 2002; Morante-Redolat et al., 2002), but no mutations have been found in this gene or its paralogs (*LGI2*, *LGI3*, *LGI4*) (Ayerdi-Izquierdo et al., 2006) in other families that are clinically identical but with lower penetrance (Michelucci et al., 2003) or in sporadic cases (Bisulli et al., 2004). Approximately 50% of families with two or more members with auditory-symptom epilepsy show a mutation in the *LGI1* gene.

The function of the *LGI1* gene is unknown. It has been described as a tumor development suppressor gene because it is expressed in low grade astrocytomas but not in glioblastomas (Gu et al., 2005), and in patients with ADLTE it is not associated with higher risk of tumor than in the general population (Brodtkorb et al., 2003). Unlike most genes related to epilepsy, *LGI1* does not code for any subunit of an ion channel or a neurotransmitter receptor, although it has been suggested that it may modify the function of presynaptic potassium channels (Schulte et al., 2006) and postsynaptic glutamate receptors (Fukata et al., 2006). It also interacts with cell receptors that modify cell reproduction and differentiation, and apoptosis and branching of the dendritic tree in such a way that the onset of epilepsy may be related to subtle changes in the establishment of neural networks. In zebrafish and mice, partial suppression of *LGI1* results in a predisposition to epileptic seizures, while its complete suppression causes abnormalities in brain development due to changes in the formation of glutamate receptors, supporting this hypothesis (Fukata et al., 2010; Teng et al., 2010).

A large Belgian family has been described with a form of occipitotemporal epilepsy associated with migraines with visual aura. Partial seizures are primarily visual, with flashes, but in other patients temporal symptoms appear, such as feelings of fear, vertigo, and auditory or autonomic symptoms. The condition is transmitted with an autosomal dominant inheritance pattern with incomplete penetrance, and has been established to be linked to chromosome 9q (Deprez et al., 2007).

Autosomal dominant mesial temporal lobe epilepsy

Berkovic et al. (1996) described another type of familial autosomal dominant epilepsy of the temporal lobe in which the characteristics of the seizures led to suspicion of mesial origin. It includes seizures with symptoms that are psychic (*déjà vu*, fear), autonomic (nausea, tachycardia), or sensorial (feeling of movement, and complex distortion of images or sound). The seizures begin in youth, are uncommon, and respond well to antiepileptic drugs, although they recur when the medication is discontinued. Only 6% of these patients have a history of febrile seizures. EEG or neuroimaging between seizures are normal. It is a heterogeneous syndrome from a genetic point of view. In one family of four generations with 21 individuals affected by focal epilepsy in which predominantly *déjà vu* seizure occurred, and was rarely a secondary generalized seizure, with no history of febrile seizure or hippocampal sclerosis, a linkage to the chromosome 4q13.2-q21.3 was found (Hedera et al., 2007). However, in the majority of these cases the genetic basis has yet to be determined, and the disease is probably of complex inherited origin, perhaps polygenic, perhaps multifactorial, with genetic and environmental factors playing a role (Crompton et al., 2010).

Subsequently, 45 families have been described with mesial temporal lobe epilepsy and hippocampal sclerosis (Kobayashi et al., 2003a). A history of febrile seizures, found in about 10% of patients with the familial form, is less common among patients with mesial epilepsy associated with sporadic hippocampal sclerosis. Complex partial seizures with oral or manual automatisms and intense postictal stupor are predominant. Most patients have a benign clinical course, and in some cases even remission of symptoms has occurred. Although many patients with hippocampal sclerosis have epilepsy that is more difficult to control with medication, some have a benign clinical course. Up to 34% of individuals with reduced hippocampal volume on magnetic resonance imaging (MRI) did not experience seizures. In refractory patients, surgery yielded results similar to those found in sporadic mesial epilepsies (Kobayashi et al., 2003b).

In a French family with febrile seizures and subsequent mesial temporal lobe epilepsy, a digenic model has been postulated, linked to chromosomes 1q25-q31 and 18qter, but the genes responsible have not been identified (Baulac et al., 2001). In another clinically similar family, linkage was found to chromosome 12q22-23.3.

Some families with mutations in the sodium channel subunits (*SCN1A* or *SCN1B*) demonstrate a homogeneous phenotype with febrile seizures in childhood and the subsequent development in some family members of mesial temporal lobe epilepsy with or without hippocampal sclerosis.

FAMILIAL PARTIAL EPILEPSY WITH VARIABLE FOCI

This is a familial epileptic syndrome that is autosomal dominant, and its most noteworthy feature is the different localization of epileptic focus in each family member, although each individual appears to have a single epileptic focus. Most patients experience seizures of frontal or temporal origin, although in some cases the origin is centroparietal or occipital. Age of onset is quite variable, ranging from the first months of life to age 50, but usually presenting in the first three decades of life, with the mean age of onset being age 10–15 years. The syndrome has a low penetrance, and its expressivity is quite variable, so that while some patients have a limited number of seizures over the course of their lives and respond very well to antiepileptic drugs, others have refractory epilepsy with very frequent seizures. Neuroimaging is normal in all cases.

The disorder is genetically heterogeneous. In an Australian family with seizures that are usually frontal or temporal and predominantly diurnal, and who often show epileptic activity on EEG between seizures, a linkage to chromosome 2q has been demonstrated (Scheffer et al., 1998). Moreover, in one Spanish (Berkovic et al., 2004), one Dutch (Callenbach et al., 2003), and three French-Canadian families (Xiong et al., 1999) that experienced primarily nocturnal seizures of generally frontal origin, with onset in the first three decades of life, with good response to drugs and EEGs between seizures that were typically normal, a linkage to chromosome 22q11-12 has been established. Despite the existence of this linkage, the low penetrance of the syndrome and the high phenotypic variability indicate that various additional factors, or other modifier genes, or environmental factors may modify the expression of the mutated gene.

BENIGN CHILDHOOD EPILEPSIES

Benign rolandic epilepsy and benign occipital epilepsy are two forms of partial epilepsy with a clear familial predisposition but with a complex inheritance pattern that makes it difficult to identify the genes involved in their onset.

Benign rolandic epilepsy is characterized by generally nocturnal seizures with hypertonia or hemifacial or upper-limb clonic twitching accompanied by salivation and guttural noises; it is of childhood onset and follows a benign course, disappearing during adolescence. It is accompanied by a typical EEG pattern with centrotemporal spikes and sharp waves, and appears to be transmitted according to an autosomal dominant pattern (Heijbel et al., 1975; Bali et al., 2007), although not all studies support this idea (Doose and Baier, 1989; Choy and Tan, 1995). Linkage of this EEG pattern has been established with the chromosome 15q14 (Neubauer et al., 1998), in the same region where linkage has been established for some families with juvenile myoclonic epilepsy. It is not known whether the gene involved is the same in both cases with differing phenotypic expressions influenced by other regulatory genes or environmental factors, or whether there are two different genes in the same region that are involved, respectively, in the appearance of each of the clinical phenotypes. In another study conducted by genomewide scanning and involving 194 individuals belonging to 34 families in the USA, linkage was found between the EEG pattern and the *hELP4* gene on chromosome 11p13, although no mutations were detected in the gene. The *hELP4* gene regulates the transcription of several genes related to cell migration and formation of the cytoskeleton (Strug et al., 2009). Moreover, a broad multinational study that included 18 twins (10 monozygotic, 8 dizygotic) found no cases of concordance, casting doubt on the importance of genetic factors in this epileptic syndrome (Vadlamudi et al., 2006).

Benign occipital epilepsy, characterized by motor seizures preceded by visual symptoms and often followed by migraine, which has a childhood onset and a benign course with spontaneous resolution in adolescence, and which shows a typical EEG pattern of occipital paroxysmal discharges, is the least well studied syndrome, but one family has been described that demonstrates a pattern of dominant inheritance, at least on EEG (Kuzniecky and Rosenblatt, 1987).

At the same time, two families in which epilepsy is associated with rolandic epilepsy with other phenotypic traits and a clear mendelian pattern of inheritance have been described. Guerrini et al. (1999) described a consanguineous family with an autosomal recessive syndrome of childhood onset in which rolandic epilepsy was associated with paroxysmal dystonia induced by exercise and writer's cramp. A linkage was found to chromosome 16p12-11.2, located in the same region as childhood seizure syndrome and autosomal dominant paroxysmal choreoathetosis, suggesting that the two entities may be allele variants. Scheffer et al. (1995b) described a family with an epileptic syndrome resembling benign rolandic epilepsy, but that was transmitted in a clearly autosomal dominant pattern with high penetrance, and possibly genetic anticipation, and was associated with oral and speech dyspraxia and cognitive impairment in recent generations. Subsequently, another family was described in which linkage has been excluded for chromosomes 11p, 15q, and 16p, and for which no candidate locus has yet been suggested (Kugler et al., 2008).

POLYGENIC EPILEPSIES

As mentioned above, the majority of epilepsies are polygenic, meaning that their onset is related to the presence of a broad collection of alleles of genes in a person that are related to membrane potentials, and that together give rise to neuronal hyperexcitability and facilitate the appearance of spontaneous epileptic seizures, or seizures that appear as the result of an injury to the brain (trauma, tumor, infection, cerebrovascular disease, etc.). Thus, no mutations exist in such cases, but instead only susceptibility polymorphisms are present, i.e., normal variants of a gene that are effective to some degree, but that have a total effect which leads to the onset of epilepsy. Studies to search for such polymorphisms are very complex, and so far the results have been disappointing, for although more than 50 potential polymorphisms that may increase susceptibility for various epileptic syndromes have been mentioned in studies, none has yet been confirmed (Tan et al., 2004; Cavalleri et al., 2005). A large study conducted by genomewide scan in populations of European origin was not able to demonstrate a significant association for any polymorphism for focal epilepsy (Kasperaviciūte et al., 2010).

NEURONAL MIGRATION DISORDERS

Neuronal migration disorders cause severe syndromes, including refractory epilepsy and major psychomotor development disorders. Several of these disorders are caused by mutations in genes encoding cytoskeleton proteins.

Lissencephaly is characterized by an absence (agyria) or decrease (pachygyria) in the convolutions of the brain. Subcortical band heterotopia is a disorder related to the above in which bands of gray matter appear interspersed in the white matter between the basal ganglia and the cerebral cortex. Mutations in either the *LIS1* or *DCX* (doublecortin) gene can cause either disorder, but most lissencephaly is caused by mutations in *LIS1*, which is transmitted with an autosomal recessive pattern, whereas most cases of subcortical band heterotopia are caused by *DCX* mutations transmitted by a recessive pattern linked to the X chromosome. Broad deletions that, along with the *LIS1* gene, include its neighboring genes are responsible for Miller–Dieker syndrome, which is associated with a predominantly posterior lissencephaly with facial dysmorphism and other malformations. Both *LIS1* and *DCX* encode microtubule proteins. *TUBA1A* is a gene that encodes a protein involved in the assembly of microtubules, and mutations of this gene can cause a particularly serious form of lissencephaly.

X-linked lissencephaly with absent corpus callosum and ambiguous genitalia (XLAG) is a serious disorder that affects only males and is caused by mutations of the X-linked Aristaless related homeobox gene (*ARX*).

Autosomal recessive lissencephaly with cerebellar hypoplasia has been associated with mutations in the *RELN* gene. It is associated with moderate lissencephaly, severe cerebellar hypoplasia, facial dysmorphism, developmental delay, and epilepsy. *RELN* encodes an extracellular matrix protein that controls cell interaction and neuronal positioning.

Periventricular nodular heterotopia is characterized by the presence of periventricular nodules of cerebral grey matter. Most patients suffer from epilepsy associated with more or less evident mental retardation. The vast majority of patients have mutations in the gene that encodes the protein filamin A (*FLNA*). Two consanguineous pedigrees have been described with a mutation in the adenosine diphosphate-ribosylation factor guanine nucleotide exchange factor 2 (ARFGEF2).

Polymicrogyria is characterized by the presence of an excessive number of small convolutions (gyri). It is a relatively common disorder that can appear in various forms and be caused by mutations in several genes. Bilateral perisylvian polymicrogyria, which is the most common form, presents with epilepsy, mild to moderate mental retardation, and oral–motor skill disorders. A patient with a mutation in the *SRPX2* gene, located on the X chromosome, has been described, but this does not seem to be the gene responsible for most forms. A linkage to 22q11.2 has been found in other patients, although the gene involved is unknown. Bilateral frontoparietal polymicrogyria (BFPP) has been associated with mutations of the G-protein-coupled receptor gene 6.

Tables 9.1 and 9.2 provide a summary of the loci and genes related to epilepsy.

Table 9.1

Focal epilepsies of genetic origin

Epileptic syndrome	Locus	Gene
Benign familial neonatal convulsions	20q13.3	*KCNQ2*
	8q24	*KCNQ3*
Benign familial infantile convulsions	19q12-13.1	
Benign familial infantile convulsions and paroxysmal choreoathetosis	16p12-11.2	
Benign neonatal/infantile seizures	2q21	*SCN2A*
Benign infantile seizures and familial hemiplegic migraine	1q23	*ATP1A2*
Autosomal dominant nocturnal frontal lobe epilepsy	20q13.3	*CHRNA4*
	15q24	
	1	*CHRNB2*
	8p12.3-8q12.3	*CHRNA2*
Autosomal dominant lateral temporal lobe epilepsy	10q24	*LGI1*
Familial temporal lobe epilepsy of mesial origin	4q13.2-q21.3	
Familial mesial temporal lobe epilepsy with hippocampal sclerosis	??	
Febrile seizures and mesial temporal lobe epilepsy	1q25-31+ 18qter	
Occipitotemporal epilepsy associated with migraine with visual aura	9q21-q22	
Familial partial epilepsy with variable foci	2q	
	22q11-q12	
Benign childhood epilepsy with rolandic paroxysmal discharges	15q14	
	11p13	*ELP4*
Autosomal dominant rolandic epilepsy with speech dyspraxia	??	
Rolandic epilepsy with paroxysmal dystonia induced by exercise and writer's cramp	16p12-11.2	

Table 9.2

Secondary epilepsies of genetic origin

Disease	Locus	Gene
Neuronal migration disorders		
Isolated lissencephaly. Subcortical band heterotopia or double cortex syndrome	17p13.3	*LIS1* or *PAFAH1B1*
	12q13.12	*TUBA1A*
	Xq22.3	*DCX*
Lissencephaly with cerebellar hypoplasia	7q22	*RELN*
Lissencephaly with abnormal genitalia	Xp22.13	*ARX*
Miller–Dieker syndrome	17p13.3	*LIS1* 14-3-3-ε and contiguous genes
Bilateral periventricular nodular heterotopia	Xq28	*FLNA*
	20q13.13	*ARFGEF2*
Bilateral perisylvian polymicrogyria	Xq28	
	11p13	*PAX6*
	Mitochondrial	*MTTL1*
Bilateral frontoparietal polymicrogyria	16q	*GPR56*
Schizencephaly	10q26.1	*EMX2*
Other neurological diseases		
Tuberous sclerosis	9p34.13	Tuberin
	16p13.3	Hamartin
Neurofibromatosis type I	17q11.2	Neurofibromin
Neurofibromatosis type II	22	
Cavernous angiomatosis	7q11-q22	
Episodic ataxia type I	12p13	Voltage-gated potassium channel
Dentatorubral–pallidoluysian atrophy	12p	
Angelman syndrome	15q11-q13	Ubiquitin-protein ligase

REFERENCES

Aridon P, Marini C, Di Resta C et al. (2006). Increased sensitivity of the neuronal nicotinic receptor alpha 2 subunit causes familial epilepsy with nocturnal wandering and ictal fear. Am J Hum Genet 79: 342–350.

Ayerdi-Izquierdo A, Stavrides G, Selles-Martinez JJ et al. (2006). Genetic analysis of the LGI/Epitempin gene family in sporadic and familial lateral temporal lobe epilepsy. Epilepsy Res 70: 118–126.

Bali B, Kull LL, Strug LJ et al. (2007). Autosomal dominant inheritance of centrotemporal sharp waves in rolandic epilepsy families. Epilepsia 48: 2266–2272.

Baulac S, Picard F, Herman A et al. (2001). Evidence for digenic inheritance in a family with both febrile convulsions and temporal lobe epilepsy implicating chromosomes 18qter and 1q25-q31. Ann Neurol 49: 786–792.

Berkovic SF, Phillips HA, Scheffer IE et al. (1995). Genetic heterogeneity in autosomal dominant nocturnal frontal lobe epilepsy. Epilepsia 36: 147.

Berkovic SF, McIntosh AM, Howell RA et al. (1996). Familial temporal lobe epilepsy: a common disorder identified in twins. Ann Neurol 40: 227–235.

Berkovic SF, Serratosa JM, Phillips HA et al. (2004). Familial partial epilepsy with variable foci: clinical features and linkage to chromosome 22q12. Epilepsia 45: 1054–1060.

Bertrand D, Picard F, Le Hellard S et al. (2002). How mutations in the nAChRs can cause ADNFLE epilepsy. Epilepsia 43: 112–122.

Bertrand D, Elmslie F, Hughes E et al. (2005). The CHRNB2 mutation I312M is associated with epilepsy and distinct memory deficits. Neurobiol Dis 20: 799–804.

Bisulli F, Tinuper P, Avoni P et al. (2004). Idiopathic partial epilepsy with auditory features (IPEAF): a clinical and genetic study of 53 sporadic cases. Brain 127: 1343–1352.

Bonati MT, Combi R, Asselta R et al. (2002). Exclusion of linkage of nine neuronal nicotinic acetylcholine receptor subunit genes expressed in brain in autosomal dominant nocturnal frontal lobe epilepsy in four unrelated families. J Neurol 249: 967–974.

Brodtkorb E, Picard F (2006). Tobacco habits modulate autosomal dominant nocturnal frontal lobe epilepsy. Epilepsy Behav 9: 515–520.

Brodtkorb E, Nakken KO, Steinlein OK (2003). No evidence for a seriously increased malignancy risk in LGI1-caused epilepsy. Epilepsy Res 56: 205–208.

Brodtkorb E, Michler RP, Gu W et al. (2005a). Speech-induced aphasic seizures in epilepsy caused by LGI1 mutation. Epilepsia 46: 963–966.

Brodtkorb E, Steinlein OK, Sand T (2005b). Asymmetry of long-latency auditory evoked potentials in LGI1-related autosomal dominant lateral temporal lobe epilepsy. Epilepsia 46: 1692–1694.

Callenbach PM, van den Maagdenberg AM, Hottenga JJ et al. (2003). Familial partial epilepsy with variable foci in a Dutch family: clinical characteristics and confirmation of linkage to chromosome 22q. Epilepsia 44: 1298–1305.

Cavalleri GL, Lynch JM, Depondt C et al. (2005). Failure to replicate previously reported genetic associations with sporadic temporal lobe epilepsy: where to from here? Brain 128: 1832–1840.

Cendes F, Lopes-Cendes I, Andermann E et al. (1998). Familial temporal lobe epilepsy: a clinically heterogeneous syndrome. Neurology 50: 554–557.

Choy YS, Tan CT (1995). Study of genetic aspects of benign rolandic epilepsy: EEG of siblings and pedigree analysis. Epilepsia 36: 27.

Combi R, Dalpra L, Ferini–Strambi L et al. (2005). Frontal lobe epilepsy and mutations of the corticotropin-releasing hormone gene. Ann Neurol 58: 899–904.

Crompton DE, Scheffer IE, Taylor I et al. (2010). Familial mesial temporal lobe epilepsy: a benign epilepsy syndrome showing complex inheritance. Brain 133: 3221–3231.

De Fusco M, Becchetti A, Patrignani A et al. (2000). The nicotinic receptor β2 subunit is mutant in nocturnal frontal lobe epilepsy. Nat Genet 26: 275–276.

Deprez L, Peeters K, Van Paesschen W et al. (2007). Familial occipitotemporal lobe epilepsy and migraine with visual aura: linkage to chromosome 9q. Neurology 68: 1995–2002.

Doose H, Baier WK (1989). Benign partial epilepsy and related conditions: multifactorial pathogenesis with hereditary impairment of brain maturation. Eur J Pediatr 149: 152–158.

Duga S, Asselta R, Bonati MT (2002). Mutational analysis of nicotinic acetylcholine receptor beta2 subunit gene (CHRNB2) in a representative cohort of Italian probands affected by autosomal dominant nocturnal frontal lobe epilepsy. Epilepsia 43: 362–364.

Fukata Y, Adesnik H, Iwanaga T et al. (2006). Epilepsy-related ligand/receptor complex LGI1 and ADAM22 regulate synaptic transmission. Science 313: 1792–1795.

Fukata Y, Lovero KL, Iwanaga T et al. (2010). Disruption of LGI1-linked synaptic complex causes abnormal synaptic transmission and epilepsy. Proc Natl Acad Sci U S A 107: 3799–3804.

Gambardella A, Annesi G, De Fusco M et al. (2000). A new locus for autosomal dominant nocturnal frontal lobe epilepsy maps to chromosome 1. Neurology 55: 1467–1471.

Godbout R, Montplaisir J, Rouleau Y (1985). Hypnogenic paroxysmal dystonia: epilepsy or sleep disorder? A case report. Clin Electroencephalogr 16: 136–142.

Gotti C, Fornasari D, Clementi F (1997). Human neuronal nicotinic receptors. Prog Neurobiol 53: 199–237.

Gu W, Brodtkorb E, Steinlein OK (2002). LGI1 is mutated in familial temporal lobe epilepsy characterized by aphasic seizures. Ann Neurol 52: 364–367.

Gu W, Brodtkorb E, Piepoli T et al. (2005). LGI1: a gene involved in epileptogenesis and glioma progression? Neurogenetics 6: 59–66.

Guerrini R, Bonanni P, Nardocci N et al. (1999). Autosomal recessive rolandic epilepsy with paroxysmal exercise-induced dystonia and writer's cramp: delineation of the syndrome and gene mapping to chromosome 16p12-11.2. Ann Neurol 45: 344–352.

Hedera P, Blair MA, Andermann E et al. (2007). Familial mesial temporal lobe epilepsy maps to chromosome 4q13.2-q21.3. Neurology 68: 2107–2112.

Heijbel J, Blom S, Rasmuson M (1975). Benign epilepsy of children with centro-temporal EEG foci: a genetic study. Epilepsia 16: 285–293.

Ito M, Kobayashi K, Fujii T et al. (2000). Electroclinical picture of autosomal dominant nocturnal frontal lobe epilepsy in a Japanese family. Epilepsia 41: 52–58.

Kalachikov S, Evgrafov O, Ross B et al. (2002). Mutations in LGI1 cause autosomal-dominant partial epilepsy with auditory features. Nat Genet 30: 335–341.

Kasperaviciūte D, Catarino CB, Heinzen EL et al. (2010). Common genetic variation and susceptibility to partial epilepsies: a genome-wide association study. Brain 133: 2136–2147.

Kobayashi E, D'Agostino MD, Lopes-Cendes I et al. (2003a). Hippocampal atrophy and T2-weighted signal changes in familial mesial temporal lobe epilepsy. Neurology 60: 405–409.

Kobayashi E, D'Agostino MD, Lopes-Cendes I et al. (2003b). Outcome of surgical treatment in familial mesial temporal lobe epilepsy. Epilepsia 44: 1080–1084.

Kugler SL, Bali B, Lieberman P et al. (2008). An autosomal dominant genetically heterogeneous variant of rolandic epilepsy and speech disorder. Epilepsia 49: 1086–1090.

Kuzniecky R, Rosenblatt B (1987). Benign occipital epilepsy: a family study. Epilepsia 28: 346–350.

Lugaresi E, Cirignotta F, Montagna P (1986). Nocturnal paroxysmal dystonia. J Neurol Neurosurg Psychiatry 49: 375–380.

Magnusson A, Stordal E, Brodtkorb E et al. (2003). Schizophrenia, psychotic illness and other psychiatric symptoms in families with autosomal dominant nocturnal frontal lobe epilepsy caused by different mutations. Psychiatr Genet 13: 91–95.

Matsushima N, Hirose S, Iwata H et al. (2002). Mutation (Ser284Leu) of neuronal nicotinic acetylcholine receptor alpha 4 subunit associated with frontal lobe epilepsy causes faster desensitization of the rat receptor expressed in oocytes. Epilepsy Res 48: 181–186.

McLellan A, Phillips HA, Rittey C et al. (2003). Phenotypic comparison of two Scottish families with mutations in different genes causing autosomal dominant nocturnal frontal lobe epilepsy. Epilepsia 44: 613–617.

Michelucci R, Poza JJ, Sofia V et al. (2003). Autosomal dominant lateral temporal epilepsy: clinical spectrum, new epitempin mutations, and genetic heterogeneity in seven European families. Epilepsia 44: 1289–1297.

Morante-Redolat JM, Gorostidi-Pagola A, Piquer-Sirerol S et al. (2002). Mutations in the LGI1/Epitempin gene on 10q24 cause autosomal dominant lateral temporal epilepsy. Hum Mol Genet 11: 1119–1128.

Neubauer BA, Fiedler B, Himmelein B et al. (1998). Centrotemporal spikes in families with rolandic epilepsy: linkage to chromosome 15q14. Neurology 51: 1608–1612.

Oldani A, Zucconi M, Asselta R et al. (1998). Autosomal dominant nocturnal frontal lobe epilepsy. A video-polysomnographic and genetic appraisal of 40 patients and delineation of the epileptic syndrome. Brain 121: 205–223.

Ottman R, Risch N, Hauser WA et al. (1995). Localization of a gene for partial epilepsy to chromosome 10q. Nat Genet 10: 56–60.

Peraita R, Piñeiro P, Diaz F et al. (1998). Epilepsia nocturna frontal autosómica dominante. Aspectos electroclínicos. Rev Neurol 26: 290.

Phillips HA, Scheffer IE, Berkovic SF et al. (1995). Localization of a gene for autosomal dominant nocturnal frontal lobe epilepsy to chromosome 20q13.2. Nat Genet 10: 117–118.

Phillips HA, Scheffer IE, Crossland KM et al. (1998). Autosomal dominant nocturnal frontal-lobe epilepsy: genetic heterogeneity and evidence for a second locus at 15q24. Am J Hum Genet 63: 1108–1116.

Phillips HA, Favre I, Kirkpatrick M et al. (2001). CHRNB2 is the second acetylcholine receptor subunit associated with autosomal dominant nocturnal frontal lobe epilepsy. Am J Hum Genet 68: 225–231.

Picard F, Chauvel P (1999). L'épilepsie frontale nocturne autosomique dominante: le syndrome. Rev Neurol (Paris) 155: 445–449.

Picard F, Bertrand S, Steinlein OK et al. (1999). Mutated nicotinic receptors responsible for autosomal dominant nocturnal frontal lobe epilepsy are more sensitive to carbamazepine. Epilepsia 40: 1198–1209.

Picard F, Baulac S, Kahane P et al. (2000). Dominant partial epilepsies. A clinical, electrophysiological and genetic study of 19 European families. Brain 123: 1247–1262.

Poza JJ, Sáenz A, Martínez-Gil A et al. (1999). Autosomal dominant lateral temporal epilepsy: clinical and genetic study of a large Basque pedigree linked to chromosome 10q. Ann Neurol 45: 182–188.

Saénz A, Galan J, Caloustian C et al. (1999). Autosomal dominant nocturnal frontal lobe epilepsy in a Spanish family with a Ser252Phe mutation in the CHRNA4 gene. Arch Neurol 56: 1004–1009.

Raggenbass M, Bertrand D (2002). Nicotinic receptors in circuit excitability and epilepsy. J Neurobiol 53: 580–589.

Rosanof MJ, Ottman R (2008). Penetrance of LGI1 mutations in autosomal dominant partial epilepsy with auditory features. Neurology 71: 567–571.

Scheffer IE, Bhatia KP, Lopes-Cendes I et al. (1994). Autosomal dominant frontal epilepsy misdiagnosed as sleep disorder. Lancet 343: 515–517.

Scheffer IE, Bhatia KP, Lopes-Cendes I et al. (1995a). Autosomal dominant nocturnal frontal epilepsy. A distinctive clinical disorder. Brain 118: 61–73.

Scheffer IE, Jones L, Pozzebon M et al. (1995b). Autosomal dominant rolandic epilepsy and speech dyspraxia: a new syndrome with anticipation. Ann Neurol 38: 633–642.

Scheffer IE, Phillips HA, O'Brien CE et al. (1998). Familial partial epilepsy with variable foci: a new partial epilepsy syndrome with suggestion of linkage to chromosome 2. Ann Neurol 44: 890–899.

Schulte U, Thumfart JO, Klocker N et al. (2006). The epilepsy-linked LGI1 protein assembles into presynaptic Kv1 channels and inhibits inactivation by Kvbeta1. Neuron 49: 697–706.

Steinlein OK, Mulley JC, Propping P et al. (1995). A missense mutation in the neuronal nicotinic acetylcholine receptor alpha4 subunit is associated with autosomal dominant nocturnal frontal lobe epilepsy. Nat Genet 11: 201–203.

Steinlein OK, Magnusson A, Stoodt J et al. (1997). An insertion mutation of the CHRNA4 gene in a family with autosomal dominant nocturnal frontal lobe epilepsy. Hum Mol Genet 6: 943–948.

Strug LJ, Clarke T, Chiang T et al. (2009). Centrotemporal sharp wave EEG trait in rolandic epilepsy maps to Elongator Protein Complex 4 (ELP4). Eur J Hum Genet 17: 1171–1181.

Tan NC, Mulley JC, Berkovic SF (2004). Genetic association studies in epilepsy: "the truth is out there". Epilepsia 45: 1429–1442.

Teng Y, Xie X, Walker S et al. (2010). Knockdown of zebrafish LGI1a results in abnormal development, brain defects and a seizure-like behavioral phenotype. Hum Mol Genet 19: 4409–4420.

Vadlamudi L, Kjeldsen MJ, Corey LA et al. (2006). Analyzing the etiology of benign rolandic epilepsy: a multicenter twin collaboration. Epilepsia 47: 550–555.

Xiong L, Labuda M, Li DS et al. (1999). Mapping of a gene determining familial partial epilepsy with variable foci to chromosome 22q11-q12. Am J Hum Genet 65: 1698–1710.

Handbook of Clinical Neurology, Vol. 107 (3rd series)
Epilepsy, Part I
H. Stefan and W.H. Theodore, Editors

Chapter 10

Inflammation and epilepsy

ANNAMARIA VEZZANI*, SILVIA BALOSSO, AND TERESA RAVIZZA
Laboratory of Experimental Neurology, Department of Neuroscience, Mario Negri Institute for Pharmacological Research, Milan, Italy

CLINICAL EVIDENCE

Clinical evidence supporting a role for inflammation in tissue epileptogenicity stems from three main findings. (1) Various markers of inflammation have been measured in epileptogenic tissue from surgically treated pharmacoresistant patients, namely in malformations of cortical development (ganglioglioma, neuroepithelial tumors, focal cortical dysplasia, tuberous sclerosis) (Maldonado et al., 2003; Ravizza et al., 2006a; Boer et al., 2008), in temporal lobe epilepsy with hippocampal sclerosis (Sheng et al., 1994; Crespel et al., 2002; Ravizza et al., 2008a) (Fig. 10.1), and in Rasmussen's encephalitis (RE) (Bien et al., 2002). Notably, in all these cases, prominent involvement of glial cells (microglia and astrocytes), macrophages, and, to a lesser extent, neurons and endothelial cells has been reported, indicating that parenchymal cells are the major common contributor to brain inflammation. Notably, adaptive immunity consisting mainly of brain invasion by T cells was significant only in some instances, such as Rasmussen's encephalitis (Bien et al., 2002) and tuberous sclerosis (Boer et al., 2008), whereas only sparse T cells, mostly intravasal, were found in temporal lobe epilepsy (TLE) (Ravizza et al., 2008a). (2) Levels of various cytokines have been shown to increase transiently in the blood and cerebrospinal fluid (CSF) of patients with epilepsy after different types of seizure (Peltola et al., 2002; Lehtimaki et al., 2004). Moreover, the cytokine concentration in CSF was higher than in blood, suggesting a brain origin. These two sets of observations suggest that brain inflammation may be caused by the intrinsic neuropathology in lesional epileptogenic tissue, by seizures, or by both. Notably, the frequency of seizures before surgery shows a positive correlation with the levels of inflammation in epileptogenic tissue (Ravizza et al., 2006a). (3) Anti-inflammatory treatments (adrenocorticotropic hormone (ACTH), steroids, intravenous immunoglobulin (IVIg), plasmapheresis, immunosuppressants, etc.) display anticonvulsant effects in epileptic syndromes (RE, West, Lennox–Gastau, and Landau–Kleffner syndromes) with seizures resistant to classical antiepileptic drugs (AEDs) (Vezzani and Granata, 2005). These findings establish a link between inflammation and seizures, and indicate that inflammation is not merely an epiphenomenon of diseased tissue but may actively contribute to the pathology.

EXPERIMENTAL STUDIES

The experimental studies addressed three main questions related to: (1) the causes of brain inflammation with a special focus on the involvement of seizures, cell death, or their association as triggering factors; (2) the possibility that a proinflammatory state in the brain can precipitate or predispose to seizures; (3) whether pharmacological or genetic interference with specific inflammatory pathways in the brain can modify seizure frequency or duration, neuronal survival, and epileptogenesis.

To address these points three main models have been used: status epilepticus induced in rodents by systemic administration of convulsant drugs or by electrical stimulation in the rat hippocampus; febrile seizures induced in immature rodents by hyperthermia; mimicking systemic infection using bacteria or bacterial components (see review Vezzani and Granata, 2005).

Status epilepticus

Seminal work by Minami et al. (1991) showed that prolonged seizures in rodents caused by kainic acid induced transcriptional activation of several proinflammatory

*Correspondence to: Annamaria Vezzani, Ph.D., Laboratory of Experimental Neurology, Department of Neuroscience, Mario Negri Institute for Pharmacological Research, Via G. La Masa 19, 20156 Milano, Italy. Tel: +39-02-39.014.410, Fax: +39-02-35.46.277, E-mail: vezzani@marionegri.it

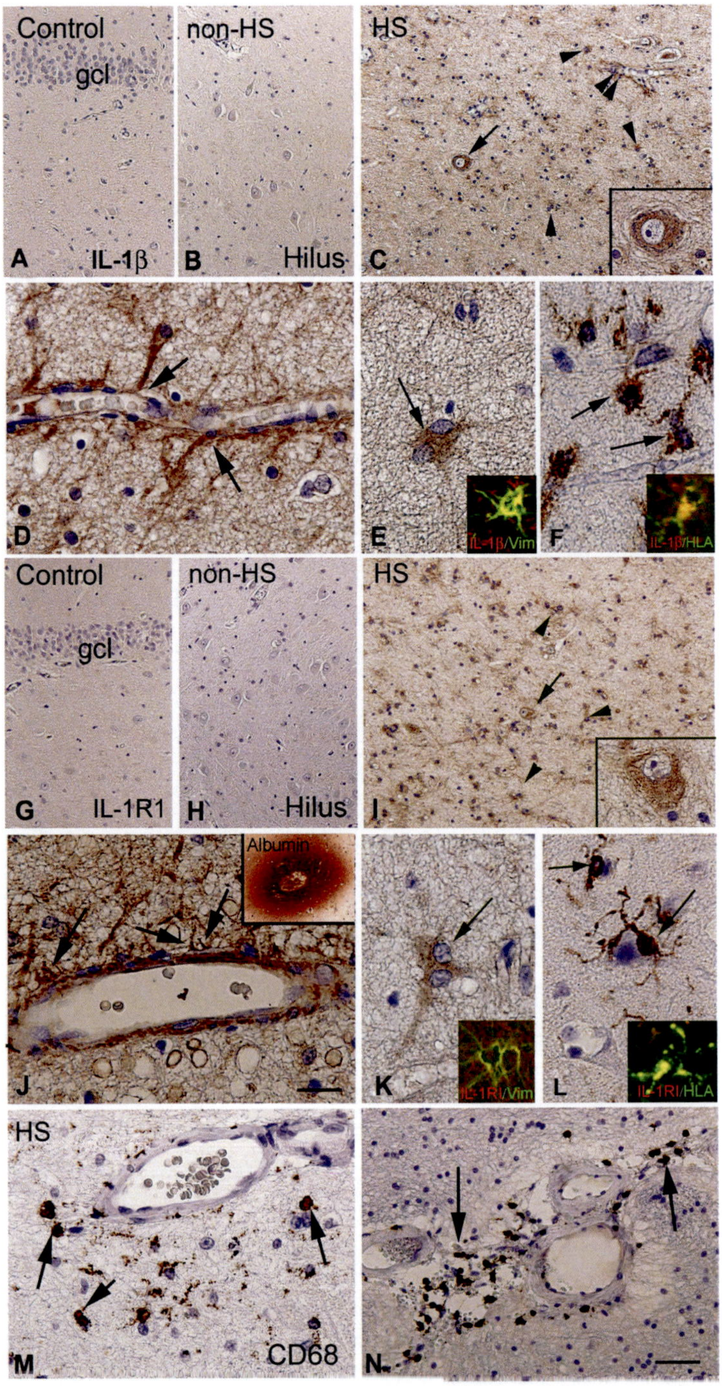

Fig. 10.1. Interleukin (IL)-1β system expression in the epileptogenic hippocampus of patients with temporal lobe epilepsy (TLE). Panels depict micrographs showing the cellular localization of IL-1β (**A–F**) and IL-1 receptor type 1 (IL-1R1) (**G–L**) in the sclerotic hippocampus (HS) of patients with TLE (**C–F; I–L**) and in control tissue obtained at autopsy from patients with no history of seizures or other neurological disease (**A,G**) or in nonsclerotic hippocampi from patients with extrahippocampal lesions (non-HS) (**B,H**). In epileptic specimens, note the strong activation of IL-1β (**C–F**) and IL-1R1 (**I–L**) in neurons (arrows in **C,I**) and in glia (arrowheads in **C,I**; high magnifications in **D–F** and **J–L**), whereas in control tissue no IL-1β (**A,B**) or IL-1R1 (**G,H**) staining was observed. Note the perivascular staining denoting IL-1β and IL-1R1 in astrocytic endfeet (**D,J**) in regions of albumin extravasation (**J**). Panels **M,N** depict monocytes/macrophages in brain parenchyma (arrows in **M**), whereas T cells are predominantly intravascular (arrows in **N**). (Adapted from Ravizza et al., 2008a.)

cytokine genes, suggesting that seizure activity *per se* could be a trigger of brain inflammation. Indeed, this evidence was confirmed by subsequent studies showing that pilocarpine-induced seizures in mice provoke a significant upregulation in brain parenchyma of a large variety of transcripts of inflammatory mediators including the transcriptional factor NFκB, proinflammatory cytokines, chemokines and cyclo-oxygenase (COX)-2 (Turrin and Rivest, 2004). A detailed time-course analysis of these changes, focusing on prototypical proinflammatory cytokines, showed that electrically provoked status epilepticus induces transcription of inflammatory genes very rapidly, within 30 minutes from its onset (De Simoni et al., 2000). This transcriptional upregulation was maximal between 6 and 12 hours, then declined to baseline expression, except for interleukin (IL)-1β. Thus, IL-1β mRNA remained increased for up to 60 days after acute status epilepticus, a time at which rats develop spontaneous recurrent seizures. These data indicate that inflammation in brain can be induced by various convulsant agents with different mechanisms of action, and can become chronic. Moreover, seizure-induced brain inflammation does not require cell death to occur because it is also provoked by nonlesional types of seizure, such as those induced by bicuculline in rats (Vezzani et al., 1999) or in mice (Vezzani et al., 2000). On the contrary, inflammation precedes seizure-induced cell loss (De Simoni et al., 2000; Ravizza and Vezzani, 2006), and in kainate-treated rats it develops following seizures in postnatal (PN) day 15 and older rats but not in PN9 rats, and thus is concomitant with the onset of seizure-induced cell loss (Rizzi et al., 2003). This evidence supports a role for inflammation as one causative factor in neurodegeneration (Viviani et al., 2003; Bernardino et al., 2005; for a review see Allan et al., 2005).

Immunohistochemical investigations were instrumental in showing the source of brain inflammation triggered by seizures (Vezzani et al., 1999; De Simoni et al., 2000; Ravizza and Vezzani, 2006; Ravizza et al., 2008a) (Fig. 10.2). Using IL-1β and its type 1 receptor (IL-1R type 1) which mediates the biological actions of this cytokine, it was possible to identify the cells expressing the cytokine and those targeted by the cytokine in a model of status epilepticus-induced epileptogenesis (Ravizza et al., 2008a). This study showed that both microglia and astrocytes were activated and showed raised levels of IL-1β during status epilepticus and in the chronic phase of spontaneous seizures; chronic inflammation in the epileptogenesis phase (before the onset of epileptiform activity leading to the occurrence of spontaneous seizures) was sustained mainly by astrocytes. We cannot exclude that other markers of inflammation may provide evidence for an additional contribution of activated microglia during the epileptogenesis phase.

Two further noteworthy observations emerged from this study: (1) the involvement of endothelial cells in the production of IL-1β in epileptogenic tissue; and (2) the occurrence of inflammation in brain regions with compromised blood–brain barrier (BBB) permeability. BBB leakage was assessed by serum albumin extravasation in brain parenchyma after status epilepticus and this feature was common to human epileptogenic tissue from patients with TLE (Rigau et al., 2007; van Vliet et al., 2007; Ravizza et al., 2008a). The finding of a strict regional association between inflammation in glia and in endothelial cells and BBB leakage suggests a reciprocal cause–effect relationship between these two events. Thus, IL-1β and other inflammatory mediators can alter the permeability properties of the BBB (Del Maschio et al., 1996; for a review see Allan et al., 2005); BBB leakage, by provoking the brain entry of albumin and IgG, can trigger immune and inflammatory processes in the surrounding tissue.

Microarray studies in rat models of TLE have highlighted the inflammatory response genes as those most significantly upregulated by status epilepticus, and during the epileptogenesis phase, suggesting that these inflammatory mediators may contribute to the progression of the disease and the occurrence of spontaneous seizures. Among these inflammatory mediators, complement factors and COX-2 have been studied in more detail.

In particular, the C1q factor of the complement cascade is upregulated by seizures in astrocytes, microglia, and neurons, and its expression is maintained in chronic epileptic tissue from animal models and human TLE (Rozovsky et al., 1994; Aronica et al., 2007). The membrane attack complex is also upregulated in microglia and surviving neurons in TLE (Aronica et al., 2007). Interestingly, when the membrane attack complex formation is induced by serial intrahippocampal injection of each component, seizures can be evoked and extensive neuronal cell loss is induced in the injected area (Xiong et al., 2003).

COX-2 has a biphasic pattern of expression following status epilepticus in mice (Lee et al., 2007), showing initial upregulation in neurons followed by increased expression in astrocytes during epileptogenesis, which persists in epileptic tissue. In tissue from patients with TLE with hippocampal sclerosis, a prominent astrocytic expression of COX-2 was also observed (Desjardins et al., 2003) (Fig. 10.3).

In summary, the expression studies of inflammatory markers in experimental models and human epileptic tissue have shown most pronounced upregulation in brain parenchymal cells, in the areas of seizure origin and their generalization; seizures induce inflammation involving glia and neurons, and astrocytes chiefly

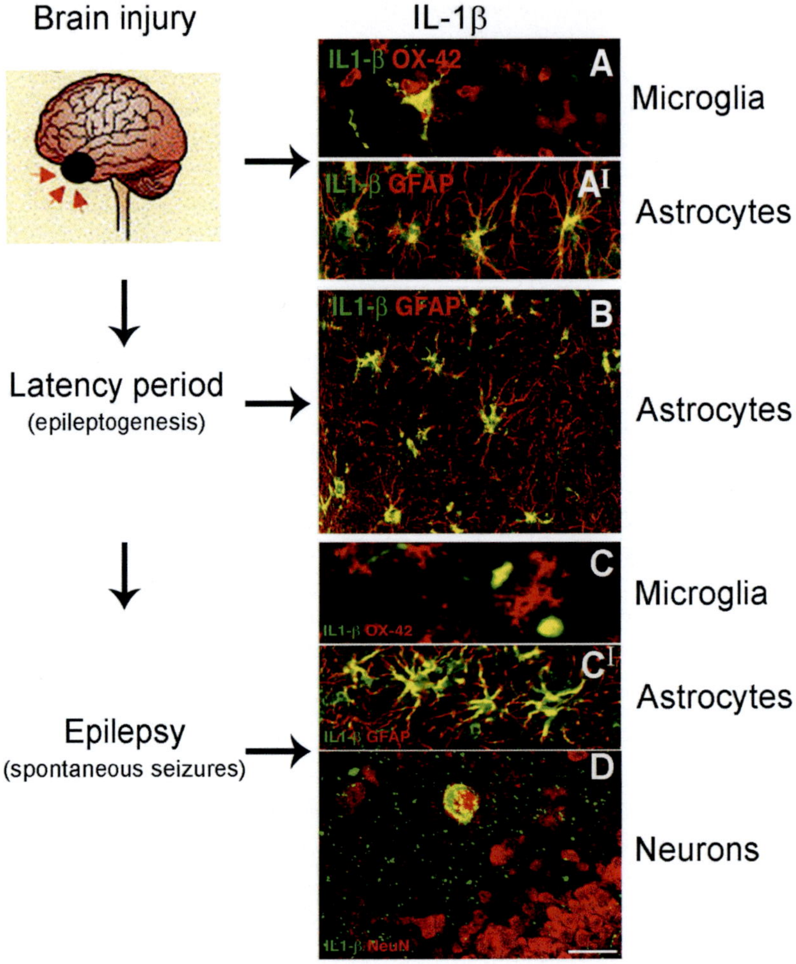

Fig. 10.2. Cellular expression of interleukin (IL)-1β in epileptogenic hippocampus from rats exposed to status epilepticus. Rats underwent electrically-induced or pilocarpine-induced status epilepticus (Ravizza et al., 2008a). Double-immunostaining with markers of glia and neurons (**A–D**) showed IL-1β production in microglia and astrocytes during status epilepticus and when rats develop spontaneous seizures, whereas astrocytes were involved predominantly in IL-1β production during epileptogenesis. Scattered neurons also showed IL-1β staining in chronic epileptic hippocampus (**D**). Thus, brain parenchymal cells sustain inflammation caused by seizures. GFAP, glial fibrillary acidic protein. (Adapted from Ravizza et al., 2008a.)

contribute to sustain chronic inflammation during epileptogenesis; inflammation is associated with areas of BBB damage and neuropathology. The evidence that inflammation precedes the development of epilepsy in experimental models of TLE suggests the possibility that it takes part in the mechanisms leading to the onset of spontaneous seizures.

Febrile seizures

Fever is a systemic response to infection, inflammation, or stress, and it can evoke febrile seizures in infants and children. Prolonged and repetitive febrile seizures are closely linked to the development of mesial TLE. However, the mechanisms by which fever induces seizures are still unknown. Several proinflammatory cytokines, including IL-1β, act as pyrogens after central or systemic administration. Recent evidence points to a prominent role for this cytokine in the onset of febrile seizures (Dubé et al., 2005). Thus, transgenic immature mice lacking IL-1R type 1 have an increased threshold of seizure induction when exposed to hyperthermia, whereas a reduction in seizure threshold is provoked by intracerebral administration of IL-1β. In another study, fever was induced by systemic lipopolysaccharide (LPS) administration in PN14 rats; at the peak of fever, the rats showed enhanced susceptibility to kainate seizures that was associated with increases in hippocampal levels of IL-1β. Intracerebral administration of IL-1 receptor antagonist (IL-1ra), the endogenous competitive antagonist of IL-1R type 1, rescued this phenotype by reversing the enhanced susceptibility to seizures at the

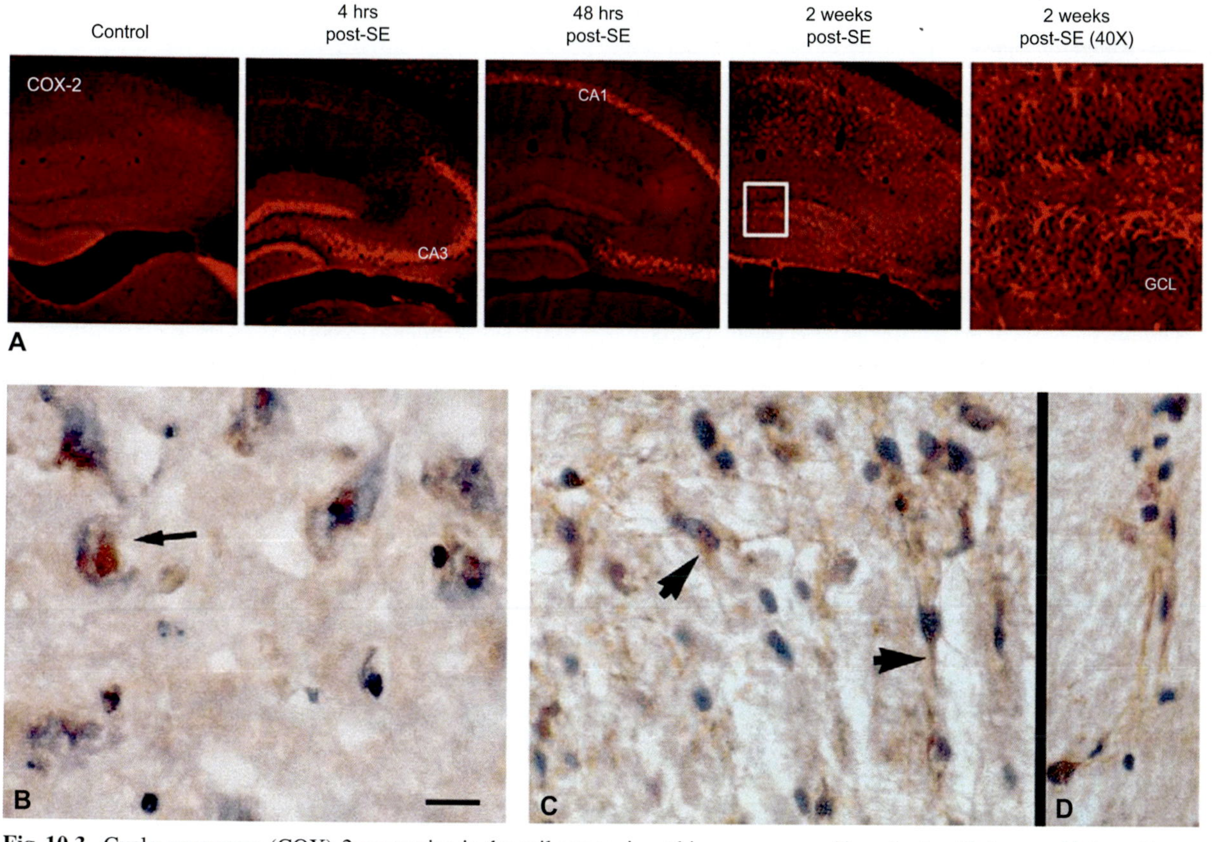

Fig. 10.3. Cyclo-oxygenase (COX)-2 expression in the epileptogenic rat hippocampus and in patients with temporal lobe epilepsy (TLE). (**A**) Immunofluorescence micrographs showing COX-2 immunoreactivity at various time points after status epilepticus (SE)-induced by pilocarpine (from 4 hours to 2 weeks). Rapid neuronal upregulation of COX-2 expression was observed from 4 to 48 hours post-SE (second and third panels in **A**). In contrast, from 2 to 14 days after SE, COX-2 was observed both in astrocytes and microglia (fourth and fifth panels in **A**). GCL, granule cell layer. (**B–D**) Photomicrographs of immunohistochemical staining for COX-2 in the hippocampus of patients with TLE. COX-2 immunostaining was found in neurons (arrow in **B**) and also in astrocytes in patients with TLE with hippocampal sclerosis (arrowheads in **C**); (**D**) depicts a COX-2-positive brain vessel. (Adapted from Desjardins et al., 2003; Lee et al., 2007.)

peak of fever (Heida and Pittman, 2005). Moreover, the induction of fever provokes a lasting upregulation of IL-1β in the brain (Dubé et al., 2010).

Pre-existing brain inflammation and epilepsy

One possible scenario is the establishment of an inflammatory substrate in the brain due to an initial precipitating event such as trauma, hypoxia/ischemia, or infection. If an injury, even when subtle, occurring at birth or during the lifetime initiates a cascade of inflammatory events, is it conceivable that this process predisposes the brain to the onset of seizures? Experimental evidence clearly shows that a large variety of insults that cause inflammation in the brain (Allan and Rothwell, 2001; Nguyen et al., 2002) also predispose to the occurrence of seizures (Pitkanen and Sutula, 2002).

In this regard, systemic administration of LPS, a component of Gram-negative bacteria that induces systemic and brain inflammation, reduces the threshold of seizure induction in mice and rats (Sayyah et al., 2003; Heida and Pittman, 2005; Galic et al., 2008), and this phenotype is rescued by the administration of anti-inflammatory drugs (Sayyah et al., 2003). LPS injection in PN7 and PN14 rats also increased neuronal cell loss after status epilepticus induced by pilocarpine (Auvin et al., 2007).

Recent evidence showed that a single peripheral administration of LPS in immature rats (at PN9 or 14) can trigger a transient brain inflammation, as assessed by measuring proinflammatory cytokines in the hippocampus, and microglia activation. Three weeks later, extracellular recordings from hippocampal slices of these rats revealed enhanced neuronal responses to afferent stimulation and to convulsant drug applications. 6–8 weeks after postnatal LPS injection, seizure susceptibility was assessed and the adult rats showed significantly greater seizure susceptibility to various convulsants, as well as increased cytokine levels and enhanced neuronal degeneration within the hippocampus after limbic seizures. These persistent increases in seizure susceptibility were dependent upon brain induction of tumor necrosis factor (TNF)-α (Galic et al., 2008). These novel results indicate that a single LPS injection during a critical postnatal period causes a long-lasting increase in seizure susceptibility. Similar findings were obtained using intracolonic administration of 2,4,6-trinitrobenzene sulfonic acid to induce intestinal inflammation (Riazi et al., 2008). These findings show that peripheral inflammation results in a number of centrally mediated physiological changes leading to a chronic increase in neuronal excitability. Moreover, a single bout of inflammation during development can program specific and persistent differences in *N*-methyl-D-aspartate (NMDA) mRNA subunit expression in the hippocampus, which are associated with behavioral and cognitive deficits in adulthood (Harré et al., 2008). These findings indicate that the immature brain can be permanently modified after a single inflammatory episode.

Clinically, central nervous system (CNS) infections occur with some frequency in young children and may be associated with an increased risk of developing seizures later in life (Herman, 2002). Therefore, these experimental findings give support to the proposed link between CNS infection and the risk of epilepsy (Annegers et al., 1988).

Pharmacological studies

Can one target inflammatory pathways to achieve anticonvulsant effects? To address this question, experimental studies have used pharmacological tools to interfere selectively with the production or biological actions of inflammatory mediators. The results obtained highlight that the outcome, either anticonvulsant or proconvulsant, depends upon the specific inflammatory pathway that is inhibited. This concept will be exemplified with a focus on IL-1β and COX-2. A more extensive review of the literature concerning other inflammatory mediators or anti-inflammatory treatments is given by Vezzani et al., (2011).

Interleukin-1β

This cytokine clearly mediates proconvulsant effects upon its release from glia during seizures, thereby representing an inflammatory molecule that contributes to ictal activity. This conclusion stems from the following evidence: (1) intracerebral application of IL-1β exerts proconvulsant actions in different seizure models (Vezzani et al., 1999, 2000) Fig. 10.4 inhibition of IL-1β synthesis using caspase-1 inhibitors (also called interleukin-1 converting enzyme) results in powerful anticonvulsant effects in kainate-treated rats (Ravizza et al., 2006b; Maroso et al., 2011) and prevents the occurrence of rapid kindling (Ravizza et al., 2008b); blockade of IL-1R type 1 using IL-1ra reduces seizures induced by kainate or bicuculline (De Simoni et al., 2000; Vezzani et al., 2000, 2002) (Fig. 10.4). The possibility of reducing seizures by the intracerebral application of these drugs supports the role of IL-1β produced by parenchymal cells in seizure activity. In accordance, transgenic mice overexpressing IL-1ra in astrocytes were less susceptible to seizures (Vezzani et al., 2000).

IL-1ra was also able to block seizures induced by pilocarpine following systemic administration (Marchi et al., 2009); this action is likely to be mediated by the ability of IL-1ra to inhibit pilocarpine-induced release of IL-1β by monocytes, an effect that appears to be instrumental for the convulsant activity of pilocarpine. Increased blood IL-1β would induce BBB damage by altering endothelial cell tight junctions (Del Maschio et al., 1996) or promoting the upregulation of adhesion molecules (Bernardes-Silva et al., 2001) and their consequent interaction with T cells (Fabene et al., 2008), thus permitting pilocarpine to enter the brain at sufficient concentrations to induce seizures. IL-1ra, by preventing these peripheral proinflammatory effects of pilocarpine, impairs the drug's ability to cause seizures.

Recent evidence also suggests the involvement of IL-1β brain overproduction in epileptogenesis, as caspase-1 inhibition was able to impair the development of fully kindled seizures in rats by a concomitant prevention of brain inflammation induced by the kindling stimulation (Ravizza et al., 2008b).

It appears, therefore, that the IL-1β-activated pathway plays an important role in contributing to seizures (Balosso et al., 2008), thus raising the possibility of using anti-IL-1β treatments, which are already in clinical use for inflammatory diseases (Randle et al., 2001; Waugh and Perry, 2005), for seizure inhibition.

Cyclo-oxygenase-2

Inhibition of this enzyme with nonsteroidal anti-inflammatory drugs provides an example of how inhibition of inflammation may result in detrimental rather than beneficial effects. Dichotomous effects of COX-2 blockade on seizures have been reported which appear to depend both on the type of seizure and on the time of pharmacological intervention. Thus, if COX-2 inhibition is achieved before the induction of status epilepticus with pilocarpine or kainate, proconvulsant effects are observed (Naffah-Mazzacoratti et al., 1995; Baik et al., 1999; Kim et al., 2008), whereas if COX-2 inhibition is achieved following status epilepticus, by injecting the selective antagonist during the epileptogenesis

Treatment		Time in seizures (min)
Vehicle+KA		26.3 ± 1.8
IL-1β+KA	1ng, i.h.	52.3 ± 4.9**
IL-1ra+KA	6μg, icv	13.4 ± 2.6**

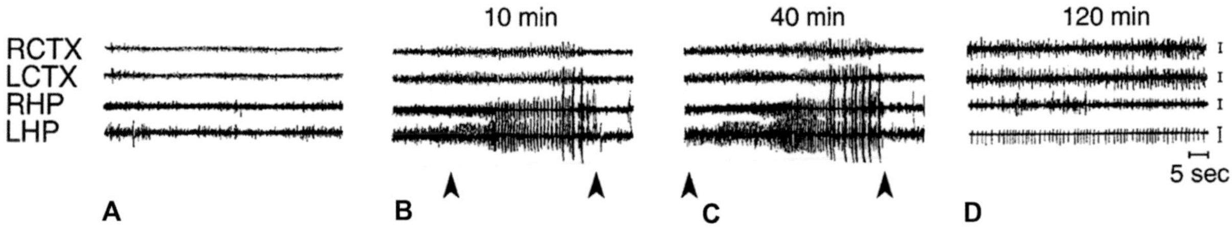

Fig. 10.4. Proconvulsant effect of interleukin (IL)-1β and anticonvulsant effect of IL-1 receptor antagonist (IL-1ra) on kainate seizures in rats. Seizures were induced by intrahippocampal application of kainic acid (KA) in rats (Vezzani et al., 1999, 2002). IL-1β or IL-1ra was applied intrahippocampally (i.h.) or intracerebroventricularly (icv), respectively, 10 minutes before injection of kainate. Seizures were monitored and quantified by electroencephalographic (EEG) analysis: panels **A–D** depict a typical EEG tracing showing preinjection baseline (**A**), ictal episodes (**B,C**), and spiking activity (**D**) after kainate injection. RCTX, LCTX, right and left cortex; RHP, LHP, right and left hippocampus. (Adapted from Vezzani et al., 1999, 2002.)

phase, then neuroprotection (Kunz and Oliw, 2001b) and reduced spontaneous seizure severity are observed (Polascheck et al., 2010; Jung et al., 2006). In contrast to status epilepticus, the anticonvulsant effects of COX-2 inhibition are observed on maximal electroshock (MES) and pentylenetetrazol seizures, when the drugs are given before the induction of seizures (Shafiq et al., 2003; Dhir and Kulkarni, 2006).

Mice overexpressing the human COX-2 in neurons show more intense seizures and increased mortality after kainate, and increased susceptibility to excitotoxic damage (Kelley et al., 1999). Moreover, COX-2-deficient mice, or mice treated with a COX-2 inhibitor, have a reduced susceptibility to kindling (Takemiya et al., 2003).

These dual effects of COX inhibitors likely depend on their specific actions on the basal production of the various prostaglandins (PGs) and on the different profiles of PG produced during seizures in the various experimental models and in the various phases of seizure (Naffah-Mazzacoratti et al., 1995). In this respect, PGE_2 has been shown to be proconvulsant and proneurotoxic (Kunz and Oliw, 2001a; Oliveira et al., 2008), whereas PGF_2 has inhibitory action on seizures (Kim et al., 2008).

Mechanistic insights into the action of inflammatory mediators

Recent investigations have addressed the mechanisms by which inflammatory molecules can alter neuronal excitability, uncovering novel pathways of communication between glia and neurons. Most of the available studies focused on TNF-α, IL-1β and PGs.

In particular, both IL-1β and TNF-α have been show to interact with the glutamatergic system by inhibiting glutamate reuptake by astrocytes (Ye and Sontheimer, 1996; Hu et al., 2000; Zou and Crews, 2005). Moreover, TNF-α induces glutamate release from astrocytes via a mechanism involving PG production (Bezzi et al., 2001), and triggers the rapid insertion of Ca^{2+}-permeable AMPA (α-amino-3-hydroxy-5-methyl-4-isoxazolepropionic acid) receptors at neuronal membranes (Ogoshi et al., 2005; Stellwagen et al., 2005); these changes are associated with enhanced excitability and excitotoxicity (Beattie et al., 2002; Leonoudakis et al., 2004; Stellwagen et al., 2005; Stellwagen and Malenka, 2006). Profound modifications in NMDA, AMPA, and kainate receptor subunits were observed in TNF-α receptor type 1 or type 2 knockout mice (Balosso et al., 2009), and these changes were associated with changes in seizure susceptibility (Balosso et al., 2005)

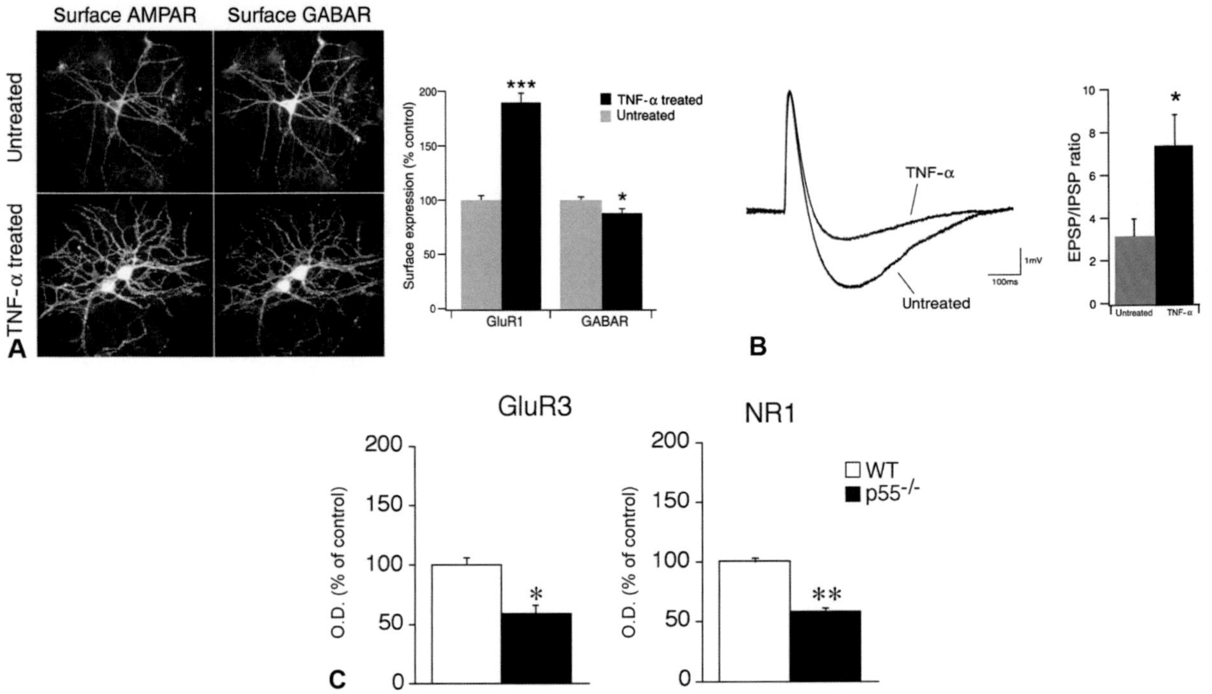

Fig. 10.5. Molecular and functional interactions between tumor necrosis factor (TNF)-α signaling and glutamate (GluR) and γ-aminobutyric acid (GABAR) receptors. (**A**) and (**B**) depict the increase induced by TNF-α in the membrane expression of AMPA receptors (AMPAR) and the reduction in $GABA_A$ receptors (**A**) and the consequent increased excitability of hippocampal CA1 pyramidal neurons to stimulation of Schaffer collaterals in slices exposed to TNF-α (**B**) (Stellwagen et al., 2005). EPSP, excitatory postsynaptic potentials; IPSP, inhibitory postsynaptic potentials. (**C**) depicts the changes in AMPA-GluR3 and NMDA-NR1 receptor subunits measured in mice lacking TNF-α type 1 (p55) receptors. These mice are less susceptible to seizures (Balosso et al., 2005). OD, optical density; WT, wild-type. (Adapted from Stellwagen et al., 2005; Balosso et al., 2009)

suggesting that TNF-α receptor signaling is involved in determining glutamate receptor subunit compositions at the membrane and the level of hippocampal excitability (Fig. 10.5).

IL-1β has been shown to increase the phosphorylation of the NR2B subunit of the NMDA receptor, thus promoting Ca^{2+} influx into neurons (Viviani et al., 2003). In particular, IL-1β induces the production of ceramide via activation of sphingomyelinase, which in turn activates the Src family of tyrosine kinases leading the NR2B phosphorylation (Balosso et al., 2008). The activation of this pathway underlies the proconvulsant effect of IL-1β (Balosso et al., 2008) (Fig. 10.6).

Interactions of these cytokines with inhibitory neurotransmission have also been reported, as TNF-α has been shown to reduce the membrane expression of γ-aminobutyric acid (GABA) type A receptors (Stellwagen et al., 2005) (see Fig. 10.5), and IL-1β has been reported to inhibit GABA-mediated Cl^- influx into neurons (Wang et al., 2000).

PGs also appear to have significant effects of neuronal excitability (Cole-Edwards and Bazan, 2005). Somatic and dendritic membrane excitability was reduced in CA1 pyramidal neurons when endogenous PGE_2 was eliminated with a selective COX-2 inhibitor. Accordingly, the exogenous application of PGE_2 produced significant increases in frequency of firing and the amplitude of excitatory postsynaptic potentials, most likely by reducing potassium currents in CA1 neurons (Chen and Bazan, 2005). In addition, COX-2 inhibition decreases basal excitatory transmission in CA1 hippocampal slices, an effect prevented by CB1 blockade and independent of inhibitory transmission (Slanina and Schweitzer, 2005). COX-2-mediated PGs synthesis also leads to the production of free radicals as intermediate products, that in turn can potentiate glutamate-mediated effects (Dawson et al., 1991). The production of PGE_2 from TNF-α-activated astrocytes can mediate astrocytic Ca^{2+}-dependent glutamate release (Bezzi et al., 2001), thus possibly contributing to ictal activity and excitotoxicity (Fellin et al., 2006; Ding et al., 2007).

Another mechanism by which inflammation can increase neuronal excitability is the breakdown of the BBB, as cytokines have been shown to increase BBB permeability by disrupting tight junctions, activating endothelial inducible nitric oxide synthase (iNOS) and matrix metaloproteinases (for a review see Allan et al., 2005).

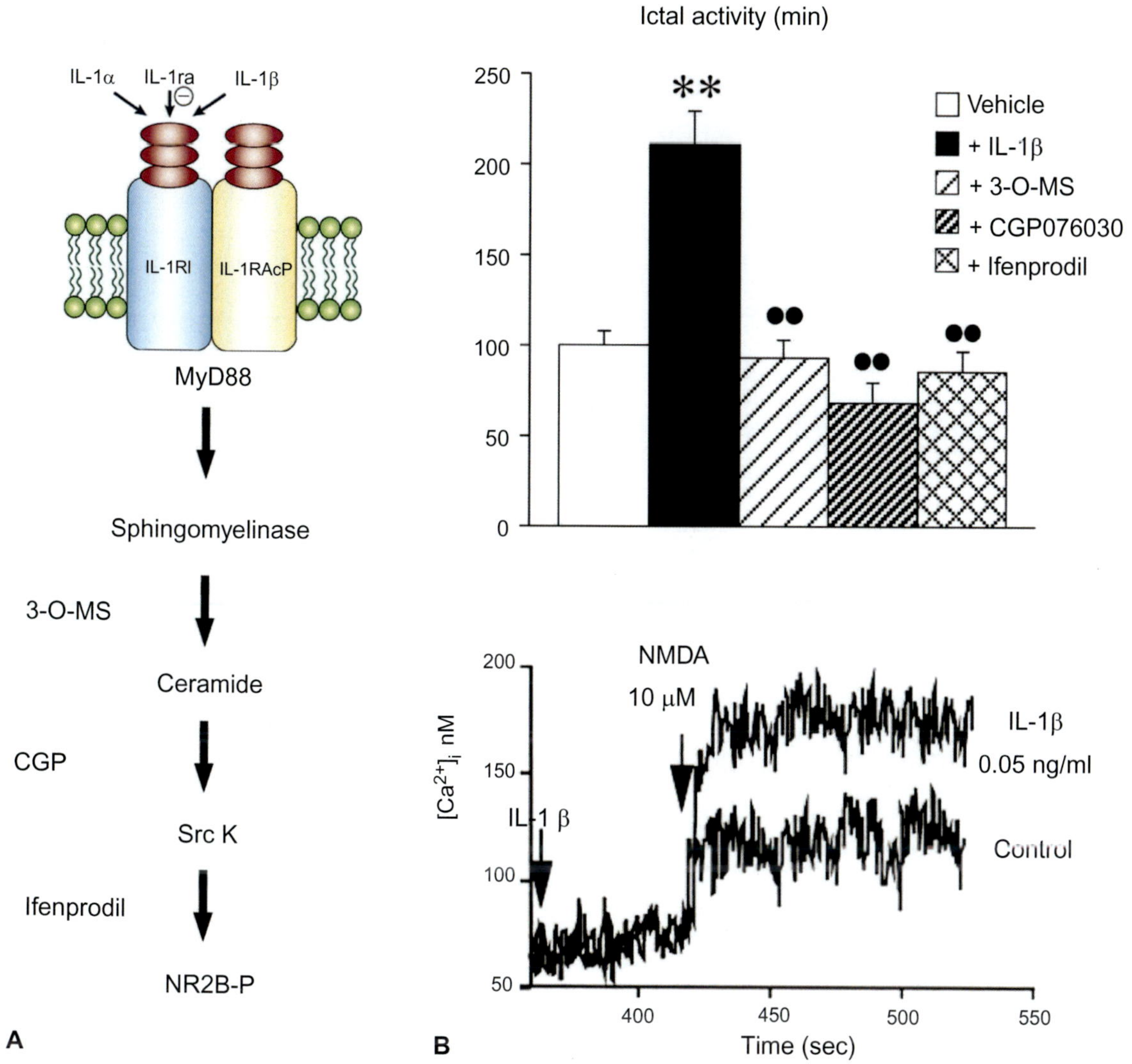

Fig. 10.6. Intracellular pathway mediating the proconvulsant effects of interleukin (IL) 1β. (**A**) depicts the sequelae of events triggered in the mouse hippocampus by the injection of IL-1β and its interaction with IL-1 receptor type 1. This pathway consists of the activation of sphingomyelinase and the production of the soluble mediator ceramide, which subsequently activates Src kinases leading to phosphorylation (P) of the NR2B subunit of the NMDA receptor (Viviani et al., 2003; Balosso et al., 2008). Pharmacological blockade of sphingomyelinase (3-*O*-methylsphingomyelin, 3-O-MS) and Src kinase (CGP76030, CGP) with selective blockers or using a specific blocker of the NR2 subunit (ifenprodil) prevents the proconvulsant activity of IL-1β. (**B**) The ultimate molecular event underlying IL-1β-induced hyperexcitability is the enhanced neuronal Ca^{2+} influx associated with NR2 subunit phosphorylation (NR2B-P) (**B**, bottom) (Viviani et al., 2003). (Adapted from Viviani et al., 2003; Balosso et al., 2008.)

It is known that BBB damage can promote epileptiform activity (Oby and Janigro, 2006; Seifert et al., 2006; Ivens et al., 2007; Marchi et al., 2007; van Vliet et al., 2007) mediated by astrocytic uptake of serum albumin, which extravasates into the brain parenchyma. The uptake of albumin impairs astrocytic function leading to altered ionic homeostasis in the extracellular space (Ivens et al., 2007); moreover, the neuronal uptake of IgG appears to contribute to cell damage (Rigau et al., 2007; Marcon et al., 2009).

CONCLUDING REMARKS

The hypothesis that brain inflammation is a significant contributor to seizures and their detrimental consequences, such as neuronal cell loss and BBB damage, is strongly supported by experimental findings and corroborated by clinical observations. Recent findings suggest that chronic inflammation may also contribute to epileptogenesis, thus predisposing the brain to the development of recurrent seizures. Ravizza et al., 2011 Importantly, several

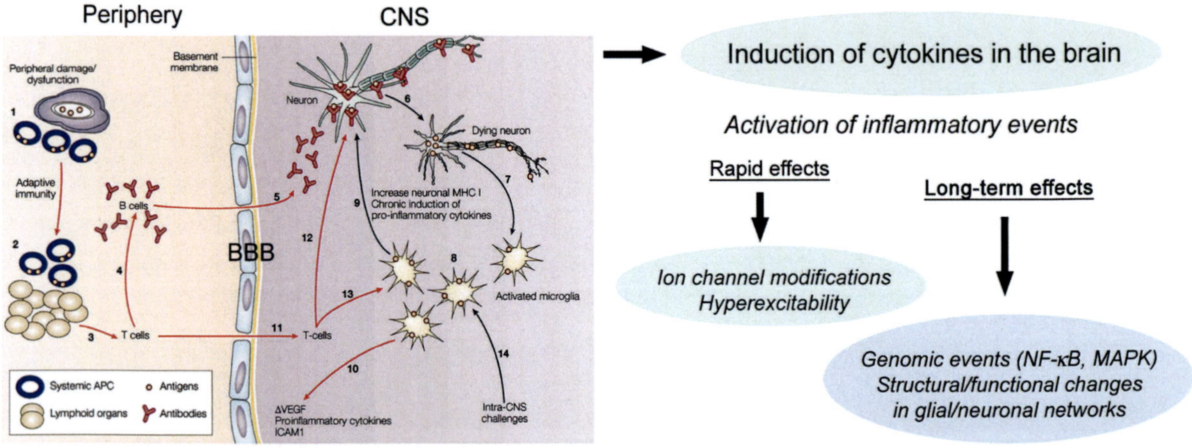

Fig. 10.7. Schematic representation of the putative triggers of brain inflammation. The initial stimulus may originate from the periphery, such as during systemic infection or in autoimmune channelopathies (Vincent et al., 2006), or in the brain such as during brain injury (Vezzani and Granata, 2005). If the initial trigger comes from the periphery then adaptive immunity mechanisms may play a major role in initiating brain inflammation. Activated T or B cells may enter the brain parenchyma and provoke microglia activation and neuronal damage, or adhesion of T lymphocytes to endothelial cells of the blood–brain barrier (BBB) activated by increased blood cytokines may contribute to BBB damage (Fabene et al., 2008). These peripheral events may subsequently lead to glial cell activation and perpetuation of brain inflammation by massive recruitment of parenchymal cells. If the first trigger originates in the brain, such as following a large variety of brain injuries (Vezzani and Granata, 2005), glial cells are first activated to produce inflammatory mediators which can lead to BBB leakage and neuronal loss, with adaptive immunity recruited as a second step. The induction of cytokines in the brain and the activation of downstream inflammatory events may result in rapid effects on neuronal excitability determined by ion channel modifications (acquired channelopathies) and in long-term effects consisting of genomic events that contribute to epileptogenesis (Vezzani and Baram, 2007). APC, antigen-presenting cells; CNS, central nervous system; ICAM, intercellular adhesion molecule; MAPK, mitogen-activated protein kinase; MHC, major histocompatibility complex; NF, nuclear factor; VEGF, vascular endothelial growth factor.

inflammatory mediators act as transcriptional activators of genes that are under NFκB and activator protein-1 (AP-1) control; thus, these genomic effects may contribute to enduring alterations in gene expression programs that underlie the epileptogenic process (Fig. 10.7). Triggers of brain inflammation include a large variety of brain injuries that have been reported to increase the risk of developing seizures and epilepsy in humans (Giroud et al., 1997; Herman, 2002; Garzon et al., 2003). In this regard, a genetic predisposition to develop sustained inflammatory reactions in response to otherwise ineffective stimuli should be taken into consideration (i.e., gene polymorphisms), as existing studies suggest this is a likely possibility (Kanemoto et al., 2000; Virta et al., 2002).

Animal studies have shown that pharmacological interference with specific inflammatory pathways can significantly reduce seizures. It is noteworthy that some of these drugs, such as caspase-1 inhibitors or IL-1ra (Anakinra), are already in clinical use for chronic inflammatory diseases. The relationship between inflammation and epilepsy highlights the possibility of using specific anti-inflammatory treatments as novel therapeutic approaches to control seizures and possibly to arrest, in individuals at risk, the cascade of pathological events induced by a brain injury and leading to epilepsy.

ACKNOWLEDGMENTS

The authors thank all colleagues who collaborated with them to originate some of the data described in this chapter, in particular Dr. T.Z. Baram, Dr. E. Aronica, Dr. T. Bartfai, Dr. S.L. Moshé, Dr. B. Viviani, and Dr. M.G. De Simoni. They also thank their sources of support: Dana Foundation, Negri-Weizmann Foundation, Epicure (LSH-CT-2006-037315).

References

Allan SM, Rothwell NJ (2001). Cytokines and acute neurodegeneration. Nat Rev Neurosci 2: 734–744.

Allan SM, Tyrrell PJ, Rothwell NJ (2005). Interleukin-1 and neuronal injury. Nat Rev Immunol 5: 629–640.

Annegers JF, Hauser WA, Beghi E et al. (1988). The risk of unprovoked seizures after encephalitis and meningitis. Neurology 38: 1407–1410.

Aronica E, Boer K, Baybis M et al. (2007). Complement activation in experimental and human temporal lobe epilepsy. Neurobiol Dis 26: 497–511.

Auvin S, Shin D, Mazarati A et al. (2007). Inflammation exacerbates seizure-induced injury in the immature brain. Epilepsia 48: 27–34.

Baik EJ, Kim EJ, Lee SH et al. (1999). Cyclooxygenase-2 selective inhibitors aggravate kainic acid induced seizure and neuronal cell death in the hippocampus. Brain Res 843: 118–129.

Balosso S, Ravizza T, Perego C et al. (2005). Tumor necrosis factor-alpha inhibits seizures in mice via p75 receptors. Ann Neurol 57: 804–812.

Balosso S, Maroso M, Sanchez-Alavez M et al. (2008). A novel non-transcriptional pathway mediates the proconvulsive effects of interleukin-1beta. Brain 131: 3256–3265.

Balosso S, Ravizza T, Pierucci M et al. (2009). Molecular and functional interactions between TNF-alpha receptors and the glutamatergic system in the mouse hippocampus: implications for seizure susceptibility. Neuroscience 161: 293–300.

Beattie EC, Stellwagen D, Morishita W et al. (2002). Control of synaptic strength by glial TNFalpha. Science 295: 2282–2285.

Bernardes-Silva M, Anthony DC, Issekutz AC et al. (2001). Recruitment of neutrophils across the blood–brain barrier: the role of E- and P-selectins. J Cereb Blood Flow Metab 21: 1115–1124.

Bernardino L, Xapelli S, Silva AP et al. (2005). Modulator effects of interleukin 1beta and tumor necrosis factor-alpha on AMPA-induced excitotoxicity in mouse organotypic hippocampal slice cultures. J Neurosci 25: 6734–6744.

Bezzi P, Domercq M, Brambilla L et al. (2001). CXCR4 activated astrocyte glutamate release via TNFalpha: amplification by microglia triggers neurotoxicity. Nat Neurosci 4: 702–710.

Bien CG, Bauer J, Deckwerth TL et al. (2002). Destruction of neurons by cytotoxic T cells: a new pathogenic mechanism in Rasmussen's encephalitis. Ann Neurol 51: 311–318.

Boer K, Jansen F, Nellist M et al. (2008). Inflammatory processes in cortical tubers and subependymal giant cell tumors of tuberous sclerosis complex. Epilepsy Res 78: 7–21.

Chen C, Bazan NG (2005). Lipid signaling: sleep, synaptic plasticity, and neuroprotection. Prostaglandins Other Lipid Mediat 77: 65–76.

Cole-Edwards KK, Bazan NG (2005). Lipid signaling in experimental epilepsy. Neurochem Res 30: 847–853.

Crespel A, Coubes P, Rousset MC et al. (2002). Inflammatory reactions in human medial temporal lobe epilepsy with hippocampal sclerosis. Brain Res 952: 159–169.

Dawson VL, Dawson TM, London ED et al. (1991). Nitric oxide mediates glutamate neurotoxicity in primary cortical cultures. Proc Natl Acad Sci U S A 88: 6368–6371.

De Simoni MG, Perego C, Ravizza T et al. (2000). Inflammatory cytokines and related genes are induced in the rat hippocampus by limbic status epilepticus. Eur J Neurosci 12: 2623–2633.

Del Maschio A, Zanetti A, Corada M et al. (1996). Polymorphonuclear leukocyte adhesion triggers the disorganization of endothelial cell-to-cell adherens junctions. J Cell Biol 135: 497–510.

Desjardins P, Sauvageau A, Bouthillier A et al. (2003). Induction of astrocytic cyclooxygenase-2 in epileptic patients with hippocampal sclerosis. Neurochem Int 42: 299–303.

Dhir A, Kulkarni SK (2006). Rofecoxib, a selective cyclooxygenase-2 (COX-2) inhibitor potentiates the anticonvulsant activity of tiagabine against pentylenetetrazol-induced convulsions in mice. Inflammopharmacology 14: 222–225.

Ding S, Fellin T, Zhu Y et al. (2007). Enhanced astrocytic Ca^{2+} signals contribute to neuronal excitotoxicity after status epilepticus. J Neurosci 27: 10674–10684.

Dubé C, Vezzani A, Behrens M et al. (2005). Interleukin-1beta contributes to the generation of experimental febrile seizures. Ann Neurol 57: 152–155.

Dubé CM, Ravizza T, Hamamura M et al. (2010). Epileptogenesis provoked by prolonged experimental febrile seizures: mechanisms and biomarkers. J Neurosci. 30: 7484–7494.

Fabene PF, Navarro Mora G, Martinello M et al. (2008). A role for leukocyte–endothelial adhesion mechanisms in epilepsy. Nat Med 14: 1377–1383.

Fellin T, Gomez-Gonzalo M, Gobbo S et al. (2006). Astrocytic glutamate is not necessary for the generation of epileptiform neuronal activity in hippocampal slices. J Neurosci 26: 9312–9322.

Galic MA, Riazi K, Heida JG et al. (2008). Postnatal inflammation increases seizure susceptibility in adult rats. J Neurosci 28: 6904–6913.

Garzon E, Fernandes RM, Sakamoto AC (2003). Analysis of clinical characteristics and risk factors for mortality in human status epilepticus. Seizure 12: 337–345.

Giroud M, Lemesle M, Madinier G et al. (1997). Stroke in children under 16 years of age. Clinical and etiological difference with adults. Acta Neurol Scand 96: 401–406.

Harré EM, Galic MA, Mouihate A et al. (2008). Neonatal inflammation produces selective behavioural deficits and alters N-methyl-D-aspartate receptor subunit mRNA in the adult rat brain. Eur J Neurosci 27: 644–653.

Heida JG, Pittman QJ (2005). Causal links between brain cytokines and experimental febrile convulsions in the rat. Epilepsia 46: 1906–1913.

Herman ST (2002). Epilepsy after brain insult: targeting epileptogenesis. Neurology 59: S21–S26.

Hu S, Sheng WS, Ehrlich LC et al. (2000). Cytokine effects on glutamate uptake by human astrocytes. Neuroimmunomodulation 7: 153–159.

Ivens S, Kaufer D, Flores LP et al. (2007). TGF-beta receptor-mediated albumin uptake into astrocytes is involved in neocortical epileptogenesis. Brain 130: 535–547.

Jung KH, Chu K, Lee ST et al. (2006). Cyclooxygenase-2 inhibitor, celecoxib, inhibits the altered hippocampal neurogenesis with attenuation of spontaneous recurrent seizures following pilocarpine-induced status epilepticus. Neurobiol Dis 23: 237–246.

Kanemoto K, Kawasaki J, Miyamoto T et al. (2000). Interleukin (IL)1beta, IL-1alpha, and IL-1 receptor antagonist gene polymorphisms in patients with temporal lobe epilepsy. Ann Neurol 47: 571–574.

Kelley KA, Winger D, Freire-Moar J et al. (1999). Potentiation of excitotoxicity in transgenic mice overexpressing neuronal cyclooxygenase-2. Am J Pathol 155: 995–1004.

Kim HJ, Chung JI, Lee SH et al. (2008). Involvement of endogenous prostaglandin F2alpha on kainic acid-induced seizure activity through FP receptor: the mechanism of proconvulsant effects of COX-2 inhibitors. Brain Res 1193: 153–161.

Kunz T, Oliw EH (2001a). Nimesulide aggravates kainic acid-induced seizures in the rat. Pharmacol Toxicol 88: 271–276.

Kunz T, Oliw EH (2001b). The selective cyclooxygenase-2 inhibitor rofecoxib reduces kainate-induced cell death in the rat hippocampus. Eur J Neurosci 13: 569–575.

Lee B, Dziema H, Lee KH et al. (2007). CRE-mediated transcription and COX-2 expression in the pilocarpine model of status epilepticus. Neurobiol Dis 25: 80–91.

Lehtimaki KA, Keränen T, Huhtala H et al. (2004). Regulation of IL-6 system in cerebrospinal fluid and serum compartments by seizures: the effect of seizure type and duration. J Neuroimmunol 152: 121–125.

Leonoudakis D, Braithwaite SP, Beattie MS et al. (2004). TNFalpha-induced AMPA-receptor trafficking in CNS neurons; relevance to excitotoxicity? Neuron Glia Biol 1: 263–273.

Maldonado M, Baybis M, Newman D et al. (2003). Expression of ICAM-1, TNF-alpha, NF kappa B, and MAP kinase in tubers of the tuberous sclerosis complex. Neurobiol Dis 14: 279–290.

Marchi N, Angelov L, Masaryk T et al. (2007). Seizure-promoting effect of blood-brain barrier disruption. Epilepsia 48: 732–742.

Marchi N, Fan Q, Ghosh C et al. (2009). Antagonism of peripheral inflammation reduces the severity of status epilepticus. Neurobiol Dis 33: 171–181.

Marcon J, Gagliardi B, Balosso S et al. (2009). Age-dependent vascular changes induced by status epilepticus in rat forebrain: implications for epileptogenesis. Neurobiol Dis 34: 121–132.

Maroso M, Balosso S, Ravizza T et al. (2011). Interleukin-1 type 1 receptor/toll-like receptor signalling in epilepsy: The importance of il-1beta and high-mobility group box 1. J Intern Med 270: 319–326.

Minami M, Kuraishi Y, Satoh M (1991). Effects of kainic acid on messenger RNA levels of IL-1 beta, IL-6, TNF alpha and LIF in the rat brain. Biochem Biophys Res Commun 176: 593–598.

Naffah-Mazzacoratti MG, Bellíssimo MI, Cavalheiro EA (1995). Profile of prostaglandin levels in the rat hippocampus in pilocarpine model of epilepsy. Neurochem Int 27: 461–466.

Nguyen MD, Julien JP, Rivest S (2002). Innate immunity: the missing link in neuroprotection and neurodegeneration? Nat Rev Neurosci 3: 216–227.

Oby E, Janigro D (2006). The blood–brain barrier and epilepsy. Epilepsia 47: 1761–1774.

Ogoshi F, Yin HZ, Kuppumbatti Y et al. (2005). Tumor necrosis-factor-alpha (TNF-alpha) induces rapid insertion of Ca^{2+}-permeable alpha-amino-3-hydroxyl-5-methyl-4-isoxazole-propionate (AMPA)/kainate (Ca-A/K) channels in a subset of hippocampal pyramidal neurons. Exp Neurol 193: 384–393.

Oliveira MS, Furian AF, Royes LF et al. (2008). Cyclooxygenase-2/PGE2 pathway facilitates pentylenetetrazol-induced seizures. Epilepsy Res 79: 14–21.

Peltola J, Laaksonen J, Haapala AM et al. (2002). Indicators of inflammation after recent tonic–clonic epileptic seizures correlate with plasma interleukin-6 levels. Seizure 11: 44–46.

Pitkanen A, Sutula TP (2002). Is epilepsy a progressive disorder? Prospects for new therapeutic approaches in temporal-lobe epilepsy. Lancet Neurol 1: 173–181.

Polascheck N, Bankstahl M, Löscher W (2010). The COX-2 inhibitor parecoxib is neuroprotective but not antiepileptogenic in the pilocarpine model of temporal lobe epilepsy. Exp Neurol 224: 219–233. Epub 2010 Mar 29.

Randle JC, Harding MW, Ku G et al. (2001). ICE/Caspase-1 inhibitors as novel anti inflammatory drugs. Expert Opin Investig Drugs 10: 1207–1209.

Ravizza T, Vezzani A (2006). Status epilepticus induces time-dependent neuronal and astrocytic expression of interleukin-1 receptor type I in the rat limbic system. Neuroscience 137: 301–308.

Ravizza T, Boer K, Redeker S et al. (2006a). The IL-1beta system in epilepsy-associated malformations of cortical development. Neurobiol Dis 24: 128–143.

Ravizza T, Lucas SM, Balosso S et al. (2006b). Inactivation of caspase-1 in rodent brain: a novel anticonvulsive strategy. Epilepsia 47: 1160–1168.

Ravizza T, Gagliardi B, Noé F et al. (2008a). Innate and adaptive immunity during epileptogenesis and spontaneous seizures: evidence from experimental models and human temporal lobe epilepsy. Neurobiol Dis 29: 142–160.

Ravizza T, Noé F, Zardoni D et al. (2008b). Interleukin converting enzyme inhibition impairs kindling epileptogenesis in rats by blocking astrocytic IL-1beta production. Neurobiol Dis 31: 327–333.

Ravizza T, Balosso S, Vezzani A (2011). Inflammation and prevention of epileptogenosis. Neurosci Lett 497: 223–230. Epub 2011 Feb 26. Review. PMID: 21362451 [PubMed - indexed for MEDLINE]

Riazi K, Galic MA, Kuzmiski JB et al. (2008). Microglial activation and TNFalpha production mediate altered CNS excitability following peripheral inflammation. Proc Natl Acad Sci U S A 105: 17151–17156.

Rigau V, Morin M, Rousset MC et al. (2007). Angiogenesis is associated with blood–brain barrier permeability in temporal lobe epilepsy. Brain 130: 1942–1956.

Rizzi M, Perego C, Aliprandi M et al. (2003). Glia activation and cytokine increase in rat hippocampus by kainic acid-induced status epilepticus during postnatal development. Neurobiol Dis 14: 494–503.

Rozovsky I, Morgan TE, Willoughby DA et al. (1994). Selective expression of clusterin (SGP-2) and complement C1qB and C4 during responses to neurotoxins in vivo and in vitro. Neuroscience 62: 741–758.

Sayyah M, Javad-Pour M, Ghazi-Khansari M (2003). The bacterial endotoxin lipopolysaccharide enhances seizure susceptibility in mice: involvement of proinflammatory factors: nitric oxide and prostaglandins. Neuroscience 122: 1073–1080.

Seifert G, Schilling K, Steinhäuser C (2006). Astrocyte dysfunction in neurological disorders: a molecular perspective. Nat Rev Neurosci 7: 194–206.

Shafiq N, Malhotra S, Pandhi P (2003). Anticonvulsant action of celecoxib (alone and in combination with sub-threshold dose of phenytoin) in electroshock induced convulsion. Methods Find Exp Clin Pharmacol 25: 87–90.

Sheng JG, Boop FA, Mrak RE et al. (1994). Increased neuronal beta-amyloid precursor protein expression in human temporal lobe epilepsy: association with interleukin-1 alpha immunoreactivity. J Neurochem 63: 1872–1879.

Slanina KA, Schweitzer P (2005). Inhibition of cyclooxygenase-2 elicits a CB1-mediated decrease of excitatory transmission in rat CA1 hippocampus. Neuropharmacology 49: 653–659.

Stellwagen D, Malenka RC (2006). Synaptic scaling mediated by glial TNF-alpha. Nature 440: 1054–1059.

Stellwagen D, Beattie EC, Seo JY et al. (2005). Differential regulation of AMPA receptor and GABA receptor trafficking by tumor necrosis factor-alpha. J Neurosci 25: 3219–3228.

Takemiya T, Suzuki K, Sugiura H et al. (2003). Inducible brain COX-2 facilitates the recurrence of hippocampal seizures in mouse rapid kindling. Prostaglandins Other Lipid Mediat 71: 205–216.

Turrin NP, Rivest S (2004). Innate immune reaction in response to seizures: implications for the neuropathology associated with epilepsy. Neurobiol Dis 16: 321–334.

van Vliet EA, da Costa Araújo S, Redeker S et al. (2007). Blood–brain barrier leakage may lead to progression of temporal lobe epilepsy. Brain 130: 521–534.

Vezzani A, Baram TZ (2007). New roles for interleukin-1 beta in the mechanisms of epilepsy. Epilepsy Curr 7: 45–50.

Vezzani A, French J, Bartfai T et al. (2011). The role of inflammation in epilepsy. Nat Rev Neurol 7: 31–40. Epub 2010 Dec 7.

Vezzani A, Granata T (2005). Brain inflammation in epilepsy: experimental and clinical evidence. Epilepsia 46: 1724–1743.

Vezzani A, Conti M, De Luigi A et al. (1999). Interleukin-1beta immunoreactivity and microglia are enhanced in the rat hippocampus by focal kainate application: functional evidence for enhancement of electrographic seizures. J Neurosci 19: 5054–5065.

Vezzani A, Moneta D, Conti M et al. (2000). Powerful anticonvulsant action of IL-1 receptor antagonist on intracerebral injection and astrocytic overexpression in mice. Proc Natl Acad Sci U S A 97: 11534–11539.

Vezzani A, Moneta D, Richichi C et al. (2002). Functional role of inflammatory cytokines and antiinflammatory molecules in seizures and epileptogenesis. Epilepsia 43: 30–35.

Vincent A, Lang B, Kleopa KA (2006). Autoimmune channelopathies and related neurological disorders. Neuron 52: 123–138.

Virta M, Hurme M, Helminen M (2002). Increased frequency of interleukin-1beta (-511) allele 2 in febrile seizures. Pediatr Neurol 26: 192–195.

Viviani B, Bartesaghi S, Gardoni F et al. (2003). Interleukin-1beta enhances NMDA receptor-mediated intracellular calcium increase through activation of the Src family of kinases. J Neurosci 23: 8692–8700.

Wang S, Cheng Q, Malik S et al. (2000). Interleukin-1beta inhibits gamma-aminobutyric acid type A (GABA(A)) receptor current in cultured hippocampal neurons. J Pharmacol Exp Ther 292: 497–504.

Waugh J, Perry CM (2005). Anakinra: a review of its use in the management of rheumatoid arthritis. BioDrugs 19: 189–202.

Xiong ZQ, Qian W, Suzuki K et al. (2003). Formation of complement membrane attack complex in mammalian cerebral cortex evokes seizures and neurodegeneration. J Neurosci 23: 955–960.

Ye ZC, Sontheimer H (1996). Cytokine modulation of glial glutamate uptake: a possible involvement of nitric oxide. Neuroreport 7: 2181–2185.

Zou JY, Crews FT (2005). TNF alpha potentiates glutamate neurotoxicity by inhibiting glutamate uptake in organotypic brain slice cultures: neuroprotection by NF kappa B inhibition. Brain Res 1034: 11–24.

Section 2

Diagnosis

Handbook of Clinical Neurology, Vol. 107 (3rd series)
Epilepsy, Part I
H. Stefan and W.H. Theodore, Editors

Chapter 11

Age-related epileptic encephalopathies

RENZO GUERRINI [1]* AND JOHN M. PELLOCK [2]

[1] *Department of Neuroscience, Pediatric Neurology Unit and Laboratories, Children's Hospital A. Meyer, University of Florence, Florence, Italy*

[2] *Division of Child Neurology, Department of Neurology, Virginia Commonwealth University, Richmond, VA, USA*

INTRODUCTION

Epileptic encephalopathies are conditions in which seizures, the epileptiform abnormalities, or both, contribute to the progressive disturbance in cerebral function (Engel, 2001). About 40% of all epilepsies occurring in the first 3 years of life fit this definition (Dalla Bernardina et al., 1983). However, the epileptic encephalopathies represent more a concept and an operational category than a syndrome spectrum. Some syndromes such as infantile spasms, Dravet syndrome (severe myoclonic epilepsy), epilepsy with continuous spike and waves during sleep, and Lennox–Gastaut syndrome always manifest as epileptic encephalopathies, irrespective of the underlying cause and severity of electroencephalographic (EEG) abnormalities. Some syndromes with usually good outcome, such as benign rolandic epilepsy, might have a complicated evolution, including learning and language impairment, when severe spike-and-wave discharges appear on the EEG. Persistent spike–wave-related anatomo-specific cortical dysfunction has been blamed for such an ominous evolution (Piccirilli et al., 1988; Shewmon and Erwin, 1988). Myoclonic–astatic epilepsy might unpredictably evolve as an epileptic encephalopathy or rapidly remit without major consequences on cognitive outcome, irrespective of its initial clinical and EEG characteristics (Guerrini and Aicardi, 2003). In such cases it is often entirely unclear which factors, clinical or EEG, can be blamed for either outcome. Finally, a particular situation is represented by epileptic encephalopathies that appear in children with a highly epileptogenic, usually developmental, brain lesion from which epileptic activity spreading to intact, remote areas interferes with their function and amplifies the clinical consequences of the malformation.

Correct diagnostic recognition and more appropriate treatment choices provide a higher chance of a better seizure outcome and reduced cognitive impairment in most epileptic encephalopathies, although this is difficult to demonstrate unequivocally. Although vigorous early treatment is often advocated in epileptic encephalopathies, for most conditions there are no established endpoints and drug choices are empirically established. Surgical treatment can be successful in selected cases. However, only in some surgically treatable syndromes does early treatment have a definite effect on long-term prognosis (Pulsifer et al., 2004). In many individuals the underlying cause, which often remains unrecognized, probably plays a greater part than is acknowledged in determining cognitive outcome.

INFANTILE SPASMS AND WEST SYNDROME

Infantile spasms are typical of the first year of life, are usually resistant to conventional antiepileptic drugs, and are associated with developmental delay, or deterioration. EEG often reveals a hypsarrhythmic pattern, which is characterized by very high-voltage (up to 500 μV) slow waves, irregularly interspersed with spikes and sharp waves that occur randomly in all cortical areas. The abnormal discharges are not synchronous over both hemispheres, so the general appearance is that of a chaotic disorganization of electrogenesis. Hypsarrhythmia is an interictal pattern and is observed mainly while the child is awake. During slow sleep, bursts of more synchronous, polyspikes and waves, often appear. In West syndrome, spasms, hypsarrhythmia, and cognitive deterioration occur together. However, infantile spasms might

*Correspondence to: Renzo Guerrini, M.D., Pediatric Neurology Unit and Laboratories, Children's Hospital A. Meyer-University of Florence, Viale Pieraccini 24, 50139 Firenze, Italy. Tel: 390555662573, Fax: 390555662329, E-mail: r.guerrini@meyer.it

occur without the typical EEG or developmental features. A cumulative incidence of 2.9 per 10 000 live births and an age-specific prevalence of 2.0 per 10 000 in 10-year-old children were observed in the USA (Trevathan et al., 1999). Epileptic spasms can persist or, rarely, appear in older children.

Infantile spasms are manifested as clusters of increasing plateau–decreasing intensity brisk (0.5–2.0 s) flexions or extensions of the neck, with abduction or adduction of the upper limbs. Clusters include a few units to several dozens of spasms and are repeated many times per day. After a series, the child is usually exhausted. Asymmetrical spasms are often associated with a lateralized brain lesion (Kramer et al., 1997), although unilateral lesions might cause symmetrical spasms. Lateralized motor phenomena, including lateral or upward eye deviation and eyebrow contraction, and abduction of one shoulder, may sometimes constitute the entire series of spasms or initiate a series that will eventually develop into bilateral phenomena. Such lateralized manifestations are usually accompanied by unilateral or asymmetric ictal EEG changes. Other seizure types can coexist.

The hypsarrhythmic EEG is often absent in severe brain lesions, such as tuberous sclerosis or lissencephaly (Dulac, 1997). Misdiagnosis of colic, startles, Moro response, or shoulder shrugs is still frequent. Duration of spasms is variable, depending both on treatment and on their tendency to remit or evolve into other seizure types. Rapid spontaneous remission is rare. In about 50% of children, spasms disappear before the age of 3 years and in 90% before the age of 5 years (Cowan and Hudson, 1991).

Developmental delay predates the onset of spasms in about 70% of children (Guerrini, 2006). Disappearance of social smile, loss of visual attention, or autistic withdrawal are often reported by the parents with the onset of spasms.

Although infantile spasms are traditionally divided into cases of *symptomatic* and *cryptogenic* origin, the meaning of these terms varies among studies and according to the extent of investigation. The specific nature of the underlying cause also implies a variable prognostic outlook. Most investigators define as symptomatic those cases in which an etiological factor can be clearly identified. Others link symptomaticity to either or both abnormal development prior to the onset of spasms and clinical or imaging evidence of a brain lesion, with brain malformations and perinatal hypoxic–ischemic encephalopathy being the most frequent causes. Cryptogenic spasms are those for which no cause can be identified, or where development was normal before clinical onset. In addition, the term *cryptogenic* does not necessarily mean that a lesion is not present; therefore, a difference of nature between cryptogenic and symptomatic cases is not clearly established. A few cases that are not included in the symptomatic group, despite increasingly accurate investigations, may belong to an "idiopathic" group (Dulac et al., 1986; Vigevano et al., 1993).

A family history of infantile spasm is found in only about 4% of the cases (Sugai et al., 2001). Familial cases are probably the expression of several genetic disorders, some of which are well characterized, including leukodystrophy (Coleman et al., 1977), tuberous sclerosis (Riikonen, 1984), X-linked lissencephaly and band heterotopia (Guerrini and Carrozzo, 2001), X-linked mental retardation, and infantile spasms due to mutations of the *ARX* gene (Stromme et al., 2002; Guerrini et al., 2007). Boys with X-linked infantile spasms due to *ARX* mutations usually have severe developmental delay and may have microcephaly. Onset of spasms is usually early and hypsarrhythmia is frequent (Stromme et al., 2002; Kato et al., 2003), although not constantly reported. Follow-up data on infantile spasms in these patients are not available. A syndrome of early-onset infantile spasms and severe quadriplegic dyskinesia, in which spasms tend to remit but episodes of status dystonicus complicate the course, has been associated with expansions in the first polyalanine tract of the *ARX* gene (Guerrini et al., 2007).

A syndrome with microcephaly and early-onset intractable seizures, including spasms with or without hypsarrhythmia, has been associated with mutations or deletions of the X-linked gene *CDKL5* (Archer et al., 2006; Elia et al., 2008; Mei et al., 2010). The syndrome is much more frequent in females. No unique EEG pattern seems to be typical for this etiology. Patients harboring deletions on chromosome 7q11.23, including the *MAGI2* gene, involved in regulation of trafficking, distribution, or function of the glutamate receptors, have infantile spasms. *MAGI2* might therefore be considered as a new gene for infantile spasms (Marshall et al., 2008).

A possibly recessive syndrome of early-onset infantile spasms, often preceded and followed by other types of seizure, associated with hypsarrhythmia, facial dysmorphism, optic atrophy, and peripheral edema, has been reported from Finland as PEHO syndrome (progressive encephalopathy with edema, hypsarrhythmia, and optic atrophy) (Riikonen, 2001). Cases exist outside Finland.

Other genetic disorders are more rare and may be of recessive (Fleiszar et al., 1977; Ciardo et al., 2001) or undetermined (Reiter et al., 2000) nature. Infantile spasms and West syndrome have also been associated with various mitochondrial disorders, inherited disorders of metabolism, chromosomal abnormalities, and copy number variations (Table 11.1).

Prognosis depends more on the cause than on treatment. Unfavorable prognostic factors include manifest symptomaticity, early onset (before 3 months),

Table 11.1

Etiologies of West and Lennox–Gastaut syndromes

Type of etiology	Specific etiology	Syndrome
Malformations of cortical development	Focal cortical dysplasia	WS
	Tuberous sclerosis *TSC1, TSC2* genes	WS, LGS
	Lissencephaly *LIS1, DCX, ARX* genes	WS, LGS
	Subcortical band heterotopia *DCX, LIS1* genes	WS, LGS
	Bilateral perisylvian polymicrogyria	WS
	Bilateral frontoparietal polymicrogyria *GPR56* gene mutations	WS
	Diffuse polymicrogyria	WS, LGS
	Hemimegalencephaly	WS
	Neurocutaneous disorders	WS
	Aicardi syndrome	IS
	Schizencephaly	IS
	Periventricular heterotopia/microcephaly *ARFGEF2* gene	IS
	Holoprosencephaly *SIX3, SHH, TGIF, ZIC2, PTCH1, GLI2* genes	WS
Pre-, peri-, or post-natal damage	Hypoxic–ischemic sequelae	WS
	Hemorrhagic	WS
	Fetal infections	WS, LGS
	Postnatal infection (encephalitis and meningitis)	WS, LGS
	Trauma	WS
	Cardiac surgery with hypothermia	WS
Chromosomal abnormalities and copy number variations	15q11.2-q13.1 duplication	LGS
	4p- (Wolf–Hirschhorn syndrome)	LGS
	invdup15	LGS
	Angelman syndrome	WS
	Down syndrome	WS, LGS
	Miller–Dieker syndrome	WS, LGS
	del1p36	WS
	del7q11.23-q21.1 (*MAGI2*)	WS
	Pallister–Killian syndrome: mosaic 12p(i[12p])	IS
Inborn errors of metabolism	Menkes disease	WS
	Phenylketonuria	WS
	Mitochondrial disease (NARP)	WS
	Complex 1 deficiency	IS
	Hypoglycemia	WS
	PEHO syndrome	WS
	Nonketotic hyperglycinemia	WS
	Other organic acid disorders	WS
	Pyridoxine dependency	IS
	Biotinidase dependency	WS
	Congenital disorders of glycosylation	WS
Vascular malformations	Sturge–Weber syndrome	WS, LGS
Brain tumors	All brain tumors	WS
Monogenic: nonmalformative, nonmetabolic	*ARX*	IS
	CDKL5	WS
	STPBX1	WS
No identifiable causes	About 40% positive family history of epilepsy	WS, LGS

West syndrome, infantile spasms, and epileptic spasms have the same etiology. The column legend indicates the prominent syndrome presentation, for example girls with Aicardi syndrome exhibit infantile spasms, rather than West syndrome; however, this distinction may not always be feasible. IS, infantile spasms; LGS, Lennox–Gastaut syndrome; NARP, neuropathy, ataxia, retinitis pigmentosa, and ptosis; PEHO, progressive encephalopathy with edema, hypsarrhythmia, and optic atrophy; WS, West syndrome.

pre-existing seizures other than spasms, asymmetrical EEG, and relapse after initial response to treatment (Guerrini, 2006). Adequate resolution requires the cessation of clinical spasms and normalization of the EEG (Pellock et al., 2010). Good prognostic indicators include cryptogenicity, normal findings on brain magnetic resonance imaging (MRI) (Saltik et al., 2002), typical hypsarrhythmia, rapid response to treatment, and no regression after onset of spasms or its short duration (Kivity et al., 2004). About 80% of patients have residual cognitive or behavioral impairment, but only one-third of cryptogenic cases do (Kivity et al., 2004). About 50% of children have other epilepsy types. Mortality rates of 5–31% have been reported, with higher rates arising from cumulative data and long-term follow-up (Riikonen, 1996).

Infantile spasms must be differentiated from rarer, earlier-onset conditions with ominous prognosis, such as early infantile epileptic encephalopathy and early myoclonic encephalopathy.

Vigabatrin and adrenocorticotropic hormone (ACTH) have proven effective in a few controlled trials, but uncertainties remain regarding the best treatment (Hancock et al., 2002; MacKay et al., 2004). In three comparative studies, vigabatrin was slightly less effective than, or as effective as, ACTH (Vigevano and Cilio, 1997; Cossette et al., 1999; Lux et al., 2004), but possibly better tolerated (Vigevano and Cilio, 1997). Two randomized trials reported a 78% responder rate (Appleton et al., 1999) and greater effectiveness with high doses (100–148 mg per kg per day) (Elterman et al., 2001). Particular efficacy has been shown in children with tuberous sclerosis (Jambaqué et al., 2000). Response to 100 mg per kg per day occurs within a few days. Many researchers regard vigabatrin as the first-line drug, despite the risk of visual field constriction (Lewis and Wallace, 2001). This side-effect appears in 30–50% of patients who receive a substantial drug load, but is not ascertainable in small children. According to the Vigabatrin Paediatric Advisory Group (2000), responders should receive vigabatrin for no more than 6 months and non-responders should be switched to ACTH within 3 weeks. Transient MRI hyperintensities of globus pallidi, thalami, dentate nuclei, and cerebral peduncles have recently been described in infants treated with vigabatrin for infantile spasms (Milh et al., 2009; Thelle et al., 2011). However, the meaning of these findings and how their report would affect treatment choices is still unclear. The UK Infantile Spasms Study (UKISS), comparing hormonal treatment with vigabatrin in the management, showed that tetracosactide (synthetic ACTH) or prednisolone controlled spasms better than vigabatrin initially, but not at 12–14 months of age (Lux et al., 2005). At 24-month follow-up, cognitive outcome was superior for the hormonal group. Tetracosactide is used in a daily dose of 20–40 IU. Nondepot ACTH has a lower risk of causing persistent hypertension. An individualized regimen allows dose-related side-effects such as hypertension, brain shrinking, adrenal hyporesponsiveness, and cardiac hypertrophy to be kept to a minimum (Heiskala et al., 1996). Infections are an ominous complication of ACTH treatment and are responsible for most deaths (Wong and Trevathan, 2001). A 4–6-week course of ACTH is advisable. Spasms may respond within days, but behavioral improvement needs several weeks. The relapse rate is 30%. A second cycle of ACTH is recommended in cases of relapse after an initial good response. ACTH proved superior to prednisone in a controlled trial (Baram et al., 1996). However, oral high-dose prednisolone has been suggested as an alternative to ACTH, providing equivalent efficacy with fewer side-effects and at considerably lower cost (Kossoff et al., 2009). Nevertheless, a recent complete review of the literature led the US Consensus report (Pellock et al., 2010) to suggest that a short course of high-dose ACTH (150 units per m^2 per day in two divided doses for 2 weeks, followed by a 2-week taper) and vigabatrin (100–150 mg per kg per day) demonstrated the best evidence for efficacy. The report stressed that a short course with higher dose led to an overall better tolerated and safer adverse event profile (Table 11.2). Pulsed intravenous methylprednisolone (Mytinger et al., 2010), valproate, topiramate, and benzodiazepines, especially nitrazepam, might represent interesting treatment alternatives. Pyridoxine is a preferred agent in Japan but its use is not supported by controlled studies (Mackay et al., 2004). Video-EEG monitoring is necessary to show that the spasms have truly disappeared (Gaily et al., 2001; Pellock et al., 2010).

Surgical treatment should be considered early when drug resistance is faced and focal epileptogenesis is shown. About 60% of children operated on become seizure-free; the best results are obtained when operating on small lesions (Asano et al., 2001). However, most children have large multilobar cortical dysplasia needing

Table 11.2

Infantile spasms: US consensus (Pellock et al., 2010)

1	Early recognition and prompt treatment are mandatory
2	Broad clinical evaluation, including detailed neurophysiology
3	ACTH and vigabatrin demonstrate efficacy to suppress spasms and abolish hypsarrhythmic EEG
4	Timely efficacy assessment recommended; longer trials (>2 weeks ACTH; >3 months vigabatrin) less successful and may lead to serious adverse effects
5	Effective treatment: cessation of spasm and resolution of EEG hypsarrhythmia – "all or none" response

ACTH, adrenocorticotropic hormone; EEG, electroencephalography.

extensive resection, with limited cognitive improvement (Pulsifer et al., 2004).

There is some evidence for use of the ketogenic diet in patients with resistant spasms (Kossoff et al., 2002; Kossoff, 2010).

LENNOX–GASTAUT SYNDROME

Lennox–Gastaut syndrome is characterized by intractable brief tonic and atonic seizures, atypical absences, and a generalized interictal EEG pattern of spike and slow-wave discharges. It accounts for 2.9% of all childhood epilepsy (Berg et al., 2000). Incidence peaks between 3 and 5 years of age. Cognitive and psychiatric impairment are frequent. About 30% of cases occur in previously healthy children; multiple etiologies are possible but most cases result from neuronal migration disorders and hypoxic brain damage. About 40% of children have previous infantile spasms (Guerrini, 2006). Persistence of seizures in adulthood is frequent.

The term Lennox–Gastaut syndrome, which was accepted by the International League Against Epilepsy in 1989, has often been used loosely to designate epilepsy syndromes of childhood featuring multiple types of intractable seizure, including falls. Epilepsy with myoclonic–astatic seizures and Dravet syndrome have likely been designated as Lennox–Gastaut syndrome in the past (Guerrini and Aicardi, 2003).

Cognitive impairment is present in most patients and is often associated with behavioral disturbances and psychiatric disorders. Many patients (20–60%) are already delayed at the onset of the syndrome, but the proportion of mentally retarded patients increases to 75–95% at 5 years from onset (Arzimanoglou et al., 2009). In primary cases (30%), the child's development seems normal before the appearance of the first seizures, but slowing of mental processing seems to be an almost constant element of the syndrome.

About 80% of patients continue to have seizures later in life, with those with symptomatic origin and early onset having the poorest outcome. Long-term follow-up studies report mortality rates of up to 17% (Guerrini, 2006).

The core seizure types of the syndrome, including tonic, atonic seizures, atypical absences, and episodes of nonconvulsive status, are not always present at onset, nor is the interictal EEG pattern of slow spike–wave. Some authors consider the presence of fast (10 Hz) rhythms associated with tonic seizures or occurring with minimal manifestations, especially during non-rapid-eye-movement (NREM) sleep, to be an essential diagnostic criterion (Beaumanoir, 1985; Genton et al., 2000).

Tonic seizures, with a "sustained increase in muscle contraction lasting a few seconds to minutes," are the most characteristic type (Blume et al., 2001). When the patient is standing, tonic seizures may forcefully throw the patient to the ground, causing sudden drop attacks. During sleep, tonic seizures may have a subtle expression with only opening of the eyes, or a short lasting apnea can be manifested as full-blown stiffening of the whole body with abduction and elevation of the limbs. Atypical absences can be difficult to identify due to their gradual onset and termination, especially in patients with cognitive impairment. Myoclonic seizures occur in a minority of patients. They are distinctly shorter (< 100 ms) than tonic events but may also lead to falls (Blume et al., 2001). Between 50% and 75% of patients also exhibit episodes of nonconvulsive status, manifested as subcontinuous atypical absences with fluctuating responsiveness that may sometimes be interspersed with recurring brief tonic seizures (Arzimanoglou et al., 2009). Episodes of nonconvulsive status seem definitely to worsen cognitive deterioration (Hoffmann-Riem et al., 2000). In addition to the main types of attack, generalized tonic–clonic seizures or focal seizures may be present in a minority of patients.

The classical EEG feature of Lennox–Gastaut syndrome is the slow spike-and-wave pattern, often repeated in bilaterally synchronous complexes at 1–2 Hz. Although slow spike-and-wave discharges are often associated with staring, confusion, or, at times, with an atonic fall, they can be interictal in many cases. Generalized bursts of "polyspikes" or fast rhythms (> 10 Hz), also called generalized paroxysmal fast activity, are recorded during slow sleep. They last from a few seconds to 15 seconds and tend to recur at relatively brief intervals (Blume et al., 1973). They occur as an interictal manifestation or are accompanied by a graded range of clinical manifestations, ranging from opening and upward deviation of the eyes, brief apnea or a mild electromyographic (EMG) axial contraction, to a typical tonic seizure. Sleep EEG recordings may be necessary to elicit their presence (Arzimanoglou et al., 2009).

The typical clinical and EEG manifestations of Lennox–Gastaut syndrome may not all be present at onset, which makes diagnosis difficult especially in cases whose onset is *de novo* (not resulting as transition from a previous different type of epilepsy). In about 20% of patients, Lennox–Gastaut syndrome evolves gradually after infantile spasms and hypsarrhythmia. Distinction between a prolonged spasm and a short tonic seizure may be arbitrary, although spasms usually appear in cluster whereas tonic seizures do so only rarely. Drop attacks are also observed in other epilepsy syndromes typical of childhood. In particular, children with myoclonic astatic epilepsy, aged 2–5 years, have prominently myoclonic or myoclonic–astatic seizures, causing drop attacks, and episodes of nonconvulsive status epilepticus (also defined as spike-and-wave stupor), interictal spike–wave, and slow spike-and-wave EEG complexes. Some also develop tonic seizures during sleep, which, however, tend to be isolated (Guerrini and Aicardi, 2003). Although myoclonic–astatic epilepsy is usually less severe than Lennox–Gastaut syndrome, it fulfils its major diagnostic criteria, making differential diagnosis difficult (Kaminska et al., 1999). Difficult problems of differential diagnosis are sometimes posed by epilepsy with continuous spike and waves during sleep (Guerrini et al., 1998b) and the atypical benign rolandic epilepsy (Aicardi and Chevrie, 1982). Children with this syndrome spectrum present with atypical and atonic absences that may cause repeated falls. Recording of continuous spike–waves during slow sleep and absence of tonic seizures usually permits differential diagnosis.

Lennox–Gastaut syndrome can appear in the absence of any obvious or suspected etiology (cryptogenic) in otherwise healthy children, or be symptomatic. As observed in West syndrome, the etiology of Lennox–Gastaut syndrome is extremely heterogeneous (see Table 11.1). The multiple causes that can be related to the syndrome can play a role in prognosis or sometimes for therapeutic strategies.

A family history of epilepsy is observed in 2.5–28% of cases (Genton and Dravet, 2008), but genetic factors, overall, appear to play a minor role. Perinatal hypoxic ischemic brain damage, intrauterine or postnatal infection, malformations of cortical development, chromosomal abnormality syndromes, head trauma, radiotherapy, acute disseminated encephalomyelitis, and brain tumors have been reported (Genton et al., 2000). Familial cases of Lennox–Gastaut syndrome have been associated with familial bilateral frontoparietal polymicrogyria due to *GPR56* gene mutations (Parrini et al., 2009) and with familial pachygyria associated with *DCX* gene mutations (Lawrence et al., 2010). In many cases, in spite of normal brain imaging, there is no obvious etiology.

The neurophysiological bases leading to the interictal and ictal EEG manifestations of Lennox–Gastaut syndrome are poorly understood. The process of secondary bilateral synchrony likely plays a major role in the generation of the seemingly generalized discharges. There is no obvious explanation for this abnormal tendency to secondary bilateral synchrony in Lennox–Gastaut syndrome. Blume (2004) hypothesized that overwhelming diffuse ictal and interictal discharges at a crucial age play a major role in diverting the brain from physiological developmental processes towards seizure control mechanisms.

The optimal treatment for Lennox–Gastaut syndrome remains uncertain, and only limited clinical trial data are available. Broad-spectrum drugs should be preferred (French et al., 2004). Only a few controlled studies are available, usually designed to evaluate the efficacy of one drug on one or two types of seizure, and no study is available investigating early overall effect of a given drug on the syndrome evolution. Randomized clinical trials in Lennox–Gastaut syndrome have been performed for lamotrigine, topiramate, felbamate, rufinamide, thyrotropin-releasing hormone (TRH) analog, and cinromide (reviewed in Arzimanoglou et al., 2009). A recent Cochrane review (Hancock and Cross, 2009) concluded that, although the optimal treatment for Lennox–Gastaut syndrome remains uncertain and no study to date has shown any one drug to be highly efficacious, rufinamide, lamotrigine, topiramate, and felbamate may be helpful as add-on therapy. A decrease in the frequency of all seizures was found for lamotrigine (Motte et al., 1997), felbamate (Felbamate Study Group, 1993), and rufinamide (Glauser et al., 2008), whereas for topiramate the decrease in total seizure frequency failed to reach statistical significance (Sachdeo et al., 1999). However, there is no guidance on how to combine these drugs and many researchers combine them with valproate, ethosuximide, or benzodiazepines, especially clobazam where available. Antiepileptic drug treatment approaches are complicated by the potential of polytherapies for adverse events and seizure aggravation (Guerrini et al., 1998a). Corticosteroids and ACTH have been used for short-term exacerbations with anecdotal reports of good results (Arzimanoglou et al., 2009). However, their role is limited by loss of efficacy and side-effects with prolonged treatment.

It has been suggested that vagus nerve stimulation and the ketogenic diet can be useful in some cases, but formal trials have not been performed (Neal et al., 2008). Corpus callosotomy might reduce seizures with drop attacks (Oguni et al., 1991), and a recent report suggests that results are superior and better tolerated when performed at a younger age (Asadi-Pooya et al., 2008). In the treatment of refractory encephalopathic epilepsy syndrome, treatment strategies need to be re-evaluated throughout the lifespan. The total quality of life may dictate therapeutic success rather than seizure freedom (Table 11.3).

LANDAU–KLEFFNER AND CONTINUOUS SPIKE AND WAVES DURING SLOW-WAVE SLEEP SYNDROMES

In Landau–Kleffner and continuous spike and waves during slow-wave sleep syndromes, frequent or persistent discharges, with or without accompanying seizures, cause impairment of cortical functions. These two syndromes, which may on occasion partially overlap, epitomize the essence of nonconvulsive age-related epileptic encephalopathies.

Table 11.3

Lennox–Gastaut syndrome

Intractable brief tonic and atonic seizures, atypical absences
Generalized interictal EEG pattern of spike and slow-wave discharges
Peak incidence between 3 and 5 years of age
Frequent neuropsychiatric comorbidities
Sleep EEG may be valuable to confirm diagnosis by showing specific features such as generalized paroxysmal fast activity
Clinical experience and studies suggest that broad spectrum AEDs (sodium valproate, benzodiazepines, and/or lamotrigine) be used early, when drop attacks predominate. They may also be effective against atypical absence seizures
Long-term treatment can be disappointing, but excessive therapy should be avoided due to risks for cognitive and behavioral toxicity
Some AEDs in combination may facilitate episodes of nonconvulsive/tonic status epilepticus
Benzodiazepines have only transitory efficacy with rapid tolerance and side-effects
Corticosteroids/ACTH may be helpful temporarily during periods of electroclinical aggravation
Carbamazepine may control tonic seizures but may aggravate atypical absences, myoclonic, nonconvulsive status
Management of Lennox–Gastaut syndrome requires a multidisciplinary medical and psychosocial team

Modified from Arzimanoglou et al., 2009.
ACTH, adrenocorticotropic hormone; AED, antiepileptic drug; EEG, electroencephalography.

Landau–Kleffner syndrome is a rare, severely disabling disorder, with an insidious, or sudden, loss of language understanding (auditory agnosia), followed by progressive or fluctuating loss of verbal expression (Deonna, 2004). Age at onset is between 3 and 7 years. Focal seizures represent the initial symptom in 60% of children, but are absent altogether in 25%. They have variable severity but remit before adulthood. EEG abnormalities predominate in the temporoparietal regions, bilaterally, or on either side (Deonna, 2004). Interference by EEG discharges with auditory-evoked responses (Seri et al., 1998) suggests epilepsy-induced dysfunction of auditory processing. The prognosis of aphasia is unpredictable but recovery without consequences is exceptional (Duran et al., 2009). However, onset before age 5 years and persistent EEG anomalies over the language areas forecast a severe evolution. Patients might be left with normal language or mild-to-severe persistent defects. No cause has been identified, although rare lesional cases have been reported.

Treatment efficacy has been investigated empirically. Large doses of ACTH or steroids for prolonged periods (>3 months) have a definite effect on EEG and language (Marescaux et al., 1990; Buzatu et al., 2009). Repeated injections several days apart might prevent major side-effects. Benzodiazepines, valproate, ethosuximide, and immunoglobulins have obtained some success (Guerrini, 2006). Surgical treatment with multiple subpial transections has produced longlasting improvement in selected cases (Grote et al., 1999), but the merit of this approach is difficult to assess and remains highly uncertain. Language therapy is indicated, and alternatives to oral language should be offered to the most severely impaired children.

In epilepsy with continuous spike-and-wave discharges during slow sleep (or electrical status epilepticus during slow sleep), continuous sleep-related EEG discharges, persisting for months to years, are associated with cognitive decline. The syndrome appears in previously healthy or in delayed children. Brain lesions, especially polymicrogyria (Guerrini et al., 1998b) and porencephaly (Tassinari et al., 2002), are found in 30–50% of patients. Onset is insidious. Seizures start at 3–5 years as nocturnal and focal attacks, and share similarities to those seen in rolandic epilepsy. After a few months, continuous spike and waves during slow-wave sleep and atypical or atonic absences appear. There is a marked decrease in intelligence quotient scores with attention deficit and hyperactivity, sometimes with language disturbances and autistic features. The long-term course of epilepsy is favorable, but cognitive impairment persists in most children. Earlier onset and long duration of continuous spike and waves during slow-wave sleep are major factors for a poor prognosis (Smith and Hoeppner, 2003). The benign atypical partial epilepsy syndrome (Aicardi and Chevrie, 1982) has a close relationship with continuous spike and waves during slow-wave sleep. Drug treatment is the same as in Landau–Kleffner syndrome, as many aspects of these syndromes truly overlap (Hughes, 2011).

DRAVET SYNDROME (SEVERE MYOCLONIC EPILEPSY IN INFANCY)

Dravet syndrome, otherwise known as severe myoclonic epilepsy of infancy (SMEI), is an increasingly recognized epileptic encephalopathy where the clinical diagnosis can be genetically confirmed in around 80% of patients. Dravet syndrome includes a spectrum of conditions with variable severity, all appearing in otherwise normal infants (Dravet et al., 2005), spanning from the classical phenotype to "borderline SMEI" (SMEB) in which patients share most but not all of the characteristic clinical features (Oguni et al., 2001).

Since its first descriptions, Dravet syndrome has been recognized increasingly worldwide, yet it remains a rare disorder with an incidence probably lower than 1 per

40 000 (Hurst, 1990). The prevalence of Dravet syndrome in children with seizure onset in the first year of life varies between 3% and 8% (Yakoub et al., 1992; Dravet et al., 2005).

The initial manifestations start before 12 months of age, with repeated *generalized or unilateral clonic* (hemiclonic with alternating side) seizures, typically triggered by fever. Seizures are often prolonged, tend to recur in clusters in the same day, and may evolve into status epilepticus. Factors that increase body temperature, such as vaccinations or hot water immersion, can precipitate seizures.

Between the ages of 1 and 4 years, other seizure types appear, including myoclonic, absences, focal, and, exceptionally, tonic seizures.

Most patients also exhibit *myoclonic seizures*, which appear between the ages of 1 and 5 years. Myoclonic jerks can be massive and involve the whole body, leading to falling, or be mild and barely visible, exhibiting a multifocal distribution. They are often precipitated by photic stimulation. Polygraphic EEG recordings show that generalized jerks are accompanied by high-voltage discharges of generalized spike and wave, or polyspike and wave discharges. However, not all myoclonic jerks are accompanied by time-locked paroxysmal EEG activity.

Absence seizures are present in 40–90% of patients (Dravet et al., 2005) and appear between ages 1 and 3 years. Absences are classified as atypical and can be associated with a prominent myoclonic component. Ictal EEG shows 2.5–3 Hz generalized spike-and-wave discharges.

About 40% of patients experience *nonconvulsive status epilepticus* or *"obtundation status,"* characterized by unresponsiveness of variable intensity, with erratic myoclonic jerks, involving the limbs or the face. These episodes may be very prolonged, lasting for days, and fluctuate in intensity, which makes them particularly insidious. Ictal EEG shows diffuse slow waves intermingled with focal or diffuse spikes, sharp waves, or spike and waves. More than 50% of patients have *focal seizures,* occurring from 4 months of age on. Focal seizures can have a main motor component – versive or clonic jerking limited to one limb or one hemiface – or be complex partial with prominent autonomic symptoms. *Convulsive seizures* tend to be present throughout as generalized clonic or tonic–clonic seizures, unilateral seizures, or "unstable seizures" (Dravet et al., 2005). *Tonic seizures* are exceptional in this syndrome.

Interictal EEG, normal at onset, subsequently shows generalized or multifocal paroxysmal activity. About 25% of children are photosensitive and may indulge in self-stimulation.

Early developmental skills and behavior are usually reported as normal. However, following seizure onset, at around the second year of life, developmental slowing or stagnation becomes obvious in most patients (Wolff et al., 2006; Ragona et al., 2011). Behavioral disturbances with hyperactivity and autistic traits are frequent. The frequency of convulsive seizures seems to correlate with the severity of developmental delay, suggesting that Dravet syndrome might be considered as a paradigmatic example of epileptic encephalopathy (Wolff et al., 2006). Early onset of absence and myoclonic seizures appears to carry a higher risk of severe cognitive impairment (Ragona et al., 2011).

A family history of epilepsy is often found. Affected relatives most often exhibit epilepsy phenotypes consistent with the generalized epilepsy with febrile seizure plus (GEFS+) spectrum (Singh et al., 1999). The initial finding that mutations of the gene coding for the α1 subunit of the sodium channel (*SCN1A*) were present in patients with GEFS+(Escayg et al., 2000) led to the subsequent discovery that an overwhelming number of *SCN1A* mutations are associated with Dravet syndrome (Claes et al., 2001; Mulley et al., 2005), including the borderline forms. The frequency of detectable mutations is around 70–80%; truncating mutations account for nearly 50% of the abnormalities with the remaining comprising splice-site and missense mutations. Intragenic deletions and whole gene deletions including only *SCN1A* and contiguous genes account for 2–3% of all cases and for about 12.5% of those exhibiting no point mutations (Marini et al., 2009). Duplications and amplifications involving *SCN1A* are additional, rare, molecular mechanisms (Marini et al., 2009). Most mutations are *de novo,* but familial *SCN1A* mutations also occur (Claes et al., 2001; Sugawara et al., 2002; Nabbout et al., 2003; Wallace et al., 2003). Somatic mosaic mutations have been reported in some patients and should be considered when estimating the recurrence (Depienne et al., 2006; Marini et al., 2006). Although mosaic *SCN1A* mutations might explain the phenotypic variability, including age of seizure onset, seizure types, and severity seen even within the same family (Guerrini et al., 2010), there certainly exist additional factors such as modifier genes, the genetic background, or environmental factors that can influence variability.

Some general genotype–phenotype correlations have been suggested: truncating, nonsense, frame-shift mutations, and partial or whole gene deletions are correlated with a classical Dravet syndrome phenotype and appear to have a significant correlation with an earlier age of seizure onset (Marini et al., 2007). The severity of the phenotypes is also correlated with *SCN1A* missense mutations falling in the pore-forming region of the sodium channel, whereas missense changes associated to the GEFS+spectrum are nearly always localized outside the pore-forming region (Meisler and Kearney, 2005).

Mutations are randomly distributed across the SCN1A protein in both Dravet syndrome and GEFS+ epilepsies.

Depienne et al. (2009) reported *PCDH19* mutations and one deletion in 12 of 74 patients (16%) with early-onset epileptic encephalopathy mimicking Dravet syndrome. *PCDH19* encodes protocadherin 19, a transmembrane protein of the cadherin family of calcium-dependent cell–cell adhesion molecules, which is strongly expressed in the central nervous system. *PCDH19* should be tested in patients with Dravet syndrome in whom no *SCN1A* abnormalities can be found. Despite intensive investigation, the etiology of about 15% of patients sharing features with Dravet syndrome remains unknown.

The definition "intractable childhood epilepsy with generalized tonic–clonic seizures (ICEGTC)" has been used to designate infants with frequent and intractable generalized tonic–clonic seizures often induced by fever and beginning before 1 year of age (Fujiwara et al., 2003). The major feature that differentiates Dravet syndrome and ICEGTC is the presence or absence of myoclonic seizures.

Neuroradiological studies are unrevealing in most patients, but structural abnormalities such as cerebral or cerebellar atrophy of various degree and focal arachnoid cysts have been reported anecdotally (Fujiwara et al., 2003; Dravet et al., 2005; Striano et al., 2007).

At onset, children are often regarded as having febrile seizures; only their frequent repetition, often as prolonged episodes with unilateral features, makes one suspect Dravet syndrome or GEFS+. Children may manifest myoclonic seizures at onset and be misdiagnosed as having benign myoclonic epilepsy of infancy. Myoclonic–astatic epilepsy should also be considered in the differential diagnosis because some children with this type of epilepsy manifest febrile seizures before the second year of life, whereas the classical myoclonic–astatic seizures occur only later on during the course.

Data on long-term evolution are sparse. Seizures persist into adulthood but are less frequent, rarely prolonged, and usually confined to sleep (Jansen et al., 2006). In the course of the disease, cognitive and motor functions may slightly improve but remain at a low level. Mortality rates are around 16% (Dravet et al., 2005), resulting mainly from sudden death or seizure-related accidents.

Valproic acid, benzodiazepines, topiramate, and levetiracetam have shown some efficacy (Dravet et al., 2005). Stiripentol, an inhibitor of the P450 cytochrome, was effective in combination with clobazam in a class I trial (Chiron et al., 2000). Stiripentol acts by increasing the concentration of norclobazam, an active metabolite of clobazam. Phenytoin, carbamazepine, and lamotrigine can worsen seizures and must be avoided (Guerrini et al., 1998a; Dravet et al., 2005).

MYOCLONIC–ASTATIC EPILEPSY

Myoclonic–astatic epilepsy is a generalized epilepsy syndrome with multiple seizure types, including myoclonic–astatic, absences, tonic–clonic, and eventually tonic seizures, appearing in a previously normal child between the ages of 18 and 60 months, with a peak around 3 years of age (Guerrini and Aicardi, 2003). The nosological limits of the disorder are difficult to determine and the course has variable severity, manifesting as an epileptic encephalopathy only in some patients.

To understand the difficulties that have surrounded the recognition of this type of epilepsy, some historical notes may be useful. Under the term "centrencephalic myoclonic–astatic petit mal," Herman Doose reported in 1970 a series of patients who shared with Lennox–Gastaut syndrome the same age of onset, generalized seizures often causing the patient to fall, cognitive delay, and generalized spike-and-wave discharges (Doose et al., 1970). These patients exhibited different combinations of generalized seizures and evolutive patterns, lacked any evidence of brain lesion, had a high incidence of familial antecedents, and thus a suspected genetic etiology. A main point raised by Doose was that of a genetic predisposition as opposed to the Lennox–Gastaut syndrome. This view, based mainly on the concept of etiology, contrasts with the syndromic approach, in which it is the combination of particular symptoms and the rather uniform prognostic outlook that determines the group, whatever the etiology. For this reason, with the purpose of assigning a prognostic outlook, in the past children with myoclonic–astatic epilepsy were often classified within the framework of syndromes with somewhat overlapping electroclinical manifestations, such as Lennox–Gastaut or Dravet syndrome.

The incidence of myoclonic–astatic epilepsy was defined by Doose and Sitepu (1983) as 1–2% of all childhood epilepsies up to age 9 years. In a hospital population of children presenting their first seizure between 1 and 10 years of age, it was estimated that myoclonic–astatic epilepsy represented 2.2% (Kaminska et al., 1999). The sex ratio has been defined as 2.7–3 : 1 in favor of males (Doose, 1992; Kaminska et al., 1999).

Genetic factors seem to play a major role. A family history of epilepsy was present in 32% of children described by Doose (1992) and in 15% in the series from Kaminska et al. (1999). Ten patients of 88 belonging to families with the GEFS+ complex had myoclonic–astatic epilepsy (Scheffer and Berkovic, 1997; Singh et al., 1999, 2001).

Myoclonic and myoclonic–astatic seizures are present in all affected children and are prominent in most. Clinically, myoclonic seizures present as brief, generalized jerks, isolated or replicated in short series of two–three events. Proximal muscles are more involved, producing a sudden flexion of the head and trunk with possible collapse to the ground (Oguni et al., 1992). A wide range of severity is observed, ranging from head nodding to falls with possible injury. The duration of these episodes is brief (0.3–1 s according to video-EEG analysis) (Oguni et al., 1992). Falls can either be the direct consequence of massive myoclonic jerks or result from the postmyoclonic silent period that may sometimes be prominent (Oguni et al., 1992). In some children, myoclonic seizures are also triggered by photic stimulation (Doose, 1992). Tonic–clonic seizures are the second most frequent seizure type, present in 75–95% of children (Doose, 1992; Kaminska et al., 1999). They are usually the first manifestation to appear. According to Doose (1992), they appear initially during daytime and later in the course of the disorder during night-time sleep. Absence seizures are present in 62–89% of patients (Doose, 1992; Kaminska et al., 1999). Most often, they present as atypical absences associated with a reduction of muscle tone (Doose, 1992). Some 14–95% of children suffer from nonconvulsive *status,* presenting as stupor and apathy associated with multifocal, arrhythmic twitching of the face and extremities. Episodes of status can last for several days and seem to be longer in children with an unfavorable evolution (Kaminska et al., 1999). They appear spontaneously or can be triggered by inappropriate treatment, especially with carbamazepine (Guerrini et al., 2002) or vigabatrin (Lortie et al., 1993). Tonic seizures have been described in 30–95% of patients (Doose, 1992; Kaminska et al., 1999). They can manifest as typical axial, tonic attacks during sleep or as tonic–vibratory seizures, especially at the end of night-time sleep, particularly between 4 and 6 a.m. (Doose, 1992). Only about one-third of children with a favorable course have tonic seizures (Kaminska et al., 1999). Febrile seizures, usually simple in type, are reported to precede nonfebrile seizures in 11–28% of children (Doose, 1992; Kaminska et al., 1999). The initial febrile seizure can appear as early as 6 weeks of age (Singh et al., 1999), but in most children it presents between 17 and 40 months (Kaminska et al., 1999).

Background EEG activity may be normal at seizure onset, although a characteristic 4–7-Hz, monomorphic theta activity with diffuse distribution, but prominent on centroparietal areas, is often observed. Interictal abnormalities consist of bursts of 2–3-Hz generalized (poly)spike-and-wave discharges, sometimes asymmetrical (Doose, 1992). Sleep is accompanied by an increase in generalized discharges. Myoclonic seizures are characterized electrographically by a generalized (poly) spike-and-wave complex, which may be isolated or repeated rhythmically at 3–4 Hz, lasting for 2–6 s (Oguni et al., 1992). Myoclonic jerks, involving mostly the proximal upper limbs, are time-locked to a spike-and-wave complex. The EMG correlate of each jerk is a burst lasting for around 100 ms, followed by a longer (200–500 ms) postmyoclonic silent period. A single jerk or a series of 2–3 jerks is observed most commonly. Neurophysiological analysis of myoclonic seizures (Bonanni et al., 2002; Guerrini et al., 2002) showed that: spike-and-wave discharges and myoclonic jerks are bilateral and synchronous, supporting a thalamocortical origin of myoclonic jerks.

The atonic component of seizures is characterized on polygraphic studies by a rhythmic discharge of (poly) spike-and-slow wave complexes at 3–4 Hz, accompanied by EMG inhibition, lasting 60–400 ms, synchronous in the recorded muscles, and time-locked to the onset of the slow wave (Oguni et al., 1992, 1997).

Tonic seizures are accompanied by 10–15-Hz polyspike discharges lasting as long as the tonic contraction on EMG.

Myoclonic status is associated to a very irregular and chaotic EEG with independent spike-and-wave discharges, sometimes resembling hypsarrhythmia (Doose, 1992). Focal, erratic, myoclonic jerks are recorded on distal and facial muscles. They are brief (30–100 ms) and are not time-locked to individual spikes on visual inspection of EEG (Guerrini et al., 2002).

The evolution of myoclonic–astatic epilepsy can be either favorable with seizure control within 3 years from onset and normal cognitive development, or unfavorable with drug-resistant seizures and cognitive impairment (Dulac et al., 1990; Kaminska et al., 1999; Guerrini and Aicardi, 2003). There is no distinguishable cluster of clinical or EEG characteristics at epilepsy onset that can help predict the outcome (Kaminska et al., 1999).

Myoclonic–astatic epilepsy must be differentiated from cryptogenic Lennox–Gastaut syndrome and atypical benign rolandic epilepsy (Aicardi and Chevrie, 1982), and from epilepsy with continuous spike–wave activity during slow sleep (Patry et al., 1971). The so-called myoclonic variant of Lennox–Gastaut syndrome shares many similarities with unfavorable myoclonic–astatic epilepsy (Kaminska et al., 1999). Atypical benign rolandic epilepsy (Aicardi and Chevrie, 1982) is observed in children with normal development who, after experiencing some sleep-related "sylvian" seizures, develop multiple seizure types including atypical absences and atonic drop attacks accompanied by very abnormal EEG showing continuous spike-and-wave activity during sleep. Differential diagnosis is sometimes necessary with the late infantile variant of ceroid-lipofuscinosis at its clinical onset.

Valproate is the first choice drug, because of its wide spectrum of action. If valproate fails, a combination of valproate with lamotrigine should be the next step. Ethosuximide can be effective, particularly when myoclonus and absence seizures are prominent in the clinical picture. Alternatively, small doses of a benzodiazepine in combination with valproate can sometimes prove effective.

Although the use of lamotrigine in epilepsies with myoclonus should be cautious, particularly in Dravet syndrome and juvenile myoclonic epilepsy (Guerrini et al., 1998a; Biraben et al., 2000), this drug seems to be of use in myoclonic–astatic epilepsy (Dulac and Kaminska, 1997).

Carbamazepine and vigabatrin should be avoided in myoclonic–astatic epilepsy, because they can increase seizure frequency and trigger episodes of myoclonic status (Lortie et al., 1993; Kaminska et al., 1999; Guerrini et al., 2002).

ENCEPHALOPATHIC CHILDHOOD EPILEPSIES ASSOCIATED WITH INHERITED METABOLIC DISORDERS

More than 50 genetically determined metabolic diseases have been described as associated with seizures or epilepsy. Most, when they present in childhood, are associated with encephalopathy. Thus, these disorders overlap with descriptions of the more classical epilepsy syndromes discussed above. However, they often present early in life with few, if any, specific findings (Nordli and DeVivo, 2008; Pellock et al., 2008). Systemic findings or dysmorphisms may be helpful for orienting diagnosis, but they are not always present. A variety of seizure types has been noted and in young infants they may be multifocal, myoclonic, or tonic in nature. Later, they may manifest as infantile spasms. As children become older, both partial and generalized mixed seizures may continue. The degree of encephalopathy depends upon the severity of the metabolic defect. This section stresses the importance of considering these possible etiologies with attention to possible specific treatments. The reader is referred to a more comprehensive review (Nordli and DeVivo, 2008). Metabolic disorder should be suspected when specific etiology or a well-recognized idiopathic syndrome is not established, or the history of the patient is more malignant than expected.

Examples of metabolic disorders with specific treatments include the following (with their treatment listed in parentheses):

- pyridoxine-responsive epilepsies (pyridoxine, pyridoxal phosphate)
- central creatinine deficiency (creatinine)
- phenylketonuria (dietary restriction)
- glucose transporter deficiency syndrome – GLUT1 DS (ketogenic diet)
- pyruvate dehydrogenase deficiency (ketogenic diet)
- disorders of lactic acidosis (thiamine, leukovorin)
- biotinidase deficiency (biotin)
- Menkes disease (copper histidinate).

As one can appreciate, the number of metabolic disorders presenting with encephalopathy and seizures continues to grow. As noted, the semiology of the events will depend upon the age of seizure onset and may change over time. The degree of encephalopathy may be progressive, or seem more static, depending upon the degree of metabolic dysfunction. Similarly, when children have relatively few seizures but then have an increase in both seizures and motor or cognitive symptoms, re-evaluation should be considered. One of the important aspects of diagnosis is not only to correct or treat existing metabolic defects but also to realize which treatments may worsen the condition. Conditions that may worsen with certain antiepileptic medications include pyruvate carboxylase deficiency worsened by ketogenic diet or ACTH, some organic acidurias worsened by the ketogenic diet, GLUT1 deficiency worsened by phenobarbital, caffeine, and other substances interfering with glucose transport across the blood–brain barrier, conditions with lactic acidosis worsened by carbonic anhydrase inhibitors, which could worsen the acidosis, and some mitochondrial disorders that may be worsened by valproate, even to the degree of life-threatening hepatotoxicity.

Abnormalities demonstrated on EEG recording may be helpful. Suppression burst pattern is noted in nonketotic hyperglycemia, phenylketonuria, maple syrup urine disease, molybdenum cofactor deficiency, and disorders of biotin metabolism. A comb-like rhythm with 7–9-Hz central activity may be demonstrated in those with maple syrup urine disease, vertex-positive spikes in sialidosis type 1, and bioccipital polymorphic delta activity in X-linked adrenal leukodystrophia, and 14–22-Hz persistent rhythm is frequently noted with infantile neuroaxonal dystrophy. However, these neurophysiological findings, along with imaging abnormalities, may vary.

Numerous mitochondrial diseases may be characterized by encephalopathy and seizures. Mitochondrial encephalomyopathies are in fact heterogeneous, but almost all that present with seizures have significant encephalopathic features. Two best known of these mitochondrial disorders are myoclonus epilepsy with ragged red fibers (MERRF) and mitochondrial encephalopathy, lactic acidosis, and stroke-like episodes (MELAS). Maternal inheritance is the rule, but symptoms may be quite variable within families. Seizures in these patients may be focal or generalized and varied depending upon the degree of mitochondrial abnormality affecting the brain. Other mitochondrial encephalopathies that are associated with nuclear mutations rather than mitochondrial DNA mutations include Leigh syndrome, Alpers syndrome, and coenzyme Q10 deficiency. These encephalopathic diseases have variable presentation with multisystemic involvement and epilepsy. A recent review discusses these disorders more comprehensively (Hirano et al., 2008). Mitochondrial disorders are treated by metabolic therapy, typically comprising cocktails containing coenzyme Q10, L-carnitine, dichloroacetate, and multivitamins, although the effects of such a treatment approach to seizure severity have not been assessed.

CONCLUSION

Nonconvulsive and convulsive age-related epileptic encephalopathies may present as a characteristic epilepsy syndrome of childhood. Alternatively, seizures may be a manifestation of underlying systemic disorders, including genetically determined metabolic defects. The clinical manifestations are of the underlying etiology, including systemic disorders, sometimes genetically determined metabolic defects. The epilepsies are typically therapy-resistant, but others are responsive to specific treatments, aggravated occasionally by classical anticonvulsants and especially polytherapy. Careful attention to the history and evolution of the clinical course of seizures and encephalopathy along with neurophysiological and imaging findings allow proper diagnosis and optimal management.

References

Aicardi J, Chevrie JJ (1982). Atypical benign partial epilepsy of childhood. Dev Med Child Neurol 24: 281–292.

Appleton RE, Peters AC, Mumford JP et al. (1999). Randomised, placebo-controlled study of vigabatrin as first-line treatment of infantile spasms. Epilepsia 40: 1627–1633.

Archer HL, Evans J, Edwards S et al. (2006). CDKL5 mutations cause infantile spasms, early onset seizures, and severe mental retardation in female patients. J Med Genet 43: 729–734.

Arzimanoglou A, French J, Blume WT et al. (2009). Lennox–Gastaut syndrome: a consensus approach on diagnosis, assessment, management, and trial methodology. Lancet Neurol 8: 82–93.

Asadi-Pooya AA, Sharan A, Nei M et al. (2008). Corpus callosotomy. Epilepsy Behav 13: 271–278.

Asano E, Chugani DC, Juhasz C et al. (2001). Surgical treatment of West syndrome. Brain Dev 23: 668–676.

Baram TZ, Mitchell WG, Tournay A et al. (1996). High-dose corticotropin (ACTH) versus prednisone for infantile spasms: a prospective, randomised, blinded study. Pediatrics 97: 375–379.

Beaumanoir A (1985). The Lennox–Gastaut syndrome. In: J Roger, M Bureau, C Dravet et al. (Eds.), Epileptic Syndromes in Infancy, Childhood, and Adolescence. John Libbey, London, pp. 89–99.

Berg AT, Shinnar S, Levy SR et al. (2000). How well can epilepsy syndromes be identified at diagnosis? A reassessment 2 years after initial diagnosis. Epilepsia 41: 1269–1275.

Biraben A, Allain H, Scarabin JM et al. (2000). Exacerbation of juvenile myoclonic epilepsy with lamotrigine. Neurology 55: 1758.

Blume WT (2004). Lennox–Gastaut syndrome: potential mechanisms of cognitive regression. Ment Retard Dev Disabil Res Rev 10: 150–153.

Blume WT, David RB, Gomez MR (1973). Generalized sharp and slow wave complexes – associated clinical features and long-term follow-up. Brain 96: 289–306.

Blume WT, Luders HO, Mizrahi E et al. (2001). ILAE Commission Report. Glossary of descriptive terminology for ictal semiology: report of the ILAE task force on classification and terminology. Epilepsia 42: 1212–1218.

Bonanni P, Parmeggiani L, Guerrini R (2002). Different neurophysiologic patterns of myoclonus characterize Lennox–Gastaut syndrome and myoclonic astatic epilepsy. Epilepsia 43: 609–615.

Buzatu M, Bulteau C, Altuzarra C et al. (2009). Corticosteroids as treatment of epileptic syndromes with continuous spike-waves during slow-wave sleep. Epilepsia 50: 68–72.

Chiron C, Marchand MC, Tran A et al. (2000). Stiripentol in severe myoclonic epilepsy in infancy: a randomised placebo-controlled syndrome-dedicated trial. STICLO study group. Lancet 11: 1638–1642.

Ciardo F, Zamponi N, Specchio N et al. (2001). Autosomal recessive polymicrogyria with infantile spasms and limb deformities. Neuropediatrics 32: 325–329.

Claes L, Del-Favero J, Ceulemans B et al. (2001). De novo mutations in the sodium-channel gene SCN1A cause severe myoclonic epilepsy of infancy. Am J Hum Genet 68: 1327–1332.

Coleman M, Hart PN, Randall J et al. (1977). Serotonin levels in the blood and central nervous system of a patient with sudanophilic leukodystrophy. Neuropadiatrie 8: 459–466.

Cossette P, Riviello JJ, Carmant L (1999). ACTH versus vigabatrin therapy in infantile spasms: a retrospective study. Neurology 52: 1691–1694.

Cowan LD, Hudson LS (1991). The epidemiology and natural history of infantile spasms. J Child Neurol 6: 355–364.

Dalla Bernardina B, Colamaria V, Capovilla G et al. (1983). Nosological classification of epilepsies in the first three years of life. In: G Nisticò, R Di Perri, H Meinardi (Eds.), Epilepsy: An Update on Research and Therapy. Alan Liss, New York, pp. 165–183.

Deonna T (2004). Cognitive and behavioral manifestations of epilepsy in children. In: SJ Wallace, K Farrell (Eds.), Epilepsy in children. 2nd edn. Arnold, London, pp. 250–257.

Depienne C, Arzimanoglou A, Trouillard O et al. (2006). Parental mosaicism can cause recurrent transmission of SCN1A mutations associated with severe myoclonic epilepsy of infancy. Hum Mutat 27: 389.

Depienne C, Bouteiller D, Keren B et al. (2009). Sporadic infantile epileptic encephalopathy caused by mutations in PCDH19 resembles Dravet syndrome but mainly affects females. PLoS Genet 5: e1000381.

Doose H (1992). Myoclonic–astatic epilepsy. Epilepsy Res Suppl 6: 163–168.

Doose H, Sitepu B (1983). Childhood epilepsy in a German city. Neuropediatrics 14: 220–224.

Doose H, Gerken H, Leonhardt R et al. (1970). Centrencephalic myoclonic–astatic petit mal. Clinical and genetic investigation. Neuropadiatrie 2: 59–78.

Dravet C, Bureau M, Oguni H et al. (2005). Severe myoclonic epilepsy in infancy: Dravet syndrome. Adv Neurol 95: 71–102.

Dulac O (1997). Infantile spasms and West syndrome. In: J Engel Jr, TA Pedley (Eds.), Epilepsy: A Comprehensive Textbook. Lippincott–Raven, Philadelphia, pp. 2277–2283.

Dulac O, Kaminska A (1997). Use of lamotrigine in Lennox–Gastaut and related epilepsy syndromes. J Child Neurol 12: S23–S28.

Dulac O, Plouin P, Jambaqué I et al. (1986). Spasmes infantiles épileptiques bénins. Rev Electroencephalogr Neurophysiol Clin 16: 371–382.

Dulac O, Plouin P, Chiron C (1990). "Benign" form of myoclonic epilepsy in children. Neurophysiol Clin 20: 115–129.

Duran MH, Guimarães CA, Medeiros LL et al. (2009). Landau–Kleffner syndrome: long-term follow-up. Brain Dev 31: 58–63.

Elia M, Falco M, Ferri R et al. (2008). CDKL5 mutations in boys with severe encephalopathy and early-onset intractable epilepsy. Neurology 71: 997–999.

Elterman RD, Shields WD, Mansfield KA et al. (2001). US Infantile Spasms Vigabatrin Study Group. Randomized trial of vigabatrin in patients with infantile spasms. Neurology 57: 1416–1421.

Engel J Jr. (2001). International League Against Epilepsy (ILAE). A proposed diagnostic scheme for people with epileptic seizures and with epilepsy: report of the ILAE Task Force on Classification and Terminology. Epilepsia 42: 796–803.

Escayg A, MacDonald BT, Meisler MH et al. (2000). Mutations of SCN1A, encoding a neuronal sodium channel, in two families with GEFS + 2. Nat Genet 24: 343–345.

Felbamate Study Group in Lennox–Gastaut Syndrome (1993). Efficacy of felbamate in childhood epileptic encephalopathy (Lennox–Gastaut syndrome). N Engl J Med 328: 29–33.

Fleiszar KA, Daniel WL, Imrey PB (1977). Genetic study of infantile spasms with hypsarrhythmia. Epilepsia 18: 55–62.

French JA, Kanner AM, Bautista J et al. (2004). Efficacy and tolerability of the new antiepileptic drugs II: treatment of refractory epilepsy: report of the Therapeutics and Technology Assessment Subcommittee of the American Academy of Neurology; Quality Standards Subcommittee of the American Academy of Neurology; American Epilepsy Society. Neurology 62: 1261–1273.

Fujiwara T, Sugawara T, Mazaki-Miyazaki E et al. (2003). Mutations of sodium channel alpha subunit type 1 (SCN1A) in intractable childhood epilepsies with frequent generalized tonic–clonic seizures. Brain 126: 531–546.

Gaily E, Liukkonen E, Paetau R et al. (2001). Infantile spasms: diagnosis and assessment of treatment response by video-EEG. Dev Med Child Neurol 43: 658–667.

Genton P, Dravet C (2008). Lennox–Gastaut syndrome. In: J Engel Jr, TA Pedley (Eds.), Epilepsy. A comprehensive textbook. 2nd edn. Lippincott, Williams and Wilkins, Philadelphia, pp. 2417–2427.

Genton P, Guerrini R, Dravet C (2000). The Lennox–Gastaut syndrome. In: H Meinardi (Ed.), The Epilepsies. Part II. Handbook of Clinical Neurology. Vol. 73. Elsevier, Amsterdam, pp. 211–222.

Glauser T, Kluger G, Sachdeo R et al. (2008). Rufinamide for generalized seizures associated with Lennox–Gastaut syndrome. Neurology 70: 1950–1958.

Grote CL, Van Slyke P, Hoeppner LA (1999). Language outcome following multiple subpial transection for Landau–Kleffner syndrome. Brain 122: 561–566.

Guerrini R (2006). Epilepsy in children. Lancet 367: 499–524.

Guerrini R, Aicardi J (2003). Epileptic encephalopathies with myoclonic seizures in infants and children (severe myoclonic epilepsy and myoclonic–astatic epilepsy). Clin Neurophysiol 20: 449–461.

Guerrini R, Carrozzo R (2001). Epileptogenic brain malformations: clinical presentation, malformative patterns and indications for genetic testing. Seizure 10: 532–547.

Guerrini R, Belmonte A, Genton P (1998a). Antiepileptic drug-induced worsening of seizures in children. Epilepsia 39: S2–S10.

Guerrini R, Genton P, Bureau M et al. (1998b). Multilobar polymicrogyria, intractable drop attack seizures and sleep-related electrical status epilepticus. Neurology 51: 504–512.

Guerrini R, Bonanni P, Rothwell J et al. (2002). Myoclonus and epilepsy. In: R Guerrini, J Aicardi, F Andermann et al. (Eds.), Epilepsy and Movement Disorders. Cambridge University Press, Cambridge, pp. 165–210.

Guerrini R, Moro F, Kato M et al. (2007). Expansion of the first polyA tract of ARX causes infantile spasms and status dystonicus. Neurology 69: 427–433.

Guerrini R, Cellini E, Mei D et al. (2010). Variable epilepsy phenotypes associated with a familial intragenic deletion of the SCN1A gene. Epilepsia 51: 2474–2477.

Hancock EC, Cross HH (2009). Treatment of Lennox–Gastaut syndrome. Cochrane Database Syst Rev 3 CD003277.

Hancock E, Osborne JP, Milner P (2002). Treatment of infantile spasms. Cochrane Database Syst Rev 2 CD001770.

Heiskala H, Riikonen R, Santavuori P et al. (1996). West syndrome: individualised ACTH therapy. Brain Dev 18: 456–460.

Hirano M, Kunz WS, Di Mauro (2008). Mitochondrial diseases. In: J Engel, TA Pedley (Eds.), Epilepsy: A Comprehensive Textbook. 2nd edn. Wolters Kluwer, Philadelphia, pp. 2621–2630.

Hoffmann-Riem M, Diener W, Benninger C et al. (2000). Nonconvulsive status epilepticus – a possible cause of mental retardation in patients with Lennox–Gastaut syndrome. Neuropediatrics 31: 169–174.

Hughes JR (2011). A review of the relationships between Landau–Kleffner syndrome, electrical status epilepticus during sleep, and continuous spike–waves during sleep. Epilepsy Behav 20: 247–253.

Hurst DL (1990). Epidemiology of severe myoclonic epilepsy of infancy. Epilepsia 31: 397–400.

Jambaqué I, Chiron C, Dumas C et al. (2000). Mental and behavioural outcome of infantile epilepsy treated by vigabatrin in tuberous sclerosis patients. Epilepsy Res 38: 151–160.

Jansen FE, Sadleir LG, Harkin LA et al. (2006). Severe myoclonic epilepsy of infancy (Dravet syndrome): recognition and diagnosis in adults. Neurology 67: 2224–2226.

Kaminska A, Ickowicz A, Plouin P et al. (1999). Delineation of cryptogenic Lennox–Gastaut syndrome and myoclonic astatic epilepsy using multiple correspondence analysis. Epilepsy Res 36: 15–29.

Kato M, Das S, Petras K et al. (2003). Polyalanine expansion of ARX associated with cryptogenic West syndrome. Neurology 61: 267–276.

Kivity S, Lerman P, Ariel R et al. (2004). Long-term cognitive outcomes of a cohort of children with cryptogenic infantile spasms treated with high-dose adrenocorticotropic hormone. Epilepsia 45: 255–262.

Kossoff EH (2010). Infantile spasms. Neurologist 16: 69–75.

Kossoff EH, Pyzik PL, McGrogan JR et al. (2002). Efficacy of the ketogenic diet for infantile spasms. Pediatrics 109: 780–783.

Kossoff EH, Hartman AL, Rubenstein JE et al. (2009). High-dose oral prednisolone for infantile spasms: an effective and less expensive alternative to ACTH. Epilepsy Behav 14: 674–676.

Kramer U, Sue W-C, Mikati M (1997). Focal features in West syndrome indicating candidacy for surgery. Pediatr Neurol 16: 213–217.

Lawrence KM, Mei D, Newton MR et al. (2010). Familial Lennox–Gastaut syndrome in male siblings with a novel DCX mutation and anterior pachygyria. Epilepsia 51: 1902–1905.

Lewis H, Wallace SJ (2001). Vigabatrin. Dev Med Child Neurol 43: 833–835.

Lortie A, Chiron C, Mumford J et al. (1993). The potential for increasing seizure frequency, relapse, and appearance of new seizure types with vigabatrin. Neurology 43: S24–S27.

Lux AL, Edwards SW, Hancock E et al. (2004). The United Kingdom Infantile Spasms Study comparing vigabatrin with prednisolone or tetracosactide at 14 days: a multicentre, randomised controlled trial. Lancet 364: 1773–1778.

Lux AL, Edwards SW, Hancock E et al. (2005). United Kingdom Infantile Spasms Study. The United Kingdom Infantile Spasms Study (UKISS) comparing hormone treatment with vigabatrin on developmental and epilepsy outcomes to age 14 months: a multicentre randomised trial. Lancet Neurol 4: 712–717.

Mackay MT, Weiss SK, Adams-Webber T et al. (2004). Practice parameter: medical treatment of infantile spasms: report of the American Academy of Neurology and the Child Neurology Society. Neurology 62: 1668–1681.

Marescaux C, Hirsch E, Finck S et al. (1990). Landau–Kleffner syndrome: a pharmacologic study of five cases. Epilepsia 31: 768–777.

Marini C, Mei D, Cross JH et al. (2006). Mosaic SCN1A mutation in familial severe myoclonic epilepsy of infancy. Epilepsia 47: 1737–1740.

Marini C, Mei D, Temudo T et al. (2007). Idiopathic epilepsies with seizures precipitated by fever and SCN1A abnormalities. Epilepsia 48: 1678–1685.

Marini C, Scheffer IE, Nabbout R et al. (2009). SCN1A duplications and deletions detected in Dravet syndrome: implications for molecular diagnosis. Epilepsia 50: 1670–1678.

Marshall CR, Young EJ, Pani AM et al. (2008). Infantile spasms is associated with deletion of the MAGI2 gene on chromosome 7q11.23-q21.11. Am J Hum Genet 83: 106–111.

Mei D, Marini C, Novara F et al. (2010). Xp22.3 genomic deletions involving the CDKL5 gene in girls with early onset epileptic encephalopathy. Epilepsia 51: 647–654.

Meisler MH, Kearney JA (2005). Sodium channel mutations in epilepsy and other neurological disorders. J Clin Invest 115: 2010–2017.

Milh M, Villeneuve N, Chapon F et al. (2009). Transient brain magnetic resonance imaging hyperintensity in basal ganglia and brain stem of epileptic infants treated with vigabatrin. J Child Neurol 24: 305–315.

Motte J, Trevathan E, Arvidsson JF et al. (1997). Lamotrigine for generalized seizures associated with Lennox–Gastaut Syndrome. N Engl J Med 337: 1807–1812.

Mulley JC, Scheffer IE, Petrou S et al. (2005). SCN1A mutations and epilepsy. Hum Mutat 25: 535–542.

Mytinger JR, Quigg M, Taft WC et al. (2010). Outcomes in treatment of infantile spasms with pulse methylprednisolone. J Child Neurol 25: 948–953.

Nabbout R, Gennaro E, Dalla Bernardina B et al. (2003). Spectrum of SCN1A mutations in severe myoclonic epilepsy of infancy. Neurology 60: 1961–1967.

Neal EG, Chaffe H, Schwartz RH et al. (2008). The ketogenic diet for the treatment of childhood epilepsy: a randomised controlled trial. Lancet Neurol 7: 500–506.

Nordli DR, DeVivo DC (2008). Inherited metabolic disorders. In: J Engel, TA Pedley (Eds.), Epilepsy: A Comprehensive Textbook. 2nd edn. Wolters Kluwer, Philadelphia, pp. 2603–2619.

Oguni H, Olivier A, Andermann F et al. (1991). Anterior callosotomy in the treatment of medically intractable epilepsies: a study of 43 patients with a mean follow-up of 39 months. Ann Neurol 30: 357–364.

Oguni H, Fukuyama Y, Imaizumi Y et al. (1992). Video-EEG analysis of drop seizures in myoclonic astatic epilepsy of early childhood (Doose syndrome). Epilepsia 33: 805–813.

Oguni H, Uehara T, Imai K et al. (1997). Atonic epileptic drop attacks associated with generalized spike-and-slow wave complexes: video-polygraphic study in two patients. Epilepsia 38: 813–818.

Oguni H, Hayashi K, Awaya Y et al. (2001). Severe myoclonic epilepsy in infants – a review based on the Tokyo Women's Medical University series of 84 cases. Brain Dev 23: 736–748.

Parrini E, Ferrari AR, Dorn T et al. (2009). Bilateral frontoparietal polymicrogyria, Lennox–Gastaut syndrome, and GPR56 gene mutations. Epilepsia 50: 1344–1353.

Patry G, Lyagoubi S, Tassinari CA (1971). Subclinical "electrical status epilepticus" induced by sleep in children. A clinical and electroencephalographic study of six cases. Arch Neurol 24: 242–252.

Pellock JM, Nordli DR, Dulac O (2008). Drug treatment in children. In: J Engel, TA Pedley (Eds.), Epilepsy: A Comprehensive Textbook. 2nd edn. Wolters Kluwer, Philadelphia, pp. 1249–1257.

Pellock JM, Hrachovy R, Shinnar S et al. (2010). Infantile spasms: a U.S. consensus report. Epilepsia 51: 2175–2189.

Piccirilli M, D'Alessandro P, Tiacci C et al. (1988). Language lateralization in children with benign partial epilepsy. Epilepsia 29: 19–25.

Pulsifer MB, Brandt J, Salorio CF et al. (2004). The cognitive outcome of hemispherectomy in 71 children. Epilepsia 45: 243–254.

Ragona F, Dalla Bernardina B, Granata T et al. (2011). Cognitive development in Dravet syndrome: a retrospective, multi center study of 26 patients. Epilepsia 52: 386–392.

Reiter E, Tiefenthaler M, Freillinger M et al. (2000). Familial idiopathic West syndrome. J Child Neurol 15: 249–252.

Riikonen R (1984). Infantile spasms: modern practical aspects. Act Paediatr Scand 73: 1–12.

Riikonen R (1996). Long-term outcome of West syndrome: a study of adults with a history of infantile spasms. Epilepsia 37: 367–372.

Riikonen R (2001). Epidemiological data of West syndrome in Finland. Brain Dev 23: 539–541.

Sachdeo RC, Glauser TA, Ritter F et al. (1999). Double-blind, randomized trial of topiramate in Lennox–Gastaut Syndrome. Neurology 52: 1882–1887.

Saltik S, Kocer N, Dervent A (2002). Informative value of magnetic resonance imaging and EEG in the prognosis of infantile spasms. Epilepsia 43: 246–252.

Scheffer IE, Berkovic SF (1997). Generalized epilepsy with febrile seizures plus. A genetic disorder with heterogeneous clinical phenotypes. Brain 120: 479–490.

Seri S, Cerquiglini A, Pisani F (1998). Spike-induced interference in auditory sensory processing in Landau–Kleffner syndrome. Electroencephalogr Clin Neurophysiol 108: 506–510.

Shewmon DA, Erwin RJ (1988). Focal spike-induced cerebral dysfunction is related to the after-coming slow wave. Ann Neurol 23: 131–137.

Singh R, Scheffer IE, Crossland K et al. (1999). Generalized epilepsy with febrile seizures plus: a common childhood-onset genetic epilepsy syndrome. Ann Neurol 45: 75–81.

Singh R, Andermann E, Whitehouse WP et al. (2001). Severe myoclonic epilepsy of infancy: extended spectrum of GEFS+? Epilepsia 42: 837–844.

Smith MC, Hoeppner TJ (2003). Epileptic encephalopathy of late childhood: Landau–Kleffner syndrome and the syndrome of continuous spikes and waves during slow-wave sleep. J Clin Neurophysiol 20: 462–472.

Striano P, Mancardi MM, Biancheri R et al. (2007). Brain MRI findings in severe myoclonic epilepsy in infancy and genotype–phenotype correlations. Epilepsia 48: 1092–1096.

Stromme P, Mangelsdorf ME, Shaw MA et al. (2002). Mutations in the human ortholog of Aristaless cause X-linked mental retardation and epilepsy. Nat Genet 30: 441–445.

Sugai K, Fukuyama Y, Yasuda K et al. (2001). Clinical and pedigree study on familial cases of West syndrome in Japan. Brain Dev 123: 558–564.

Sugawara T, Mazaki-Miyazaki E, Fukushima K et al. (2002). Frequent mutations of SCN1A in severe myoclonic epilepsy in infancy. Neurology 58: 1122–1124.

Tassinari CA, Rubboli G, Volpi L et al. (2002). Electrical status epilepticus during slow sleep (ESES or CSWS) including acquired epileptic aphasia (Landau–Kleffner syndrome). In: J Roger, M Bureau, C Dravet et al. (Eds.), Epileptic Syndromes in Infancy, Childhood and Adolescence. 3rd edn. John Libbey, London, pp. 69–79.

Thelle T, Gammelgaard L, Hansen JK et al. (2011). Reversible magnetic resonance imaging and spectroscopy abnormalities in the course of vigabatrin treatment for West syndrome. Eur J Paediatr Neurol 15: 260–264.

Trevathan E, Murphy CC, Yeargin-Allsopp M (1999). The descriptive epidemiology of infantile spasms among Atlanta children. Epilepsia 40: 748–751.

Vigabatrin Paediatric Advisory Group (2000). Guideline for prescribing vigabatrin in children has been revised. BMJ 320: 1404–1405.

Vigevano F, Cilio MR (1997). Vigabatrin versus ACTH as first-line treatment for infantile spasms: a randomized prospective study. Epilepsia 38: 1270–1274.

Vigevano F, Fusco L, Cusmai R et al. (1993). The idiopathic form of West syndrome. Epilepsia 34: 743–746.

Wallace RH, Hodgson BL, Grinton BE et al. (2003). Sodium channel alpha1-subunit mutations in severe myoclonic epilepsy of infancy and infantile spasms. Neurology 61: 765–769.

Wolff M, Cassè-Perrot C, Dravet C (2006). Severe myoclonic epilepsy of infants (Dravet syndrome): natural history and neuropsychological findings. Epilepsia 47: 45–48.

Wong M, Trevathan E (2001). Infantile spasms. Pediatr Neurol 24: 89–98.

Yakoub M, Dulac O, Jambaqué I et al. (1992). Early diagnosis of severe myoclonic epilepsy in infancy. Brain Dev 14: 299–303.

Handbook of Clinical Neurology, Vol. 107 (3rd series)
Epilepsy, Part I
H. Stefan and W.H. Theodore, Editors

Chapter 12

Epileptic syndromes with focal seizures of childhood and adolescence

TOBIAS LODDENKEMPER [1,2], ELAINE WYLLIE [1]*, AND EDOUARD HIRSCH [3]
[1] *Pediatric Neurology Center, Department of Neurology, Cleveland Clinic, Cleveland, OH, USA*
[2] *Division of Epilepsy and Clinical Neurophysiology, Children's Hospital Boston, Boston, MA, USA*
[3] *Department of Neurology, University Hospitals of Strasburg, Strasburg, France*

INTRODUCTION

The first description of "benign" focal epilepsy of childhood (BFEC) likely dates back to Martinus Rulandus in the 16th century (van Huffelen, 1989). Further delineation over the past 60 years led to the identification "benign" rolandic epilepsy (Nayrac and Beaussart, 1958) and subsequently of occipital subtypes and variants (Tassinari et al., 1985; Panayiotopoulos, 1989c). The pattern of spontaneous occurrence and resolution with age has led to the term of benign seizure susceptibility syndromes.

Recognition of the first benign localization related epilepsy syndromes also triggered a revision of the International League Against Epilepsy (ILAE) epilepsy classification at that time, as no idiopathic focal epilepsies were known until then (Commission on Classification and Terminology of the ILAE, 1989; Panayiotopoulos, 1989c). Since then, further symptoms and features have been characterized. In this chapter we will outline the three main forms of epileptic syndrome with focal seizures of childhood, including focal epilepsy with centrotemporal spikes and focal epilepsy with occipital spikes of the Gastaut and Panayiotopoulos type.

BENIGN FOCAL EPILEPSY WITH CENTROTEMPORAL SPIKES (BECTS)

Epidemiology

BECTS is the most frequent focal epilepsy syndrome among children, accounting for up to 23% of new-onset epilepsy (Cavazzuti, 1980; Eriksson and Koivikko, 1997; Chahine and Mikati, 2006). Incidence among children under 16 years has been estimated to be 21 per 100 000 (Heijbel et al., 1975a). There is a mild male predominance with a male to female ratio of approximately 3 : 2 (Beaussart, 1972; Ma and Chan, 2003). Patients have a predisposition to febrile seizures (16%) and present more frequently with seizures in infancy (1–8%) (Chahine and Mikati, 2006).

Clinical presentation and seizure semiology

Age of onset

Average age of onset is around 8 years, and a range of 3–13 years has been described (Gobbi et al., 2006). In almost all patients the condition remits around the age of 16 years (Kriz and Gazdik, 1978; Bouma et al., 1997).

Circadian pattern

Seizures frequently present at night, predominantly at the transition from wakefulness to sleep or from sleep to wakefulness (Wirrell, 1998). In 55%, seizures occur solely out of sleep and in 30% they occur only out of wakefulness. In the remaining 15%, seizures are seen during wakefulness and sleep (Beaussart, 1972; Wirrell, 1998).

Duration

Duration of seizures is seconds to minutes. Status epilepticus occurs in up to 17% (Wirrell, 1998).

Frequency

Seizure frequency ranges from single seizures (13%) to rare seizure recurrences within 1 year (66%) and frequent seizures (21%) (Lerman and Kivity, 1975).

*Correspondence to: Elaine Wyllie, M.D., Head, Pediatric Neurology Center, Cleveland Clinic, 9500 Euclid Ave, Cleveland, OH 44195, USA. E-mail: wylliee@ccf.org

Semiology

Clinical semiology frequently presents with a hemifacial sensory aura, such as perioral or intraoral paresthesias (tingling) or numbness, jaw and tongue stiffness, and at times a sensation of choking. Based on the age of the patient and on onset out of sleep, auras may be missed.

Unilateral face and limb motor features including clonic, tonic, or tonic–clonic seizures are present in 34% (Chahine and Mikati, 2006). These motor features specifically involve the lips, face, tongue, and limbs. The oropharynx and larynx are involved in up to 40%, and oropharyngeal motor features may present with guttural noises, gargling, grunting, or even a "death rattle"(Panayiotopoulos et al., 2008).

Additional features include drooling; parents frequently highlight this as the most prominent ictal clinical feature. Speech arrest or inability to talk occurs in 40% and this has been ascribed to laryngeal and oropharyngeal ictal features. Comprehension and sign language is frequently preserved. Patients remain conscious during the initial phase of the seizure unless seizures become secondarily generalized. Evolution into generalized tonic–clonic seizures occurs in 54% (Ma and Chan, 2003). Occasionally, postictal emesis occurs.

Neuroimaging

Imaging studies are not routinely recommended unless atypical features are present (Wirrell, 1998). In an unmatched case–control study, magnetic resonance imaging (MRI) abnormalities in patients with benign focal epilepsy of childhood and migraine patients were compared. Two independent blinded examiners rated the MRIs for abnormalities and found no significant differences between the two groups (Boxerman et al., 2007). A number of central nervous system (CNS) abnormalities have been reported in patient with BECTS, but these findings do not seem to alter the disease course.

EEG findings and sleep activation

Interictal EEG is characterized by a high-voltage, diphasic spike followed by a prominent slow wave (Holmes, 1992). These spikes usually present with a horizontal dipole and have a negative maximum at C3/T3 or C4/T4 and a positive frontal maximum (Graf et al., 1990) (Figs 12.1 & 12.2). Location of spiking may vary and may be located centrally (38%), centrotemporally (30%), centroparietally (16%), midtemporally (8%), or parietally (8%) (Holmes, 1992). In follow-up studies foci may shift towards or away from the centrotemporal area (Wirrell, 1998). A single generator tangential to the surface in the rolandic region has been suspected (Blom and Heijbel, 1975; Gregory and Wong, 1984).

Lateralization of spikes may be unilateral (60%) or bilateral (40%). Bilateral spikes vary in synchrony and symmetry (Holmes, 1992). Distribution between both hemispheres is equal (Loddenkemper et al., 2007). Background activity is normal in most cases. Bilateral or

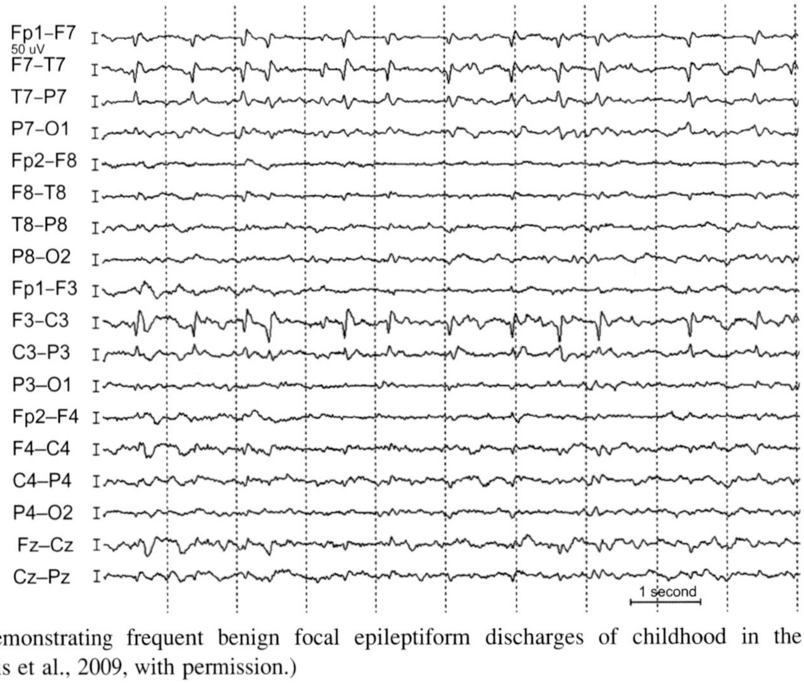

Fig. 12.1. EEG demonstrating frequent benign focal epileptiform discharges of childhood in the left centrotemporal region. (From Sarkis et al., 2009, with permission.)

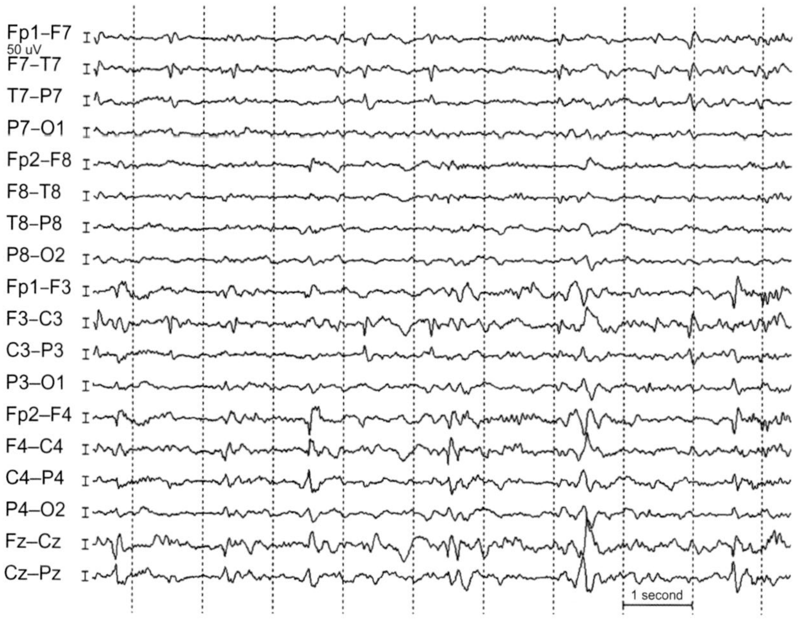

Fig. 12.2. EEG demonstrating independent benign focal epileptiform discharges in the left and right centrotemporal region. (From Sarkis et al., 2009, with permission.)

bisynchronous spike-and-wave complexes and associated "absence seizure"-like behavior can be seen (Sarkis et al., 2009).

Spikes are frequently activated by non-rapid eye movement (NREM) sleep (Blom and Heijbel, 1975; Dalla et al., 1975; Rose and Duron, 1984; Holmes, 1992) and decrease during REM sleep (Rose and Duron, 1984). Occasional interictal spikes during wakefulness may develop into almost continuous spiking, and bilateral spiking may be unmasked by NREM sleep. About 30% of patients have spikes only during sleep (Blom and Heijbel, 1975). Spike frequency does not correlate with severity, duration, or frequency of seizures (Blom and Heijbel, 1975; Holmes, 1992).

Ictal EEG has rarely been described. Although BFEC is one of the most common childhood epilepsies, few ictal recordings have been reported (Fig. 12.3) (Sarkis et al., 2009). This may be attributed to the fact that nocturnal seizures frequently occur unnoticed by the parents. Seizures are actually focal in origin. The generalized tonic phase occurs during secondary generalization of the EEG seizure pattern. Most cases in the literature report a focal onset of the seizure, predominantly in the centrotemporal region (Sarkis et al., 2009), although a few cases with a parietal origin have been reported (Saint-Martin et al., 2001a). Ictal EEG and clinical symptoms can be classified into three major categories: classical focal seizures, spike-and-wave-related symptoms, and paraictal symptoms. *Classical focal seizures* constitute the electroclinical expression of the development and the propagation of a focal cortical neuronal discharge. *Spike-and-wave-related symptoms* are brief neurological or neuropsychological phenomena having a relatively strict temporal relation with individual components of isolated focal or generalized spikes and waves. *Paraictal symptoms* consist of acquired progressive and fluctuating motor or cognitive deficits and are not directly correlated with Todd paralysis. Variability in clinical expression probably reflects the implication of different pathophysiological mechanisms, which in turn could explain differences in sensitivity to treatment (Saint-Martin et al., 2001a).

Neuropsychological manifestations

Up to up 53% of children with BECTS may present with neuropsychological abnormalities (Vinayan et al., 2005). Specific neuropsychological impairments are seen in auditory–verbal and visuospatial memory tasks, executive function, language, attention, learning, and behavior (Wirrell, 1998; Croona et al., 1999; Deonna, 2000; Ong and Wyllie, 2000; Saint-Martin et al., 2001b; Vinayan et al., 2005; Chahine and Mikati, 2006; Metz-Lutz and Filippini, 2006; Pinton et al., 2006; Sart et al., 2006; Fejerman, 2009; Volkl-Kernstock et al., 2009). Lateralization of interictal abnormalities is related to the type of cognitive deficit. More severe abnormalities are seen in patients with more severe and bilateral spiking (Chahine and Mikati, 2006).

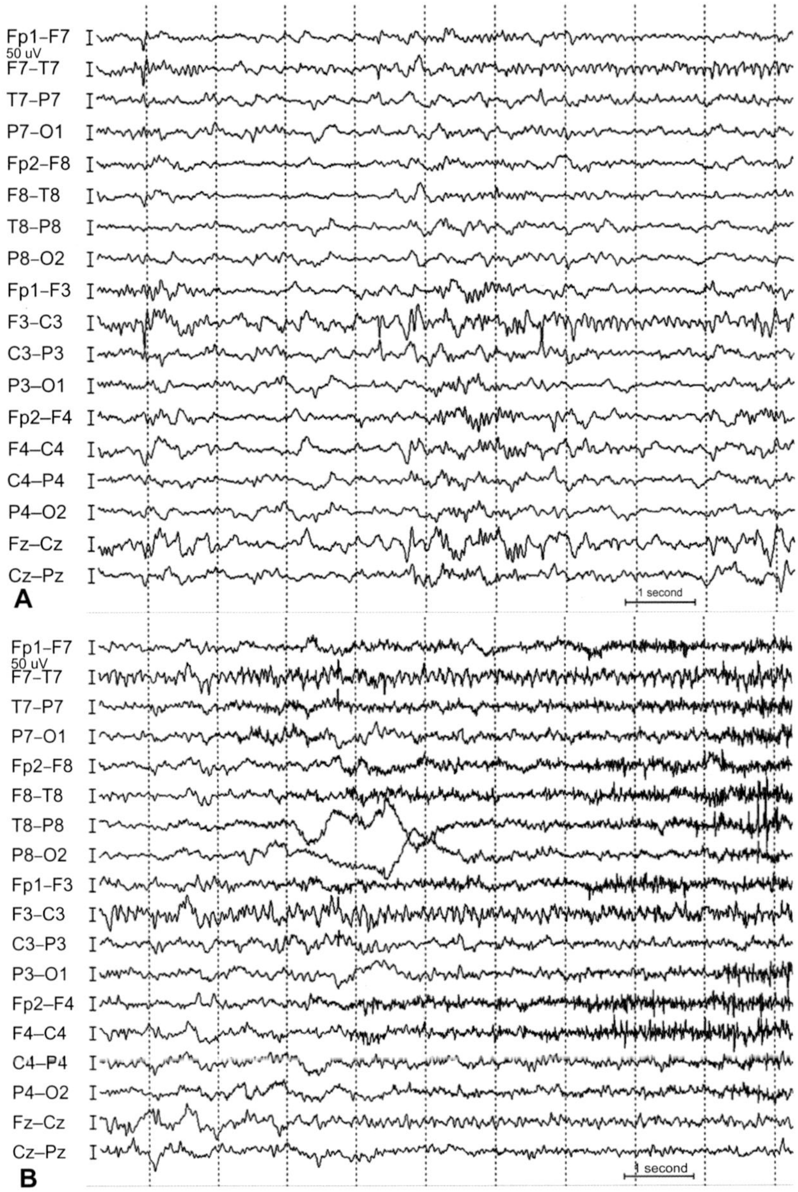

Fig. 12.3. EEG demonstrating the onset (**A**) and evolution (**B**) of a left centrotemporal EEG seizure in a patient with benign focal epilepsy of childhood with left centrotemporal spikes preceding the seizure onset. (From Sarkis et al., 2009, with permission.)

Genetics and pathophysiology

Linkage to a locus on chromosome 15q14 has been described (Neubauer et al., 1998). Additionally, increased prevalence of BECTS has been described in family members of affected children (Heijbel et al., 1975b; Doose et al., 1997; Wirrell, 1998). Segregation ratio analysis of centrotemporal spikes in rolandic epilepsy families suggested a highly penetrant autosomal dominant trait (Bali et al., 2007). A series of eight twin pairs did not show cotwin concordance (Vadlamudi et al., 2004), suggesting possible environmental or epigenetic influences (Rudolf et al., 2009). Metrakos and Metrakos (1961) also suggested variable penetrance based on age.

Pathophysiologically, the age-dependent presentation, the self-limiting course with resolution around puberty, and the familial clustering suggest a "hereditary impairment of brain maturation" (Doose and Baier, 1989; Holmes, 1992). The localization explains hemifacial as well as laryngeal and pharyngeal clonic seizures and somatosensory auras. Recent results from a genomewide linkage study suggested linkage to the elongator protein complex 4 gene (*ELP4*) (Strug et al., 2009).

Management and prognosis

After discussion of risks, benefits, and alternatives, treatment with antiepileptic drugs (AEDs) may be withheld in case of rare seizures, if seizures are mild and only nocturnal. Treatment may be indicated in children with seizure onset at age less than 4 years, in patients with daytime seizures, repeated generalized tonic–clonic seizures, or status epilepticus (Wirrell, 1998; Chahine and Mikati, 2006). Medication treatment options include clobazam, clonazepam, sultiame, levetiracetam, oxcarbazepine, carbamazepine, phenytoin, valproate, and phenobarbital among others (Chahine and Mikati, 2006). Seizures may be controlled in up to 65% of patients (Wirrell, 1998; Chahine and Mikati, 2006), although treatment at times does not affect seizure frequency and duration of the disorder (Ambrosetto and Tassinari, 1990). Despite medical intractability in 30–35% of cases, the condition usually remits by 18 years of age (Wirrell and Hamiwka, 2006).

Aggravation of BECTS caused by some AEDs (carbamazepine, phenytoin, valproate, and phenobarbital) happens only rarely. There is a small risk that drug-induced aggravation may occur only during certain periods, coinciding with spontaneous worsening of BECTS (Corda et al., 2001). The occurrence of atypical evolutions and risk of aggravation with some AEDs could be significantly higher in patients with combinations of at least three of six distinctive interictal EEG patterns (intermittent slow-wave focus, multiple asynchronous spike–wave foci, long spike–wave clusters, generalized 3-cycles/second "absence-like" spike–wave discharges, conjunction of interictal paroxysms with negative or positive myoclonia, and abundance of interictal abnormalities during wakefulness and sleep (Massa et al., 2001).

BENIGN FOCAL EPILEPSY WITH OCCIPITAL SPIKES OF GASTAUT

Epidemiology

Gastaut syndrome is seen in 0.15% of all focal epilepsies (Oguni et al., 1999). About 20% of patients present with a family history of epilepsy (Caraballo et al., 2008). Febrile seizures, migraine, and a history of BECTS have also been reported (Caraballo et al., 2008).

Clinical presentation and semiology

Age of onset

Age of first afebrile seizure ranges from 3 to 16 years, with a mean onset at around 8 years (Chahine and Mikati, 2006; Covanis, 2006; Caraballo et al., 2008).

Frequency

Seizures occur on average 1–2 times per month, and 20% have multiple seizures per week whereas 10% have fewer than 2 seizures per year (Caraballo et al., 2008).

Duration

Seizure duration is 1–2 minutes in the majority of patients (Covanis, 2006), but up to 40% of children have seizures lasting for 10–15 minutes (Panayiotopoulos, 1999; Tsai et al., 2001; Caraballo et al., 2008).

Circadian pattern

Patients usually have seizures out of wakefulness, but one-third may also have seizures out of sleep (Kivity et al., 2000; Covanis, 2006; Caraballo et al., 2008).

Semiology

Visual auras are the initial presentation in over 80% of patients (Caraballo et al., 2008). These present usually as stereotyped simple elementary visual pattern, such as circles or light flashes. Visual patterns may move through the visual field. Within patients, visual auras are usually stereotyped in morphology, pattern, location, and movement. Additionally, complex visual auras (9%) and ictal (51%) or postictal (21%) blindness may occur (Gastaut, 1982; Panayiotopoulos, 1999; Chahine and Mikati, 2006; Caraballo et al., 2008).

Motor manifestations include tonic eye deviation and head deviation (60%), and this frequently occurs after the visual auras. About 20% of patients also present with eyelid blinking. Additional features include evolution into unilateral motor seizures (45%) and generalized tonic–clonic seizures (20%) (Chahine and Mikati, 2006; Caraballo et al., 2008).

Autonomic features, such as ictal emesis and pallor, have also been described (Panayiotopoulos, 1999; Chahine and Mikati, 2006; Caraballo et al., 2008).

Ictal and postictal headache, associated with nausea, emesis, and photophobia, is a predominant feature in up to 50% of patients, and this occurs more frequently during or after prolonged seizures (Panayiotopoulos, 1999; Caraballo et al., 2008).

EEG findings

Interictal EEG presents with occipital sharp waves (Fig. 12.4). These are frequently attenuated by eye opening, but rarely occipital sharp waves nonreactive to eye opening are seen (12%) (Caraballo et al., 2008). Concomitant generalized (27%) as well as centrotemporal (24%) sharp waves have also been noted (Caraballo et al., 2008). Occipital spikes are sleep potentiated, and concomitant

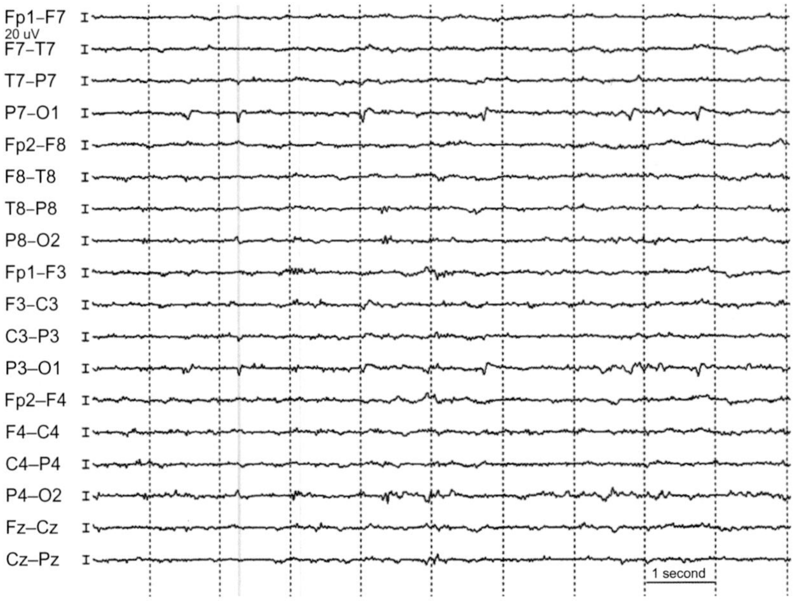

Fig. 12.4. EEG showing left occipital epileptiform discharges in a patient with benign focal occipital lobe epilepsy.

centrotemporal spikes are frequently activated and unmasked by sleep.

Ictal EEG has rarely been recorded, and presents in the few reported cases with an occipital EEG seizure pattern (Caraballo et al., 2008).

Neuropsychological manifestations

Neuropsychological manifestations of Gastaut-type benign childhood epilepsy with occipital paroxysms (BCEOP) have not been investigated. Previous papers did not mention major abnormalities.

Pathophysiology and genetics

Familial presentation of Gastaut-type BCEOP has been described (Nagendra and Rossiter, 1990; Kellerman, 1993), but no single gene has been identified.

Management and prognosis

Carbamazepine has been the most frequently recommended antiepileptic medication, although oxcarbazepine, valproic acid, phenobarbital, and clobazam have also been used (Gastaut, 1982; Verrotti et al., 2000; Chahine and Mikati, 2006).

Gastaut reported a remission rate of 92% by the age of 19 years in his series, and 53% remitted with the initiation of antiepileptic therapy (Gastaut, 1982). Response rates of up to 90% have been reported with treatment (Panayiotopoulos, 1999; Tsai et al., 2001). Although Gastaut-type BCEOP is generally considered more difficult to control than the Panayiotopoulos type, one trial did not find a statistical difference between the two (Tsai et al., 2001).

BENIGN FOCAL EPILEPSY WITH OCCIPITAL SPIKES OF PANAYIOTOPOULOS

Epidemiology

Based on results of a 15-year prospective study, Panayiotopoulos defined a more common subtype of benign focal occipital lobe epilepsy of childhood with onset under the age of 8 years (Panayiotopoulos, 1988, 1989a, b, 2001). He proposed a separation into early-onset (Panayiotopoulos) and late-onset (Gastaut) benign focal epilepsy of childhood (BFEC) (Table 12.1).

Panayiotopoulos syndrome is seen in 6% in 1–15-year-old and in 13% 3–6-year-old pediatric patients with focal epilepsy (Oguni et al., 1999; Lada et al., 2003). Based on these figures, the estimated incidence is 2–3 per 1000 children in the general population. Febrile seizures have been reported in 5–25% of patients (Caraballo et al., 2000, 2007; Lada et al., 2003), and patients may suffer from migraine in up to 15% of cases (Oguni et al., 1999).

Seizure semiology and clinical presentation

Age of onset

Age of onset may range from 1 to 14 years with a peak at 4–5 years (Caraballo et al., 2000; Kivity et al., 2000; Covanis, 2006).

Table 12.1

Comparison of benign childhood epilepsies with occipital paroxysms (BCEOP) of Gastaut and Panayiotopoulos type (modified after Chahine and Mikati, 2006, with permission)

	Gastaut-type BCEOP	Panayiotopoulos-type BCEOP
Epidemiology	0.15% of focal epilepsies in childhood	13% of focal epilepsies in childhood
Clinical presentation		
Age of onset (years)	3–16 (mean 8)	2–12 (mean 5)
Seizure semiology	Visual aura followed by automotor seizure, unilateral clonic, and versive seizure, with and without evolution into a generalized tonic–clonic seizure; postictal headache with or without nausea; rarely status epilepticus	Ictal emesis and eye versive seizure followed by autonomic seizures; subsequently unilateral clonic or generalized tonic–clonic seizure in 50%; frequently status epilepticus
Seizure timing	80% diurnal	80% nocturnal
Seizure frequency	Multiple seizures, frequently monthly or daily	Isolated seizures in up to 50%; variable
Seizure duration	Usually less than 5 min	Seizure duration 2–10 min in one-third; autonomic status lasting 30 min or more in up to 50%
Electrophysiology		
Interictal EEG	Occipital spikes; spikes can be blocked by fixation	Frequently occipital, but may be multiregional
Ictal EEG	Occipital α or β frequencies that slow down to the theta range	Semirhythmic occipital δ or theta frequencies
Dipole	Superficial	Deep
Prognosis	Remission in late teens in 60%; ongoing seizures in 40%	Remission in 60% within 1–2 years of seizure onset; most patients remit by 12 years of age

Circadian patterns

At least two-thirds of seizures occur at night, although concomitant daytime seizures may be seen in up to 30% (Caraballo et al., 2000, 2007; Lada et al., 2003).

Frequency

In a prospective series of 190 patients, 44% had a single seizure, 41% had 2–5 seizures, 10% had seizures every few months, and 5% had several seizures per month (Caraballo et al., 2007).

Duration

Seizures are frequently prolonged, lasting atleast 5 minutes, and up to one-third have status epilepticus lasting longer than 30 minutes (Caraballo et al., 2007). Status epilepticus may be the first presentation of this epilepsy in up to 20% of patients (Caraballo et al., 2007)

Semiology

Auras are seen in 15–20% of patients. Up to 10–20% of seizures may be preceded by a visual aura (Caraballo et al., 2000, 2007; Panayiotopoulos, 2001). Abdominal auras may occur in 15% of patients.

Autonomic features include pallor, ictal emesis, retching, nausea, and rarely incontinence or syncope. Ictal emesis is frequently the first semiological seizure manifestation and occurs in about 40–80% of patients (Oguni et al., 1999; Kivity et al., 2000; Panayiotopoulos, 2001; Koutroumanidis, 2002; Lada et al., 2003; Chahine and Mikati, 2006; Caraballo et al., 2007), and in 15–20% is accompanied or preceded by retching and nausea (Caraballo et al., 2007). Other associated ictal autonomic features include pallor in up to 90% of patients (Caraballo et al., 2007). Additional autonomic features may include urinary and fecal incontinence, syncope-like fainting episodes, and hypersalivation (Ferrie and Grunewald, 2001; Koutroumanidis, 2002; Lada et al., 2003; Chahine and Mikati, 2006; Caraballo et al., 2007).

Motor features include tonic eye deviation and unilateral clonic seizures. Tonic eye deviation occurs in 80–90% of all seizures and is frequently associated with tonic head deviation (Oguni et al., 1999; Kivity et al., 2000; Chahine and Mikati, 2006; Caraballo et al., 2007). Secondary generalization with evolution into a generalized tonic–clonic seizure is seen in one-third of all patients (Panayiotopoulos, 2001; Koutroumanidis, 2002; Lada et al., 2003; Caraballo et al., 2007).

Consciousness is usually preserved at the onset of seizures, although confusion may occur and up to 80% have partial obtundation or impairment of consciousness at the end of seizures (Panayiotopoulos, 1999; Caraballo et al., 2000, 2007, 2008).

A second "rolandic" seizure type with typical features of speech arrest and unilateral facial motor seizure was seen in 12.5% of patients, and these were seen either after resolution of seizures with ictal emesis and eye deviation, or at the same time, occasionally presenting with simultaneous symptoms within the same seizure (Koutroumanidis, 2002; Covanis, 2006; Caraballo et al., 2007).

Neuroimaging

Neuroimaging is usually normal (Caraballo et al., 2007), and abnormal neuroimaging is frequently used as an exclusion criterion for studies.

EEG findings

Interictal EEG presents with occipital spikes in 75%, extraoccipital spikes in 23%, and normal interictal EEGs in up to 2% (Caraballo et al., 2007). Patients with occipital spikes also had temporal (26%) and frontal (10%) spikes. Patients with extraoccipital interictal EEG findings only had predominantly temporal or frontal spikes (Caraballo et al., 2007). Sleep potentiation of spiking is frequent and has been described in up to 90% of cases (Gastaut, 1982; Lada et al., 2003; Caraballo et al., 2007).

Few *ictal EEG* recordings have been reported. Typical seizures may start with rhythmic spiking in the occipital regions, and then spread into temporal and frontal areas (Caraballo et al., 2007).

Neuropsychological manifestations

Patients may perform worse on neuropsychological tasks of global visual perception, visual-motor integration, and visual attention compared with age-matched controls (Germano et al., 2005). Patients may also present with lower IQ during the active phase of the disease (Oguni et al., 2001). There are no detailed information on neuropsychological features in Panayiotopoulos syndrome.

Pathophysiology and genetics

No genetic linkage has been described to date. A family history of seizures was found in 7–32% of patients, suggesting an underlying genetic predisposition (Oguni et al., 1999, 2001; Caraballo et al., 2000, 2007; Lada et al., 2003). Additionally, the high incidence of febrile seizures may be related to genetic predisposition (Caraballo et al., 2000, 2007; Lada et al., 2003). Abnormalities during birth may also play a role.

Management and prognosis

Most patients are treated with AEDs. Carbamazepine, valproic acid, phenobarbital, oxcarbazepine, and clobazam have been tried successfully (Chahine and Mikati, 2006). Up to 90% of patients become seizure-free after initiation of treatment (Caraballo et al., 2007). Rarely, exacerbation during carbamazepine treatment has been reported (Kikumoto et al., 2006).

In almost all patients, seizures remit within 1–6 years after onset, and the mean duration is 3 years (Panayiotopoulos, 1999). Evolution into another BFEC (Caraballo et al., 2007), and on one occasion into generalized absence epilepsy (Caraballo et al., 2004), has rarely been seen.

BFEC WITH OTHER LESIONS, BFEC VARIANTS AND ATYPICAL PRESENTATIONS

In addition to these classical and better delineated benign focal epilepsy syndromes of childhood, several authors recognize atypical benign focal epilepsies of childhood.

Definitions and delineation of these atypical variants vary and there is a significant overlap between different subcategories (Table 12.2). Atypical features may include changes in seizure semiology and frequency, sleep potentiation, and localization of interictal epileptiform discharges, as well as associated clinical symptoms and neurological or neuropsychological deficits. The following overview will be limited to major variations of this spectrum including atypical benign rolandic epilepsy, Landau–Kleffner syndrome, and continuous spike and waves during slow-wave sleep.

Atyical benign focal epilepsy of childhood

Atypical features may include early onset, occurrence of seizures during daytime only, different seizure semiology, frequency, and duration, and variations in neuropsychological, electrophysiological, or imaging findings (Table 12.2). Clinical presentation of BECTS may vary, and may include atypical features, such as leg clonic seizures and versive seizures, status epilepticus, seizures only during daytime, and postictal Todd's palsy (Wirrell et al., 1995; Vinayan et al., 2005) or BFEC with myoclonic seizures. Additional overlap may exist with acquired epileptic opercular syndrome presenting with prolonged episodes of drooling and oromotor apraxia (Roulet et al., 1989), continuous spike–waves during sleep syndrome (Tassinari et al., 1985, 2000), atypical benign partial epilepsy, pseudo-Lennox syndrome, and early-onset benign childhood seizure susceptibility syndrome with occipital or extraoccipital spikes (Gobbi et al., 2006). Additional subcategories that have been

Table 12.2

Clinical variations in benign focal epilepsies of childhood

Clinical features	Clinical syndrome variation
Clinical presentation	
Age of onset	BECTS with early onset
Circadian pattern	BECTS with seizures during daytime only
Seizure semiology	BECTS with myoclonia/negative myoclonus
Seizure frequency and duration	Status epilepticus of benign rolandic epilepsy
	Status epilepticus of benign occipital lobe epilepsy
Neurological and neuropsychological deficits	Landau–Kleffner syndrome
	Acquired epileptic opercular syndrome
	Early developmental dysphasia
	BECTS with affective symptoms/behavioral disorders
	BECTS with specific transient cognitive deficits
	ECTS/ESES with autistic regression
EEG findings	
Location of spiking	Benign parietal lobe epilepsy
	BECTS and absence-like spike–wave discharges
Morphology of interictal spiking	
Abnormal background	
Photosensitivity	Benign occipital lobe epilepsy with photosensitivity
	Occipital evoked spike epilepsy in childhood
Sleep activation	ESES
Imaging findings	
Structural lesion	BECTS with structural lesion

This table is not meant as a comprehensive list, but rather a list of examples. Additional variations in the clinical presentation are likely depending on delineation criteria.
(B)ECTS, (benign) focal epilepsy with centrotemporal spikes; ESES, electrical status epilepticus in sleep.

characterized by a variation include benign focal epilepsies that differ based on location of the discharge: benign parietal lobe epilepsy and benign childhood focal seizures associated with frontal and midline spikes, and others. Severe ends of this spectrum may be represented by Landau–Kleffner syndrome (Landau and Kleffner, 1957) and continuous spike-and-wave discharges during slow-wave sleep (Patry et al., 1971).

Landau–Kleffner syndrome (LKS) and continuous spiking during slow-wave sleep (CSWS)

In 1957, William Landau and Frank Kleffner described an epilepsy syndrome presenting with acquired language regression (Landau and Kleffner, 1957). Even then, they suspected that epileptiform discharges led to incapacitation of cortical areas important for language development. In a second landmark publication, Patry et al. (1971) described an epilepsy syndrome defined by generalized and almost continuous electrical status epilepticus during slow-wave sleep of at least 85% (Fig. 12.5). Subsequently, it became apparent that both syndromes share progressive cognitive dysfunction as a common feature (Van Bogaert and Paquier, 2009) and they were subsequently considered to be part of the same spectrum of a single syndrome by the ILAE Commission (Engel, 2006).

LKS is a rare epileptic encephalopathy that presents with regression in developmental language milestones, in particular comprehension, after the first 2 years of life. Age of onset may range from 2 to 14 years (Bishop, 1985; Steinlein, 2009). In addition to this acquired aphasia, other neuropsychological and behavioral abnormalities may arise, including hyperactivity and attention deficit, developmental motor deficits, and autism spectrum disorder as well as global developmental delay (Metz-Lutz and Filippini, 2006). About 30% of patients do not have any seizures, and clinical seizures frequently present with focal motor features and preserved consciousness (Beaumanoir, 1992). Seizures usually remit between 20 and 30 years of age, but cognitive deficits remain (Beaumanoir, 1992). EEG reveals sleep-potentiated centrotemporal spiking and slowing in this region. Neuroimaging is usually normal (Beaumanoir, 1992; Steinlein, 2009).

Epilepsy with continuous spike-and-wave activity during slow-wave sleep (Patry et al., 1971) is part of

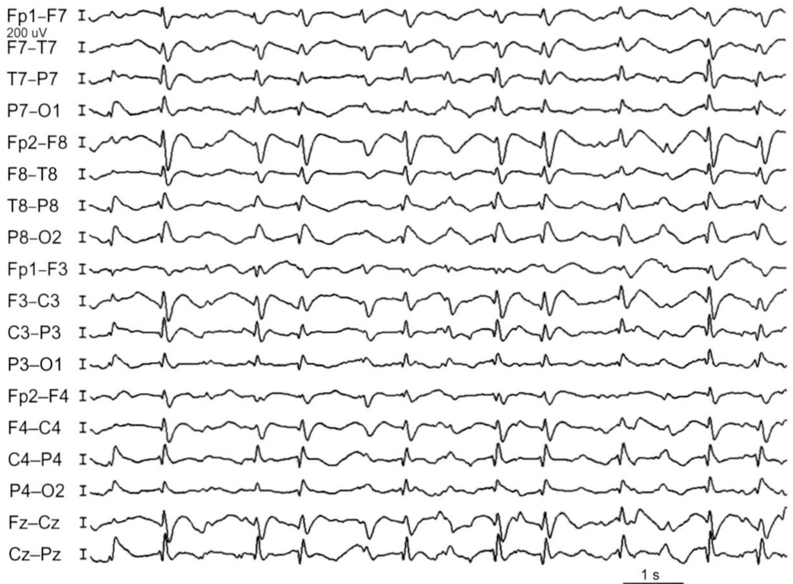

Fig. 12.5. EEG showing electrical status epilepticus during slow-wave sleep presenting with high-amplitude, generalized, 1–2-Hz continuous sharp-wave complexes. (From Loddenkemper et al., 2009, with permission.)

the LKS spectrum (Landau and Kleffner, 1957; Aicardi and Chevrie, 1982; Nass and Petrucha, 1990; Gobbi et al., 2006). Despite different clinical presentations, many of the above-mentioned epileptic encephalopathies can present with electrical status epilepticus in sleep (ESES) or sleep-potentiated spiking. A 0.5% incidence of CSWS among 12 854 children with epilepsy has been reported (Morikawa et al., 1989). Seizures start between the age of 2 months and 12 years, present with focal motor or generalized tonic–clonic seizures, and frequently occur at night (Tassinari et al., 1985, 2000). Many children experience developmental regression, lose developmental milestones, and present with deficits in language, socialization skills, memory, global intellect, and motor function (Tassinari et al., 2000). Although seizures and ESES remit with age, persistent and often severe cognitive deficits remain. Severity and persistence of neuropsychological deficits are thought to correlate with the duration of the ESES (De Negri, 1997). EEG presents with generalized sleep-potentiated spiking during 85% of slow-wave sleep (Tassinari et al., 1985), although some authors tend to include patients with regional sleep-potentiated spiking. Early developmental lesions, at times involving the thalamus, in particular periventricular leucomalacia, strokes, and malformation of cortical development, may be related to CSWS (Hirtum-Das et al., 2006; Loddenkemper et al., 2009). It has been suspected that abnormal epileptic EEG activity occurring during sleep may contribute to developmental delay and regression due to interference with sleep-related processes such as plasticity, learning, and memory consolidation (Tassinari et al., 2009).

Treatment of CSWS and LKS

No clear consensus on the optimal treatment of LKS and CSWS exists. As neuropsychological regression and continuous status epilepticus during slow-wave sleep, as well as frequent interictal epileptiform discharges, seem to be related, the EEG pattern has been targeted with AED treatment, including valproic acid, ethosuximide, and high-dose diazepam (Ohtsuka et al., 1992; De Negri et al., 1995; Ribacoba et al., 1997; Inutsuka et al., 2006). However, it remains unclear whether frequent spiking is cause of regression, just a surface phenomenon of regression and developmental delay, or an additional clinical presentation of a common underlying cause of epileptic activity and regression. Speech and occupational therapy are extremely important. In addition to anticonvulsants for seizures, encephalopathy has been treated with a 6–12-week trial of corticosteroids (Buzatu et al., 2009). Furthermore, intravenous immunoglobulin application has been tried (Arts et al., 2009). Medical treatment may provide some improvement in more than 50% of cases, but patients usually do not return to baseline. It remains unclear whether treatment can influence the long-term outcome with language and cognitive delay (Arts et al., 2009; Buzatu et al., 2009).

Multiple subpial transections (MSTs) provide a surgical treatment option (Morrell et al., 1995). MST consists of sectioning of the intracortical transverse fibers with sparing of the vertically directed pathways, and has been found to be a useful application in eloquent cortex (Devinsky et al., 1994). Because of the self-limiting process in many cases, surgical treatment has been controversial. Nonetheless, the devastating developmental outcome from Landau–Kleffner spectrum has prompted the use of multiple subpial transections as a surgical option (Morrell et al., 1995). Based on indications of a focal origin (Morikawa et al., 1989; Hirsch et al., 1995), resective epilepsy surgery has also recently been attempted (Loddenkemper et al., 2009). Data on treatment outcome are limited, and no data on neuropsychological outcome are available to date.

OUTLOOK FOR A UNIFYING CONCEPT OF BENIGN FOCAL EPILEPSY AND BENIGN EPILEPTIC ENCEPHALOPATHIES OF CHILDHOOD: BENIGN SEIZURE SUSCEPTIBILITY SYNDROMES

It has been suggested that febrile seizures, benign occipital epilepsies, and benign focal epilepsy with centrotemporal spikes are an age-related continuum. The clinical symptom complex has therefore also been termed benign seizure susceptibility syndrome (Panayiotopoulos, 1999). Interactions between brain development and maturation processes, as well as genetic influences, may play a role in the development of various childhood epileptic syndromes associated with language and cognitive deficits (Rudolf et al., 2009). Recent discoveries of the involvement of *ELP4* and other genes with possible roles in cell motility, migration, and adhesion have provided first insights into the complex molecular bases of childhood focal epilepsies (Roll et al., 2006; Strug et al., 2009). Maturation-related cortical hyperexcitability has been suspected and may be regulated by genetic influences as well as early developmental lesions involving subcortical neuronal migration (Rudolf et al., 2009).

The hypothesis of a spectrum is also supported by interesting interrelations with evolution of BECTS into BCEOP (Caraballo et al., 2008), concomitant presentation of BECTS and BCEOP Panayiotopoulos (Caraballo et al., 2004), evolution of BCEOP Gastaut into generalized absence epilepsy (Caraballo et al., 2008), as well as interrelations between generalized absence epilepsy and BECTS (Sarkis et al., 2009), and between BECTS and ESES (Chahine and Mikati, 2006; De Tiège et al., 2006). Further evidence is needed to determine underlying pathophysiological and genetic causes of this unique group of developmental epileptic encephalopathies.

REFERENCES

Aicardi J, Chevrie JJ (1982). Atypical benign partial epilepsy of childhood. Dev Med Child Neurol 24: 281–292.

Ambrosetto G, Tassinari CA (1990). Antiepileptic drug treatment of benign childhood epilepsy with rolandic spikes: is it necessary? Epilepsia 31: 802–805.

Arts WF, Aarsen FK, Scheltens-de Boer M et al. (2009). Landau–Kleffner syndrome and CSWS syndrome: treatment with intravenous immunoglobulins. Epilepsia 50: 55–58.

Bali B, Kull LL, Strug LJ et al. (2007). Autosomal dominant inheritance of centrotemporal sharp waves in rolandic epilepsy families. Epilepsia 48: 2266–2272.

Beaumanoir A (1992). The Landau–Kleffner syndrome. In: J Roger, M Bureau, C Dravet et al. (Eds.), Epileptic Syndromes in Infancy, Childhood and Adolescence. 2nd edn. John Libbey, London, pp. 231–244.

Beaussart M (1972). Benign epilepsy of children with Rolandic (centro-temporal) paroxysmal foci. A clinical entity. Study of 221 cases. Epilepsia 13: 795–811.

Bishop DV (1985). Age of onset and outcome in 'acquired aphasia with convulsive disorder' (Landau–Kleffner syndrome). Dev Med Child Neurol 27: 705–712.

Blom S, Heijbel J (1975). Benign epilepsy of children with centro-temporal EEG foci. Discharge rate during sleep. Epilepsia 16: 133–140.

Bouma PA, Bovenkerk AC, Westendorp RG et al. (1997). The course of benign partial epilepsy of childhood with centrotemporal spikes: a meta-analysis. Neurology 48: 430–437.

Boxerman JL, Hawash K, Bali B et al. (2007). Is Rolandic epilepsy associated with abnormal findings on cranial MRI? Epilepsy Res 75: 180–185.

Buzatu M, Bulteau C, Altuzarra C et al. (2009). Corticosteroids as treatment of epileptic syndromes with continuous spike-waves during slow-wave sleep. Epilepsia 50: 68–72.

Caraballo R, Cersosimo R, Medina C et al. (2000). Panayiotopoulos-type benign childhood occipital epilepsy: a prospective study. Neurology 55: 1096–1100.

Caraballo RH, Sologuestua A, Granana N et al. (2004). Idiopathic occipital and absence epilepsies appearing in the same children. Pediatr Neurol 30: 24–28.

Caraballo R, Cersosimo R, Fejerman N (2007). Panayiotopoulos syndrome: a prospective study of 192 patients. Epilepsia 48: 1054–1061.

Caraballo RH, Cersosimo RO, Fejerman N (2008). Childhood occipital epilepsy of Gastaut: a study of 33 patients. Epilepsia 49: 288–297.

Cavazzuti GB (1980). Epidemiology of different types of epilepsy in school age children of Modena, Italy. Epilepsia 21: 57–62.

Chahine LM, Mikati MA (2006). Benign pediatric localization-related epilepsies. Epileptic Disord 8: 243–258.

Commission on Classification and Terminology of the International League Against Epilepsy (1989). Proposal for revised classification of epilepsies and epileptic syndromes. Epilepsia 30: 389–399.

Corda D, Gelisse P, Genton P et al. (2001). Incidence of drug-induced aggravation in benign epilepsy with centrotemporal spikes. Epilepsia 42: 754–759.

Covanis A (2006). Panayiotopoulos syndrome: a benign childhood autonomic epilepsy frequently imitating encephalitis, syncope, migraine, sleep disorder, or gastroenteritis. Pediatrics 118: e1237–e1243.

Croona C, Kihlgren M, Lundberg S et al. (1999). Neuropsychological findings in children with benign childhood epilepsy with centrotemporal spikes. Dev Med Child Neurol 41: 813–818.

Dalla BB, Pajno-Ferrara F, Beghini G (1975). Proceedings: Rolandic spike activation during sleep in children with and without epilepsy. Electroencephalogr Clin Neurophysiol 39: 537.

De Negri M (1997). Electrical status epilepticus during sleep (ESES). Different clinical syndromes: towards a unifying view? Brain Dev 19: 447–451.

De Negri M, Baglietto MG, Battaglia FM et al. (1995). Treatment of electrical status epilepticus by short diazepam (DZP) cycles after DZP rectal bolus test. Brain Dev 17: 330–333.

De Tiège X, Goldman S, Verheulpen D et al. (2006). Coexistence of idiopathic rolandic epilepsy and CSWS in two families. Epilepsia 47: 1723–1727.

Deonna T (2000). Rolandic epilepsy: neuropsychology of the active epilepsy phase. Epileptic Disord 2: S59–S61.

Devinsky O, Perrine K, Vazquez B et al. (1994). Multiple subpial transections in the language cortex. Brain 117: 255–265.

Doose H, Baier WK (1989). Benign partial epilepsy and related conditions: multifactorial pathogenesis with hereditary impairment of brain maturation. Eur J Pediatr 149: 152–158.

Doose H, Brigger-Heuer B, Neubauer B (1997). Children with focal sharp waves: clinical and genetic aspects. Epilepsia 38: 788–796.

Engel J Jr (2006). Report of the ILAE classification core group. Epilepsia 47: 1558–1568.

Eriksson KJ, Koivikko MJ (1997). Prevalence, classification, and severity of epilepsy and epileptic syndromes in children. Epilepsia 38: 1275–1282.

Fejerman N (2009). Atypical rolandic epilepsy. Epilepsia 50: 9–12.

Ferrie CD, Grunewald RA (2001). Panayiotopoulos syndrome: a common and benign childhood epilepsy. Lancet 357: 821–823.

Gastaut H (1982). A new type of epilepsy: benign partial epilepsy of childhood with occipital spike-waves. Clin Electroencephalogr 13: 13–22.

Germano E, Gagliano A, Magazu A et al. (2005). Benign childhood epilepsy with occipital paroxysms: neuropsychological findings. Epilepsy Res 64: 137–150.

Gobbi G, Boni A, Filippini M (2006). The spectrum of idiopathic Rolandic epilepsy syndromes and idiopathic occipital epilepsies: from the benign to the disabling. Epilepsia 47: 62–66.

Graf M, Lischka A, Gremel K (1990). Benign Rolandic epilepsy in children. Topographic EEG analysis. Wien Klin Wochenschr 102: 206–210.

Gregory DL, Wong PK (1984). Topographical analysis of the centrotemporal discharges in benign rolandic epilepsy of childhood. Epilepsia 25: 705–711.

Heijbel J, Blom S, Bergfors PG (1975a). Benign epilepsy of children with centrotemporal EEG foci. A study of incidence rate in outpatient care. Epilepsia 16: 657–664.

Heijbel J, Blom S, Rasmuson M (1975b). Benign epilepsy of childhood with centrotemporal EEG foci: a genetic study. Epilepsia 16: 285–293.

Hirsch E, Pierre M, Metz-Lutz MN et al. (1995). The eponym "Landau–Kleffner syndrome" should not be restricted to childhood-acquired aphasia with epilepsy. In: A Beaumanoir, M Bureau, T Deonna et al. (Eds.), Continuous Spikes and Waves During Slow Sleep. Electrical Status Epilepticus During Slow Sleep. John Libbey, London, pp. 57–62.

Hirtum-Das M, Licht EA, Koh S et al. (2006). Children with ESES: variability in the syndrome. Epilepsy Res 70: S248–S258.

Holmes GL (1992). Rolandic epilepsy: clinical and electroencephalographic features. Epilepsy Res Suppl 6: 29–43.

Inutsuka M, Kobayashi K, Oka M et al. (2006). Treatment of epilepsy with electrical status epilepticus during slow sleep and its related disorders. Brain Dev 28: 281–286.

Kellerman K (1993). Benign epilepsy of childhood with occipital paroxysms: familial occurrence with three affected children. Epilepsia 34: 65.

Kikumoto K, Yoshinaga H, Oka M et al. (2006). EEG and seizure exacerbation induced by carbamazepine in Panayiotopoulos syndrome. Epileptic Disord 8: 53–56.

Kivity S, Ephraim T, Weitz R et al. (2000). Childhood epilepsy with occipital paroxysms: clinical variants in 134 patients. Epilepsia 41: 1522–1533.

Koutroumanidis M (2002). Panayiotopoulos syndrome. BMJ 324: 1228–1229.

Kriz M, Gazdik M (1978). Epilepsy with centrotemporal (Rolandic) spikes. A peculiar seizure disorder of childhood. Neurol Neurochir Pol 12: 413–419.

Lada C, Skiadas K, Theodorou V et al. (2003). A study of 43 patients with Panayiotopoulos syndrome, a common and benign childhood seizure susceptibility. Epilepsia 44: 81–88.

Landau W, Kleffner F (1957). Syndrome of acquired aphasia with convulsive disorder in children. Neurology 7: 523–530.

Lerman P, Kivity S (1975). Benign focal epilepsy of childhood. A follow-up study of 100 recovered patients. Arch Neurol 32: 261–264.

Loddenkemper T, Burgess RC, Syed T et al. (2007). Lateralization of interictal EEG findings. J Clin Neurophysiol 24: 379–385.

Loddenkemper T, Cosmo G, Kotagal P et al. (2009). Epilepsy surgery in children with electrical status epilepticus in sleep. Neurosurgery 64: 328–337.

Ma CK, Chan KY (2003). Benign childhood epilepsy with centrotemporal spikes: a study of 50 Chinese children. Brain Dev 25: 390–395.

Massa R, Saint-Martin A, Carcangiu R et al. (2001). EEG criteria predictive of complicated evolution in idiopathic rolandic epilepsy. Neurology 57: 1071–1079.

Metrakos K, Metrakos JD (1961). Genetics of convulsive disorders. II. Genetic and electroencephalographic studies in centrencephalic epilepsy. Neurology 11: 474–483.

Metz-Lutz MN, Filippini M (2006). Neuropsychological findings in Rolandic epilepsy and Landau–Kleffner syndrome. Epilepsia 47: 71–75.

Morikawa T, Seino M, Osawa T et al. (1989). Clinical relevance of continuous spike-wave discharges during sleep. In: Advances in Epileptology. Vol. 17. Raven Press, New York, NY, pp. 359–363.

Morrell F, Whisler WW, Smith MC et al. (1995). Landau–Kleffner syndrome. Treatment with subpial intracortical transection. Brain 118: 1529–1546.

Nagendra K, Rossiter M (1990). Benign occipital epilepsy of childhood: a family study. J R Soc Med 83: 804–805.

Nass R, Petrucha D (1990). Acquired aphasia with convulsive disorder: a pervasive developmental disorder variant. J Child Neurol 5: 327–328.

Nayrac P, Beaussart M (1958). Les pointes-ondes prerolandiques: expression EEG très particulière: étude electroclinique de 21 cas. Rev Neurol 99: 201–206.

Neubauer BA, Fiedler B, Himmelein B et al. (1998). Centrotemporal spikes in families with rolandic epilepsy: linkage to chromosome 15q14. Neurology 51: 1608–1612.

Oguni H, Hayashi K, Imai K et al. (1999). Study on the early-onset variant of benign childhood epilepsy with occipital paroxysms otherwise described as early-onset benign occipital seizure susceptibility syndrome. Epilepsia 40: 1020–1030.

Oguni H, Hayashi K, Funatsuka M et al. (2001). Study on early-onset benign occipital seizure susceptibility syndrome. Pediatr Neurol 25: 312–318.

Ohtsuka Y, Amano R, Mizukawa M et al. (1992). Treatment of intractable childhood epilepsy with high-dose valproate. Epilepsia 33: 158–164.

Ong HT, Wyllie E (2000). Benign childhood epilepsy with centrotemporal spikes: is it always benign? Neurology 54: 1182–1185.

Panayiotopoulos CP (1988). Vomiting as an ictal manifestation of epileptic seizures and syndromes. J Neurol Neurosurg Psychiatry 51: 1448–1451.

Panayiotopoulos CP (1989a). Benign childhood epilepsy with occipital paroxysms: a 15-year prospective study. Ann Neurol 26: 51–56.

Panayiotopoulos CP (1989b). Benign childhood epilepsy with occipital paroxysms: a 15-year prospective study. Ann Neurol 26: 51–56.

Panayiotopoulos CP (1989c). Benign nocturnal childhood occipital epilepsy: a new syndrome with nocturnal seizures, tonic deviation of the eyes, and vomiting. J Child Neurol 4: 43–49.

Panayiotopoulos CP (1999). Early-onset benign childhood occipital seizure susceptibility syndrome: a syndrome to recognize. Epilepsia 40: 621–630.

Panayiotopoulos CP (2001). Panayiotopoulos syndrome. Lancet 358: 68–69.

Panayiotopoulos CP, Michael M, Sanders S et al. (2008). Benign childhood focal epilepsies: assessment of established and newly recognized syndromes. Brain 131: 2264–2286.

Patry G, Lyagoubi S, Tassinari CA (1971). Subclinical "electrical status epilepticus" induced by sleep in children. A clinical and electroencephalographic study of six cases. Arch Neurol 24: 242–252.

Pinton F, Ducot B, Motte J et al. (2006). Cognitive functions in children with benign childhood epilepsy with centrotemporal spikes (BECTS). Epileptic Disord 8: 11–23.

Ribacoba R, Salas-Puig J, Solar DM et al. (1997). The efficacy of the valproic acid–ethosuximide combination in the continuous slow point wave syndrome during sleep. Neurologia 12: 335–338.

Roll P, Rudolf G, Pereira S et al. (2006). SRPX2 mutations in disorders of language cortex and cognition. Hum Mol Genet 15: 1195–1207.

Rose D, Duron B (1984). Prognostic value of EEG abnormalities observed during sleep in epilepsy with rolandic spikes (RSE). Rev Electroencephalogr Neurophysiol Clin 14: 217–226.

Roulet E, Deonna T, Despland PA (1989). Prolonged intermittent drooling and oromotor dyspraxia in benign childhood epilepsy with centrotemporal spikes. Epilepsia 30: 564–568.

Rudolf G, Valenti MP, Hirsch E et al. (2009). From rolandic epilepsy to continuous spike-and-waves during sleep and Landau–Kleffner syndromes: insights into possible genetic factors. Epilepsia 50: 25–28.

Saint-Martin AD, Carcangiu R, Arzimanoglou A et al. (2001a). Semiology of typical and atypical Rolandic epilepsy: a video-EEG analysis. Epileptic Disord 3: 173–182.

Saint-Martin AD, Seegmuller C, Carcangiu R (2001b). Cognitive consequences of rolandic epilepsy. Epileptic Disord 3: SI59–SI65.

Sarkis RA, Loddenkemper T, Burgess RC et al. (2009). Childhood absence epilepsy in patients with benign focal epileptiform discharges. Pediatr Neurol 41: 428–434.

Sart ZH, Demirbilek V, Korkmaz B et al. (2006). The consequences of idiopathic partial epilepsies in relation to neuropsychological functioning: a closer look at the associated mathematical disability. Epileptic Disord 8: 24–31.

Steinlein OK (2009). Epilepsy–aphasia syndromes. Expert Rev Neurother 9: 825–833.

Strug LJ, Clarke T, Chiang T et al. (2009). Centrotemporal sharp wave EEG trait in rolandic epilepsy maps to Elongator Protein Complex 4 (ELP4). Eur J Hum Genet 17: 1171–1181.

Tassinari CA, Bureau M, Dravet C et al. (1985). Epilepsy with continuous spikes and waves during slow sleep. In: J Roger, M Bureau, C Dravet et al. (Eds.), Epileptic Syndromes in Infancy, Childhood and Adolescence. John Libbey, London, pp. 194–204.

Tassinari CA, Rubboli G, Volpi L et al. (2000). Encephalopathy with electrical status epilepticus during slow sleep or ESES syndrome including the acquired aphasia. Clin Neurophysiol 111: S94–S102.

Tassinari CA, Cantalupo G, Rios-Pohl L et al. (2009). Encephalopathy with status epilepticus during slow sleep: "the Penelope syndrome". Epilepsia 50: 4–8.

Tsai ML, Lo HY, Chaou WT (2001). Clinical and electroencephalographic findings in early and late onset benign childhood epilepsy with occipital paroxysms. Brain Dev 23: 401–405.

Vadlamudi L, Harvey AS, Connellan MM et al. (2004). Is benign rolandic epilepsy genetically determined? Ann Neurol 56: 129–132.

Van Bogaert P, Paquier PF (2009). Landau–Kleffner syndrome: 50 years after. Epilepsia 50: 1–2.

van Huffelen AC (1989). A tribute to Martinus Rulandus. A 16th-century description of benign focal epilepsy of childhood. Arch Neurol 46: 445–447.

Verrotti A, Domizio S, Guerra M et al. (2000). Childhood epilepsy with occipital paroxysms and benign nocturnal childhood occipital epilepsy. J Child Neurol 15: 218–221.

Vinayan KP, Biji V, Thomas SV (2005). Educational problems with underlying neuropsychological impairment are common in children with benign epilepsy of childhood with centrotemporal spikes (BECTS). Seizure 14: 207–212.

Volkl-Kernstock S, Bauch-Prater S, Ponocny-Seliger E et al. (2009). Speech and school performance in children with benign partial epilepsy with centro-temporal spikes (BCECTS). Seizure 18: 320–326.

Wirrell EC (1998). Benign epilepsy of childhood with centro-temporal spikes. Epilepsia 39: S32–S41.

Wirrell EC, Hamiwka LD (2006). Do children with benign rolandic epilepsy have a higher prevalence of migraine than those with other partial epilepsies or nonepilepsy controls? Epilepsia 47: 1674–1681.

Wirrell EC, Camfield PR, Gordon KE et al. (1995). Benign rolandic epilepsy: atypical features are very common. J Child Neurol 10: 455–458.

Handbook of Clinical Neurology, Vol. 107 (3rd series)
Epilepsy, Part I
H. Stefan and W.H. Theodore, Editors

Chapter 13

Idiopathic generalized epilepsies

AMY KAO [1]* AND POOJA M. RAO [2]

[1] *Division of Neurophysiology, Epilepsy, and Critical Care, Center for Neuroscience and Behavioral Medicine, Children's National Medical Center, Washington, DC, USA*

[2] *Division of Child Neurology, Center for Neuroscience and Behavioral Medicine, Children's National Medical Center, Washington, DC, USA*

INTRODUCTION

The term "idiopathic" by definition refers to a state that is of "spontaneous origin, neither sympathetic nor traumatic" (Dorland's Illustrated Medical Dictionary, 26th edition, 1981). It refers to a condition that is a primary disorder, with its own independent pathogenesis and pathology. It is now further understood that idiopathic generalized epilepsies (IGEs) are genetically determined.

Overall, the different types of IGE manifest relatively early in life with the same seizure types, including absence, myoclonic, generalized tonic–clonic (GTC), and potentially atonic and tonic seizures. They are associated with normal neurological examination, intelligence, and magnetic resonance imaging (MRI) findings. They have similar electroencephalogram (EEG) findings, namely generalized epileptiform abnormalities with no abnormal background slowing. Based upon age of onset and predominant seizure type, individual syndromes within IGE are defined; however, the IGEs can be seen as a continuum of disorders that evolve into one another and have potentially overlapping genetic origins. Clinically speaking, differentiating among the specific subtypes of IGE is somewhat less important than diagnosing IGE from localization-related epilepsy or symptomatic/cryptogenic generalized epilepsy, as it has implications on treatment options and prognosis (Benbadis, 2005) as well as molecular research endeavors.

Prior to the first International League against Epilepsy (ILAE) classification in 1960, IGEs were classified as primary generalized epilepsies, including patients with various clinical seizures, as long as there was an absence of brain lesion, regardless of EEG features. Their current classification, as updated in 1989 and 2006, is based on strict clinical and EEG features. The list of syndromes is unchanged in the most recent revision by the 2005–2009 term of the Commission on Classification and Terminology of the ILAE, although modifications of terminology and approach to classification are recommended, based on the consideration of contributions from neuroscientific advances. The ILAE now includes a broad group of entities viewed as genetic epilepsies, characterized by seizures that have generalized (as opposed to partial) onset. The term "idiopathic" must now be supported by documentation of a genetic basis, or the understanding that the syndrome is a "direct result of known or presumed genetic defect." The Commission has proposed that instead of classification of epilepsies into *idiopathic, symptomatic, and cryptogenic* syndromes, that *genetic, structural/metabolic, and unknown cause* be terms used. The reader is referred to their report for a more extensive and interesting discussion of revised concepts (Berg et al., 2010).

Keeping in mind these ongoing changes in classification, Table 13.1 lists syndromes that can be considered IGEs and are currently recognized, as well as syndromes that likely fulfill criteria for IGE but are not yet recognized by ILAE (Nordli, 2005; Panayiotopoulos, 2005). This chapter limits its review to those recognized syndromes, and their clinical characteristics, EEG features, associated symptoms, and prognosis. In addition, recent genetic and neuroradiological findings are reviewed, and their impact on our understanding of underlying pathophysiological mechanisms discussed.

EPIDEMIOLOGY

The frequency of IGEs is high, making them an important subclassification of epilepsy. Keeping in mind the

*Correspondence to: Amy Kao, M.D., Attending Neurologist, Pediatric Neurology, Children's National Medical Center, Washington, DC, USA. Tel: +1-202-476-2120, Fax: +1-202-476-2676, E-mail: akao@childrensnational.org

Table 13.1

Syndromes of idiopathic generalized epilepsies (IGEs) recognized by the International League against Epilepsy (ILAE) (listed based upon approximate age of onset), of probable IGEs not recognized by the ILAE

Recognized IGEs
Myoclonic epilepsy in infancy (formerly benign myoclonic epilepsy in infancy)
Generalized epilepsy with febrile seizures plus
Epilepsy with myoclonic absences
Epilepsy with myoclonic–astatic seizures (Doose syndrome)
Childhood absence epilepsy
Juvenile absence epilepsy
Juvenile myoclonic epilepsy
Epilepsy with generalized tonic–clonic seizures
IGEs not recognized
Idiopathic generalized epilepsy with absences of early childhood
Perioral myoclonia with absences
Idiopathic generalized epilepsy with phantom absences
Jeavons syndrome (eyelid myoclonia with absences)
Autosomal dominant cortical tremor, myoclonus, and epilepsy
Familial infantile myoclonic epilepsy

problems of past epidemiological studies, including differences in classification and the inclusion of cryptogenic epilepsies, lack of EEG data, and lack of prevalence/incidence data, the general frequency is approximately 15–20% in cohorts of adults and children, and approximately 20% in children alone. However, the reported range, based on several studies from various countries, is 6.4–35.8%, as shown in Tables 13.2 and 13.3.

Table 13.3

Frequency of generalized idiopathic epilepsies in children cohort studies (adapted from Jallon and Latour, 2005)

Country	Population	Distribution (%)
Japan	1872	20.6
Sweden	155	26.5
USA	613	20.6
Lithuania	378	18.8
Finland	157	23
Norway	198	12.1
Norway	157	22
India	470	15.3
China	309	32

GENERAL MANAGEMENT OF IDIOPATHIC GENERALIZED EPILEPSY

The broad-spectrum drugs commonly used in the management of IGE are discussed immediately below. Data and practice specific to each syndrome are discussed later, in the individual syndrome elaborations.

Valproic acid (VPA)

VPA is effective against all three seizure types in IGE; absence, myoclonic, and GTC. The exact mechanism of action is not known, although the suggested mechanisms include an increased concentration of γ-aminobutyric acid (GABA), by blocking its metabolism, and an alteration of calcium T-channels and sodium channels.

The most serious idiosyncratic side-effects of VPA include hepatic failure, encephalopathy, aplastic anemia, pancreatitis, and bleeding disorders. Risk factors for

Table 13.2

Frequency of generalized idiopathic epilepsies in some adult and pediatric cohort studies (adapted from Jallon and Latour, 2005)

Authors	Country	Population	Frequency (%)	Comments
Gastaut (1975)	France	4591	28.4	Included "primary generalized epilepsies"
Joensen (1986)	Faroe Islands	194 (pediatric only)	34.5	Included "primary generalized epilepsies"
Loiseau (1991)	France	1006	16.3 vs 35.8	University hospital vs private practice
Manford (1992)	England	567	6.8	
King (1998)	Australia	300	22.3	Consecutive cases
Zarelli (1999)	Rochester	157	15.7	4-year inclusion
Jallon (2001)	France	1942	16 vs 27.4	Single seizure vs index seizures
Senanayake (1993)	Sri Lanka	1250	17.2	
Murthy (1998)	South India	2531	6.4	
Danesi (1985)	Nigeria	945	20.4	

fulminant hepatotoxicity include young age (particularly less than 3 years of age), polytherapy, and underlying metabolic disorder (particularly mutation in *POLG1*, which encodes mitochondrial DNA polymerase γ). Dose-related tremor, sedation, and thrombocytopenia are seen frequently. Other effects include increased appetite/weight gain, menstrual irregularities, polycystic ovaries, hyperammonemia, hypocarnitinemia, hyperinsulinism, hair loss, brain atrophy, and teratogenicity (Bourgeois, 2008b).

Ethosuximide (ETX)

Approved in 1957 in the USA, ETX is one of the oldest antiseizure drugs, and was determined to be the optimal first-line medication against childhood absence epilepsy in a recent National Institutes of Health-sponsored, multicenter, randomized, controlled trial comparing ETX, VPA, and lamotrigine.

ETX is effective mainly against absence seizures and is considered not to be effective against GTC seizures. The mechanism of action is not clearly known; the most accepted theory is that it blocks calcium T-channels in thalamic neurons.

A common side-effect is gastrointestinal upset; administration with food may minimize this. Other side-effects include headaches, sedation, and dose-related reversible granulocytopenia (Bourgeois, 2008a).

Lamotrigine

Approved in 1994 in the USA, the indications for lamotrigine include as adjunctive therapy for generalized seizures of Lennox–Gastaut syndrome and for primary GTC seizures in patients age 2 years and older. There are reports that it may worsen myoclonic seizures, especially in juvenile myoclonic epilepsy (JME) and severe myoclonic epilepsy of infancy/Dravet syndrome. There is suggestion of synergy when lamotrigine and VPA are administered together, with increased efficacy.

The mechanism of action is likely inhibition of voltage-activated sodium channels.

Side-effects include rash with rapid titration. This is most often benign, but may indicate Stevens–Johnson syndrome. Other adverse effects can include dizziness, diplopia, headache, nausea, blurred vision, and insomnia, although in general lamotrigine is well tolerated (Pellock, 2008).

Levetiracetam

Approved in the USA in 2000, levetiracetam's indications include adjunctive therapy in the treatment of primary GTC seizures in patients 6 years or older with IGE, and adjunctive therapy for myoclonic seizures in patients 12 years and older with JME. This drug has shown minimal drug interactions. Its mechanism of action seems to be related to modulation of a synaptic vesicle protein (Chaves and Sander, 2005).

Side-effects include mood disturbances such as aggression, anxiety, and psychosis, potentially with greater frequency in patients who are otherwise predisposed to psychological issues. It is generally well tolerated (Sankar and Shields, 2008).

Topiramate

Approved in the USA in 1996, topiramate's indications include adjunctive therapy for primary GTC seizures in patients aged 2 years and older, and initial monotherapy for primary GTC seizures in patients 10 years and older. Topiramate has shown minimal drug interactions with other antiseizure medications. Various mechanisms include sodium ion channel blockade, inhibition of excitatory glutamate-mediated neurotransmission, enhancement of GABAergic inhibitory synaptic transmission, enhancement of potassium channel conductance, and carbonic anhydrase inhibition.

Side-effects include paresthesia, anorexia, and nephrolithiasis, potentially via acidosis. Hypohidrosis or oligohidrosis may be asymptomatic or may present as heat intolerance. Cognitive deficits have also been reported (Glauser, 2008).

Clonazepam

Clonazepam is one of the most common benzodiazepines prescribed and has been found to be effective in controlling absence seizures, myoclonic and atonic seizures. Its main mechanism of action is by enhancing the inhibitory action of GABA.

Side-effects include drowsiness, ataxia, behavioral changes, excessive salivation (Farrell and Michoulas, 2008).

Zonisamide

Zonisamide has been used in Asia since 1989 as both monotherapy and adjunctive therapy in the treatment of partial, generalized, and combined seizures, but has approval in the USA only for adjunctive therapy of partial seizures. Because of several mechanisms of action, a broad-spectrum effect is suspected. However, there are no evidence-based data supporting its efficacy in IGE (Bergey, 2005).

Studies have found efficacy for zonisamide in absence seizures and seizures of JME, specifically myoclonic seizures. A survey of pediatric epilepsy specialists in the USA suggested that zonisamide may be used as a first-line drug for initial monotherapy in children with GTC seizures if the child also has myoclonic seizures (Wheless et al., 2005).

The exact mechanism of action remains unknown, although various mechanisms have been proposed, including blocking of T-type voltage-dependent calcium channels, inhibiting potassium-mediated glutamate release, and altering gene expression of neurotransmitter transporter proteins. Zonisamide is chemically related to acetazolamide, a carbonic anhydrase inhibitor, similar to topiramate. Although its antiseizure effects do not necessarily involve carbonic anhydrase inhibition, its side-effects do relate to this. There is also suggestion that zonisamide has the capacity to protect the brain from free radical-mediated injury.

Side-effects include hyperthermia related to oligohidrosis, renal calculi, behavioral effects such as aggression, agitation, anxiety, and hyperactivity, and metabolic acidosis (Kerrigan and Pellock, 2008).

Antiseizure medications to avoid

Antiseizure medications that target focal-onset seizures may be ineffective and actually exacerbate the seizures of IGE. There has been published evidence on carbamazepine, phenytoin, oxcarbazepine, and tiagabine in IGE, as well as gabapentin in childhood absence epilepsy. Use of these medications could create "pseudointractability" of a case of IGE (Benbadis, 2005).

GENETICS OF IDIOPATHIC GENERALIZED EPILEPSY

The recurrence risk of IGE for first-degree relatives is 5–8%, which is 10–15 times greater than in the general population.

A genetic component to the etiology of IGE is well recognized, but the mechanism of inheritance and specific genes involved are yet to be fully understood. Numerous candidate susceptibility genes, and single gene mutations that produce mendelian-inherited forms of idiopathic epilepsy have been found in some families; however, these have often not been replicated in the general population of patients with IGE subtypes. The majority of idiopathic epilepsies likely have complex inheritance. The model considered most likely at this time is a *polygenic* model, in which a number of loci interact to produce specific subtypes of IGE. To elaborate, a specific syndrome would be due to the interaction of a variation at a gene that is specific to the syndrome, and a group of susceptibility loci common to all IGEs that induce the general lowering of seizure threshold (Cavalleri et al., 2007).

Those monogenic familial syndromes have largely autosomal dominant transmission with reduced penetrance, and are associated with mutations in genes encoding for voltage- and ligand-gated ion channels. For instance, $GABA_A$ receptors are ligand-gated channels formed by several classes of subunits; mutations in $GABA_A$ receptor subunit genes (*GABRA1* encoding the $\alpha 1$ subunit, *GABRB3* encoding the $\beta 3$ subunit, *GABRG2* encoding the $\gamma 2$ subunit, and *GABRD* encoding the δ subunit) have been associated with a number of phenotypes of IGE, including childhood absence epilepsy, JME, febrile seizures, and generalized epilepsy with febrile seizures plus.

Specific susceptibility loci and mutations are discussed within the syndrome-specific sections.

CLINICAL SYNDROMES

Myoclonic epilepsy in infancy

Myoclonic epilepsy in infancy (previously known as benign myoclonic epilepsy) is a rare syndrome, representing 1% of epilepsies. It affects developmentally normal children, boys more than girls. Brief generalized myoclonus typically begins between ages 4 months and 3 years (up to 5 years), causing head-drop and upward/outward movement of the arms with flexion of the legs. The movement tends to be mild, with more subtle manifestations including a brief forward movement of the head, upward eye deviation, eye rolling, or eye closure. More severe manifestations are less common, but may involve throwing of objects from the hands or a fall. The myoclonus is brief (1–3 seconds), but may be longer in older children, with repeated jerks lasting 5–10 seconds. Some are stimulus-induced, by sudden noise or touch.

Although they occur more during drowsiness, the seizures do not tend to occur upon awakening, and should not occur in prolonged clusters as infantile spasms do. Patients may have rare simple febrile seizures, and there have been reports of GTC seizures during adolescence, although this may be exclusionary criterion for this diagnosis. In general, patients should not develop other seizure types.

EEG

The interictal EEG is usually normal, though focal (usually frontocentral and vertex areas) or generalized discharges (in rapid eye movement (REM) sleep) have been reported. Ictal EEG during the myoclonias shows fast generalized spike or polyspike waves at higher than 3 Hz. Photosensitivity may also be seen.

Genetics

There is suggestion of a genetic contribution, as a family history of febrile seizures or epilepsy is common, but exact genetic abnormalities have not been found.

Treatment

Valproic acid is the drug of choice, with seizures often easily controlled. Benzodiazepines and ethosuximide can also be used.

Prognosis

Myoclonic seizures in most patients last for less than a year. Duration greater than 6 years has been reported in patients who have not been treated appropriately. With long-term follow-up, few patients have mild to moderate degrees of cognitive impairment. Patients who respond quickly to treatment have a better outcome. Patients should be followed for development of other seizure types, in order to confirm the diagnosis, and to ensure that a different, more ominous, epilepsy syndrome is not present (Dravet and Bureau, 2005; Nordli, 2005).

Genetic epilepsy with febrile seizures plus (GEFS+)

Formerly "generalized" epilepsy with febrile seizures plus, GEFS+ is not a single clinical epilepsy syndrome, but is instead a designation that encompasses several phenotypes with shared genetic susceptibility. This diagnosis exemplifies the process by which the identification of mutations is defining clinical boundaries of a syndrome. At the mildest end of the spectrum of syndromes encompassed by GEFS+ is typical *febrile seizures,* characterized by brief (< 15 minutes) GTC seizures occurring in children between ages 6 months and 5–6 years. Also at the mild end of the spectrum is *febrile seizures plus*, in which febrile seizures continue beyond the limits of that typical age range, and afebrile tonic–clonic seizures also may occur. The GEFS+ spectrum also includes conditions in which other seizure types are present with febrile seizures or febrile seizures plus, namely absence, myoclonic, atonic, and partial. The more severe end of the spectrum includes myoclonic–astatic epilepsy and Dravet syndrome (severe myoclonic epilepsy of infancy). Patients with the phenotypes within GEFS+ usually have seizure onset within the first decade of life, with the majority beginning with febrile seizures. A clinical diagnosis is made on the basis of at least two persons with GEFS+ phenotypes in a family.

This diagnosis was originally recognized in large families demonstrating autosomal dominant transmission with low penetrance. However, most cases occur in small families, or sporadically. Family history may be significant for seizures on both sides of the family; complex inheritance and interaction of several genes is supported. Although this has obvious implications for genetic research, clinically this also implies low risk to siblings of affected patients.

It is in those families that abnormalities have been identified in genes encoding both voltage-gated (sodium channel) and ligand-gated ($GABA_A$ receptor) ion channel subunits (Scheffer et al., 2005):

1. *SCN1A* – gene for the $\alpha 1$ subunit of the neuronal sodium channel; more than 600 sequence variants, associated with mild to severe phenotypes, including severe myoclonic epilepsy of infancy
2. *SCN1B* – gene for the $\beta 1$ subunit of the neuronal sodium channel; associated in particular with phenotypes involving temporal lobe epilepsy
3. *GABRG2* – gene for the $\gamma 2$ subunit of the $GABA_A$ receptor, which forms part of the benzodiazepine binding site and mediates a link between the $GABA_A$ receptor and dopamine D5 receptor
4. *GABRD* – gene for the δ subunit of the $GABA_A$ receptor.

Despite the ongoing discovery of numerous mutations within these genes, association of genotype to phenotype has not been straightforward, and continues to be pursued. Modification by other genetic loci and environmental factors also must be contributing factors (Burgess, 2005). However, recently it has been discovered that missense mutations are found more often than truncating mutations in milder phenotypes (FS+); patients with truncating mutations have earlier age of onset of seizures than those with missense mutations, and patients in whom there is greater physiochemical differences between amino acids are more likely to have myoclonic seizures and earlier onset of seizures (Zuberi et al., 2011).

Clinical characteristics continue to be refined. In general, neurological examination and intellect are normal in the mild phenotypes. Neuroimaging is normal. EEG shows normal background with generalized epileptiform activity. Genetic testing is commercially available in the USA; however, the impact of positive results on treatment, prognosis, and counseling also remains to be refined.

Epilepsy with myoclonic absences

Epilepsy with myoclonic absences is a rare subtype as it may affect only 0.5% of all people with epilepsy. Past classifications likely combined symptomatic and idiopathic cases, as chromosomal anomalies, specifically Angelman syndrome, and prematurity, perinatal injury, congenital hemiparesis, and brain malformations have been reported associations in the past.

Onset occurs in infancy to early adolescence, at a median age of 7 years. Seizures typically occur several times per day and consist of alteration of consciousness of variable severity, with rhythmic myoclonic jerks which can be asymmetrical, and tonic contractions of predominantly the proximal arms resulting in elevation of the arms. When muscles of the face are involved, they tend to be around the chin and mouth as opposed to the eyelids. Duration has been reported as ranging from 8 to 60 seconds. The seizures are often provoked by hyperventilation or may occur during light sleep, awakening the patient. In some cases, autonomic manifestations such as a change or arrest of respiration and loss of urine have been reported. Other associated seizure types have been reported, including GTC, convulsive clonic, and atonic seizures.

EEG

Ictal recordings demonstrate a 3-Hz generalized rhythmic spike–wave which is bilateral, synchronous and symmetrical. Polyspikes may be intermixed. Interictal EEG shows generalized, focal, or multifocal discharges. The onset and the end of the discharges are typically abrupt, although there are cases in which the discharges end progressively with sometimes asymmetrical frontal δ waves.

Neuroimaging

Neuroimaging has been reported to be abnormal in 17% of the cases, most commonly demonstrating mild diffuse atrophy, without focal lesions. However, these reports may have included symptomatic cases.

Treatment

If only myoclonic absence seizures are present, valproic acid and ethosuximide may be useful. Addition of lamotrigine can be considered. In some cases, phenobarbital and benzodiazepines are effective.

Prognosis

Patients in whom myoclonic absence seizures are the only or predominant type of seizure have a better prognosis than patients in whom other seizure types occur, particularly GTC. Myoclonic absences will often cease within 5 years of diagnosis. Half of patients, although neurologically normal prior to the onset of the epilepsy, show cognitive difficulties later (Bureau and Tassinari, 2005; Nordli, 2005).

Childhood absence epilepsy (CAE)

This syndrome was earlier termed *pyknolepsy*, derived from the Greek term *pyknos*, meaning "clusters," referring to the tendency for the seizures to occur frequently throughout the day, in clusters. This is a fairly common subtype of IGE, with recent population/community-based studies finding a prevalence of 5.9–12.3% of children with epilepsy younger than 16 years. Girls constitute 60–70% of patients with CAE. Epidemiological data, of course, are influenced by the level of strictness of diagnostic criteria and differences in classification of patients into syndromes along the continuum of IGE.

CAE onset is usually between 4 and 10 years of age (peak 5–7 years) in children with normal intellect and normal findings on neurological examination. The condition is characterized by typical absence seizures which present as periods of abrupt loss of consciousness and arrest of activity, lasting 4–20 seconds, followed by abrupt cessation and return to previous activity. Although patients may take a few seconds to return to normal behavior, and may recognize that a lapse of time has occurred, there is no dramatic postictal alteration of consciousness. Random eye blinking or clonus of the eyelids, slight upward deviation of the eyes, mild myoclonic activity around the eyes, and mild motor automatisms may occur during the ictus; however, predominant eyelid/perioral/body myoclonus should not occur.

The typical absence seizures of CAE are provoked by hyperventilation (in 95–100% of patients); 3 minutes is the typical duration performed clinically. Interestingly, the seizures tend not to occur when the patient is stimulated by cognitive activity or attention, or physical activity.

Comorbidities

Although intelligence is normal, issues with attention and school performance may occur in many children with CAE. Reaction time and sustained attention have been found to be abnormal during brief discharges, which are not obviously correlated with clinical change. A history of febrile seizures has been noted in 20–23% of cases.

EEG

The seizure is associated with 3-Hz (2.7–4 Hz) generalized high-amplitude spike and slow-wave complexes, usually most prominent in the frontal regions. These discharges have a very regular appearance, although the first 1–2 seconds of the onset may be unusually fast. The frequency of the discharges may be fastest in the beginning of the seizure. Abrupt onset and offset on EEG correlates with the clinical symptoms. Background is normal, although some patients may show runs of high-amplitude 3-Hz slow activity in the posterior regions, decreased by eye opening and increased by hyperventilation, consistent with the named pattern, occipital intermittent rhythmic delta activity (OIRDA). Interictal discharges consist of single or brief generalized spike and slow waves, particularly during sleep. Asymmetries, which are not persistent or consistent, can be seen during ictal and interictal discharges; if persistently asymmetrical or focal discharges are seen in a frontal region, differential diagnosis of frontal lobe-onset seizures should be considered. Fragments of generalized discharges can also be seen interictally. See Figures 13.1–13.3 for examples of EEG findings.

Continuous video-EEG monitoring is necessary if the exact frequency of absence seizures needs to be determined, as parental report underestimates the frequency, due to the relative subtlety of clinical manifestations (Hirsch and Panayiotopoulos, 2005). Video-EEG is also helpful for determining whether there is a clinical correlate to the abnormal discharges seen.

Genetics

A family history of epilepsy is found in 15–44% of cases. There is clearly a genetic determination, although the exact mechanism of inheritance of CAE and the genes involved are unclear. Linkage analyses of families in which both childhood absence and other seizure types occur have found potential loci on chromosome 1 and

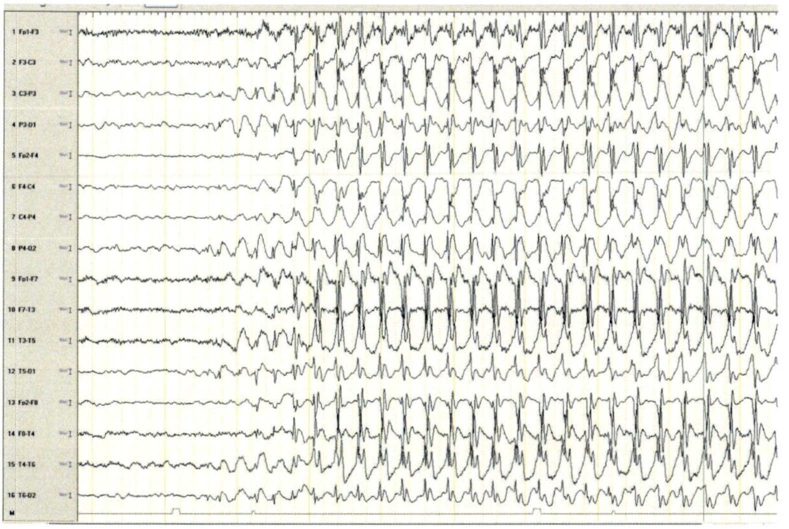

Fig. 13.1. EEG from a 7-year-old with staring, activity arrest after 20 seconds of hyperventilation. Biposterior onset is seen to the burst of regular 3-Hz generalized spike and slow wave (20 microvolts/mm sensitivity).

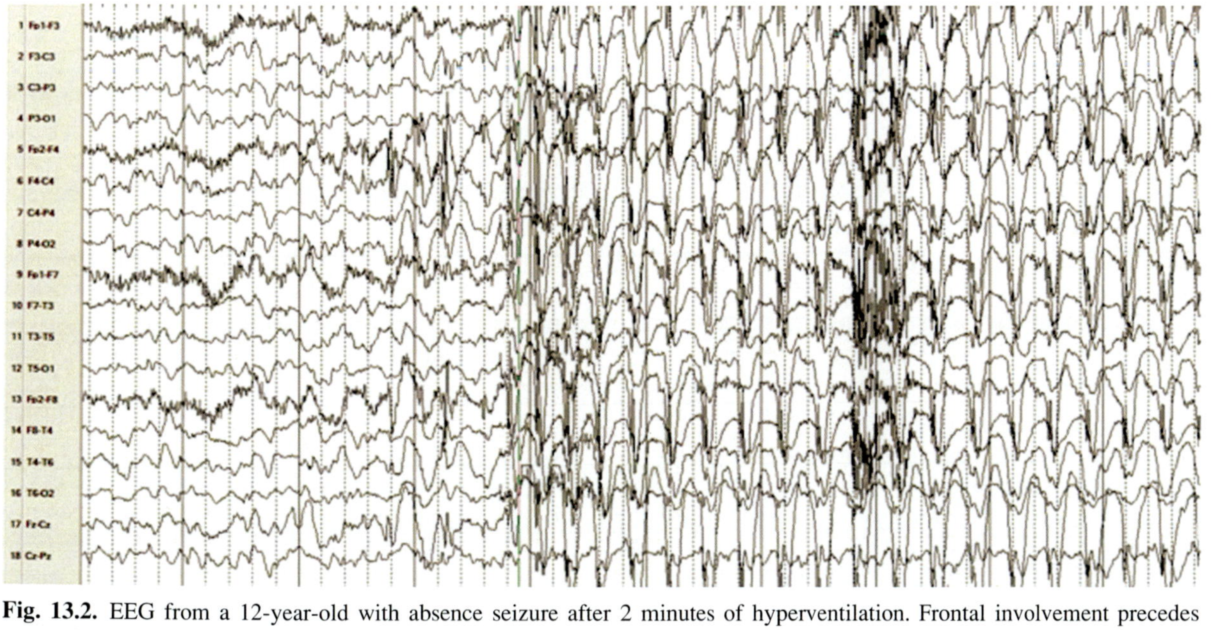

Fig. 13.2. EEG from a 12-year-old with absence seizure after 2 minutes of hyperventilation. Frontal involvement precedes generalized discharges.

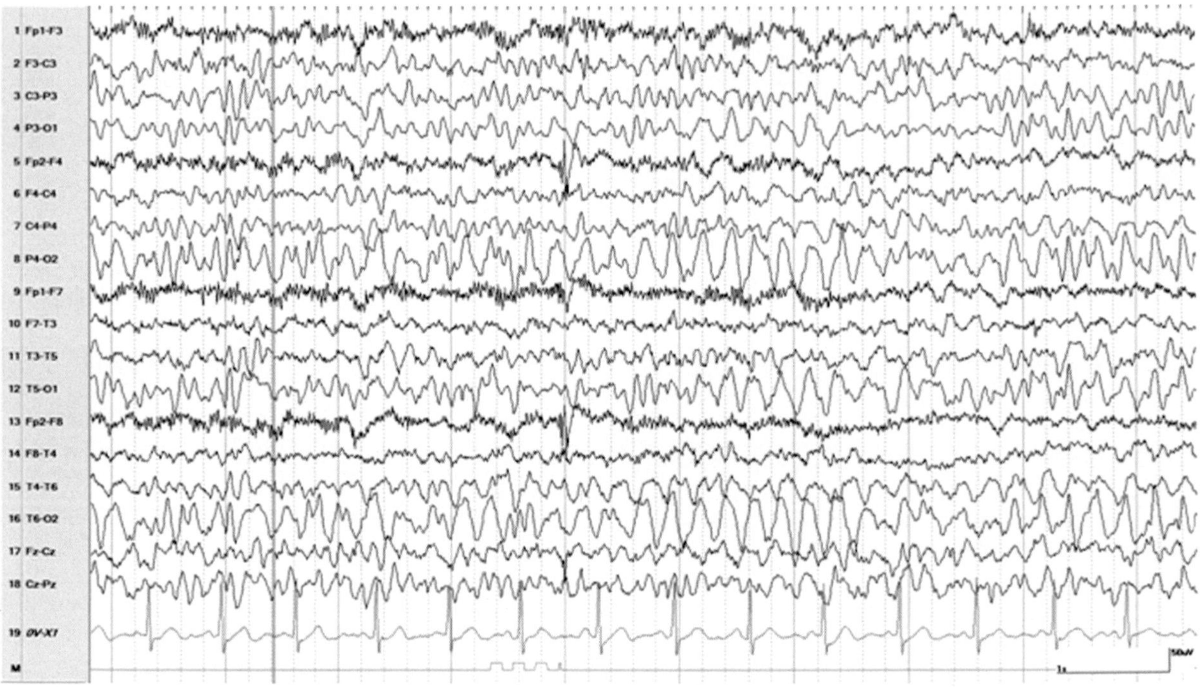

Fig. 13.3. Bioccipital rhythmic slowing (occipital intermittent rhythmic delta activity) in an 8-year-old with normal background and childhood absence epilepsy.

8q24. On 3q26, candidate gene *CLCN2* encodes voltage-gated chloride channel CLC-2, which may act in maintaining the low intracellular chloride concentration needed for inhibitory GABA responses. Mutations in *CLCN2* have been identified in families in which members had any of a number of phenotypes, including CAE, juvenile absence epilepsy, JME, and epilepsy with generalized seizures on awakening (Gardiner, 2005). Chromosomes 5q31.1 and 19p13.2 have also been implicated (Hirsch and Panayiotopoulos, 2005). As mentioned above, mutations in genes *GABRG2* on chromosome 5 and *GABRB3* on chromosome 15q11 have been described (Lachance-Touchette et al., 2010).

Missense mutations in the calcium channel *CACNA1H* gene have been found, occurring in the highly conserved residues of the T-type calcium channel gene. Other candidate genes include *CHRNB2* (encoding a subunit of the nicotinic acetylcholine receptor) and *ADAR* (encoding adenosine deaminase) on chromosome 1q21.3, as found in a boy with a family history of both parents with CAE and himself with onset of absence seizures at age 9 months (Muhle et al., 2010a), and *TRAK1* and *CACNA2D2* on 3p23-p14 (Gardiner, 2005; Chioza et al., 2009; Mullen et al., 2010).

Recent analysis of five consanguinous families with members with CAE, some with GTC seizures, looked at candidate genes *CACNG2*, *CACNA1A*, *CACNB4*, and *CACNA2D2*, which encode T-type calcium channels, but was negative (Abouda et al., 2010).

Pathophysiology and neuroimaging studies

Our understanding of the pathophysiological mechanisms behind the seizures and other features of IGE can be based largely on studies examining absence seizures. Historically, there have been a number of theories of the neuroanatomical origin of absence and primary generalized seizures. The *centrencephalic* theory hypothesizes that generalized spike and slow-wave discharges originate in the thalamus and upper brainstem. The *cortical* theory postulates that foci in the frontal lobes trigger seizures. Lastly, the *cortico-reticular* theory speculates that both cortex and thalamic processes are necessary (Szaflarski et al., 2010).

Many animal model studies have localized the processes behind absence seizures to the network of thalamocortical circuitry. This network consists of glutamatergic synapses between cortical pyramidal cells and nucleus reticularis thalami and of GABAergic synapses from nucleus reticularis thalami (NRT) to $GABA_A$ and $GABA_B$ receptors on thalamic relay neurons, in addition to recurrent GABAergic fibers from NRT neurons to $GABA_A$ receptors on adjacent NRT neurons. Low voltage-activated calcium channels (*T-channels*) are present in this network, and maintain the rhythmic burst ("oscillatory") firing of the NRT cells that, under normal conditions, generate activities such as sleep spindles. During absence seizures, excessive abnormal oscillatory rhythms generate spike and slow-wave discharges; these abnormal rhythms may be due to abnormalities of T-channels or increased $GABA_B$ function, leading to prolonged depolarization or deinactivation of T-channels. The pharmacological correlate is that valproic acid and ethosuximide suppress T-currents. Interestingly, however, when ethosuximide is administered directly into the thalami of the genetic rat model of absence seizure, the firing rate of NRT cells decreases, but at a slower and lower rate than when administered systemically, suggesting that the thalamus is not the only source of the spike and slow-wave discharges (Pearl and Holmes, 2008). In addition, lidocaine administered into the frontoparietal cortex of absence rats decreases the discharges (Szaflarski et al., 2010), suggesting a significant role for the cortex. For an inclusive discussion of calcium channel and thalamocortical physiology, the reader is referred to Khosravani and Zamponi (2006).

Neuroimaging provides a noninvasive, albeit indirect, means to study the localization of absence seizures in humans. Many studies support localization to a network of cortical and subcortical/thalamic regions. Increased cerebral blood flow in the thalamus and decreased flow in the cortex during absence seizures have been seen by Doppler studies. $H_2{}^{15}O$-positron emission tomography (PET) found broadly decreased blood flow to the cortex and increased flow in the thalami (Prevett et al., 1995).

Functional MRI (fMRI) using simultaneous EEG and blood oxygenated level-dependent (BOLD) signal as representation of metabolic activity has shown more specific, but generally similar, findings during absence seizures, despite many studies including patients with varied phenotypes of IGE. These have demonstrated BOLD signal increase in the thalamus and varied cortical regions, with a symmetrical decrease in signal in the frontal cortex, lateral and medial parietal cortex, cingulated, lateral frontal cortex, and basal ganglia (Berman et al., 2010). There have also been findings of increased BOLD signal in the ventrobasal thalamus and sensory cortex at onset of absence seizure, with decrease in BOLD signal in the temporal and motor cortices (Duncan, 2005).

With recent attempts to apply more stringent diagnostic criteria and limit subjects to those with CAE, studies have shown signal increases in the thalamus, frontal cortex, primary visual, auditory, somatosensory, and motor cortex, and decreases in medial and lateral parietal cortex, cingulate, and basal ganglia, suggesting a network involved in attention and sensorimotor and information processing, with dysfunction contributing to the impaired consciousness in absence seizures (Berman et al., 2010). Another study showed increased BOLD signal in the thalamus, with decreased signal in the parietal cortex, caudate nuclei, and dorsal pontine reticular structures of the brainstem. Those authors postulated that the variability in cortical regions involved in various studies might relate to phenotypic and genetic variability (Carney et al., 2010).

In another recent study, brief BOLD signal increases in the prefrontal and dorsolateral (frontal/parietal) cortex preceded signal increases in the thalamus, suggesting that the cortex initiates the spike and slow-wave discharges in absence seizures, and the thalamus maintains them (Szaflarski et al., 2010). Further studies will help to refine understanding of pathophysiological mechanisms; however, the current data have established that CAE is a systems or network disorder.

Treatment

In the past, there was a conspicuous lack of evidence-based data regarding the most effective treatment in CAE. The Cochrane Review found only four randomized controlled trials that looked at lamotrigine versus placebo or valproate versus ethosuximide, enrolling small numbers of patients and providing inadequate evidence (Posner et al., 2005). Thus, choice of medication was, as in many cases, founded upon experiential and anecdotal information. Based on a survey of 39 pediatric epileptologists in the USA in 2005, consensus was that ethosuximide was the treatment of choice, and that valproic acid and lamotrigine were also first-line options if ethosuximide failed. Open-label trials also have suggested efficacy for zonisamide and topiramate (Wheless et al., 2005). A similar survey of 42 pediatric epileptologists in Europe in 2007 found that European consensus ranked valproic acid as the treatment of choice, followed by ethosuximide, and finally lamotrigine (Wheless et al., 2007).

In 2010, however, the short-term (16–20 weeks), double-blind, randomized, controlled study by Glauser and colleagues was published. It investigated the effectiveness, tolerability, and neuropsychological effects of ethosuximide, valproic acid, and lamotrigine in children with previously untreated CAE. The study determined that ethosuximide (at a mean dose of 33.5 ± 15.3 mg per kg per day and mean trough level of 93 μg/mL) and valproic acid (at a mean dose of 34.9 ± 15.8 mg per kg per day and mean trough level 94 μg/mL) were significantly more effective than lamotrigine (mean dose 9.7 ± 6.3 mg per kg per day and mean trough level 7.8 μg/mL) in controlling seizures without intolerable side-effects. It also showed that valproic acid had significantly greater negative effects on attentional measures than ethosuximide or lamotrigine. These outcomes together suggest that ethosuximide is the optimal initial medication for monotherapy of CAE.

However, freedom from treatment failure due primarily to lack of seizure control or intolerable side-effects was only 58% for ethosuximide and 66% for valproic acid, demonstrating that even the determined best medication fails in a significant number of patients (albeit using strict failure criteria, including definition of seizure as spike–wave bursts lasting ≥3 seconds). Long-term follow-up of subjects is planned, particularly to monitor for development of GTC seizures and the effectiveness of ethosuximide in that situation (Glauser et al., 2010).

Thus, ethosuximide is the treatment of choice, but for patients in whom GTC seizures occur, valproic acid is indicated. Patients with seizures that do not respond to monotherapy can be tried on combination therapy. Other broad-spectrum medications used include topiramate, zonisamide, lamotrigine, levetiracetam, and clonazepam.

Prognosis

The average age of cessation of absence seizures has been noted to be 10.5 or 14 years. Some children may continue to have absence seizures beyond puberty. Typical absence seizures generally have a favorable prognosis; of patients with absence seizures only, more than 90% remit over time. However, GTC seizures may occur in 36–60% of patients with typical absence seizures in the age range of CAE; they occur 5–10 years after onset of the absence seizures, less frequently in those patients with onset of absence seizures before 9 years of age than in older patients. The presence of GTC seizures confers a somewhat worse prognosis, one study finding 77% of patients with absence plus GTC seizures remitting. Earlier age of onset and rapid response to medication also are favorable prognostic factors. Ultimate remission is more likely when the initial drug is successful than when it is not (Hirsch and Panayiotopoulos, 2005).

Unfavorable prognostic factors include features that are often considered exclusionary criteria for the diagnosis of CAE. These include cognitive impairment at diagnosis, abnormal EEG background, history of absence status epilepticus, presence of GTC or myoclonic seizures in the active stage of absences, eyelid or perioral myoclonia. A family history of generalized seizures in first-degree relatives also is a negative risk factor. The persistence of spike and slow-wave discharges, however, does not necessarily correlate with persistence of clinical seizures.

When strict diagnostic criteria for CAE (age of onset as described above, normal development, typical absence characteristics as above, typical EEG discharges as above) are followed, however, rates of seizure control are better, rates of remission are greater, GTC seizures occur in fewer patients, and treatment duration is shorter, with fewer patients receiving polytherapy (Grosso et al., 2005).

Juvenile absence epilepsy (JAE)

JAE illustrates in particular the view that IGEs are a continuum of syndromes that evolve into one another. In fact, there is some debate over whether JAE should be considered a separate syndrome, distinct from CAE. Differentiation from CAE is largely based on age of onset; other, more slight, clinical differences are also noted.

Onset of seizures in JAE peaks around the time of puberty, between 9 and 13 years, with no preponderance in either sex. Absence seizures tend to be less frequent but of longer duration than those in CAE. A case series examining video-EEGs in patients with JAE found milder or less rapid impairment of language, consciousness, and activity during absence seizures compared with during those in CAE. Absence seizures are often not triggered by hyperventilation.

There are also clinical similarities with JME. A large number of patients also have GTC seizures, often preceding the recognition of absence seizures. These tonic–clonic seizures are infrequent and tend to occur in the morning. Myoclonic seizures also occur in approximately 15–20% of patients.

EEG

Background activity is normal. Generalized, frontally predominant, spike or polyspike and slow-wave discharges occur interictally and ictally, with frequency faster (3.5–4 Hz) than in CAE. In general, more regularity is seen than in JME, but more fragmentation than in CAE. Duration of ictal discharges may also be longer than in CAE and JME.

Genetics

Patients with JAE frequently have a family history of epilepsy. It has been observed that a family history of CAE is more commonly seen than a family history of JME, suggesting the greater likelihood of a shared genetic etiology between JAE and CAE than between JAE and JME. Relationship of JAE to mutations in the kainite-selective glutamate receptor gene *GRIK1* and calcium channel subunit genes has been suggested, but not consistently supported.

Treatment

JAE has a good response to therapy even with the presence of GTC seizures. However, in a cross-sectional study of adults and teenagers with absence seizures and continued treatment, all patients who had absence seizures only were seizure-free, compared with 87% of those who had fewer than 10 GTC seizures and 76% of those with more than 10 GTC seizures.

The presence of myoclonic seizures did not affect response to treatment.

US and European expert opinion has found valproic acid and lamotrigine to be first-line options, reflecting efficacy for both absence and GTC seizures. If valproic acid fails, experts would then treat with lamotrigine. Topiramate and zonisamide are also considered "high" second-line options in the USA (Wheless et al., 2005, 2007). Carbamazepine and oxcarbazepine may aggravate seizures in JAE.

Prognosis

Seizure control is achieved in most patients, although patients may require long-term treatment (Nordli, 2005; Wolf and Inoue, 2005).

Epilepsy with myoclonic–astatic seizures (Doose syndrome)

This syndrome was first proposed by Doose as "myoclonic astatic petit mal," implying the presence of several seizure types. The name was ultimately changed to myoclonic–astatic epilepsy (MAE), referring to the presence of its major and unique seizure type. MAE was originally classified as a cryptogenic epilepsy, but now is considered an IGE. It has been estimated that MAE accounts for 1–2% of all childhood epilepsies. There is a male predominance. Age of onset is between 1.5 and 5 years.

The seizures in this syndrome are characterized by symmetrical, brief, generalized myoclonic jerks, occurring in an isolated fashion or in a short series of two or three jerks, then followed by a quick period of loss of muscle tone, which causes a drop. The seizures often present with a sudden fall. If the child is sitting, he or she falls forward or backward depending on the center of gravity. Proximal muscles are more involved by the myoclonus; a mild manifestation can be a head nod. The child recovers immediately from the seizure. However, in some cases, the seizures may recur repeatedly, constituting status epilepticus, lasting for hours or days. Later in the course, seizures may occur not only during wakefulness but also during nighttime sleep.

Tonic–clonic and absence seizures also occur in the majority of patients with MAE. Tonic–clonic seizures are often the first seizure type to manifest, sometimes preceding myoclonic seizures by months to years. Febrile seizures specifically may occur before afebrile seizures present. Atypical absence seizures occur, involving loss of muscle tone. Patients with MAE are at risk of absence/nonconvulsive status epilepticus, during which they may be encephalopathic with frequent myoclonus. Atonic and tonic seizures may also occur. Tonic seizures occur particularly during sleep or as tonic–vibratory seizures at the end of nighttime sleep. Some authors, however, have used the presence of tonic seizures as exclusion criteria for MAE, in order to differentiate it from other "catastrophic" or symptomatic epilepsy syndromes, namely Lennox–Gastaut syndrome, which is characterized by mixed seizure types, slow spike and wave on EEG, and mental retardation.

Comorbidities

Mild behavioral disorders, such as hyperactivity, are frequently associated. The majority (up to 80%) of patients have normal IQ on long-term follow-up. However, some have deterioration of cognitive abilities with development of mental retardation, as discussed more below.

EEG

The EEG initially shows a normal EEG background but may develop background slowing as the disease progresses. The myoclonic jerks are correlated with a single generalized spike or polyspike and slow-wave discharge. During the subsequent astatic or atonic phase, rhythmic 2–4-Hz spike or polyspike and slow-wave discharges occur. During the tonic phase of a tonic–clonic seizure, there is diffuse rhythmic fast activity (10–15 Hz) that may then evolve into rhythmic runs of sharp, spike, or polyspike–wave discharges during the subsequent clonic phase.

Genetics

Up to one-third of patients with MAE have a family history of epilepsy or seizures, including febrile seizures and Dravet syndrome. Some members in GEFS+ families have myoclonic–astatic seizures, suggesting that these various phenotypes and syndromes share susceptibility genes. No definite monogenic etiology has been found for MAE thus far.

Treatment

Historically, the first drug of choice is valproic acid. Other broad-spectrum choices include valproic acid plus lamotrigine, valproic acid plus benzodiazepine, ethosuximide (especially for the myoclonic and absence seizures), and felbamate. Phenobarbital has been suggested as effective acute treatment for frequent GTC seizures. Steroids have been suggested for the epileptic encephalopathy seen with refractory myoclonic–astatic seizures or nonconvulsive status epilepticus. Carbamazepine and vigabatrin may exacerbate seizures and even trigger myoclonic status epilepticus.

A nonpharmacological option that is quite effective in MAE in particular is the ketogenic diet; seizures may be controlled on the ketogenic diet alone or a combination of ketogenic diet and medication (Guerrini et al., 2005; Nordli, 2005).

Prognosis

The prognosis is variable and difficult to predict, relating both to seizure remission and to development of cognitive and behavioral issues. Development is normal prior to the onset of seizures. At least half continue to have normal IQ, but others develop mental retardation. In general, if the seizures cease, cognitive outcome is good. If seizures continue, cognitive outcome is guarded. However, although electroclinical abnormalities (e.g., myoclonic status epilepticus) may cause temporary cognitive and behavioral decline, this is not necessarily associated with negative prognosis. The ultimate outcome may be influenced by the length and frequency of these periods of worsening. In this way, early and effective treatment thus may improve cognitive outcome (Filippini et al., 2006).

Seizure remission also occurs in greater than 50% of patients within 3 years (age 3–8 years), and may be found even when seizures occur in multiple types and with high frequency. The occurrence of nocturnal tonic/tonic vibratory seizures is considered to be a negative prognostic factor; however, this is not consistent (Guerrini et al., 2005; Nordli, 2005). Other potentially unfavorable features include duration of seizures of 3 years or more and EEG with long periods of epileptiform discharges and loss of normal background rhythms over several minutes (Filippini et al., 2006).

Juvenile myoclonic epilepsy (JME)

JME is a common type of epilepsy that bridges the patient populations of pediatric and adult neurologists. It accounts for 5–10% of all epilepsy cases and 20–27% of all IGE cases. Studies conflict as to gender predominance; data and anecdotal experience support a female predominance. As mentioned previously, clinical overlap with JAE is noted. JME presents in the majority of patients between 12 and 18 years of age (range 8–26 years), and is characterized by typical absence, myoclonic, and GTC seizures. Absence seizures begin earlier (mean 11.5 years) than myoclonic and GTC seizures (mean 15.5 years) (Nordli, 2005). Patients often are referred to the neurologist after first GTC seizure. A history of simple febrile seizures is also seen in 5–10% of patients with JME.

The defining seizures tend to occur more in the mornings within the first half-hour of sleep, or after waking from a nap, and are described as bilateral, single or repetitive, arrhythmic, irregular myoclonic jerks, primarily in the arms (Commission on Classification and Terminology of the ILAE, 1989), which can lead to dropping or flinging of objects, or rarely to a sudden fall if more severe. There is, however, no associated loss of consciousness, even during episodes of myoclonic status epilepticus, which have been reported in 7% of patients. Myoclonic jerks are sometimes considered to be asymmetrical.

GTC seizures occur in 80–95% of patients with JME. They are typically preceded by a cluster of myoclonic jerks which evolve with increasing amplitude and frequency into a GTC seizure, with a sequence described as clonic–tonic–clonic. Absence seizures have been described in 10–38% of patients with JME.

Seizures are commonly triggered by sleep deprivation, stress, and alcohol consumption, factors that adolescents and young adults may likely subject themselves to. Photosensitivity manifesting with a photoparoxysmal response on EEG has been noted in one-third to one-half of patients with JME, although clinical photosensitivity (i.e., triggering of seizures by visual stimuli in the environment) is less frequent. In up to half of patients with JME, seizures have also been precipitated by activities such as writing, reading, and mental/written calculation, suggesting a connection between JME and reflex epilepsies. In particular, perioral myoclonic jerks of the mouth, tongue, or face, similar to those characterizing reading epilepsy, can be seen in JME, but more commonly with talking than with reading (Thomas et al., 2005).

Comorbidities

It has been speculated that the presence of clinical or subclinical discharges over time can lead to structural changes in the neural network, in turn causing neuropsychological issues. In contrast, it has also been hypothesized that both neuropsychological issues and seizures are caused by the same underlying genetically determined neurobiological dysfunction. This has been questioned in IGE, in particular in JME.

In studies of cognitive function, patients with JME have been found to have normal intelligence but a high frequency of impairment in frontal and memory functions, including concept formation, abstract reasoning, verbal fluency, mental flexibility, cognitive speed, planning, and organization.

Patients with JME have also been observed to have particular personality traits, including emotional instability, suggestibility, and immaturity, as well as lack of discipline and indifference toward their disease. Personality disorders have been found in JME, most commonly borderline personality (Beghi et al., 2006). Patients also tend to have a sleep cycle in which they fall asleep late and get up late in the morning, with impaired function in the mornings; it is theorized both that these are related to clinical or subclinical epileptic activity, or that they both represent the underlying subcortical/cortical abnormality in JME (Pung and Schmitz, 2006).

EEG

The EEG background is normal. Generalized polyspike and slow-wave discharges may be seen interictally, and may be asymmetrical or involving only the anterior regions, occurring more frequently during sleep. The interictal discharges may be irregular and tend to be faster than 2.5–3.5 Hz.

During myoclonic seizures, there is a burst of irregular, generalized, frontocentral, maximal 10–16-Hz polyspike and slow-wave discharges. Slow waves of 3–4 Hz follow the polyspikes, resulting in a complex that has longer duration than the actual myoclonic jerk (Thomas et al., 2005). Figure 13.4 illustrates EEG findings in JME, including photosensitivity.

Neuroimaging

PET scans have found reduced fluorodeoxyglucose levels in the dorsolateral prefrontal cortex during a working memory task and magnetic resonance spectroscopy has shown reduced *N*-acetyl aspartate levels in the prefrontal cortex (Pung and Schmitz, 2006). Up to 40% of patients may have minor structural abnormalities on MRI (Szaflarski et al., 2010).

Genetics

A family history of epilepsy is noted in one-third of patients, and a family history of seizure in a first- and second-degree relative has been seen in up to half of patients. Approximately 15% of first-degree relatives are noted to have isolated EEG abnormalities.

EFHC1 nonsense mutations were identified in a study of familial JME; the gene encodes a protein that regulates calcium channel activity and affects programmed cell death. It is located at 6p11-p12. Other gene mutations/polymorphisms have also been identified; however, they are not seen in only JME, but are associated with a variety of IGE phenotypes. These have included the *BRD2* locus at 6p21, which likely regulates nuclear transcription. *GRM4*, which encodes metabotropic glutamate receptor 4, is also located at 6p21.3; a mild association between JME and other IGE phenotypes and polymorphisms has also been found (Muhle et al., 2010b). Associations have also been seen between JME and polymorphisms of the α4-subunit gene of the neuronal nicotinic acetyl receptor (*CHRNA4*) (Rozycka et al., 2009). The study of a family in which JME was inherited in an autosomal dominant pattern identified a mutation in the *GABRA1* gene on 5q34. Other candidate genes include *GABRD* and *CLCN2* (encoding voltage-dependent chloride channel).

Treatment

Avoidance of lifestyle-related precipitants is necessary. Patients should be counseled regarding the need for regular and sufficient sleep, minimizing of alcohol intake, avoiding visual stimuli, and avoiding driving soon after awakening.

Regarding medications, expert opinion in the USA is that valproic acid and lamotrigine are the treatment of choice in adolescent males with JME; topiramate is also a first-line option. However, in adolescent females with JME, lamotrigine is the treatment of choice; topiramate

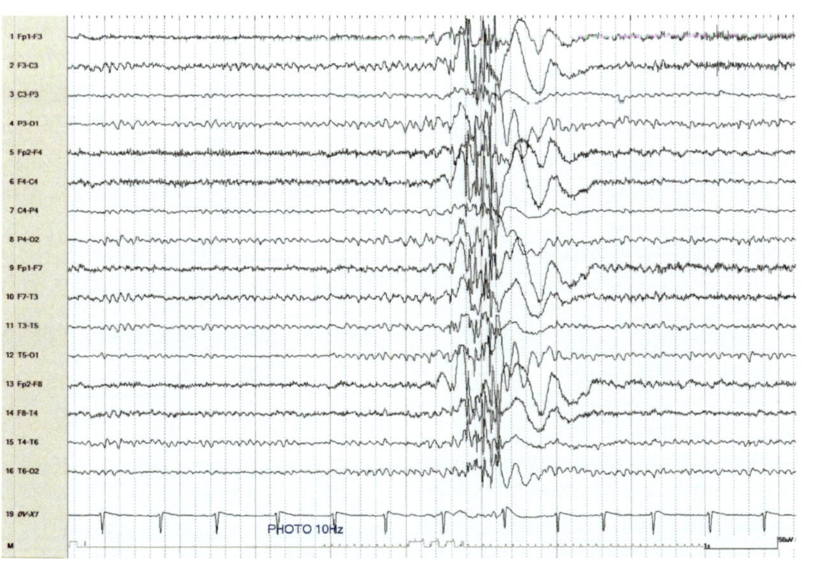

Fig. 13.4. EEG from 17-year-old girl with episodes of shoulder shaking and dropping a cup. Bilateral arm myoclonus seen with polyspike and slow-wave discharge during 10-Hz photic stimulation (10 microvolts/mm). Diagnosis is juvenile myoclonic epilepsy.

and valproic acid are first-line options, reflecting the concern of teratogenicity with valproic acid. Studies examining these three medications suggest that valproic acid has the greatest efficacy (Wheless et al., 2005).

Double-blind placebo-controlled trials have shown significantly higher seizure freedom rates with levetiracetam versus placebo for JME as well as JAE and GTC seizures on awakening (Rosenfeld et al., 2009). It has also been shown on EEGs that levetiracetam decreases epileptiform discharges and photoparoxysmal response of patients with JME (Specchio et al., 2008). Levetiracetam received US Food and Drug Administration approval as adjunctive therapy for myoclonic seizures in patients 12 years and older with JME. Reduction in EEG abnormalities have also been demonstrated with zonisamide. Other drugs that have been used are clonazepam, acetazolamide, and methosuximide (Thomas et al., 2005). The combination of valproic acid and lamotrigine may also offer synergy.

Prognosis

JME in general has an excellent response to treatment (80–90% of patients are fully controlled), although it may be a persistent condition, requiring lifelong treatment (Thomas et al., 2005). However, a few studies have found the potential for remission. A population-based cohort of 23 patients with JME who were interviewed up to 25 years after diagnosis found that one-third of patients had remission of all seizure types or the presence of only myoclonic seizures. Another study found that 54% of patients had cessation of myoclonic seizures after a mean age of 33 years, with the majority of the remainder having decrease in myoclonic seizures over a similar time period (Baykan et al., 2008). Neurological and intellectual outcome is also good, other than subtle comorbidities as described above. Persistence of interictal EEG changes does not appear to have a bad prognostic significance. However, those patients with difficult-to-control JME tend to have greater frequencies of all seizure types (myoclonic, absence, GTC) than patients who respond readily to antiseizure medications, and are more likely to demonstrate psychiatric issues suggesting frontal lobe dysfunction (Szaflarski et al., 2010).

Epilepsy with generalized tonic–clonic seizures (GTCS) only

This designation, listed as a "special epilepsy condition" by the ILAE classification core group in 2006 (Engel, 2006), includes what was previously referred to as "epilepsy with grand mal on awakening" (EGMA), as well as less specific cases in which seizures occur at any time of day without association with sleep. EGMA was characterized by GTCS occurring predominantly shortly after awakening, regardless of the time of day. Peak age of onset was 16–17 years, with a range from 6 years to middle age. Precipitating factors, similar to JME, were sleep deprivation, alcohol intake, and premenstrual syndrome. Photosensitivity, absence seizures, and myoclonic seizures were seen, although the diagnosis was suspected most when GTCS occurred upon awakening *without* myoclonic jerks. The EEG shows irregular spike and polyspike and slow-wave discharges, with frequencies between 3 and 4 Hz. Prognosis is positive, as seizures are rare and treatment response good. This discussion will remain short, as further definition and clarification of this entity will occur over time (Genton et al., 2005; Nordli, 2005).

CONCLUSION

The IGEs are a group of common epilepsy syndromes, consisting of varied phenotypes, including age-dependent manifestations of absence, myoclonic, atonic, and GTC seizures. They afflict children and adolescents of normal intelligence, although subtle neuropsychological and personality differences are seen. Prognosis is in general favorable, with some idiopathic generalized epilepsies having an excellent chance of complete seizure control and remission, and, importantly, significantly lower mortality rates compared with symptomatic epilepsies (Sillanpaa and Shinnar, 2010).

Progress in best treatment options is being made, and will be influenced by research regarding underlying etiological mechanisms. Neuroimaging performed in clinical care is normal, although specific techniques are finding morphometric and metabolic features that are helping to clarify pathophysiological mechanisms. Etiology of the idiopathic generalized epilepsies is obviously genetically influenced, although mechanisms of inheritance, which are likely complex, need to be elucidated. As genetic etiologies are further understood, ongoing changes in the classification of idiopathic generalized epilepsies will surely be further refined.

ACKNOWLEDGMENTS

The authors would like to thank Dr. William D. Gaillard and Dr. Phillip L. Pearl for their thoughtful review of the manuscript.

References

Abouda H, Hizem Y, Garbouri A et al. (2010). Familial form of typical childhood absence epilepsy in a consanguineous context. Epilepsia 51: 1889–1893.

Baykan B, Altindag EA, Bebek N et al. (2008). Myoclonic seizures subside in the fourth decade in juvenile myoclonic epilepsy. Neurology 70: 2123–2129.

Beghi M, Beghi E, Cornaggia CM et al. (2006). Idiopathic generalized epilepsies of adolescence. Epilepsia 47: 107–110.

Benbadis SR (2005). Practical management issues for idiopathic generalized epilepsies. Epilepsia 46: 125–132.

Berg AT, Berkovic SF, Brodie MJ et al. (2010). Revised terminology and concepts for organization of seizures and epilepsies: report of the ILAE commission on classification and terminology 2005–2009. Epilepsia 51: 676–685.

Bergey GK (2005). Evidence-based treatment of idiopathic generalized epilepsies with new antiepileptic drugs. Epilepsia 46: 161–168.

Berman R, Negishi M, Vestal M et al. (2010). Simultaneous EEG, fMRI, and behavior in typical childhood absence seizures. Epilepsia 51: 2011–2022.

Bourgeois BFD (2008a). Ethosuximide, methosuximide, and trimethadione. In: JM Pellock, BFD Bourgeois, WE Dodson (Eds.), Pediatric Epilepsy: Diagnosis and Therapy. 3rd edn. Demos Medical Publishing, New York, pp. 579–584.

Bourgeois BFD (2008b). Valproate. In: JM Pellock, BFD Bourgeois, WE Dodson (Eds.), Pediatric Epilepsy Diagnosis and Therapy. 3rd edn. Demos Medical Publishing, New York, pp. 685–697.

Bureau M, Tassinari CA (2005). The syndrome of myoclonic absences. In: J Roger, M Bureau, C Dravet et al. (Eds.), Epileptic Syndromes in Infancy, Childhood and Adolescence. 4th edn. John Libbey Eurotext, Montrouge, pp. 77–88.

Burgess DL (2005). Neonatal epilepsy syndromes and GEFS+: mechanistic considerations. Epilepsia 46: 51–58.

Carney PW, Masterton RAJ, Harvey AS et al. (2010). The core network in absence epilepsy. Differences in cortical and thalamic BOLD response. Neurology 75: 904–911.

Cavalleri GL, Walley NM, Soranzo N et al. (2007). A multicenter study of BRD2 as a risk factor for juvenile myoclonic epilepsy. Epilepsia 48: 706–712.

Chaves J, Sander JW (2005). Seizure aggravation in idiopathic generalized epilepsies. Epilepsia 46: 133–139.

Chioza BA, Aicardi J, Aschauer H et al. (2009). Genome wide high density SNP-based linkage analysis of childhood absence epilepsy identifies a susceptibility locus on chromosome 3p23-p14. Epilepsy Res 87: 247–255.

Commission on Classification and Terminology of the International League Against Epilepsy (1989). Proposal for revised classification of epilepsies and epileptic syndromes. Epilepsia 30: 389–399.

Danesi MA (1985). Classification of the epilepsies: an investigation of 945 patients in a developing country. Epilepsia 26: 131–136.

Dorland's Illustrated Medical Dictionary (1981). 26th edn. WB Saunders, Philadelphia.

Dravet C, Bureau M (2005). Benign myoclonic epilepsy in infancy. In: J Roger, M Bureau, C Dravet et al. (Eds.), Epileptic Syndromes in Infancy, Childhood and Adolescence. 4th edn. John Libbey Eurotext, Montrouge, pp. 77–88.

Duncan JS (2005). Brain imaging in idiopathic generalized epilepsies. Epilepsia 46: 108–111.

Engel J (2006). Report of the ILAE classification core group. Epilepsia 47: 1558–1568.

Farrell K, Michoulas A (2008). Benzodiazepines. In: JM Pellock, BFD Bourgeois, WE Dodson (Eds.), Pediatric Epilepsy: Diagnosis and Therapy. 3rd edn. Demos Medical Publishing, New York, pp. 557–566.

Filippini M, Boni A, Dazzani G et al. (2006). Neuropsychological findings: myoclonic astatic epilepsy (MAE) and Lennox–Gastaut syndrome (LGS). Epilepsia 47: 56–59.

Gardiner M (2005). Genetics of idiopathic generalized epilepsies. Epilepsia 46: 15–20.

Gastaut H, Gastaut JL, Goncalves e Silva GE et al. (1975). Relative frequency of different types of epilepsy: a study employing the classification of the International League Against Epilepsy. Epilepsia 16: 457–461.

Genton P, Gonzalez Sanchez MS et al. (2005). Epilepsy with grand mal on awakening. In: J Roger, M Bureau, C Dravet et al. (Eds.), Epileptic Syndromes in Infancy, Childhood and Adolescence. 4th edn. John Libbey Eurotext, Montrouge, pp. 389–394.

Glauser TA (2008). Topiramate. In: JM Pellock, BFD Bourgeois, WE Dodson (Eds.), Pediatric Epilepsy: Diagnosis and Therapy. 3rd edn. Demos Medical Publishing, New York, pp. 671–683.

Glauser TA, Cnaan A, Shinnar S et al. (2010). Ethosuximide, valproic acid, and lamotrigine in childhood absence epilepsy. N Engl J Med 362: 790–799.

Grosso S, Galimberti D, Vezzosi P et al. (2005). Childhood absence epilepsy: evolution and prognostic factors. Epilepsia 46: 1796–1801.

Guerrini R, Parmeggiani L, Bonanni P et al. (2005). Myoclonic astatic epilepsy. In: J Roger, M Bureau, C Dravet et al. (Eds.), Epileptic Syndromes in Infancy, Childhood and Adolescence. 4th edn. John Libbey Eurotext, Montrouge, pp. 115–124.

Hirsch E, Panayiotopoulos C (2005). Childhood absence epilepsy and related syndromes. In: J Roger, M Bureau, C Dravet et al. (Eds.), Epileptic Syndromes in Infancy, Childhood and Adolescence. 4th edn. John Libbey Eurotext, Montrouge, pp. 315–335.

Jallon P, Latour P (2005). Epidemiology of idiopathic generalized epilepsies. Epilepsia 46: 10–14.

Jallon P, Loiseau P, Loiseau J (2001). Newly diagnosed unprovoked epileptic seizures: presentation at diagnosis in CAROLE study Coordination Active du Reseau Observatoire Longitudinal de l'Epilepsi. Epilepsia 42: 464–475.

Joensen P (1986). Prevalence, incidence, and classification of epilepsy in the Faroes. Acta Neurol Scand 74: 150–155.

Kerrigan JF, Pellock JM (2008). Zonisamide. In: JM Pellock, BFD Bourgeois, WE Dodson (Eds.), Pediatric Epilepsy: Diagnosis and Therapy. 3rd edn. Demos Medical Publishing, New York, pp. 727–738.

Khosravani H, Zamponi GW (2006). Voltage-gated calcium channels and idiopathic generalized epilepsies. Physiol Rev 86: 941–966.

King MA, Newton MR, Jackson GD et al. (1998). Epileptology of the first seizure presentation: a clinical, electroencephalographic, and magnetic resonance imaging study of 300 consecutive patients. Lancet 352: 1007–1011.

Lachance-Touchette P, Martin C, Poulin C et al. (2010). Screening of GABRB3 in French-Canadian families with idiopathic generalized epilepsy. Epilepsia 51: 1894–1897.

Loiseau P, Duche B, Loiseau J (1991). Classification of epilepsies and epileptic syndromes in two different samples of patients. Epilepsia 32: 303–309.

Manford M, Hart YM, Sander JW et al. (1992). The National General Practice Study of Epilepsy. The syndromic classification of the International League Against Epilepsy applied to epilepsy in a general population. Arch Neurol 49: 801–808.

Muhle H, Steinich I, von Spiczak S et al. (2010a). A duplication in 1q21.3 in a family with early onset and childhood absence epilepsy. Epilepsia 51: 2453–2456.

Muhle H, von Spiczak S, Gaus V et al. (2010b). Role of GRM4 in idiopathic generalized epilepsies analysed by genetic association and sequence analysis. Epilepsy Res 89: 319–326.

Mullen SA, Suls A, De Jonghe P et al. (2010). Absence epilepsies with widely variable onset are a key feature of familial GLUT1 deficiency. Neurology 75: 432–440.

Murthy JMK, Yangala R, Srinivas M (1998). The syndromic classification of the International League Against Epilepsy: a hospital-based study from South India. Epilepsia 39: 48–54.

Nordli DR (2005). Idiopathic generalized epilepsies recognized by the International League Against Epilepsy. Epilepsia 46: 48–56.

Panayiotopoulos CP (2005). Syndromes of idiopathic generalized epilepsies not recognized by the International League Against Epilepsy. Epilepsia 46: 57–66.

Pearl PL, Holmes GL (2008). Childhood absence epilepsies. In: JM Pellock, BFD Bourgeois, WE Dodson (Eds.), Pediatric Epilepsy: Diagnosis and Therapy. 3rd edn. Demos Medical Publishing, New York, pp. 323–334.

Pellock JM (2008). Lamotrigine. In: JM Pellock, BFD Bourgeois, WE Dodson (Eds.), Pediatric Epilepsy Diagnosis and Therapy. 3rd edn. Demos Medical Publishing, New York, pp. 603–610.

Posner EB, Mohamed K, Marson AG (2005). A systematic review of treatment of typical absence seizures in children and adolescents with ethosuximide, sodium valproate or lamotrigine. Seizure 14: 117–122.

Prevett MC, Duncan JS, Jones T et al. (1995). Demonstration of thalamic activation during typical absence seizures using $H_2(15)O$ and PET. Neurology 45: 1396–1402.

Pung T, Schmitz B (2006). Circadian rhythm and personality profile in juvenile myoclonic epilepsy. Epilepsia 47: 111–114.

Rosenfeld WE, Benbadis S, Edrich P et al. (2009). Levetiracetam as add-on therapy for idiopathic generalized epilepsy syndromes with onset during adolescence: analysis of two randomized, double-blind, placebo-controlled studies. Epilepsy Res 85: 72–80.

Rozycka A, Steinborn B, Trzeciak WH (2009). The 1674 + 11 C > T polymorphism of CHRNA4 is associated with juvenile myoclonic epilepsy. Seizure 18: 601–603.

Sankar R, Shields WD (2008). Levetiracetam. In: JM Pellock, BFD Bourgeois, WE Dodson (Eds.), Pediatric Epilepsy Diagnosis and Therapy. 3rd edn. Demos Medical Publishing, New York, pp. 611–619.

Scheffer IE, Harkin LA, Dibbens LM et al. (2005). Neonatal epilepsy syndromes and generalized epilepsy with febrile seizures plus (GEFS +). Epilepsia 46: 41–47.

Senanayake N, Roman GC (1993). Epidemiology of epilepsy in developing countries. Bull World Health Organ 71: 247–258.

Sillanpaa M, Shinnar S (2010). Long-term mortality in childhood-onset epilepsy. N Engl J Med 363: 2522–2529.

Specchio N, Boero G, Michelucci G et al. (2008). Effects of levetiracetam on EEG abnormalities in juvenile myoclonic epilepsy. Epilepsia 49: 663–669.

Szaflarski JP, DiFrancesco M, Hirschauer T et al. (2010). Cortical and subcortical contributions to absence seizure onset examined with EEG/fMRI. Epilepsy Behav 18: 404–413.

Thomas P, Genton P, Gelisse P et al. (2005). Juvenile myoclonic epilepsy. In: J Roger, M Bureau, C Dravet et al. (Eds.), Epileptic Syndromes in Infancy, Childhood and Adolescence. 4th edn. John Libbey Eurotext, Montrouge, pp. 367–388.

Wheless JW, Clarke DF, Carpenter D (2005). Treatment of pediatric epilepsy: expert opinion, 2005. J Child Neurol 20: S1–S56.

Wheless JW, Clarke DF, Arzimanoglou A et al. (2007). Treatment of pediatric epilepsy: European expert opinion, 2007. Epileptic Disord 9: 353–412.

Wolf P, Inoue Y (2005). Juvenile absence epilepsy. In: J Roger, M Bureau, C Dravet et al. (Eds.), Epileptic Syndromes in Infancy, Childhood and Adolescence. 4th edn. John Libbey Eurotext, Montrouge, pp. 363–366.

Zarrelli MM, Beghi E, Rocca WA et al. (1999). Incidence of epileptic syndromes in Rochester, Minnesota: 1980–1984. Epilepsia 40: 1708–1714.

Zuberi SM, Brunklaus A, Brich R et al. (2011). Genotype–phenotype associations in SCN1A-related epilepsies. Neurology 76: 594–600.

Handbook of Clinical Neurology, Vol. 107 (3rd series)
Epilepsy, Part I
H. Stefan and W.H. Theodore, Editors

Chapter 14

Temporal lobe epilepsy

MARIA THOM[1] AND EDWARD H. BERTRAM[2]*

[1]*Institute of Neurology, National Hospital for Neurology and Neurosurgery, University College London, London, UK*

[2]*F.E. Dreifuss Comprehensive Epilepsy Program, Department of Neurology, University of Virginia, Charlottesville, VA, USA*

INTRODUCTION

The term temporal lobe epilepsy (TLE) has different meanings to different people. In the broadest sense, TLE encompasses all epilepsy with the seizures arising anywhere in the temporal lobe, irrespective of the location or the pathology. To others, TLE means specifically seizures arising in the mesial structures of the hippocampus, amygdala, and entorhinal cortex, and this form of epilepsy is more precisely called mesial temporal lobe epilepsy (MTLE) or limbic epilepsy (because it arises in the limbic structures of the temporal lobe). Because the non-MTLE forms of TLE result from a number of associated pathologies (dysplasias, hamartomas, trauma, vascular malformations) that also are associated with epilepsy in other neocortical regions, we will leave the discussion of these forms of epilepsy to other chapters and focus on MTLE.

Although most consider MTLE as a distinct syndrome, a completely agreed upon definition has not been achieved. In 2002, the International League Against Epilepsy held a meeting to review the existing information about MTLE including the natural history, pathology, neurophysiology, clinical features, and surgical outcomes. At the end of the meeting there was no clear agreement, but the general consensus was that it was not a single disorder, but a collection of different syndromes with variations in pathology and etiology although with a likely common feature of involvement of one or more of the mesial limbic structures at seizure onset (Wieser, 2004). In this chapter we will not enter into that discussion. Rather, it is our intention to provide a broad introduction to the nature of the disorder, its clinical features, and the variations in the associated pathology, as well as theoretical frameworks for the functional anatomy of the seizure circuits and the potential contributors to the pathophysiology. The information is far from complete, but with the development in the last two decades of animal models that have many features in common with human MTLE, our insight into the potential pathophysiology has grown exponentially.

CLINICAL FEATURES

Auras are a common clinical feature of MTLE. The most common description by patients is of an epigastric or substernal rising sensation, or a sensation that is difficult to describe is often noted by patients with the syndrome. Other subjective symptoms described by patients include sudden fear or anxiety, a sense of familiarity, autonomic symptoms, and, less often, olfactory or gustatory sensations (Fried et al., 1995). Auras are not experienced by all patients, but with nondominant temporal lobe seizures there may not be a complete alteration of consciousness, as the patient may interact and respond even in the midst of automatisms. With or without alteration of awareness there is typically an arrest of behavior. The automatisms seen most commonly are oral, with lip smacking or chewing. Motor symptoms are less common, but dystonic posturing of the arm contralateral to the side of seizure onset is often encountered and may be considered a lateralizing feature. As the seizures progress, head deviation and clonic and tonic activity may develop, at times culminating in a convulsion. Convulsions, especially in patients on medical therapy, are uncommon. The postictal period can be quite variable, ranging from minimal, especially with nondominant temporal lobe onset, to a number of minutes of postictal aphasia. Less well recognized is postictal memory impairment in which

*Correspondence to: Edward H. Bertram, Department of Neurology, University of Virginia, P.O. Box 800394, Charlottesville, VA 22908-0394, USA. Tel: +1-434-924-0369, Fax: +1-434-982-1726, E-mail: ehb2z@virginia.edu

the patient appears to be acting normally but for a significant period has no subsequent recollection. This period of amnesia, which can last for several hours, is not always recognized unless formally tested.

Making the diagnosis of MTLE as an outpatient is largely presumptive. Although, as noted above, there are common symptoms that are seen in patients during seizures, none is pathognomonic. On interictal scalp EEG there may be temporal-lobe spike and sharp waves, as well as focal slowing. The spikes may be ipsilateral or contralateral to the site of onset, but the slowing is more common on the side of the focus (Williamson et al., 1993). On routine magnetic resonance imaging (MRI), relative qualitative atrophy of the affected hippocampus on T1 imaging and unilateral increase signal on T2 or fluid-attenuated inversion-recovery (FLAIR) imaging are the most common findings (Berkovic et al., 1991; Jackson et al., 1991), and, in combination with supporting clinical history and electroencephalography (EEG) findings, will support the diagnosis. However, because the MRI changes are subtle, and there is often bilateral involvement, the qualitative asymmetries that are used to support the diagnosis are not seen. Thus, in the absence of definitive pathology, a definite diagnosis cannot always be made, which makes understanding the true incidence of this syndrome difficult.

NATURAL HISTORY

The exact cause of hippocampal sclerosis (HS) associated with MTLE is unknown. The most widely accepted theory is still based on Meyer's original hypothesis, proposed in the 1950s, that an early insult, typically a complex febrile convulsion or other initial precipitating injury (IPI) occurring usually in the first 4–5 years of life, culminates in HS and the development of MTLE (Meyer et al., 1954; Cavanagh and Meyer, 1956; Mathern et al., 2002). Other theories that have been argued include a pre-existing hippocampal developmental abnormality or abnormal maturation that predisposes to both temporal lobe seizures and hippocampal atrophy (Blumcke et al., 2002). More recent studies have explored the potential role of inflammatory processes including viral limbic encephalitis such as caused by human herpesvirus 6 (Theodore et al., 2008). The contribution of mitochondrial dysfunction (Kudin et al., 2009) is also under speculation and investigation. More recently, the onset of intractable MTLE has been associated with an autoimmune limbic encephalitis with antibodies directed, amongst other targets, to potassium channels, glutamic acid decarboxylase, γ-aminobutyric acid type B ($GABA_B$) receptors and *N*-methyl-D-aspartate receptors (Bien et al., 2007; Lai et al., 2010; Lancaster et al., 2010; Liimatainen et al., 2010; Vincent et al., 2010).

Although IPIs may contribute to the eventual development of MTLE, there is a high proportion of patients with this syndrome who have no recognizable IPI that precedes the onset of the habitual seizures. Most cases of MTLE appear to be sporadic, but there are reports of familial forms of MTLE in which there are hippocampal abnormalities in the MRIs of asymptomatic family members of patients with the syndrome (Cendes et al., 1998). These observations raise the possibility that, at least in some cases, there may be a genetic component in the development of MTLE (Kobayashi et al., 2002). This hypothesis is supported in part by studies that have suggested that mutations in the sodium channel, voltage-gated, type I, α subunit (SCN1A) are associated with a familial generalized epilepsy with febrile seizures syndrome (GEFS+) in some family members with MTLE, at least one of whom had HS (Abou-Khalil et al., 2001). Studies of transgenic mice with human epilepsy-associated sodium channel mutations have also found spontaneous seizures, but the genetic background (mouse strain) had a major influence on the development of seizures (Kearney et al., 2001). Overall, it may be concluded that there may be a variety of etiologies for the disorder, but that an interaction between an individual's genetic makeup and environmental factors likely plays a significant role in many, but not all, cases.

In patients with an identifiable IPI, as in most other forms of acquired epilepsy such as post-traumatic, there is a silent or latent period between the presumed inducing injury and the first spontaneous seizure. Typically, the first seizures of MTLE begin in late childhood or early adolescence, but they may first appear earlier or much later. Although there is some evidence that seizures appear earlier if there is a defined IPI (Mathern et al., 1995), there does not seem to be a strong correlation with seizure history and the severity of the HS (Mathern et al., 2002). Patients, however, do sometimes note the occurrence of repeated transient subjective sensations (auras) long before they were officially diagnosed with epilepsy after the more overt seizures that are associated with alterations of consciousness and obvious automatisms began. This observation of evolving duration and severity (i.e., from seizures without alterations of awareness to seizures in which the patient is overly impaired) has raised the issue of MTLE as a progressive disorder, a term that implies changes in the substrate of the brain that supports the seizure. There are several interpretations of this concept of "progressive." One interpretation is that the neuronal loss and atrophy seen in HS worsens over time. Although there are some imaging studies and animal studies that raise the possibility of progressive atrophy over time (Cavazos and Sutula, 1990; Bernhardt et al., 2009), there are many other studies from surgical pathology and animal studies that suggest that there is little neuronal loss over time (Bertram et al., 1990; Mathern et al., 1997a, 2002; Gorter et al., 2003; Liu et al., 2005). There are some imaging reports that indicate there is progressive atrophy in the hippocampus over time, but these studies do not control for the development of depression, a common comorbidity of MTLE, or the use of medications that are associated with volume loss (Guerrini et al., 1998; Bernhardt et al., 2009).

Perhaps the strongest support for the idea that MTLE is a progressive disorder is supported by its natural history, in which the seizures appear to worsen over time. The apparent development of intractability in which the seizures are no longer completely controlled by the medications is also cited as evidence for progression. It is unclear whether patients who are destined to develop intractable epilepsy are really intractable from the beginning, regardless of the treatment, or whether drug resistance appears because of recurrent seizures. At present there is no clear answer, which lies in a tangle of not understanding the pathophysiology of the disorder, the varying pathologies found in patients with MTLE, and not knowing the true untreated natural history of the disorder. The natural history issue revolves around the possibility that some patients are naturally going to have only a few seizures, whereas others will have seizures that increase in frequency and severity over time. Animal studies have provided good support for the idea that there are separate populations of patients with MTLE, some of whom remain stable over time and others that progress (Bertram and Cornett, 1994; Gorter et al., 2001; Williams et al., 2009). There is some epidemiological evidence that some patients with MTLE have seizures that are quite readily managed whereas others are rapidly identified as therapy resistant (Stephen et al., 2001).

FUNCTIONAL ANATOMY OF MESIAL TEMPORAL LOBE EPILEPSY

There is general agreement that the seizures of MTLE involve the limbic structures of the medial temporal lobe because the structures are anatomically abnormal and because removal of this region at surgery usually controls the seizures (and, at times, cures). However, the role of the hippocampus, entorhinal cortex, and amygdala in the process of seizure initiation and spread is mostly the subject of speculation. In some models of the functional anatomy of MTLE, the seizures arise in local circuits from which the seizures break out and spread to other regions of the brain by recruitment of adjacent regions. In other models, this region takes the initial seizure generated elsewhere and spreads it to the rest of the brain, serving as a critical amplifier for the seizure. More recent models suggest that any of the regions is able to generate seizures independently and recruit other areas through an interaction between limbic and subcortical structures. We will not include in this discussion seizures in which the limbic system is clearly involved secondarily. In such cases the region is really a passive participant, and its removal has little impact on the seizures.

With regard to the model in which the seizures develop first in local circuits, several hypotheses have been developed to explain how seizures arise. One focuses on the well-known trisynaptic (actually more) pathway from the entorhinal cortex, to the dentate gyrus, to Ammon's horn (CA3 and CA1), and back to the entorhinal cortex. This circuit has been well described anatomically, all components support seizure activity quite well (Goddard et al., 1969), and all are involved in limbic seizure activity (Bertram, 1997). The hypothesis proposes that the seizure develops in this reverberatory circuit, where it is maintained until it breaks out to other regions through the broad connections of the entorhinal cortex (Lothman et al., 1991) (Fig. 14.1). The proposal makes good sense of well-known biological activities and circuits, but it runs into trouble with several clinical realities. First, it does not take into consideration the observation from some patients of "amygdala only" seizures (Hudson et al., 1993). Although not commonly seen, they have been described, and their existence suggests that the entorhinal–hippocampal circuit is not essential to seizure generation in the limbic system. The second observation against the trisynaptic circuit hypothesis is from surgical outcomes. If the trisynaptic circuit were the critical basis for limbic seizure initiation, simply interrupting transmission from one part of the circuit to another would be sufficient to prevent the amplification of the seizure (e.g., cutting the pathway between the entorhinal cortex and the dentate gyrus, or removal of the entorhinal cortex). The clinical observation is that all or most of the regions, as well as the amygdala and parahippocampal gyrus (including the subiculum), must be removed to ensure a good outcome. This issue is also true for the hypothesis in which a focus outside the limbic structures has an obligate pathway that uses the trisynaptic components to amplify a focal seizure The failure of the removal of a single component of the trisynaptic circuit to control the seizures raises the possibility that each of the sites is capable of initiating seizure activity independently, which raises the alternative hypothesis for the functional anatomy of limbic seizures: the multiple independent generator hypothesis.

In the multiple independent generator concept of the seizure onset zone, each region is capable of initiating the seizure and subsequently recruiting the other regions into the seizure. Although not proved, this hypothesis

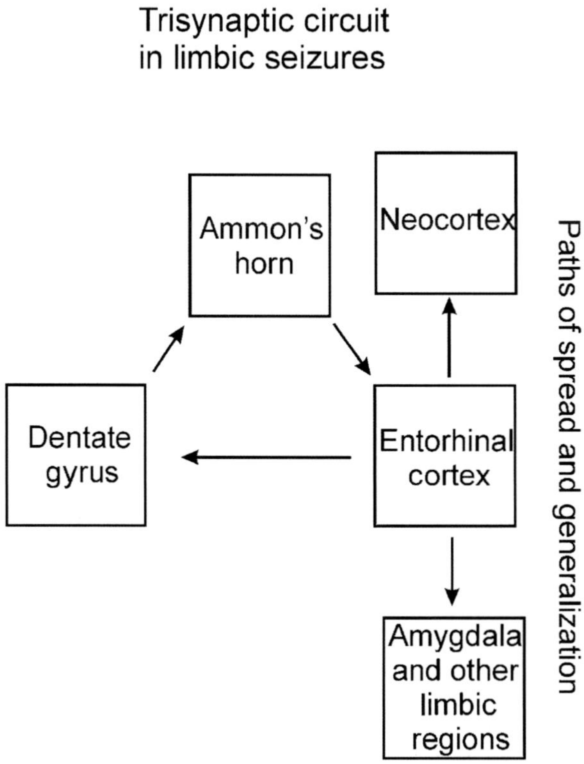

Fig. 14.1. Trisynaptic seizure circuit. Hypothetical circuit within the limbic system for initiating circuit. By this theory, seizure activity would reverberate within the confines of the entorhinal cortex–dentate gyrus–Ammon's horn, eventually spreading to other limbic sites and the neocortex through the entorhinal cortex. Although there is anatomical and some physiological evidence to support this proposed seizure circuit, the observation that removal of one of the components alone (e.g., the entorhinal cortex) does not control the seizures suggests that this circuit is not a major component of limbic seizures.

fits many of the observations from the clinical and laboratory worlds (Fig. 14.2). As noted in the section on pathology, the neuronal loss and gliosis is spread throughout the mesial limbic structures as well as to several subcortical regions, such as specific thalamic nuclei, as well as in the hypothalamus (Meyer et al., 1954; Margerison and Corsellis, 1966; Bertram and Scott, 2000; Moran et al., 2001). Intracranial recordings have revealed a common pattern of regional onset involving synchronized onset across multiple limbic regions, although individual seizures have had a more focal onset in a single site such as the amygdala or the hippocampus (So, 1991; Spencer and Spencer, 1994; Bertram, 1997). As we will describe later, studies from animal models have shown that the neurons in all of these regions have an enhanced excitability, with lower thresholds for firing action potentials, with more action potentials with each discharge. These observations suggest that the entire network is hyperexcitable and each region is prone to initiating a seizure. The question may arise whether, in reality, all sites are capable of initiating a seizure successfully. Although not a model with many spontaneous seizures, the kindling model, in which seizures are induced by electrical stimulation of a specific structure, may give us some insight. In the kindling model, all of the limbic sites (hippocampus, entorhinal cortex, amygdala, piriform cortex) are capable of initiating seizures that involve all of the other regions (Goddard et al., 1969). This finding indicates that the limbic system is broadly connected and that any site within it is capable of initiating seizures throughout the system. This broad potential for inducing seizures is supported by the clinical observation that extensive resection of multiple limbic sites provides the best seizure control over time. At present, there is good, although circumstantial, support for the multiple independent generator hypothesis.

Much of the attention regarding the functional anatomy of MTLE has been given to the traditional mesial temporal focus of the amygdala, hippocampus, and their neighbors, with good reason: there is clear pathology, seizures arise there, and removal of those structures frequently controls the seizures. However, over the last 10–20 years, there has been growing evidence that there are subcortical structures that play a significant role in seizure initiation and spread. Two of these regions are the pars reticulata of the substantia nigra

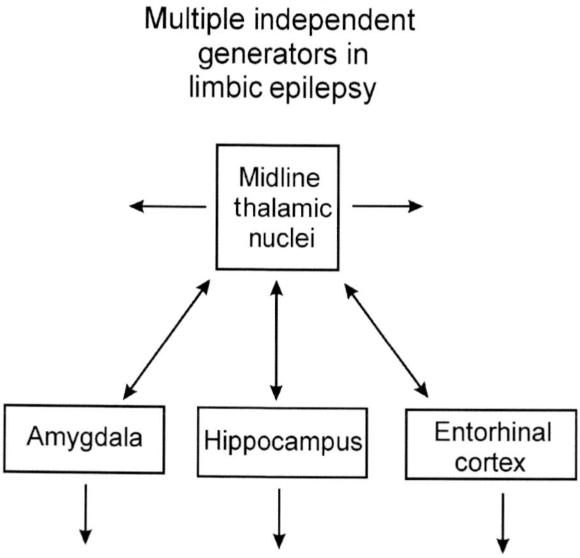

Fig. 14.2. Multiple independent seizure generators. This proposed circuit suggests that any one region of the mesial temporal lobe is capable of initiating a seizure and spreading it to other regions either directly or through subcortical structures such as the thalamus. There is anatomical evidence for this model for seizure initiation and spread, and the persistence of seizures following partial mesial temporal resections supports this model.

(a GABAergic projection nucleus) and the midline thalamic nuclei, which includes the medial dorsal nucleus. In the kindling model it was shown by several laboratories that manipulation of the substantia nigra with GABAergic agents significantly altered the behavioral expression of the seizures, and at times would block the convulsions (McNamara et al., 1984; Gale, 1992; Moshé et al., 1995). Because EEGs were not always performed, it was not clear whether this intervention altered the spread of seizures to other sites, or whether the seizure duration was altered, so that the exact role the pars reticulata of the substantia nigra plays in limbic seizures (modulating duration or the recruitment of other regions) is unclear.

There are more data about the role of the midline thalamic nuclei. As with the substantia nigra, the original observations were behavioral, in which suppression of activity in the medial dorsal nucleus reduced the behavioral severity (from convulsive to nonconvulsive) (Miller and Ferrendelli, 1990; Cassidy and Gale, 1998; Bertram et al., 2008). As work progressed, evidence appeared that the medial dorsal nucleus was an active participant in the electrographic seizure activity from the beginning of the seizure in the peripheral limbic structures. Suppression of activity in the medial dorsal region shortened the duration of the seizure on EEG in the limbic structures as well as in the thalamus (Bertram et al., 2008). The behavioral severity of the seizures is lessened as well. Anatomically, the medial dorsal nucleus is well connected to the amygdala, hippocampus, and entorhinal cortex, so that it is easy to construct a reciprocal circuit between the thalamus and the limbic structures in which seizures could develop and spread (Su and Bentivoglio, 1990; van Groen and Wyss, 1990; Turner and Herkenham, 1991; Van der Werf et al., 2002). Several recordings from people have demonstrated involvement of the medial dorsal nucleus and the hippocampus at seizure onset (Guye et al., 2006). Studies of the pathology of human MTLE, as well as from animal models of limbic epilepsy, have shown neuronal loss and gliosis similar to hippocampal sclerosis. In addition, imaging studies have shown atrophy in this region on quantitative MRI, and functional imaging (positron emission tomography; PET) have suggested involvement of this region as well (Juhász et al., 1999; Natsume et al., 2003). Although further evaluation is necessary, there is a growing body of evidence that the thalamus plays a significant role in the onset of limbic seizures and that it might be a critical control point for these seizures. There is a recent report that suggests that the medial dorsal nucleus of the thalamus plays the critical role in seizure initiation and spread by serving as an additional excitatory input to a region involved in seizure initiation and spread as part of a divergent convergent circuit that amplifies and prolongs the excitatory drive on a target population (Fig. 14.3) (Sloan et al., 2011). Attenuating the additional excitatory input from the thalamus lessens the chance of pushing the target regions into a seizure. This role of the thalamus fits well into the multiple independent generator model as these limbic regions have broad connections among themselves as well as the medial dorsal region.

In summary, current data support the hypothesis that each region is capable of initiating a seizure independently. Although it is still too early to determine how critical the subcortical structures are in seizure initiation and spread, the evidence suggests that they play an important role as well. It is most important, however, as we try to understand the pathophysiology of the disorder, to determine the roles that the different regions play so that we can identify those regions, and the changes in them, that are most critical to seizure initiation and spread.

STRUCTURAL BASIS FOR MESIAL TEMPORAL LOBE EPILEPSY: NEUROPATHOLOGY

Histological examination of resected surgical specimens carried out for the treatment of refractory temporal lobe epilepsy (including *en bloc* temporal lobectomy or selective amygdalohippocampectomy) allows further

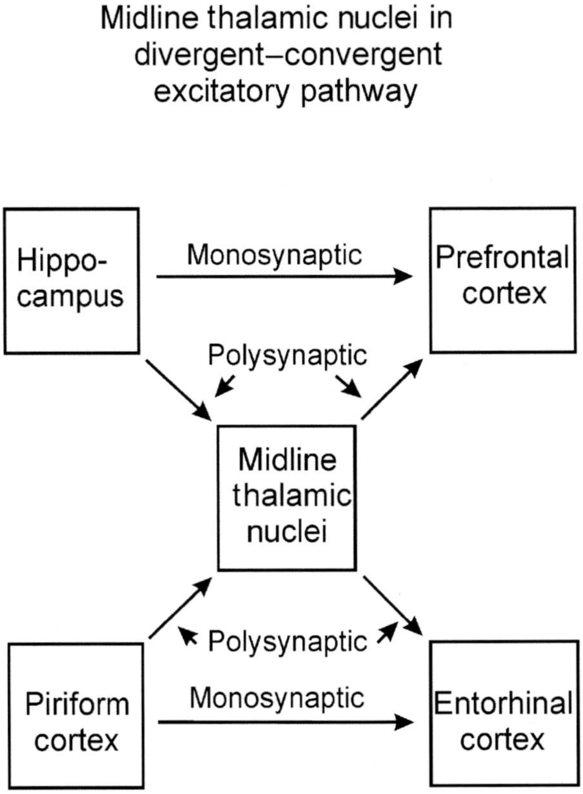

Fig. 14.3. Thalamic circuits in limbic seizures, based on anatomical and physiological evidence. Each limbic region connects to other areas through monosynaptic direct connections and a polysynaptic path involving the midline thalamic nuclei. This polysynaptic connection prolongs the duration of excitation on the target site (in this figure the entorhinal cortex and the prefrontal cortex) as the polysynaptic signal arrives at the end of the monosynaptic response.

characterization of any abnormality identified on MRI. The main pathology groups are outlined in Table 14.1, with sclerosis of the medial temporal lobe structures being the commonest pathology group. In a minor proportion of patients in most series, no distinct or specific pathological lesion is identified (also referred to as paradoxical or "cryptogenic" TLE). In a further group, HS is seen in combination with a second distinct pathology in the resected material; this is termed a dual pathology.

Mesial temporal lobe sclerosis

Brief history, nomenclature, and patterns of hippocampal sclerosis

The principal neurons of the hippocampus are vulnerable to a variety of insults including hypoxia–ischemia, trauma, and hyperglycemia, and are also involved early in many neurodegenerative disease processes, particularly Alzheimer disease with subsequent atrophy of the hippocampal formation. The association of hippocampal pathology in patients with epilepsy was first noted through the detailed post-mortem studies of Sommer (1880) and Bratz (1899) more than 100 years ago, where pathological features of HS (also termed Ammon's horn sclerosis) were delineated (for review see Thom, 2009). Neuronal loss centered on the CA1 sector, with less complete loss of neurons from the CA4 region, and a resistant sector corresponding to CA2 forming the classical type of the pathology. These changes are accompanied by a cellular and fibrous gliosis and tissue volume contraction and hardening. There is no single explanation for the regional selectivity of pyramidal cell loss between subfields; excitatory pathways, altered inhibitory input, and the effectiveness of endogenous neuroprotective mechanisms are likely to be involved.

From the outset, as noted in the earliest surgical temporal lobectomy series for the treatment of epilepsy (Bruton and Institute of Psychiatry, University of London, 1988), it was appreciated that the severity and distribution of neuronal loss could vary between cases. This resulted in the introduction of several grading or classification schemes to define subtypes of hippocampal sclerosis; some of these are outlined in Table 14.2. These subtypes appear to be of clinical relevance in that they may identify distinct pathoetiological factors, epileptogenic mechanisms or pathways, and have differing

Table 14.1

Frequency of main pathology types identified in larger surgical series (from Greenfield et al., 2008)

Common pathological categories identified in surgical epilepsy specimens	Approximate average (range) percentages based on large surgical series
Mesial temporal lobe sclerosis/hippocampal sclerosis	37% (14–63%)
Low-grade tumors (particularly glioneuronal tumors; dysembryoplastic neuroepithelial tumors, ganglioglioma)	32% (10–75%)
Cortical malformations (e.g., focal cortical dysplasia, FCD)	20% (6–56%)
Vascular malformations	6% (1–15%)
Old scars (including perinatal infarcts, old traumatic lesions)	18% (1–53%)
Inflammatory pathologies	4% (1.5–13%)
No specific pathology identified	12% (4.3–17%)
Dual pathology: hippocampal sclerosis plus a second lesional pathology	6–16%

Types of surgical resection, inclusion of pediatric patients, and other selection criteria, as well as diagnostic criteria for focal cortical dysplasias, likely cause the variation in incidence of reporting pathologies between centers.

Table 14.2

Qualitative and quantitative classification schemes introduced for the evaluation of subtypes of hippocampal sclerosis

	Classification scheme		
	Based on Bruton et al. (1988)*	Wyler grading scheme for HS (1992)†	Blumcke et al. (2007)‡
Histological method	Qualitative	Qualitative	Quantitative with IHC
No HS	No HS	Grade 0–1 (33%): no HS or neuronal loss	No HS (19%): no significant neuronal loss in any subfield (19%)
Atypical HS patterns	End folium HS (4%)	Grade 2 (7%): moderate neuronal loss in CA4 and/or CA1/3	MTS type 3 (4%): significant neuronal loss restricted to CA4
	CA1 predominant HS*		MTS type 2 (6%): significant neuronal loss in CA1
Classical HS patterns	Classical HS (57%): neuronal loss in CA1 and CA4	Grade 3 (48%): severe neuronal loss in CA1, CA3, and CA2 but sparing of CA2	MTS type 1a (19%): severe neuronal loss in CA1, moderate loss in other subfields except CA2
	Total HS (39%): neuronal loss in all subfields including CA2 and dentate gyrus	Grade 4 (12%): marked neuronal loss in all sectors including dentate gyrus	MTS type 1b (53%): severe neuronal loss in all subfields

*This pattern was not in Bruton's original series but was described by Sagar and Oxbury (1987) and De Lanerolle et al. (2003).
†Wyler score as utilized in the series reported by Davies et al. (1996).
‡Categorization of MTS type in Blumcke's series is based on quantitative analysis of NeuN-stained sections.
The percentages of cases in each group are shown.
HS, hippocampal sclerosis; IHC, immunohistochemistry; MTS, mesial temporal sclerosis.

responses to surgery. For example, nonclassical or atypical patterns of sclerosis, including end-folium sclerosis pattern and CA1-predominant patterns identified in 4% and 6–8% of patients respectively, have been linked to poorer outcomes in terms of postoperative seizure freedom in some reports (Bruton and Institute of Psychiatry, University of London, 1988; de Lanerolle et al., 2003; Blumcke et al., 2007; Van Paesschen et al., 1997). Poorer outcomes are also seen in patients where no HS (or other pathology) is identified, with only 44–58% of patients becoming seizure-free compared with around 70–80% in patients with classical HS (de Lanerolle et al., 2003; Blumcke et al., 2007) (Fig. 14.4). These studies highlight that HS is unlikely to be a single entity or condition.

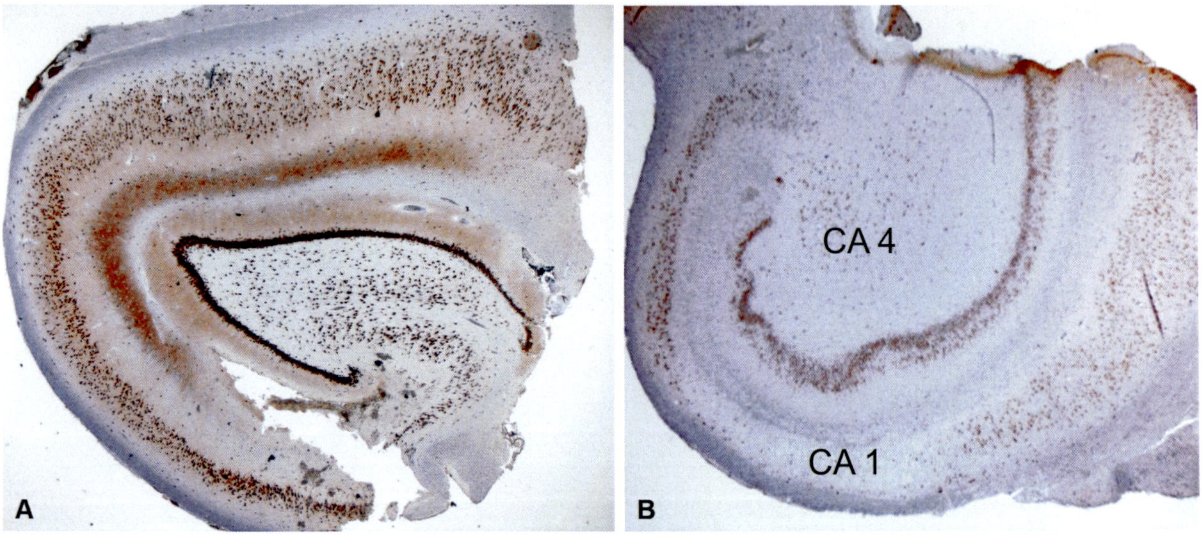

Fig. 14.4. NeuN-stained sections of (**A**) a patient with temporal lobe epilepsy and no hippocampal sclerosis, in contrast to (**B**) a patient with classical hippocampal sclerosis (neuronal loss from CA1 and CA4 regions). Note that the granule cell layer is broadened in the patient with sclerosis.

There is also little evidence that one subtype or grade of HS progresses to another. It is likely in the future that atypical patterns of HS will be diagnosed preoperatively with more advanced MRI sequences (Eriksson et al., 2008); this could influence planning of surgery.

Additional pathology features noted in HS in surgical cases

Dispersion of granule cells of the dentate gyrus into the molecular layer (Houser, 1990) is a phenomenon peculiar to seizure-induced HS and encountered in 40–50% of the surgical cases (Lurton et al., 1997, 1998; Thom et al., 2002; Wieser, 2004). In the presence of dispersion, granule cells often appear enlarged and more fusiform in shape, with increased cytoplasm and neuropil separating neurons. Granule cell dispersion is almost invariably associated with gliosis in the granule cell layer. Other patterns of dispersion include distinct clusters of granule cells in the molecular layer, or a bilaminar granule cell layer (Blumcke et al., 2009). The extent and pattern of dispersion may vary within cases, may preferentially involve either the internal and external blades of the dentate gyrus, and may alternate with regions of granule cell depletion. Definitions of granule cell dispersion include a granule cell layer more than 10 cells wide (Wieser, 2004) or of more than 120 mm (Fig. 14.5).

Dispersion of granule cells has also been demonstrated in experimental models of TLE, being noted as early as 4 days following experimental seizures (Suzuki et al., 2005). Dispersion in human tissue appears to be associated with the presence of hilar neuronal loss (Mathern et al., 1997b) and is less dramatic in patients with CA1 sclerosis alone (Blumcke et al., 2007). It may be a manifestation of early seizures or insult on the developing and maturing dentate gyrus (Lurton et al., 1998). Local deficiencies in reelin proteins have been proposed as a mechanism for the dispersion (Frotscher et al., 2003), or alternatively it may be an effect of seizures on local progenitor cell populations. A relationship between granule cell changes in HS and memory performance in patients with TLE has been shown (Pauli et al., 2006; Stefan et al., 2009), but there is no reported independent influence of the extent of granule cell dispersion on outcome following surgery. In post-mortem specimens from patients with epilepsy

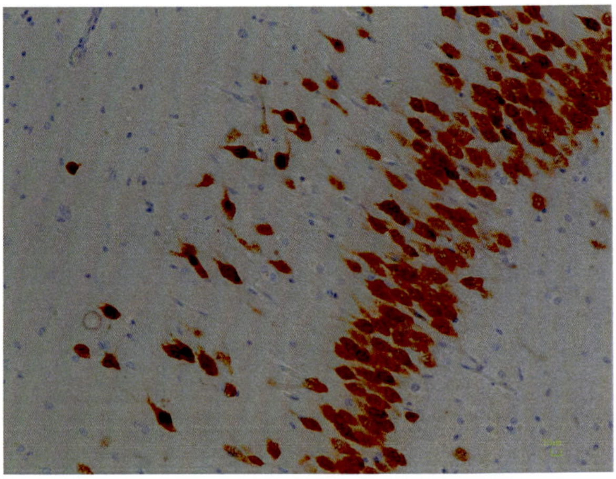

Fig. 14.5. NeuN-stained section through the granule cell layer in a patient with hippocampal sclerosis showing dispersion of neurons away from the main layer into the molecular layer.

and HS, granule cell dispersion may be observed bilaterally and appears to persist with a long lifetime of seizures (Thom et al., 2009b).

Mechanisms for epilepsy

Elucidating the cellular mechanisms for epileptogenesis associated with HS remains a challenge. Not all patients with the MRI features (Auer et al., 2008) or pathology features of HS will have epilepsy. Histological studies of HS in epilepsy surgical series have aimed to decipher which cellular alterations distinguish patients with epilepsy that could promote abnormal excitatory pathways and seizures. Abnormal axonal sprouting, selective loss, or alteration to inhibitory neurons, gliosis, inflammatory reactions, and altered vasculature are potential candidates (Pitkanen and Lukasiuk, 2009).

Mossy fiber sprouting

In animal models of MTLE (e.g., the kainate model), as well as human surgical tissues, recurrent projection of mossy fiber axon collaterals into the molecular layer of the dentate gyrus is a common observation (Sutula et al., 1989; Nadler, 2003). This process is more commonly known as mossy fiber sprouting. The sprouted mossy fibers make excitatory synaptic contact (Cavazos et al., 2003) with apical dendrites and spines of other granule cells in the inner molecular layer, and a smaller proportion with inhibitory interneurons. Mossy fiber sprouting is best visualized by either the Timm sulfide silver method or dynorphin immunohistochemistry (Houser et al., 1990). Dynorphin is an opioid neuropeptide that is normally present in the granule cells, their axons, and the terminal fields of the mossy fibers. Mossy fiber sprouting may be observed in all subtypes of HS, including end folium gliosis (Fig. 14.6). At autopsy, it may be bilateral and can be observed in epilepsy syndromes other than TLE (Thom et al., 2009b). Therefore, whether it is a network change in response to seizures or is directly promoting seizures remains to be resolved.

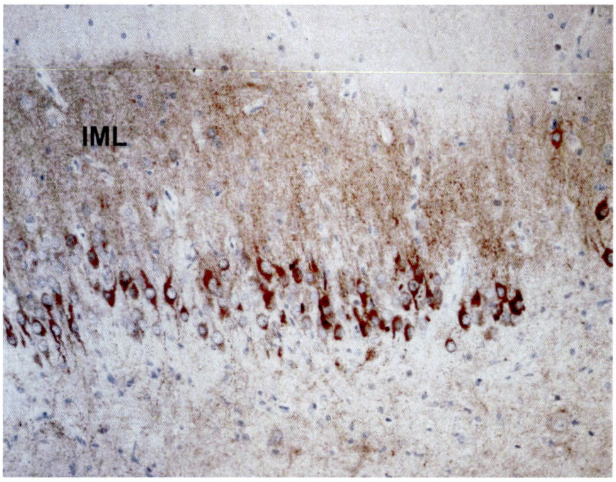

Fig. 14.6. Dynorphin staining confirming positivity of labeling of granule cell bodies and their axons (mossy fibers) which project in the internal molecular layer (IML) more than the hilus. This pattern confirms mossy fiber sprouting.

Alteration to inhibitory neurons

Structural and functional changes to inhibitory networks have been demonstrated in HS and animal models of MTLE that could support a deficit of inhibitory synaptic transmission. This includes altered number and morphology of inhibitory neurons. The challenge is to distinguish changes that directly influence epileptogenesis from those that represent adaptive phenomena in response to seizures or indeed to pharmacological treatments. Loss of hilar mossy excitatory cells may be an early event in the process of HS. Loss of hilar peptidergic neurons, including neuropeptide Y-positive neurons, has also been shown (de Lanerolle et al., 2003). These neurons are likely to mediate feedback inhibition on principal neurons. Loss of calbindin expression in granule cells, as well as altered morphology, sprouting, and complexity of terminals of parvalbumin and calbindin-positive inhibitory neurons in the dentate gyrus as well as CA1, has been reported (Magloczky et al., 2000; Wittner et al., 2002, 2005) (Fig. 14.7).

Glial cell populations and microvasculature in HS

Cellular and reactive gliosis in HS has commonly been regarded as a structural or reparative cellular reaction in response to neuronal loss. However, research is beginning to address the functional contribution of glial cells to excitability. Alterations to astrocytic, microglial, oligodendroglial, and polydendrocyte populations may be involved in human epilepsies (Pitkanen and Lukasiuk, 2009). For example, astrocytes have roles in glutamate transport, and through gap junctions may have roles in synchronizing neuronal activity. In addition, there is a capacity for proliferation and some glial cells may acquire a stem cell-like phenotype, as has been shown in epilepsy tissues (Martinian et al., 2009). Liberation of cytokines from astrocytes and microglia, including proinflammatory cytokines, may have a role in the process of sclerosis as well as influencing seizures (Vezzani et al., 2008). Alterations in microvascular networks have been reported in HS, including angiogenesis and loss of microvessels in CA1 (Rigau et al., 2007; Kastanauskaite et al., 2009), which may be relevant to dysfunction in blood–brain barrier permeability.

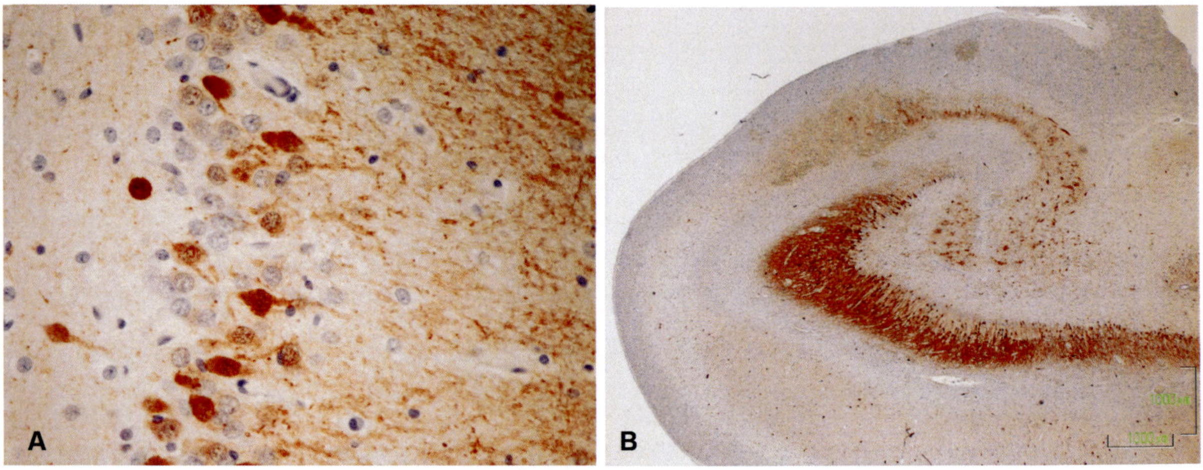

Fig. 14.7. Calbindin immunohistochemistry in hippocampal sclerosis showing loss of expression in a proportion of granule cells (**A**). (**B**) Low-power image confirms residual calbindin in the granule cells and their projection to CA4 and CA3 neurons.

More widespread pathology in related structures

In patients with HS, gliosis and neuronal loss (sclerosis) in adjacent mesial temporal structures (including amygdala and parahippocampal gyrus) as well as the lateral temporal neocortex may be observed. The term mesial temporal lobe sclerosis (MTS) may be reserved for when neuropathological involvement of these mesial structures in addition to the hippocampus is confirmed, but there is no strict definition for this term and it is often used when HS alone is confirmed. Involvement of nuclei in the lateral and basal nuclear complex of the amygdala (neuronal loss, gliosis) have been reported in TLE (Yilmazer-Hanke et al., 2000). However, from a practical viewpoint, detailed examination of the extent and distribution of amygdala structures is hampered by its incomplete and piecemeal removal during temporal lobe surgery, making precise delineation of anatomical subregions difficult. Of interest, recently abnormal voltage properties of satellite glial cells in amygdala specimens from patients with epilepsy have been reported, suggesting a functional importance of amygdala gliosis/sclerosis (Faber-Zuschratter et al., 2009) (Fig. 14.8).

The entorhinal cortex, which is the anterior part of the parahippocampal gyrus, is at the junction between hippocampus and neocortex, and acts as a conduit for incoming afferent information and reciprocal efferent signals. There is evidence that this region may be of importance in the initiation of seizures, and neuroimaging studies have reported volume reduction in this region in patients with HS, although neuropathology reports are less consistent (Cavanagh and Meyer, 1956; Du et al., 1993; Yilmazer-Hanke et al., 2000).

In around 11% of patients with HS, sclerosis may also extend to the superficial layers of the adjacent neocortex, particularly cortical layers II and III of the anterior temporal lobe. This process may be extensive throughout the lobe or preferentially involve the pole (Thom et al., 2009a). Temporopolar involvement has also been shown on neuroimaging studies of patients with HS (Moran et al., 2001; Coste et al., 2002). The temporal pole has connections with the hippocampus and may play a role in seizure initiation in EEG studies (Chabardes et al., 2005). The additional neuropathological findings of disorganization of residual neurons in outer cortical layers in temporal lobe sclerosis suggest that there is a superimposed acquired dysplasia or "dysmaturation." In many cases there is an early onset of seizures, which could indicate an age-related vulnerability to this pathology (Thom et al., 2009a) (Fig. 14.9). In Bruton's series, the presence of temporal lobe sclerosis was more often associated with more severe HS (total sclerosis) (Bruton (1988) and Institute of Psychiatry, University of London). As yet, there is no certain evidence that the presence of this more extensive pathology in the temporal lobe has any effect on outcome following surgery.

Pathophysiology

As described in the previous section, much is known about the larger structural changes in MTLE, but far less is known about how those changes lead to epilepsy. There is an obvious limit to how much can be learned from human tissue, but much progress has been made in the last two decades, in large part because of the availability of animal models that closely mimic the human condition. The development of the animal models has

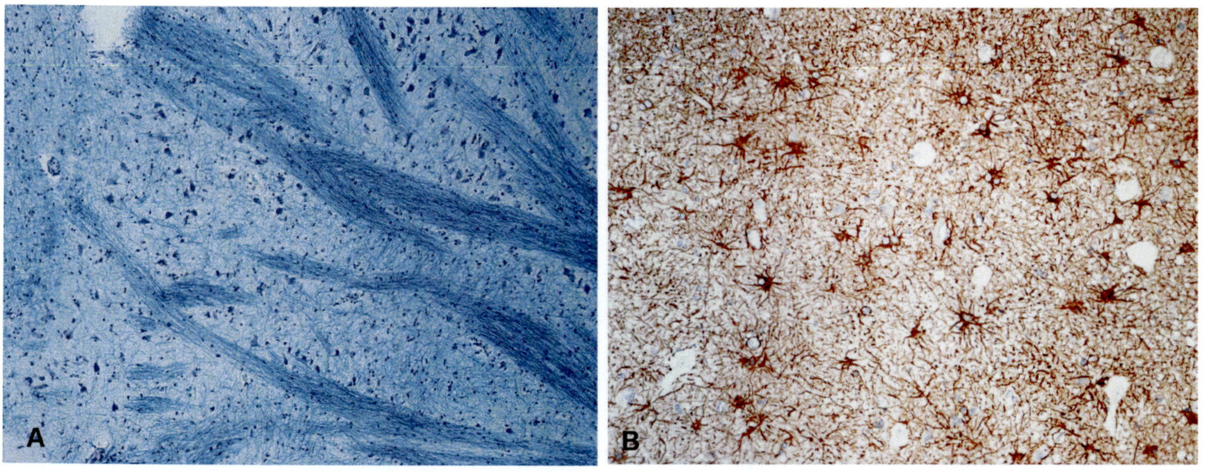

Fig. 14.8. Surgical specimen from a patient with classical hippocampal sclerosis. (**A**) The specimen from the amygdala is often fragmented (cavitron ultrasonic surgical aspiratory (CUSA) specimen), but within this material regions of lateral nucleus with typical myeloarchitecture are recognizable. (**B**) A glial fibrillary acidic protein (GFAP)-stained section confirms a reactive gliosis.

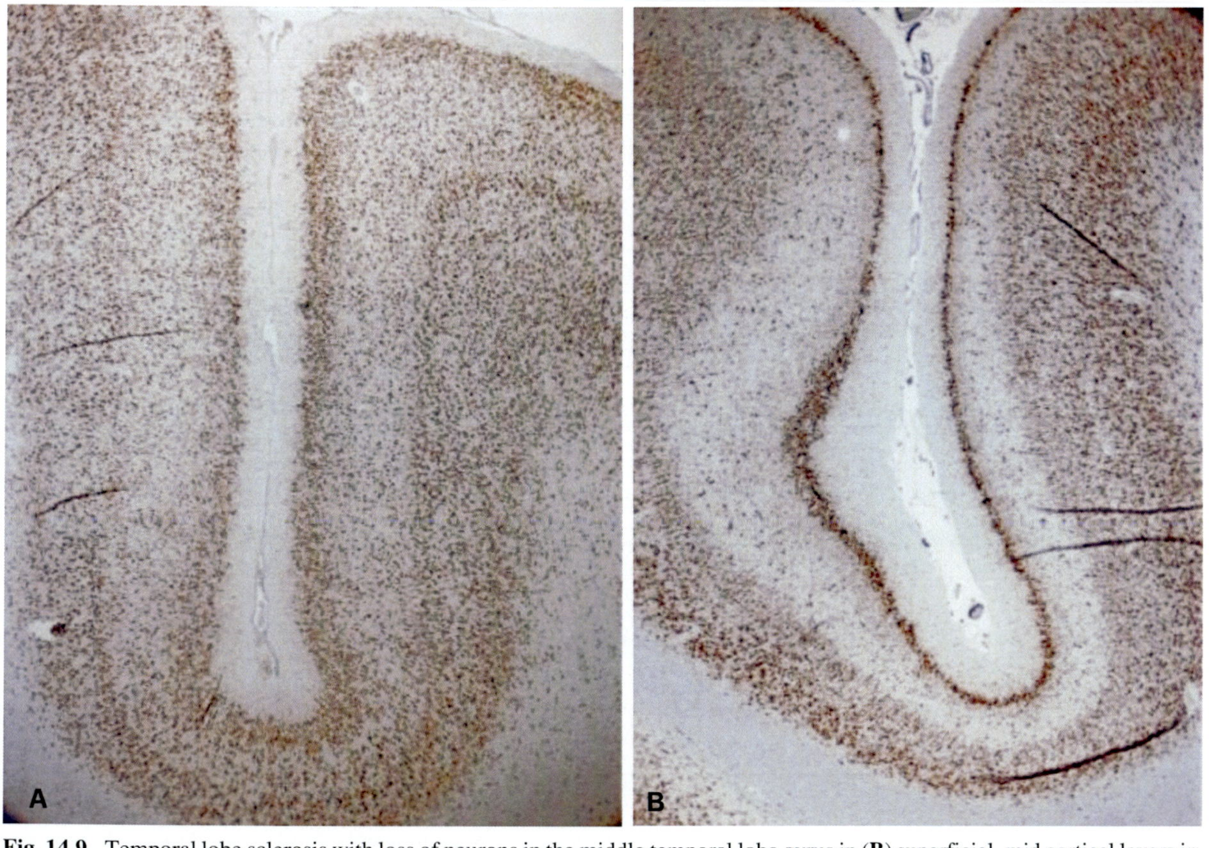

Fig. 14.9. Temporal lobe sclerosis with loss of neurons in the middle temporal lobe gyrus in (**B**) superficial–mid cortical layers in the case compared with (**A**) normal cortex.

paralleled the growth in genetics and molecular biology that has led to an explosion in our understanding of the structure and function of receptors and channels, especially as it relates to how slight variations in the structure of channel and receptor isoforms significantly alter the physiology and pharmacology. These discoveries have provided new directions in epilepsy research and insights into the basis of MTLE as well as drug resistance.

Research into the pathophysiology of epilepsy has been an examination of the balances between excitation and inhibition. With the development of the animal models of MTLE, it has become clear that there are changes on both sides of the balance that would tilt the cell towards a hyperexcitable state. In several regions in the limbic system, the inhibitory potentials are reduced with clear reductions in $GABA_A$ and $GABA_B$ components of the response (Mangan and Lothman, 1996; Mangan and Bertram, 1997, 1998). This reduction enhances the excitatory response of the neurons (Fig. 14.10). Of further note, there is a change in the expression of the receptors themselves, with a different composition of the $GABA_A$ subunits (Nishimura et al., 2005) and in the overall expression of the $GABA_B$ subunit (Billinton et al., 2001; Furtinger et al., 2003a, b). There are also changes in the expression of the glutamate receptors (Mathern et al., 1997b; Aronica et al., 2000).

More recently there has been a renewed focus on alterations in voltage-gated sodium channels. This reexamination of the potential changes in sodium channel expression has come about because of the discovery of multiple isoforms of the voltage-gated sodium channels, the recognition that a number of sodium channel mutations are associated with epilepsy (including some familial forms of TLE associated with HS), and because a number of the effective drugs presumably work on the sodium channel. It has become clear that there is a major shift in the expression of sodium channels in the hippocampus and entorhinal cortex (Aronica et al., 2001; Hargus et al., 2011) with a consequent shift in the voltage-gated sodium channel physiology (Ketelaars et al., 2001; Hargus et al., 2011) and, perhaps just as important, pharmacology (Remy and Beck, 2006; Jones et al., 2009). The shifts in physiology result in sodium channels that have a lower threshold for firing and tend to fire in bursts, thus making the neurons far more likely to have bursts of action potential to less intense stimulation. This shift in sodium channel expression also has therapeutic implications because, just as is the case for the $GABA_A$ receptor, the expression of alternative sodium channels alters (usually reduces) sensitivity to the currently available antiepileptic drugs. This shift in pharmacosensitivity to these drugs may contribute to the drug resistance that is often associated with MTLE (Remy and Beck, 2006).

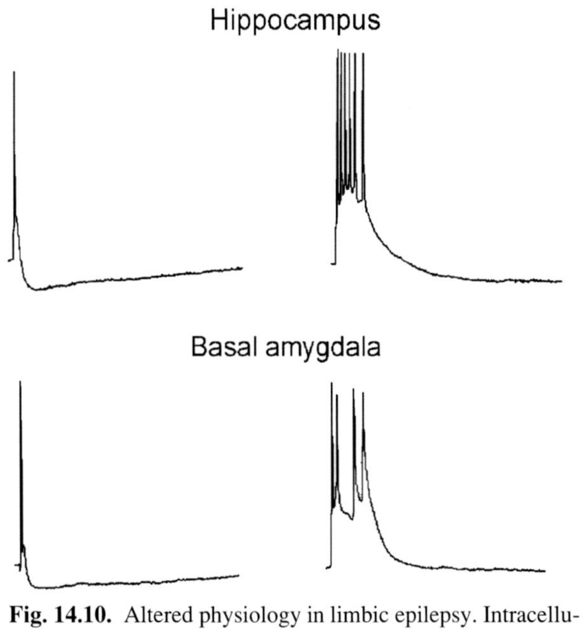

Fig. 14.10. Altered physiology in limbic epilepsy. Intracellular neuronal evoked responses from normal (left) and epileptic (right) rats from the hippocampus (area CA1) and the amygdala (basolateral nucleus). Neurons from normal rats show brief excitatory responses, a single action potential, and a period of hyperpolarization. Neurons from epileptic rats have a prolonged excitatory response with multiple action potentials and no subsequent hyperpolarization.

There has been much focus on changes in expression of the primary channels and receptors, but there are also a number of changes in the modulators of neuronal excitability such as neuropeptide Y (Vezzani and Sperk, 2004) or brain-derived neurotrophic factor (BDNF) (Tongiorgi et al., 2006). Changes in the expression of the primary receptor subtypes, such as $GABA_A$, also affect the sensitivity of the receptors to other neuromodulators, such as the neurosteroids (Mtchedlishvili et al., 2001). The neuromodulators are underappreciated for their potential role in seizure onset. The changes in receptors and channels are fixed and present all the time, but seizures do not happen all of the time. It has been shown that the seizures of MTLE are much more likely to occur during the day, especially in the afternoon (Quigg et al., 1998). This diurnal pattern of seizure occurrence implies that there are variations of system excitability and that the initiation of seizures might be the result of rises and falls in the levels of neuromodulators. Of some note, this pattern of diurnal seizure preference appears to be unique for MTLE, which also suggests that the pathophysiology of the different types of epilepsy is unique to the particular syndrome.

SUMMARY

In the last two decades our understanding of MTLE and its pathophysiology has grown remarkably. Perhaps the most important recognition is that it is not a single entity with a uniform pathology. Rather, it is associated with significant variations in pathology that, in turn, are likely associated with different causes, functional anatomies, physiologies, and outcomes to treatment (medical and surgical). There are numerous changes in the expression of channels and receptors that contribute to the development of epilepsy and, perhaps, drug resistance. This progress in our understanding has also been aided immeasurably by the development of animal models with many parallels to the human condition. These models have allowed us to look at changes in anatomy and physiology and to dissect the circuits in ways that have not been possible in humans. The animal models have also allowed us to create hypotheses about the pathophysiology of the disorder that we have started to examine with the new imaging tools. At present, it is best to summarize our understanding of MTLE by saying there are multiple changes in multiple sites that contribute to the development of the chronic condition. For this reason alone, we should consider MTLE to be a systems disorder.

References

Abou-Khalil B, Ge Q, Desai R et al. (2001). Partial and generalized epilepsy with febrile seizures plus and a novel SCN1A mutation. Neurology 57: 2265–2272.

Aronica E, van Vliet EA, Mayboroda OA et al. (2000). Upregulation of metabotropic glutamate receptor subtype mGluR3 and mGluR5 in reactive astrocytes in a rat model of mesial temporal lobe epilepsy. Eur J Neurosci 12: 2333–2344.

Aronica E, Yankaya B, Troost D et al. (2001). Induction of neonatal sodium channel II and III alpha-isoform mRNAs in neurons and microglia after status epilepticus in the rat hippocampus. Eur J Neurosci 13: 1261–1266.

Auer T, Barsi P, Bone B et al. (2008). History of simple febrile seizures is associated with hippocampal abnormalities in adults. Epilepsia 49: 1562–1569.

Berkovic SF, Andermann F, Oliver A et al. (1991). Hippocampal sclerosis in temporal lobe epilepsy demonstrated by magnetic resonance imaging. Ann Neurol 29: 175–182.

Bernhardt BC, Worsley KJ, Kim H et al. (2009). Longitudinal and cross-sectional analysis of atrophy in pharmacoresistant temporal lobe epilepsy. Neurology 72: 1747–1754.

Bertram EH (1997). The functional anatomy of spontaneous seizures in a rat model of chronic limbic epilepsy. Epilepsia 38: 95–105.

Bertram EH, Cornett J (1994). The evolution of a rat model of chronic limbic epilepsy. Brain Res 661: 157–162.

Bertram EH, Scott C (2000). Pathological substrate for limbic epilepsy: is the medial dorsal thalamic nucleus the unifying abnormality. Epilepsia 41: S3–S9.

Bertram E, Lothman E, Lenn N (1990). The hippocampus in experimental chronic epilepsy: a morphometric analysis. Ann Neurol 27: 43–48.

Bertram EH, Zhang DX, Williamson JM (2008). Multiple roles of midline dorsal thalamic nuclei in induction and spread of limbic seizures. Epilepsia 49: 256–268.

Bien CG, Urbach H, Schramm J et al. (2007). Limbic encephalitis as a precipitating event in adult-onset temporal lobe epilepsy. Neurology 69: 1236–1244.

Billinton A, Baird VH, Thom M et al. (2001). $GABA_B$ receptor autoradiography in hippocampal sclerosis associated with human temporal lobe epilepsy. Br J Pharmacol 132: 475–480.

Blumcke I, Thom M, Wiestler OD (2002). Ammon's horn sclerosis: a maldevelopmental disorder associated with temporal lobe epilepsy. Brain Pathol 12: 199–211.

Blumcke I, Pauli E, Clusmann H et al. (2007). A new clinicopathological classification system for mesial temporal sclerosis. Acta Neuropathol 113: 235–244.

Blumcke I, Kistner I, Clusmann H et al. (2009). Towards a clinico-pathological classification of granule cell dispersion in human mesial temporal lobe epilepsies. Acta Neuropathol 117: 535–544.

Bratz E (1899). Ammonshornbefunde bei epileptikern. Arch Psychiatr Nervenkr 32: 820–835.

Bruton CJ (1988). The Neuropathology of Temporal Lobe Epilepsy. Oxford University Press, Oxford.

Cassidy RM, Gale K (1998). Mediodorsal thalamus plays a critical role in the development of limbic motor seizures. J Neurosci 18: 9002–9009.

Cavanagh JB, Meyer A (1956). Aetiological aspects of Ammon's horn sclerosis associated with temporal lobe epilepsy. Br Med J 2: 1403–1407.

Cavazos JE, Sutula TP (1990). Progressive neuronal loss induced by kindling: a possible mechanism for mossy fiber synaptic reorganization and hippocampal sclerosis. Brain Res 527: 1–6.

Cavazos JE, Zhang P, Qazi R et al. (2003). Ultrastructural features of sprouted mossy fiber synapses in kindled and kainic acid-treated rats. J Comp Neurol 458: 272–292.

Cendes F, Lopes-Cendes I, Andermann E et al. (1998). Familial temporal lobe epilepsy: a clinically heterogeneous syndrome. Neurology 50: 554–557.

Chabardes S, Kahane P, Minotti L et al. (2005). The temporopolar cortex plays a pivotal role in temporal lobe seizures. Brain 128: 1818–1831.

Coste S, Ryvlin P, Hermier M et al. (2002). Temporopolar changes in temporal lobe epilepsy: a quantitative MRI-based study. Neurology 59: 855–861.

Davies KG, Hermann BP, Dohan FC Jr et al. (1996). Relationship of hippocampal sclerosis to duration and age of onset of epilepsy, and childhood febrile seizures in temporal lobectomy patients. Epilepsy Res 24: 119–126.

de Lanerolle NC, Kim JH, Williamson A et al. (2003). A retrospective analysis of hippocampal pathology in human temporal lobe epilepsy: evidence for distinctive patient subcategories. Epilepsia 44: 677–687.

Du F, Whetsell WO Jr, Abou-Khalil B et al. (1993). Preferential neuronal loss in layer III of the entorhinal cortex in patients with temporal lobe epilepsy. Epilepsy Res 16: 223–233.

Eriksson SH, Thom M, Bartlett PA et al. (2008). PROPELLER MRI visualizes detailed pathology of hippocampal sclerosis. Epilepsia 49: 33–39.

Faber-Zuschratter H, Huttmann K, Steinhauser C et al. (2009). Ultrastructural and functional characterization of satellitosis in the human lateral amygdala associated with Ammon's horn sclerosis. Acta Neuropathol 117: 545–555.

Fried I, Spencer DD, Spencer SS (1995). The anatomy of epileptic auras: focal pathology and surgical outcome. J Neurosurg 83: 60–66.

Frotscher M, Haas CA, Forster E (2003). Reelin controls granule cell migration in the dentate gyrus by acting on the radial glial scaffold. Cereb Cortex 13: 634–640.

Furtinger S, Bettler B, Sperk G (2003a). Altered expression of $GABA_B$ receptors in the hippocampus after kainic-acid-induced seizures in rats. Brain Res Mol Brain Res 113: 107–115.

Furtinger S, Pirker S, Czech T et al. (2003b). Increased expression of gamma-aminobutyric acid type B receptors in the hippocampus of patients with temporal lobe epilepsy. Neurosci Lett 352: 141–145.

Gale K (1992). Subcortical structures and pathways involved in convulsive seizure generation. J Clin Neurophysiol 9: 264–277.

Goddard GV, McIntyre DC, Leech CK (1969). A permanent change in brain function resulting from daily electrical stimulation. Exp Neurol 25: 295–330.

Gorter JA, van Vliet EA, Aronica E et al. (2001). Progression of spontaneous seizures after status epilepticus is associated with mossy fibre sprouting and extensive bilateral loss of hilar parvalbumin and somatostatin-immunoreactive neurons. Eur J Neurosci 13: 657–669.

Gorter JA, Goncalves Pereira PM, van Vliet EA et al. (2003). Neuronal cell death in a rat model for mesial temporal lobe epilepsy is induced by the initial status epilepticus and not by later repeated spontaneous seizures. Epilepsia 44: 647–658.

Greenfield JG, Love S, Louis DN et al. (2008). Greenfield's Neuropathology. 8th edn. Hodder Arnold, London.

Guerrini R, Belmonte A, Canapicchi R et al. (1998). Reversible pseudoatrophy of the brain and mental deterioration associated with valproate treatment. Epilepsia 39: 27–32.

Guye M, Regis J, Tamura M et al. (2006). The role of corticothalamic coupling in human temporal lobe epilepsy. Brain 129: 1917–1928.

Hargus NJ, Merrick EC, Nigam A et al. (2011). Temporal lobe epilepsy induces intrinsic alterations in Na channel gating in layer II entorhinal cortex neurons. Neurobiol Dis 41: 361–376.

Houser CR (1990). Granule cell dispersion in the dentate gyrus of humans with temporal lobe epilepsy. Brain Res 535: 195–204.

Houser CR, Miyashiro JE, Swartz BE et al. (1990). Altered patterns of dynorphin immunoreactivity suggest mossy fiber reorganization in human hippocampal epilepsy. J Neurosci 10: 267–282.

Hudson LP, Munoz DG, Miller L et al. (1993). Amygdaloid sclerosis in temporal lobe epilepsy. Ann Neurol 33: 622–631.

Jackson GD, Duncan JS, Connelly A et al. (1991). Increased signal in the mesial temporal region on T2 weighted MRI: a quantitative study of hippocampal sclerosis. Neurology 41 (suppl 1): 170–171.

Jones PJ, Merrick EC, Hargus NJ et al. (2009). Modulation of sodium channel inactivation gating by a novel lactam: implications for seizure suppression in chronic limbic epilepsy. J Pharmacol Exp Ther 328: 201–212.

Juhász C, Nagy F, Watson C et al. (1999). Glucose and [C-11] flumazenil positron emission tomography abnormalities of thalamic nuclei in temporal lobe epilepsy. Neurology 53: 2037–2045.

Kastanauskaite A, Alonso-Nanclares L, Blazquez-Llorca L et al. (2009). Alterations of the microvascular network in sclerotic hippocampi from patients with epilepsy. J Neuropathol Exp Neurol 68: 939–950.

Kearney JA, Plummer NW, Smith MR et al. (2001). A gain-of-function mutation in the sodium channel gene Scn2a results in seizures and behavioral abnormalities. Neuroscience 102: 307–317.

Ketelaars SO, Gorter JA, van Vliet EA et al. (2001). Sodium currents in isolated rat CA1 pyramidal and dentate granule neurones in the post-status epilepticus model of epilepsy. Neuroscience 105: 109–120.

Kobayashi E, Li LM, Lopes-Cendes I et al. (2002). Magnetic resonance imaging evidence of hippocampal sclerosis in asymptomatic, first-degree relatives of patients with familial mesial temporal lobe epilepsy. Arch Neurol 59: 1891–1894.

Kudin AP, Zsurka G, Elger CE et al. (2009). Mitochondrial involvement in temporal lobe epilepsy. Exp Neurol 218: 326–332.

Lai M, Huijbers MG, Lancaster E et al. (2010). Investigation of LGI1 as the antigen in limbic encephalitis previously attributed to potassium channels: a case series. Lancet Neurol 9: 776–785.

Lancaster E, Lai M, Peng X et al. (2010). Antibodies to the GABA(B) receptor in limbic encephalitis with seizures: case series and characterisation of the antigen. Lancet Neurol 9: 67–76.

Liimatainen S, Peltola M, Sabater L et al. (2010). Clinical significance of glutamic acid decarboxylase antibodies in patients with epilepsy. Epilepsia 51: 760–767.

Liu RSN, Lemieux L, Bell GS et al. (2005). Cerebral damage in epilepsy: a population-based longitudinal quantitative MRI study. Epilepsia 46: 1482–1494.

Lothman EW, Bertram EH, Stringer J (1991). Functional anatomy of hippocampal seizures. Prog Neurobiol 37: 1–82.

Lurton D, Sundstrom L, Brana C et al. (1997). Possible mechanisms inducing granule cell dispersion in humans with temporal lobe epilepsy. Epilepsy Res 26: 351–361.

Lurton D, El Bahh B, Sundstrom L et al. (1998). Granule cell dispersion is correlated with early epileptic events in human temporal lobe epilepsy. J Neurol Sci 154: 133–136.

Magloczky Z, Wittner L, Borhegyi Z et al. (2000). Changes in the distribution and connectivity of interneurons in the epileptic human dentate gyrus. Neuroscience 96: 7–25.

Mangan PS, Bertram EH (1997). Shortened-duration GABA (A) receptor-mediated synaptic potentials underlie enhanced CA1 excitability in a chronic model of temporal lobe epilepsy. Neuroscience 80: 1101–1111.

Mangan PS, Bertram EH (1998). Ontogeny of altered synaptic function in a rat model of chronic temporal lobe epilepsy. Brain Res 799: 183–196.

Mangan PS, Lothman EW (1996). Profound disturbances of pre- and postsynaptic $GABA_B$-receptor-mediated processes in region CA1 in a chronic model of temporal lobe epilepsy. J Neurophysiol 76: 1282–1296.

Margerison JH, Corsellis JA (1966). Epilepsy and the temporal lobes. A clinical, electroencephalographic and neuropathological study of the brain in epilepsy, with particular reference to the temporal lobes. Brain 89: 499–530.

Martinian L, Boer K, Middeldorp J et al. (2009). Expression patterns of glial fibrillary acidic protein (GFAP)-delta in epilepsy-associated lesional pathologies. Neuropathol Appl Neurobiol 35: 394–405.

Mathern GW, Pretorius JK, Babb TL (1995). Influence of the type of initial precipitating injury and at what age it occurs on course and outcome in patients with temporal lobe seizures. J Neurosurg 82: 220–227.

Mathern GW, Bertram EH, Babb TL et al. (1997a). In contrast to kindled seizures, the frequency of spontaneous epilepsy in the limbic status model correlates with greater fascia dentata excitatory and inhibitory axon sprouting and increased staining for NMDA, AMPA and GABA-A receptors. Neuroscience 77: 1003–1019.

Mathern GW, Kuhlman PA, Mendoza D et al. (1997b). Human fascia dentata anatomy and hippocampal neuron densities differ depending on the epileptic syndrome and age at first seizure. J Neuropathol Exp Neurol 56: 199–212.

Mathern GW, Adelson PD, Cahan LD et al. (2002). Hippocampal neuron damage in human epilepsy: Meyer's hypothesis revisited. Prog Brain Res 135: 237–251.

McNamara JO, Galloway MT, Rigsbee LC et al. (1984). Evidence implicating substantia nigra in regulation of kindled seizure threshold. J Neurosci 4: 2410–2417.

Meyer A, Falconer MA, Beck E (1954). Pathological findings in temporal lobe epilepsy. J Neurol Neurosurg Psychiatry 17: 276–285.

Miller JW, Ferrendelli JA (1990). Characterization of GABAergic seizure regulation in the midline thalamus. Neuropharmacology 29: 649–655.

Moran NF, Lemieux L, Kitchen ND et al. (2001). Extrahippocampal temporal lobe atrophy in temporal lobe epilepsy and mesial temporal sclerosis. Brain 124: 167–175.

Moshé SL, Garant DS, Sperber EF et al. (1995). Ontogeny and topography of seizure regulation by the substantia nigra. Brain Dev 17: 61–72.

Mtchedlishvili Z, Bertram EH, Kapur J (2001). Diminished allopregnanolone enhancement of $GABA_A$ receptor currents in a rat model of chronic temporal lobe epilepsy. J Physiol 537: 453–465.

Nadler JV (2003). The recurrent mossy fiber pathway of the epileptic brain. Neurochem Res 28: 1649–1658.

Natsume J, Bernasconi N, Andermann F et al. (2003). MRI volumetry of the thalamus in temporal, extratemporal, and idiopathic generalized epilepsy. Neurology 60: 1296–1300.

Nishimura T, Schwarzer C, Gasser E et al. (2005). Altered expression of GABA(A) and GABA(B) receptor subunit mRNAs in the hippocampus after kindling and electrically induced status epilepticus. Neuroscience 134: 691–704.

Pauli E, Hildebrandt M, Romstock J et al. (2006). Deficient memory acquisition in temporal lobe epilepsy is predicted by hippocampal granule cell loss. Neurology 67: 1383–1389.

Pitkanen A, Lukasiuk K (2009). Molecular and cellular basis of epileptogenesis in symptomatic epilepsy. Epilepsy Behav 14: 16–25.

Quigg M, Straume M, Menaker M et al. (1998). Temporal distribution of partial seizures: comparison of an animal model with human partial epilepsy. Ann Neurol 43: 748–755.

Remy S, Beck H (2006). Molecular and cellular mechanisms of pharmacoresistance in epilepsy. Brain 129: 18–35.

Rigau V, Morin M, Rousset MC et al. (2007). Angiogenesis is associated with blood–brain barrier permeability in temporal lobe epilepsy. Brain 130: 1942–1956.

Sagar HJ, Oxbury JM (1987). Hippocampal neuron loss in temporal lobe epilepsy: correlation with early childhood convulsions. Ann Neurol 22: 334–340.

Sloan DM, Zhang D, Bertram EM, 3rd. (2011). Increased GABAergic inhibition in the midline thalamus affects signaling and seizure spread in the hippocampus–prefrontal cortex pathway. Epilepsia 52: 523–530.

So NK (1991). Depth electrode studies in mesial temporal lobe epilepsy. In: H Luders (Ed.), Epilepsy Surgery. Raven Press, New York, pp. 371–384.

Sommer W (1880). Erkrankung des Ammonshornes als aetiologisches Moment der Epilepsie. Arch Psychiatr Nervenkr 10: 631–675.

Spencer SS, Spencer DD (1994). Entorhinal–hippocampal interactions in medial temporal lobe epilepsy. Epilepsia 35: 721–727.

Stefan H, Hildebrandt M, Kerling F et al. (2009). Clinical prediction of postoperative seizure control: structural, functional findings and disease histories. J Neurol Neurosurg Psychiatry 80: 196–200.

Stephen LJ, Kwan P, Brodie MJ (2001). Does the cause of localisation related epilepsy influence the response to antiepileptic drug treatment? Epilepsia 42: 357–382.

Su H-S, Bentivoglio M (1990). Thalamic midline cell populations projecting to the nucleus accumbens, amygdala, and hippocampus in the rat. J Comp Neurol 297: 582–593.

Sutula T, Cascino G, Cavazos J et al. (1989). Mossy fiber synaptic reorganization in the epileptic human temporal lobe. Ann Neurol 26: 321–330.

Suzuki F, Heinrich C, Boehrer A et al. (2005). Glutamate receptor antagonists and benzodiazepine inhibit the progression of granule cell dispersion in a mouse model of mesial temporal lobe epilepsy. Epilepsia 46: 193–202.

Theodore WH, Epstein L, Gaillard WD et al. (2008). Human herpes virus 6B: a possible role in epilepsy? Epilepsia 49: 1828–1837.

Thom M (2009). Hippocampal sclerosis: progress since Sommer. Brain Pathol 19: 565–572.

Thom M, Sisodiya SM, Beckett A et al. (2002). Cytoarchitectural abnormalities in hippocampal sclerosis. J Neuropathol Exp Neurol 61: 510–519.

Thom M, Eriksson S, Martinian L et al. (2009a). Temporal lobe sclerosis associated with hippocampal sclerosis in temporal lobe epilepsy: neuropathological features. J Neuropathol Exp Neurol 68: 928–938.

Thom M, Martinian L, Catarino C et al. (2009b). Bilateral reorganization of the dentate gyrus in hippocampal sclerosis: a postmortem study. Neurology 73: 1033–1040.

Tongiorgi E, Domenici L, Simonato M (2006). What is the biological significance of BDNF mRNA targeting in the dendrites? Clues from epilepsy and cortical development. Mol Neurobiol 33: 17–32.

Turner BH, Herkenham M (1991). Thalamoamygdaloid projections in the rat: a test of the amygdala's role in sensory processing. J Comp Neurol 313: 295–325.

Van der Werf YD, Witter MP, Groenewegen HJ (2002). The intralaminar and midline nuclei of the thalamus. Anatomical and functional evidence for participation in processes of arousal and awareness. Brain Res Rev 39: 107–140.

van Groen T, Wyss JM (1990). Extrinsic projections from area CA_1 of the rat hippocampus: olfactory, cortical, subcortical, and bilateral hippocampal formation projections. J Comp Neurol 302: 515–528.

Van Paesschen W, Revesz T, Duncan JS (1997). Quantitative neuropathology and quantitative magnetic resonance imaging of the hippocampus in temporal lobe epilepsy. Ann Neurol 42: 756–766.

Vezzani A, Sperk G (2004). Overexpression of NPY and Y2 receptors in epileptic brain tissue: an endogenous neuroprotective mechanism in temporal lobe epilepsy? Neuropeptides 38: 245–252.

Vezzani A, Balosso S, Ravizza T (2008). The role of cytokines in the pathophysiology of epilepsy. Brain Behav Immun 22: 797–803.

Vincent A, Irani SR, Lang B (2010). The growing recognition of immunotherapy-responsive seizure disorders with autoantibodies to specific neuronal proteins. Curr Opin Neurol 23: 144–150.

Wieser HG (2004). ILAE Commission Report. Mesial temporal lobe epilepsy with hippocampal sclerosis. Epilepsia 45: 695–714.

Williams PA, White AM, Clark S et al. (2009). Development of spontaneous recurrent seizures after kainate-induced status epilepticus. J Neurosci 29: 2103–2112.

Williamson PD, French JA, Thadjani VM et al. (1993). Characteristics of medial temporal lobe epilepsy. II: interictal and ictal scalp electroencephalography, neuropsychological testing, neuroimaging, surgical results and pathology. Ann Neurol 34: 781–787.

Wittner L, Eross L, Szabo Z et al. (2002). Synaptic reorganization of calbindin-positive neurons in the human hippocampal CA1 region in temporal lobe epilepsy. Neuroscience 115: 961–978.

Wittner L, Eross L, Czirjak S et al. (2005). Surviving CA1 pyramidal cells receive intact perisomatic inhibitory input in the human epileptic hippocampus. Brain 128: 138–152.

Yilmazer-Hanke DM, Wolf HK, Schramm J et al. (2000). Subregional pathology of the amygdala complex and entorhinal region in surgical specimens from patients with pharmacoresistant temporal lobe epilepsy. J Neuropathol Exp Neurol 59: 907–920.

Handbook of Clinical Neurology, Vol. 107 (3rd series)
Epilepsy, Part I
H. Stefan and W.H. Theodore, Editors

Chapter 15

Extratemporal epilepsies

SEBASTIAN BAUER[1]* AND HAJO M. HAMER[2]

[1]*Interdisciplinary Epilepsy Center, Department of Neurology, UKGM Marburg, Philipps University, Marburg, Germany*

[2]*Epilepsy Center, Department of Neurology, University Hospital Erlangen, Erlangen, Germany*

INTRODUCTION

Focal extratemporal epilepsies comprise different syndromes according to the location of the epileptogenic zone. This chapter focuses on neocortical frontal lobe epilepsy (FLE), parietal lobe epilepsy (PLE), and occipital lobe epilepsy (OLE). Infrequent syndromes, such as insular epilepsy and gelastic epilepsy due to hypothalamic hamartomas, are beyond the scope of this chapter. Plenty of studies are available for FLE, whereas data regarding PLE and OLE are sparse. Clinical features, diagnostic evaluation, therapy, and outcome are reviewed separately for FLE, PLE, and OLE.

FRONTAL LOBE EPILEPSIES

Anatomy of the frontal lobe

To understand the seizure semiology that is seen in frontal lobe seizures, knowledge of the structural and functional anatomy is important.

STRUCTURAL ANATOMY

Macroscopically, the frontal lobe extends from the central sulcus to the frontal pole and is separated from the temporal lobe by the lateral sulcus. Due to its functional connectivity, the area between the precentral and the postcentral sulcus is referred to as the central lobe by some authors (Brun, 1999).

The frontal lobe can be divided into:

- the lateral part, which comprises the precentral gyrus, the lateral part of the superior frontal gyrus, and the middle and inferior frontal gyrus
- the mesial (or medial) part, which consists of the medial part of the superior frontal gyrus and the cingulated gyrus
- the orbital (or basal) part, composed of the lateral, medial, anterior, and posterior orbital gyrus as well as the gyrus rectus.

Microscopically, the frontal lobe consists of neocortex with six layers of neurons. Brodmann subdivided and numerated 52 areas of different cytoarchitectural patterns. However, there is considerable variability of these cytoarchitectural areas in relation to macroanatomical landmarks (Amunts et al., 1999; Geyer et al., 2000; Brett et al., 2002).

FUNCTIONAL ANATOMY

Beginning in the 19th century, the function of different frontal lobe areas has been determined by lesion studies on primates and by electrical stimulation. The most obvious function of the frontal lobe is motor function. Therefore, the functional frontal lobe areas are usually subdivided into "primary" motor cortex, "premotor" cortex, and "prefrontal" cortex.

The *primary motor cortex (or M1)* is located on the precentral gyrus and in the central sulcus. It is consistent with Brodmann area 4 and topically organized as a "homunculus" according to the results of electrical stimulation studies (Penfield and Boldrey, 1937).

The *premotor cortex* can be defined as "the region or regions in the frontal lobe that project directly to M1 in primates" (Dum and Strick, 2002). It is located rostrally to the precentral gyrus within parts of the lateral and mesial surface, and contains at least six "premotor"

*Correspondence to: S. Bauer, M.D., Interdisciplinary Epilepsy Center, Department of Neurology, UKGM Marburg, Philipps University, Baldingerstrasse, 35033 Marburg, Germany. Tel: +49-6421-5862850, Fax: +49-6421-586 7055, E-mail: bauer-se@med.uni-marburg.de regions including the supplementary motor area (SMA). Each of these regions is thought to control specific aspects of motor tasks via projection into M1 and direct projection to spinal cord neurons (Dum and Strick, 2002). Furthermore, the frontal eye field (Brodmann area 8 at the intersection of the precentral and superior frontal sulcus) and Broca's language region (Brodmann areas 44 and 45 at the opercular and triangular parts of the inferior frontal gyrus in the dominant hemisphere) belong to the premotor cortex. The main function of the frontal eye field is the control of intentional saccades. Therefore, it receives input from occipital and parietal lobes. Broca's language area is connected with Wernicke's temporal speech area and the primary motor cortex to enable its function in speech production.

The remaining parts of the frontal lobe that belong neither to the primary motor nor to the premotor cortex are referred to as *prefrontal cortex*. An alternative (and equivalent) proposal defines the prefrontal cortex as the part of the cerebral cortex that receives projections from the mediodorsal nucleus of the thalamus. Its function is rather vaguely defined and covers executive control, monitoring in working memory, learning, temporal structuring of behavior, and control of behavior by context (Duncan and Owen, 2000). Few specific regions have been identified that are recruited by different demands indicating a "prefrontal" network involved in the solution of diverse cognitive problems.

Epidemiology of frontal lobe epilepsies

Few data are available on the incidence and prevalence of FLE. If the localization of seizure onset is estimated mainly on the basis of the clinical semiology, frontal lobe involvement is frequently overrated owing to the fact that motor signs are usually the most impressive features of an epileptic seizure. For instance, the National General Practice Study of Epilepsy (NGPSE) (Manford et al., 1992a, b) enrolled 594 patients with newly diagnosed epilepsy in a prospective manner. About 40% of these patients suffered from partial epilepsy. The NGPSE investigators found a clinically localizable seizure onset in 27% of the patients. Within this group, the clinical seizure onset was "frontal" in 22.5%, "central sensorimotor" in 32.5%, and "frontotemporal" in 5.6%. This would suggest FLE in about 60% of all patients with partial epilepsy and localizable seizure onset, which is obviously contrary to clinical experience. Indeed, electroencephalography (EEG) and computed tomography (CT) findings were frequently discordant with the seizure semiology in this study.

On the other hand, FLE is probably underrepresented in hospital-based studies because patients with extratemporal epilepsies may be referred less frequently to presurgical video-EEG monitoring compared with patients with temporal lobe epilepsies due to unclear results in seizure semiology and interictal EEG and magnetic resonance imaging (MRI) findings that make eligibility for surgery difficult. FLE was found in 10–27% of adult patients (Brekelmans et al., 1998; Ryvlin et al., 1998; Semah et al., 1998; Dobesberger et al., 2004) and in 18–21% of children (Ohtsuka et al., 2001; Lawson et al., 2002; Fujiwara and Shigematsu, 2004) referred to epilepsy centers.

Not only the patient population but also the method of epilepsy classification has an influence on the identification of epilepsy prevalence. This has been shown by using a newly proposed five-dimensional epilepsy classification (Loddenkemper et al., 2005) instead of the International League Against Epilepsy (ILAE) classification. The epileptogenic zone was found to be localized in the frontal lobe in 4% and in the perirolandic area in 3% of 94 randomly selected adult patients of a tertiary epilepsy center; in 7% of 91 children the epileptogenic zone could be localized to the perirolandic area, and no child with frontal lobe epilepsy was identified (Kellinghaus and Luders, 2004).

As fewer patients with FLE are good surgical candidates compared with patients with temporal lobe epilepsy (TLE), FLE is underrepresented in surgical series. Of a series of 2177 patients who had epilepsy surgery, 7% had central lobe epilepsy and 18% had epilepsy of the (remaining) frontal lobe (Rasmussen, 1991). Another study included 124 consecutive patients and found FLE in 15% of the patients (Inoue and Mihara, 1998).

In conclusion, frontal lobe epilepsies appear to be the second most frequent partial epilepsy syndromes after temporal lobe epilepsies (Kellinghaus et al., 2004) and account for 20–40% of all partial epilepsies.

Etiology of frontal lobe epilepsies

Available data on the etiology of symptomatic FLE are summarized in Table 15.1. Newer studies tend to report cortical dysplasias more frequently, probably due to improving neuroimaging capabilities (Fig. 15.1).

Moreover, there are two types of idiopathic focal epilepsy related to the frontal and central lobe: benign epilepsy with centrotemporal spikes (BECTS) and autosomal dominant nocturnal frontal lobe epilepsy (ADNFLE). ADNFLE is genetically heterogeneous and can be caused by mutations of genes coding for subunits of the neuronal nicotinic acetylcholine receptor (Combi et al., 2004). BECTS has been classified as idiopathic (and thus a presumed genetic etiology) by the ILAE (Commission on Classification and Terminology of the ILAE, 1989), although there was a lack of concordance in twin studies (Vadlamudi et al., 2006).

Table 15.1

Etiology of symptomatic frontal lobe epilepsies

Etiology	Frequency in FLE (%)
Focal cortical dysplasia (FCD)	20–84
Tumor	
Total	13–35
Astrocytoma	10
Ganglioglioma	5–10
Oligodendroglioma	3–10
Dysembryoplastic neuroepithelial tumor (DNET)	1–6
Vascular malformations	
Total	≤15
Arteriovenous malformation (AVM)	6
Cavernoma	9
Gliosis including post-traumatic and postischemic lesions	10–28
Postinflammatory scars	≤10
Birth trauma	≤8
Unknown	≤20

Sources: Ferrier et al., 1999; Frater et al., 2000; Janszky et al., 2000a; Jobst et al., 2000; Schramm et al., 2002; Jeha et al., 2007; Lee et al., 2008

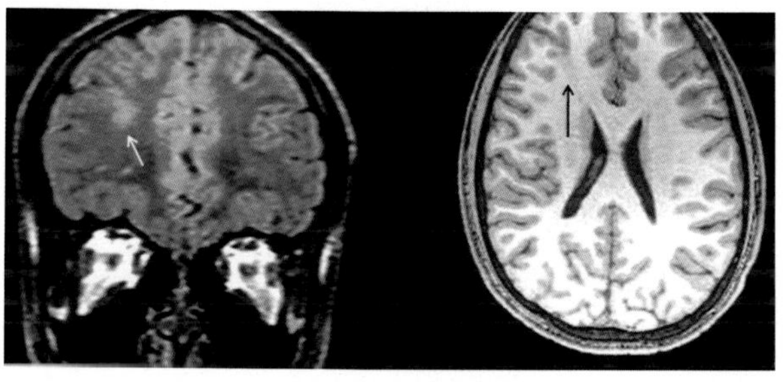

Fig. 15.1. Magnetic resonance image of a 14-year-old patient with right frontal lobe epilepsy. Note focal cortical dysplasia right frontal (arrows). The patient remained seizure-free after resection of dysplasia. © 2012 H.M. Hamer.

Clinical features

Seizure semiology in frontal lobe epilepsy

Central lobe seizures are accompanied by focal somatosensory auras and focal motor signs (Manford et al., 1996; Fogarasi et al., 2001):

- *Focal somatosensory auras* are specific for involvement of the central lobe. However, these auras have to be distinguished from nonspecific auras that occur in the majority of patients with FLE (Jobst et al., 2000; Jobst and Williamson, 2005).
- *Focal motor signs* comprise tonic, dystonic, clonic, and complex motor symptoms. Using electromyography (EMG) and subdural EEG electrodes, it has been shown that clonic seizures are preceded by a tonic phase which is sometimes too subtle to be recognized clinically (Hamer et al., 2003). Repetitive EEG spiking in primary motor areas during the initial tonic phase is followed by spike–wave complexes and synchronous clonic contraction of both agonistic and antagonistic contralateral muscles. EEG spiking matches muscle contractions, whereas relaxation occurs in synchrony with EEG slow waves.

Seizures involving the *"premotor" cortex* may present with the following symptoms (Manford et al., 1996; Kotagal and Arunkumar, 1998; Janszky et al., 2001):

- *Contralateral version* that precedes secondary generalization in half of the seizures (Bonelli and Baumgartner, 2002; Rheims et al., 2005).
- Version must be distinguished from the infrequent unforced *ipsilateral or contralateral head-turning* of unknown pathophysiology without any clonic or pronounced tonic component, which frequently appears at seizure onset (Rheims et al., 2005). Both forms can appear successively in the same seizure.
- *Aphasia, dysphasia, or vocalization* occurs if Broca's language area is involved. Pure vocalization other than those caused by cloni or apnea was seen in 40% (Janszky et al., 2000a). Surprisingly, prolonged postictal dysphasia occurred in less than 10% of 118 complex partial frontal lobe seizures in 24 patients (Goldberg-Stern et al., 2004). The dysphasia was of short duration even when the seizure onset zone was located in the dominant hemisphere. However, seizures starting in the frontal lobe of the dominant side and spreading to the ipsilateral temporal lobe caused long-lasting postictal dysphasia in more than 90% of cases. A short distance between the seizure onset zone and the anatomical location of Broca's speech area (determined by electrical cortical mapping) did not correlate with the appearance of postictal language disturbances. This finding suggests a disruption of temporal speech networks rather than a direct influence on cortical speech areas as the cause for dysphasia.
- Seizures starting in the supplementary sensorimotor area (SSMA) located in the mesial frontal lobe are usually of short duration (10–40 s) and are attended by a rapid bilateral asymmetrical tonic posturing (Laich et al., 1997).

Seizures involving the *"prefrontal" cortex* can present with complex motor seizures including dialeptic (sometimes also referred to as "frontal lobe absences"), automotor, hypermotor, and gelastic seizures (Luders et al., 1998). Hypermotor seizures (complex movements involving trunk and proximal limb segments, such as bicycling movements, as well as screaming, jumping, running around, or aggressive sexual automatisms), which are considered to be specific for FLE with special relation to lesions of frontopolar and orbitofrontal cortex (Manford et al., 1996), occur frequently at night and tend to cluster (Jobst et al., 2000). It can be difficult to distinguish hypermotor seizures from psychogenic seizures. Behavioral symptoms such as mood change, unexpected quietness, subtle change of awareness, or awakening are other features of "prefrontal" seizures (Fohlen et al., 2004). Unlike seizures that involve primary motor or sensory areas, the complex semiology of prefrontal seizures may be caused more by disruption of neuronal synchrony between different brain regions than by excitation of single cortical areas (Bartolomei et al., 2005).

Table 15.2 summarizes the frequency and lateralizing value of seizure signs in FLE.

Table 15.2

Frequency and lateralizing value of some seizure symptoms and signs in frontal lobe epilepsy (FLE)

Symptom	Frequency in patients with FLE (%)	Lateralizing value (positive predictive value)	References
Postictal headache	41–53	None (in contrast to TLE)	Ito et al., 2004; Yankovsky et al., 2005
Vocalization	37–77	Probably none (contradictory data)	Janszky et al., 2000a; Bonelli and Baumgartner, 2002; Bonelli et al., 2007
Unilateral tonic posturing	32–48	Contralateral (67–100%)	Bleasel et al., 1997; Werhahn et al., 2000; Janszky et al., 2001; Bonelli and Baumgartner, 2002
Unilateral grimacing	32	Contralateral (100%)	Bonelli et al., 2007
Sign of figure 4*	32	None (in contrast to TLE)	Bonelli et al., 2007
Postictal paresis	27–37	Contralateral (100%)	Jobst et al., 2000; Bonelli and Baumgartner, 2002
Unilateral clonic seizure	23–52	Contralateral (81–100%)	Quesney et al., 1990; Jobst et al., 2000; Janszky et al., 2001; Bonelli and Baumgartner, 2002; Jobst and Williamson, 2005; Bonelli et al., 2007
Head version	21–60	Contralateral (66–100%)	Quesney et al., 1990; Jobst et al., 2000; Janszky et al., 2001; Bonelli and Baumgartner, 2002; Rheims et al., 2005; Bonelli et al., 2007; Lee et al., 2008
Complete loss of consciousness	19	Nondominant	Inoue and Mihara, 1998
Focal somatosensory auras	16–31	Contralateral (100%)	Janszky et al., 2001; Bonelli and Baumgartner, 2002
Unilateral automatisms	16–19	Contradictory data: ipsilateral (67%) or none	Bonelli and Baumgartner, 2002; Bonelli et al., 2007
Asymmetrical ending of the clonic phase of sGTCS	16	Ipsilateral to the side of the last clonic jerk (80%)	Bonelli et al., 2007
Asymmetrical tonic seizure	15–30	None	Jeha et al., 2007; Lee et al., 2008
Hypermotor seizures	11–38	None	Janszky et al., 2000a; Jobst et al., 2000; Fogarasi et al., 2001; Bonelli and Baumgartner, 2002; Jeha et al., 2007; Lee et al., 2008
Early unforced head-turning	11–31	None	Janszky et al., 2001; Bonelli and Baumgartner, 2002; Rheims et al., 2005; Bonelli et al., 2007
Postictal nose wiping	3–37	None (in contrast to TLE)	Geyer et al., 1999; Janszky et al., 2001; Bonelli et al., 2007
Unilateral eye blinking	3	None	Bonelli et al., 2007
Unilateral dystonic posturing	0–26	Contralateral (75–100%)	Bleasel et al., 1997; Janszky et al., 2001; Bonelli and Baumgartner, 2002; Bonelli et al., 2007

*The "sign of figure 4" is an asymmetry of limb posturing in the beginning tonic phase of secondarily generalized tonic–clonic seizures whereby one elbow is extended while the other is flexed.

sGTCS, secondarily generalized tonic–clonic seizure; TLE, temporal lobe epilepsy.

Cluster analysis of seizure evolution

Seizure signs as described above frequently do not appear in isolation. Hence, an analysis of characteristic clusters has been performed (Manford et al., 1996). Four seizure patterns have been found to be of localizing value in frontal or central lobe epilepsy:

- Somatosensory aura with or without a Jacksonian march, often followed by tonic posturing and head version or clonic seizures. Automatisms and vocalization are rare in this seizure pattern. As expected, there is a strong association with central lobe lesions.
- Focal (tonic–)clonic seizures with a Jacksonian march without secondary generalization, usually accompanied by ipsilateral head version and followed by postictal paresis. This seizure pattern is also associated with central lobe lesions.
- Version or posturing occurring early during the seizure evolution, frequently followed by other motor manifestations such as simple automatisms. This seizure sequence is associated with lesions of the "premotor" cortex.
- Hypermotor seizures with vocalizations and rapid postictal recovery. This seizure pattern is associated with orbitofrontal or frontopolar lesions.

General features of frontal lobe seizures

Seizure frequency in FLE shows wide variation. At least in surgical series, a high frequency of several seizures per day is not rare in FLE (Jobst et al., 2000), but in patients with newly diagnosed epilepsy no significant differences in average seizure frequency were found between various partial epilepsies (Manford et al., 1992b).

Frontal lobe seizures tend to *cluster*, especially at night times. More than half of patients have experienced status epilepticus at some point in their history, and this may even appear periodically in some patients (Jobst et al., 2000).

The *duration* of partial seizures arising from the frontal lobe is reported to be significantly shorter than the duration of temporal lobe seizures, and is usually not more than 1 minute (Jobst et al., 2000; Jobst and Williamson, 2005). Another study did not confirm these results concerning the average seizure duration, but noted also that extremely short seizures (< 10 s) were more likely to occur in FLE (Manford et al., 1996).

Secondary generalization occurs in up to 70% of the patients during their lifetime (Jobst et al., 2000). However, the hypothesis that secondary generalization was more frequent in FLE than in other epilepsies could not be confirmed in more recent studies (Jobst and Williamson, 2005).

Frontal lobe seizures were found to occur more frequently during nonrapid eye movement (NREM) sleep than temporal lobe seizures (Crespel et al., 1998). However, this feature is of little clinical value in distinguishing between these syndromes in individual patients, because patients who develop seizures during sleep are seen in both epilepsy syndromes (Bazil and Walczak, 1997; Crespel et al., 1998).

Postictal headache (migraine-type, tension-type, or unclassified) occurred in 41–53% of patients after frontal lobe seizures (Ito et al., 2004; Yankovsky et al., 2005). The more posteriorly the seizures started, the more frequent was the migraine-type postictal headache (occipital lobe 20%, temporal lobe 10%, frontal lobe 5%) (Ito et al., 2004). In contrast to TLE, in which the side of the headache was found to be ipsilateral to the seizure onset zone in 90%, there seems to be no lateralizing value of postictal headache in frontal and central lobe epilepsy (Yankovsky et al., 2005).

In *children* with FLE, the immature cortex architecture might influence seizure semiology. The lack of automatisms and secondary generalization has been attributed to this feature (Fogarasi et al., 2001).

Diagnostic evaluation

The epileptogenic zone is "the area of cortex indispensable for the generation of clinical seizures" (Rosenow and Luders, 2001). Complete resection of the epileptogenic zone will lead to seizure freedom. Its definition is therefore essential for the assessment of surgical therapy chances. However, the epileptogenic zone cannot be defined directly by any diagnostic investigation. Rather, there are different tools that help to estimate the localization of the epileptogenic zone. The diagnostic value of these tools is described below.

EEG

Interictal EEG reveals spikes or sharp waves in 60–80% of patients with FLE; these epileptiform discharges are of less localizing value than in TLE because they can be bilateral, lateralized, or even generalized (Salanova et al., 1993; Laskowitz et al., 1995; Mosewich et al., 2000; Wetjen et al., 2002; Kellinghaus and Luders, 2004; Beleza et al., 2009). The localizing value of both interictal and ictal EEG findings is higher when the epileptogenic zone is located in the lateral frontal lobe compared with the mesial or basal frontal lobe (Bautista et al., 1998). Concordance of the epileptogenic zone with the irritative zone was found in 72% of patients with lateral FLE compared with 33% of those with mesial FLE (Vadlamudi et al., 2004). Possible reasons for this difference are the smaller distance between lateral cortex areas and scalp electrodes, and the fact that tangential dipoles in mesial FLE cannot be detected by EEG. The use of closely spaced surface electrodes (according to the 10-10 system) can improve localization of the irritative zone, but neither increased EEG sensitivity in 23 patients with frontal or central lobe epilepsy nor helped in lateralizing the irritative zone in those patients who had bilateral epileptic discharges on conventional EEG (Gross et al., 2000). The sensitivity of interictal EEG is greater in intracranial subdural than in scalp recordings. Due to their closer distance to the cortex, subdural electrodes may reveal a smaller extent of the irritative zone in some patients than surface electrodes do. However, a sampling bias remains in invasive monitorings (Salanova et al., 1993). Pre-excision epileptiform activity during intraoperative electrocorticography recorded from more than two lateral frontal lobe gyri and from the central lobe predicts a poorer surgical outcome, whereas postresection absence of spikes or sharp waves other than those at the resection borders strongly correlates with a favorable surgical result (Wennberg et al., 1998, 1999).

Interictal rhythmic midline theta (RMT) during wake state (5–7 Hz, duration 3–12 s, located over vertex (Cz) or frontocentral midline (Fz), occurrence 2–10 times per day) could be found in about 50% of patients with FLE, but in only 4% of patients with TLE (Beleza et al., 2009). Moreover, RMT appeared more often in patients with mesial FLE and in patients without interictal epileptiform discharges. Thus, RMT can be helpful to distinguish FLE from TLE and adds to the localization of the epileptogenic zone. However, drowsiness and mental activation are other reasons for the appearance of RMT and have to be excluded.

Short seizure duration, fast cortical spreading, and frequent muscle artefact in seizures with early motor signs, as well as the large portion of frontal lobe cortex that is "hidden" to scalp electrodes due to its distance and orientation, restrict the value of ictal EEG recordings in FLE (Lee et al., 2000). Again, this restriction applies more to mesial than to lateral FLE: seizures originating in the mesial frontal lobe were found to propagate faster than dorsolateral frontal seizures (Blume et al., 2001). Ictal scalp EEG in 127 seizures of 15 patients with lateral FLE showed correct localization of the epileptogenic zone in 65% of patients, whereas 26% of the seizures started with generalized EEG activity and 3% were mislateralized in the EEG analysis (Foldvary et al., 2001). Only 1.5% of the seizures were obscured by artifacts or did not show EEG changes at all. The most frequent EEG patterns at seizure onset were repetitive epileptiform activity (36%), rhythmic delta (26%), and EEG suppression (14%). Rhythmic theta activity, the most frequent seizure pattern in TLE, was seen in only 9%. A smaller study of 9 patients, also comparing medial and lateral FLE, found that absence of focal electrographic seizure activity excluded the possibility of dorsolateral frontal lobe seizures with a negative predictive value of 93% (Bautista et al., 1998). Although scalp electrodes showed a widespread seizure onset and the MRI was read as normal or nonlocalizing, the use of subdural grid electrodes that covered frontal areas extensively were reported to localize the seizure onset zone in more than 90% by several authors (Blume et al., 2001; Cukiert et al., 2001b).

MRI

Surgical series showed lesions on MRI in 46–97% of the patients (Cascino et al., 1992; Laskowitz et al., 1995; Lorenzo et al., 1995; Menzel et al., 1997; Janszky et al., 2000b; Jobst et al., 2000; Schramm et al., 2002). In 38 children, the rate of lesions detected by MRI was found to be only 32% compared with 97% in 17 children with mesial TLE (Lawson et al., 2002). Presence of a lesion on MRI strongly correlates with a good surgical outcome: 25–41% of patients without lesions on MRI became seizure-free or had only nondisabling seizures after surgery, compared with 67–72% of patients with MRI-positive findings (Cascino et al., 1992; Lorenzo et al., 1995; Mosewich et al., 2000). According to the frequent etiologies of FLE, inclusion of fluid-attenuated inversion-recovery (FLAIR) and proton-weighted series for detection of dysplasias and blood products is recommended (Marusic et al., 2002; Ruggieri et al., 2004; Jobst and Williamson, 2005). The use of 3 T MRI improves the diagnostic yield by 20% (Duncan, 2009). Furthermore, MRI review by experienced neuroradiologists can remarkably improve the sensitivity (Von Oertzen et al., 2002).

Neuropsychological evaluation

The published studies on neuropsychological deficits in FLE do not differentiate between certain cortical areas. Impaired motor programming and coordination together with reduced response inhibition can be found in about two-thirds of patients with FLE and may contribute to differentiate them from patients suffering from TLE, whereas speed, attention, and memory span do not differ between the epilepsy syndromes (Helmstaedter et al., 1996). An exception might be patients with right-sided FLE and early seizure onset (<6 years) in whom motor skills were found to be less impaired than those of patients with left-sided FLE or later onset (Upton and Thompson, 1997).

Single-photon computed tomography (SPECT) and positron emission tomography (PET)

Interictal ^{99}Tc-HMPAO-SPECT is of little value in neocortical epilepsy; areas of hypoperfusion have been found in only 24% of patients without abnormalities on MRI, and these areas did not match the epileptogenic or seizure onset zone (Siegel et al., 2002). Of 22 children with FLE, only 2 had interictal localized hypoperfusion that was concordant with clinical, EEG, MRI, and pathological findings (Harvey et al., 1993). Therefore, performance of interictal SPECT seems to be reasonable only together with ictal SPECT.

An early report on exploration of seizure onset zone in 22 children with FLE using *ictal* ^{99}*Tc-HMPAO-SPECT* showed hyperperfusion in 91% and correct localization in 95% of cases (Harvey et al., 1993). However, newer data on adults have not confirmed these promising data. Localization of the seizure onset was found in only 33–43% of patients with FLE (Kaiboriboon et al., 2002; Lee et al., 2002, 2005). Seizures that started in supplementary motor areas were mislocalized to the anterior cingulate cortex by ictal SPECT in 4 of 4 patients (Fukuda et al., 2006). In FLE, the digital subtraction method is superior to side-by-side visual comparison of interictal and ictal SPECT (Lee et al., 2006).

Subtraction ictal SPECT coregistered to MRI (SISCOM), as well as the combination of ictal SPECT with near-infrared spectroscopy (NIRS), has increased diagnostic sensitivity (O'Brien et al., 1998; Watanabe et al., 2002; Cascino, 2004), but sufficient data on frontal lobe seizures are not yet available.

The overall sensitivity of *[*^{18}*F]fluorodeoxyglucose-PET (FDG-PET)* scans in FLE was reported to be 46–96% (Mauguiere and Ryvlin, 2004). There is a correlation between MRI lesions and pathological results in FDG-PET: hypometabolism was found in about 75% of patients with unilateral FLE and abnormalities on MRI (Ryvlin et al., 1998; Kim et al., 2002). However, localizing hypometabolism was seen on FDG-PET in only 29–45% of patients with no MRI-detectable lesion but electroclinical features of unilateral FLE (Ryvlin et al., 1998; Kim et al., 2002; Lee et al., 2005). In a prospective study, PET revealed pathological findings in no patient with bifrontal epilepsy and normal MRI findings (Ryvlin et al., 1998). *Flumazenil-PET* for detection of low benzodiazepine receptor density showed only a slightly higher sensitivity to lateralize cryptogenic unilateral FLE. The method did not contribute significantly to localization of the epileptogenic zone. The sensitivity for FDG-PET was 92% in children with FLE, whereas the specificity for frontal lobe lesions was only 62% and additional hypometabolism outside frontal regions was detected frequently (da Silva et al., 1997). Hence, the value of FDG-PET and flumazenil-PET seems to be restricted in FLE compared with TLE (Ryvlin et al., 1998), although the sensitivity can be slightly increased by use of statistical parametrical mapping (Plotkin et al., 2003). α-[^{11}C]methyl-L-tryptophan-PET also revealed focal abnormalities in MRI-negative patients; the method showed a high specificity of 97–100% and may become a helpful diagnostic tool (Duncan., 2009).

Other diagnostic tools

Registration and localization of interictal discharges using *magnetoencephalography* (MEG) and *magnetic source imaging* (MSI; MEG coregistered with MRI) has been shown to be of predictive value for surgical outcome in some patients with FLE (Genow et al., 2004). Of 21 patients who were considered for invasive monitoring, 9 had no epileptic EEG discharges (Knake et al., 2006). In 3 of these patients, MEG showed interictal epileptic discharges. In particular, patients with lateral neocortical localization of the irritative zone and patients whose epilepsy was caused by focal cortical dysplasia seemed to benefit from investigation with MEG. Hence, the combination of MEG and EEG can be helpful for tailoring the placement of invasive electrodes.

Despite its low spatial resolution, *magnetic resonance spectroscopy (MRS)* can help to lateralize and even localize epileptogenic frontal and central lobe lesions detecting reduced *N*-acetylaspartate levels (Stanley et al., 1998; Lundbom et al., 2001). The area of decreased *N*-acetylaspartate concentration frequently exceeds the epileptogenic lesion as seen on MRI (Li et al., 2000).

Diffusion tensor imaging may be helpful for detection of the epileptogenic lesion in patients without structural changes on conventional MRI, especially in patients with focal cortical dysplasia (Eriksson et al., 2001; Rugg-Gunn et al., 2001; Ito et al., 2004). Furthermore, multiplanar reconstruction and curvilinear reformating improves the localization of focal cortical dysplasias in the frontal lobe (Montenegro et al., 2002).

Unlike in mesial TLE, postictal *diffusion-weighted MRI* may be helpful in detection of the seizure onset zone in selected patients with FLE (Oh et al., 2004).

In conclusion, ictal EEG, seizure semiology, and MRI are most important for determining the localization and extent of the epileptogenic zone in FLE. If seizure semiology, MRI, PET, and SPECT results are concordantly pointing to the same frontal lobe region, intracranial EEG may be dispensable (Mariottini et al., 2001). In MR-positive cases, pure lesionectomy without further attempt to localize the epileptogenic zone led to a seizure reduction of at least 95% in 13 of 14 patients with central lobe epilepsy (Sandok and Cascino, 1998). However, invasive EEG monitoring is frequently required:

- if noninvasive investigations reveal ambiguous results
- in patients with no MRI-detectable lesion
- in patients with a close relationship between the epileptogenic zone and eloquent cortex
- in patients with focal cortical dysplasia because of ill-defined lesion margins (Brekelmans et al., 1998; Chung et al., 2005).

Therapy and outcome

Antiepileptic drugs

There are few studies on medical therapy of FLE. Randomized studies comparing the efficacy of different antiepileptic drugs (AEDs) in FLE do not exist. AED treatment led to seizure freedom in 37% of 200 patients with difficult-to-treat FLE who were referred to a tertiary epilepsy center (Semah et al., 1998). In an open-label nonrandomized study, a combination of valproate and lamotrigine was used in 21 patients (McCabe et al., 2001). The use of additional AEDs was allowed. After 1 year of treatment, 48% of the patients were seizure-free and a further 29% experienced seizure reduction of at least 50%. A similar seizure freedom rate of 50% was seen in 22 retrospectively observed children with FLE (Sinclair et al., 2004). Treatment with topiramate led to seizure freedom in 38% of patients with newly diagnosed FLE and in 10% of patients with difficult-to-treat FLE; a further 31% of newly diagnosed patients and 8% in the difficult-to-treat group experienced seizure reduction of 50% or more without major side-effects (Verrotti et al., 2007).

Surgical treatment

Presurgical identification of eloquent cortex

The detection of eloquent cortical areas is crucial prior to and during resection of central lobe cortex due to the motor and language representation in this area.

Preoperative and intraoperative localization of the central sulcus by use of somatosensory evoked potentials is possible in more than 90% of cases; however, the method may fail in patients with tumor etiology in which the anatomical cortex structure is deranged (Salanova et al., 1993; Cedzich et al., 1996; Romstock et al., 2002). MEG responses evoked by electrical stimulation of the median nerve can also help to locate the central sulcus (Ossenblok et al., 2003). Electrical cortical stimulation via implanted grid or strip electrodes has the highest validity for cortical mapping, especially with respect to motor and language areas. Reproducibility of seizure symptoms during cortical stimulation was associated with a good outcome in extratemporal epilepsy, if these areas were included in the resection (Foldvary et al., 2001).

Seizure outcome after resectional surgery and prognostic factors

In older series, 13–41% of patients with FLE became seizure-free after surgery (Rasmussen, 1991). A meta-analysis of studies that included at least 20 patients of any age showed an overall long-term seizure freedom rate of 27% (Tellez-Zenteno et al., 2005). However, as diagnostic capabilities (especially neuroimaging) improved, seizure freedom or an outcome with nondisabling or very rare seizures was reported in 52–66% (Jobst et al., 2000; Kral et al., 2001; Schramm et al., 2002; Jeha et al., 2007; Elsharkawy et al., 2008; Lee et al., 2008). However, seizure freedom rates decreased to 30–47% after 5 years (Jeha et al., 2007; Elsharkawy et al., 2008). In patients without MRI-detectable lesions, Engel class I outcome was achieved in 43% of 35 patients with FLE (Lee et al., 2005). Another meta-analysis summarized data for 40 children aged 17 years or less with FLE; the authors found an Engel class I outcome in 27.5% (Ansari et al., 2010).

A retrospective study that included 223 patients with extratemporal epilepsy focused on the hazard of seizure recurrence after postsurgical AED withdrawal (Park et al., 2010). In this study, each 27% of the patients became seizure-free with and without medication within a mean observation period of 84 months.

Acute seizures within the first week after resection occur in 25–40% of patients after surgery for FLE, particularly in patients who develop intracerebral hematomas (Tigaran et al., 2003; Jeha et al., 2007); a correlation with poor outcome is debatable.

During 5 postoperative years, seizure outcome improved in 15% and deteriorated in 5% of patients with FLE (Ficker et al., 1999). In this study, late improvement after surgery occurred significantly more frequently in FLE than in TLE.

Neuropsychological benefits (e.g., improvement in short-term memory) may occur in patients who become seizure-free after frontal lobe resection (Helmstaedter et al., 1998).

Prognostic factors for surgical outcome are summarized in Table 15.3. However, the prognostic value of several above-mentioned features found in some studies has not been corroborated by other authors. For example, most studies revealed a strong correlation between the presence of MRI-detectable lesions and a favorable seizure outcome (Smith et al., 1997; Ferrier et al., 1999; Kral et al., 2001), whereas other data showed no correlation (Swartz et al., 1998; Zaatreh et al., 2002) or even better results in patients with normal MRI findings (Jobst et al., 2000).

Complications of surgery

Neurological deficits after lesionectomy (paresis, hypesthesia, dysphasia, abulia, incontinence) occurred in 15–40% after frontal lobe resection, although only 1–3% of the deficits persisted (Swartz et al., 1998; Schramm et al., 2002; Kellinghaus and Luders, 2004).

Table 15.3

Clinical factors with and without correlation with surgical outcome in frontal lobe epilepsy (FLE)

	Prognostic factors
Correlation with good outcome	Tumor or posttraumatic etiology Occurrence of complex partial seizures Focal MRI lesion Focal lesion or normal result in FDG-PET Ipsilateral IEDs in preoperative EEG Focal ictal β-activity in EEG at seizure onset Slow spreading of EEG seizure pattern Localization of the resection in lateral frontal lobe Seizure control within first year after resection
Correlation with poor outcome	Autonomic seizure symptoms Tonic seizures Nonspecific aura Contralateral head version Eye deviation (any direction) History of childhood febrile seizures Etiology of cortical dysplasia (especially if not detectable on MRI) Generalized slowing or generalized IEDs in presurgical EEG EEG seizure onset nonlocalizable/generalized Need for subdural EEG recording Additional extrafrontal lesions Localization of the resection in medial frontal lobe Incomplete resection Postoperative auras Acute postoperative seizures Postsurgical IEDs in scalp EEG
No correlation with outcome, or contradictory data	Family history of epilepsy Gender Age at operation Age at onset Epilepsy duration Seizure frequency Seizure duration Side of surgery Generalized tonic–clonic seizures Multiple clinical seizure types

Sources: Cukiert et al., 1996; Kazemi et al., 1997; Smith et al., 1997; Swartz et al., 1998; Ferrier et al., 1999; Kutsy, 1999; Janszky et al., 2000b; Mosewich et al., 2000; Kral et al., 2001; Worrell et al., 2002; Zaatreh et al., 2002; Chung et al., 2005; Lee et al., 2005; Elsharkawy et al., 2008; Ansari et al., 2010.

EEG, electroencephalography; FDG-PET, [^{18}F]fluorodeoxyglucose-positron emission tomography; IED, interictal epileptiform discharge; MRI, magnetic resonance imaging.

Resection of primary hand and arm motor cortex leads to contralateral paresis. Functional recovery starts within 1–3 weeks, but fine motor skills may not recover completely (Lehman et al., 1994). Due to crossing fibers leading to bilateral representation, resection of the supplementary motor area and axial, face, and tongue motor areas usually recovers completely, and so does sensory function after removal of postcentral cortex (Lehman et al., 1994; Cukiert et al., 2001a).

Other surgical methods

If resectional surgery is impossible due to overlap of the epileptogenic zone and eloquent cortex, multiple subpial transections (MSTs) and callosotomy remain as further surgical approaches. Some 3 months after MST in the frontal lobe, 30% of the patients were seizure-free in one study (Helmstaedter et al., 1998). However, the long-term seizure freedom rate is probably far lower (Tellez-Zenteno et al., 2005). In patients without localizing diagnostic results, callosotomy can be performed as a palliative procedure that prevents secondary generalization of seizures by inhibiting the spread of seizure activity to the contralateral hemisphere (Zimmerman and Sirven, 2003). Freedom from most disabling astatic seizures can be achieved by this procedure in 35% of cases (Tellez-Zenteno et al., 2005).

Vagus nerve stimulation (VNS) reduces seizure frequency by at least 50% in 30–40% of patients, and efficacy increases over time (Guberman, 2004). No specific data are available on VNS therapy in patients with FLE.

Other methods, such as deep brain or cortical stimulation or focal cortical cooling, are still experimental.

OCCIPITAL LOBE EPILEPSY

Seizure semiology

Signs and symptoms of seizures arising from the occipital area can be divided into phenomena of occipital lobe origin and those induced by ictal spreading to adjacent areas. In contrast to children, the majority of adults with OLE report visual auras (Salanova et al., 1992; Blume and Wiebe, 2000; Fogarasi et al., 2003; Kun et al., 2005; Jobst et al., 2010). They usually start in the contralateral visual field and propagate quickly if the patient is able to give a detailed report (Boesebeck et al., 2002). Visual phenomena comprise elementary visual hallucinations, such as flashing colors or rotating lights or shapes, complex visual hallucinations, and ictal blindness. Other occipital manifestations include blinking, contralateral nystagmus, and contralateral eye pulling (Salanova et al., 1992). Infrasylvian seizure spread to the temporal lobe produces alteration of awareness and automatisms. Suprasylvian spread to the mesial frontal lobe produces asymmetrical tonic posturing, whereas propagation laterally results in focal motor or sensory seizures.

EEG

The great majority of patients with OLE have abnormal interictal or ictal EEG findings, but scalp EEG may fail to detect epileptiform activity generated by an irritative zone on the inferior and mesial occipital surfaces. The most frequent interictal epileptiform discharges (IEDs) in OLE are spikes and sharp waves in temporal or temporo-occipital regions with shifting maxima in some patients (Williamson et al., 1992b; Sveinbjornsdottir and Duncan, 1993; Aykut-Bingol et al., 1998; Taylor et al., 2003). Widespread and bilateral IEDs, including secondary bilateral synchrony, are common, and isolated epileptiform activity restricted to the occipital lobe is infrequent (Williamson and Spencer, 1986; Salanova et al., 1992; Williamson et al., 1992b; Aykut-Bingol et al., 1998). Rarely, IEDs can be recorded with greatest amplitude in the contralateral occipital region in the sense of a paradoxical lateralization if their dipole is oriented in such a way that contralateral occipital electrodes best detect it (Blume, 2001). Patients with focal epilepsies generally have a low incidence of photosensitivity of 0.7–3.0% (Wolf and Goosses, 1986; Kasteleijn-Nolst Trenite, 1989; Shiraishi et al., 2001). Among these patients, however, patients with OLE have the highest incidence, ranging from 6% to 13% (Ludwig and Marsan, 1975; Shiraishi et al., 2001; Taylor et al., 2003). In contrast to TLE, where the lack of contralateral IED is predictive for a seizure-free postoperative outcome (Schulz et al., 2000), this correlation is under discussion in posterior epilepsies (Aykut-Bingol et al., 1998; Bösebeck et al., 2002; Kun et al., 2005).

Like the clinical signs and symptoms, ictal electrographic manifestations of occipital lobe seizures reflect also different patterns of propagation (Salanova et al., 1992; Williamson et al., 1992b). Invasive recordings demonstrate propagation from the occipital region to the mesial temporal structures, the supplementary motor area, or dorsolateral frontal convexity before generalization (Williamson et al., 1992b). Ictal recordings may show diffuse suppression or rhythmic activity that is usually generalized but may be lateralized or maximal over the temporo-occipital region (Salanova et al., 1992; Williamson et al., 1992b; Aykut-Bingol et al., 1998). In a small series of 6 patients who were seizure-free after resectional surgery, nearly 70% of seizures had localizing features (Foldvary et al., 2001). However, the ictal onset was typically generalized and only 21% of seizures were localized to the occipital region at onset. Mislocalization occurred in 28% of seizures. Among these seizures, occipital ictal discharges were mislateralized to the contralateral occipital lobe, although mislocalization to the ipsilateral frontotemporal region was also observed.

Surgical therapy

Etiology includes a broad variety of epileptogenic lesions. Postoperative outcome can vary and correlates significantly with the concordance of the different presurgical testing, such as EEG and MRI (Kun et al., 2005; Jobst et al., 2010).

Panayiotopoulos syndrome and idiopathic childhood occipital epilepsy of Gastaut (ICOE-G)

Both of these syndromes are classified as focal idiopathic epilepsies in childhood. Panayiotopoulos syndrome is defined as an idiopathic epilepsy syndrome with an excellent prognosis and normal findings on MRI characterized by a clinical ictal triad of nocturnal seizures, tonic deviation of the eyes, and autonomic manifestations including vomiting (Lada et al., 2003; Covanis, 2006; Caraballo et al., 2007; Panayiotopoulos et al., 2008; Specchio et al., 2010). The EEG shows shifting and/or multiple foci, often with occipital predominance. Education about Panayiotopoulos syndrome is the cornerstone of management. Prophylactic treatment with antiepileptic medication may not be needed for most patients (Covanis, 2006).

ICOE-G reveals typical visual seizures that typically consist of brief elementary visual hallucinations, ictal blindness, or deviation of the eyes (Caraballo et al., 2008, 2009). Many children suffer from migraine-like symptoms. The seizures are usually frequent and diurnal. The EEG often shows occipital IEDs, demonstrating fixation-off sensitivity. Patients usually respond well to AEDs and about two-thirds remit by the age of 16 years (Caraballo et al., 2009). One possible misdiagnosis may be migraine with visual aura or acephalgic or basilar migraine.

PARIETAL LOBE EPILEPSY

Seizure semiology

The relative frequency of PLE is generally considered low and data for this patient group are limited (Sveinbjornsdottir and Duncan, 1993; Salanova et al., 1995). Many patients experience auras which can consist of a variety of symptoms, such as somatosensory (paresthetic, painful, thermal, sexual, apraxia, disturbances of body image), visual (amaurotic, elementary and complex hallucinations, illusions), and other phenomena (anosognosia, apraxia, acalculia, alexia, aphemia, confusional states, gustatory, vertiginous, adversive, oculoclonic and eyelid flutter) (Sveinbjornsdottir and Duncan, 1993; Kim et al., 2004). The symptoms can be contralateral or bilateral. The auras evolve typically into asymmetrical tonic posturing, unilateral clonic activity, or contralateral version when the ictal discharges activate the frontal region (Williamson et al., 1992a). Propagation to the temporal lobe produces alteration of awareness and automatisms (Williamson et al., 1992a; Salanova et al., 1995).

EEG

The majority of patients with PLE show IEDs. The IEDs are usually widespread and multifocal, and can be bilateral suggesting an extent of the irritative zone far beyond the epileptogenic zone (Blume et al., 1991; Cascino et al., 1993; Sveinbjornsdottir and Duncan, 1993; Salanova et al., 1995; Bösebeck et al., 2002). Secondary bilateral synchrony can be recorded in up to 30% of cases, especially with parasagittal lesions (Salanova et al., 1995; Bösebeck et al., 2002). In general, extracranial interictal EEG findings are an unreliable indicator of PLE. The ictal EEG varies with the pathway of propagation and may erroneously suggest temporal or frontal lobe origin. Simple partial seizures of parietal lobe origin frequently have no EEG correlate (Devinsky et al., 1988; Cascino et al., 1993; Foldvary et al., 2001). Other seizure types are most commonly associated with diffuse suppression or nonlateralized rhythmic activity or lateralized changes (Williamson et al., 1992a; Cascino et al., 1993; Salanova et al., 1995). Therefore, electrophysiological studies should be addressed carefully if there is disagreement between scalp-recorded EEG and neuroimaging findings.

Surgical treatment

The etiology of parietal lobe seizures varies and a good postoperative outcome relies on the concordance of neuroimaging, EEG findings, and clinical manifestations.

CONCLUSION

FLE is the most frequent extratemporal epilepsy. Knowledge of structural and functional anatomy is a prerequisite for understanding the seizure semiology of extratemporal epilepsies, especially in FLE. Established diagnostic methods (EEG and MRI) are the basis of diagnostic workup; however, in selected cases additional methods (e.g., SPECT or PET) can be helpful. The diagnostic value of newer methods such as MEG and MRS is not yet clear. Extratemporal epilepsy syndromes differ mainly in seizure semiology and suitability and characteristics regarding epilepsy surgery, but share a similar prognosis. Despite development of new diagnostic tools, the surgical outcome is still less favorable than for TLE.

References

Amunts K, Schleicher A, Burgel U et al. (1999). Broca's region revisited: cytoarchitecture and intersubject variability. J Comp Neurol 412: 319–341.

Ansari SF, Maher CO, Tubbs RS et al. (2010). Surgery for extratemporal nonlesional epilepsy in children: a meta-analysis. Childs Nerv Syst 26: 945–951.

Aykut-Bingol C, Bronen RA, Kim JH et al. (1998). Surgical outcome in occipital lobe epilepsy: implications for pathophysiology. Ann Neurol 44: 60–69.

Bartolomei F, Trebuchon A, Gavaret M et al. (2005). Acute alteration of emotional behaviour in epileptic seizures is related to transient desynchrony in emotion-regulation networks. Clin Neurophysiol 116: 2473–2479.

Bautista RE, Spencer DD, Spencer SS (1998). EEG findings in frontal lobe epilepsies. Neurology 50: 1765–1771.

Bazil CW, Walczak TS (1997). Effects of sleep and sleep stage on epileptic and nonepileptic seizures. Epilepsia 38: 56–62.

Beleza P, Bilgin O, Noachtar S (2009). Interictal rhythmical midline theta differentiates frontal from temporal lobe epilepsies. Epilepsia 50: 550–555.

Bleasel A, Kotagal P, Kankirawatana P et al. (1997). Lateralizing value and semiology of ictal limb posturing and version in temporal lobe and extratemporal epilepsy. Epilepsia 38: 168–174.

Blume WT (2001). Interictal electroencephalography in neocortical epilepsy. In: HO Lüder, Y Comair (Eds.), Epilepsy Surgery. Lippincott Williams & Wilkins, Philadelphia, pp. 403–412.

Blume WT, Wiebe S (2000). Occipital lobe epilepsies. Adv Neurol 84: 173–187.

Blume WT, Whiting SE, Girvin JP (1991). Epilepsy surgery in the posterior cortex. Ann Neurol 29: 638–645.

Blume WT, Ociepa D, Kander V (2001). Frontal lobe seizure propagation: scalp and subdural EEG studies. Epilepsia 42: 491–503.

Boesebeck F, Schulz R, May T et al. (2002). Lateralizing semiology predicts the seizure outcome after epilepsy surgery in the posterior cortex. Brain 125: 2320–2331.

Bonelli SB, Baumgartner C (2002). Frontal lobe epilepsy – clinical seizure semiology. Wien Klin Wochenschr 114: 334–340.

Bonelli SB, Lurger S, Zimprich F et al. (2007). Clinical seizure lateralization in frontal lobe epilepsy. Epilepsia 48: 517–523.

Bösebeck F, Schulz R, May T (2002). Lateralizing semiology predicts the seizure outcome after epilepsy surgery in the posterior cortex. Brain 125: 2320–2331.

Brekelmans GJ, van Emde BW, Velis DN et al. (1998). Comparison of combined versus subdural or intracerebral electrodes alone in presurgical focus localization. Epilepsia 39: 1290–1301.

Brett M, Johnsrude IS, Owen AM (2002). The problem of functional localization in the human brain. Nat Rev Neurosci 3: 243–249.

Brun A (1999). The emergence of the frontal lobe and its morbidity, as opposed to the central lobe. Dement Geriatr Cogn Disord 10: 3–5.

Caraballo R, Cersosimo R, Fejerman N (2007). Panayiotopoulos syndrome: a prospective study of 192 patients. Epilepsia 48: 1054–1061.

Caraballo RH, Cersosimo RO, Fejerman N (2008). Childhood occipital epilepsy of Gastaut: a study of 33 patients. Epilepsia 49: 288–297.

Caraballo R, Koutroumanidis M, Panayiotopoulos CP et al. (2009). Idiopathic childhood occipital epilepsy of Gastaut: a review and differentiation from migraine and other epilepsies. J Child Neurol 24: 1536–1542.

Cascino GD (2004). Surgical treatment for extratemporal epilepsy. Curr Treat Options Neurol 6: 257–262.

Cascino GD, Jack CR Jr, Parisi JE et al. (1992). MRI in the presurgical evaluation of patients with frontal lobe epilepsy and children with temporal lobe epilepsy: pathologic correlation and prognostic importance. Epilepsy Res 11: 51–59.

Cascino GD, Hulihan JF, Sharbrough FW et al. (1993). Parietal lobe lesional epilepsy: electroclinical correlation and operative outcome. Epilepsia 34: 522–527.

Cedzich C, Taniguchi M, Schafer S et al. (1996). Somatosensory evoked potential phase reversal and direct motor cortex stimulation during surgery in and around the central region. Neurosurgery 38: 962–970.

Chung CK, Lee SK, Kim KJ (2005). Surgical outcome of epilepsy caused by cortical dysplasia. Epilepsia 46: 25–29.

Combi R, Dalpra L, Tenchini ML et al. (2004). Autosomal dominant nocturnal frontal lobe epilepsy – a critical overview. J Neurol 251: 923–934.

Commission on Classification and Terminology of the International League Against Epilepsy (1989). Proposal for revised classification of epilepsies and epileptic syndromes. Epilepsia 30: 389–399.

Covanis A (2006). Panayiotopoulos syndrome: a benign childhood autonomic epilepsy frequently imitating encephalitis, syncope, migraine, sleep disorder, or gastroenteritis. Pediatrics 118: e1237–e1243.

Crespel A, Baldy-Moulinier M, Coubes P (1998). The relationship between sleep and epilepsy in frontal and temporal lobe epilepsies: practical and physiopathologic considerations. Epilepsia 39: 150–157.

Cukiert A, Olivier A, Andermann F (1996). Post-traumatic frontal lobe epilepsy with structural changes: excellent results after cortical resection. Can J Neurol Sci 23: 114–117.

Cukiert A, Buratini JA, Machado E et al. (2001a). Seizure's outcome after cortical resections including the face and tongue rolandic areas in patients with refractory epilepsy and normal MRI submitted to subdural grids' implantation. Arq Neuropsiquiatr 59: 717–721.

Cukiert A, Buratini JA, Machado E et al. (2001b). Results of surgery in patients with refractory extratemporal epilepsy with normal or nonlocalizing magnetic resonance findings investigated with subdural grids. Epilepsia 42: 889–894.

da Silva EA, Chugani DC, Muzik O et al. (1997). Identification of frontal lobe epileptic foci in children using positron emission tomography. Epilepsia 38: 1198–1208.

Devinsky O, Kelley K, Porter RJ et al. (1988). Clinical and electroencephalographic features of simple partial seizures. Neurology 38: 1347–1352.

Dobesberger J, Walser G, Unterberger I et al. (2004). Genital automatisms: a video-EEG study in patients with medically refractory seizures. Epilepsia 45: 777–780.

Dum RP, Strick PL (2002). Motor areas in the frontal lobe of the primate. Physiol Behav 77: 677–682.

Duncan J (2009). The current status of neuroimaging for epilepsy. Curr Opin Neurol 22: 179–184.

Duncan J, Owen AM (2000). Common regions of the human frontal lobe recruited by diverse cognitive demands. Trends Neurosci 23: 475–483.

Elsharkawy AE, Alabbasi AH, Pannek H et al. (2008). Outcome of frontal lobe epilepsy surgery in adults. Epilepsy Res 81: 97–106.

Eriksson SH, Rugg-Gunn FJ, Symms MR et al. (2001). Diffusion tensor imaging in patients with epilepsy and malformations of cortical development. Brain 124: 617–626.

Ferrier CH, Engelsman J, Alarcon G et al. (1999). Prognostic factors in presurgical assessment of frontal lobe epilepsy. J Neurol Neurosurg Psychiatry 66: 350–356.

Ficker DM, So EL, Mosewich RK et al. (1999). Improvement and deterioration of seizure control during the postsurgical course of epilepsy surgery patients. Epilepsia 40: 62–67.

Fogarasi A, Janszky J, Faveret E et al. (2001). A detailed analysis of frontal lobe seizure semiology in children younger than 7 years. Epilepsia 42: 80–85.

Fogarasi A, Boesebeck F, Tuxhorn I et al. (2003). A detailed analysis of symptomatic posterior cortex seizure semiology in children younger than seven years. Epilepsia 44: 89–96.

Fohlen M, Bulteau C, Jalin C et al. (2004). Behavioural epileptic seizures: a clinical and intracranial EEG study in 8 children with frontal lobe epilepsy. Neuropediatrics 35: 336–345.

Foldvary N, Klem G, Hammel J et al. (2001). The localizing value of ictal EEG in focal epilepsy. Neurology 57: 2022–2028.

Frater JL, Prayson RA, Morris HH, 3rd. et al. (2000). Surgical pathologic findings of extratemporal-based intractable epilepsy: a study of 133 consecutive resections. Arch Pathol Lab Med 124: 545–549.

Fujiwara T, Shigematsu H (2004). Etiologic factors and clinical features of symptomatic epilepsy: focus on pediatric cases. Psychiatry Clin Neurosci 58: S9–S12.

Fukuda M, Masuda H, Honma J et al. (2006). Ictal SPECT in supplementary motor area seizures. Neurol Res 28: 845–848.

Genow A, Hummel C, Scheler G et al. (2004). Epilepsy surgery, resection volume and MSI localization in lesional frontal lobe epilepsy. Neuroimage 21: 444–449.

Geyer JD, Payne TA, Faught E et al. (1999). Postictal nose-rubbing in the diagnosis, lateralization, and localization of seizures. Neurology 52: 743–745.

Geyer S, Matelli M, Luppino G et al. (2000). Functional neuroanatomy of the primate isocortical motor system. Anat Embryol (Berl) 202: 443–474.

Goldberg-Stern H, Gadoth N, Cahill W et al. (2004). Language dysfunction after frontal lobe partial seizures. Neurology 62: 1637–1638.

Gross DW, Dubeau F, Quesney LF et al. (2000). EEG telemetry with closely spaced electrodes in frontal lobe epilepsy. J Clin Neurophysiol 17: 414–418.

Guberman A (2004). Vagus nerve stimulation in the treatment of epilepsy. CMAJ 171: 1165–1166.

Hamer HM, Luders HO, Knake S et al. (2003). Electrophysiology of focal clonic seizures in humans: a study using subdural and depth electrodes. Brain 126: 547–555.

Harvey AS, Hopkins IJ, Bowe JM et al. (1993). Frontal lobe epilepsy: clinical seizure characteristics and localization with ictal ^{99m}Tc-HMPAO SPECT. Neurology 43: 1966–1980.

Helmstaedter C, Kemper B, Elger CE (1996). Neuropsychological aspects of frontal lobe epilepsy. Neuropsychologia 34: 399–406.

Helmstaedter C, Gleissner U, Zentner J et al. (1998). Neuropsychological consequences of epilepsy surgery in frontal lobe epilepsy. Neuropsychologia 36: 681–689.

Inoue Y, Mihara T (1998). Awareness and responsiveness during partial seizures. Epilepsia 39: 7–10.

Ito M, Adachi N, Nakamura F et al. (2004). Characteristics of postictal headache in patients with partial epilepsy. Cephalalgia 24: 23–28.

Janszky J, Fogarasi A, Jokeit H et al. (2000a). Are ictal vocalisations related to the lateralisation of frontal lobe epilepsy? J Neurol Neurosurg Psychiatry 69: 244–247.

Janszky J, Jokeit H, Schulz R et al. (2000b). EEG predicts surgical outcome in lesional frontal lobe epilepsy. Neurology 54: 1470–1476.

Janszky J, Fogarasi A, Jokeit H et al. (2001). Lateralizing value of unilateral motor and somatosensory manifestations in frontal lobe seizures. Epilepsy Res 43: 125–133.

Jeha LE, Najm I, Bingaman W et al. (2007). Surgical outcome and prognostic factors of frontal lobe epilepsy surgery. Brain 130: 574–584.

Jobst BC, Williamson PD (2005). Frontal lobe seizures. Psychiatr Clin North Am 28: 635–639.

Jobst BC, Siegel AM, Thadani VM et al. (2000). Intractable seizures of frontal lobe origin: clinical characteristics, localizing signs, and results of surgery. Epilepsia 41: 1139–1152.

Jobst BC, Williamson PD, Thadani VM et al. (2010). Intractable occipital lobe epilepsy: clinical characteristics and surgical treatment. Epilepsia 51: 2334–2337.

Kaiboriboon K, Lowe VJ, Chantarujikapong SI et al. (2002). The usefulness of subtraction ictal SPECT coregistered to MRI in single- and dual-headed SPECT cameras in partial epilepsy. Epilepsia 43: 408–414.

Kasteleijn-Nolst Trenite DG (1989). Photosensitivity in epilepsy. Electrophysiological and clinical correlates. Acta Neurol Scand Suppl 125: 3–149.

Kazemi NJ, So EL, Mosewich RK et al. (1997). Resection of frontal encephalomalacias for intractable epilepsy: outcome and prognostic factors. Epilepsia 38: 670–677.

Kellinghaus C, Luders HO (2004). Frontal lobe epilepsy. Epileptic Disord 6: 223–239.

Kellinghaus C, Loddenkemper T, Najm IM et al. (2004). Specific epileptic syndromes are rare even in tertiary epilepsy centers: a patient-oriented approach to epilepsy classification. Epilepsia 45: 268–275.

Kim YK, Lee DS, Lee SK et al. (2002). (18)F-FDG PET in localization of frontal lobe epilepsy: comparison of visual and SPM analysis. J Nucl Med 43: 1167–1174.

Kim DW, Lee SK, Yun CH et al. (2004). Parietal lobe epilepsy: the semiology, yield of diagnostic workup, and surgical outcome. Epilepsia 45: 641–649.

Knake S, Halgren E, Shiraishi H et al. (2006). The value of multichannel MEG and EEG in the presurgical evaluation of 70 epilepsy patients. Epilepsy Res 69: 80–86.

Kotagal P, Arunkumar GS (1998). Lateral frontal lobe seizures. Epilepsia 39: S62–S68.

Kral T, Kuczaty S, Blumcke I et al. (2001). Postsurgical outcome of children and adolescents with medically refractory frontal lobe epilepsies. Childs Nerv Syst 17: 595–601.

Kun LS, Young LS, Kim DW et al. (2005). Occipital lobe epilepsy: clinical characteristics, surgical outcome, and role of diagnostic modalities. Epilepsia 46: 688–695.

Kutsy RL (1999). Focal extratemporal epilepsy: clinical features, EEG patterns, and surgical approach. J Neurol Sci 166: 1–15.

Lada C, Skiadas K, Theodorou V et al. (2003). A study of 43 patients with Panayiotopoulos syndrome, a common and benign childhood seizure susceptibility. Epilepsia 44: 81–88.

Laich E, Kuzniecky R, Mountz J et al. (1997). Supplementary sensorimotor area epilepsy. Seizure localization, cortical propagation and subcortical activation pathways using ictal SPECT. Brain 120: 855–864.

Laskowitz DT, Sperling MR, French JA et al. (1995). The syndrome of frontal lobe epilepsy: characteristics and surgical management. Neurology 45: 780–787.

Lawson JA, Cook MJ, Vogrin S et al. (2002). Clinical, EEG, and quantitative MRI differences in pediatric frontal and temporal lobe epilepsy. Neurology 58: 723–729.

Lee SK, Kim JY, Hong KS et al. (2000). The clinical usefulness of ictal surface EEG in neocortical epilepsy. Epilepsia 41: 1450–1455.

Lee DS, Lee SK, Kim YK et al. (2002). The usefulness of repeated ictal SPET for the localization of epileptogenic zones in intractable epilepsy. Eur J Nucl Med Mol Imaging 29: 607–614.

Lee SK, Lee SY, Kim KK et al. (2005). Surgical outcome and prognostic factors of cryptogenic neocortical epilepsy. Ann Neurol 58: 525–532.

Lee SK, Lee SY, Yun CH et al. (2006). Ictal SPECT in neocortical epilepsies: clinical usefulness and factors affecting the pattern of hyperperfusion. Neuroradiology 48: 678–684.

Lee JJ, Lee SK, Lee SY et al. (2008). Frontal lobe epilepsy: clinical characteristics, surgical outcomes and diagnostic modalities. Seizure 17: 514–523.

Lehman R, Andermann F, Olivier A et al. (1994). Seizures with onset in the sensorimotor face area: clinical patterns and results of surgical treatment in 20 patients. Epilepsia 35: 1117–1124.

Li LM, Cendes F, Andermann F et al. (2000). Spatial extent of neuronal metabolic dysfunction measured by proton MR spectroscopic imaging in patients with localization-related epilepsy. Epilepsia 41: 666–674.

Loddenkemper T, Kellinghaus C, Wyllie E et al. (2005). A proposal for a five-dimensional patient-oriented epilepsy classification. Epileptic Disord 7: 308–316.

Lorenzo NY, Parisi JE, Cascino GD et al. (1995). Intractable frontal lobe epilepsy: pathological and MRI features. Epilepsy Res 20: 171–178.

Luders H, Acharya J, Baumgartner C et al. (1998). Semiological seizure classification. Epilepsia 39: 1006–1013.

Ludwig BI, Marsan CA (1975). Clinical ictal patterns in epileptic patients with occipital electroencephalographic foci. Neurology 25: 463–471.

Lundbom N, Gaily E, Vuori K et al. (2001). Proton spectroscopic imaging shows abnormalities in glial and neuronal cell pools in frontal lobe epilepsy. Epilepsia 42: 1507–1514.

Manford M, Hart YM, Sander JW et al. (1992a). National General Practice Study of Epilepsy (NGPSE): partial seizure patterns in a general population. Neurology 42: 1911–1917.

Manford M, Hart YM, Sander JW et al. (1992b). The National General Practice Study of Epilepsy. The syndromic classification of the International League Against Epilepsy applied to epilepsy in a general population. Arch Neurol 49: 801–808.

Manford M, Fish DR, Shorvon SD (1996). An analysis of clinical seizure patterns and their localizing value in frontal and temporal lobe epilepsies. Brain 119: 17–40.

Mariottini A, Lombroso CT, DeGirolami U et al. (2001). Operative results without invasive monitoring in patients with frontal lobe epileptogenic lesions. Epilepsia 42: 1308–1315.

Marusic P, Najm IM, Ying Z et al. (2002). Focal cortical dysplasias in eloquent cortex: functional characteristics and correlation with MRI and histopathologic changes. Epilepsia 43: 27–32.

Mauguiere F, Ryvlin P (2004). The role of PET in presurgical assessment of partial epilepsies. Epileptic Disord 6: 193–215.

McCabe PH, McNew CD, Michel NC (2001). Effect of divalproex–lamotrigine combination therapy in frontal lobe seizures. Arch Neurol 58: 1264–1268.

Menzel C, Grunwald F, Ostertun B et al. (1997). Incidence of lesions described by magnetic resonance imaging in the clarification of focal epilepsy of frontal and temporal origin. Nuklearmedizin 36: 187–193.

Montenegro MA, Li LM, Guerreiro MM et al. (2002). Focal cortical dysplasia: improving diagnosis and localization with magnetic resonance imaging multiplanar and curvilinear reconstruction. J Neuroimaging 12: 224–230.

Mosewich RK, So EL, O'Brien TJ et al. (2000). Factors predictive of the outcome of frontal lobe epilepsy surgery. Epilepsia 41: 843–849.

O'Brien TJ, Zupanc ML, Mullan BP et al. (1998). The practical utility of performing peri-ictal SPECT in the evaluation of children with partial epilepsy. Pediatr Neurol 19: 15–22.

Oh JB, Lee SK, Kim KK et al. (2004). Role of immediate postictal diffusion-weighted MRI in localizing epileptogenic foci of mesial temporal lobe epilepsy and non-lesional neocortical epilepsy. Seizure 13: 509–516.

Ohtsuka Y, Yoshinaga H, Kobayashi K et al. (2001). Predictors and underlying causes of medically intractable localization-related epilepsy in childhood. Pediatr Neurol 24: 209–213.

Ossenblok P, Leijten FS, de Munck JC et al. (2003). Magnetic source imaging contributes to the presurgical identification of sensorimotor cortex in patients with frontal lobe epilepsy. Clin Neurophysiol 114: 221–232.

Panayiotopoulos CP, Michael M, Sanders S et al. (2008). Benign childhood focal epilepsies: assessment of established and newly recognized syndromes. Brain 131: 2264–2286.

Park KI, Lee SK, Chu K et al. (2010). Withdrawal of antiepileptic drugs after neocortical epilepsy surgery. Ann Neurol 67: 230–238.

Penfield W, Boldrey E (1937). Somatic motor and sensory representation in the cerebral cortex of man as studied by electrical stimulation. Brain 60: 389–443.

Plotkin M, Amthauer H, Merschhemke M et al. (2003). Use of statistical parametric mapping of (18)F-FDG-PET in frontal lobe epilepsy. Nuklearmedizin 42: 190–196.

Quesney LF, Constain M, Fish DR et al. (1990). The clinical differentiation of seizures arising in the parasagittal and anterolaterodorsal frontal convexities. Arch Neurol 47: 677–679.

Rasmussen T (1991). Tailoring of cortical excisions for frontal lobe epilepsy. Can J Neurol Sci 18: 606–610.

Rheims S, Demarquay G, Isnard J et al. (2005). Ipsilateral head deviation in frontal lobe seizures. Epilepsia 46: 1750–1753.

Romstock J, Fahlbusch R, Ganslandt O et al. (2002). Localisation of the sensorimotor cortex during surgery for brain tumours: feasibility and waveform patterns of somatosensory evoked potentials. J Neurol Neurosurg Psychiatry 72: 221–229.

Rosenow F, Luders H (2001). Presurgical evaluation of epilepsy. Brain 124: 1683–1700.

Rugg-Gunn FJ, Symms MR, Barker GJ et al. (2001). Diffusion imaging shows abnormalities after blunt head trauma when conventional magnetic resonance imaging is normal. J Neurol Neurosurg Psychiatry 70: 530–533.

Ruggieri PM, Najm I, Bronen R et al. (2004). Neuroimaging of the cortical dysplasias. Neurology 62: S27–S29.

Ryvlin P, Bouvard S, Le Bars D et al. (1998). Clinical utility of flumazenil-PET versus [^{18}F]fluorodeoxyglucose-PET and MRI in refractory partial epilepsy. A prospective study in 100 patients. Brain 121: 2067–2081.

Salanova V, Andermann F, Olivier A et al. (1992). Occipital lobe epilepsy: electroclinical manifestations, electrocorticography, cortical stimulation and outcome in 42 patients treated between 1930 and 1991. Surgery of occipital lobe epilepsy. Brain 115: 1655–1680.

Salanova V, Morris HH, 3rd., Van Ness PC et al. (1993). Comparison of scalp electroencephalogram with subdural electrocorticogram recordings and functional mapping in frontal lobe epilepsy. Arch Neurol 50: 294–299.

Salanova V, Andermann F, Rasmussen T et al. (1995). Parietal lobe epilepsy. Clinical manifestations and outcome in 82 patients treated surgically between 1929 and 1988. Brain 118: 607–627.

Sandok EK, Cascino GD (1998). Surgical treatment for perirolandic lesional epilepsy. Epilepsia 39: S42–S48.

Schramm J, Kral T, Kurthen M et al. (2002). Surgery to treat focal frontal lobe epilepsy in adults. Neurosurgery 51: 644–654.

Schulz R, Luders HO, Hoppe M et al. (2000). Interictal EEG and ictal scalp EEG propagation are highly predictive of surgical outcome in mesial temporal lobe epilepsy. Epilepsia 41: 564–570.

Semah F, Picot MC, Adam C et al. (1998). Is the underlying cause of epilepsy a major prognostic factor for recurrence? Neurology 51: 1256–1262.

Shiraishi H, Fujiwara T, Inoue Y et al. (2001). Photosensitivity in relation to epileptic syndromes: a survey from an epilepsy center in Japan. Epilepsia 42: 393–397.

Siegel A, Lewis P, Siegel AM (2002). The value of interictal brain SPECT in epilepsy patients without mesial-temporal sclerosis. Clin Nucl Med 27: 716–720.

Sinclair DB, Wheatley M, Snyder T (2004). Frontal lobe epilepsy in childhood. Pediatr Neurol 30: 169–176.

Smith JR, Lee MR, King DW et al. (1997). Results of lesional vs. nonlesional frontal lobe epilepsy surgery. Stereotact Funct Neurosurg 69: 202–209.

Specchio N, Trivisano M, Di Ciommo V et al. (2010). Panayiotopoulos syndrome: a clinical, EEG, and neuropsychological study of 93 consecutive patients. Epilepsia 51: 2098–2107.

Stanley JA, Cendes F, Dubeau F et al. (1998). Proton magnetic resonance spectroscopic imaging in patients with extratemporal epilepsy. Epilepsia 39: 267–273.

Sveinbjornsdottir S, Duncan JS (1993). Parietal and occipital lobe epilepsy: a review. Epilepsia 34: 493–521.

Swartz BE, Gado-Escueta AV, Walsh GO et al. (1998). Surgical outcomes in pure frontal lobe epilepsy and foci that mimic them. Epilepsy Res 29: 97–108.

Taylor I, Scheffer IE, Berkovic SF (2003). Occipital epilepsies: identification of specific and newly recognized syndromes. Brain 126: 753–769.

Tellez-Zenteno JF, Dhar R, Wiebe S (2005). Long-term seizure outcomes following epilepsy surgery: a systematic review and meta-analysis. Brain 128: 1188–1198.

Tigaran S, Cascino GD, McClelland RL et al. (2003). Acute postoperative seizures after frontal lobe cortical resection for intractable partial epilepsy. Epilepsia 44: 831–835.

Upton D, Thompson PJ (1997). Age at onset and neuropsychological function in frontal lobe epilepsy. Epilepsia 38: 1103–1113.

Vadlamudi L, So EL, Worrell GA et al. (2004). Factors underlying scalp-EEG interictal epileptiform discharges in intractable frontal lobe epilepsy. Epileptic Disord 6: 89–95.

Vadlamudi L, Kjeldsen MJ, Corey LA et al. (2006). Analyzing the etiology of benign rolandic epilepsy: a multicenter twin collaboration. Epilepsia 47: 550–555.

Verrotti A, Sofia V, Franzoni E et al. (2007). Topiramate in frontal lobe epilepsy. Acta Neurol Scand 115: 132–135.

Von Oertzen J, Urbach H, Jungbluth S et al. (2002). Standard magnetic resonance imaging is inadequate for patients with refractory focal epilepsy. J Neurol Neurosurg Psychiatry 73: 643–647.

Watanabe E, Nagahori Y, Mayanagi Y (2002). Focus diagnosis of epilepsy using near-infrared spectroscopy. Epilepsia 43: 50–55.

Wennberg R, Quesney F, Olivier A et al. (1998). Electrocorticography and outcome in frontal lobe epilepsy. Electroencephalogr Clin Neurophysiol 106: 357–368.

Wennberg R, Quesney LF, Lozano A et al. (1999). Role of electrocorticography at surgery for lesion-related frontal lobe epilepsy. Can J Neurol Sci 26: 33–39.

Werhahn KJ, Noachtar S, Arnold S et al. (2000). Tonic seizures: their significance for lateralization and frequency in different focal epileptic syndromes. Epilepsia 41: 1153–1161.

Wetjen NM, Cohen-Gadol AA, Maher CO et al. (2002). Frontal lobe epilepsy: diagnosis and surgical treatment. Neurosurg Rev 25: 119–138.

Williamson PD, Spencer SS (1986). Clinical and EEG features of complex partial seizures of extratemporal origin. Epilepsia 27: S46–S63.

Williamson PD, Boon PA, Thadani VM et al. (1992a). Parietal lobe epilepsy: diagnostic considerations and results of surgery. Ann Neurol 31: 193–201.

Williamson PD, Thadani VM, Darcey TM et al. (1992b). Occipital lobe epilepsy: clinical characteristics, seizure spread patterns, and results of surgery. Ann Neurol 31: 3–13.

Wolf P, Goosses R (1986). Relation of photosensitivity to epileptic syndromes. J Neurol Neurosurg Psychiatry 49: 1386–1391.

Worrell GA, So EL, Kazemi J et al. (2002). Focal ictal beta discharge on scalp EEG predicts excellent outcome of frontal lobe epilepsy surgery. Epilepsia 43: 277–282.

Yankovsky AE, Andermann F, Bernasconi A (2005). Characteristics of headache associated with intractable partial epilepsy. Epilepsia 46: 1241–1245.

Zaatreh MM, Spencer DD, Thompson JL et al. (2002). Frontal lobe tumoral epilepsy: clinical, neurophysiologic features and predictors of surgical outcome. Epilepsia 43: 727–733.

Zimmerman RS, Sirven JI (2003). An overview of surgery for chronic seizures. Mayo Clin Proc 78: 109–117.

Handbook of Clinical Neurology, Vol. 107 (3rd series)
Epilepsy, Part I
H. Stefan and W.H. Theodore, Editors

Chapter 16

Reflex epilepsies

PETER WOLF[1]* AND MATTHIAS KOEPP[2]
[1]*Danish Epilepsy Center Filadelfia, Dianalund, Denmark*
[2]*Department of Clinical and Experimental Epilepsy, UCL Institute of Neurology, London, UK*

DEFINITION AND CLASSIFICATION

The terminology reflex epilepsy is not uniform, and often the distinction between epilepsy and seizures is not clearly made. In a broader sense, the term is used in cases where the seizures can be triggered reproducibly and immediately by some well-defined sensory or cognitive stimulus. In a stricter sense, a diagnosis of reflex epilepsy is given when a patient has no spontaneous seizures but only in response to specific stimuli or tasks.

The term does not include the facilitation of seizures by nonspecific factors such as alcohol or sleep deprivation.

There is at present no generally accepted classification of reflex epilepsies but a useful distinction, which is also applied in this chapter, is according to the type of precipitating stimulus: simple, usually sensory (including proprioceptive), or complex, usually cognitive. It must be realized, however, that some triggers (e.g., toothbrushing and hot water) cannot easily be categorized in this rather simplistic dichotomy.

At present only one type of reflex epilepsy, primary reading epilepsy, is recognized as a separate epilepsy syndrome (Commission on Classification and Terminology of the International League Against Epilepsy (ILAE), 1989). In other types (e.g., photosensitivity), the relationship between specific stimulus and epilepsy syndromes has been established (e.g., Wolf and Goosses, 1986), and the reflex epileptic phenomena can be considered as traits that are present in some, but not all, of the patients affected with these syndromes.

In this chapter much attention is given, beyond electroencephalography (EEG), to functional imaging and related methods because recently they have contributed much to our understanding of how seizures arise in reflex epilepsies. Functional neuroimaging, using functional magnetic resonance imaging (fMRI), single-photon emission computed tomography (SPECT), and positron emission tomography (PET), allows for localization of the changes in cerebral blood flow, metabolism, and neurotransmitter levels that accompany changes in neural activity.

In epilepsy in general, ictal investigations other than EEG are difficult to perform owing to the paroxysmal nature of the epilepsies, but reflex epilepsies have attracted a recent surge in such investigations; reflex epilepsies are an ideal model to examine peri-ictal changes, the neuronal systems that underlie the specific seizure-provoking trigger and its relationship to epileptiform activity because of the possibility of reliably inducing seizures within the scanner environment.

Functional imaging techniques can contribute to an understanding of the metabolic and perfusion changes associated with both ictal and interictal EEG discharges in patients with reflex epilepsies. These patients are ideal candidates for *in vivo* measurements, as their EEG and clinical phenomena usually have a localized onset and occur with minimal head motion.

SIMPLE TRIGGERS

Seizure precipitation by simple sensory stimuli is characterized by the following features:

- The stimulus is well defined, uniform, and at least to some extent quantitative.
- The response follows immediately upon the stimulus, usually within a definable time interval.
- The clinical, or at least the epileptiform, EEG response is anatomically related to the primary sensory field, which is activated by the stimulus.
- With repetitive stimulation, the epileptic response may both habituate or augment; this depends to some extent on the mode of repetition, and after

*Correspondence to: Professor Peter Wolf, Danish Epilepsy Center Filadelfia, Kolonivej 1, DK–4293 Dianalund, Denmark, E-mail: pwl@filadelfia.dk a provoked seizure there may be a brief refractory period.

- The response depends to some extent upon the state of activation of the neuronal system involved; it may be conditioned and deconditioned.

The vast majority of sensory stimuli that may provoke a seizure are related to the visual system. Among these, "photosensitivity" (i.e., sensitivity to intermittent light stimuli) is the most common.

Photosensitivity

Photosensitivity is the commonest reflex epileptic trait but it is not homogeneous. In humans, two major varieties exist, plain photosensitivity and photosensitivity to single and low-frequency light stimuli.

Plain photosensitivity

This is the type that is usually thought of, and written about, when photosensitivity is mentioned, and it has been amply written about (for a recent comprehensive review see Kasteleijn-Nolst Trenité et al., 2005). It consists of seizure precipitation or epileptiform EEG discharge brought on by intermittent light stimulation (ILS) in a more or less restricted frequency band with the maximum response typically between 14 and 30 Hz. The EEG findings are known as the "photoparoxysmal response" (PPR). The seizures precipitated by ILS are bilateral myoclonic, absences or generalized tonic–clonic, with myoclonic seizures being the most common type. In a small number of patients, the seizures are of focal, occipital type, with visual symptoms usually starting in one hemifield, and may be accompanied by an ipsilateral version of the eyes (and head), or version as the only symptom. The lateralization may be constant or alternating.

Photosensitive seizures are provoked by flickering sunlight (e.g., sun shining through trees, through fences, reflected by car bumpers, or on a glittering water surface) or by intermittent artificial lights (e.g., stroboscopes in discotheques, flickering neon tubes). The most common triggers today are related to television and computer screens, especially when seen from a close distance, when flickering lines appear due to poor functioning or during a program with strong light contrasts. Seizures during video games may be caused by a combination of photosensitivity and praxis induction (see below).

Self-induction of photosensitive seizures is a well-known phenomenon and was first described by Radovici et al. (1932). In earlier reports, patients looked at a bright light and rapidly waved a hand with spread fingers before their eyes, or they blinked rapidly while looking at a light source. Self-induction by looking at a television screen seems now to have become more common, more so in children than in adults. Patients are usually reluctant to talk about this, but self-induction seems to result in pleasure or relaxation.

Syndromes

Photosensitive patients with only reflex seizures and no spontaneous seizures are relatively rare. It is probably because of their rarity that the condition is usually not separated out as a syndrome. However, it is worth noting that such patients exist and can be treated by sensory protection alone, without the need for drugs.

Of the major epilepsy syndromes, photosensitivity is closely related to the idiopathic generalized epilepsies (IGE) and observed in up to 50% of patients with juvenile myoclonic epilepsy (JME) (Wolf and Goosses, 1986). Probably most cases with occipital lobe seizures belong to the category of idiopathic photosensitive occipital lobe epilepsy, which was proposed by Guerrini et al. (1995).

Photosensitivity is also seen in various generalized epilepsy syndromes of childhood. These include benign myoclonic epilepsy in infancy (Dravet et al., 1992), Dravet syndrome (Dravet et al., 2005), and myoclonic–astatic epilepsy (Doose, 1992). Of the idiopathic occipital lobe epilepsies of childhood, photosensitivity does not feature in the Gastaut type and only exceptionally in the Panayiotopoulos type (Covanis et al., 2005).

As a separate genetic trait, photosensitivity may occur coincidentally with any other syndrome, more frequently with idiopathic epilepsies, for example in 9% of patients with primary reading epilepsy (Wolf, 1992).

Photosensitivity is a genetically determined, probably genotypically inhomogeneous, trait (Stephani et al., 2004) and is more frequent in females (Kasteleijn-Nolst Trenité et al., 2005).

Photosensitivity is an age-dependent trait related to adolescence. Of the 454 patients of Harding and Jeavons (1994), the mean $\pm$ SD age of onset was 13.7 ± 5.1. In the study of 1062 consecutive adult patients investigated in a video-EEG laboratory in Berlin (Wolf and Goosses, 1986), the mean $\pm$ SD age of epilepsy onset in 103 photosensitive patients was 14.4 ± 5.1, compared with 19.9 ± 7.6 for the nonphotosensitive subjects.

This age dependence implies that individuals who present with PPR in the most sensitive period may later lose it. This issue was studied in longitudinal investigations by Harding and Jeavons (1994), who concluded that the majority of patients remain photosensitive. However, they rarely followed their patients beyond the third decade of life, and about 30% who remained unmedicated had lost the PPR by the age of about 25 years. Regesta and Tanganelli (1989) also followed 53 patients for between 6 and 14 years and found remission of seizures and PPR in all 8 patients with only provoked seizures and in 24 (PPR: 22) of 32 patients with provoked and spontaneous clinical seizures, but in none of 13 patients with PPR and only spontaneous seizures. Their patients were older at study onset, and therefore followed up to a later age, which may explain their more optimistic results.

Treatment

Valproic acid (VPA) seems to be the most effective of the available antiepileptic drugs (AEDs) for photosensitivity. Beyond pharmacotherapy, the defined seizure trigger opens the possibility of alternative protective approaches. Forster (1977) successfully applied several methods of deconditioning (e.g., by starting ILS with subthreshold flicker frequencies or with reduced light intensity), but the success was not sustained. Protection against environmental flickering stimuli by dark glasses is a useful therapeutic approach. In patients with pure photosensitivity and no spontaneous seizures, this has been applied successfully without concomitant use of AEDs (Wolf and Okujava, 1999). Capovilla et al. (2006) and Takahashi et al. (2004) reported enhanced protective effects with colored glasses.

As a long-term strategy, it is useful to adjust the patient to a dose that fully controls the seizures but does not completely abolish the PPR. This allows the PPR to be kept under observation, and its possible remission to be detected. If the PPR disappears under longitudinal observation, the AED dose can be reduced and the EEG controlled. In the case of PPR reappearance, the reduced dose is continued for an unlimited period or until the PPR remits again and the procedure is repeated.

Sensitivity to slow flicker and single light flashes

This variant of photosensitivity is observed in various types of progressive myoclonus epilepsy, such as the ceroid lipofuscinoses, Unverricht–Lundborg disease, myoclonic epilepsy with ragged red fibers (MERRF), and others (Kasteleijn-Nolst Trenité et al., 2005).

Photosensitivity in animals

There are two genetic types of photosensitivity in two very different animals – baboons and chicken. Photosensitive baboons belong to the species *Papio papio* and live in the Casamance region of Senegal. Photosensitive chickens belong to the Fayumi breed. Their similarities and dissimilarities compared with each other and with human photosensitivity have been discussed by Naquet and Batini (2004).

Functional imaging in photosensitivity

The problem that functional imaging is expected to solve was formulated in one of the earliest papers on photosensitivity (Bickford et al., 1953). The stimulation is to the visual cortex, but the most specific response, that of myoclonic jerks, is in the motor system. What is the circuitry behind this? They proposed three possibilities: a corticocortical mechanism; activation of the motor area from the striate cortex via the thalamus; or activation of the thalamocortical system via the lateral geniculate body in parallel with the activation of the visual area.

It had long been noted that the distribution of "generalized" spike-wave activity in the PPR and in eye closure sensitivity in most cases deviates from the usual frontoprecentral dominance by an occipitoparietal accentuation. This indicated involvement of the parieto-occipital area, but further quantification of this effect is necessary.

In a PET study of a patient with MERRF, stimulation with 3 Hz produced only epileptiform EEG activity, whereas a flash rate of 5 Hz also induced myoclonic jerks (Träff et al., 2000). The PET scans showed increased metabolism in the thalamus with left preference at both frequencies, with additional activation of the supplementary motor cortex when myocloni were induced.

A few magnetoencephalography (MEG) studies have attempted to study the neuromagnetic origin of the PPR in patients with epilepsy. Ricci et al. (1990) performed neuromagnetic measurements by using four sensors with simultaneous two-channel EEG recording in 12 patients with PPR identified in routine studies. Their results supported a cortical origin of the PPR, with a regional sensitivity and occasional asymmetries. These authors concluded that the erratic cortical involvement suggested the existence of a general instability of cortical excitability.

Recently, MEG has been used to study the phase synchronization properties of the driving response preceding the onset of the PPR (Kalitzin et al., 2002). This study found an enhanced synchrony in the γ-band harmonics when IPS triggered a PPR. This was not seen in controls or in subjects in whom no PPR was elicited. Thus, it seems that properties of the phase spectrum, especially in MEG recordings, can characterize the dynamics of underlying neuronal networks more specifically than can amplitude spectra. These findings may reflect a loss of control of the brain over a fast-frequency oscillatory process that normally operates transiently to connect neural assemblies involved (e.g., in perceptual mechanisms). The possibility of anticipating the onset of a PPR may lead to new diagnostic evaluation of photosensitive patients, eventually resulting in improved safety of the IPS procedure, decreasing the risk of unnecessarily provoking seizures.

Novel methods of simultaneous acquisition of EEG and fMRI have been developed recently. They capitalize on the relative merits of strength of the individual methods, achieving an unprecedented time and spatial resolution. Some of the initial technological difficulties were related to the effect of strong magnetic fields on the EEG apparatus. Artifact correction algorithms and specific hardware design have now overcome these initial limitations, allowing clinical studies to be undertaken (Iannetti et al., 2002; Jager et al., 2002). A recent study using simultaneous EEG and fMRI acquisition during pattern stimulation was able to localize sources of visual evoked responses *in vivo* in the calcarine area with unprecedented spatiotemporal resolution, demonstrating that the largest cortical activation corresponds to the N75 and P100 components of the visual evoked potential (VEP) (Bonmassar et al., 2001).

Moeller et al. (2009a) studied 30 photosensitive subjects with EEG-triggered fMRI and elicited the PPR in 6 (4 with IGE and 2 with tension headache). Apart from the obvious activation of the visual areas, they found activation of the parietal cortex close to the intraparietal sulcus and of the frontal premotor cortex 3 seconds before the onset of PPR, i.e., at the time of synchronization of cortical γ oscillations preceding the PPR. At the onset of PPR, the same areas were deactivated. Only one patient showed, in addition, activation of the thalamus. The authors concluded that the PPR is predominantly a cortical phenomenon involving parietal and frontal areas.

One patient was excluded from this study because during the investigation he had a complex visual aura that evolved into a generalized tonic–clonic seizure. This case was published separately (Moeller et al., 2009b). During the visual aura, there was activation of the thalamus, colliculi superiores, and lateral geniculate bodies, whereas frontal and parietal cortex were deactivated, as with the PPR. At present, no absences or myoclonic responses to photosensitivity have been identified.

Eye closure sensitivity

This trait was first noted in the EEGs of some photosensitive patients by Bickford et al. (1953). It can also be seen, without being mentioned specifically, in some EEG figures of Janz and Christian's original paper on JME (Janz and Christian, 1957). In the EEG it is obvious (but remains often unreported), whereas clinically it is mostly overlooked unless patients use it for self-induction of seizures. Eye closure sensitivity is defined by seizures or epileptiform EEG activity triggered by eye closure and identified by the appearance of spikes and waves, usually as a brief subclinical volley, within 2 seconds of eye closure. Often, the response is different with voluntary and involuntary eye closure. Newmark and Penry (1979) reviewed the early reports that investigated the effect of eye closure in light or dark, passive eye closure, and attempted closure of eyes forcibly held open. The findings were inconclusive, indicating that this trait comprises a motor and a visual component, the importance of which varies between individuals.

There is some overlap with photosensitivity where the PPR is usually augmented by eye closure. However, the two traits are not identical (Fabian and Wolf, 1987; Sevgi et al., 2007).

According to Guirao Bringas et al. (1987), syndrome-wise eye closure sensitivity is related to IGE and seizure-wise to absences with eyelid myocloni. Of 459 consecutive prospective epileptic patients in an EEG laboratory, a minimum of 19 (4.1%) presented eye closure sensitivity, and of these 15 had IGE (Fischer et al., 1989). Sevgi et al. (2007) found eye closure sensitivity mostly in eyelid myoclonia with absence (or Jeavons syndrome; Striano et al., 2009), JME, IGE with GTC seizures, and idiopathic occipital lobe epilepsy. All cited authors agree that the trait is more common in females.

Self-induction by rapid blinking at a light source is a well-known feature, especially with eye closure sensitivity, and may be applied by those photosensitive patients who are also eye closure sensitive. As eyelid myoclonus is the seizure type provoked by eye closure, it may be difficult to determine whether self-induction is taking place or not.

Fixation-off sensitivity

The presumed first observation of eye closure sensitivity reported in a case by Robinson (1939) is much more likely to be a case of fixation-off sensitivity (Panayiotopoulos, 1994). This is a rare type of reflex epilepsy which, in the older literature, was not clearly distinguished from eye closure sensitivity. Characteristically for fixation-off sensitivity, epileptiform activity is present on the EEG as long as the eyes remain closed or out of focus. Clinically it is related to the idiopathic occipital childhood epilepsies, both the Panayiotopoulos and the Gastaut type (Covanis et al., 2005).

Parra et al. (2000) studied the fixation-off phenomenon and its relations with the α rhythm. This condition denotes a variety of EEG abnormalities elicited by elimination of central vision and fixation, which include high-amplitude runs of repetitive occipital spike–wave or rhythmical slow activity in the EEG or even generalized discharges (Panayiotopoulos, 1994). Their findings indicated that abnormalities related to fixation-off sensitivity could emerge in thalamocortical networks, with larger and more anterior cortical distribution than those that generate α rhythm. Thus, the transition in the type of oscillation appears not only to depend on a change in cellular dynamics but also to be reflected in a different spatial distribution of the underlying neuronal networks (Parra et al., 2000).

Pattern sensitivity

Bickford et al. (1953) first reported a case of pattern sensitivity in a paper on the convulsive effects of light stimulation. Many aspects of this trigger mechanism were clarified by Chatrian et al. (1970a, b), who meticulously investigated four typical cases. These patients respond to patterns of contrasting vertical parallel stripes. The typical responses are absence seizures. Pattern sensitivity often coexists with photosensitivity, and Harding and Jeavons (1994) proposed that patients with a combination of both sensitivities were most likely to have television-induced seizures. As in other visually induced seizures, self-induction of trance-like states, presumably representing absence status, is also known from pattern sensitivity. Provocative environmental patterns reported by patients include wallpapers, garments, tablecloths, radiators, window screens, and grids of escalators.

Radhakrishnan et al. (2005) reported on 73 patients who were identified at the Mayo Clinic from 1950 to 2000. All but 8 patients were also photosensitive, and television was the most common precipitant. Pattern sensitivity was found in 59 patients (81%) with IGE (14 with JME, 19%), 7 (10%) with symptomatic generalized epilepsies, and 7 (10%) with localization-related epilepsies. The spike-wave discharges elicited by pattern stimulation were "all generalized" in two-thirds of the patients, and restricted to the posterior region in one-third. Self-induction in this long-term follow-up study seemed not to present a major problem, and the prognosis of these patients was in general favorable.

Inoue et al. (1999) studied 15 patients with photosensitive and pattern-sensitive epilepsy with seizures induced by electronic screen games, and compared them with 14 nonphotosensitive patients while they were playing videogames in the MEG environment. They estimated equivalent current dipoles of the MEG spikes and found that, whereas in pattern-sensitive patients dipoles had a posterior predominance, in nonphotosensitive patients the estimated sources of these epileptiform spikes tended to cluster over the anterior part of the brain. They concluded that factors involving functions of the anterior regions of the brain other than photo- or pattern sensitivity may play a role in the induction of seizures during the playing of electronic video games. Furthermore, the changes in spike frequency in specific brain areas may correspond to their involvement in praxis activity and emotional changes during these games.

Sensitivity to touch and movement

Sensitivity to touch and movement seems to be rare but may be underreported. According to Biraben et al. (2004), sensitivity to touch and movement appears to form a continuum and has been described especially with symptomatic focal perirolandic epilepsies of variable etiology. The seizure-precipitating movements typically are specific for the individual case, and the triggering touch needs to be applied to a specific trigger zone contralateral to the lesion. There is no element of surprise, and self-induction of seizures is sometimes possible (Forster, 1977; Wolf and Dockweiler, 1989; Biraben et al., 2004). Precipitation by mere imagination of the triggering movement was reported by Forster (1977) and by Biraben et al. (2004). The seizures are simple focal motor, often with a somatosensory component or aura (Biraben et al., 2004). This reflex epileptic trait appears as a relatively frequent feature in epilepsia partialis continua, reported in 24 of 65 retrospective cases (37%) of different etiologies (Mameniskiene et al., 2011), but no systematic study has been undertaken so far.

Eye movements

As mentioned above, eye closure sensitivity seems to include both a visual and a motor component. Shanzer et al. (1965) reported a patient with seizures precipitated by lateral gaze, and Vignaendra and Lim (1978) described convergence of the eyes as a trigger.

Apart from startle epilepsy (see below), the most important differential diagnosis of movement-induced seizures is paroxysmal kinesigenic choreoathetosis (Revol et al., 1989), a type of paroxysms that in the early descriptions was considered a form of reflex epilepsy (Lishman et al., 1962) and the epileptic or nonepileptic nature of which is still under discussion (Ohmori et al., 2002; Kato et al., 2006).

Treatment

Pharmacological and surgical treatments of focal epilepsies with movement- and touch-induced seizures are not fundamentally different from those of other symptomatic focal epilepsies. The identification of a specific trigger allows again for possible preventive intervention; preparation for movement and slow initiation of action tend to reduce or abort seizures (Biraben et al., 2004). A patient of Falconer et al. (1963) was able to defer seizures by voluntary relaxation of the quadriceps muscle, and Wolf and Dockweiler (1989) described successful deconditioning therapy in a patient with touch-induced focal motor seizures.

Seizures precipitated by toothbrushing

Starting with Forster (1977), several authors have described seizures precipitated by toothbrushing (Holmes et al., 1982; Benabou et al., 1996 (five cases); O'Brien et al., 1996; Koutroumanidis et al., 2001). The trigger mechanism in some patients is quite specific, even regarding which teeth are brushed or with which hand, but a broader range of precipitation including other oral activities such as eating or drinking has also been reported (Benabou et al., 1996; D'Souza et al., 2007). Local irritation by a palatal plate was an important pathogenic factor in the patient described by Holmes et al. (1982), in whom, however, touching the zone in different ways as well as performing a similar movement sequence without actually brushing the teeth, as in some other patients, was not effective. The hand movements seemed to be an important part of the trigger mechanism in several patients, but not in the patient described by Haytac et al. (2008), in whom the seizures were triggered by a powered toothbrush.

The provoked seizures usually are simple focal motor or sensorimotor at onset and may evolve into complex partial or generalized tonic–clonic seizures. Some patients only have provoked seizures, and others also have spontaneous seizures. The seizures start between 15 seconds and up to 10 minutes of toothbrushing, which in some cases needs to be vigorous. Spontaneous seizures may or may not occur.

The majority of the 13 hitherto reported patients had cryptogenic focal epilepsies. Recently, three patients were reported with reflex toothbrushing-induced epilepsy associated with small circumscribed structural lesions in the primary somatosensory cortex in close proximity to the hand and speech motor areas (D'Souza et al., 2007). Sensory symptoms were observed at clinical onset with localizing focal ictal and interictal epileptiform discharges on EEG. Findings in these patients refine the localization of this type of reflex epilepsy and suggest possible mechanisms of ictogenesis and classification of this reflex epilepsy. Toothbrushing is a complex programmed task involving motor, proprioception, and somatosensory networks with stimuli of variable frequency, duration, and intensity probably required for neuronal synchronization to provoke the seizures. Seizure generation may require excitation of a critical mass of an already hyperexcitable area within the somatosensory cortex of the parietal operculum. The respective role of somatosensory, proprioceptive, and motor components, however, is sufficiently variable, and the time required to build up the epileptic response is often sufficiently long to argue for considering induction by toothbrushing a complex trigger.

Divergent cases include a patient of Navarro et al. (2006) in whom, in addition to the act of toothbrushing, seeing a toothbrush and toothpaste or thinking of these was sufficient to elicit seizures. This patient had temporal lobe epilepsy, and the seizures started with a *jamais vécu* experience. A patient described by Chuang et al. (2004), whose seizures started with sexual arousal and an orgasm-like experience, also had (right) temporal lobe epilepsy with hippocampal atrophy.

With respect to treatment, patients with a slow precipitation only by vigorous toothbrushing were able to avoid the seizures by adjusting their toothbrushing accordingly.

Startle epilepsy

Startle epilepsy, first described by Alajouanine and Gastaut (1955), refers to a heterogeneous trait associated with different seizure types and epilepsies (Lancman et al., 1993). Startle epilepsy is most frequently observed in lesional epilepsies with infantile hemiplegia (Aguglia et al., 1984), but also in other types of severe brain damage (Lancman et al., 1993). Seizures are predominantly tonic and can be generalized or focal. These patients are quite resistant to AEDs. An idiopathic variant in infants with myoclonic seizures has been described by Ricci et al. (1995) and by Zafeiriou et al. (2003), and its excellent treatment response and prognosis was confirmed by Plouin and Vigevano (2004). García-Morales et al. (2009) recently published a series of four patients with normal findings on MRI with video-EEG and MEG suggesting a right frontocentral seizure origin. Tibussek et al. (2006) concluded in a series of 22 patients that startle epilepsy comprises a number of highly diverse subentities with distinct clinical, semiological, and EEG features, unlikely to have a common underlying pathophysiological mechanism.

However, in all variants, the most typical trigger is a sudden, unexpected loud noise that produces a startle response, which may be normal or exaggerated. The movement may evolve directly into a tonic seizure, but in other cases there is a short interval and the seizure appears to be a reflex response to the movement. Because of the frequent role of an acoustic trigger, startle seizures are sometimes mistaken for audiogenic seizures. The epileptic response in startle epilepsy may also be triggered by an unexpected touch and may then likewise be mistaken for a somatosensory reflex seizure. More rarely, a sudden visual stimulus can precipitate the seizure.

In many patients, two or all three of these modalities can be demonstrated, and the common denominator of all triggers is the element of surprise leading to a motor start.

The most important differential diagnosis is the exaggerated startle response of hyperekplexia (Andermann et al., 1980), which was described in the same paper as startle epilepsy (Alajouanine and Gastaut, 1955) and is not epileptic. Both may look similar to an untrained observer, and a video registration may be required to make the distinction.

Treatment

Startle epilepsy is often pharmacoresistant, apart from the benign infantile myoclonic variety which may even spontaneously remit and otherwise responds well to VPA (Plouin and Vigevano, 2004). Of the traditional AEDs, carbamazepine appears to be the most effective, although newer AEDs have not been tried systematically. Initial good responses to clonazepam and clobazam typically wear off after some time (Aguglia et al., 1984). Mayer and Specht (1995) reported good effects for propranolol in some patients, the mechanism probably being attenuation of the startle response. With focal lesional etiologies, surgical treatments are considered (García-Morales et al., 2009).

Hot water epilepsy

Two different varieties of seizure precipitation through a hot bath have been described, one in infants (Plouin and Vigevano, 2004) and one in adolescents and adults (Satishchandra, 2003).

Infants

The onset is before 1 year of age, there are no spontaneous seizures, and the reflex seizures stop spontaneously after the age of 3 years. There is no family history, and the mental and physical development and neurological findings are normal. Seizures are precipitated when the child is sat in water with a temperature above 37.5°C. The seizures are complex partial, and no drug treatment is required because the seizures can be effectively prevented by bathing the child in water of lower temperature. The precise precipitating mechanism is unknown and may include two somatosensory components (temperature and touch) and a rise in body temperature. Visual stimulation by light reflected from the water surface has also been discussed (Plouin and Vigevano, 2004).

Adolescents and adults

The quite different adult type was first described by Allen (1945). Most cases were found in southern India, where it accounts for almost 7% of all epilepsies in Bangalore (Satishchandra et al., 2004) and has a lifetime prevalence of 0.285% in Yelandur (Mani et al., 1998). It has been studied extensively by Satishchandra and coworkers, who also developed an animal model (Satishchandra et al., 2004). Typically, hot water needs to be poured over the head to become a trigger, and it has been shown that these patients have a defect in thermoregulation resulting in a systemic rise of body temperature when hot water is poured over the head (Satishchandra, 2003). The seizures usually are complex partial, sometimes evolving into secondarily generalized tonic–clonic seizures. Up to 10% of the patients experience intense pleasure and continue to pour water over their heads after seizure onset (Satishchandra et al., 2004). A positive family history is reported in up to 22.6% (Satishchandra et al., 2004). Two gene loci have recently been described in families with autosomal dominant hot water epilepsy (Ratnapriya et al., 2009a, b).

There may be a motor component, as bathing in these parts is typically done using a pail and, in a succession of rapid movements, throwing hot water from a bucket over one's head. At least in these cases, the trigger mechanism could be complex.

Spontaneous seizures in addition to reflex seizures occur in a minority of patients. Adult hot water epilepsy often responds well to treatment with classical AEDs such as phenytoin and carbamazepine. Alternative approaches are the use of lukewarm water for head bathing or sponging the head with hot towels. Dhanaraj and Jayavelu (2003) reported successful monotherapy with intermittent clobazam applied prophylactically before a head bath.

Audiogenic and vestibulogenic seizures

Whereas genetic audiogenic seizures in rodents are frequent, seizures precipitated by simple auditive stimuli without a startle mechanism seem to be extremely rare in humans. Isolated cases were described by Zagury et al. (1989) in a 59-year-old woman, who appears to have a variant of migraine epilepsy, and by Grosso et al. (2007) in a patient with Aicardi syndrome. One of the present authors (P.W.) has seen an unpublished case, a professional church musician with mesiotemporal lobe epilepsy due to hippocampal sclerosis, who has undergone successful surgery. He knew, during his active epilepsy, that he had to avoid modes where the high C appears frequently because its repetition would provoke a seizure. To discover this kind of trigger requires that the patient has perfect pitch, so it may be more frequent but remain undiscovered.

Seizures precipitated by vestibular stimulation ("reflex vestibular epilepsy") were reviewed by Karbowski (1989), who found several reports in the older, mainly

German, literature. He exposed 62 patients with epilepsy to caloric stimulation and observed the appearance or increase of EEG anomalies in 22 patients, with seizures being provoked in two.

Sensitivity to taste and smell

Apart from a possible role of tastes in the complex ictogenesis of eating seizures, gustatory seizure precipitation seems not to have been reported. In addition, reports of seizures precipitated by smell are scarce, which is surprising considering the close relationship of the temporal lobe to olfactory functions. On the other hand, seizure inhibition by olfactory stimuli has been studied repeatedly (Gowers, 1881; Efron, 1956, 1957; Betts, 2003; Jaseja, 2008). Servit et al. (1981), however, reported that activation of epileptiform EEG discharge by hyperventilation was enhanced with nasal compared with oral hyperventilation, because the former adds an olfactory stimulation to the seizure-inducing hypocapnia produced by overbreathing. This distinction became a tradition in the Czech school and was reviewed by Komarek (1994).

Conclusion for reflex epilepsy with simple triggers

Reflex epileptic traits can be found in idiopathic and symptomatic epilepsies, both generalized and localization-related. The most common types involve the visual system and are related to IGE, especially to JME. In several of these epilepsies, self-induced seizures have been reported. Specific treatments have been developed that are based upon protection against, avoidance or attenuation of the trigger mechanisms, usually applied as a supplement to pharmacotherapy. Sometimes these treatments have been used successfully without the need for drugs in patients who have no spontaneous seizures.

COMPLEX TRIGGERS

There is greater variability of reflex epilepsy with complex than with simple triggers. Unlike simple triggers, where the effect is usually seen immediately or with a delay of some seconds, most complex triggers become active after a phase of "warming up" or "tuning," which can last for several minutes.

The absence of interictal epileptiform EEG abnormalities in complex reflex epilepsies is a common finding, not unusual in idiopathic epilepsies. The ongoing activity is normal. Unlike simple triggers, some of which are part of the standard EEG investigation (eye closure, intermittent light stimulation) and routinely yield ictal EEGs, individually tailored provocation methods need to be applied to obtain ictal EEG in response to complex triggers.

The majority of functional imaging studies have focused on complex reflex epilepsies, such as musicogenic and reading epilepsy. In complex reflex epilepsies, seizures are elicited by intricate stimuli in which a specific pattern, sometimes just the expectation of the provoking stimulus, is the triggering factor, suggesting the involvement of higher cortical function. Functional imaging techniques have a low temporal resolution; for PET or SPECT, it is at best 2 minutes, and even with fMRI the resolution is in the order of seconds rather than milliseconds as in neurophysiological investigations. Still, this delay from the stimulus to the beginning of the seizure allows the seizure-provoking activity (listening to music or reading) to be studied separately from the effects that the seizure itself has on blood flow, metabolism, or neurotransmitter release. The best designed studies allow for this differentiation to be made. It is of particular importance to ascertain whether the cognitive activity leading to the seizure is in any way different from physiological activity.

Praxis induction and thinking seizures

Praxis induction is a reflex epileptic mechanism defined by the precipitation of seizures through cognition-guided complex motor tasks, typically requiring complex visuomotor coordination and decision-making. Emotional involvement with the performed task seems to enhance the triggering effect. Typically, after an individually variable time of exposition to the precipitating task, the affected patients develop jerks in the activated musculature (e.g., right hand in writing or both upper extremities with playing piano), which may evolve into a secondary generalized tonic–clonic seizure.

The history of the concept and the related terminology has been reviewed by Inoue and Zifkin (2004). The term was first used by Daniele et al. (1989), and adopted by Inoue et al. (1994). Earlier case reports used multiple terms such as epilepsia arithmetices, chess playing epilepsy, card playing epilepsy, or seizures at drawing or decision-making. Matsuoka et al. (2000) developed a neuropsychological battery with which they tested a series of 480 unselected patients with epilepsy for praxis-induced epileptiform activity and seizures. They found praxis induction in 38 patients (7.9%), 36 of whom had IGE. Of their 45 patients with JME, 22 (48.9%) had praxis induction.

The concept of seizures precipitated by thinking was developed in parallel (Goossens et al., 1990), focusing on abstract cognitive activities including spatial tasks (Andermann et al., 1998). The question of whether the two terms, praxis induction and thinking-induced seizures, really describe the same or two separate trigger mechanisms was discussed controversially by Inoue and Zifkin (2004), who concluded that, if there were differences at all, they would be minimal. The findings of Guaranha et al. (2009) confirmed that the mere planning of the precipitating actions was a trigger by itself, the difference being only quantitative.

Outside Japan, praxis induction in JME seems to be less frequent, but it still occurs in 25–35% of the patients (Mayer et al., 2006; Guaranha et al., 2009).

Orofacial reflex myocloni

Small, lightning-like, single or arrhythmic myocloni in the perioral muscles, tongue, throat, and jaw, precipitated by language-related activities, particularly by reading and talking, are related to two different epilepsy syndromes.

Primary reading epilepsy (PRE)

In the International Classification of Epilepsies and Epileptic Syndromes (Commission on Classification and Terminology of the ILAE, 1989), PRE appears as the only syndrome that is characterized by a reflex mechanism, and the only idiopathic localization-related syndrome starting in adolescence and adulthood.

PRE was first described by Bickford et al. in 1956, and the syndrome was delineated in detail by Wolf (1992) in a meta-analysis of all 111 published cases. It is a syndrome with a frequent specific hereditary background, with an age of onset between 12 and 25 years and no tendency of deterioration. Seizures are precipitated by reading, whereas spontaneous seizures are absent in 95% and very rare in 5%. Reading aloud is more provocative than silent reading. The content of the text is irrelevant (it may be nonsense or a text in a foreign language that the patient does not understand), but it is the more provocative the more difficult the text is to read. After a delay of typically some minutes, orofacial reflex myocloni start in full consciousness and may rapidly evolve into a generalized tonic–clonic seizure if the patient continues to read. Some patients experience a visual disturbance, which seems to consist mostly of a brief dyslexia, and very rarely this aura replaces the reflex myoclonus. Other language-related activities are additional triggers in subgroups of patients: talking (27%), writing (11%), and reading figures (4–7%). Occasionally, reading musical scores and reading Braille were additional triggers and produced manual myocloni (Stevens, 1957; Forster and Daly, 1973). In individual cases, language-related activities other than reading and talking prevail, for instance writing (Chifari et al., 2004). Stress and emotion are possible modifiers (Wolf et al., 1998).

Ictal EEG

Ictally, PRE is characterized by evoked paroxysmal rhythmic theta activity or spikes over either one or both frontocentral, centroparietal, or temporoparietal regions in spite of the rather uniform clinical correlate. They are most commonly bilateral with unilateral accentuation, whereas unilateral or focal discharges are seen less frequently. Lateralization to the language-dominant hemisphere is more common than to the nondominant side. Prolonged partial seizures are associated with a wide variety of activity, either with bursts of slow activity over the left temporal area (Koutroumanidis et al., 1998), with left occipital transients (Chavany et al., 1956), or with fast rhythmic discharge localized at the left parieto-occipital region (Gastaut and Tassinari, 1966).

Ictal EEGs of variable quality of secondarily generalized tonic–clonic seizures were available for 6 of 111 patients in the meta-analysis of Wolf (1992), an unusually high number considering that the reviewed literature was from before the era of intensive monitoring. The reason is probably that seizures induced by reading are easily testable in the EEG laboratory, and that in some patients the transition from the reflex myocloni to a tonic–clonic seizure is rapid. In the four patients with unequivocal reports, the seizure onsets were localized, but with individual patterns. One patient reported by Gastaut and Tassinari (1966) had two partial seizures registered with different semiology, one evolving to a generalized tonic–clonic seizure. One started in the left parietal and the other in the right parietal region.

Treatment

Many patients manage to stop reading when the reflex myocloni appear, thus preventing convulsive seizures. These patients have no need to take AEDs. Pharmacotherapy is indicated in patients in whom the reflex epileptic response develops rapidly or in those who need to read a lot. In these cases, VPA is the drug of first choice, although positive results have also been reported with clonazepam.

Juvenile myoclonic epilepsy

Orofacial reflex myocloni also occur in JME, where they are always precipitated by talking and in about 40% by reading (Mayer and Wolf, 1997). Of 65 patients of Mayer et al. (2006) who responded to a questionnaire, 33 (51%) reported some reflex epileptic phenomenon, which was orofacial myocloni with talking in 17 (26%, 9 of them also with reading). Of these 33 patients with a history of seizure triggers, 25 were available for neuropsychological testing under video-EEG monitoring and were compared with a control group of patients with focal epilepsy. The investigation used the modified test protocol of Matsuoka et al. (2000) with more extensive linguistic tasks. Language-provoked spikes were found in 9 patients with JME, compared with 2 in the control group.

These findings were supported by the group in Sao Paolo using the same protocol as Mayer et al. (2006), with linguistic tasks triggering seizures or epileptiform discharges in 19% of 76 patients with JME (Guaranha et al., 2009).

The phenotype is indistinguishable from PRE, and the genetics of orofacial reflex myocloni have not yet been studied in either syndrome.

Functional imaging investigation in PRE

PRE is probably the best suited and studied of the reflex epilepsies. Seizures (i.e., reflex myocloni) can be triggered reliably with minimal movement artifact in the scanner environment. Structural neuroimaging findings are usually normal. However, one group reported a local structural abnormality in 2 of 3 patients with an unusual gyrus branching anteriorly off the left central sulcus, suggesting that the spikes in PRE spread from working memory areas into adjacent motor cortex, activating a cortical subcortical circuit (Archer et al., 2003). In a more recent study, Salek-Haddadi et al. (2009) did not find any structural abnormalities, either individually or in a group analysis of 9 patients with PRE.

A spike-triggered fMRI study in a 16-year-old girl with PRE showed increased activity, related to individual spikes in the left posterior middle frontal gyrus, that colocalized with the brain regions activated by the working memory component of the reading task, and also bilateral motor cortical and subcortical activity in the bilateral inferior central sulcus and bilateral globus pallidus (Archer et al., 2003).

In the largest series of fMRI studies to date in 9 patients with PRE (Salek-Haddadi et al., 2009), ictal fMRI revealed activations within cortical (right medial frontal gyrus) and subcortical (left putamen) areas during reading-induced seizures. Although there were no gross abnormalities in cognitive or motor organization, most of the cortical areas were either in close proximity with or directly overlapped the areas activated by cognitive and motor functions. These subcortical areas may be closely linked to areas of hyperexcitable cortex, which constitute part of the normal reading network or physiological motor function.

Salek-Haddadi and colleagues also observed bilateral blood oxygen-level dependent (BOLD) increases in the hand area of a patient previously diagnosed with JME. In this case, primary motor areas are presumably part of the hyperexcitable cortex providing a functional link for the often noticed association of PRE and JME in the same individual, and the recently reported observation of orofacial reflex myocloni triggered by reading and talking in JME (Mayer et al., 2006).

The ictal fMRI data have also provided further evidence for involvement of the putamen, caudate, and pallidum in the modulation of seizure activity. In both fMRI studies (Archer et al., 2003; Salek-Haddadi et al., 2009), spike-triggered fMRI data analysis revealed a significant activation pattern in the left precentral gyrus, near or directly in area BA6, and bilaterally in the central sulcus and globus pallidus. In one patient in the Salek-Haddadi series who presented with frequent seizures on silent reading with clear EEG correlates, but very little movement, the area of maximal BOLD response was also functionally connected to a network of cortical and subcortical regions. Connectivity analysis in this patient suggested that, during reading-provoked seizures, the neuronal state of both left piriform cortex and left BA6 were driving the activity within the thalamus, claustrum, and right inferior frontal gyrus. This connectivity analysis supports the important role of deep cortical structures, and particularly the frontal piriform cortex (or the primary olfactory cortex), as key regions in facilitating seizure occurrence. These regions are involved in the propagation and modulation of seizure activity, as previously established in animals (Piredda and Gale, 1985) and humans (Blumenfeld et al., 2004).

In PRE, BA6 appears to be the area relating the particular cognitive activation (grapheme-to-phoneme transition) to seizure activity. The importance of this area is supported by MEG analysis of the above-mentioned patient in the Salek Haddadi series. Predominantly frontal MEG findings were confirmed by concomitant EEG localization results, revealing activity extending precentrally into BA6 (Fig. 16.1).

Ictal radioisotope studies are limited by the low temporal resolution in SPECT and PET. Ictal SPECT with [^{99m}Tc]hexamethylpropylene amine oxide (HMPAO) in a 14-year-old Japanese boy revealed hyperperfusion in both frontal lobes, more notable in the left, and also within the left temporal lobe. (Miyamoto et al., 1995). Meaningful interpretation of the findings were difficult as the healthy control also showed left frontotemporal hyperperfusion, albeit to a lesser degree and extent. The ictal EEG in this patient was characterized by bilateral spike–wave complexes with a left frontotemporal predominance and in a similar distribution to the ictal SPECT findings.

Koepp et al. (1998a) found direct *in vivo* PET evidence for the dynamic multifocal release of endogenous opioids during and after reading-induced partial seizures in areas known to be involved in reading, visual

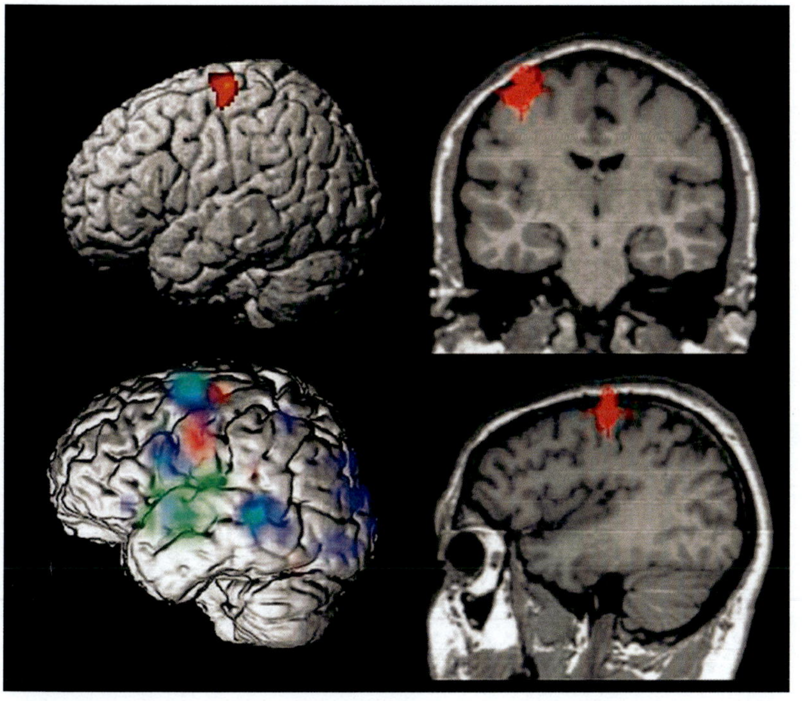

Fig. 16.1. Functional imaging in primary reading epilepsy. *Top left:* Blood oxygen level-dependent functional magnetic resonance imaging (fMRI BOLD) activation in a patient with reading-induced orofacial reflex myocloni, indicating maximum BOLD response at Brodman area (BA) 6. *Bottom left:* Spike-related BOLD changes (red) coregistered with language-related activations (blue) and motor jaw movements (green). *Right side of image:* Predominant frontal magnetoencephalography (MEG) findings revealing activity extending precentrally into BA6 (*top:* coronal view; *bottom:* sagittal view).

processing, and word recognition. The most significant affected areas during reading-induced seizures were in close proximity to areas found to be hypoactive in the same patients in areas of the brain involved in normal reading (Salek-Haddadi et al., 2009). These cortical and subcortical areas may both represent hyperexcitable cortex and constitute part of the normal reading network. This led to the hypothesis that there are networks of cortical areas concurrently subserving both physiological cognitive functions and epileptic activity.

"Secondary reading epilepsy"

The term was proposed by Bickford et al. (1956) for occasional patients whose seizures are sometimes precipitated by reading but who also have spontaneous seizures. No syndrome has emerged because the few reported cases present a rather random selection of different syndromes, seizure types, and etiologies, and no common pathomechanism has been proposed.

Complex audiogenic seizures

Musicogenic epilepsy

Musicogenic epilepsy is categorized as a complex reflex epilepsy and is characterized by seizures induced typically by hearing music (Critchley, 1977). Like scripture, music belongs to the most cherished cultural accomplishments of humankind whose involvement in epilepsy was unexpected. Since the first case report by Merzheevsky in 1884 (Janz, 1969) and the detailed description by Critchley in 1937, musicogenic epilepsy has fascinated many authors. When Janz (1969) reviewed 72 cases, including 4 of his own patients, the relationship with temporal lobe epilepsy was well established, and it was known that the patients usually did not react to any kind of music but to certain styles or composers, specific instruments, or even one particular musical piece. Often it is music with a particular emotional load. A musical stimulus has at least five components: melody, harmony, rhythm, emotional effect, and memory. Each of these different components might be epileptogenic for a particular patient (Tayah et al., 2006), but it is often difficult to isolate the effective stimulus.

Wieser (2004) based his meta-analysis on 83 cases (36 male and 43 female patients; sex unknown for 4 patients), including 7 of his own observations. He tried to relate the ictogenesis in musicogenic epilepsy to the functional anatomy of musical perception. The different components of a musical stimulus are elaborated by different cortical areas and the cerebral structures involved in processing a musical stimulus are part of a complex network that encompasses the auditory cortex (Peretz and Coltheart, 2003; Zatorre et al., 2007). The auditory cortex is considered to consist of a core of primary cortex that receives thalamic projections. It has tonotopically organized sections and is especially sensitive to pure tones (Johnsrude et al., 2002). The primary auditory cortex is surrounded by and linked to several belt areas that show more sensitivity to complex stimuli than to pure tones and have a less structured tonotopicity (Rauschecker and Tian, 2000).

Functional imaging in musicogenic epilepsy

The pathophysiology of musicogenic epilepsy is not well understood. Numerous functional neuroimaging studies (Zatorre, 2002, 2004) in subjects with unilateral cortical lesions (Johnsrude et al., 2000; Samson et al., 2002) have demonstrated predominant involvement of right hemisphere structures in networks involved in the processing of musical information. The majority of reports are case reports or small series of patients. In one of the most comprehensive case reports, a 36-year-old right-handed man was studied who had experienced partial seizures since the age of 24 every time he played or listened to music with a strong emotional charge (Pittau et al., 2008). This patient underwent videopolygraphic recording including autonomic variables and a brain fMRI study, during which he listened to both "neutral" and "emotionally charged" music. Three right temporal seizures recorded during videopolygraphic monitoring were elicited by listening to the triggering song. The fMRI study disclosed activation in right acoustic areas during "neutral music," whereas an "emotionally charged melody" provoked widespread activation over the right frontotemporo-occipital area before seizure onset. In the associated comprehensive literature review, Pittau and colleagues summarized findings from 110 published cases of musicogenic epilepsy that seemed to suggest a right-sided predominance of the epileptogenic zone. Their case report supported the role of the right temporal lobe in musicogenic epilepsy and demonstrated that the cerebral areas activated during the period of strong emotion leading to the seizures encompass the auditory cortex activated by neutral music. A strong emotional feeling provoked by specific melodies seems to have been the triggering stimulus in this patient, as his seizures were preceded for several seconds by increased heart rate and blood pressure suggestive of a mesial temporal discharge not yet visible on the scalp EEG. Another possibility is that autonomic activation is an expression of the emotional component that an individual has in response to a certain stimulus, which can then facilitate the reflex epileptic seizure. However, this would not explain why the seizures are evoked only by music and not by other otherwise moving or touching events (e.g., reading a poem or watching a show).

The possible lateralizing value of musicogenic seizures is controversial. A dominant role of the right temporal lobe in this kind of epilepsy has been suggested, and right temporal predominance and right anterior and mesial hyperperfusion have been demonstrated on ictal SPECT (Wieser et al., 1997; Genc et al., 2001; Gelisse et al., 2003; Cho et al., 2007).

Right temporal involvement has also been shown on subdural EEGs (Tayah et al., 2006).

Another interesting topic is the predisposition of highly musical individuals for this kind of epilepsy (Scott, 1977; Wieser et al., 1997).

One valid tool for studying the role of the musical stimuli is fMRI. There are only a few descriptions of patients with musicogenic epilepsy who underwent fMRI both during the evoked seizure and while simply listening to the epileptogenic music (Morocz et al., 2003; Pittau et al., 2008). In the Morocz fMRI study, an epileptogenic song was repeated eight times and the paradigm was the playing of epileptogenic music until the patient experienced an aura, whereas Pittau and coworkers repeated the epileptogenic song only three times (lower habituation) and stopped the music before the start of the seizure. The length of the epileptogenic music played during the fMRI study was too short to produce a clinical seizure. To avoid artifacts resulting from the seizure, their goal was limited to recalling the subjective feelings that consistently preceded the seizure in this particular patient. The cortical activation appears to reflect the initial involvement of the cortical areas leading to the beginning of the paroxysmal discharge, not evident on EEG scalp electrodes. However, the fronto-orbital structures could be linked to the emotional component induced by the musical stimulus (Blood et al., 1999).

Other

Forster et al. (1969) reported the unusual case of a 53-year-old woman with post-traumatic left temporal lobe epilepsy with seizures reproducibly precipitated by listening to the voices of three particular radio announcers, independently of the texts. No other voices could provoke a seizure. Extensive studies did not conclusively clarify the nature of the trigger mechanism. The authors believe, however, that an element of prosody may have played a role. The patient was treated successfully by deconditioning.

Possible complex auditory triggers are so ubiquitous that they can easily be overlooked. Interestingly in this context, Ramani (1991) reported a very similar case of a 45-year-old woman with cryptogenic right temporal lobe seizures triggered by a particular female cohost in a popular television entertainment program. Systematic testing revealed that the patient was sensitive to the performer's voice and not to visual stimulation, emotional anticipation, or background music, nor to other programs or other female voices.

Many patients with familial temporal lobe epilepsy with aphasic seizures linked to chromosome 10q22-q24 have a particular kind of reflex seizures precipitated by hearing language (being spoken to, answering the phone, turning on the radio; Brodtkorb et al., 2002). The seizures typically include aphasia or more or less complex auditory hallucinations. Ramani's case might belong here, as well as the three very similar patients of Michelucci et al. (2004).

Complex visual stimuli

Although visual stimuli are predominant among the simple triggers of reflex seizures, complex visual stimuli rarely appear to precipitate seizures and only anecdotal reports exist. Klass (1989) reported a child with self-induction of atonic, video-EEG-documented seizures by looking at his own hand. This behavior lasted from age 14 months to 3 years, whereafter it disappeared, and the patient was still seizure-free without drugs when last contacted at age 30. Mitchell et al. (1954) described a patient who, by looking at a safety pin, induced pleasurable feelings that would evolve into a complex partial seizure.

One of the present authors (P.W.) knows of a young woman with cryptogenic right parietal lobe epilepsy and simple focal seizures that started with the perception of whitish filaments moving in her left visual hemifield. These were habitually provoked by complex visual stimuli such as the scanning of complex graphs at her workplace, portraits of family members and friends, and a particular painting by Salvador Dalí, which gives a strong illusion of three-dimensional space.

Complex vegetative stimuli

Eating as a trigger of seizures

After the first report by Scollo-Lavizzari and Hess (1967), many other cases were published but the seizure types and the relation to various epilepsy syndromes have remained rather obscure.

The majority of case reports with this peculiar type of reflex epilepsy are from the Indian subcontinent. Senanayake (1990a) reported 120 cases from Sri Lanka, and Koul et al. (1989) described 50 patients from Kashmir, where it was the commonest form of reflex epilepsy (5% of all epilepsies). All Sri Lankan patients, and 48 of 50 from Kashmir had some kind of partial seizure, with no apparent relation to any specific localization. The two populations seem to be different. In Sri Lanka, similar to the report of Scollo-Lavizzari and Hess (1967), eating-induced seizures could occur in different phases during the act of eating, sometimes even before starting to eat or within 30 minutes after the meal (Senanayake, 1990a). However, 49 of the 50 patients from Kashmir had seizures during mastication (Koul et al., 1989). The Sri Lankan cohort included 9 families where multiple members were affected, whereas no familial cases were reported from Kashmir.

Rémillard et al. (1989) reported on 10 surgically treated patients and proposed the existence of two subtypes, one with temporal and another with perisylvian seizure onset. In the temporal group, the activation of seizures by eating was present from the onset of epilepsy, and spontaneous seizures were infrequent. In the second group, the trigger mechanism developed later in the course of the disorder, and spontaneous seizures were more frequent.

According to Senanayake (1990a), eating seizures are three times more frequent in males. Sex ratios were not given by Koul et al. (1989) or Rémillard et al. (1989). Both symptomatic and idiopathic eating epilepsies seem to exist, and familial occurrence of eating epilepsy has been described in Sri Lanka (Senanayake, 1990b) and Brazil (Yacubian et al., 2004).

Sexual activity

Marquis d'Harville, a literary character with epilepsy in the novel *The Mysteries of Paris* by Eugène Sue (1842/43; Fig. 16.2), has a convulsive seizure on the night of the wedding, immediately the marriage is consummated, to his bride's horror. The writer, who grew up in a family of surgeons and was himself a surgeon, may have based the scene on a real event that had come to his knowledge. In the medical literature, seizures triggered by sexual activity have rarely been described, but may be underreported.

Hoenig and Hamilton (1960) gave the first detailed report of a female patient who had complex partial seizures with left-sided myocloni and, in the ictal EEG, right frontotemporal rhythmic theta waves. Seizures occurred habitually immediately after orgasm but sometimes also spontaneously. Özkara (2006) reviewed the literature and added six of his own cases. Precipitation by orgasm seems to occur predominantly in females with mostly right-sided temporal lobe epilepsy. The above-mentioned patient of Mitchell et al. (1954) may also belong here, as his "fits occurred soon after awakening when, with a full bladder, adult sexual outlets were sought but refused by a frigid wife."

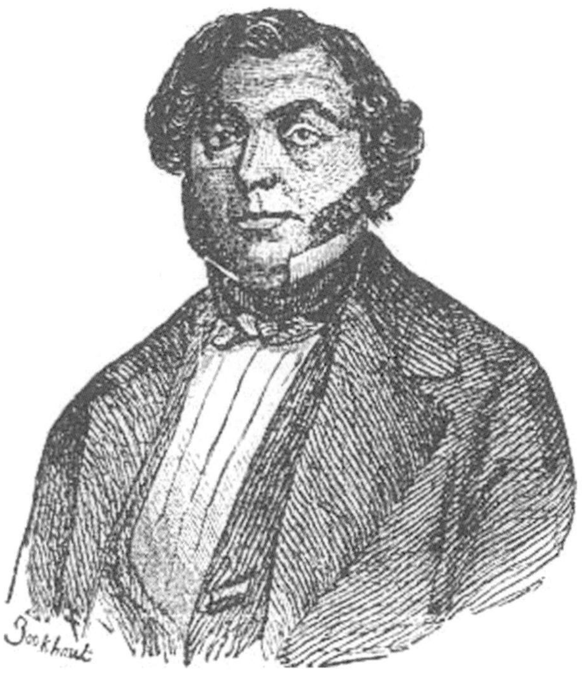

Fig. 16.2. Eugène Sue (1805–1957).

Emotional triggers, psychogenic epileptic seizures

Emotions are involved frequently in musicogenic epilepsy, and emotional involvement or context is a known modifier of other complex trigger mechanisms such as praxis induction, reading, and language-induced orofacial myocloni. Emotions are also part of sexual activity. Can emotions be triggers of seizures in their own right? It is one of the most common public beliefs about epilepsy, and explanations from patients insist that strong affects and emotional stress result in epileptic seizures. In a survey conducted by Mattson (1991), 58% of 177 patients with epilepsy considered "emotional states" as a trigger for their seizures. The closely related issue of psychogenic epileptic seizures was discussed by Fenwick (1994), including possible underlying neuronal mechanisms. The mediating role of sleep deprivation and hyperventilation was investigated by Mattson (1991). Important methodological problems are related to these aspects, as reviewed and discussed by Schöndienst (2004). There can be little doubt that emotions and affect can substantially contribute to ictogenesis. However, these seem at present to belong primarily to the facilitating factors that increase seizure susceptibility in a general way rather than interfering with specific ictogenic substrates and thus fulfilling the definition of reflex seizures. This view may change as these aspects become better investigated.

Conclusion of reflex epilepsy with complex triggers

Like reflex epilepsy with simple triggers, this is not a homogeneous group and the interindividual variability seems here to be even greater. However, some common features exist. Seizure precipitation by complex triggers, as by simple triggers, appears more common in idiopathic than in symptomatic epilepsies. Self-induction occurs, and treatment by avoidance or modification of the trigger is sometimes possible.

The prominent place of the visual system in the former group, however, seems here to be replaced by the important role of complex cognitive performances, and the reflex epileptic response rarely appears immediately but typically with some delay. In many of these reflex epilepsies, this delay appears to be due to a two-phase development, which is discussed below.

REFLEX SEIZURES, HUMAN ICTOGENESIS, AND THE NOSOLOGY OF THE EPILEPSIES

Reflex seizures have for a long time been mostly regarded as a kind of curiosity, an arabesque in the otherwise stern and sinister realm of epilepsy. This has started to change only recently, and we have begun to understand that they are a kind of natural experiment that can give us valuable *in vivo* information about ictogenesis, the generation of seizures in human epilepsies. This information is qualitative to start with, but probably quantifiable in many instances. It is not yet available for all reflex epilepsies, because it requires solid information about stimulation parameters, time, and details of the epileptic response. These relations are discussed here to the extent they are currently known.

Photosensitivity

The ictogenic system in photosensitivity appears to involve an occipitofrontoparietal cortical network generating the subclinical EEG response. The corticothalamic system becomes secondarily activated with the evolution to clinical seizures.

Eye closure sensitivity (ECS)

The trigger is a proprioceptive afference from the eyelid musculature, and the resulting seizures typically consist of or include myocloni of the same musculature indicating a short-loop ictogenic circuit. Other factors, however, are involved. Often, a difference appears to exist between voluntary and involuntary eye closure, but this has not yet been studied in greater detail. Both types do not use exactly the same neuronal networks.

Sensitivity to touch and movement

This sensitivity is seen in focal epilepsies with local ictogenic networks expected rather than widespread bihemispheric circuits. Interestingly, this phenomenon is often seen in epilepsia partialis continua, which can be understood as a condition in equilibrium on the edge of ictogenesis, with incoming proprioceptive or exteroceptive stimulus resulting in a spread of the locally restricted ongoing minimal paroxysmal activity. Often a single stimulus is sufficient, whereas in photosensitivity repetitive stimuli are required to trigger the epileptic response.

Praxis induction

There are two phases in the ictogenesis of praxis induction. In the first phase a complex cognitive visuomotor task involving decision-making is performed. There are no indications that task performance is in any way different from that in healthy subjects, so it is assumed that physiological functional–anatomical networks are activated, resulting in a state of hyperexcitability or upregulation of a complex central ictogenic system. Once this stage is reached, in the second phase myocloni are produced in brief peripheral reflex loops consisting of a proprioceptive afference, and an efference in the same sensorimotor segment.

Orofacial reflex myocloni

Ictogenesis appears to occur in a two-step process analogous to praxis induction, starting with activation of a complex functional–anatomical network that is followed by the generation of myocloni in a peripheral reflex loop (Wolf, 1994). The myocloni appear in the muscles that are active in the task, the musculature involved in speech. However, there is plasticity and the ictogenic reflex loop may also be activated elsewhere. Forster and Daly (1973) described a patient with PRE who taught herself Braille to avoid the orofacial reflex myocloni but instead developed manual myocloni at finger reading. In a patient with PRE of Stevens (1957), in whom playing music from a sheet was one of the possible triggers, the resulting myocloni occurred in the hands together with the orofacial muscles.

An interesting difference to praxis induction is that the functional–anatomical system used in reading epilepsy is not a preformed physiological system but one acquired by learning. It comprises (Wolf, 1992) the visual cortex (primary visual perception), right parietal (recognition of words and groups of words, "kanji processing") and left parietal (recognition of graphemes, "kana processing") cortex, auditory cortex (evocation of phonemes), motor cortex (pronunciation and program for writing), and language areas (semantic control).

Recruitment of a "critical mass" of language-related areas with synchronization and subsequent spreading of excitation in response to the epileptogenic stimulus precipitates a clinical seizure. Increasing the complexity of epileptogenic stimuli may facilitate such recruitment. Task difficulty, complexity, emotional content, and duration enhance the chances of electrographic or clinical activation in reading epilepsy, suggesting maximal neuronal interaction to be at least a facilitating factor (Koepp et al., 1998b). This recruitment may involve the participation and interaction of several cortical and subcortical structures activated by reading or the emotional content of the reading material (mesiotemporal, amygdala, limbic structures).

Nosological considerations

The prevalent nosological concept of the epilepsies, as it is expressed in the International Classification of Epilepsy Syndromes and Epilepsies (Commission on Classification and Terminology of the ILAE, 1989), is based upon a double dichotomy of idiopathic versus symptomatic, and of localization-related versus generalized epilepsies. In recent years, most of these concepts have come under critical scrutiny (Wolf, 2006).

It is especially the concept of generalized seizures and generalized epilepsies that seems no longer to be tenable. "Generalized" in its present definition is based primarily on the EEG finding of a widespread bilateral symmetrical and synchronous epileptiform discharge, which is typical for this group of epilepsies. The different regional distributions of this discharge were never paid much attention to. However, when the newer functional and more sophisticated morphological investigations such as SPECT, PET, fMRI, EEG-triggered fMRI, MEG, and MR spectroscopy discovered a multitude of deviant regional and local findings in these epilepsies, it became clear that there is nothing homogeneously generalized about them. They rather are characterized by widely distributed deviations of brain function. These observations are consistent with the concept of variable hyperexcitability at multiple cortical and subcortical levels, potentially allowing for any combination of asymmetrical or symmetrical, generalized, regional, and focal discharges. The difference to idiopathic localization-related epilepsies, such as idiopathic childhood epilepsy with centrotemporal spikes, appears to be gradual rather than fundamental, as these also display bilateral seizure generation. The notion that the ictogenic mechanisms relate to functional–anatomical subsystems of the central nervous system, thus suggesting a concept of "system epilepsies," has been discussed by Wolf (2006) and Avanzini et al. (2012).

The study of reflex epilepsies, applying both anatomical analysis of ictogenesis and advanced functional investigations as reported in this chapter, has contributed significantly to this new nosological understanding. The information provided about interactions of local stimulation and local epileptic discharge in the ictogenesis of idiopathic generalized epilepsies made it possible to develop initial hypotheses regarding the pathological functional–anatomical circuits involved. They indicate that commonly pre-existing systems subserving normal function are used, and that these include both natural pre-established programs and others, as in the case of reading epilepsy, that are culture-dependent results of learning.

The occurrence of identical perioral reflex myocloni in PRE and JME – two syndromes belonging to either side of the traditional dichotomy – highlights the fundamental pathophysiological similarities between the various syndromes of idiopathic epilepsies that stand united in the concept of system epilepsies.

WIDENING OF THE CONCEPT: EPILEPSIES WITH EXTERNAL MODIFICATION OF ICTOGENESIS

Reflex epilepsies are conditions where stimulation of the ictogenic system by some external (i.e., sensory, motor, or cognitive) input can precipitate a seizure. The reverse of seizure precipitation is seizure inhibition, of which much fewer reports exist. However, Gowers (1881) wrote extensively about the "arrest" of seizures by sensory, motor, and other stimuli, and the interruption of incipient seizures by olfactory stimulation has been described in detail by Efron (1956, 1957), Betts (2003), and Jaseja (2008). Yanagisawa et al. (2009) reported the suppression of interictal spikes by movement in neocortical sensorimotor epilepsy. Both Gowers (1881) and Efron (1956) noted the importance of timing, of not delivering the arresting stimulus too late to stop the commencing seizure.

Of particular interest are conditions where the same stimulus delivered to the same patient can sometimes produce a provocative and sometimes an inhibitory effect (Guaranha et al., 2009; Mameniskiene et al., 2011). This was used as a therapeutic approach in a patient with seizures precipitated by touch by Wolf and Dockweiler (1989). Here again, the right timing was crucial for treatment success.

It would seem that, at least in these patients, seizure inhibition and precipitation are two exchangeable modes of response whose common denominator is the strong reactivity of the ictogenic system to external influences. The stimulus is the same, and the stimulated system is the same. The difference in response depends on the state of the stimulated system at the moment it is stimulated. To understand the role of timing, more investigations are necessary that focus on this particular aspect, which has received little research attention. Where it has been studied in detail (Efron, 1956; Wolf and Dockweiler, 1989), it was clearly related to the amount of buildup of seizure activity that had been reached, within the individual ictogenic system, when the stimulus was applied. Further research will clarify to what extent this ambiguity of response is a special case or, rather, a general quality of the epilepsies that, as "reflex epilepsies," are currently considered under only one of the two aspects.

ACKNOWLEDGMENTS

The authors thank Professor Hermann Stefan, Erlangen, for the MEG image included in Figure 16.1.

REFERENCES

Aguglia U, Tinuper P, Gastaut H (1984). Startle-induced epileptic seizures. Epilepsia 25: 712–720.

Alajouanine T, Gastaut H (1955). La syncinésie-sursaut et l'épilepsie sursaut à déclenchement sensoriel ou sensitif inopiné. Les faits anatomo-cliniques (15 observations). Rev Neurol 93: 29–41.

Allen IM (1945). Observations on cases of reflex epilepsy. N Z Med J 44: 135–142.

Andermann F, Keene DL, Andermann E et al. (1980). Startle disease or hyperekplexia. Further delineation of the syndrome. Brain 103: 985–997.

Andermann F, Zifkin BG, Andermann E et al. (1998). Epilepsy induced by thinking and spatial tasks. Adv Neurol 75: 263–272.

Archer JS, Briellmann RS, Syngeniotis A et al. (2003). Spike-triggered fMRI in reading epilepsy: involvement of left frontal cortex working memory area. Neurology 60: 415–421.

Avanzini G, Manganotti P, Meletti S et al. (2012). The system epilepsies: a pathophysiological hypothesis. Epilepsia in press.

Benabou R, Reutens DC, Andermann F et al. (1996). Toothbrushing seizures: reflex epilepsy originating in the face area. Epilepsia 37: 29.

Betts T (2003). Use of aromatherapy (with or without hypnosis) in the treatment of intractable epilepsy – a two-year follow-up study. Seizure 12: 534–538.

Bickford RG, Daly D, Keith DW (1953). Convulsive effects of light stimulation in children. Am J Dis Child 86: 179–183.

Bickford RG, Whelan JL, Klass DW et al. (1956). Reading epilepsy: clinical and electroencephalographic studies of a new syndrome. Trans Am Neurol Assoc 81: 100–102.

Biraben A, Doury E, Scarabin JM (2004). Motor reflex epilepsy induced by touch and movement. In: P Wolf, Y Inoue, B Zifkin (Eds.), Reflex Epilepsies: Progress in Understanding. J. Libbey Eurotext, Montrouge, pp. 135–142.

Blood AJ, Zatorre RJ, Bermudez P et al. (1999). Emotional responses to pleasant and unpleasant music correlate with activity in paralimbic brain regions. Nat Neurosci 2: 382–387.

Blumenfeld H, McNally KA, Vanderhill SD et al. (2004). Positive and negative network correlations in temporal lobe epilepsy. Cereb Cortex 14: 892–902.

Bonmassar G, Schwartz DP, Liu AK et al. (2001). Spatiotemporal brain imaging of visual-evoked activity using interleaved EEG and fMRI recordings. Neuroimage 13: 1035–1043.

Brodtkorb E, Gu W, Nakken KO et al. (2002). Familial temporal lobe epilepsy with aphasic seizures and linkage to chromosome 10q22-q24. Epilepsia 43: 228–235.

Capovilla G, Gambardella A, Rubboli G et al. (2006). Suppressive efficacy by a commercially available blue lens on PPR in 610 photosensitive epilepsy patients. Epilepsia 47: 529–533.

Chatrian GE, Lettich E, Miller LH et al. (1970a). Pattern-sensitive epilepsy. Part 1. An electrographic study of its mechanisms. Epilepsia 11: 125–149.

Chatrian GE, Lettich E, Miller LH et al. (1970b). Pattern-sensitive epilepsy. Part 2. Clinical changes, tests of responsiveness and motor output, alterations of evoked potentials and therapeutic measures. Epilepsia 11: 151–162.

Chavany JA, Fischgold H, Messimy R et al. (1956). Clinical and EEG aspects of a case of epilepsy electively induced by reading. Rev Neurol 95: 381–387.

Chifari R, Piazzini A, Turner K et al. (2004). Reflex writing seizures in two siblings with juvenile myoclonic epilepsy. Acta Neurol Scand 109: 232–235.

Cho JW, Seo DW, Joo EY et al. (2007). Neural correlates of musicogenic epilepsy: SISCOM and FDG-PET. Epilepsy Res 77: 169–173.

Chuang YC, Lin TK, Lui CC et al. (2004). Tooth-brushing epilepsy with ictal orgasms. Seizure 13: 179–182.

Commission on Classification and Terminology of the ILAE (1989). Proposal for revised classification of epilepsies and epileptic syndromes. Epilepsia 30: 389–399.

Covanis A, Ferrie CD, Koutroumanidis M et al. (2005). Panayiotopoulos syndrome and Gastaut type idiopathic childhood occipital epilepsy. In: J Roger, M Bureau, C Dravet et al. (Eds.), Epileptic Syndromes in Infancy, Childhood and Adolescence. 4th edn. J. Libbey Eurotext, Montrouge, pp. 227–253.

Critchley M (1937). Musicogenic epilepsy. Brain 60: 13–27.

Critchley M (1977). Musicogenic epilepsy. In: M Critchley, RA Henson (Eds.), Music and the Brain: Studies in the Neurology of Music. Heineman, London, pp. 344–353.

Daniele O, Raieli V, Mattaliano A et al. (1989). Seizures precipitated by unusual epileptogenic tasks. In: A Beaumanoir, H Gastaut, R Naquet (Eds.), Reflex Seizures and Reflex Epilepsies. Editions Médecine & Hygiène, Geneva, pp. 333–336.

Dhanaraj M, Jayavelu A (2003). Prophylactic use of clobazam in hot water epilepsy. J Assoc Physicians India 51: 43–44.

Doose H (1992). Myoclonic astatic epilepsy of early childhood. In: J Roger, M Bureau, C Dravet et al. (Eds.), Epileptic Syndromes in Infancy, Childhood and Adolescence. 2nd edn. . J. Libbey, London, pp. 103–114.

Dravet C, Bureau M, Roger J (1992). Benign myoclonic epilepsy in infants. In: J Roger, M Bureau, C Dravet et al. (Eds.), Epileptic Syndromes in Infancy, Childhood and Adolescence. 2nd edn. . J. Libbey, London, pp. 67–74.

Dravet C, Bureau M, Oguni H et al. (2005). Severe myoclonic epilepsy in infancy (Dravet syndrome). In: J Roger, M Bureau, C Dravet et al. (Eds.), Epileptic Syndromes in Infancy, Childhood and Adolescence. 4th edn. J. Libbey Eurotext, Montrouge, pp. 89–113.

D'Souza WJ, O'Brien TJ, Murphy M et al. (2007). Tooth-brushing-induced epilepsy with structural lesions in the primary somatosensory area. Neurology 68: 769–771.

Efron R (1956). The effect of olfactory stimuli in arresting uncinate fits. Brain 79: 267–281.

Efron R (1957). The conditioned inhibition of uncinate fits. Brain 80: 251–262.

Fabian A, Wolf A (1987). Epileptic discharge after eye closure: relation to photosensitivity. In: P Wolf, M Dam, D Janz et al. (Eds.), Advances in Epileptology. XVIth Epilepsy International Symposium. Raven, New York, pp. 259–264.

Falconer MA, Driver MV, Serafetinides EA (1963). Seizures induced by movement: report of a case relieved by operation. J Neurol Neurosurg Psychiatry 26: 300–307.

Fenwick P (1994). Psychogenic epileptic seizures and behavioural treatment of epilepsy. In: P Wolf (Ed.), Epileptic Seizures and Syndromes, with Some of their Theoretical Implications. J. Libbey, London, pp. 657–665.

Fischer R, Noachtar S, Wolf P (1989). Lidschlußempfindlichkeit. Konstanz dieses Phänomens und seine Abhängigkeit von Reizvariationen. In: P Wolf (Ed.), Epilepsie. 88. Einhorn-Presse, Reinbek, pp. 233–235.

Forster FM (1977). Reflex Epilepsy, Behavioral Therapy and Conditional Reflexes. Thomas, Springfield.

Forster FM, Daly RF (1973). Reading epilepsy in identical twins. Trans Am Neurol Assoc 98: 186–188.

Forster FM, Hansotia P, Cleeland CS et al. (1969). A case of voice-induced epilepsy treated by conditioning. Neurology 19: 325–331.

García-Morales I, Maestú F, Pérez-Jiménez FA et al. (2009). A clinical and magnetoencephalography study of MRI-negative startle epilepsy. Epilepsy Behav 16: 166–171.

Gastaut H, Tassinari CA (1966). Triggering mechanisms in epilepsy. The electroclinical point of view. Epilepsia 2: 85–138.

Gelisse P, Thomas P, Padovani R et al. (2003). Ictal SPECT in a case of pure musicogenic epilepsy. Epileptic Disord 5: 133–137.

Genc BO, Genc E, Tastekin G et al. (2001). Musicogenic epilepsy with ictal single photon emission computed tomography (SPECT): could these cases contribute to our knowledge of music processing? Eur J Neurol 8: 191–194.

Goossens L, Andermann F, Andermann E et al. (1990). Reflex seizures induced by calculation, card or board games, and spatial tasks: a review of 25 patients and delineation of the epileptic syndromes. Neurology 40: 1171–1176.

Gowers WR (1881). Epilepsy and Other Chronic Convulsive Diseases. Wood, London.

Grosso S, Farnetani MA, Bernardoni E et al. (2007). Intractable reflex audiogenic seizures in Aicardi syndrome. Brain and Development 29: 243–246.

Guaranha MS, Da Silva Sousa P, de Araujo-Filho GM et al. (2009). Provocative and inhibitory effects of a video-EEG neuropsychologic protocol in juvenile myoclonic epilepsy. Epilepsia 50: 2446–2455.

Guerrini R, Dravet Ch, Genton P et al. (1995). Idiopathic photosensitive occipital lobe epilepsy. Epilepsia 36: 883–891.

Guirao Bringas IP, Behl I, Wolf P (1987). Epileptic discharge after eye closure: relation to epileptic syndromes. In: P Wolf, M Dam, D Janz et al. (Eds.), Advances in Epileptology. XVIth Epilepsy International Symposium. Raven, New York, pp. 255–258.

Harding GFA, Jeavons PM (1994). Photosensitive Epilepsy. MacKeith, London.

Haytac MC, Aslan K, Ozcelik O et al. (2008). Epileptic seizures triggered by the use of a powered toothbrush. Seizure 17: 288–291.

Hoenig J, Hamilton CM (1960). Epilepsy and sexual orgasm. Acta Psychiatr Neurol Scand 35: 448–456.

Holmes GL, Blair S, Eisenberg E et al. (1982). Tooth-brushing induces epilepsy. Epilepsia 23: 657–661.

Iannetti GD, Di Bonaventura C, Pantano P et al. (2002). fMRI/EEG in paroxysmal activity elicited by elimination of central vision and fixation. Neurology 58: 976–979.

Inoue Y, Zifkin BG (2004). Praxis induction and thinking induction: one or two mechanisms? A controversy. In: P Wolf, Y Inoue, B Zifkin (Eds.), Reflex Epilepsies: Progress in Understanding. J. Libbey Eurotext, Montrouge, pp. 41–55.

Inoue Y, Seino M, Tanaka M et al. (1994). Epilepsy with praxis-induced seizures. In: P Wolf (Ed.), Epileptic Seizures and Syndromes. John Libbey, London, pp. 81–91.

Inoue Y, Fukao K, Araki T et al. (1999). Photosensitive and nonphotosensitive electronic screen game induced seizures. Epilepsia 40: 8–16.

Jager L, Werhahn KJ, Hoffmann A et al. (2002). Focal epileptiform activity in the brain: detection with spike-related functional MR imaging: preliminary results. Radiology 223: 860–869.

Janz D (1969). Die Epilepsien. Spezielle Pathologie und Therapie. Thieme, Stuttgart.

Janz D, Christian W (1957). Impulsiv-petit mal. Dtsch Z Nervenheilkd 176: 346–386.

Jaseja H (2008). Scientific basis behind traditional practice of application of "shoe-smell" in controlling epileptic seizures in the eastern countries. Clin Neurol Neurosurg 110: 535–538.

Johnsrude IS, Penhune VB, Zatorre RJ (2000). Functional specificity in the right human auditory cortex for perceiving pitch direction. Brain 123: 155–163.

Johnsrude IS, Giraud AL, Frackowiak RS (2002). Functional imaging of the auditory system: the use of positron emission tomography. Audiol Neurootol 7: 251–276.

Kalitzin S, Parra J, Velis DN et al. (2002). Enhancement of phase clustering in the EEG/MEG gamma frequency band anticipates transitions to paroxysmal epileptiform activity in epileptic patients with known visual sensitivity. IEEE Trans Biomed Eng 49: 1279–1286.

Karbowski K (1989). Epileptic seizures induced by vestibular and auditory stimuli. In: A Beaumanoir, H Gastaut, R Naquet (Eds.), Reflex Seizures and Reflex Epilepsies. Editions Médecine & Hygiène, Geneva, pp. 255–260.

Kasteleijn-Nolst Trenité D, Pinto D, Hirsch E et al. (2005). Photosensitivity, visual induced seizures and epileptic syndromes. In: J Roger, M Bureau, C Dravet et al. (Eds.), Epileptic Syndromes in Infancy, Childhood and Adolescence. 4th edn. . J. Libbey Eurotext, Montrouge, pp. 395–420.

Kato N, Sadamatsu M, Kikuchi T et al. (2006). Paroxysmal kinesigenic choreoathetosis: from first discovery in 1892 to genetic linkage with benign familial infantile convulsions. Epilepsy Res 70: S174–S184.

Klass DW (1989). Self-induced seizures: long-term follow-up of two unusual cases. In: A Beaumanoir, H Gastaut, R Naquet (Eds.), Reflex Seizures and Reflex Epilepsies. Editions Médecine & Hygiène, Geneva, pp. 369–376.

Koepp MJ, Hansen ML, Pressler RM et al. (1998a). Comparison of EEG, MRI and PET in reading epilepsy: a case report. Epilepsy Res 29: 251–257.

Koepp MJ, Richardson MP, Brooks DJ et al. (1998b). Focal cortical release of endogenous opioids during reading-induced seizures. Lancet 352: 952–955.

Komarek V (1994). Olfactory activation in epilepsy. In: P Wolf (Ed.), Epileptic Seizures and Syndromes, with Some of their Theoretical Implications. J. Libbey, London, pp. 107–114.

Koul R, Koul S, Razdan S (1989). Eating epilepsy. Acta Neurol Scand 86: 78–80.

Koutroumanidis M, Koepp MJ, Richardson MP et al. (1998). The variants of reading epilepsy. A clinical and video-EEG study of 17 patients with reading-induced seizures. Brain 121: 1409–1427.

Koutroumanidis M, Pearce R, Sadoh DR et al. (2001). Tooth brushing-induced seizures: a case report. Epilepsia 42: 686–688.

Lancman ME, Asconapé JJ, Penry JK (1993). Startle epileptic seizures: clinical and imaging findings. J Epilepsy 6: 215–219.

Lishman WA, Symonds CP, Whitty GWM et al. (1962). Seizures induced by movement. Brain 85: 93–108.

Mameniskiene R, Bast T, Bentes C et al. (2011). Clinical course and variability of non-Rasmussen, non-stroke motor and sensory epilepsia partialis continua: a European survey and analysis of 65 cases. Epilepsia 52: 1168–1176.

Mani KS, Rangan G, Srinivas HV et al. (1998). The Yelandur study: a community based approach to epilepsy in rural south India. Epidemiological aspects. Seizure 7: 281–288.

Matsuoka H, Takahashi T, Sasaki M et al. (2000). Neuropsychological EEG activation in patients with epilepsy. Brain 123: 318–330.

Mattson R (1991). Emotional effects on seizure occurrence. In: DB Smith, DM Treiman, MR Trimble (Eds.), Neurobehavioral Problems in Epilepsy. Raven, New York, pp. 453–460.

Mayer T, Specht U (1995). Propranolol in startle induced epileptic seizures. J Neurol Neurosurg Psychiatry 58: 382–383.

Mayer T, Wolf P (1997). Reading epilepsy: related to juvenile myoclonic epilepsy? Epilepsia 38: 18–19.

Mayer TA, Schroeder F, May TW et al. (2006). Perioral reflex myoclonias: a controlled study in patients with JME and focal epilepsies. Epilepsia 47: 1059–1067.

Michelucci R, Gardella E, de Haan GJ et al. (2004). Telephone-induced seizures: a new type of reflex epilepsy. Epilepsia 45: 280–283.

Mitchell W, Falconer MA, Hill D (1954). Epilepsy with fetishism relieved by temporal lobectomy. Lancet 264: 626–630.

Miyamoto A, Takahashi S, Tokumitsu A et al. (1995). Ictal HMPAO-single photon emission computed tomography findings in reading epilepsy in a Japanese boy. Epilepsia 36: 1161–1163.

Moeller F, Siebner HR, Ahlgrimm N et al. (2009a). fMRI activation during spike and wave discharges evoked by photic stimulation. Neuroimage 48: 682–695.

Moeller F, Siebner HR, Wolff S et al. (2009b). Mapping brain activity on the verge of a photically induced generalized tonic–clonic seizure. Epilepsia 50: 1632–1637.

Morocz IA, Karni A, Haut S et al. (2003). fMRI of triggerable aurae in musicogenic epilepsy. Neurology 60: 705–709.

Naquet R, Batini C (2004). Varieties of photosensitivity in man ("plain" and progressive myoclonus epilepsies), in baboon and fowl. In: P Wolf, Y Inoue, B Zifkin (Eds.), Reflex Epilepsies: Progress in Understanding. J. Libbey Eurotext, Montrouge, pp. 15–26.

Navarro V, Adam C, Petitmengin C et al. (2006). Toothbrush-thinking seizures. Epilepsia 47: 1971–1973.

Newmark ME, Penry JK (1979). Photosensitivity and Epilepsy: A Review. Raven Press, New York.

O'Brien TJ, Hogan RE, Sedal L et al. (1996). Tooth-brushing epilepsy: a report of a case with structural and functional imaging and electrophysiology demonstrating a right frontal focus. Epilepsia 37: 694–697.

Ohmori I, Ohtsuka Y, Ogino T et al. (2002). The relationship between paroxysmal kinesigenic choreoathetosis and epilepsy. Neuropediatrics 33: 15–20.

Özkara C, Özdemir S, Yilmaz A et al. (2006). Orgasm-induced seizures: a study of six patients. Epilepsia 47: 2193–2197.

Panayiotopoulos CP (1994). Fixation-off-sensitive epilepsies: clinical and EEG characteristics. In: P Wolf (Ed.), Epileptic Seizures and Syndromes. J. Libbey, London, pp. 55–66.

Parra J, Meeren HKM, Kalitzin S et al. (2000). Magnetic source imaging in fixation-off sensitivity: relationship with alpha rhythm. J Clin Neurophysiol 17: 212–223.

Peretz I, Coltheart M (2003). Modularity of music processing. Nat Neurosci 6: 688–691.

Piredda S, Gale K (1985). A crucial epileptogenic site in the deep prepiriform cortex. Nature 317: 623–625.

Pittau F, Tinuper P, Bisulli F et al. (2008). Videopolygraphic and functional MRI study of musicogenic epilepsy. A case report and literature review. Epilepsy Behav 13: 685–692.

Plouin P, Vigevano F (2004). Reflex seizures in infancy. In: P Wolf, Y Inoue, B Zifkin (Eds.), Reflex Epilepsies: Progress in Understanding. J. Libbey Eurotext, Montrouge, pp. 115–122.

Radhakrishnan K, Louis EKS, Johnson JA et al. (2005). Pattern-sensitive epilepsy: electroclinical characteristics, natural history, and delineation of the epileptic syndrome. Epilepsia 46: 48–58.

Radovici A, Misirliou V, Gluckmann M (1932). Epilepsie réflexe provoquée par excitations optiques des rayons solaires. Rev Neurol (Paris) 1: 1305–1308.

Ramani V (1991). Audiogenic epilepsy induced by a specific television performer. N Engl J Med 325: 134–135.

Ratnapriya R, Satishchandra P, Dilip S et al. (2009a). Familial autosomal dominant reflex epilepsy triggered by hot water maps to 4q24-q28. Hum Genet 126: 677–683.

Ratnapriya R, Satishchandra P, Kumar SD et al. (2009b). A locus for autosomal dominant reflex epilepsy precipitated by hot water maps at chromosome 10q21.3-q22.3. Hum Genet 125: 541–549.

Rauschecker JP, Tian B (2000). Mechanisms and streams for processing of "what" and "where" in auditory cortex. Proc Natl Acad Sci U S A 97: 11800–11806.

Regesta G, Tanganelli P (1989). The evolution and prognosis of photosensitive epilepsies. A study of 53 patients. In: A Beaumanoir, H Gastaut, R Naquet (Eds.), Reflex Seizures and Reflex Epilepsies. Editions Médecine & Hygiène, Geneva, pp. 175–177.

Rémillard GM, Andermann F, Zifkin BG et al. (1989). Eating epilepsy: a study of ten surgically treated patients suggests the presence of two separate syndromes. In: A Beaumanoir, H Gastaut, R Naquet (Eds.), Reflex Seizures and Reflex Epilepsies. Editions Médecine & Hygiène, Geneva, pp. 289–300.

Revol M, Moreau T, Isnard H et al. (1989). Paroxysmal kinesigenic choreoathetosis. In: A Beaumanoir, H Gastaut, R Naquet (Eds.), Reflex Seizures and Reflex Epilepsies. Editions Médecine & Hygiène, Geneva, pp. 131–138.

Ricci GB, Chapman RM, Erné SN et al. (1990). Neuromagnetic topography of photoconvulsive response in man. Electroencephalogr Clin Neurophysiol 75: 1–12.

Ricci S, Cusmai R, Fusco L et al. (1995). Reflex myoclonic epilepsy in infancy: a new age-dependent idiopathic epilepsy syndrome related to startle reaction. Epilepsia 36: 342–348.

Robinson LJ (1939). Induction of seizures by closing the eyes, or by ocular pressure, in a patient with epilepsy. Case report. J Nerv Ment Dis 90: 333–336.

Salek-Haddadi A, Mayer T, Hamandi K et al. (2009). Imaging seizure activity: a combined EEG/EMG–fMRI study in reading epilepsy. Epilepsia 50: 256–264.

Samson S, Zatorre RJ, Ramsay JO (2002). Deficits of musical timbre perception after unilateral temporal-lobe lesion revealed with multidimensional scaling. Brain 125: 511–523.

Satishchandra P (2003). Hot water epilepsy. Epilepsia 44: 29–32.

Satishchandra P, Ullal GR, Shankar SK (2004). Trigger mechanisms in hot-water epilepsy. In: P Wolf, Y Inoue, B Zifkin (Eds.), Reflex Epilepsies: Progress in Understanding. J. Libbey Eurotext, Montrouge, pp. 105–114.

Schöndienst M (2004). Emotional seizure precipitation and psychogenic epileptic seizures. In: P Wolf, Y Inoue, B Zifkin (Eds.), Reflex Epilepsies: Progress in Understanding. J. Libbey Eurotext, Montrouge, pp. 93–104.

Scollo-Lavizzari G, Hess R (1967). Sensory precipitation of epileptic seizures. Report on two unusual cases. Epilepsia 8: 157–161.

Scott D (1977). Musicogenic epilepsy. In: M Critchley, RA Henson (Eds.), Music and the Brain: Studies in the Neurology of Music. Heinemann, London, pp. 344–353.

Senanayake N (1990a). "Eating epilepsy" – a reappraisal. Epilepsy Res 5: 74–79.

Senanayake N (1990b). Familial eating epilepsy. J Neurol 237: 388–391.

Servit Z, Kristof M, Kolinova M (1981). Activating effect of nasal and oral hyperventilation on epileptic electrographic phenomena: reflex mechanisms of nasal origin. Epilepsia 22: 321–329.

Sevgi EB, Saygı S, Ciger A (2007). Eye closure sensitivity and epileptic syndromes: a retrospective study of 26 adult cases. Seizure 16: 17–21.

Shanzer S, April R, Atkin A (1965). Seizures induced by eye deviation. Arch Neurol 13: 621–626.

Stephani U, Tauer U, Koeleman B et al. (2004). Genetics of photosensitivity (photoparoxysmal response): a review. Epilepsia 45: 19–23.

Stevens H (1957). Reading epilepsy. N Engl J Med 257: 165–170.

Striano S, Capovilla G, Sofia V et al. (2009). Eyelid myoclonia with absences (Jeavons syndrome): a well-defined idiopathic generalized epilepsy syndrome or a spectrum of photosensitive conditions? Epilepsia 50: 15–19.

Sue E (1989). (1842/43). Les Mystères de Paris. Reprint Robert Laffont, Paris.

Takahashi Y, Fujiwara S, Matsuo N et al. (2004). Prevention of photosensitive seizures by optical filters. In: P Wolf, Y Inoue, B Zifkin (Eds.), Reflex Epilepsies: Progress in Understanding. J. Libbey Eurotext, Montrouge, pp. 27–40.

Tayah TF, Abou-Khalil B, Gilliam FG et al. (2006). Musicogenic seizures can arise from multiple temporal lobe foci: intracranial EEG analyses of three patients. Epilepsia 47: 1402–1406.

Tibussek D, Wohlrab G, Boltshauser E et al. (2006). Proven startle-provoked epileptic seizures in childhood: semiologic and electrophysiologic variability. Epilepsia 47: 1050–1058.

Träff J, Petrovic P, Ingvar M (2000). Thalamic activation in photic myoclonus. Acta Neurol Scand 101: 339–343.

Vignaendra V, Lim CL (1978). Epileptic discharges triggered by eye convergence. Neurology 28: 589–591.

Wieser HG (2004). Musicogenic seizures and findings on the anatomy of musical perception. In: P Wolf, Y Inoue, B Zifkin (Eds.), Reflex Epilepsies: Progress in Understanding. J. Libbey Eurotext, Montrouge, pp. 79–91.

Wieser HG, Hungerbuhler H, Siegel AM et al. (1997). Musicogenic epilepsy: review of the literature and case report with ictal single photon emission computed tomography. Epilepsia 38: 200–207.

Wolf P (1992). Reading epilepsy. In: J Roger, M Bureau, C Dravet et al. (Eds.), Epileptic Syndromes in Infancy, Childhood and Adolescence. 2nd edn. . J. Libbey, London, pp. 281–298.

Wolf P (1994). Reading epilepsy. In: P Wolf (Ed.), Epileptic Seizures and Syndromes, with Some of their Theoretical Implications. J. Libbey, London, pp. 67–73.

Wolf P (2006). Basic principles of the ILAE syndrome classification. Epilepsy Res 70: 20–26.

Wolf P, Dockweiler U (1989). Deconditioning therapy in a patient with versive seizures precipitated by touch. In: A Beaumanoir, H Gastaut, R Naquet (Eds.), Reflex Seizures and Reflex Epilepsies. Editions Médecine & Hygiène, Geneva, pp. 447–451.

Wolf P, Goosses R (1986). Relation of photosensitivity to epileptic syndromes. J Neurol Neurosurg Psychiatry 49: 1386–1391.

Wolf P, Okujava N (1999). Possibilities of non-pharmacological conservative treatment of epilepsy. Seizure 8: 45–52.

Wolf P, Mayer T, Reker M (1998). Reading epilepsy: report of five new cases and further considerations on the pathophysiology. Seizure 7: 271–279.

Yacubian EM, Skaff R, Garzon E et al. (2004). Seizures induced by eating in a family. In: P Wolf, Y Inoue, B Zifkin (Eds.), Reflex Epilepsies: Progress in Understanding. J. Libbey Eurotext, Montrouge, pp. 123–134.

Yanagisawa T, Hirata M, Kishima H et al. (2009). Movement induces suppression of interictal spikes in sensorimotor neocortical epilepsy. Epilepsy Res 87: 12–17.

Zafeiriou D, Vargiami E, Kontopoulos E (2003). Reflex myoclonic epilepsy in infancy: a benign age dependent idiopathic startle epilepsy. Epileptic Disord 5: 121–122.

Zagury S, Haury JA, Jomini-Jalanti RM (1989). Partial sensitive epilepsy triggered by a pure sound. A case report. In: A Beaumanoir, H Gastaut, R Naquet (Eds.), Reflex Seizures and Reflex Epilepsies. Editions Médecine & Hygiène, Geneva, pp. 251–253.

Zatorre RJ, Bouffard M, Ahad P et al. (2002). Where is "where" in the human auditory cortex? Nat Neurosci 5: 905–909.

Zatorre RJ, Bouffard M, Belin P (2004). Sensitivity to auditory object features in human temporal neocortex. J Neurosci 24: 3637–3642.

Zatorre RJ, Chen JL, Penhune VB (2007). When the brain plays music: auditory–motor interactions in music perception and production. Nat Rev Neurosci 8: 547–558.

Handbook of Clinical Neurology, Vol. 107 (3rd series)
Epilepsy, Part I
H. Stefan and W.H. Theodore, Editors

Chapter 17

Psychogenic nonepileptic seizures

PETER WIDDESS-WALSH [1,2]*, BARBARA MOSTACCI [3], PAOLO TINUPER[3], AND ORRIN DEVINSKY [1,2]

[1]*Comprehensive Epilepsy Center, Institute of Neurology and Neurosurgery at St. Barnabas, Livingston, NJ, USA*

[2]*Comprehensive Epilepsy Center, NYU Langone School of Medicine, New York, NY, USA*

[3]*IRCCS Istituto delle Scienze Neurologiche, University of Bologna, Bologna, Italy*

DEFINITION AND INTRODUCTION

Psychogenic nonepileptic seizures (PNES) are paroxysmal episodes of altered consciousness, behavior, or repetitive movement. They appear similar to seizures but do not result from excessive neuronal discharges, in contrast to epileptic or acute symptomatic seizures. They are a subset of neurological somatoform disorders that includes psychogenic movement disorders and paralysis. Symptoms are highly variable but usually consist of either positive (shaking, posturing) or negative (collapse, unresponsiveness) components. They must be differentiated from *physiological* nonepileptic events such as convulsive syncope or sleep attacks.

The nomenclature has changed over the years and has included pseudoseizures, hysterical seizures, and nonepileptic attack disorder (NEAD). Some authors avoid the use of the term "seizures" to reduce the connection with epilepsy. The term "pseudoseizure" is no longer used as it implies falseness. Dichotomies based on semiology, psychological profiles, and mechanisms have been suggested, but not established (Griffith and Szaflarski, 2010).

PNES have occurred throughout history and across cultures (Veith, 1965). In other cultures and times, hysteria/PNES were interpreted as demonic possession, and often resulted in exorcism or execution. In the 19th century, Carter, Briquet, and Charcot (Carter, 1853; Briquet, 1859; Janet, 1895) introduced modern concepts of unconscious conversion symptoms caused by repression of (usually sexual) conflicts. Janet, Kraepelin, and Freud expanded the role of hysteria, but channeled interest in PNES within dynamic psychiatry rather than neurology until the last few decades (Devinsky, 1998).

EPIDEMIOLOGY AND RELEVANCE

The prevalence of PNES in the general population is unclear, as the literature contains series based on referrals to epilepsy centers, where up to 10–20% of children and 10–22% of adults have PNES (Gates et al., 1985; Wyllie et al., 1990; Benbadis and Allen Hauser, 2000; Reuber and Elger, 2003; Wood et al., 2004). Up to 10% of patients with PNES may have comorbid epilepsy (Widdess-Walsh et al., 2010). Patients with PNES often present to epilepsy centers due to lack of effect of antiepileptic drugs (AEDs); up to 50% of patients with refractory seizures may have PNES (Lesser, 1996; Hovorka et al., 2007). Historically, in Charcot's "Quartier des Epileptiques," 46 (12%) of 385 women in a ward of epileptic patients were found to have what was *thought to be* PNES (Temkin, 1994). An estimated calculation of prevalence based on known epidemiological data is 2–33 per 100 000 (Benbadis and Allen Hauser, 2000). The annual incidence of PNES is between 0.91 and 3.03 per 100 000 (Table 17.1). These numbers are probably underestimated; somatoform disorders are common and almost 6% of patients with anxiety disorders have somatoform symptoms (Rogers et al., 1996). "Hysterical symptoms" account for 1% of neurological diagnoses (Marsden, 1986). The most common age group is 20–30 years (Krumholz and Niedermeyer, 1983; Gumnit and Gates, 1986). Misdiagnosis is common: PNES was misdiagnosed as status epilepticus in 27% of patients with PNES who then received treatment for prolonged seizures. Prolonged events (> 30 min) were seen in 77.6% of patients with PNES (Reuber et al., 2003c). Unless correctly diagnosed, these patients suffer iatrogenic

*Correspondence to: Peter Widdess-Walsh, M.B., M.R.C.P.I., Institute of Neurology and Neurosurgery at St. Barnabas, Suite 101, 200 South Orange Avenue, Livingston, NJ 07039, USA. Tel: +1-973-3227117, Fax: +1-973-3227505, E-mail: pwiddesswalsh@barnabashealth.org

Table 17.1

Incidence of psychogenic nonepileptic seizures

Reference	Details of study	No. of patients	Incidence	Sex	Age (years)
Sigurdardottir and Olafsson, 1998	Homogeneous population, single center, Iceland – 5% of all new-onset seizures	14	1.4 per 100 000	F 79%	Range 15–24
Szaflarski et al., 2000	Hamilton county, Ohio, USA – 6.8% of all seizures	77	3.03 per 100 000	F 73%	Range 25–44
O'Sullivan et al., 2007	Homogeneous population, Cork, Ireland	50	0.91 per 100 000	F 61%	Average 32.4

adverse events such as respiratory arrest, unnecessary procedures, and drug reactions. (Howell et al., 1989).

PNES are the most common type of conversion reaction in many countries including India, Turkey, and Oman, where the estimated prevalence may be as high as 3–4% (Martínez-Taboas et al., 2010). The advent and availability of video-EEG have influenced the reporting of PNES.

PNES are 3–4 times more common in females, except for patients before puberty and the elderly (Wyllie et al., 1999; Duncan et al., 2006). Females are more likely to suffer and report sexual abuse, physical abuse, and self-harm (Oto et al., 2005). A history of abuse (particularly sexual) is a common feature of PNES and is discussed in more detail below. Subjective and/or functional complaints are more common in women than in men. In addition, there are physiological differences between women and men from exposure of the brain and hypothalamus to sex hormones, which influence this dichotomy.

Patients with low IQ are at 5–7 times greater risk for developing PNES (Reuber and Elger, 2003). In a series of 288 patients with PNES, 8.6% had a learning disability (Duncan and Oto, 2008a). Patients with PNES and learning disabilities have lower rates of sexual abuse or female gender. They have more situational triggers and a higher proportion of epilepsy (Duncan and Oto, 2008b).

PNES are not confined to young adults. In one series, 13 of 128 (10.2%) patients were over 55 years of age (Acar and Salinsky, 2010). Patients aged over 65 years represented 9.6% (9 of 94) of patients with PNES in another series, with 8 of the 9 being women (Behrouz et al., 2006).

The personal, social, and economic cost of PNES cannot be underestimated. The lifetime dollar cost of PNES is estimated to be $100 000 per patient. The total cost per year could be up to $900 million in the USA alone (Martin et al., 1998). The cost is magnified by the average delay in diagnosis of up to 7 years, often until inpatient video-EEG is performed (Reuber et al., 2002a). Costs are similar to those for patients with refractory epilepsy, who, while representing 10–15% of all patients with epilepsy, account for over 50% in costs (Begley et al., 1994). One study showed that diagnosis with video-EEG monitoring and multidisciplinary management reduced healthcare costs in patients with PNES (emergency room visits, outpatient clinic visits, and diagnostic tests) by 70% (Martin et al., 1998). Poor quality of life is associated with PNES, particularly if the events are frequent (Al Marzooqi et al., 2004; Lawton et al., 2009).

PATHOGENESIS

The most common basis for PNES is the conversion disorder, a subconscious "conversion" of internal conflicts into physical symptoms. Controversies exist as to whether somatization (Brown and Trimble, 2000; Akyuz et al., 2004) or dissociation (Kuyk et al., 1997; Reuber and House, 2002; Bowman, 2006), or both, is the underlying mechanism. The International Classification of Diseases, 9th revision (ICD-9), classifies conversion under dissociative disorders, whereas the Diagnostic and Statistical Manual of Mental Disorders, 4th edition (DSM-IV), classifies it under somatoform disorders. In addition, controversy exists as to whether PNES should be a separate disease entity or just a symptom of an underlying psychiatric disorder (Reuber and Elger, 2003).

Modern theories of PNES emerged in the 19th century. In 1853, Carter suggested three etiological factors for hysteria: temperament, circumstantial triggers, and concealment (repression) of the exciting cause. Charcot argued against intentional symptom production. Janet first attributed PNES to dissociation; he felt that the traumatized individual enters a state of self-hypnosis involving a dissociation of sensory and/or motor functions as a reaction to overwhelming or childhood traumatic events (Moene and Kuyk, 2010). PNES related to post-traumatic stress disorder (PTSD) was first described by Janet in war trauma survivors (Janet, 1889). According to Freud, "these fits are nothing but pantomimically interpreted phantasies, translated into the motor system, projected into motility" (Strachey, 1955).

A minority of apparent cases of PNES may be produced intentionally, such as with malingering (if motivated by obvious external gains), factitious disorder/Munchausen syndrome (if motivated in order to attain the "sick role"; Savard et al., 1988), or Munchausen syndrome by proxy (such as an attempt by a parent or caregiver to create the impression that the person has seizures, when they do not). It should also be determined that events are not directly caused by a primary psychiatric disorder such as panic attacks, agitation, or hallucinations. Video-EEG may not fully exclude coexisting epileptic seizures (ES) if the events in question are not captured or if ES are scalp EEG-negative.

Some evidence exists that the nondominant hemisphere may have a role in the development of PNES. Abnormalities on magnetic resonance imaging (MRI) or epileptiform EEG abnormalities in patients with PNES were found to be more common (72%) in the right hemisphere (Devinsky et al., 2001). Functional MRI (fMRI) of psychogenic tremor due to a conversion reaction showed hypoactivity of the right temporoparietal junction during the tremor. The authors theorized that the associated lack of sensory feedback to movement removes "self-agency" (experience that one is the cause of one's own actions), so that the patient perceives the movements as involuntary (Voon et al., 2010). Inhibitory centers such as the ventromedian prefrontal cortex showed increased activation on fMRI motor imagery in conversion paralysis compared with the unaffected limb (de Lange et al., 2008). Single-photon emission computed tomography (SPECT) and fMRI studies have shown abnormalities in the anterior cingulate gyrus and orbitofrontal cortex in patients with conversion disorder. No fMRI data exist for PNES.

Basal hypercortisolism and an abnormal hypothalamic–pituitary axis have been described in patients with PNES, particularly in those with a history of sexual trauma, compared with normal controls (Simeon et al., 2007; Bakvis et al., 2010).

A variety of models and theories exist for PNES. Precipitants of PNES include abuse, trauma, neglect, bereavement, family dysfunction, health anxiety, social stress, and a history of insecure attachments (Duncan and Oto, 2008a; Bowman, 2010). One model of PNES describes predisposing factors (genetic/biological, childhood events or abuse, trauma, comorbid conditions), then precipitating events (sickness, emotional stressor, major life events) triggering the PNES, then perpetuating events resulting in recurrent PNES (i.e., conditioning (primary or secondary gain), emotional disorder, illness belief) (Stone et al., 2005). Classical and operant conditioning theory explain how PNES persists over time. PNES has been modeled as a dissociative response to arousal ("panic without panic") (Goldstein, 2004). LaFrance and Devinsky (2002) divided PNES into etiological subsets: 1, anxious; 2a, abused – borderline personality; 2b, abused afraid (PTSD); 3, somatic; 4, dysthymic/depressed; 5, mentally retarded. According to Bowman (1999), there are four pathways to the development of PNES: a history of sexual or physical abuse, recent sexual assault, multiple life stressors that overwhelm coping abilities, and panic attacks mistaken for PNES.

Some 66% of patients with PNES had witnessed a seizure prior to their symptom onset, implying a role for symptom modeling (Bautista et al., 2008). Symptom modeling involves the mimicking of another person's (or the person themselves') symptoms to satisfy primary and secondary gains. This study excluded patients with comorbid PNES and epilepsy. Only 9 of the 27 patients had other family members with seizures.

The psychodynamic theory of PNES reflects the conflict between the components of personality; the id, the ego, and the superego. Offensive thoughts and memories are repressed in order not to be aware of them. These repressed thoughts may find an outlet in physical symptoms that allow the patient to relieve their unconscious selves (i.e., the id) and to keep the offending content or thoughts further repressed – the primary gain. The primary pathology is the unresolved intrapsychic conflict. Eventually this leads to secondary gain from obtaining attention, and avoiding responsibility.

PNES in children are often accompanied by abnormal family dynamics such as enmeshment, impaired conflict resolution, and parental conflict. The physical symptoms may reduce responsibility for family conflicts. It may also relieve the child of going to school, resulting in secondary gain and worsening the severity of the problem. The PNES becomes an expression of what is wrong within the family rather than the individual. There may be modeling of parental somatizing behaviors (Plioplys et al., 2007).

CLINICAL FEATURES

History and comorbidities

There has been a previous psychological trauma in 44–100% of patients with PNES (Fleisher et al., 2002; Fiszman et al., 2004; Duncan and Oto, 2008a). A history of sexual or physical abuse is particularly common, with a wide range of prevalence (9–77%) in various studies (Alper et al., 1993; Rechlin et al., 1997; Reuber et al., 2000; Abubakr et al., 2003; Binzer et al., 2004; Fiszman et al., 2004; Duncan and Oto, 2008a). Studies using careful interviews with psychologists rather than self-reports found an overall lifetime risk of 84–90% (Bowman and Markand, 1999; Dikel et al., 2003). Sexual abuse is more common in female patients (Dworetzky et al., 2005; Duncan and Oto, 2008a; Selkirk et al., 2008). Patients with a history of abuse have poorer mental health, earlier-onset PNES, and their spells are more severe (Selkirk et al., 2008). One study reported incest in 30% of the patients (Binzer et al., 2004); other traumatic events include bereavement and bullying (Duncan and Oto, 2008a). The exact role of abuse or trauma in the development of PNES remains to be elucidated, although putative dissociative mechanisms exist.

Childhood factors have also been implicated, and perceived parental rearing mean scores showed significant differences from those in patients with ES. In particular, in one series, patients with PNES recollected less parental warmth and more paternal rejection (Binzer et al., 2004).

The overall number of life events, especially negative, unexpected events related to personal health issues and with adjustment problems in the year preceding disease onset, is significantly higher in patients with PNES than in those with ES (Binzer et al., 2004). Health-related traumatic experiences are particularly common in late-onset PNES (Duncan et al., 2006).

Psychiatric comorbidities are reported in 50–100% of patients with PNES (Rechlin et al., 1997; Reuber et al., 2000; Fiszman et al., 2004; O'Sullivan et al., 2007). Personality disorders, prominently borderline type, are reported in up to 65% of patients (Smith et al., 1992; Jawad et al., 1995; Binzer et al., 2004). Depression is significantly more common than in the general population, but its prevalence is comparable to that of patients with ES (Rechlin et al., 1997; Binzer et al., 2004; Dworetzky et al., 2005; O'Sullivan et al., 2007; Asmussen et al., 2009). However, depression in PNES is more likely to present with prominent physiological symptoms (Asmussen et al., 2009). Conversion disorder was diagnosed in all patients with pseudostatus in one series (Rechlin et al., 1997). PTSD is significantly more common than in ES and occurs in 9–100% of patients with PNES (Fiszman et al., 2004; Dworetzky et al., 2005). Anxiety and somatoform disorders were also reported (Binzer et al., 2004; Dworetzky et al., 2005; O'Sullivan et al., 2007). The prevalence of suicide attempts was 11–46% in PNES (Meierkord et al., 1991; Peguero et al., 1995; Lesser, 1996; Binzer et al., 2004) and up to 60–67% in pseudostatus (Rechlin et al., 1997; Reuber et al., 2000).

A history of unexplained medical symptoms has been reported in 37–80% of patients (Meierkord et al., 1991; De Wet et al., 2003; Mellers, 2005; O'Sullivan et al., 2007). Chronic pain is very common (Dworetzky et al., 2005), and a history of chronic pain and fibromyalgia was highly predictive of PNES in a population of patients with refractory epilepsy (Benbadis, 2005). Asthma, of possible psychogenic origin, was reported in 26.5% of patients in one study (De Wet et al., 2003).

Although the absence of risk factors for ES may be reassuring, their presence may be misleading: family history of epilepsy, learning disability, and head trauma are not uncommon in these patients (Mellers, 2005; O'Sullivan et al., 2007; Duncan and Oto, 2008a).

Of particular complexity is the co-occurrence of PNES and epilepsy in the same patient, estimated to occur in up to 10% of patients with PNES (Lesser et al., 1983; Benbadis et al., 2001). This co-occurrence is more common in the learning disabled population (Duncan and Oto, 2008a, b). The PNES will typically start after the ES, and may present as a new seizure type or as "pseudoresistance" to AEDs and in association with psychiatric instability. There is often a longer time to diagnosis and higher use of AEDs. There are few characteristic features compared with those in patients with PNES alone, and the seizure types often appear similar. Clinicians, patients, and families must differentiate PNES from ES, as the treatments are divergent. In these cases, video-EEG or home video analysis is extremely valuable. Sitting down to review events with family and caregivers can help them determine which ones are true PNES; when they subsequently call to report events, the physician is more likely to make the correct management decision. Although PNES and ES occur at separate times, PNES may occur in the early phase of an epileptic seizure, or the epileptic seizure can facilitate PNES. This group is at risk for overtreatment of pseudostatus, due to the established diagnosis of epilepsy and assumption that the PNES is actually an epileptic seizure (Widdess-Walsh et al., 2010). PNES can occur *de novo* after epilepsy surgery, and need to be differentiated from recurrent ES and presumed surgical failure (Parra et al., 1998).

Ictal features

PNES presents in various forms, and some authors classify them according to their resemblance to different epileptic seizure types. Others question this division, claiming that the processes underlying PNES are distinct from those of epilepsy and that classification based on superficial resemblance to ES is misleading (Leis et al., 1992). Several authors have grouped PNES according to semiology, the most consistent division being prominent limpness or collapse versus prominent motor behavior (Meierkord et al., 1991; Chen and Izadyar, 2010). Attacks with only subjective symptoms can occur (DeToledo and Ramsay, 1996; Hovorka et al., 2007), but are more difficult to diagnose definitely as they are frequently excluded from video-EEG semiological studies because their nonepileptic origin cannot be demonstrated – the EEG is often normal during simple partial seizures with sensory symptoms. Therefore, we focus on PNES presenting with objective alterations in consciousness and/or motor behavior.

The onset of PNES is usually gradual, contrasting with the abrupt onset of ES (Gulick et al., 1982; Meierkord et al., 1991; Lesser, 1996; Mellers, 2005) and usually or exclusively occurs during wakefulness (Gowers, 1901; Luther et al., 1982; Kanner et al., 1990; Saygi et al., 1992; Raymond et al., 1999) (Table 17.2). However, one study described PNES arising from stage II–III sleep or a few seconds after awakening (Orbach et al., 2003). Moreover, PNES may occur during behavioral sleep, with EEG revealing normal waking activity. Benbadis et al. (1996) named this condition "pseudosleep," a very specific feature of PNES (Thacker et al., 1993; Benbadis et al., 1996; Hovorka et al., 2007).

Precipitating factors implicating anxiety and stress situations are commonly found in PNES (Luther et al., 1982; Slater et al., 1995; Lesser, 1996) as well as ES, although stress is less prominent as a provocative factor (Slater et al., 1995; Lesser, 1996). PNES tend to

Table 17.2

Clinical features of psychogenic nonepileptic seizures (PNES) versus epileptic seizures (ES)

Clinical features	PNES	ES
Precipitants	Common	Possible but less obvious
Occurrence in presence of significant others	Common	Not associated
Occurrence during sleep	Rarely reported; pseudosleep	Common
Onset	Gradual	Abrupt
Duration	Variable, often >2 min	Up to 1–2 min
Response to verbal stimulus	Common	Never preserved in GTCS. Rarely and only partially preserved in CPS
Motor phenomena		
Movements of upper and lower extremities	Out of phase	In-phase in GTCS
Opisthotonic posturing, "*arc de cercle*"	Occasional	Absent
Thrashing, violent movements of the body	Occasional/common	Occasional/common in FLS; very rare in other types
Side-to-side head/body movements	Occasional/common	Occasional/common in FLS; rare in other types
Unilateral head turning	Rare/occasional	Common before GTCS
Pelvic thrusting forward	Occasional/common (especially in female patients)	Occasional/common in FLS; very rare in other types
Whole-body rigidity	May be absent in PNES "mimicking" GTCS	Always present in the tonic phase of GTCS
Fluctuating course; pauses in motor activity	Common	Very rare
Prolonged unresponsiveness without prominent motor features	Occasional	Very rare (absence status)
Vocalization features	Emotional: moans, screams, gasps, "ictal weeping"; understandable statements	Monotonous epileptic cry in GTCS; continuous, moans, animal-like noises, uttering in FLS
Eye closure	Common/very common, sustained, forceful, with opposition to opening	Very rare, partial, never forceful, never throughout the spell
Incontinence	Very uncommon, but may be reported	Common, especially in GTCS
Self-injury	Very uncommon, but may be reported	Occasional/common
Bite to the tongue	Very rare, on the tip	Occasional/common in GTCS, on the side
Postictal symptoms		
Abrupt recovery	Common	Very rare
Confusion	Occasional/common	Common/very common
Headache	Very rare	Common
Fatigue or lethargy	Occasional	Common

Continued

Table 17.2

Continued

Clinical features	PNES	ES
Postictal memory	Common	Very rare
Breathing pattern	Rapid, shallow, irregular, with pauses, never stertorous	Deep, prolonged, regular, loud, snoring (stertorous breathing) in GTCS
Inappropriate events sequence	Common	Absent
Induction		
Hypnosis, placebo, suggestion	May be induced	Not inducible
Cognitive assessment (PNES versus partial seizures)		
Impaired responsiveness	Very common	Very common
Any response	Common	Occasional
Recall of memory items	Very common and commonly > 50%	Rare and always < 50%
Corneal reflex	Present	May be impaired
Avoidance behavior	Common	Rare (depending on kind of seizure)
Visual fixation	Present	Absent
Extensor plantar response after seizure	Absent	Common after GTCS

Values for the frequency of these features are approximate: very common, > 70%; common, 30–70%; occasional, 10–30%; rare, 5–10%; very rare, < 5%.
CPS, complex partial seizures; FLS, frontal lobe seizures; GTCS, generalized tonic–clonic seizures.

occur in the presence of "significant" others (Luther et al., 1982) and the occurrence of a paroxysmal behavioral change during a clinic visit predicts PNES (Benbadis, 2005).

Prodromal feelings are frequent, generally neither specific nor lateralized, and include dizziness or funny feelings, as well as olfactory, auditory, visual, or complex sensations and focal numbness (Gulick et al., 1982; Luther et al., 1982; Hovorka et al., 2007). Symptoms suggesting hyperventilation include lightheadedness, acral paresthesias, and palpitations (Lesser, 1996).

PNES usually last for more than 2 minutes and may be longer than 30 minutes, which is very unusual for ES (Gulick et al., 1982; Gates et al., 1985; Kanner et al., 1990; Meierkord et al., 1991; Saygi et al., 1992; Raymond et al., 1999; Hovorka et al., 2007; Azar et al., 2008).

A motor behavior is frequently reported as part of the attack. The features most often reported include asynchronous out-of-phase limb movements, or absence of in-phase limb movements in attacks resembling generalized tonic–clonic seizures (GTCS) (Gates et al., 1985; Leis et al., 1992; Hovorka et al., 2007; Azar et al., 2008). The absence of whole-body rigidity during the entire duration of an attack "mimicking" GTCS is highly specific for PNES according to Gates et al. (1985). Side-to-side head/body turning is common in PNES, whereas these patients seldom show unilateral head turning, as may occur at the beginning of a partial secondary generalized seizure (Gates et al., 1985; Leis et al., 1992; Saygi et al., 1992). Pelvic thrusting is commonly described (Gates et al., 1985; Leis et al., 1992; Saygi et al., 1992; Flügel et al., 1996; Geyer et al., 2000; Abubakr et al., 2003; Hovorka et al., 2007; Azar et al., 2008), especially in women (Meierkord et al., 1991; Abubakr et al., 2003), and according to some authors it is typically forwards, whereas when it occurs during GTCS it is generally backwards (Gates et al., 1985). Thrashing and grabbing behavior is another typical feature (Gulick et al., 1982; Kanner et al., 1990; Raymond et al., 1999; Abubakr et al., 2003). In contrast to supplementary motor area (frontal lobe) seizures (FLS), the movements in PNES generally involve the head and neck, whereas FLS are generalized or mainly involve the lower limbs and trunk (Kanner et al., 1990). All of the motor patterns reported in PNES can occur in FLS, especially those involving the mesial structures, including maintenance of consciousness during bilateral motor attacks, lack of postictal signs, and normal ictal EEGs (Kanner et al., 1990; Saygi et al., 1992; Geyer et al., 2000; Azar et al., 2008). Therefore, the differential diagnosis of PNES and FLS can be challenging. Features that strongly suggest FLS include: turning to a prone position (Saygi et al., 1992), tonic posturing in abduction of upper extremities (Kanner et al., 1990), short duration, highly stereotyped pattern, and frequent or exclusive occurrence during sleep (Kanner et al., 1990; Mellers, 2005). Tonic posturing and opisthotonus can occur with PNES (Gulick et al., 1982; Luther et al., 1982; Kanner et al., 1990; Hovorka et al., 2007), even though the "*arc de cercle*" considered pathognomonic for psychogenic disorder by Charcot and Richer (1887) is seldom encountered nowadays. PNES often exhibit a discontinuous pattern with motor activity alternated with brief periods of rest, in contrast to the epileptic pattern (Gulick et al., 1982; Meierkord et al., 1991; Mellers, 2005).

Figure 17.1 shows frames of several psychogenic seizures recorded in the video-EEG laboratory of IRCCS Istituto delle Scienze Neurologiche, University of Bologna, Bologna, Italy.

Semipurposeful behavior can occur with PNES (Gulick et al., 1982; Luther et al., 1982; Meierkord et al., 1991) and occurs *de novo*, unlike ES in which patients can continue purposeful activity begun before the attack. The activity is generally goal-directed with a dramatic or violent element (Gulick et al., 1982). Less frequent features of PNES include alimentary phenomena (Gulick et al., 1982), trembling (Gulick et al., 1982; Hovorka et al., 2007), whole-body flaccidity (Gates et al., 1985; Lcis et al., 1992), grimacing (Gulick et al., 1982), and jerking (Gulick et al., 1982; Raymond et al., 1999).

Vocalization is common in both PNES and ES, but differs in quality. Vocalization in GTCS is invariably the typical "epileptic cry," whereas vocalization during FLS is continuous and monotonous, mimicking moaning or animal noises and sometimes containing understandable words. Vocalization during PNES is variable and may consist of words, moans, or screams, often evoking emotional sadness or pain (Gulick et al., 1982; Luther et al., 1982; Gates et al., 1985; Kanner et al., 1990; Saygi

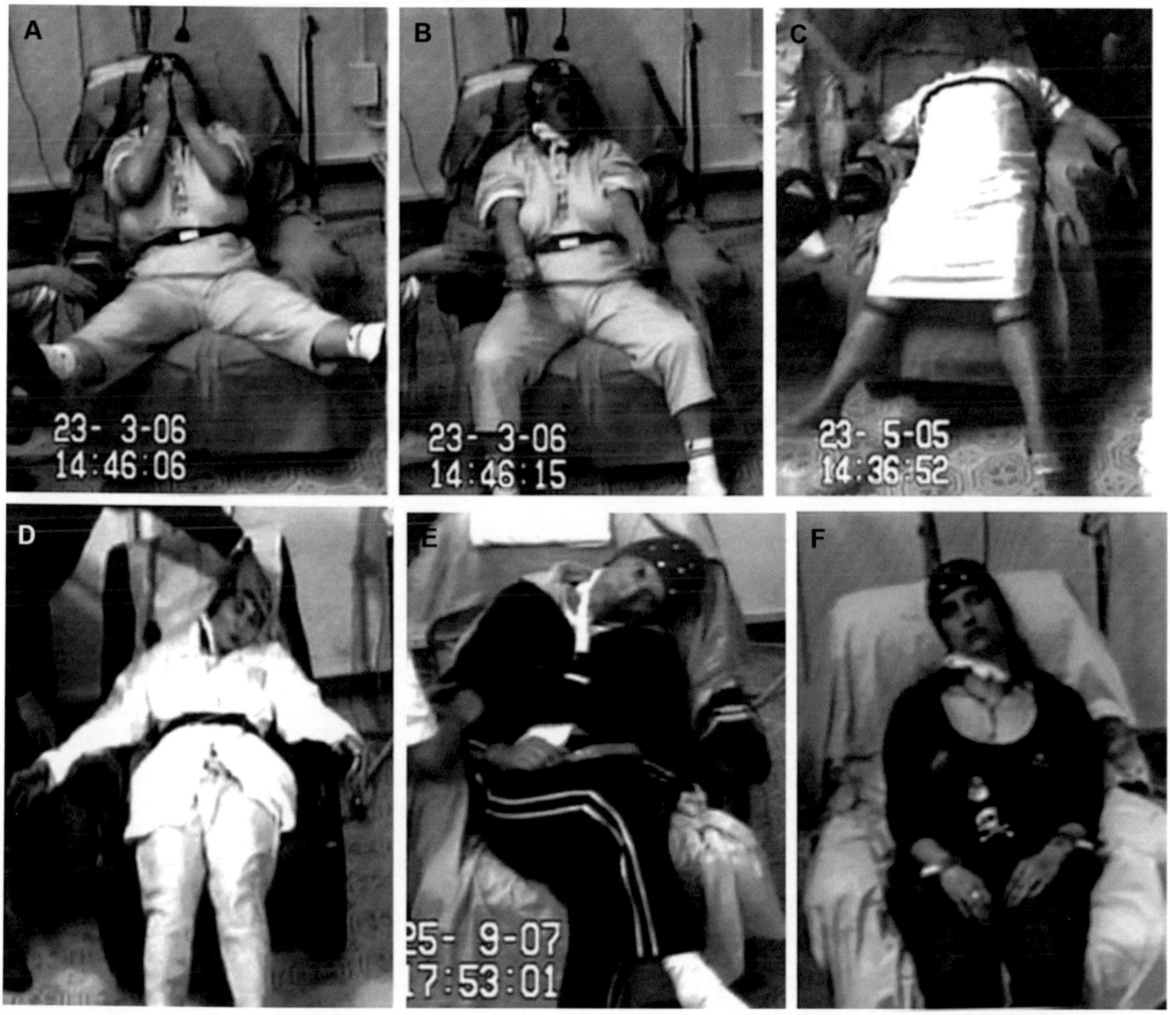

Fig. 17.1. (**A**) Patient covering her face with her hands. Pseudodystonic posture of the inferior limbs. (**B**) Tonic posturing and facial grimace. (**C**) Opisthotonic posture. (**D**) Prolonged unresponsiveness without prominent motor features, resistance to eye opening. (**E**) Pseudodystonic posturing of the neck. (**F**) Prolonged unresponsiveness without prominent motor features.

et al., 1992; Slater et al., 1995; Hovorka et al., 2007; Azar et al., 2008). Note that many ES can include similar vocalizations, but they are usually stereotypical and consistent between seizures. Ictal stuttering was described in 8.5% of patients with PNES but in no patients with ES in a large series (Vossler et al., 2004). Some degree of verbal responsiveness can occur in PNES resembling complex partial seizures (CPS) (Bell et al., 1998) and, when present during apparent GTCS, is pathognomonic for PNES (Gulick et al., 1982). However, FLS can cause bilateral motor phenomena with preserved consciousness, leading to the misdiagnosis of PNES.

Several video-EEG studies have found that the eyes are closed during 55–96% of PNES (Gulick et al., 1982; DeToledo and Ramsay, 1996; Flügel et al., 1996; Alhalabi and Verma, 1994; Chung et al., 2006; Hovorka et al., 2007; Azar et al., 2008; Syed et al., 2008). Conversely, the eyes are open at the beginning or throughout 92–100% of ES, including episodes arising from sleep (Alhalabi and Verma, 1994; DeToledo and Ramsay, 1996; Chung et al., 2006; Azar et al., 2008). The eyes are characteristically forcefully closed with active opposition to opening in PNES (DeToledo and Ramsay, 1996; Hovorka et al., 2007). Purely sensory PNES probably constitute an exception: in one series, eyes were closed in 11% and patients always opened their eyes when told to do so (DeToledo and Ramsay, 1996). Some studies found that most (82–88%) patients with PNES have no ictal eye manifestation (Gates et al., 1985; Leis et al., 1992); in one series this was significantly different from GCTS (Gates et al., 1985). Notably, self and observer reports of eye closure were unreliable in one study, identifying only half of the events correctly (Syed et al., 2008).

Prolonged limpness without motor symptoms often accompanied by apparent atonia is another common form of PNES (Gulick et al., 1982; Luther et al., 1982; Meierkord et al., 1991; Leis et al., 1992; Raymond et al., 1999; Abubakr et al., 2003; Hovorka et al., 2007). In some of these prolonged atonic PNES, there is intermittent eye blinking, swallowing, or mouthing movements (Gulick et al., 1982), slumping forward (Gulick et al., 1982), staring (Hovorka et al., 2007), or avoidance behavior (Luther et al., 1982). This PNES pattern does not parallel any seizure type other than absence status, but atonia is rare in this epileptic seizure type. Other etiologies are also unlikely, as episodes lasting more than 5 minutes that completely reverse suggest PNES, not other organic disorders (Meierkord et al., 1991; Mellers, 2005).

Urinary incontinence is very rare during video-EEG recorded PNES (Luther et al., 1982; Meierkord et al., 1991; Slater et al., 1995; Abubakr et al., 2003; Hovorka et al., 2007; Oliva et al., 2008), although it may be self-reported (44% in one study) (Peguero et al., 1995; Dworetzky et al., 2005).

Self-injury was uncommon during video-EEG recordings of PNES (Meierkord et al., 1991; Benbadis et al., 1995; Abubakr et al., 2003; Hovorka et al., 2007; Oliva et al., 2008), although it is more commonly self-reported (Luther et al., 1982; Peguero et al., 1995). In one study, 40% of patients with PNES reported some kind of injury, including injuries requiring sutures, causing bone fracture, or tongue biting. Interestingly burns were never reported by patients with PNES, but only by patients with epilepsy (Peguero et al., 1995). Tongue biting is rare in PNES (Luther et al., 1982; Meierkord et al., 1991; Benbadis et al., 1995; Hovorka et al., 2007; Oliva et al., 2008) and, when it occurs, is typically on the tip (Hovorka et al., 2007) and not in the lateral or anterolateral tongue as in GTCS (DeToledo and Ramsay, 1996; Oliva et al., 2008).

Uncommon but relatively specific features of PNES include ictal weeping (Bergen and Ristanovic, 1993), the "teddy bear sign" of age-inappropriate behavior, such as bringing a teddy bear or similar item to the epilepsy monitoring unit (Burneo et al., 2003), and responding to questions in a whispering voice and to commands with partial motor responses postictally (Chabolla and Shih, 2006).

The postictal breathing pattern after PNES is often rapid, shallow and soft, irregular, and associated with pauses. Snoring and stertorous breathing are rare, unlike in GTCS when postictal breathing is deep, with prolonged inspiratory and expiratory phases, regular, loud, usually with snoring ("stertorous"), and impaired for longer, and in FLS when it is usually shallow, regular, and quiet (Sen et al., 2007; Azar et al., 2008).

Postictal agitation, confusion, headache, and fatigue are uncommon after PNES (Ettinger et al., 1999a; Azar et al., 2008). Ability to recall the seizure is frequent in PNES, contrasting with GCTS and CPS (Leis et al., 1992; Bell et al., 1998; Mellers, 2005).

Although stereotypy is usually considered specific for ES, stereotyped events were recorded in 67–90% of video-EEG studies recording multiple PNES in the same patient (Gulick et al., 1982; Meierkord et al., 1991; Raymond et al., 1999; Hovorka et al., 2007).

Individual ictal features occasionally mimic a specific epileptic seizure type, but rarely does a complete PNES closely resemble a single epileptic seizure type (Luther et al., 1982; Meierkord et al., 1991; Leis et al., 1992). Thus, the precise temporal sequence of events should always be elicited, and variable, random, or nonphysiological (e.g., thumb jerking followed by toe jerking followed by eye jerking) sequences should raise the suspicion of PNES.

A dangerous complication of PNES is psychogenic status. Patients may present with all the features described above without returning to normal state for a long time. Psychogenic status may be the first manifestation or complicate a history of PNES, and a single episode of "status" occurred in up to 78% of patients with PNES (Reuber et al., 2003b).

Ictal testing during video-EEG recording or observed PNES can be helpful. Corneal reflex is usually impaired after GTCS (Leis and Ross, 1992; Mellers, 2005) but normal after PNES. Unilateral or bilateral extensor plantar response, common within 5 minutes of GTCS is not seen in PNES (Walczak and Rubinsky, 1994).

Avoidance maneuvers consist of evaluating the patient's resistance to eye opening, avoiding placing his or her hand on the face, or avoiding placing a heel on the opposite shin. Avoidance can occur in up to 100% of PNES (Luther et al., 1982). When eyes are open, searching for evidence of fixation can be useful. One maneuver consists of rolling the patient onto his or her side: if fixation is maintained, the patient's eyes are generally deviated to the ground; when the patient is rolled onto the other side, the eyes should be directed on the ground again ("Henry and Woodruff sign"). Alternatively the examiner may place a mirror in front of the patient and look for evidence of convergence and fixation (Henry and Woodruff, 1978; Mellers, 2005).

NEUROPSYCHOLOGICAL MEASURES

Personality testing

Much of the psychological research in patients with PNES has used the Minnesota Multiphasic Personality Inventory (MMPI) and MMPI-2, where patients score higher on scales related to hypochondriasis, hysteria, and, to a lesser extent, schizophrenia and depression. A frequent finding is the high prevalence of "conversion V" profile among patients with PNES (Griffith et al., 2007; LaFrance, 2008). Patients with "motor" events generally have more severe psychopathology than those with "catatonic" events (Wilkus and Dodrill, 1989; Griffith et al., 2007). MMPI-2 outcomes coupled with clinical variables yielded 48–80% sensitivity and 68–80% specificity for a diagnosis of PNES (Cragar et al., 2003; Schramke et al., 2007). The MMPI alone or with other measures can help identify personality or etiology-based PNES subtypes, suggesting potential therapeutic approaches. Results are equivocal and will not be considered here (Gumnit and Gates, 1986; Barrash et al., 1989; Cragar et al., 2005).

Harden et al. (2009) compared patients with PNES to patients with ES with respect to personality clusters, using the Structured Clinical Interview Personality Disorders Modules for DSM-IV-TR (SCID-II). Overall, personality disorders were common in both groups: 75% in patients with ES and 81% in those with PNES. Patients with PNES were more likely to meet criteria for a personality disorder in Cluster A (paranoid, schizoid, schizotypal) or B (antisocial, borderline, histrionic, narcissistic) compared with patients with ES, who were more likely to have Cluster C criteria (avoidant, dependent, obsessive–compulsive). The difference was statistically significant.

Intelligence measures and cognitive testing

Binder et al. (1998) found no significant differences between patients with ES and PNES on several IQ tests of intelligence or learning and memory, but scores were significantly inferior to those of control subjects. Another study found that performance IQ ranged from deficient to very superior in patients with PNES, but the distribution was skewed toward the low normal range and 41.5% of the patients had full-scale IQ scores in the low average or borderline range. Scores on the Halstead Reitan Neuropsychological Test Battery showed impairment in 63% of patients with PNES. Impaired performance involved diverse cognitive functions such as mental flexibility and ease of learning in novel problem-solving situations, spatial localization memory, auditory perception and discrimination, motor speed, and coordination. However, the sample considered had a high incidence of closed head injury and substance abuse, which could account for the abnormal findings (Kalogjera-Sackellares and Sackellares, 1999).

Abnormal neuropsychological performance in patients with PNES was positively correlated with the degree of psychopathology on the MMPI-2, suggesting that impaired cognition may be linked to emotional rather than organic factors in these patients (Cragar et al., 2005).

Psychomotor measures

Reduced motor speed and grip strength were found in patients with PNES compared with healthy controls (Sackellares and Sackellares, 2001), although these features could be signs of lack of motivation (LaFrance, 2008).

Motivational measures

Patients with PNES score lower than those with ES on some motivational measures, although not necessarily in an intentional manner, and this could affect neuropsychological test results (Brown et al., 1991; Binder et al., 1994, 1998; Drane et al., 2006). This finding is controversial, as others failed to find impaired motivational effort, claiming that patients with PNES produce trustworthy findings in neuropsychological tests (Cragar et al., 2006; Dodrill, 2008).

Health-related quality of life (HRQoL)

HRQoL, measured with different validated scales, is lower in patients with PNES than in patients with epilepsy or depression. Low scores are due mainly to depression, AED side-effects, somatization, and psychological distress (Szaflarski et al., 2003; Szaflarski and Szaflarski, 2004; Testa et al., 2007; LaFrance and Syc, 2009). Seizure frequency is not independently related to quality of life, but its influence is mediated by psychological distress and other physical symptoms (LaFrance and Syc, 2009).

LINGUISTIC ANALYSIS

Patients with epilepsy and those with PNES talked differently about their seizures in studies conducted in German- and English-speaking patients. Thus, interactional and linguistic analysis of patients' description of their seizures allows a correct diagnosis of ES or PNES in 85–100% of cases (Schwabe et al., 2007; Plug et al., 2009a; Reuber et al., 2009). Patients with ES discuss subjective symptoms in detail and focus more easily on description, whereas patients with PNES discuss sparingly and with difficulty; patients with ES attempt to fill gaps and are willing to know what happens during periods of reduced consciousness, whereas those with PNES name unconsciousness without further description. Patients with PNES tend to concentrate on the circumstances in which the seizure presented rather than on the seizure itself. Moreover, patients with ES often give self-initiated hints at strategies they use to interrupt or prevent seizures, such as focusing on a particular thought, whereas patients with PNES do not.

There are also differences in the use of the metaphoric conceptualization of seizures, which are likely to reflect differences in subjective seizure experience between patients with PNES and those with epilepsy: ES are conceptualized as a more external, self-directed entity (i.e., an enemy or threat) than PNES, which are depicted as a state or place patients go through (Plug et al., 2009b).

Studies in languages other than English or German are lacking.

DIAGNOSTIC MEASURES

Electroencephalography (EEG)

EEG alone cannot diagnose PNES, as it may not make nor exclude the diagnosis of epilepsy. A single routine EEG is normal in 30% of patients with ES (Chadwick, 1994; Mellers, 2005). In addition, up to 15% of the normal population have nonspecific abnormalities and less than 1% have epileptiform discharges on EEG. Abnormalities are more common in patients with PNES independent of comorbid epilepsy (Reuber et al., 2002b; Woollacott et al., 2010), as well as in borderline personality disorder and in relatives of patients with epilepsy, which are common conditions in PNES (Luther et al., 1982; Lesser, 1996; De la Fuente et al., 1998; Mellers, 2005). Up to 37% of patients with PNES had a report of an epileptiform baseline EEG, generally made by neurologists who were not epileptologists or electroencephalographers (Benbadis and Tatum, 2003; Lobello et al., 2006). When tracings were re-evaluated at an epilepsy center, the epileptiform abnormalities were found to be normal variants (Benbadis and Tatum, 2003).

Stable rhythmic artifacts on the EEG in PNES records can be due to a stable frequency of rhythmic movements contrasting with a true epileptic pattern, characterized by rhythms in the frequency of delta and beta range evolving from one to the other during the course of the seizure. Brief pauses in rhythmic movement during a seizure, followed by resumption of movement at the same frequency, were highly specific for PNES ("on–off–on" pattern) (Vinton et al., 2004).

Video-EEG telemetry

Video-EEG monitoring remains the "gold standard" investigation for PNES: the patient undergoes a prolonged simultaneous EEG and video recording to record the habitual event. Notably, one study showed only a moderate interrater reliability of video-EEG for PNES (Benbadis et al., 2009). The combination of observed semiology and normal background EEG before, during, and after the attack is usually diagnostic. There are some important limitations. First, motion artifacts can obscure the EEG or be mistaken for ictal discharges. Second, ictal scalp-EEG often shows no epileptic features during simple partial seizures and FLS, a type that can easily be clinically mistaken for PNES. Third, as many patients may have both ES and PNES, it is very important for diagnosis that the captured event is the habitual one, so the video should always be shown to someone who has witnessed the patient's attacks before establishing a diagnosis. For similar reasons, if more than one type of seizure is reported, try to record each type. Fourth, generalized epileptiform discharges can occur during drug withdrawal (especially barbiturates) even in patients with PNES. Finally, in patients with rare attacks, it may be very difficult to record a spontaneous seizure.

A typical event occurred within the first 48 hours of video-EEG monitoring in 88–98.5% of patients with PNES (Lobello et al., 2006; Woollacott et al., 2010). This suggests that outpatient monitoring can be cost-effective. When a spontaneous episode is not recorded, induction procedures prove useful. Methods have included compression of body parts, photic stimulation, hyperventilation, verbal suggestion, placing a tuning fork or moistened patches on the skin, intravenous administration of saline or other placebo, and hypnosis. However, the use of these techniques is controversial, mainly due to ethical concerns, especially when a placebo is used, and some have questioned their specificity (Devinsky and Fisher, 1996; Gates, 2001). However, induction can reduce the time to diagnosis, contributing substantially to the wellbeing of the patient and avoiding the hazards of an inappropriate diagnosis of epilepsy (Benbadis, 2001). Moreover, when the procedure was disclosed to the patient in a supportive manner after successful induction, the physician–patient relationship was not altered and patients agreed to further interventions (Lancman et al., 1994; Walczak et al., 1994). Induction maneuvers have a high sensitivity and a specificity approaching 100% for PNES (Slater et al., 1995; Barry et al., 2000; Benbadis et al., 2000; Benbadis et al., 2004; Lancman et al., 1994; Walczak et al., 1994). Hypnosis may be used also for children (Olson et al., 2008).

Home video recording

Video alone may have a high specificity and sensitivity in selected patients when reviewed by experienced observer (respectively 94% and 93% in a recent study) (Chen et al., 2008). However, the onset of the seizure is generally missed in home videos. Caregivers should also be instructed to capture limb and face movements in order to obtain useful information. Nevertheless, home video recording may be helpful for screening before video-EEG recording, especially in patients with few events.

Serum prolactin assay

Serum prolactin levels rise to concentrations greater than 500 IU/mL in more than 90% of patients after GCTS and 60% of patients after CPS, 10–20 minutes after the attack (Trimble, 1986; Mellers, 2005). Positive results are possible in PNES and are commonly found after syncope (Trimble, 1986; Oribe et al., 1996; Alving, 1998; Shukla et al., 2004). Little is known about prolactin levels after other organic imitators of seizures. The use of serum prolactin assay has not been established in the evaluation of status epilepticus, repetitive seizures, and seizures different from CPS and GTCS. A baseline prolactin test should be available to exclude from evaluation conditions associated with hyperprolactinemia. Finally, the criteria for abnormal levels of prolactin after a seizure are not standardized and different authors have used different cutoffs. Despite these limits, serum prolactin assay is a useful adjunctive test for the differentiation of GCTS or CPS from PNES (Chen et al., 2005)

SPECT

Data on SPECT in PNES are limited. The few studies are small and usually retrospective, and often lack a control group. Moreover, timing and method of analyzing the examinations are not standardized, probably affecting the results. When available, the specificity of a negative SPECT study in PNES was 70–73%, sensitivity 64–80% (Varma et al., 1996; Ettinger et al., 1998).

Subtraction ictal SPECT coregistered to MRI (SISCOM) has been used in cases of probable PNES when other procedures were insufficient for diagnosis (Neiman et al., 2009). As expected, SISCOM demonstrated no localizing or lateralizing hyperperfusion or hypoperfusion changes in 85% of PNES cases. Sensitivity was 70%. The authors also reported that, combining their data with those of the previous studies, 89% of patients with PNES had a negative SPECT examination. Therefore, SPECT scans can help in diagnosing challenging cases of PNES.

TREATMENT

There are few evidence-based reports on the treatment of PNES (Baker et al., 2007; Brooks et al., 2007). In one large study 71 of 187 patients (38%) became "spell-free" just with communication of the diagnosis (McKenzie et al., 2010). The way that the diagnosis is presented is of paramount importance (Shen et al., 1990). The data on this topic thus far support that early diagnosis and intervention are important to avoid PNES becoming a chronic "way of life" (Lempert and Schmidt, 1990; Betts and Boden, 1992; Mace and Trimble, 1996).

Once the diagnosis is established, usually by video-EEG, the patient can be told that there is "good news" regarding the seizures. These events are not due to abnormal or harmful brain activity and are not the result of brain damage. The importance of knowing what the events are not, should be reiterated as a positive finding. In a supportive manner, the patient should be informed that the episodes are not volitional and no one believes that they are "faking." The patient should be told that these episodes usually have a psychological basis despite the patient's lack of awareness of coexistent stress or emotional upset. This serves to dispel some of the common arguments presented by patients or their families that these seizures are absolutely not psychological. With this information the patient can be told that they will not require potentially harmful antiepileptic medications. The use of AEDs by patients with PNES is common, and elimination of these medications and their side-effects is a critical part of the treatment plan (Hantke et al., 2007). The patient should be reassured that he or she can continue to work together with the physician on eliminating these spells so that the physician–patient relationship is maintained. The patient can then be told that further help may be needed by a psychiatrist, as this type of physician is an expert in dealing with upsetting emotions, a frequently discovered cause for these events. The power of suggestion can be used as part of the cure. The patient should be told that these spells may resolve spontaneously and that they can take an active role in the resolution process by consciously trying to abort the event when they feel one is coming on. The patient should be advised not to become discouraged if breakthrough events occur. Healthcare utilization after video-EEG diagnosis reduced emergency room visits by 97%, outpatient visits by 80%, and diagnostic tests by 76% in the short term (Martin et al., 1998).

Comorbidities, such as major depressive disorder, PTSD, personality disorder, trauma, and family disorders, should be diagnosed and treated. Any suicidal risk should be identified and treated appropriately. There is a high prevalence of comorbid epilepsy and this should be evaluated thoroughly even if current events are clearly nonepileptic. The family should be advised on how to manage events after discharge. It is often helpful to show patients or family the video of the events to improve insight and recognition. Visits to the emergency room should be avoided as they can reinforce dysfunctional seizure-related beliefs and behaviors. Healthcare personnel not familiar with PNES may provide excessive or inappropriate treatment; practitioners who see these patients in their outpatient office or the emergency room must make decisions based on only history or fragmentary descriptions from family, nurses or caregivers. The follow-up should include the neurologist, psychiatrist, and psychotherapist, in close collaboration with an epilepsy center (Aboukasm et al., 1998). Seeing patients regularly can reduce the need for the patient to produce more or severe symptoms to get medical attention, reduce emergency room admission or inappropriate testing, and reduce patient feelings of abandonment. Treatment is often limited, however, by the resources available to the team, and the team's experience. National resource centers for PNES treatment and referral are needed.

Psychodynamic psychotherapy can reduce shame, explore trauma, and identify emotions raised by trauma. The symptoms can be understood, for instance that shaking represents a release of energy, unresponsiveness represents a "freezing" response, and falling can represent "sham death." Group therapy with a psychodynamic focus reduced PNES in 12 patients (Barry et al., 2008). However, some patients require alternate methods because they are poor candidates for insight-oriented therapy due to borderline intelligence, lack of motivation or introspection capabilities, important secondary gains, or a tendency for behavioral acting out.

Cognitive behavioral therapy (CBT) can address avoidance behavior, deal with the sequelae of prior traumatic experiences, and reduce health and symptom anxiety (Deary et al., 2007). In this form of treatment, PNES are viewed as a learned maladaptive behavior that is reinforced by the environment. The inappropriate behavior (i.e., PNES) is no longer rewarded or may even be punished. An advantage of this method is that neither normal intelligence nor insight is necessary for success. A disadvantage is that behavioral therapy relies on controlling environmental conditions, which may be impossible to monitor. In the LaFrance study, 11 of 17 patients were seizure-free at the end of a 12-week course of CBT. CBT and family therapy can improve quality-of-life measures (LaFrance, 2008; LaFrance et al., 2008, 2009a, b). CBT reduced PNES by 20% after a 4-month course in a group of 64 patients randomized to CBT or standard medical care (Goldstein et al., 2010).

Family therapy is beneficial in many cases because PNES may largely result from problems related to the dysfunctional family (LaFrance and Bjørnaes, 1993). In this form of therapy, the dysfunction of the family, rather than the individual patient, is emphasized. Family therapy can follow different approaches including psychoanalytical, structural, or a strategic/systems approach.

Biofeedback was helpful at preventing events in one adolescent (Pop-Jordanova et al., 2005). Eye movement desensitization and reprocessing (EMDR) can reduce PNES, particularly if there is a history of PTSD or an abusive experience (Chemali and Meadows, 2004). Hypnosis may also have an adjunctive role (Glenn and Simonds, 1977; Miller, 1983), especially if the PNES is part of a dissociative disorder (Kluft, 1992).

Psychoactive medication

Psychiatric medications may be indicated for Axis I disorders. Selective serotonin reuptake inhibitors (SSRIs) have been used for somatization or dissociation (O'Malley et al., 1999) with some success. A pilot randomized controlled trial of sertraline in 38 patients with PNES showed seizure reduction of 45% from baseline compared with 8% in the placebo group, although the result was not statistically significant (LaFrance et al., 2010). Neuroleptics and propranolol can be effective for severe dissociative disorders (Soloff, 1998).

Summary

Treatment for PNES must be individualized. A combination of approaches is probably the most beneficial for improvement. Treatment should not simply emphasize removing maladaptive PNES behavior, but should also focus on learning new coping skills and removing secondary gains. If PNES persist, therapy should be reevaluated.

PROGNOSIS

Limited information is available on the outcome after diagnosis and treatment of PNES. Many studies have a short follow-up, and a considerable proportion of the patients are lost to follow-up. Moreover, few studies included social issues and psychiatric comorbidities as measures of outcome, although these are more strongly associated with a poor quality of life and disability than the seizures themselves (Walczak et al., 1995; Reuber et al., 2005). Rates of remission have ranged from 16% to 51% in different adult series (Walczak et al., 1995; Ettinger et al., 1999c; Jongsma et al., 1999; Kanner et al., 1999; Reuber et al., 2003a; Thompson et al., 2005; Arain et al., 2007; Bodde et al., 2007; O'Sullivan et al., 2007) and are much higher (up to 82%) in children and adolescents (Gudmundsson et al., 2001). An improvement in symptoms has been reported in 55–80% of patients (Walczak et al., 1995; Ettinger et al., 1999b; Jongsma et al., 1999).

Seizure reduction was related to an improvement in different levels of psychological function: reduction in psychological distress and in feelings of dissatisfaction and passive avoidant behavior, a more active attitude towards social contact, a reduction in dissociative features such as amnesia, and an increase in self-control (Bodde et al., 2007). However, at follow-up, unemployment, dependence on social security, and psychiatric comorbidities are often still present irrespective of seizure remission (Reuber et al., 2003a, 2005; Arain et al., 2007). The mean proportion of patients living independently in a range of outcome studies was 43% (Reuber et al., 2005).

Favorable predictors of outcome are younger age at onset and diagnosis, higher IQ, educational and social status, being accompanied to the first clinic visit, attacks with less dramatic features or motionless spells, a lower level of negativism (self-avoidant behavior), fewer additional somatoform complaints, lower dissociation scores, and lower scores of the personality dimensions "inhibitedness," "emotional dysregulation," and "compulsivity" (Selwa et al., 2000; Reuber et al., 2003a; Arain et al., 2007; Bodde et al., 2007). In children and adolescents favorable predictors are younger age at presentation, female sex, having more types of seizure (possibly because they allow an earlier suspicion of PNES), and not receiving both inpatient and outpatient treatment (possibly reflecting minor severity) (Gudmundsson et al., 2001).

Longer duration and older age at PNES onset and diagnosis are associated with poor outcome, as are higher rates of psychiatric comorbidity, in particular, according to Kanner et al. (1999), a history of chronic abuse, recurrent major depression, dissociative and personality disorder (Lempert and Schmidt, 1990; Buchanan and Snars, 1993; Walczac et al., 1995; Kanner et al., 1999; Selwa et al., 2000; Reuber et al., 2003a). Head injury was associated with poor long-term outcome, including long-lasting disability, despite being relatively mild (Westbrook et al., 1998). Semiological features associated with poor outcome are positive motor features, tongue biting, and incontinence (Selwa et al., 2000; Reuber et al., 2003a). Other negative prognostic factors include abnormal findings on MRI (Kanner et al., 1999) and recurrent pseudostatus (Reuber et al., 2003a).

Comorbid epilepsy, if present, does not significantly affect outcome (Walczak et al., 1995; Jongsma et al., 1999; Kanner et al., 1999; Reuber et al., 2003a).

It is difficult to assess the role of therapy, which has been associated with improved PNES outcome in several, but not all, outcome studies, also due to the fact that presentation of a diagnosis is sometimes sufficient and removes the need for any specific intervention to the individual patient. Acceptance of psychotherapy ranges from 12.5% to 47% (Arain et al., 2007; O'Sullivan et al., 2007), and is related to acceptance of diagnosis, the most important step towards a favorable outcome both in adults and in children and adolescents. In this sense, a definitive and expert diagnosis, good and respectful information, and a specific educational approach are of great value (Gudmundsson et al., 2001; Thompson et al., 2005; Bodde et al., 2009).

CONCLUSION

The significance of PNES should not be underestimated. These episodes can significantly impair quality of life, and lead to unnecessary therapies and invasive diagnostic studies that can be dangerous and expensive. Unrecognized PNES, particularly pseudostatus, may have very serious consequences, mainly due to iatrogenic injury, and can be fatal (Reuber et al., 2004). Early detection utilizing video-EEG monitoring can avoid misdiagnosis and direct the patient towards appropriate care.

References

Aboukasm A, Mahr G, Gahry BR et al. (1998). Retrospective analysis of the effects of psychotherapeutic interventions on outcomes of psychogenic nonepileptic seizures. Epilepsia 39: 470–473.

Abubakr A, Kablinger A, Caldito G (2003). Psychogenic seizures: clinical features and psychological analysis. Epilepsy Behav 4: 241–245.

Acar G, Salinsky MC (2010). Demographic and historical backgrounds of the elderly with nonepileptic seizures: a comparative study. Neurol India 58: 48–52.

Akyuz G, Kugu N, Akyuz A et al. (2004). Dissociation and childhood abuse history in epileptic and pseudoseizure patients. Epileptic Disord 6: 187–192.

Al Marzooqi SM, Baker GA, Reilly J et al. (2004). The perceived health status of people with psychologically derived non-epileptic attack disorder and epilepsy: a comparative study. Seizure 13: 71–75.

Alhalabi MS, Verma NP (1994). Closure of eyes is a frequent and reliable sign of pseudoepileptic seizures. Epilepsia 35: 15.

Alper K, Devinsky O, Perrine K et al. (1993). Nonepileptic seizures and childhood sexual and physical abuse. Neurology 43: 1950–1953.

Alving J (1998). Serum prolactin levels are elevated also after pseudo-epileptic seizures. Seizure 7: 85–89.

Arain AM, Hamadani AM, Islam S et al. (2007). Predictors of early seizure remission after diagnosis of psychogenic nonepileptic seizures. Epilepsy Behav 11: 409–412.

Asmussen SB, Kirlin KA, Gale SD et al. (2009). Differences in self-reported depressive symptoms between patients with epileptic and psychogenic nonepileptic seizures. Seizure 18: 564–566.

Azar NJ, Tayah TF, Wang L et al. (2008). Postictal breathing pattern distinguishes epileptic from nonepileptic convulsive seizures. Epilepsia 49: 132–137.

Baker GA, Brooks JL, Goodfellow L et al. (2007). Treatments for non-epileptic attack disorder. Cochrane Database Syst Rev 1: CD006370.

Bakvis P, Spinhoven P, Giltay EJ et al. (2010). Basal hypercortisolism and trauma in patients with psychogenic nonepileptic seizures. Epilepsia 51: 752–759.

Barrash J, Gates JR, Heck DG et al. (1989). MMPI subtypes among patients with nonepileptic events. Epilepsia 30: 730.

Barry JJ, Atzman O, Morrell MJ (2000). Discriminating between epileptic and nonepileptic events: the utility of hypnotic seizure induction. Epilepsia 41: 81–84.

Barry JJ, Wittenberg D, Bullock KD et al. (2008). Group therapy for patients with psychogenic nonepileptic seizures: a pilot study. Epilepsy Behav 13: 624–629.

Bautista RE, Gonzales-Salazar W, Ochoa JG (2008). Expanding the theory of symptom modeling in patients with psychogenic nonepileptic seizures. Epilepsy Behav 13: 407–409.

Begley CE, Annegers JF, Lairson DR et al. (1994). Cost of epilepsy in the United States: a model based on incidence and prognosis. Epilepsia 35: 1230–1243.

Behrouz R, Heriaud L, Benbadis SR (2006). Late-onset psychogenic nonepileptic seizures. Epilepsy Behav 8: 649–650.

Bell WL, Park YD, Thompson EA et al. (1998). Ictal cognitive assessment of partial seizures and pseudoseizures. Arch Neurol 55: 1456–1459.

Benbadis SR (2001). Provocative techniques should be used for the diagnosis of psychogenic nonepileptic seizures. Arch Neurol 58: 2063–2064.

Benbadis SR (2005). A spell in the epilepsy clinic and a history of "chronic pain" or "fibromyalgia" independently predict a diagnosis of psychogenic seizures. Epilepsy Behav 6: 264–265.

Benbadis SR, Allen Hauser WA (2000). An estimate of the prevalence of psychogenic non-epileptic seizures. Seizure 9: 280–281.

Benbadis S, Tatum W (2003). Overinterpretation of EEGs and misdiagnosis of epilepsy. J Clin Neurophysiol 20: 42–44.

Benbadis SR, Wolgamuth BR, Goren H et al. (1995). Value of tongue biting in the diagnosis of seizures. Arch Intern Med 155: 2346–2349.

Benbadis SR, Lancman ME, King LM et al. (1996). Preictal pseudosleep: a new finding in psychogenic seizures. Neurology 47: 63–67.

Benbadis SR, Johnson K, Anthony K et al. (2000). Induction of psychogenic nonepileptic seizures without placebo. Neurology 55: 1904–1905.

Benbadis SR, Agrawal V, Tatum WO (2001). How many patients with psychogenic nonepileptic seizures also have epilepsy? Neurology 57: 915–917.

Benbadis SR, Siegrist K, Tatum WO et al. (2004). Short-term outpatient EEG video with induction in the diagnosis of psychogenic seizures. Neurology 63: 1728–1730.

Benbadis SR, LaFrance WC Jr, Papandonatos GD et al. (2009). NES Treatment Workshop. Interrater reliability of EEG-video monitoring. Neurology 73: 843–846.

Bergen D, Ristanovic R (1993). Weeping as a common element of pseudoseizures. Arch Neurol 50: 1059–1060.

Betts T, Boden S (1992). Diagnosis, management and prognosis of a group of 128 patients with non-epileptic attack disorder. Part II. Previous childhood sexual abuse in the aetiology of these disorders. Seizure 1: 27–32.

Binder LM, Salinsky MC, Smith SP (1994). Psychological correlates of nonepileptic seizures. J Clin Exp Neuropsychol 16: 524–530.

Binder LM, Kindermann SS, Heaton RK et al. (1998). Neuropsychologic impairment in patients with nonepileptic seizures. Arch Clin Neuropsychol 13: 513–522.

Binzer M, Stone J, Sharpe M (2004). Recent onset pseudoseizures – clues to aetiology. Seizure 13: 146–155.

Bodde NMG, Janssena MAJ, Theunsa C et al. (2007). Factors involved in the long-term prognosis of psychogenic nonepileptic seizures. J Psychosom Res 62: 545–551.

Bodde NM, Brooks JL, Baker GA et al. (2009). Psychogenic non-epileptic seizures—definition, etiology, treatment and prognosis issues: a critical review. Seizure 18(8): 543–553.

Bowman ES (1999). Nonepileptic seizures: psychiatric framework, treatment, and outcome. Neurology 53: S84–S88.

Bowman E (2006). Why conversion seizures should be classified as a dissociative disorder. Psychiatr Clin North Am 29: 185–211.

Bowman ES (2010). Posttraumatic stress disorder, abuse, and trauma: relationships to psychogenic nonepileptic seizures. In: SC Schachter, WC LaFrance Jr (Eds.), Gates and Rowan's Nonepileptic Seizures. 3rd edn. Cambridge University Press, Cambridge, pp. 213–224.

Bowman ES, Markand ON (1999). The contribution of life events to pseudoseizure occurrence in adults. Bull Menninger Clin 63: 70–88.

Briquet P (1859). Traite Clinique et Therapeutique de l' Hysterie. Baillière, Paris.

Brooks JL, Goodfellow L, Bodde NM et al. (2007). Nondrug treatments for psychogenic nonepileptic seizures: what's the evidence? Epilepsy Behav 11: 367–377.

Brown RJ, Trimble MR (2000). Dissociative psychopathology, non-epileptic seizures, and neurology. J Neurol Neurosurg Psychiatry 69: 285–289.

Brown MC, Levin BE, Ramsay DE et al. (1991). Characteristics of patients with nonepileptic seizures. J Epilepsy 4: 225–229.

Buchanan N, Snars J (1993). Pseudoseizures (non-epileptic attack disorder): clinical management and outcome in 50 patients. Seizure 2: 141–146.

Burneo JG, Martin R, Powell T et al. (2003). Teddy bears: an observational finding in patients with non-epileptic events. Neurology 61: 714–715.

Carter RB (1853). On the Pathology and Treatment of Hysteria. John Churchill, London.

Chabolla DR, Shih JJ (2006). Postictal behaviors associated with psychogenic nonepileptic seizures. Epilepsy Behav 9: 307–311.

Chadwick D (1994). Epilepsy. J Neurol Neurosurg Psychiatry 57: 264–277.

Charcot JM, Richer P (1887). In: A Delahaye, E Lescrosnier (Eds.), Les Demoniaques dans l'Art. Avec 67 figures intergalées dans le texte. Paris.

Chemali Z, Meadows ME (2004). The use of eye movement desensitization and reprocessing in the treatment of psychogenic seizures. Epilepsy Behav 5: 784–787.

Chen DK, Izadyar S (2010). Characteristics of psychogenic nonepileptic events among veterans with posttraumatic stress disorder: an association of semiology with the nature of trauma. Epilepsy Behav 17: 188–192.

Chen DK, So YT, Fisher RS (2005). Use of serum prolactin in diagnosing epileptic seizures: report of the Therapeutics and Technology Assessment Subcommittee of the American Academy of Neurology. Neurology 65: 668–675.

Chen DK, Graber KD, Anderson CT et al. (2008). Sensitivity and specificity of video alone versus electroencephalography alone for the diagnosis of partial seizures. Epilepsy Behav 13: 115–118.

Chung SS, Gerber P, Kirlin KA (2006). Ictal eye closure is a reliable indicator for psychogenic nonepileptic seizures. Neurology 66: 1730–1731.

Cragar DE, Schmitt FA, Berry DT et al. (2003). A comparison of MMPI-2 decision rules in the diagnosis of nonepileptic seizures. J Clin Exp Neuropsychol 25: 793–804.

Cragar DE, Berry DTR, Schmitt FA et al. (2005). Cluster analysis of normal personality traits in patients with psychogenic nonepileptic seizures. Epilepsy Behav 6: 593–600.

Cragar DE, Fakhoury TA, Berry DTR et al. (2006). Performance of patients with epilepsy or psychogenic non-epileptic seizures on four measures of effort. Clin Neuropsychol 20: 552–566.

De la Fuente JM, Tugendhaft P, Mavroudakis N (1998). Electroencephalographic abnormalities in borderline personality disorder. Psychiatry Res 77: 131–138.

de Lange F, Roelofs K, Toni I (2008). Motor imagery: a window into the mechanisms and alterations of the motor system. Cortex 44: 494–506.

De Wet CJ, Mellers JDC, Gardner WN et al. (2003). Pseudoseizures and asthma. J Neurol Neurosurg Psychiatry 74: 639–641.

Deary V, Chalder T, Sharpe M (2007). The cognitive behavioural model of medically unexplained symptoms: a theoretical and empirical review. Clin Psychol Rev 27: 781–797.

DeToledo JC, Ramsay RE (1996). Patterns of involvement of facial muscles during epileptic and nonepileptic events: review of 654 events. Neurology 47: 621–625.

Devinsky O (1998). Nonepileptic psychogenic seizures: quagmires of pathophysiology, diagnosis, and treatment. Epilepsia 39: 458–462.

Devinsky O, Fisher R (1996). Ethical use of placebos and provocative testing in diagnosing nonepileptic seizures. Neurology 47: 866–870.

Devinsky O, Mesad S, Alper K (2001). Nondominant hemisphere lesions and conversion nonepileptic seizures. J Neuropsychiatry Clin Neurosci 13: 367–373.

Dikel TN, Fennell EB, Gilmore RL (2003). Posttraumatic stress disorder, dissociation, and sexual abuse history in epileptic and nonepileptic seizure patients. Epilepsy Behav 4: 644–650.

Dodrill CB (2008). Do patients with psychogenic nonepileptic seizures produce trustworthy findings on neuropsychological tests? Epilepsia 49: 691–695.

Drane DL, Williamson DJ, Stroup ES et al. (2006). Cognitive impairment is not equal in patients with epileptic and psychogenic nonepileptic seizures. Epilepsia 47: 1879–1886.

Duncan R, Oto M (2008a). Predictors of antecedent factors in psychogenic nonepileptic attacks: multivariate analysis. Neurology 71: 1000–1005.

Duncan R, Oto M (2008b). Psychogenic nonepileptic seizures in patients with learning disability: comparison with patients with no learning disability. Epilepsy Behav 12: 183–186.

Duncan R, Oto M, Martin E et al. (2006). Late onset psychogenic nonepileptic attacks. Neurology 66: 1644–1647.

Dworetzky BA, Strahonja-Packard A, Shanahan CW et al. (2005). Characteristics of male veterans with psychogenic nonepileptic seizures. Epilepsia 46: 1418–1422.

Ettinger AB, Coyle PK, Jandord L et al. (1998). Postictal SPECT in epileptic versus nonepileptic seizures. J Epilepsy 11: 67–73.

Ettinger AB, Weisbrot DM, Nolan E et al. (1999a). Postictal symptoms help distinguish patients with epileptic seizures from those with non-epileptic seizures. Seizure 8: 149–151.

Ettinger AB, Dhoon A, Weisbrot DM et al. (1999b). Predictive factors for outcome of nonepileptic seizures after diagnosis. J Neuropsychiatry Clin Neurosci 11: 458–463.

Ettinger AB, Devinsky O, Weisbrot DM et al. (1999c). A comprehensive profile of clinical, psychiatric, and psychosocial characteristics of patients with psychogenic nonepileptic seizures. Epilepsia 40: 1292–1298.

Fiszman A, Vieira Alves-Leon S, Gomes Nunes R et al. (2004). Traumatic events and posttraumatic stress disorder in patients with psychogenic nonepileptic seizures: a critical review. Epilepsy Behav 5: 818–825.

Fleisher W, Staley D, Krawetz P et al. (2002). Comparative study of trauma-related phenomena in subjects with pseudoseizures and subjects with epilepsy. Am J Psychiatry 159: 660–663.

Flügel D, Bauer J, Käseborn U et al. (1996). Closed eyes during a seizure indicate psychogenic etiology: a study with suggestive seizure provocation. J Epilepsy 9: 165–169.

Gates JR (2001). Provocative testing should not be used for nonepileptic seizures. Arch Neurol 58: 2065.

Gates JR, Ramani V, Whalen S et al. (1985). Ictal characteristics of pseudoseizures. Arch Neurol 42: 1183–1187.

Geyer JD, Payne TA, Drury I (2000). The value of pelvic thrusting in the diagnosis of seizures and pseudoseizures. Neurology 54: 227–229.

Glenn TJ, Simonds JF (1977). Hypnotherapy of a psychogenic seizure disorder in an adolescent. Am J Clin Hypn 19: 245–249.

Goldstein LH (2004). Assessment of patients with psychogenic non-epileptic seizures. J Neurol Neurosurg Psychiatry 75: 667–668.

Goldstein LH, Chalder T, Chigwedere C et al. (2010). Cognitive behavioural therapy for psychogenic nonepileptic seizures: a pilot RCT. Neurology 74: 1986–1994.

Gowers WR (1901). Epilepsy and Other Chronic Convulsive Disorders. JA Churchill, London.

Griffith NM, Szaflarski JP (2010). Epidemiology and classification of psychogenic nonepileptic seizures. In: SC Schachter, WC LaFrance Jr (Eds.), Gates and Rowan's Nonepileptic seizures. 3rd edn. Cambridge University Press, Cambridge, pp. 3–16.

Griffith NM, Szaflarski JP, Schefft BK et al. (2007). Relationship between semiology of psychogenic nonepileptic seizures and Minnesota Multiphasic Personality Inventory profile. Epilepsy Behav 11: 105–111.

Gudmundsson O, Prendergast M, Foreman D et al. (2001). Outcome of pseudoseizures in children and adolescents: a 6-year symptom survival analysis. Dev Med Child Neurol 43: 547–551.

Gulick TA, Spinks IP, King DW (1982). Pseudoseizures: ictal phenomena. Neurology 32: 24–30.

Gumnit RT, Gates JR (1986). Psychogenic seizures. Epilepsia 27(S2): S124–S129.

Hantke NC, Doherty MJ, Haltiner AM (2007). Medication use profiles in patients with psychogenic nonepileptic seizures. Epilepsy Behav 10: 333–335.

Harden CL, Jovine L, Burgut FT et al. (2009). A comparison of personality disorder characteristics of patients with nonepileptic psychogenic pseudoseizures with those of patients with epilepsy. Epilepsy Behav 14: 481–483.

Henry JA, Woodruff GH (1978). A diagnostic sign in states of apparent unconsciousness. Lancet 2: 920–921.

Hovorka J, Nezada T, Herman E et al. (2007). Psychogenic nonepileptic seizures, prospective clinical experience: diagnosis, clinical features, risk factors, psychiatric comorbidity, treatment outcome. Epileptic Disord 9: S52–S58.

Howell SJ, Owen L, Chadwick DW (1989). Pseudostatus epilepticus. Q J Med 71: 507–519.

Janet PJM (1889). L'Automatisme Psychologique. Alcan, Paris.

Janet PJM (1895). Charcot, son oeuvre psychologiue. Rev Philos 39: 569–604.

Jawad SS, Jamil N, Clarke EJ et al. (1995). Psychiatric morbidity and psychodynamics of patients with convulsive pseudoseizures. Seizure 4: 201–206.

Jongsma MJ, Mommers JM, Renier WO et al. (1999). Follow-up of psychogenic, non-epileptic seizures: a pilot study–experience in a Dutch special centre for epilepsy. Seizure 8: 146–148.

Kalogjera-Sackellares D, Sackellares JC (1999). Intellectual and neuropsychological features of patients with psychogenic pseudoseizures. Psychiatr Res 86: 73–84.

Kanner AM, Morris HH, Lüders H et al. (1990). Supplementary motor seizures mimicking pseudoseizures: some clinical differences. Neurology 40: 1404–1407.

Kanner AM, Parra J, Frey M et al. (1999). Psychiatric and neurologic predictors of psychogenic pseudoseizure outcome. Neurology 53: 933–938.

Kluft RP (1992). The use of hypnosis with dissociative disorders. Psychiatr Med 10: 31–46.

Krumholz A, Niedermeyer E (1983). Psychogenic seizures: a clinical study with follow-up data. Neurology 33: 498–502.

Kuyk J, Leijten F, Meinardi H et al. (1997). The diagnosis of psychogenic non-epileptic seizures: a review. Seizure 6: 243–253.

LaFrance WC Jr (2008) Psychogenic nonepileptic seizures. Curr Opin Neurol 21: 195–201.

LaFrance WC, Bjørnæs H (1993). Designing treatment plans based on etiology of psychogenic nonepileptic seizures. In: SC Schachter, WC LaFrance Jr (Eds.), Gates and Rowan's Nonepileptic seizures. 3rd edn. Cambridge University Press, Cambridge, pp. 266–280.

LaFrance WC Jr, Devinsky O (2002). Treatment of nonepileptic seizures. Epilepsy Behav 3: 19–23.

LaFrance WC Jr, Syc S (2009). Depression and symptoms affect quality of life in psychogenic nonepileptic seizures. Neurology 73: 366–371.

LaFrance WC Jr, Rusch MD, Machan JT (2008). What is "treatment as usual" for nonepileptic seizures? Epilepsy Behav 12: 388–394.

LaFrance WC Jr, Blum AS, Ryan CE et al. (2009a). Comorbidities in patients with psychogenic nonepileptic seizures. Neurology 72: 328.

LaFrance WC Jr, Miller IW, Ryan CE et al. (2009b). Cognitive behavioral therapy for psychogenic nonepileptic seizures. Epilepsy Behav 14: 591–596.

LaFrance WC Jr, Keitner GI, Papandonatos GD et al. (2010). Pilot pharmacologic randomized controlled trial for psychogenic nonepileptic seizures. Neurology 75: 1166–1173.

Lancman ME, Asconape JJ, Craven WJ et al. (1994). Predictive value of induction of psychogenic seizures by suggestion. Ann Neurol 35: 359–361.

Lawton GR, Mayor J, Howlett S et al. (2009). Psychogenic nonepileptic seizures and health-related quality of life: the relationship with psychological distress and other physical symptoms. Epilepsy Behav 14: 167–171.

Leis AA, Ross MA (1992). Psychogenic seizures. Neurology 42: 1128–1129.

Leis AA, Ross MA, Summers AK (1992). Psychogenic seizures: ictal characteristics and diagnostic pitfalls. Neurology 42: 95–99.

Lempert T, Schmidt D (1990). Natural history and outcome of psychogenic seizures: a clinical study in 50 patients. J Neurol 237: 35–38.

Lesser RP (1996). Psychogenic seizures. Neurology 46: 1499–1507.

Lesser RP, Lueders H, Dinner DS (1983). Evidence for epilepsy is rare in patients with psychogenic seizures. Neurology 33: 502–504.

Lobello K, Morgenlander JC, Radtke JA et al. (2006). Video/EEG monitoring in the evaluation of paroxysmal behavioral events: duration, effectiveness and limitations. Epilepsy Behav 8: 261–266.

Luther JS, McNamara JO, Carwile S et al. (1982). Pseudoepileptic seizures: methods and video analysis to aid diagnosis. Ann Neurol 12: 458–462.

Mace CJ, Trimble MR (1996). Ten-year prognosis of conversion disorder. Br J Psychiatry 169: 282–288.

Marsden CD (1986). Hysteria – a neurologist's view. Psychol Med 16: 277–288.

Martin RC, Gilliam FG, Kilgore M et al. (1998). Improved health care resource utilization following video-EEG-confirmed diagnosis of nonepileptic psychogenic seizures. Seizure 7: 385–390.

Martínez-Taboas A, Lewis-Fernández R, Sar V et al. (2010). Cultural aspects of psychogenic nonepileptic seizures. In: SC Schachter, WC LaFrance Jr (Eds.), Gates and Rowan's Nonepileptic seizures. 3rd edn. Cambridge University Press, Cambridge, pp. 121–130.

McKenzie P, Oto M, Russell A et al. (2010). Early outcomes and predictors in 260 patients with psychogenic nonepileptic attacks. Neurology 74: 64–69.

Meierkord H, Will B, Fish D et al. (1991). The clinical features and prognosis of pseudoseizures diagnosed using video-EEG telemetry. Neurology 41: 1643–1646.

Mellers JDC (2005). The approach to patients with "non-epileptic seizures". Postgrad Med J 81: 498–504.

Miller HR (1983). Psychogenic seizures treated by hypnosis. Am J Clin Hypn 25: 228–252.

Moene FC, Kuyk J (2010). Hypnosis in the treatment of psychogenic nonepileptic seizures. In: SC Schachter, WC LaFrance Jr (Eds.), Gates and Rowan's Nonepileptic Seizures. 3rd edn. Cambridge University Press, Cambridge, pp. 297–306.

Neiman ES, Noe KH, Drazkowski JF et al. (2009). Utility of subtraction ictal SPECT when video-EEG fails to distinguish atypical psychogenic and epileptic seizures. Epilepsy Behav 15: 208–212.

Oliva M, Pattison C, Carino J et al. (2008). The diagnostic value of oral lacerations and incontinence during convulsive "seizures". Epilepsia 49: 962–967.

Olson DM, Howard N, Shaw RJ (2008). Hypnosis-provoked nonepileptic events in children. Epilepsy Behav 12: 456–459.

O'Malley PG, Jackson JL, Santoro J et al. (1999). Antidepressant therapy for unexplained symptoms and symptom syndromes. J Fam Pract 48: 980–990.

Orbach D, Ritaccio A, Devinsky O (2003). Psychogenic, nonepileptic seizures associated with video-EEG-verified sleep. Epilepsia 44: 64–68.

Oribe E, Amini R, Nissenbaum E et al. (1996). Serum prolactin concentrations are elevated following syncope. Neurology 47: 60–62.

O'Sullivan SS, Spillane JE, McMahon EM et al. (2007). Clinical characteristics and outcome of patients diagnosed with psychogenic nonepileptic seizures: a 5-year review. Epilepsy Behav 11: 77–84.

Oto M, Conway P, McGonigal A et al. (2005). Gender differences in psychogenic non-epileptic seizures. Seizure 14: 33–39.

Parra J, Iriarte J, Kanner AM et al. (1998). De novo psychogenic nonepileptic seizures after epilepsy surgery. Epilepsia 39: 474–477.

Peguero E, Abou-Khalil B, Fakhoury T et al. (1995). Self-injury and incontinence in psychogenic seizures. Epilepsia 36: 586–591.

Plioplys S, Asato MR, Bursch B et al. (2007). Multidisciplinary management of pediatric nonepileptic seizures. J Am Acad Child Adolesc Psychiatry 46: 1491–1495.

Plug L, Sharrack B, Reuber M (2009a). Conversation analysis can help to distinguish between epilepsy and non-epileptic seizure disorders: a case comparison. Seizure 18: 43–50.

Plug L, Sharrack B, Reuber M (2009b). Seizure metaphors differ in patients' accounts of epileptic and psychogenic nonepileptic seizures. Epilepsia 50: 994–1000.

Pop-Jordanova N, Zorcec T, Demerdzieva A (2005). Electrodermal biofeedback in treating psychogenic nonepileptic seizures. Prilozi 26: 43–51.

Raymond AA, Gilmore WV, Scott CA et al. (1999). Video-EEG telemetry: apparent manifestation of both epileptic and non-epileptic attacks causing potential diagnostic pitfalls. Epileptic Disord 1: 101–106.

Rechlin T, Loew TH, Joraschky P (1997). Pseudoseizure "status". J Psychosom Res 42: 495–498.

Reuber M, Elger CE (2003). Psychogenic nonepileptic seizures: review and update. Epilepsy Behav 4: 205–216.

Reuber M, House AO (2002). Treating patients with psychogenic non-epileptic seizures. Curr Opin Neurol 15: 207–211.

Reuber M, Enright SM, Goulding PJ (2000). Postoperative pseudostatus: not everything that shakes is epilepsy. Anaesthesia 55: 74–78.

Reuber M, Fernandez G, Bauer J et al. (2002a). Diagnostic delay in psychogenic nonepileptic seizures. Neurology 58: 493–495.

Reuber M, Fernández G, Bauer J et al. (2002b). Interictal EEG abnormalities in patients with psychogenic nonepileptic seizures. Epilepsia 43: 1013–1020.

Reuber M, Pukrop R, Bauer J et al. (2003a). Outcome in psychogenic nonepileptic seizures: 1 to 10-year follow-up in 164 patients. Ann Neurol 53: 305–311.

Reuber M, Pukrop R, Mitchell AJ et al. (2003b). Clinical significance of recurrent psychogenic nonepileptic seizure status. J Neurol 250: 1355–1362.

Reuber M, Qurishi A, Bauer J et al. (2003c). Are there physical risk factors for psychogenic non-epileptic seizures in patients with epilepsy? Seizure 12: 561–567.

Reuber M, Baker GA, Gill R et al. (2004). Failure to recognize psychogenic nonepileptic seizures may cause death. Neurology 62: 834–835.

Reuber M, Mitchell AJ, Howlett S et al. (2005). Measuring outcome in psychogenic nonepileptic seizures: how relevant is seizure remission? Epilepsia 46: 1788–1795.

Reuber M, Monzoni C, Sharrack B et al. (2009). Using interactional and linguistic analysis to distinguish between epileptic and psychogenic nonepileptic seizures: a prospective, blinded multirater study. Epilepsy Behav 16: 139–144.

Rogers MP, Weinshenker NJ, Warshaw MG et al. (1996). Prevalence of somatoform disorders in a large sample of patients with anxiety disorders. Psychosomatics 37: 17–22.

Sackellares DK, Sackellares JC (2001). Impaired motor function in patients with psychogenic pseudoseizures. Epilepsia 42: 1600–1606.

Savard G, Andermann F, Teitelbaum J et al. (1988). Epileptic Munchausen's syndrome: a form of pseudoseizures distinct from hysteria or malingering. Neurology 38: 1628–1629.

Saygi S, Katz A, Marks DA et al. (1992). Frontal lobe partial seizures and psychogenic seizures: comparison of clinical and ictal characteristics. Neurology 42: 1274–1277.

Schramke CJ, Valeri A, Valeriano JP et al. (2007). Using the Minnesota Multi-phasic Inventory 2, EEGs, and clinical data to predict nonepileptic events. Epilepsy Behav 11: 343–346.

Schwabe M, Howell SJ, Reuber M (2007). Differential diagnosis of seizure disorders: a conversation analytic approach. Soc Sci Med 65: 712–724.

Selkirk M, Duncan R, Oto M et al. (2008). Clinical differences between patients with nonepileptic seizures who report antecedent sexual abuse and those who do not. Epilepsia 49: 1446–1450.

Selwa LM, Geyer L, Nikakhtar N (2000). Nonepileptic seizure outcome varies by type of spell and duration of illness. Epilepsia 41: 1330–1334.

Sen A, Scott C, Sisodiya SM (2007). Stertorous breathing is a reliably identified sign that helps in the differentiation of epileptic from psychogenic non-epileptic convulsions: an audit. Epilepsy Res 77: 62–64

Shen WE, Bowman S, Markand ON (1990). Presenting the diagnosis of pseudoseizure. Neurology 40: 756–759.

Shukla G, Bhatia M, Vivekanandhan S et al. (2004). Serum prolactin levels for differentiation of nonepileptic versus true seizures: limited utility. Epilepsy Behav 5: 517–521.

Sigurdardottir KR, Olafsson E (1998). Incidence of psychogenic seizures in adults: a population-based study in Iceland. Epilepsia 39: 749–752.

Simeon D, Knutelska M, Yehuda R et al. (2007). Hypothalamic-pituitary-adrenal axis function in dissociative disorders, post-traumatic stress disorder, and healthy volunteers. Biol Psychiatry 61: 966–973.

Slater JD, Brown MC, Jacobs W et al. (1995). Induction of pseudoseizures with intravenous saline placebo. Epilepsia 36: 580–585.

Smith S, Ruthven D, Salinsky M et al. (1992). Psychiatric diagnoses in patients with epilepsy or pseudoseizures referred for diagnostic neurotelemetry. Epilepsia 33: 17.

Soloff PH (1998). Algorithms for pharmacological treatment of personality dimensions: symptom-specific treatments for cognitive-perceptual, affective, and impulsive-behavioral dysregulation. Bull Menninger Clin 62: 195–214.

Stone J, Carson A, Sharpe M (2005). Functional symptoms and signs in neurology: assessment and diagnosis. J Neurol Neurosurg Psychiatry 76: i2–i12.

Strachey J (Ed.), (1955). The Standard Edition of the Complete Psychological Works of Sigmund Freud, Volume II (1893–1895): Studies on Hysteria. The Hogarth Press and the Institute of Psycho-Analysis, London.

Syed TU, Arozullah AM, Suciu GP et al. (2008). Do observer and self-reports of ictal eye closure predict psychogenic nonepileptic seizures? Epilepsia 49: 898–904.

Szaflarski JP, Szaflarski M (2004). Seizure disorders, depression, and health-related quality of life. Epilepsy Behav 5: 50–57.

Szaflarski JP, Ficker DM, Cahill WT et al. (2000). Four-year incidence of psychogenic nonepileptic seizures in adults in Hamilton county, OH. Neurology 55: 1561–1563.

Szaflarski JP, Hughes C, Szaflarski M et al. (2003). Quality of life in psychogenic nonepileptic seizures. Epilepsia 44: 236–242.

Temkin O (1994). The Falling Sickness. 2nd edn. Johns Hopkins University Press, Baltimore.

Testa SM, Schefft BK, Szaflarski JP et al. (2007). Mood, personality, and health-related quality of life in epileptic and psychogenic seizure disorders. Epilepsia 48: 973–982.

Thacker K, Devinsky O, Perrine K et al. (1993). Nonepileptic seizures during apparent sleep. Ann Neurol 33: 414–418.

Thompson NC, Osorio I, Hunter EE (2005). Nonepileptic seizures: reframing the diagnosis. Perspect Psychiatr Care 41: 71–78.

Trimble MR (1986). Pseudoseizures. Neurol Clin 4: 531–547.

Varma AR, Moriarty J, Costa DC et al. (1996). HMPAO SPECT in non-epileptic seizures: preliminary results. Acta Neurol Scand 94: 88–92.

Veith I (1965). Hysteria: The History of a Disease. University of Chicago Press, Chicago.

Vinton A, Carino J, Vogrin S et al. (2004). "Convulsive" nonepileptic seizures have a characteristic pattern of rhythmic artifact distinguishing them from convulsive epileptic seizures. Epilepsia 45: 1344–1350.

Voon V, Gallea C, Hattori N et al. (2010). The involuntary nature of conversion disorder. Neurology 74: 223–228.

Vossler DG, Haltiner AM, Schepp SK et al. (2004). Ictal stuttering: a sign suggestive of psychogenic nonepileptic seizures. Neurology 63: 516–519.

Walczak TS, Rubinsky M (1994). Plantar responses after epileptic seizures. Neurology 44: 2191–2193.

Walczak TS, Williams DT, Berten W (1994). Utility and reliability of placebo infusion in the evaluation of patients with seizures. Neurology 44: 394–399.

Walczak TS, Papacostas S, Williams DT et al. (1995). Outcome after diagnosis of psychogenic nonepileptic seizures. Epilepsia 36: 1131–1137.

Westbrook LE, Devinsky O, Geocadin R (1998). Nonepileptic seizures after head injury. Epilepsia 39: 978–982.

Widdess-Walsh P, Nadkarni S, Devinsky O (2010). Comorbidity of epileptic and psychogenic nonepileptic seizures: diagnostic considerations. In: SC Schachter, WC LaFrance Jr (Eds.), Gates and Rowan's Nonepileptic seizures. 3rd edn. Cambridge University Press, Cambridge, pp. 51–61.

Wilkus RJ, Dodrill CB (1989). Factors affecting the outcome of MMPI and neuropsychological assessments of psychogenic and epileptic seizure patients. Epilepsia 30: 339–347.

Wood BL, Haque S, Weinstock A et al. (2004). Pediatric stress-related seizures: conceptualization, evaluation, and treatment of nonepileptic seizures in children and adolescents. Curr Opin Pediatr 16: 523–531.

Woollacott IOC, Scott C, Fish DR et al. (2010). When do psychogenic nonepileptic seizures occur on a video/EEG telemetry unit? Epilepsy Behav 17: 228–235.

Wyllie E, Friedman D, Rothner AD et al. (1990). Psychogenic seizures in children and adolescents: outcome after diagnosis by ictal video and electroencephalographic recording. Pediatrics 85: 480–484.

Wyllie E, Glazer JP, Benbadis S et al. (1999). Psychiatric features of children and adolescents with pseudoseizures. Arch Pediatr Adol Med 153: 244–248.

Handbook of Clinical Neurology, Vol. 107 (3rd series)
Epilepsy, Part I
H. Stefan and W.H. Theodore, Editors

Chapter 18

Syncope

BERNT A. ENGELSEN*

Epilepsy Unit, Institute of Clinical Medicine, University of Bergen, and Department of Neurology, Haukeland University Hospital, Bergen, Norway

INTRODUCTION

As a cause of transient loss of consciousness (LOC), syncope is important in the differential diagnosis of epileptic seizures. As the prognostic risk stratification of syncope depends on the specific cause (e.g., cardiac disease), a correct diagnose of transient LOC with classification of any syncope is mandatory for treatment and prognosis. This chapter examines the classification, diagnosis, and treatment of syncope in the clinical context of an epilepsy unit based in a neurological department of a university hospital. Cases are presented that reflect the complexity of the topic. Recommended recent overviews for further reading are by Brignole et al. (2001), Strickberger et al. (2006), and Benditt et al. (2007).

NOMENCLATURE, DEFINITION, AND PATHOPHYSIOLOGY

Syncope is derived from the Greek *syn*, meaning "with," and *koptein*, to cut or "to interrupt."

In a medical context, the term syncope refers to an abrupt and transient LOC and muscle tone, due to global impairment of cerebral perfusion. A recently proposed definition excludes loss of postural tone because this is not of particular value in differentiating syncope from the transient LOC encompassing the differential diagnostic conditions such as epileptic seizures, hypoglycemia, metabolic disorders, toxic insults, etc. This definition suggests that syncope be defined as "a transient spontaneous loss of consciousness with a rapid onset, and a self limited, complete, and usually prompt recovery in which the underlying mechanism is a transient global cerebral hypo perfusion" (Blanc, 2007, pp.5–6).

Cerebral perfusion pressure is largely dependent on systemic arterial pressure, which again depends on cardiac output and total peripheral vascular resistance. Cardiac output may be impaired due to lack of venous filling, bradyarrhythmia or tachyarrhythmia, valvular disease, and other reasons for pump failure. Moreover, vascular dilatation, for example when hot, or impaired capacity to increase vascular resistance, such as during prolonged standing, may contribute to either reflex syncope or orthostatic syncope. Vasoactive drugs and autonomic neuropathies are two important contributing factors in such occurrences (Table 18.1).

Cessation of cerebral blood flow for 6–8 seconds (Rossen et al., 1943) or a decrease in systolic blood pressure to 60 mmHg may be sufficient to cause transient LOC (Sheldon and Killam, 1992). A 20% decrease in cerebral oxygen delivery may result in transient LOC (Rossen et al., 1943), and regardless of symptoms orthostatic hypotension may be defined as a decrease in systolic blood pressure of 20 mmHg or more within 3 minutes of standing or tilting (Consensus Committee, 1996).

Vasovagal syncope may occur when the cardiac output has decreased by about 50%. Thus, a "classical" response during tilt-table testing (see below) in a young subject would be a vasodilatation with a concurrent vagally mediated bradycardia with a rapid fall in blood pressure.

CLASSIFICATION

Cardiac syncope is by definition related to cardiac disturbance. Cardiac ischemia or arrhythmia-related syncope may be confirmed by electrocardiographic (ECG) changes. Exertional syncope may result from heart disease where a fixed output does not increase with exercise; this can arise from coronary artery anomalies, and arrhythmic or neurocardiogenic disorders. Neurogenic or reflex syncope refers to a reflex that, when triggered, gives rise to vasodilatation and bradycardia.

*Correspondence to: Bernt A. Engelsen, Professor of Neurology, Department of Neurology, Haukeland University Hospital, Helse-Bergen, HF. N-5021 Bergen, Norway. E-mail: bernt.engelsen@helse-bergen.no

Table 18.1

Causes of syncope

Type of syncopy	Etiology
Cardiac syncope	Impaired filling or outflow (e.g., pump failure)
Cardiac arrhythmias	Bradyarrhythmias Tachyarrhythmias Long QT syndrome: familial, spontaneous, drug induced
Structural cardiac or cardiopulmonary disease	Cardiac valvular disease Acute myocardial infarction/ischemia Obstructive cardiomyopathy Atrial myxoma Idiopathic hypertrophic subaortic stenosis Pulmonary embolus/pulmonary hypertension
Neurally mediated reflex syncopal syndromes (disorders of vascular tone or volume)	Vasovagal/neurocardiogenic syncope Orthostatic syncope Carotid hypersensitivity
Situational syncope	Acute hemorrhage Acute gastrointestinal stimulation (swallowing, defecation, visceral pain) Other stimulus-induced: breath-holding in children; coughing, sneezing; micturition
Drug-induced syncope	
Cerebrovascular	Subclavian steal syndrome
Multifactorial	
Others, including transient neurological dysfunction	Epileptic syncope (secondarily to seizure-induced arrhythmia) (see Fig. 18.1B,C) Basilar migraine

It is defined by the lack of an established cause such as vasovagal faints, situational and other syncope events. Vasovagal syncope is diagnosed when precipitating events such as fear, severe pain, emotional distress, instrumentation, or prolonged standing are associated with typical prodromal symptoms (Brignole et al., 2001). Situational syncope occurs following urination, defecation, coughing, or swallowing (see Table 18.1). Orthostatic syncope is associated with orthostatic hypotension, i.e. failure of vasoconstrictor mechanisms during or prior to LOC.

DRUG-INDUCED (IATROGENIC) SYNCOPE

Drugs may induce syncope by orthostatic hypotension, volume or blood loss, or by cardiac conduction changes such as a prolonged QT interval. Alpha- and beta-blockers, L-dopa, dopa agonists, diuretics, monoamine oxidase inhibitors, sympatholytics, sympathomimetics, tricyclic antidepressants, serotonin reuptake inhibitors, narcotics, sedatives, vasodilators (e.g., sildenafil), and alcohol may all elicit syncope, especially in elderly patients. Moreover, erythromycin, haloperidol, lithium, methylphenidate, procainamide, and venlafaxine may prolong the QT interval. The list of medications is long, and even antiepileptic drugs have been known to influence heart rate, for instance by atrioventricular blockage (Beermann et al., 1975).

EPIDEMIOLOGY

The frequency of syncope may vary between 15% to 25% in different populations (Brignole et al., 2001), making it far more frequent than epileptic seizures. Of approximately 3000 airforce personnel averaged 29 years, 7% had experienced at least one episode of syncope (Dermkasian and Lamb, 1958). However, syncope accounts for less than 3%, possibly 1–2%, of visits to emergency departments (Day et al., 1982; Brignole et al., 2001; Blanc et al., 2002; Colman et al., 2004). The cumulative recollected lifetime incidence of reflex syncope may be in the order of 17–34% in young people (Colman et al., 2004). In general, syncope is more frequent in women than men (Sheldon and Serletis, 2007). In the first Framingham study of 5029 adults, aged 30–62 years, followed for 26 years, only 3.0% of men and 3.5% of women admitted to having had a syncopal event during the course of the study (Savage et al., 1985). Approximately 35% of patients with syncope had a recurrence after 3 years of follow-up (Kapoor et al., 1987; Kapoor, 1990).

The statistics demonstrate that there is major uncertainty as to the community prevalence of syncope. The age distribution of syncope is bimodal, with peaks in adolescents and in the elderly (Colman et al., 2004). In general, patients with syncope in emergency wards are older, with a mean age of about 60 years. About 50% probably have vasovagal syncope, 5–20% have cardiac syncope, approximately 5% each may have carotid sinus syncope or orthostatic hypotension, and 10–20% may not have syncope (Sheldon and Serletis, 2007). Based on a review of over 800 patients from three publications, Bleck (1997) estimated that approximately 19% of syncope frequency was due to vasovagal occurrences, 18% to cardiac dysfunction, and 34% of unknown cause, whereas seizures made up 8% of occurrences of transient LOC.

CLINICAL SYMPTOMS

Often, transient LOC occurs without warning and is brief, usually up to 20 seconds in duration. In a videometric analysis of 56 episodes without premonitory symptoms, more than 90% occurred with myoclonic jerks and the mean duration was 12 (range 5–22) seconds (Lempert et al., 1994). Other motor phenomena may be brief convulsion-like movements, irregular muscle twitching or tonic movements, and muscle atonia. Rarely duration may be longer, and unconsciousness lasting several minutes has been recorded. Premonitory symptoms may be lightheadedness, dizziness, nausea, sweating, weakness, dyspnea, chest pain, palpitations, visual disturbances, "greying out," etc. (Brignole et al., 2001; Sheldon et al., 2002). Patients may be ashen (grey) or pale, become diaphoretic, have dilated pupils, with "eyes rolling back into the head." Clinical features may suggest specific causes of syncope; for example, throat or facial pain suggest neuralgia. Syncope within 1 hour after a meal suggests autonomic failure and postprandial syncope. Nausea and vomiting may suggest vasovagal syncope, and syncope associated with vertigo, dysarthria, and diplopia points to brainstem transient ischemic attacks.

Signs or symptoms suggestive of seizures rather than syncope are tongue biting, abnormal behavior, postictal confusion, prodromal *déjà vu* or *jamais vu*, etc. (Sheldon et al., 2002).

PROGNOSIS

Cardiac causes of syncope may be associated with the highest mortality rate (Kapoor, 1990; Soteriades et al., 2002). The 5-year outcome of 433 patients revealed a mortality rate of more than 50% in patients with a cardiac cause, compared with 30% in patients with a noncardiac cause and 22% in those with an unknown cause (Kapoor, 1990; Bleck, 1997). The occurrence of arrhythmias or death within 1 year was 4–7% in patients with no risk factor, and increased progressively to 58–80% in those with three or more factors, i.e. age above 45 years, history of congestive heart failure, history of ventricular arrhythmias, and abnormal ECG findings (Martin et al., 1997). However, it was shown recently that the mortality rate was not increased in patients with syncope when compared to matched controls with a similar degree of heart disease (Kapoor and Hanusa, 1996). Noticeably, in 3 of 4 patients the cause of syncope may be established (Blanc et al., 2002). An approximately 5% first-year mortality rate in patients with unexplained syncope has been reported in several investigations (Brignole et al., 2001).

Of patients with syncope seen by physicians, 16–36% may have injuries with minor lacerations, bruises, etc. to the hip or face, or limb fractures (Day et al., 1982; Kapoor, 1990).

INVESTIGATIONS

Medical history and routine tests

Few syncopal events are observed by medical personnel, and a clear description from friends or family is an essential contribution to correct diagnosis, sometimes with a very high sensitivity or specificity (Sheldon et al., 2002). Family history may be important. Routine laboratory tests are seldom of specific value in differential diagnoses; however, in suspected or ascertained cases of hypertrophic cardiomyopathy molecular genetic testing may be relevant. Alcohol or drugs may unmask pathology and trigger syncope in cardiac disease such as the Brugada syndrome (Rossenbacker and Priori, 2007).

Supine and standing blood pressure should be examined after 5 minutes of supine position, and after 1–5 minutes of standing. Delayed measurements for more than 10 minutes after rising may sometimes be warranted (Consensus Committee, 1996). Heart murmur, differences in blood pressure between extremities, scarring after gastric surgery (dumping syndrome), etc. may be relevant for diagnosis. Clinical neurological examination may be warranted in elderly patients in order to diagnose Parkinson's disease, multiple system atrophy, autonomic neuropathy, or other conditions predisposing for syncope.

Carotid sinus massage

Carotid sinus massage with continuous ECG and blood pressure monitoring is indicated in patients with syncope occurring during neck turning or in patients aged over 40 years with syncope of unknown etiology after the initial evaluation. Pressure is applied at the side of the common carotid bifurcation, and a ventricular pause over 3 seconds or more and a fall in systolic blood pressure of 50 mmHg or more is considered abnormal (Brignole et al., 2001).

Electrocardiography, including long-term ECG monitoring

An initial ECG is commonly normal in patients with syncope, whereas a pathological baseline ECG is an independent predictor of cardiac syncope and increased mortality risk (Brignole et al., 2001). In some conditions, such as the Romano–Ward syndrome, it is important to perform exercise ECG. Noninvasive or even invasive monitoring is indicated when the initial evaluation suggests an arrhythmic cause of syncope.

Echocardiography

In patients with suspected heart disease or palpitations associated with syncope, echocardiography is indicated, and may contribute to stratify the risk.

Tilt testing

Although procedures may vary, a tilting to an angle of 60° for 45–60 minutes is applied and may lead to hypotension and/or bradycardia. In patients with no response after a defined time interval (e.g., a minimum of 20 min and maximum of 45 min), intravenous isoproterenol or isoprenaline or sublingual nitroglycerine can be given for additional provocation. The drug phase should last for 15–20 minutes. The endpoint is defined as induction of syncope. Testing is warranted in single unexplained syncopal episodes in high-risk settings or in recurrent episodes in the absence of obvious cardiac disease. Tilt testing may be useful not only as a discriminator of transient LOC, but also for therapy in the form of tilt training (daily tilting to a 60° angle until syncope or a maximum of 45–90 min) (Petkar and Fitzpatrick, 2008).

EEG in syncope

As syncope may be diagnosed during video-EEG monitoring, it is worth mentioning that syncope classically is associated with an attenuation or loss of electrocerebral activity (Aminoff et al., 1988). The EEG may be flat or associated with movement artifacts or muscle artifacts (i.e., during phases of atonia (head dropping, etc.) or tonic muscle activity).

ESTABLISHING A DIAGNOSIS

A detailed history, physical examination, supine and upright blood pressure measurements, and standard ECG comprise the initial diagnostic workup (Linzer et al., 1997; Brignole et al., 2001). Subsequently, cardiology examinations with long-term ECG, echocardiography, and tilt testing with isoproterenol or nitroglycerine may follow.

DIFFERENTIAL DIAGNOSES

Strictly speaking, conditions causing transient LOC are the major differential diagnoses, such as epileptic seizures, hypoglycemia, basilar migraine, and, rarely, transient ischemic attacks.

Many conditions may, however, mimic a syncope or epileptic LOC, such as cataplexy, a fall due to alcohol intoxication, various psychogenic conditions with anxiety, panic, conversion, or somatization disorders.

TREATMENT

Treatment of syncope depends on the nature of the underlying cause, and thus the establishment of a correct diagnosis.

In cardiac syncope, arrhythmias may be treated with drugs, different cardiac pacemaker therapies, transcatheter ablation, etc., and in structural disease revascularization procedures or corrective surgery are appropriate treatments.

In neurally mediated reflex syncopal syndromes, tilt training may be performed, or drugs may be added, such as beta-blockers (e.g., metoprolol – although this drug may not be effective in preventing vasovagal or neurally mediated reflex syncope) (Sutton, 2007). First-line treatment in vasovagal syncope with prodromal symptoms may be simple counterpressure maneuvers such as leg crossing, hand gripping, arm tensing, etc. In some patients, increased fluid and salt intake may help.

Isolated vasovagal syncope may not need specific treatment or any restrictions of driving. Recurrent syncope may need specific treatment, or prevention of specific triggering stimuli. In such cases, tilt-training techniques may be applied or beta-blockers used, although several trials of such medication have been negative (Sutton, 2007). Specifically, antihypertensive or other medication may be stopped or modified. In some patients, cardiac pacing may be a key treatment (Sutton, 2007). Most important for treatment is a correct diagnosis, but in the present context one should remember that epilepsy and syncope of various causes may coexist.

CASE EXAMPLES

Case 1

An 18-year-old man woke up at high altitude and experienced impaired vision and amnesia for a 45-minute period together with disorientation, headache, and nausea. He was admitted to hospital, but discharged with a diagnosis of a probable stress reaction. Two months later he was readmitted with five complex partial seizures (CPS) with visual hallucinations including flashes in the left visual hemifield, and a continuous bilateral frontal headache. Computed tomography (CT) revealed a possible right temporal–occipital tumor, although subsequent magnetic resonance imaging revealed this to be right temporal–occipital heterotopy (Fig. 18.1A). In 2003, seizure frequency increased despite treatment with carbamazepine. At least one episode was accompanied by a fall and was considered to be a possible atonic seizure or syncope. Seizures occurred with a frequency of once a week to once every second week. A video-EEG analysis was performed (Fig. 18.1B,C), and revealed a clear epileptic seizure during which the patient developed asystole (Fig. 18.1C). Retrospective evaluation of the history suggested that he had had other syncopal episodes, and he was treated with a pacemaker. CPS and a few generalized tonic–clonic seizures persisted, but the patient's syncopal events disappeared.

Case 2

A 70-year-old, previously healthy man suddenly experienced numbness of his left arm and fingers followed by 10–15 minutes loss of power in the left arm. CT revealed a right, medially situated parietal(-frontal) meningioma. The tumor was surgically removed, leaving the patient with a mild left-sided hemiplegia and minor seizures considered to be somatosensory, with jacksonian march. He was treated with lamotrigine, developed an exanthematous reaction, and was switched to oxcarbazepine. He continued to have focal sensory seizures and a few probable atonic seizures of the left side. Once he had a left-sided dystonic seizure. Impaired motor performance in the patient's left hand following the sensory seizures curtailed the patient's abilities to play the piano. Some of his seizures developed after showering in hot water. He had a "drop attack" or syncope 6 months after an increase in the oxcarbazepine dose, and had persisting episodic sensory symptoms. Subsequently, the patient was seizure-free for 2 years, until he developed classical symptoms of a cardiac infarction with T-wave elevation in V3–V6. The oxcarbazepine dosage was increased and he had no focal sensory symptoms or convulsive seizures, but was readmitted to hospital after two episodes of suspected syncope. ECG revealed a total AV block and the patient was given a pacemaker. Since then he has been free of episodes of transient LOC, although the EEG still shows focal medial parietal epileptic activity.

DISCUSSION

Although syncope is an important differential diagnosis for epilepsy, both conditions may coexist (see Fig. 18.1B, C). Treatment with anticonvulsant drugs may even be a precipitating factor, as witnessed in a patient with a defective Purkinje fiber system, who developed ventricular asystole and subsequent Adams–Stokes attacks

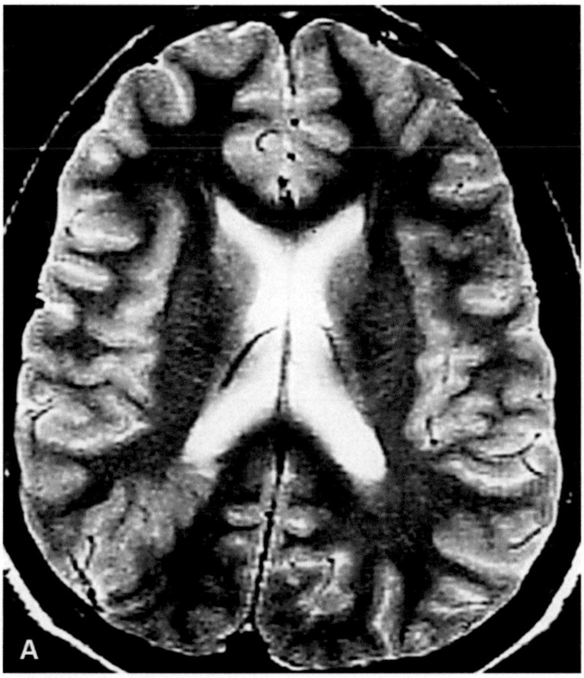

Fig. 18.1. (A) Magnetic resonance imaging (MRI) scan of the patient in Case 1.

Continued

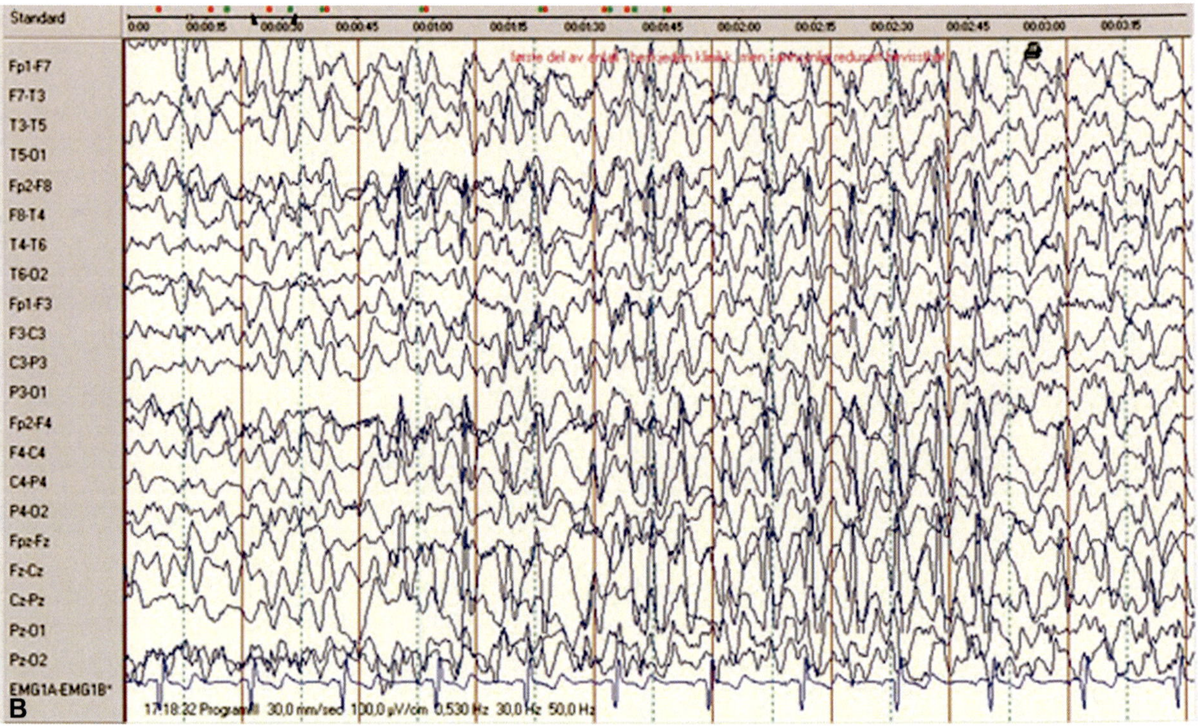

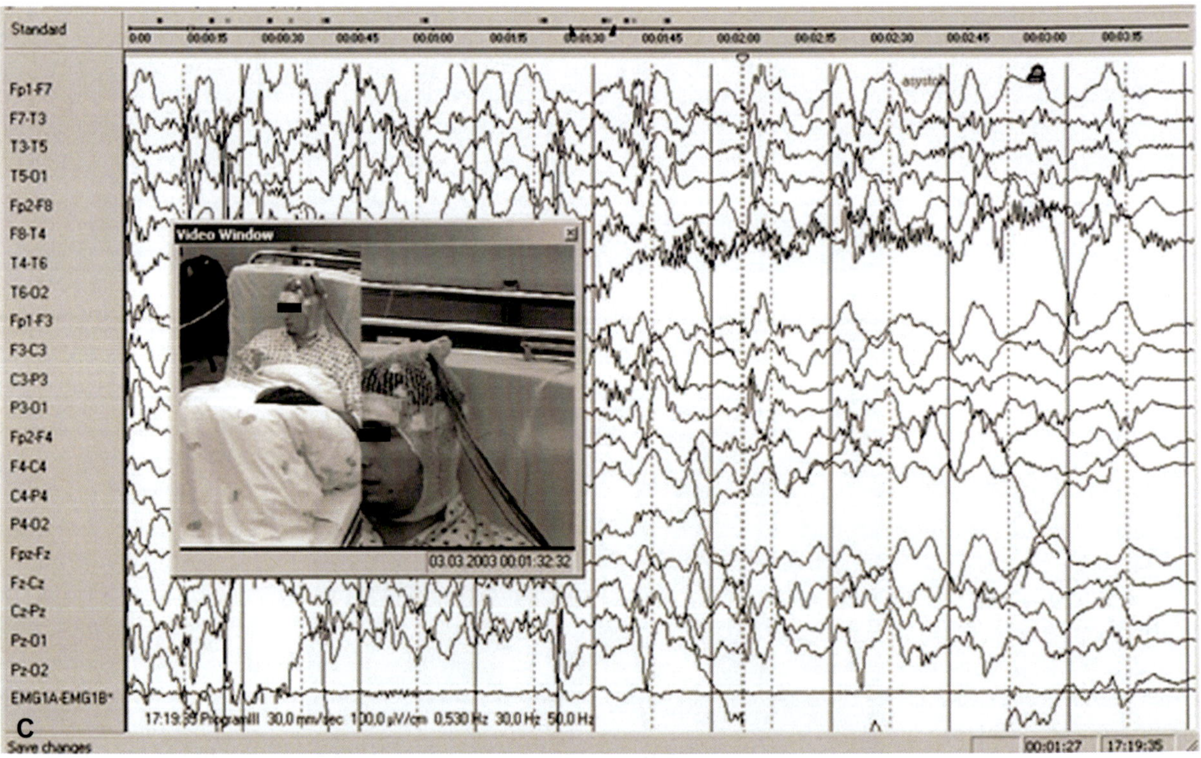

Figure 18.1—cont'd (**B**) The patient had simple partial and complex partial seizures every second week, 10–20% with distinct simple formed visual hallucinations. Some seizures were described as being combined with an inability to "store memory" (CPS?). The figure shows the initial epileptic activity in a CPS developing into an asystolic EEG (2/0613/03). (**C**) Tonic extension of the neck during asystole of duration 20 seconds, starting approximately 1 minute after seizure initiation (EEG 2/0613/03).

following treatment with carbamazepine (Beermann et al., 1975; Hamilton, 1978).

The most important element in the management of patients with syncope is risk stratification based on correct diagnosis. Isolated neurogenic syncope is associated with a good prognosis, whereas cardiac syncope often has a worse prognosis and can even result in sudden death (Kapoor, 1990). Studies in the 1980s showed a 1-year mortality rate in patients with cardiac syncope of 18–33%, whereas the mortality rate in patients with a noncardiac cause was 0–12% and the rate in those with unexplained syncope was 6% (Brignole et al., 2001). The most important risk factors appear to be age over 45 years, a history of congestive heart failure or ventricular arrhythmia, and abnormal ECG (Martin et al., 1997). Thus, if a cardiac etiology for syncopal events is suspected, rigorous diagnostic workup is warranted. As well as a thorough medical history, ECG is the best screening test to detect a cardiac cause of syncope, being diagnostic in 30% of arrhythmias (Kapoor, 1990). The author advocates aggressive diagnostic workup in patients with serious symptoms, including falls with physical injury, or where occupational hazards are present. Repeated tilt testing may be required, although even tilt tests may have variable sensitivity and specificity (Strickberger et al., 2006; Petkar and Fitzpatrick, 2008). In cases of suspected orthostatic syncope, delaying blood pressure testing for 10 minutes or more, or the use of tilt testing, may be warranted, because delayed orthostatic hypotension may occur in more than 50% of patients with milder abnormalities of sympathetic adrenergic function (Gibbons and Freeman, 2006). EEG is not warranted as a routine screen in syncope (Linzer et al., 1997). Cerebrovascular investigations are generally not indicated in patients with syncope, with the exception of patients with suspected subclavian, or other, steal syndromes.

So, how does one know that transient LOC in a syncopal event is not a seizure? Prodromal symptoms, the context of the transient LOC, brief motor symptoms, rapid recovery without amnesia, or postictal confusion of less than 30 seconds in duration would suggest a syncope. However, if the patient is kept upright more pronounced motor symptoms may occur, and if a patient falls to the ground or against a hard object various degrees of concussion with amnesia or confusion may be present.

Important differential diagnoses are epileptic seizures, migraine, cataplexy, hypoglycemia, drug effects or intoxication, hypocapnia or hyperventilation, and, importantly, panic disorder and conversion or somatization disorders. Transient ischemic attacks may very rarely cause transient LOC.

Patients with seizures are more likely to have had tongue biting, bedwetting, prodromal *déjà vu*, preoccupation, mood changes, and hallucinations or trembling before transient LOC, and postictal confusion, muscle pain, headache, head turning, cyanosis, and observed convulsive movements during syncope. Bladder emptying may occur with LOC of any cause and is a poor differentiator of syncope and seizure. Patients with syncope are more likely to experience symptoms such as diaphoresis, dyspnea, chest pain, palpitations, warmth,

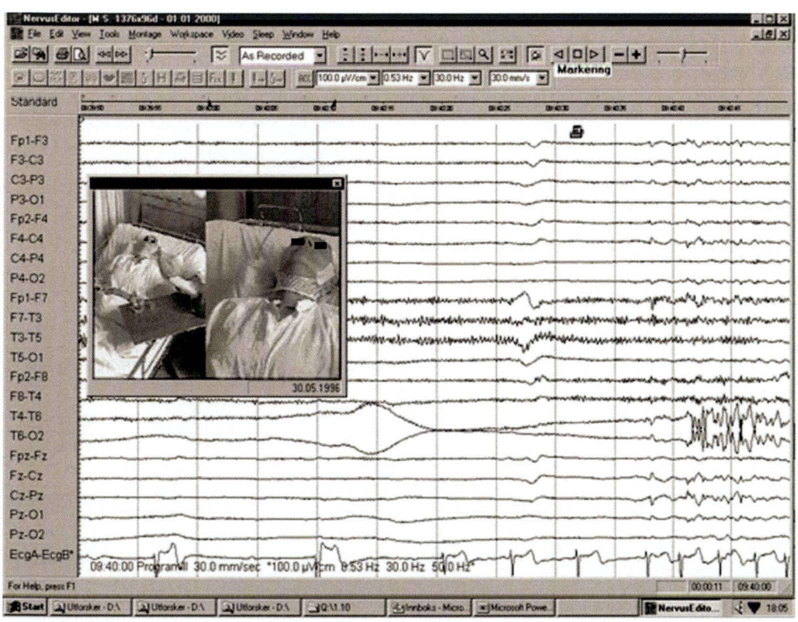

Fig. 18.2. Loss of electrocerebral activity in EEG during a 20-second asystole, with tonic extension of the neck and muscle artifacts in EEG. Cerebral EEG activity gradually recurs, as does heart frequency.

nausea, vertigo, and "presyncope" symptoms prior to a spell (Sheldon et al., 2002).

CONCLUSION

Close observation or a thorough medical history will often allow good differentiation between an epileptic seizure and syncope. The most important prognostic risk stratification is the establishment of any underlying specific cause, notably cardiac disease. When in doubt, the author has a low threshold for video-EEG monitoring (Fig. 18.2) and additional tests such as tilt-table testing.

ACKNOWLEDGMENT

The author would like to thank Dr. Bjørn Karlsen, M.D., for video-EEG analyses.

REFERENCES

Aminoff MC, Schenman MM, Griffin JC et al. (1988). Electrocerebral accompaniments of syncope associated with malignant ventricular arrhythmias. Ann Intern Med 108: 791–796.

Beermann B, Edhag O, Vallin H (1975). Advanced heart block aggravated by carbamazepine. Br Heart J 37: 668–671.

Benditt DG, Brignole M, Raviele A et al. (Eds.), (2007). Syncope and Transient Loss of Consciousness: Multidisciplinary Management. Blackwell Publishing, Oxford.

Blanc J-J (2007). Definition and classification of syncope and transient loss of consciousness. In: DG Benditt, M Brignole, A Raviele et al. (Eds.), Syncope and Transient Loss of Consciousness: Multidisciplinary Management. Blackwell Publishing, Oxford, pp. 3–7.

Blanc J-J, L'Her C, Touiza A et al. (2002). Prospective evaluation and outcome of patients admitted for syncope over a 1 year period. Eur Heart J 23: 815–820.

Bleck TP (1997). Syncope. In: J Engel Jr, TA Pedley (Eds.), Epilepsy: A Comprehensive Textbook. Lippincott-Raven, Philadelphia, pp. 2649–2659.

Brignole M, Alboni P, Benditt DG et al. Task Force on Syncope, European Society of Cardiology (2001). Guidelines on management (diagnosis and treatment) of syncope. Eur Heart J 22: 1256–1306.

Colman N, Nahm K, Ganzeboom KS et al. (2004). Epidemiology of reflex syncope. Clin Auton Res 14: 9–17.

Consensus Committee of the American Autonomic Society and the American Academy of Neurology (1996). Consensus statement on the definition of orthostatic hypotension, pure autonomic failure and multiple system atrophy. Neurology 46: 1470.

Day SC, Cook EF, Funkenstein H et al. (1982). Evaluation and outcome of emergency room patients with transient loss of consciousness. Am J Med 73: 15–23.

Dermkasian G, Lamb LE (1958). Syncope in a population of healthy young adults. JAMA 168: 1200–1207.

Gibbons CH, Freeman R (2006). Delayed orthostatic hypotension. A frequent cause of orthostatic intolerance. Neurology 67: 28–32.

Hamilton DV (1978). Carbamazepine and heart block. Lancet 1: 1365.

Kapoor WN (1990). Evaluation and outcome of patients with syncope. Medicine 69: 160–175.

Kapoor WN, Hanusa BH (1996). Is syncope a risk factor for poor outcomes? Comparison of patients with and without syncope. Am J Med 100: 646–655.

Kapoor W, Peterson J, Wieand HS et al. (1987). Diagnostic and prognostic implications of recurrences in patients with syncope. Am J Med 83: 700–708.

Lempert T, Bauer M, Schmidt D (1994). Syncope: a videometric analysis of 56 episodes of transient cerebral hypoxia. Ann Neurol 36: 233–237.

Linzer M, Yang EH, Mark Estes NA, III et al. (1997). Clinical guideline: Diagnosing syncope: Part 1: Value of history, physical examination, and electrocardiography. Ann Intern Med 126: 989–996.

Martin TP, Hanusa BH, Kapoor WN (1997). Risk stratification of patients with syncope. Ann Emerg Med 29: 459–466.

Petkar S, Fitzpatrick A (2008). Tilt-table testing: transient loss of consciousness discriminator or epiphenomenon? Europace 10: 747–750.

Rossen R, Kabat H, Anderson JP (1943). Acute arrest of cerebral circulation in man. Arch Neurol Psychiatry 50: 510–528.

Rossenbacker T, Priori SG (2007). The Brugada syndrome. Curr Opin Cardiol 22: 163–170.

Savage DD, Corwin L, McGee DL et al. (1985). Epidemiologic features of isolated syncope: the Framingham study. Stroke 16: 626–629.

Sheldon R, Killam S (1992). Methodology of isoproterenol-tilt table testing in patients with syncope. J Am Coll Cardiol 19: 773–779.

Sheldon RS, Serletis A (2007). Epidemiologic aspects of transient loss of consciousness/syncope. In: DG Benditt, M Brignole, A Raviele et al. (Eds.), Syncope and Transient Loss of Consciousness: Multidisciplinary Management. Blackwell Publishing, Oxford, pp. 8–14.

Sheldon R, Rose S, Ritchie D et al. (2002). Historical criteria that distinguish syncope from seizures. J Am Coll Cardiol 40: 142–148.

Soteriades ES, Evans JC, Larson MG et al. (2002). Incidence and prognosis of syncope. N Engl J Med 347: 878–885.

Strickberger SA, Benson DW, Biaggioni I et al. (2006). AHA/ACCF scientific statement on the evaluation of syncope. Circulation 113: 316–327.

Sutton R (2007). Treatment strategies in neurally-mediated reflex syncope: effectiveness of drugs, pacing and physical maneuvers. In: DG Benditt, M Brignole, A Raviele et al. (Eds.), Syncope and Transient Loss of Consciousness: Multidisciplinary Management. Blackwell Publishing, Oxford, pp. 83–88.

Handbook of Clinical Neurology, Vol. 107 (3rd series)
Epilepsy, Part I
H. Stefan and W.H. Theodore, Editors

Chapter 19

Sleep and epilepsy

PÉTER HALÁSZ*
Department of Neurology, National Institute of Neuroscience, Budapest, Hungary

INTRODUCTION

It is well known that ictal and interictal epileptic manifestations have a complex relationship with sleep. Several studies have tried to search for correlations between epilepsy syndrome characteristics or seizure localization and their modulation by different states of vigilance (Dinner and Lüders, 2001; Mendez and Radtke, 2001; Bazil, 2002; Foldvary-Schaefer and Grigg-Damberger, 2006). It has become more and more evident that epileptic events are modulated on one hand by the ongoing vigilance state (tonic influence), and on the other hand by arousal-related dynamic changes (phasic influence). Analysis of the microstructure of sleep by detection of phasic events, the cyclic alternating pattern (CAP), and frequency specific sleep oscillations has made it possible to study the relationship of interictal epileptiform discharges (IEDs) and seizures with arousal-dependent dynamic changes of sleep (Parrino et al., 2000).

Epilepsies reflect abnormalities of neuronal networks related more or less to functional brain systems (Spencer, 2002). These networks show a strong correlation with neuronal circuits underlying the sleep process and sleep oscillations. Several cortical association areas and subcortical structures responsible for cognitive functions overlap with these epilepsy and sleep circuits. Accordingly, epileptic manifestations in sleep may be associated with cognitive dysfunction as well.

This chapter explores the intimate relationship between epilepsy and sleep in idiopathic generalized epilepsy (IGE) as an example of an epileptic alteration of the thalamocortical network; in Lennox–Gastaut syndrome (LGS), showing early involvement of the thalamocortical network; in the perisylvian epileptic network as a continuum of rolandic epilepsy with centrotemporal spikes–Landau–Kleffner syndrome (RECTS–LKS) and electrical status epilepticus in sleep (ESES), syndromes in the temporolimbic network; and in nocturnal frontal lobe epilepsy (NFLE), representing the anterior frontomediobasal epileptic network (Fig. 19.1).

From a practical point of view, sleep provides an excellent diagnostic tool to activate epileptic interictal and ictal manifestations. Another aim of the chapter is to show the specific sleep profiles of different epileptic manifestations and to provide guidance on how to use sleep in evaluation of epilepsy.

SEIZURE AND SPIKE PROPENSITY IN RELATION TO REM AND NREM SLEEP STAGES IN DIFFERENT EPILEPSIES

The relationship between sleep and epilepsy covers two related aspects: ictal (seizures and ictal EEG) and interictal (EEG) manifestations.

Nonrapid eye movement (NREM) sleep permits, and sometimes promotes, generalized tonic–clonic seizures (GTCS), promotes complex partial seizures (CPS) in mesial temporal lobe epilepsy (MTLE) (mildly) and in frontal lobe epilepsy (FLE) (strongly); seizures of benign *focal childhood epilepsies,* tonic axial seizures in LGS and focal interictal discharges, especially in MTLE and rolandic epilepsy, as well as generalized paroxysmal fast activity (GPFA). Extension and spread of discharges are facilitated, including interhemispheric transmission. Expression of suppression burst activity of infantile epilepsies is also increased by NREM sleep. Rapid eye movement (REM) sleep permits complex partial seizures in MTLE and interictal discharges in temporal lobe and extratemporal lobe epilepsies (Mendez and Radtke, 2001; Bazil, 2002; Foldvary-Schaefer and Grigg-Damberger, 2006).

The awake state permits every type of seizure, promotes complex partial seizures in MTLE, inhibits complex partial seizures in FLE, and tonic axial seizures in LGS.

*Correspondence to: Péter Halász, M.D., Ph.D., D.Sci., Institute of Experimental Medicine, Hungarian Academy of Sciences, 1026 Budapest, Lotz K. Street, 18 Budapest, Hungary. Tel: +3670 370 8401, Fax: +361 200 8610, E-mail: halasz35@gmail.com

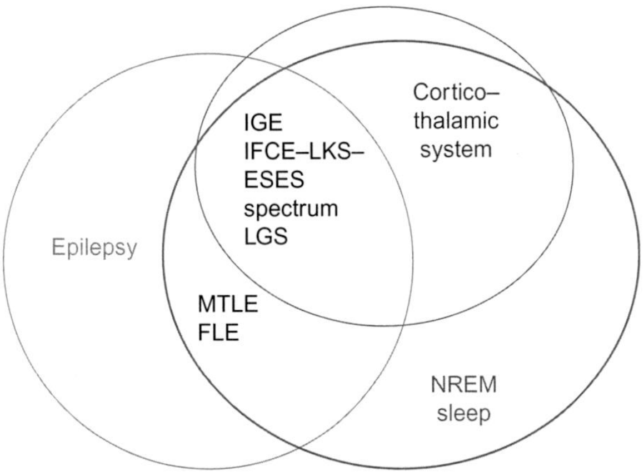

Fig. 19.1. Relationships of the epilepsies considered in this chapter, activated by nonrapid eye movement (NREM) sleep, with and without involvement of the thalamocortical system. ESES, electrical status epilepticus in sleep; FLE, frontal lobe epilepsy; IFCE, idiopathic focal childhood epilepsy; IGE, idiopathic generalized epilepsy; LGS, Lennox–Gastaut syndrome; LKS, Landau–Kleffner syndrome; MTLE, mesial temporal lobe epilepsy.

Transition from awake and REM sleep toward NREM sleep, and vice versa, promotes, in IGE, various absence-type seizures, myoclonic seizures in juvenile myoclonic epilepsy (JME) and awakening GTCS, and infantile spasms in West syndrome (Tables 19.1–19.3).

The work of the Steriade group has shown systemically that NREM sleep is characterized by a synchronous thalamocortical bursting mode, whereby discharges of cortical neurons are highly synchronized, driven by the

Table 19.1

Seizure propensity in different vigilance states

	Awake	NREM	REM	TRANS
Generalized tonic–clonic	+	+		?
Complex partial, FLE	+	+++		
Complex partial, TLE	+	+	+	
Simple partial, RECTS	+	+++		
Tonic axial	+	+++		
Infantile spasm	++	+		+?
Absence	+	+ (?stage 1)		+++
Myoclonic	+			+++

FLE, frontal lobe epilepsy; RECTS, rolandic epilepsy with centrotemporal spikes; TLE, temporal lobe epilepsy; TRANS, transitional states between awake, nonrapid eye movement (NREM) and rapid eye movement (REM) sleep.

Table 19.2

Propensity of displaying different types of interictal epileptiform discharges in vigilance states

	Awake	NREM	REM	TRANS
TLE spike	++	+++	+	
ETLE spike	+	+	+	
GSWD	++	++		++
Absence-like SW	+			+++
GPFA	+	+++		
Suppression burst discharges	+	+++		
ESES		+++		

ESES, electrical status epilepticus in sleep; ETLE, extratemporal lobe epilepsy; GPFA, generalized paroxysmal fast activity; GSWD, generalized spike–wave discharge; SW, spike–wave; TLE, temporal lobe epilepsy; TRANS, transitional states between awake, nonrapid eye movement (NREM) and rapid eye movement (REM) sleep.

γ-aminobutyric acid (GABA)ergic gating machine of the nucleus reticularis thalami (Steriade, 2003). This working mode provides, depending on the degree of hyperpolarization of thalamic cell membranes, lasting spindling and delta oscillations throughout wide bilateral fields of the cortical mantle belonging to association cortex. These synchronous synaptic effects, regardless of their excitatory or inhibitory nature, augment the amplitude and propagation possibilities of every postsynaptic response promoting epileptic discharges. All the influences that synchronize the EEG promote the appearance of IEDs (Shouse et al., 2004).

Research starting in the last decade of the 20th century provided convincing evidence that high-frequency oscillation (HFO) within the 200–500-Hz range is related topographically to the seizure onset zone (SOZ), during both interictal and preictal periods (Akiyama et al., 2005; Worrell et al., 2008; Khosravani et al., 2009). Congruently, surgical removal of the SOZ where HFOs were localized resulted in good seizure control (Khosravani et al., 2009; Jacobs et al., 2010). Thus, HFO increasingly became a surrogate marker of epilepsy. HFO activity proved to be maximal during slow-wave sleep (upstates) (Grenier et al., 2001; Staba et al., 2004; Worrell et al., 2008), and this provides an additional powerful explanation for the activation and distribution of epileptic discharges in sleep and for seizure and discharge-promoting effect of NREM sleep. In contrast, REM sleep is characterized by desynchronized EEG, and is not conducive to the initiation and propagation of epileptic discharges.

However, the possibility of motor seizure manifestations during sleep depends on the excitatory–inhibitory balance on the motor neurons in different sleep stages. The well-known downstream inhibition of motor

Table 19.3

Influence of vigilance states on syndrome-dependent interictal epileptiform discharges (IEDs)

	Awake seizure	Awake IED	NREM seizure	NREM IED	REM seizure	REM IED
IGE/absence	++	++	+++ (stage 1–2)	+++	–	–
IGE/awakening GTC	++ (around awakening	+	–	+	–	–
IGE/JME	++ (morning)	±+	–	+++ (around awakening	–	–
MTLE	++ (GTC < CP)	+	++ (GTC > CP)	+++	+	+
NFLE	–	±	+++	±	–	–
Partial epilepsy	+	+	+	++	+	+
IFCE	–	+	++	+++	–	+
LKS/ESES	–	++	–	++++	–	+
LGS	++	++	+++	++++	–	–
West syndrome	++ (around awakening)	++	++	+++	+	+

CP, complex partial seizure; ESES, electrical status epilepticus in sleep; GTC, generalized tonic–clonic seizures; IED, interictal epileptiform discharges; IFCE, idiopathic focal childhood epilepsies; IGE, idiopathic generalized epilepsy; JME, juvenile generalized myoclonic epilepsy; LGS, Lennox–Gastaut syndrome; LKS, Landau–Kleffner syndrome; MTLE, medial temporal lobe epilepsy; NFLE, frontal lobe epilepsy, prefrontal, basomedial origin.

Table 19.4

Physiological factors of seizure propensity in different vigilance states (after Shouse et al., 2004)

	NREM	REM	Awake
Cortical afferentation	Synchronized sigma/delta oscillation in thalamocortical system [+++]	Ventral type cholinergic reticular activation (asynchronous cellular discharges)[‡]	Diffuse cholinergic reticular activation (asynchronous cellular discharges)[‡]
Efferent muscular innervation	Diminished muscular tone*	Loss of muscular tone (active inhibition)[†]	Full muscular tone*
Aminergic system	Diminished cortical innervation	Loss of cortical innervation [+] (?)	Full cortical innervation

[+]Factor promoting epileptiform discharge
*factor allowing seizure
[†]factor inhibiting motor seizure manifestation
[‡]factor inhibiting epileptiform discharge.

neurons by brainstem structures and the absence of antigravitational muscle tone contributes to limitation of the motor manifestations of epileptic seizures during REM sleep. During NREM sleep, postural muscle tone is not entirely absent, although diminished, allowing manifestations of GTCS and other motor seizures (Table 19.4).

In NREM sleep beyond the sleep phases, the CAP and arousal-related phasic responses represent further changes, with a proven dynamic influence on the appearance and distribution of epileptiform discharges and seizures (Parrino et al., 2000). Mounting evidence is showing that cortical slow and infraslow oscillations (up-and-down states) provide cyclic regulation of cortical excitability, creating gates for epileptiform activity (Vanhatalo et al., 2004; Csercsa et al., 2010).

SLEEP ACTIVATION IN EPILEPTIC NETWORKS AND SYNDROMES

Idiopathic generalized epilepsies and the thalamocortical network

Seizures, EEG, and vigilance

The three different types of seizure within the IGE spectrum show different relationships to vigilance level:

- *Absences* occur in the awake state, promoted by monotonous, drowsy periods, clustering around awakening in the morning, before going to sleep in the evening, and postlunch dips. Their occurrence increases in transitional periods between the waking state, NREM and REM sleep.
- *GTCS* may occur in every state, but are promoted by transitions from NREM sleep to awakening, or immediately after awakening. GTCS are often preceded by absence-type spike–wave discharge series. In the tonic phase of GTCS, wave components break down and are replaced by continuous spiking.
- *Myoclonic seizures* are most common after morning awakening (Dinner and Lüders, 2001). Synchronously with the jerks, polyspike discharges, terminated by a slow-wave component, occur.

The EEG of the three seizure manifestations appears to reflect the degree of depolarization of pyramidal cells; in absences, recurrent waves ensure inhibition with no, or only minor, motor symptoms. During the myoclonic jerks, excitation increases above the threshold of pyramidal output, but upcoming inhibition interrupts further excitation. During GTCS, recurrent inhibition does not continue and there is continuous pyramidal cell excitation.

Epileptic phenomena related to sleep EEG features

Generalized spike–wave (GSW) activity is a well-known common EEG marker in all forms of IGE. However, the morphology of GSW activity is not uniform and shows some syndrome-specific characteristics. There is a very close relationship between the level of vigilance and the expression of spike–wave paroxysms. Absence-type ictal discharges appear in the wake state, in the transitional states between wakefulness and NREM sleep, and in the transitions between NREM and REM sleep.

The ictal type of discharge seems to be inhibited by full REM sleep and by the aroused awake state (Halász and Dévényi, 1974). While falling asleep, moving across different stages of NREM sleep, characteristic transformations are seen in the morphology of GSW activity (Ross et al., 1966; Kotagal, 2001). The awake-like pure absence-type regular 3-Hz paroxysms are present or even activated by somnolence and stage 1. In stage 2, fragmentation and distortion of the regular pattern begins: paroxysms become shorter and the regular sequence of spikes and waves is less clear. In stages 3 and 4, only fragments of the spike–wave series are present, but these may have higher amplitude and sharper or more abundant spike components compared with the awake counterpart, and may be more frequent. In some cases they form groups, interrupted only by short periods of background activity.

In JME, the multiple spike–wave groups show less morphological variability and their distribution during different states of vigilance is more uniform, except for transitions from NREM sleep to wakefulness, especially during morning awakening, when their frequency increases.

In other patients with IGE without absences and myoclonic jerks, usually with rare GTCS, the amount of GSW activity may be small and limited to the awakening period of a whole night's sleep record. The specific diagnostic features (GSW discharges in sleep) are frequently missed by the routine use of short sleeps after sleep deprivation. In these patients, EEG diagnosis is especially difficult because the waking state is frequently free of discharges.

Relationship of interictal GSW discharges with sleep phasic events

Another interesting aspect is the strong link of GSW activity with phasic events in superficial NREM sleep.

If sensory stimuli applied in NREM sleep – usually in stage 2 – elicit GSW discharge, this is linked with the "synchronization type" (K-complexes, spindles, and delta waves) reaction and never with the "desynchronization type" (decrease in amplitude and increase in frequency response), identical with the *phase d'activation transitoire* of the Strasburg group (Halász, 1991a; Halász et al., 2004a).

The association of GSW activity with synchronization-type oscillations in NREM sleep was further confirmed by studies based on the CAP phenomenon. The occurrence of GSW discharges in patients with IGE was shown to be linked to the synchronized part (containing slow waves, K-complexes) of the CAP oscillation (linked to the so-called A phase) (Terzano et al., 2000). Later, once the A phase had been separated into A1, A2, and A3 types (Parrino et al., 2000), further studies showed a strong link to A1 phase but not to the A3 phase (Halász et al., 2002b).

Delineation of the epileptic network

Delineation of the network basis of the IGE, or more specifically the absence type of IGE, has a long story. Gloor and coworkers proposed a "mild cortical excitatory state" by which the thalamic impulses produced in normal situation spindles evokes GSW activity. According to the original suggestion of Gloor et al. (1990), elaborated later by Kostopoulos (2000), the transformation of sleep spindling into a 3-Hz spike–wave pattern is the main assumed mechanism in the generation of GSW activity, shown in cats by Steriade et al. (1994). The pharmacological block of $GABA_A$ receptors in ferret geniculate slices results in the transformation of spindle waves into paroxysmal activity, such that both thalamocortical and perigeniculate neurons have a greatly increased intensity of burst discharges and become phase-locked into a 2–4-Hz rhythm (von Krosigk et al., 1993; Bal et al., 1995a, b). Bal et al. (1995a, b) suggested that this shift from normal to paroxysmal activity resulted from the disinhibition of perigeniculate neurons, resulting in increased discharges of these cells and a large increase in the postsynaptic activation of $GABA_B$ receptors in thalamocortical neurons (see Huguenard and Prince, 1994; Sanchez-Vives et al., 1995). GSW activity seems to share a common substrate with NREM sleep phasic events, in the bursting mode action of thalamocortical networks. The role of the cortex in initiating seizures has also become more and more convincing (Meeren et al., 2005).

The thalamocortical network in the awake state serves to transmit sensory inflow to the cortex (relay function). During NREM sleep, owing to GABAergic inhibition by the reticular thalamic nuclei, this kind of transmission suffers disruption. The network oscillates between cortical facilitation and dysfacilitation (bursting mode) (Steriade, 2003). Cortical sleep oscillations, including sigma (sleep) spindles and delta activity, are the product of this bursting mode. The level of thalamic relay cell membrane hyperpolarization determines the oscillation time constant and regulates the appearance of spindles and/or delta activity.

GSW discharges seem to reflect an epileptic transformation of the physiological burst-firing mode of the thalamocortical system, and therefore GSW activity is greatly activated by NREM sleep.

Sleep deprivation increases the delta power and also the strength of reactive delta bouts (Borbely et al., 1981). This might explain why the activation propensity of GSW discharges after sleep deprivation increases so significantly.

Relation to cognitive function

Transitory cognitive deficits occur during absence seizures. The cognitive function of the cortex seems to be altered in a widespread way, including comprehension, execution of cognitive tasks, memory, sensation, and motor functions (Blumenfeld, 2005).

Recent functional imaging results providing single-photon emission computed tomography (SPECT), positron emission tomography (PET), and functional magnetic resonance imaging (fMRI) data in animal and human absences strongly support the presence of cortical disconnection during absences. In several independent studies, SPECT showed widespread cortical hypoperfusion, and fMRI also showed a widespread cortical, mainly fronto-parietal, negative blood oxygen level-dependent (BOLD) response during absences seizures (Salek-Haddadi et al., 2003; Aghakhani et al., 2004).

In cellular recordings with cortical and thalamic electrodes in animals, EEG spikes coincide with neuronal discharges, whereas during the "wave" component a dysfacilitation (lack of discharges) has been observed (Avoli et al., 1983; Steriade et al., 1994; Steriade, 2003), in good agreement with the neuroimaging observations. Thus, dysfacilitation during the wave component is probably responsible for the cortical disconnection.

Impairment of cognitive function can be graded in terms of differences among individuals and within the same individual's seizures. As discussed above, cortical dysfacilitation (disconnection) explains why sensorimotor functions and cognition are absent during an absence. In the case of myoclonic jerks, the polyspike component is overwhelming, corresponding to short cortical excitatory cycles interrupted by the wave component, again representing dysfacilitation. Owing to the shortness of events in absences and myoclonic jerks, dysfacilitation is transient and thus permanent cognitive impairment does not develop.

During interictal single or multiple GSW discharges, a transient cognitive impairment is detectable (Aarts et al., 1984; Kasteleijn-Nolst Trenite, 1995; Binnie, 1996; Fonseca et al., 2005), but these are floating, superficial events, inducing permanent disorder only if they are very frequent.

Transient cognitive impairment during absences may also be related both to cortical dysfacilitation conjoined with the wave component of GSW activity, and to distortion of the thalamic relay function for sensory transmission.

Spectrum of idiopathic focal childhood epilepsies (IFCE), Landau–Kleffner syndrome, and electrical status epilepticus in sleep

An overlap between IFCE, LKS, and ESES, creating a spectrum of disorders, is increasingly recognized. Atypical cases with transitional characteristics bearing the features of more than one syndrome, and cases showing an evolution in time between syndromes, provide evidence for this phenomenon (Nieto-Barrera et al.,

1997; Fejerman et al., 2000; Massa et al., 2000; Hahn et al., 2001; Halász et al., 2005).

Rolandic epilepsy with centrotemporal spikes

Epileptic symptoms

Nowadays, IFCE are also seen as a spectrum of epileptic disorders constituting the most frequent, genetically based, nonlesional epilepsies of childhood (Kellaway, 2000). The most well-known variant is RECTS. Seizures are characterized by sensorimotor manifestations in the face, tongue, and throat originating from the lower part of the rolandic strip, usually in sleep or at awakening. Frequent interictal focal spike–wave discharges with a wide frontotemporal projection field are a typical finding in the interictal EEG. There is great diversity in the topography of centrotemporal spikes. Patients with RECTS frequently have bilateral independent or bilateral synchronous discharges. The spikes in RECTS may be ipsilateral or contralateral to the epileptogenic hemisphere. Furthermore, discharges are frequently multifocal. Posterior variants show a shift towards more anterior fields during the course of illness, with changing clinical features (Guerrini et al., 1997). All of these observations tend to change the concept of focal epilepsy towards a more widespread, genetically based, condition of increased cortical excitability with shifting predominance, underlain by a hereditary impairment of brain maturation (Doose et al., 2000).

An important group of patients with IFCE exhibit GSW discharges modulated by sleep and arousal, similar to the GSW discharges of absence epilepsy. The occurrence of GSW bursts in RECTS has been reported by most authors as 13–40% (Beaussart, 1972; Beaumanoir et al., 1974; Dalla Bernardina et al., 1984). Degen and Degen (1990) found this pattern in 28 (65%) of 43 children with rolandic epilepsy, and GSW discharges were present in 32% of the siblings of their patients.

Underlying circuit

The semiology of seizures and the EEG mapping studies (van der Meij et al., 2001) show that both the epileptic pacemaker area and the irritative zone lie in the inner part of the sylvian fissure (Fig. 19.2).

However, the presence of GSW discharges, activated by sleep in a proportion of the children, indicates involvement of the thalamocortical system. There are some experimental studies supporting the possibility of activation limited to regional subsystems (a sector) of the thalamocortical system (Huguenard, 2000). The theory of partial involvement of thalamocortical system in RECTS helps to reconcile the differences between the partial (local spike–wave) versus generalized (generalized spike–wave) features in the EEG of patients with RECTS.

Sleep characteristics

NREM sleep characteristically increases the occurrence rate, amplitude, and distribution field of IEDs (Pan and Lüders, 2000). In some cases, the IEDs persist in REM sleep. In such cases they are restricted to the region exhibiting discharges in the awake state.

Some studies have found that maximum spike/min ratios were related to slow sleep stages, especially delta sleep, and in general to the first cycle (Clemens and Majoros, 1987). A relationship between spikes and spindle sleep was shown more than a decade ago (Nobili et al., 1999; Ferrillo et al., 2000; Kellaway, 2000).

Cognitive impairment

Neuropsychological studies of children with benign epilepsy with centrotemporal spikes (BECTS) show that in general they have normal intelligence but often have particular weaknesses in abilities localized to the anterior opercular perisylvian region: graphomotor skill, verbal expression, language comprehension, memory. These weaknesses could interfere with learning important skills at a critical period, but in the majority of children seem to be subtle and transient, disappearing in parallel with the EEG discharges (Nicolai et al., 2006; Pinton et al., 2006). The direct role of epileptic discharges during sleep in causing these transient cognitive deficits has not been proved, and another possibility is that the IEDs are trait markers of the genetic disposition underlying neuropsychological deficits as well. This possibility is supported by the increased frequency of rolandic spikes in patients with attention-deficit/hyperactivity disorder (ADHD), who display similar neuropsychological deficit profiles (Holtmann et al., 2006).

"Atypical" and transitional RECTS

In recent years several studies have described less benign, "atypical," progressive cases with seizures not responding to antiepileptic drug treatment, showing abundant bilateral spike activity during NREM sleep and cognitive deficit symptoms, and also patients with transition from RECTS to LKS and/or ESES (Deonna, 1991; Deonna and Roulet, 1995; Fejerman et al., 2000; Halász et al., 2005; Saltik et al., 2005; Fejerman, 2009; Deonna and Roulet-Perez, 2010).

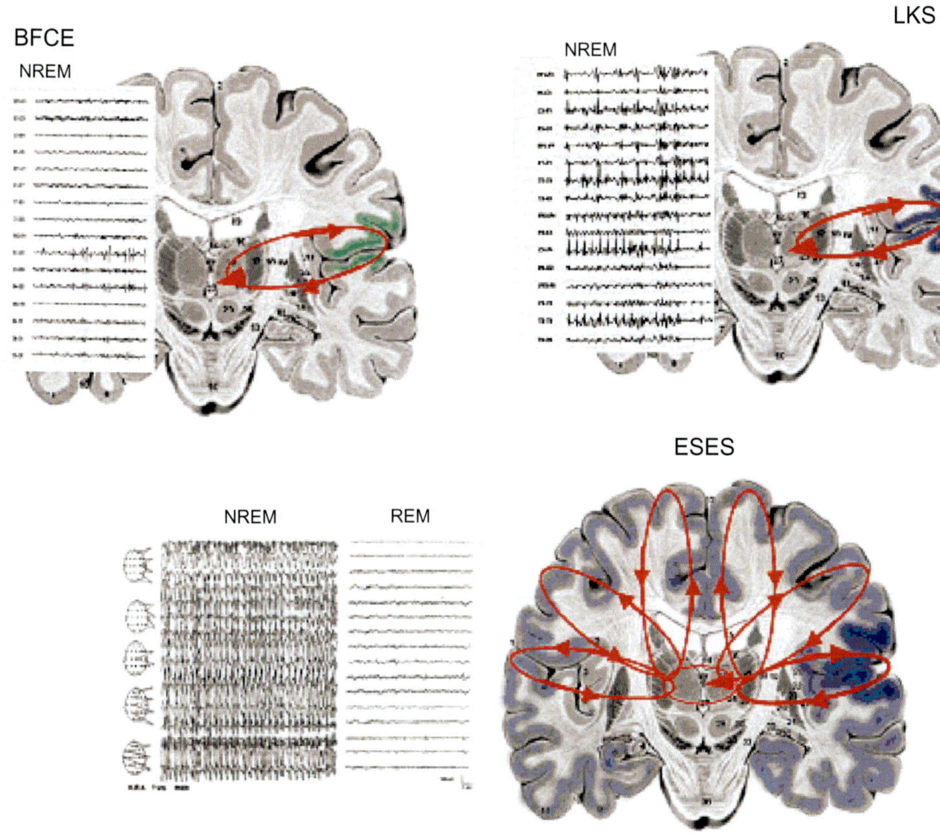

Fig. 19.2. Circuitry, epileptic, and cognitive involvement in the benign focal childhood epilepsy–Landau–Kleffner syndrome–electrical status epilepticus in sleep (BFCE–LKS–ESES) spectrum. In BFCE, only a sector of the thalamocortical system is involved (red) with perisylvian epileptic interictal and ictal symptoms and mild neuropsychological dysfunction (green). In LKS, involvement of the posterior perisylvian structures (blue), responsible for speech functions, is more severe. EEG findings, probably due to secondary bilateral synchrony, are bilateral (shown by red only on the primary side). In ESES by secondary synchrony the whole (bilateral) thalamocortical system (red) and wide associative cortical areas (blue) are involved (speech functions may or may not be altered; darker blue).

Landau–Kleffner syndrome (LKS)

Epileptic symptoms

LKS is a childhood disorder arising in previously normal children, characterized by the loss of language skills, acquired verbal auditory agnosia, multifocal spikes, and spike–wave discharges localized mainly over the centrotemporal regions, continuously or subcontinuously during sleep. Epileptic seizures (usually rare), behavioral disorders, and hyperkinesia are observed in about two-thirds of the patients. "The prognosis is favorable, with remission of seizures and EEG abnormalities before the age of 15 years" (Rossi et al., 1999). No evidence of associated focal brain lesions has been documented. In a recent review, Deonna and Roulet-Peret (2010, p.747) emphasized that "Landau–Kleffner is now seen as the rare and severe end of a spectrum of cognitive–behavioral symptoms that can be seen in idiopathic (genetic) focal epilepsies of childhood, the benign end being the more frequent typical rolandic epilepsy."

At an early stage of the disorder, unilateral IEDs are more common, resembling discharges seen in IFCE, localized to a wide area around the sylvian fissure. Bilateral "generalized" spike–wave discharges are also common. Later, bilateral focal discharges are prevalent in roughly homologous areas.

Involved circuits

In LKS, the speech disorder is related to dysfunction of the perisylvian opercular structures and/or the posterior part of the first temporal convolution. There is an important circumscribed continuous deficit of the perisylvian network, which is affected only mildly in BECTS.

Sleep activation

NREM sleep has a strong activating effect. The transition from LKS to ESES during long-term clinical and EEG follow-up has been described (Dulac et al., 1983; Hirsch et al., 1990; Marescoux et al., 1990). Usually REM sleep shows no discharges, and in all cases described no GSW discharges were present during REM sleep. Methohexital studies performed by Morrell's group (Ford et al., 1982) showed that one hemisphere is "driving" the other in bilateral discharges. There are some data suggesting that the locus of the discharges lies in the auditory cortex in the depth of the sylvian fissure (Paetau et al., 1991; Seri et al., 1998).

Sleep and cognitive profile

The most serious cognitive deficit characterizing this syndrome is the aphasic disorder, which affects children who have already developed speech. The onset may be quite abrupt; the degree of the speech disorder may fluctuate with the degree of concomitant spiking. When aphasia persists for more than 2–3 years, complete recovery is rarely seen and a proportion of patients are unable to achieve a normal social life (Massa et al., 2000). The relationship between local spiking in sleep and evolution of the aphasia is supported by the good results following surgical resection of the spiking area (Morrell et al., 1995; Massa et al., 2000).

Electrical status epilepticus in sleep (ESES)

Epileptic symptoms

This is a rare condition characterized by the following coexistent aspects: (1) ESES pattern in NREM sleep occurring in at least 85% of NREM sleep and persisting on three or more records over a period of at least 1 month; (2) cognitive impairment, in the form of global or selective regression of cognitive function; (3) motor impairment (ataxia, dyspraxia, dystonia, or unilateral pyramidal deficit); (4) rare epileptic seizures (particularly in the period of ESES) with focal and/or generalized seizures (unilateral or bilateral clonic, GTCS, and complex partial seizures or epileptic falls – tonic seizures never occur). The EEG abnormalities disappear around puberty, and the epilepsy shows a benign outcome too, but the cognitive impairment is not completely reversible in all cases, and some residual impairment remains. LKS and ESES are separate entities, but the two conditions show a wide overlap.

Involved circuit

The overlap between LKS and ESES is probably due to shared perisylvian pathology. However, the bilateral widespread EEG abnormality, mental deterioration, and behavior disorders suggest a more widespread involvement of the cortical mantle. Possibly this widespread involvement is manifest through the thalamocortical system, involving cortical association areas. The role of the thalamic structures is supported by case reports showing a relationship between particular early thalamic lesions involving the mediodorsal nucleus and ESES phenomena (Kelemen et al., 2006).

A series of Japanese studies have provided data favoring the proposal that the mechanism of ESES is secondary bilateral synchrony (Morikawa et al., 1989; Kobayashi et al., 1992), and functional neuroimaging studies in accordance with the focal clinical signs have shown local seizure activity underlying ESES (Guerrini et al., 1998).

Sleep and cognitive features

NREM sleep activation is the most characteristic feature, in the form of 1.5–2-Hz GSW discharges presenting continuously across all sleep stages, beginning immediately with the onset of NREM sleep (Michelucci et al., 1987; Veggiotti et al., 1999).

All patients exhibit severe deterioration during ESES. The pattern of cognitive impairment may differ from patient to patient; the proportion of speech dysfunction is also variable; and the type of impairment seems to depend on the localization of the field exhibiting GSW activity (Billiard et al., 1981; Tassinari et al., 1985; Roulet-Perez et al., 1993; Tassinari et al., 2001).

There is a close temporal relationship between ESES and the neuropsychological deterioration, and parallels between the duration of ESES and the neuropsychological outcome. ESES is a kind of status epilepticus leading to nonconvulsive seizure symptoms hidden in sleep, manifested repeatedly during sleep, causing prolonged interference with cognitive function (Tassinari et al., 2001).

Common features of IFCE–LKS–ESES spectrum epilepsies

All three syndromes are characterized by a transient, age-dependent, nonlesional, genetically based, epileptogenic abnormality, although ESES may develop on the basis of structural damage as well. The brain tissue responsible for the disorder is localized around the sylvian fissure, and strongly correlated with speech function and cognition (Siniatchkin et al., 2010). The interictal discharges are partially localized to this perisylvian area, and partially show different degrees of generalization and secondary bilateral synchrony. Discharges in all syndromes appear in the form of a focal or generalized spike–wave pattern. The amount and persistence of interictal discharges seems to correlate with the degree of cognitive deficit, and there is a correlation between the degree of spiking (during sleep) and the degree of cognitive deficit across syndromes.

The epileptic discharges are accompanied by a slow-wave components, associated with cognitive deficit rather than frequent seizures. This characteristic situation has been called "cognitive epilepsy." The slow-wave components of the GSW discharges may protect against conventional, sustained, depolarization-based seizures, but on the other hand interfere with normal cortical functioning. This assumption is strongly supported by several recent results showing that sleep has a use-dependent homeostatic function, connected with sleep slow-wave activity, needed for the frontal lobe plastic functions and impaired when abundant epileptic discharges interfere with it (Massimini et al., 2009; Tassinari et al., 2009).

Lennox–Gastaut syndrome (LGS) as a developmental epilepsy with early involvement of the corticothalamic system

Epileptic symptoms

LGS is an age-dependent syndrome beginning before the age of 4 years, although the upper age limit of onset is not clear. Patients may have a persistent syndrome during adulthood; there may also be a "late-onset LGS" (Lipinski, 1977; Bauer et al., 1983; Stenzel and Panteli, 1983; Roger et al., 1987).

The coexistence of several seizure types is typical. The most characteristic are tonic axial seizures occurring more frequently during NREM sleep, causing drop attacks in the awake state. Atypical absence with irregular GSW paroxysms is the other characteristic seizure form. The EEG shows frequent slow spike–wave paroxysms emerging from a slow and irregular background. Mental retardation is the rule. LGS is assumed to develop through "secondary generalization," based on early involvement of the thalamocortical network (Blume, 2001).

Involved circuits

One of the most important features of LGS is that interictal and ictal epileptic manifestations appear during brain development, suggesting that "excitation-producing etiologies and/or genetically induced aberrant cortical development and physiology during a sensitive window of enhanced epileptogenicity in the immature central nervous system induces synaptic remodeling leading to homotopic and thalamic epileptic discharge propagation and a diffuse bisynchronous epileptogenic process, with excess cortical excitation and increased cortico-thalamic oscillation" (Blume, 2001).

Sleep and cognitive features

NREM sleep importantly activates slow GSWs, but their frequency does not reach the level seen in ESES. Another very characteristic feature of NREM sleep in LGS is the presence of runs of generalized paroxysmal fast activity (GPFA). The appearance of GPFA shows a strong correlation with the third and fourth stages of NREM sleep. These runs are bilaterally synchronous, with frontal predominance; their frequency is around 10 Hz. Very frequent in NREM sleep, they never occur in REM sleep, and are rare in the awake state. Polygraphic recording reveals some ictal involvement in most of them. The most regularly observed somatic concomitant of the discharge is acceleration or deceleration of the heart and/or respiration rate, and increase of axial tone, most noticeably in the neck muscles with a slight elevation of the head and slight opening of the eyelids.

The slow GSW activity so characteristic of LGS has a frontal predominance and belongs to the category of secondary bilateral synchrony (Halász, 1991a; Ohtahara et al., 1995). This kind of pattern is believed to be the result of focal epileptic activity propagating to the contralateral hemisphere through the corpus callosum, driving widespread corticothalamic entrainment (Kobayashi et al., 1992; Ohtahara et al., 1995).

The frequent occurrence of GPFA and its morphology raises the possibility of a relationship with sleep spindles. There is a relationship between the presence of slow spike–wave discharges and GPFA. In our material, the association of GSW discharges and GPFA was more than 90% in both ictal and interictal states.

In Doose syndrome, where GPFA is not present, mental deterioration is less frequent and not so severe as in LGS (Doose, 1992a, b). Recently, we reported exceptional cases where typical paroxysmal fast activity was present without mental deterioration and intractability in difficult-to-treat patients with IGE (Halász et al., 2004b).

The influence of the frequent discharges mainly in sleep might have an effect on mental development. A possible effect could be interference with memory consolidation during NREM sleep (Peigneux et al., 2001). Distortion of physiological spindling by GPFA leading to giant pathological spindles may have a special worsening effect on memory consolidation (Clemens et al., 2005).

Epilepsy with unilateral or bilateral involvement of the temporolimbic network

Epileptic symptoms

Temporolimbic network epilepsy (TLNE) is the most frequent epilepsy type in adulthood (Wieser, 1993; Engel, 1996). The most frequent etiology is hippocampal sclerosis preceded by an "initial precipitatory insult" (atypical febrile seizure or status epilepticus) damaging the hippocampus and initiating an epileptogenic synaptic reorganization of this structure, which may lead to epilepsy only after a long interval (Mathern et al., 1996). Synaptic reorganization of the hippocampal network is a key point in the evolution of temporolimbic epilepsies (Babb et al., 1991; Maglóczky et al., 2000; Sutula and Dudek, 2007). Other frequent etiological factors are tumors (gangliogliomas, embryoplastic neuroepitheliomas, oligodendrogliomas), cortical dysgenetic malformations, cavernomas, posttraumatic and postencephalitic lesions.

Involved circuits

The main substrate of TLNE is held to be the hippocampus; however, more widespread temporal structural damage apparently plays a role (Bernasconi et al., 2004; Bernhardt et al., 2008). In the majority of patients with TLNE, interictal EEG (mainly during sleep) or other diagnostic categories (neuropsychology, MRI, fluorodeoxyglucose (FDG)-PET, MR spectroscopy, pathological workup) show bilateral involvement and frequent contralateral spread of seizures.

Sleep and cognitive impairment

Temporal lobe epilepsies associated with hippocampal damage display memory disturbances being proportional to the degree of the damage. (Alessio et al., 2006) The role of epileptic discharges altering the normal functions of the temporomedial structures is a less investigated issue, However the role of ripples in the medial temporal lobe in memory consolidation is increasingly supported (Axmacher et al., 2008), therefore epileptic discharges in the hippocampus confirmed to having a leading role in temporo-limbic epilepsies probably contributes to loss of memory by interfering with memory consolidation during NREM sleep.

Sleep features

Complex partial and secondarily generalized seizures originating from the TLNE are frequently apparent during sleep as well as waking. Sleep seizures are more frequent in NREM sleep and secondarily generalized seizures tend to be more prominent in sleep.

Discharges in sleep appear at a higher rate and in a more explicit form compared with the awake-state findings. NREM sleep is associated with an increased spiking rate, extension of the electrical field, and rate of bilateral independent discharges, whereas in REM sleep a restriction of the electrical field was observed (Lieb et al., 1980; Rowan et al., 1982; Rossi et al., 1984; Sammaritano et al., 1991). The propensity to express bilateral discharges is particularly reflected in sleep records. Residual bilateral spiking after surgery proved to be associated with a bad postoperative outcome (Halász et al., 2004c). Within NREM sleep the activation of temporal spiking is greatest in stage 3–4 (Lieb et al., 1980), increasing as patients move to deeper stages of NREM sleep (Malow et al., 1998). Temporomesial compared with temporolateral cortical structures may display spiking at different sleep levels (Clemens et al., 2003).

A small number of patients show activation during REM sleep, localizing the primary epileptogenic focus better than spike activity in either waking or NREM sleep.

Nocturnal frontal lobe epilepsy (NFLE) and the prefrontal mediobasal network

Characterization of the epilepsy syndrome

Since the early 1980s a series of studies have reported on patients with peculiar short motor seizures and dystonic–dyskinetic features, usually involving both sides of the body, clustering during NREM sleep, and often accompanied with strange vocalization, under different headings (Lugaresi et al., 1986; Scheffer et al., 1995; Oldani et al., 1996). The attacks recur (with multiple episodes during the night) almost every night, at least in certain periods during the course of the disease. Consciousness is preserved or regained very quickly. Approximately one-third of patients exhibit some kind of IED localized to the frontal region. Ictal scalp EEG recording reveals epileptic features only exceptionally. The motor pattern is highly stereotyped for each individual with slight variation, but may have highly variable patterns across patients. Almost half of the patients exhibit occasional GTCS in the awake state or in sleep.

The seizures vary with the character of the hypermotor pattern. In some seizures the asymmetrical tonic postural component is more prominent, resembling those originating from the supplementary sensorimotor area (SSMA). The higher occurrence rate of SSMA seizure in sleep compared with wakefulness has been demonstrated by Anan and Dudley (1998).

In the mid 1990s, Berkovic and coworkers (Scheffer et al., 1995) described a familial variant of NFLE with autosomal dominant inheritance (ADNFLE).

Epileptic phenomena related to sleep EEG features

As well as the association of NFLE seizures with sleep, there is also a characteristic link with NREM sleep arousal dynamics. Seizures are always preceded by microarousals. Terzano and colleagues (1997) demonstrated that motor events are closely related to periods of unstable NREM sleep, and began during a CAP A-phase. The overall CAP rate in their patients was increased, and when attacks were suppressed the CAP rate decreased. In this kind of epilepsy the association of clinical (motor) epileptic events with NREM sleep arousal events is evident.

Relation to cognitive function

Patients with NFLE do not show cognitive disturbances, either ictally or interictally. The lack of scalp EEG involvement is an interesting characteristic of NFLE, partially due to the localization of epileptogenic areas in the hidden frontomedial and orbital surfaces. The interictal discharges do not show any GSW characteristics. This supports the assumption that the spike–wave-generating thalamocortical system is not involved in NFLE. We have to assume that in NFLE arousal activation has direct access to frontal cortical circuitry involving the basal ganglia, responsible for hyperkinetic motor paroxysms. Greater involvement in motor functions contrasts with epilepsies related to the corticothalamic network, which is more involved in sensory information processing and cognition. Moreover, a striking contrast can be established between IGE and NFLE: whereas IGE may represent the epilepsy of the NREM sleep trophotropic network, the NFLE represents the ergotropic frontal cholinergic arousal/alarm network (Table 19.5).

Summary

Both clinical and EEG manifestations of many epilepsy syndromes are linked to aspects of sleep, and epileptic EEG manifestations in sleep are strongly associated with the presence of cognitive dysfunction (see Fig. 19.1).

It is clear that in epilepsies involving the corticothalamic network, long-lasting as in the perisylvian group, or in LGS, interictal epileptiform discharges are harmful for cognitive function independently of the epileptic seizures. Interference with cognition seems to parallel the amount and extension of spike–wave discharges in NREM sleep. Discharges originating from one part of the thalamocortical associative areas can interfere with functions represented in that part of the network. For example, in LKS, discharges in the perisylvian, mainly posterior, part of the first temporal convolution interfere with certain aspects of speech function (Honbolygo et al., 2006). A more extensive functional deficit may be related to cortical dysfacilitatory effects of the wave component of GSW discharges demonstrated by electrophysiological (Steriade and Contreras, 1998) and fMRI (Aghakhani et al., 2004) methods. A third component of cognitive impairment may be the interference of GSW discharges with the increasingly evidenced restorative functions of NREM sleep. In the last 10–15 years local aspects of homeostatic regulation have received more and more attention. The frontal preponderance of sleep slow-wave activity and, further, the frontal dominance of the recovery increase after sleep deprivation and dominant hemisphere preponderance was emphasized in several studies (Cajochen et al., 1999; Finelli et al., 2001). Recent studies have shown that procedures presumably leading to local plastic changes in the cerebral cortex can lead to a local increase in slow-wave activity during subsequent sleep (Kattler et al., 1994; Stickgold et al., 2000; Vyazovskiy et al., 2000; Huber et al., 2004, 2006). Daytime utilization of a function (e.g., a cognitive task) led to an increase in the intensity of delta sleep over the cortical representation of the function. Furthermore, this increase was accompanied by an improvement in the same cognitive functioning. In this way, day and night (sleep and awake state) are strongly interconnected, and sleep ensures the process by which training provides us with learning. The tool that sleep employs for this is slow-wave activity. If delta activity is lost as a result of acoustic stimulation (Aeschbach et al., 2008), the subsequent improvement after daytime training will be lost.

Thus, we have more and more evidence supporting the view that NREM sleep (especially delta sleep) homeostatic regulation is governed by use-dependent plastic processes. In other words, delta homeostasis and use-dependent plasticity are two different sides of the same coin, probably representing the biological function of slow-wave sleep (Massimini et al., 2009). Probably, the full-blown development of these intermingled regulations is a human neoformation that became necessary for the recuperation of vulnerable frontal cognitive functions.

The occupation of a considerable amount of slow-wave sleep by spike–wave discharges, as in ESES and LKS, or even in a more circumscribed way by rolandic discharges, and also in LGS, clearly interferes with restorative function, resulting in the exhaustion of cognitive capacity.

In the group of epilepsies where the corticothalamic system seems not to be involved, such as in NFLE and TLNE, such cognitive consequences do not develop. However, in NTLE the development of secondary bilateral synchrony probably involves the thalamocortical system and may be responsible for certain cognitive decline, and the local involvement of hippocampal memory circuits interferes with memory consolidation during sleep. In addition, structural lesions due to the etiological factors (tumor, trauma, encephalitis, etc.)

Table 19.5

Contrasting differences between epilepsies with generalized spike–wave activity and nocturnal frontal lobe epilepsy (NFLE)

	Seizures	Participation of autonomic system	Participation of thalamocortical system	Vigilance dependency	Cognitive consequences	Network substrate
IGE and slow spike–wave encephalopathies	No purposeful movements or emotions	Minimal if any parasympathetic	NREM burst-firing; working mode	Transition of NREM and awake state	In IGE: only during seizures In encephalopathic variations: serious cognitive decline	NREM sleep system, thalamocortical part; trophotropic functions
NFLE	Hypermotor, agitation, escape, fear	High, sympathetic	No ictal epileptiform activity; no spike–wave activity	NREM sleep; elicitability by microarousals	No cognitive impairment even during seizures	Cholinergic frontal arousal/alarm system; ergotropic functions (flight, fear, fight)

IGE, idiopathic generalized epilepsy; NREM, nonrapid eye movement; NFLE, nocturnal frontal lobe epilepsy.

may also contribute to local cognitive dysfunction. The NFLE syndrome, without the entrainment of the spike–wave discharge generator corticothalamic system, is relatively free from cognitive deficits, in striking contrast to the well-known importance of the frontal lobe in cognitive functioning.

Sleep seems to be a key factor in determining how epilepsy induces cognitive impairment. Generalized or segmental thalamocortical epileptogenesis, producing spike–wave discharges and interfering with restorative frontal sleep function, might be the executive agent in this process.

SLEEP AS A DIAGNOSTIC TOOL

The place of sleep activation in EEG evaluation of epilepsy

NREM sleep has a strong activation effect in almost all epilepsies. These brain events are hidden by the darkness of the night, and without sleep studies we would never detect them.

Sleep activation provides a sleep profile characteristic for the epilepsy syndromes and can show the extent of epileptic involvement in terms of spread, lateralization, and generalization in a particular individual. Sleep characteristics should be explored in every epileptic patient during the diagnostic evaluation procedure. The importance of sleep studies in epilepsy today is strongly supported by the close correlation of epileptic activity in NREM sleep and cognitive impairment (demonstrated in the syndromic part of this chapter). Thus, the detection of abundant epileptiform activity in sleep is an important diagnostic and hopefully preventive task. The most frequent situations where sleep activation can answer specific diagnostic questions are summarized in Table 19.6 and particular epileptic EEG patterns detectable exclusively in sleep are shown in Table 19.7.

Table 19.6

The place of sleep activation in the epilepsy diagnostic algorithm

Activation of interictal epileptiform discharges (by traditional EEG or by mobile long-term EEG) • when awake recording do not provide diagnostic information • when the diagnostic value of awake recording is uncertain (to provide proof when suggestive) • for early diagnosis of epilepsy type/syndrome • to see the whole spectrum (in spatial dimension and electromorphology) of epileptiform activity • in temporal lobe epilepsy with unilateral spiking, to explore the involvement of the other side • when clinical symptoms are suggestive of generalized epilepsy with no supportive awake EEG signs, to look for generalized spike–wave bursts
Activation/observation of subclinical and clinical ictal manifestations with an electroclinical correlation of the event (by mobile long-term EEG or video-EEG monitoring)
Differentiation between epileptic and nonepileptic (parasomnias) nocturnal events (by video-EEG)

Table 19.7

Strongly sleep-related EEG patterns

Electrical status epilepticus in sleep (ESES) – exclusively during sleep
Generalized paroxysmal fast activity (GPFA) with polygraphic subtle ictal signs – almost always during sleep
Generalized spike–wave bursts in the awakening GTC form – almost exclusively during sleep in the awakening period
Focal sharps/spikes in frontal lobe epilepsies – frequently only during sleep
Bilateral independent spiking in temporal lobe epilepsy – compared with wakefulness more frequently during sleep
Centrotemporal unilateral or bilateral spiking in rolandic epilepsy – compared with wakefulness, more frequently

How to get a sleep record: minimal requirements of sleep EEG and polysomnographic recordings

The easiest and natural way to get a sleep record is to allow a nap in the laboratory. However, not everybody is able to sleep under artificial circumstances. The most likely subjects for this procedure are children, together with their parent. In most laboratories, morning sleep after partial or total sleep deprivation is the most common way to obtain a sleep record. Many studies report increased epileptiform discharge activity following sleep deprivation (SD) (Mattson et al., 1965; Rowan et al., 1982; Degen and Degen, 1991; Fountain et al., 1998; Malow, 2004).

There is no general agreement whether the provocative effect of SD is caused merely by inducing sleep, or whether SD has an independent activating effect. Sleep propensity decreases in the morning. A genuine morning activating effect of SD might be due to the "clash" between sleep-promoting (by sleep deprivation) and sleep-inhibiting (time of day effect) factors, leading to epileptiform discharges. Although SD could have an activation effect without sleep, the most essential component of activation is sleep *per se* (Halász et al., 2002a). Therefore it is very important to obtain a sleep record after sleep deprivation in the EEG laboratory. There are two drawbacks to SD. The first is the risk of provoking generalized tonic–clonic seizures. Patients with JME may be especially at risk. The second is the difficulty falling asleep in the laboratory, and of providing a good environment and sufficient time (usually a minimum of 1 hour to record at least one sleep cycle).

Recording during a whole night provides the opportunity to record more than one sleep cycle, superficial and deep sleep, both NREM and REM sleep, and all the transitional periods between wakefulness, NREM, and REM sleep. This method requires overnight personnel, and the evaluation is also time-consuming. Mobile long-term EEG techniques allow patients to sleep naturally at home.

Video-EEG monitoring over several days provides maximal advantages to observe both EEG and the behavioral concomitant of subclinical and clinical epileptic manifestations. It is the most expensive method among the sleep registration possibilities, usually reserved for diagnostic dilemmas and presurgical evaluation.

References

Aarts JH, Binnie CD, Smit AM et al. (1984). Selective cognitive impairment during focal and generalized epileptiform EEG activity. Brain 107: 293–308.

Aeschbach D, Cutler AJ, Ronda JM (2008). A role for non-rapid-eye-movement sleep homeostasis in perceptual learning. J Neurosci 28: 2766–2772.

Aghakhani Y, Bagshaw AP, Benar CG et al. (2004). fMRI activation during spike and wave discharges in idiopathic generalized epilepsy. Brain 127: 1127–1144.

Akiyama T, Otsubo H, Ochi A et al. (2005). Focal cortical high-frequency oscillations trigger epileptic spasms: confirmation by digital video subdural EEG. Clin Neurophysiol 116: 2819–2825.

Alessio A, Bonilha L, Rorden C (2006). Memory and language impairments and their relationships to hippocampal and perirhinal cortex damage in patients with medial temporal lobe epilepsy. Epilepsy Behav 8 (3): 593–600.

Anan I, Dudley SD (1998). Relation of supplementary motor area epilepsy and sleep. In: Epilepsy and Sleep Symposium, June 22, Cleveland, OH, Abstract 16.

Avoli M, Gloor P, Kostopoulos G et al. (1983). An analysis of penicillin-induced generalized spike and wave discharges using simultaneous recordings of cortical and thalamic single neurons. J Neurophysiol 50: 819–837.

Axmacher N, Elger CE, Fell J (2008). Ripples in the medial temporal lobe are relevant for human memory consolidation. Brain 131 (Pt 7): 1806–1817.

Babb TL, Kupfer WR, Pretorius JK et al. (1991). Synaptic reorganization by mossy fibers in human epileptic fascia dentata. Neuroscience 42: 351–363.

Bal T, von Krosigk M, McCormick DA (1995a). Synaptic and membrane mechanisms underlying synchronized oscillations in the ferret lateral geniculate nucleus in vitro. J Physiol 483: 641–663.

Bal T, von Krosigk M, McCormick DA (1995b). Role of the ferret perigeniculate nucleus in the generation of synchronized oscillations in vitro. J Physiol 483: 665–685.

Bauer G, Aichner F, Saltuari L (1983). Epilepsies with diffuse slow spikes and waves of late onset. Eur Neurol 22: 344–350.

Bazil CW (2002). Sleep and epilepsy. Semin Neurol 22: 321–327.

Beaumanoir A, Ballis T, Varfis G et al. (1974). Benign epilepsy of childhood with Rolandic spikes. A clinical, electroencephalographic, and telencephalographic study. Epilepsia 15: 301–315.

Beaussart M (1972). Benign epilepsy of children with Rolandic (centro-temporal) paroxysmal foci. A clinical entity. Study of 221 cases. Epilepsia 13: 795–811.

Bernasconi N, Duvhesne S, Janke A et al. (2004). Whole brain voxel-based statistical analysis of gray matter in temporal lobe epilepsy. Neuroimage 23: 17–23.

Bernhardt BC, Worsley KJ, Besson P et al. (2008). Mapping limbic network organization in temporal lobe epilepsy using morphometric correlations insights on the relation between mesiotemporal connectivity and cortical atrophy. Neuroimage 42: 515–524.

Billiard C, Autret A, Laffont F (1981). Aphasie acquise de l'enfant avec epilepsie. A purpos de 4 observations avec etat de mal infraclinique du sommeil. Rev Electroencephalogr Neurophysiol Clin 11: 457–467.

Binnie CD (1996). Cognitive effects of subclinical EEG discharges. Neurophysiol Clin 26: 138–142.

Blume WT (2001). Pathogenesis of Lennox–Gastaut syndrome: considerations and hypotheses. Epileptic Disord 3: 183–196.

Blumenfeld H (2005). Consciousness and epilepsy: why are patients with absence seizures absent? Prog Brain Res 150: 271–286.

Borbely AA, Baumann F, Brandeis D et al. (1981). Sleep deprivation: effect on sleep stages and EEG power density in man. Electroencephalogr Clin Neurophysiol 51: 483–495.

Cajochen C, Foy R, Dijk DJ (1999). Frontal predominance of a relative increase in sleep delta and theta EEG activity after sleep loss in humans. Sleep Res Online 2: 65–69.

Clemens B, Majoros E (1987). Sleep studies in benign epilepsy of childhood with rolandic spikes. II. Analysis of discharge frequency and its relation to sleep dynamics. Epilepsia 28: 24–27

Clemens Z, Janszky J, Szucs A et al. (2003). Interictal epileptic spiking during sleep and wakefulness in mesial temporal lobe epilepsy: a comparative study of scalp and foramen ovale electrodes. Epilepsia 44: 186–192.

Clemens Z, Fabó D, Halász P (2005). Overnight verbal memory retention correlates with the number of sleep spindles. Neuroscience 132: 529–535.

Csercsa R, Dombovári B, Fabó D et al. (2010). Laminar analysis of slow wave activity in humans. Brain 133: 2814–2829.

Dalla Bernardina B, Colamaria V, Capovilla G et al. (1984). Sleep and benign partial epilepsies of childhood.

In: R Degen, E Niedermeyer (Eds.), Epilepsy: Sleep and Sleep Deprivation. Elsevier, Amsterdam, pp. 119–133.

Degen R, Degen HE (1990). Some genetic aspects of rolandic epilepsy: waking and sleep EEGs in siblings. Epilepsia 31: 795–801.

Degen R, Degen HE (1991). Sleep and sleep deprivation in epileptology. Epilepsy Res Suppl 2: 235–260.

Deonna T (1991). Acquired epileptiform aphasia in children (Landau–Kleffner syndrome). J Clin Neurophysiol 8: 288–298.

Deonna T, Roulet E (1995). Acquired epileptic aphasia (AEA): definition of the syndrome and current problems. In: A Beaumanoir, M Bureau, T Deonna et al. (Eds.), Continuous Spike and Waves During Slow Sleep: Electrical Status Epilepticus During Slow Sleep. John Libbey, London, pp. 37–45.

Deonna T, Roulet-Perez E (2010). Early-onset acquired epileptic aphasia (Landau–Kleffner syndrome, LKS) and regressive autistic disorders with epileptic EEG abnormalities: the continuing debate. Brain Dev 32: 746–752.

Dinner DS, Lüders HO (2001). Epilepsy and Sleep. Academic Press, San Diego.

Doose H (1992a). Myoclonic–astatic epilepsy. Epilepsy Res Suppl 6: 163–168.

Doose H (1992b). Myoclonic astatic epilepsy of early childhood. In: J Roger, M Bureau, C Dravet et al. (Eds.), Epileptic Syndromes in Infancy, Childhood and Adolescence. (2nd edn). John Libbey, London, pp. 103–114.

Doose H, Neubauer BA, Petersen B (2000). The concept of hereditary impairment of brain maturation. Epileptic Disord 2: S45–S49.

Dulac O, Billard C, Arthuis M (1983). Electroclinical and developmental aspects of epilepsy in the aphasia-epilepsy syndrome. Arch Fr Pediatr 40: 299–308.

Engel J Jr. (1996). Introduction to temporal lobe epilepsy. Epilepsy Res 26: 141–150.

Fejerman N (2009). Atypical rolandic epilepsy. Epilepsia 50: 9–12.

Fejerman N, Caraballo R, Tenembaum SN (2000). Atypical evolutions of benign localization-related epilepsies in children: are they predictable? Epilepsia 41: 380–390.

Ferrillo F, Beelke M, Nobili L (2000). Sleep EEG synchronization mechanisms and activation of interictal epileptic spikes. Clin Neurophysiol 111: 565–573.

Finelli LA, Borbély AA, Achermann P (2001). Functional topography of the human nonREM sleep electroencephalogram. Eur J Neurosci 13: 2282–2290.

Foldvary-Schaefer N, Grigg-Damberger M (2006). Sleep and epilepsy: what we know, don't know, and need to know. J Clin Neurophysiol 23: 4–20.

Fonseca LC, Tedrus GM, Lalloni DT et al. (2005). Transient cognitive impairment during generalized or diffuse epileptiform EEG discharges. Arq Neuropsiquiatr 63: 817–824.

Ford EW, Morrell F, Whisler WW (1982). Methohexital anaesthesia in the surgical treatment of uncontrollable epilepsy. Anesth Analg 61: 997–1001.

Fountain NB, Kim JS, Lee SI (1998). Sleep deprivation activates epileptiform discharges independent of the activating effects of sleep. J Clin Neurophysiol 15: 69–75.

Gloor P, Avoli M, Kostopoulos G (1990). Thalamocortical relationships in generalized epilepsy with bilaterally synchronous spike-and-wave discharge. In: M Avoli, P Gloor, G Kostopoulos et al. (Eds.), Generalized Epilepsy: Neurobiological Approaches. Birkhauser, Boston, pp. 190–212.

Grenier F, Timofeev I, Steriade M (2001). Focal synchronization of ripples (80–200 Hz) in neocortex and their neuronal correlates. J Neurophysiol 86: 1884–1898.

Guerrini R, Belmonte A, Veggiotti P et al. (1997). Delayed appearance of interictal EEG abnormalities in early onset childhood epilepsy with occipital paroxysms. Brain Dev 19: 343–346.

Guerrini R, Genton P, Bureau M et al. (1998). Multilobar polymicrogyria, intractable drop attack seizures, and sleep-related electrical status epilepticus. Neurology 51: 504–512.

Hahn A, Pisthol J, Neubauer BA et al. (2001). Atypical "benign" partial epilepsy or pseudo-Lennox syndrome. Part I: Symptomatology and long-term prognosis. Neuropediatrics 32: 1–8.

Halász P (1991a). Runs of rapid spikes in sleep: a characteristic EEG expression of generalized malignant epileptic encephalopathies. A conceptual review with new pharmacological data. Epilepsy Res Suppl 2: 49–71.

Halász P, Dévényi É (1974). Petit mal absence in night-sleep with special reference to transitional sleep and REM periods. Acad Med Hung 31: 31–45.

Halász P, Filakovszky J, Vargha A et al. (2002a). Effect of sleep deprivation on spike-wave discharges in idiopathic generalised epilepsy: a 4 × 24 h continuous long term EEG monitoring study. Epilepsy Res 51: 123–132.

Halász P, Terzano MG, Parrino L (2002b). Spike-wave discharge and the microstructure of sleep-wake continuum in idiopathic generalised epilepsy. Neurophysiol Clin 32: 38–53.

Halász P, Terzano M, Parrino L et al. (2004a). The nature of arousal in sleep. J Sleep Res 13: 1–23.

Halász P, Janszky J, Barcs G et al. (2004b). Generalized paroxysmal fast activity (GPFA) is not always a sign of malignant epileptic encephalopathy. Seizure 13: 270–276.

Halász P, Janszky J, Rásonyi GY et al. (2004c). Postoperative interictal spikes during sleep contralateral to the operated side is associated with unfavourable surgical outcome in patients with preoperative bitemporal spikes. Seizure 13: 460–466.

Halász P, Kelemen A, Clemens B et al. (2005). The perisylvian epileptic network. A unifying concept. Ideggyogy Sz 58: 21–31.

Hirsch E, Marescoux C, Maquet P et al. (1990). Landau–Kleffner syndrome: a clinical and EEG study of five cases. Epilepsia 31: 756–767.

Holtmann M, Matei A, Hellmann U et al. (2006). Rolandic spikes increase impulsivity in ADHD – a neuropsychological pilot study. Brain Dev 28: 633–640.

Honbolygo F, Csepe V, Fekeshazy A et al. (2006). Converging evidences on language impairment in Landau–Kleffner syndrome revealed by behavioral and brain activity measures: a case study. Clin Neurophysiol 117: 295–305.

Huber R, Ghilardi MF, Massimini M et al. (2004). Local sleep and learning. Nature 430: 78–81.

Huber R, Ghilardi MF, Massimini M et al. (2006). Arm immobilization causes cortical plastic changes and locally decreases sleep slow wave activity. Nat Neurosci 9: 1169–1176.

Huguenard JR (2000). Circuit mechanisms of spike-wave discharge: are there similar underpinnings for centrotemporal spikes? Epilepsia 41: 1076–1077.

Huguenard JR, Prince DA (1994). Intrathalamic rhythmicity studied in vitro: nominal T-current modulation causes robust antioscillatory effects. J Neurosci 14: 5485–5502.

Jacobs J, Zijlmans M, Zelmann R et al. (2010). High-frequency electroencephalographic oscillations correlate with outcome of epilepsy surgery. Ann Neurol 67: 209–220.

Kasteleijn-Nolst Trenite DG (1995). Transient cognitive impairment during subclinical epileptiform electroencephalographic discharges. Semin Pediatr Neurol 2: 246–253.

Kattler H, Dijk DJ, Borbely AA (1994). Effect of unilateral somatosensory stimulation prior to sleep on the sleep EEG in humans. J Sleep Res 3: 159–164.

Kelemen A, Barsi P, Gyorsok Z et al. (2006). Thalamic lesion and epilepsy with generalized seizures, ESES and spike-wave paroxysms – report of three cases. Seizure 15: 454–458.

Kellaway P (2000). The electroencephalographic features of benign centrotemporal (Rolandic) epilepsy of childhood. Epilepsia 41: 1053–1056.

Khosravani H, Mehrotra N, Rigby M et al. (2009). Spatial localization and time-dependent changes of electrographic high frequency oscillations in human temporal lobe epilepsy. Epilepsia 50: 605–616.

Kobayashi K, Ohtsuka Y, Oka E et al. (1992). Primary and secondary bilateral synchrony in epilepsy: differentiation by estimation of interhemispheric small time differences during short spike-wave activity. Electroencephalogr Clin Neurophysiol 83: 93–103.

Kostopoulos GK (2000). Spike-and-wave discharges of absence seizures as a transformation of sleep spindles: the continuing development of a hypothesis. Clin Neurophysiol 111: S27–S38.

Kotagal P (2001). Sleep deprivation and epilepsy. In: DS Dinner, HO Lüders (Eds.), Epilepsy and Sleep. Academic Press, San Diego, pp. 63–74.

Lieb J, Joseph JP, Engle J Jr et al. (1980). Sleep state and seizure foci related to depth spike activity in patients with temporal lobe epilepsy. Electroencephalogr Clin Neurophysiol 49: 538 557.

Lipinski CG (1977). Epilepsies with astatic seizures of late onset. Epilepsia 18: 13–20.

Lugaresi E, Cirignotta F, Montagna P (1986).HYPERLINK "http://www.ncbi.nlm.nih.gov/pubmed/2939199" Nocturnal paroxysmal dystonia. J Neurol Neurosurg Psychiatry 49 (4): 375–380.

Maglóczky Z, Wittner L, Borhegyi Z et al. (2000). Changes in the distribution and connectivity of interneurons in the epileptic human dentate gyrus. Neuroscience 96: 7–25.

Malow BA (2004). Sleep deprivation and epilepsy. Epilepsy Curr 4: 193–195.

Malow BA, Lin X, Kushwaha R et al. (1998). Interictal spiking increases with sleep depth in temporal lobe epilepsy. Epilepsia 39: 1309–1316.

Marescoux C, Hirsch E, Finck S et al. (1990). Landau–Kleffner syndrome: a pharmacologic study of five cases. Epilepsia 31: 768–777.

Massa R, de Saint-Martin A, Hirsch E et al. (2000). Landau–Kleffner syndrome: sleep EEG characteristics at onset. Clin Neurophysiol 111: S87–S93.

Massimini M, Tononi G, Huber R (2009). Slow waves, synaptic plasticity and information processing: insights from transcranial magnetic stimulation and high-density EEG experiments. Eur J Neurosci 29: 1761–1770.

Mathern GW, Babb TL, Leite JP et al. (1996). The pathogenic and progressive features of chronic human hippocampal epilepsy. Epilepsy Res 26: 151–161.

Mattson RH, Pratt KL, Calverley JR (1965). Electroencephalograms of epileptics following sleep deprivation. Arch Neurol 13: 310–315.

Meeren H, van Luijtelaar G, Lopes da Silva F et al. (2005). Evolving concepts on the pathophysiology of absence seizures: the cortical focus theory. Arch Neurol 62: 371–376.

Mendez M, Radtke RA (2001). Interactions between sleep and epilepsy. J Clin Neurophysiol 18: 106–127.

Michelucci R, Rubboli G, Plasmati R (1987). Clinical relevance of various EEG features of electrical status epilepticus during slow sleep. In: Epilepsy International Congress, Book of Abstracts. John Libbey, London, pp. 229–242.

Morikawa T, Seino M, Watanabe Y et al. (1989). Clinical relevance of continuous spike-waves during slow wave sleep. In: S Manelis, E Bental, JN Loeber et al. (Eds.), Advances in Epileptology. Raven Press, New York, pp. 359–363.

Morrell F, Whisler WW, Smith MC et al. (1995). Landau–Kleffner syndrome. Treatment with subpial intracortical transection. Brain 118: 1529–1546.

Nicolai J, Aldenkamp AP, Arends J et al. (2006). Cognitive and behavioral effects of nocturnal epileptiform discharges in children with benign childhood epilepsy with centrotemporal spikes. Epilepsy Behav 8: 56–70.

Nieto-Barrera M, Aguilar-Quero F, Montes E et al. (1997). Epileptic syndromes which show continuous spike and wake complexes during slow wave sleep. Rev Neurol 25: 1045–1051.

Nobili L, Ferrillo F, Baglietto MG et al. (1999). Relationship of sleep interictal epileptiform discharges to sigma activity (12–16 Hz) in benign epilepsy of childhood with rolandic spikes. Clin Neurophysiol 110: 39–46.

Ohtahara S, Ohtsuka Y, Kobayashi K (1995). Lennox–Gastaut syndrome: a new vista. Psychiatry Clin Neurosci 49: S179–S183.

Oldani A, Zucconi M, Ferini-Strambi L et al. (1996). Autosomal dominant nocturnal frontal lobe epilepsy: electroclinical picture. Epilepsia 37: 964–976.

Pan A, Lüders HO (2000). Epileptiform discharges in benign focal epilepsy of childhood. Epileptic Disord 2: S29–S36.

Parrino L, Smerieri A, Spaggiari MC et al. (2000). Cyclic alternating pattern (CAP) and epilepsy during sleep: how a physiological rhythm modulates a pathological event. Clin Neurophysiol 111: S39–S46.

Paetau R, Kajola M, Korkman M et al. (1991). HYPERLINK "http://www.ncbi.nlm.nih.gov/pubmed/1716495" Landau-Kleffner syndrome: epileptic activity in the auditory cortex. Neuroreport 2 (4): 201–204.

Peigneux P, Laureys S, Delbeuck X et al. (2001). Sleeping brain, learning brain. The role of sleep for memory systems. Neuroreport 12: A111–A1124.

Pinton F, Ducot B, Motte J et al. (2006). Cognitive functions in children with benign childhood epilepsy with centrotemporal spikes (BECTS). Epileptic Disord 8: 11–23.

Roger J, Remy C, Bureau M et al. (1987). Lennox–Gastaut syndrome in the adult. Rev Neurol 143: 401–405.

Ross J, Johnson LC, Walter RD (1966). Spike and wave discharges during stages of sleep. Arch Neurol 14: 399–407.

Rossi GF, Colicchio G, Pola P (1984). Interictal epileptic activity during sleep: a stereo-EEG study in patients with partial epilepsy. Electroencephalogr Clin Neurophysiol 58: 97–106.

Rossi PG, Parmeggiani A, Posar A et al. (1999). Landau–Kleffner syndrome (LKS) long-term follow-up and links with electrical status epilepticus during sleep (ESES). Brain Dev 21: 90–98.

Roulet-Perez E, Daviddoff V, Despland PA et al. (1993). Mental and behavioural deterioration of children with epilepsy and ESES: acquired epileptic frontal syndrome. Dev Med Child Neurol 35: 661–674.

Rowan AJ, Veldhuisen RJ, Nagelkerke NJ (1982). Comparative evaluation of sleep deprivation and sedated sleep EEGs as diagnostic aids in epilepsy. Electroencephalogr Clin Neurophysiol 54: 357–364.

Salek-Haddadi A, Lemieux L, Merschhemke M et al. (2003). Functional magnetic resonance imaging of human absence. Ann Neurol 53: 663–667.

Saltik S, Uluduz D, Cokar O et al. (2005). A clinical and EEG study on idiopathic partial epilepsies with evolution into ESES spectrum disorders. Epilepsia 46: 524–533.

Sammaritano M, Gigli GL, Gotman J (1991). Interictal spiking during wakefulness and sleep and the localization of foci in temporal lobe epilepsy. Neurology 41: 290–297.

Sanchez-Vives MV, Bal T, McCormick DA (1995). Properties of GABAergic inhibition in the ferret lateral geniculate nucleus contributing to the generation of synchronized oscillations. Soc Neurosci Abstr 21: 11.

Scheffer IE, Bhatia KP, Lopes-Cendes I et al. (1995). Autosomal dominant nocturnal frontal lobe epilepsy. A distinctive clinical disorder. Brain 118: 61–73.

Seri S, Cerquiglini A, Pisani F (1998). Spike-induced interference in auditory sensory processing in Landau–Kleffner syndrome. Electroencephalogr Clin Neurophysiol 108: 506–510.

Shouse MN, Scordato JC, Farber PR (2004). Sleep and arousal mechanisms in experimental epilepsy: epileptic components of NREM and antiepileptic components in REM sleep. Ment Retard Dev Disabil Res Rev 10: 117–121.

Siniatchkin M, Groening K, Moehring J et al. (2010). Neuronal networks in children with continuous spikes and waves during slow sleep. Brain 133: 2798–2813.

Spencer SS (2002). Neural networks in human epilepsy: evidence of and implications for treatment. Epilepsia 43: 219–227.

Staba RJ, Wilson CL, Bragin A et al. (2004). High-frequency oscillations recorded in human medial temporal lobe during sleep. Ann Neurol 56: 108–115.

Stenzel E, Panteli C (1983). Lennox–Gastaut-Syndome des 2. Lebensjahrzehntes. In: H Hemschmidt, R Rentz, J Jungmann (Eds.), Epilepsie. Thieme, Stuttgart, pp. 99–107.

Steriade M (2003). The corticothalamic system in sleep. Front Biosci 8: 878–899.

Steriade M, Contreras D (1998). Spike-wave complexes and fast components of cortically generated seizures. I. Role of neocortex and thalamus. J Neurophysiol 80: 1439–1455.

Steriade M, Contreras D, Amzica F (1994). Synchronized sleep oscillations and their paroxysmal developments. Trends Neurosci 17: 199–208.

Stickgold R, James L, Hobson JA (2000). Visual discrimination learning requires sleep after training. Nat Neurosci 3: 1237–1238.

Sutula TP, Dudek FE (2007). Unmasking recurrent excitation generated by mossy fiber sprouting in the epileptic dentate gyrus an emergent property of a complex system. Prog Brain Res 163: 541–563.

Tassinari CA, Bureau M, Dravet C et al. (1985). Epilepsy with continuous spike and waves during slow sleep. In: J Roger, M Bureau, C Dravet et al. (Eds.), Epileptic Syndromes in Infancy, Childhood and Adolescence. John Libbey, London, pp. 194–204.

Tassinari CA, Rubboli G, Volpi L et al. (2001). Encephalopathy with electrical status epilepticus during slow wave sleep or ESES syndrome including the acquired aphasia. Clin Neurophysiol 111: S94–S102.

Tassinari CA, Cantalupo G, Rios-Pohl L et al. (2009). Encephalopathy with status epilepticus during slow sleep: "The Penelope syndrome". Epilepsia 50: 4–8.

Terzano MG, Monge-Strauss MF, Mikol F et al. (1997). Cyclic alternating pattern as a provocative factor in nocturnal paroxysmal dystonia. Epilepsia 38: 1015–1025.

Terzano MG, Parrino L, Boselli M et al. (2000). CAP components and EEG synchronization in the first 3 sleep cycles. Clin Neurophysiol 111: 283–290.

van der Meij W, Huiskamp GJ, Rutten GJ et al. (2001). The existence of two sources in rolandic epilepsy, confirmation with high resolution EEG, MEG and fMRI. Brain Topogr 13: 275–282.

Vanhatalo S, Palva JM, Holmes MD et al. (2004). Infraslow oscillations modulate excitability and interictal epileptic activity in the human cortex during sleep. Proc Natl Acad Sci U S A 101: 5053–5057.

Veggiotti P, Beccaria R, Guerrini R et al. (1999). Continuous spike-and-wave activity during slow-wave sleep: syndrome or EEG pattern? Epilepsia 34: S37–S53.

von Krosigk M, Bal T, McCormick DA (1993). Cellular mechanisms of a synchronized oscillation in the thalamus. Science 261: 361–364.

Vyazovskiy V, Borbély AA, Tobler I (2000). Unilateral vibrissae stimulation during waking induces interhemispheric EEG asymmetry during subsequent sleep in the rat. J Sleep Res 9: 367–371.

Wieser HG (1993). Surgically remediable temporal lobe syndromes. In: J Engel Jr (Ed.), Surgical Treatment of the Epilepsies. 2nd edn. Raven Press, New York, pp. 49–63.

Worrell GA, Gardner AB, Stead SM et al. (2008). High-frequency oscillations in human temporal lobe: simultaneous microwire and clinical macroelectrode recordings. Brain 131: 928–937.

Handbook of Clinical Neurology, Vol. 107 (3rd series)
Epilepsy, Part I
H. Stefan and W.H. Theodore, Editors

Chapter 20

Electroencephalography and video-electroencephalography

ANTONIO GIL-NAGEL[1] AND BASSEL ABOU-KHALIL[2]*

[1]*Epilepsy Program, Department of Neurology, Hospital Ruber Internacional, Madrid, Spain*

[2]*Epilepsy Division, Department of Neurology, Vanderbilt University Medical Center, Nashville, TN, USA*

INTRODUCTION

An electroencephalogram (EEG) is a graphic representation of voltage changes over time comparing two points on the scalp. Video-electroencephalography (V-EEG) monitoring involves the simultaneous recording of EEG and video, which allows the correlation of electrical function of the brain with clinical manifestations. In patients with epilepsy, the EEG may record characteristic abnormalities; specific interictal abnormalities are referred to as epileptiform discharges, and specific ictal abnormalities are called ictal discharges or seizure patterns. EEG and V-EEG are at the same time readily available, relatively inexpensive, noninvasive, and suitable for prolonged study. Because of this, EEG and V-EEG are used extensively in the evaluation and clinical management of epilepsy, where they provide several applications. In patients with episodic impairment of neurological function in whom seizures are suspected, EEG helps support the diagnosis of epilepsy and V-EEG can resolve the differential diagnosis when typical events are recorded. In patients diagnosed with epilepsy, EEG is indispensable in the classification of epilepsy into partial or generalized, and may provide information to help diagnose specific epileptic syndromes. V-EEG can identify subtle seizures or seizures that the patient is not aware of; it allows an assessment of the severity of the episodes, in order to assess risk for accidents; and it is necessary in the localization of the epileptogenic zone prior to epilepsy surgery. This chapter reviews basic methodology and clinical applications of EEG and V-EEG.

METHODOLOGY OF ELECTROENCEPHALOGRAPHY

Technical recommendations

The American Electroencephalographic Society has published guidelines for the performance of routine EEG (American Electroencephalographic Society, 1994; American Clinical Neurophysiology Society, 2006a). Silver–silver chloride or gold disk electrodes are recommended. For prolonged recordings, these should be held on with collodion and placed according to the International 10/20 System (Fig. 20.1A,B) (Jasper, 1983), so that results can be compared with other published findings and in the same patient over time. During recording, the low-frequency filter (LFF) should be no higher than 1 Hz, preferably 0.3 Hz, and the high-frequency filter (HFF) should be no lower than 70 Hz. The 60-Hz (50 Hz in Europe), or notch filter, should be avoided during acquisition; this can be done by adequate isolation of the EEG unit and grounding of the equipment. The notch filter should be used only when other measures against stray current interference fail, a situation that often occurs in the intensive care unit (ICU) and operating room. The notch filter should not be used for focal 60/50-Hz artifact, which is usually due to impedance imbalance. Electrode impedance should be checked at the beginning of recording and regularly during the study, and should not exceed 5 kohms throughout the recording. Additional electrodes using the 10/10 System can be helpful for studies on topography and source analysis (Fig. 20.1C) (Oostenveld and Praamstra, 2001; American Clinical Neurophysiology Society, 2006b), and in the search of restricted scalp fields over a suspected area.

*Correspondence to: Bassel Abou-Khalil, M.D., Department of Neurology, Epilepsy Division, Vanderbilt University Medical Center, Nashville, Tennessee, USA. E-mail:bassel.abou-khalil@vanderbilt.edu

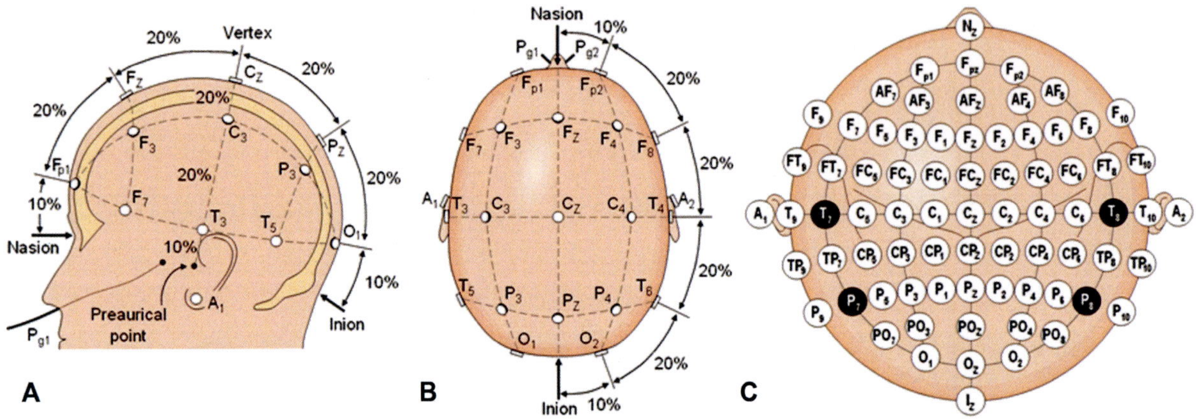

Fig. 20.1. Scalp electrode placement in the 10/20 International System (**A,B**) and 10/10 System (**C**). (Reproduced with permission from Schalk and Mellinger (2010). © Springer.)

Standard equipment includes one or two cameras for video recording already synchronized with the EEG. Cameras should focus on areas of major interest or the entire body. The use of two cameras allows close-up focus on the face, as well as wider coverage of the whole body for analysis of ictal semiology, and reduces the risk of missing clinical information due to visual obstruction by personnel or visitors. Technologists must be trained in the detection and correction of artifacts, the identification of wakefulness and sleep, and identification of seizure discharges and other EEG abnormalities. When antiepileptic drugs are reduced or discontinued, permanent observation by trained personnel is mandatory, in order to identify seizures and administer rescue medication if seizure frequency or severity requires prompt intervention. Because patients admitted in epilepsy units may have antiepileptic medication discontinued, and may suffer from cardiac disorders, V-EEG personnel must also be trained regularly in the detection of cardiac arrest and in cardiorespiratory resuscitation.

Duration and timing of studies

Outpatient routine EEG should have a minimum of 20 minutes of technically satisfactory recording, including recording in eyes-open and eyes-closed conditions, and standard activation procedures, such as hyperventilation (Patel and Maulsby, 1987) and photic stimulation (Kasteleijn-Nolst Trenite et al., 1999). In adults and older children most studies have a duration of 30 minutes, whereas in infants the duration is usually more than an hour. The routine EEG is the most commonly performed diagnostic procedure in patients suspected of having seizures (Marsan and Zivin, 1970). In association with a careful clinical history, routine EEG allows the diagnosis of epileptic seizures in most patients, and classification of the epilepsy type after the first seizure in more than 75% of patients (King et al., 1998). Sleep deprivation can increase the probability of recording interictal epileptiform activity (Leach et al., 2006). However, excessive indiscriminate use of home sleep deprivation may result in a seizure prior to the recording, on the way to the hospital. In juvenile myoclonic epilepsy, a morning recording has superior yield of epileptiform activity (Labate et al., 2007). Ideally, most of the recording will be obtained immediately after awakening from sleep. A sleep recording is essential in several forms of epilepsy; for example, the waking EEG may be completely normal in benign epilepsy with centrotemporal spikes, with very frequent epileptiform discharges recorded during sleep. Nonrapid eye movement (NREM) sleep is known to activate epileptiform activity in temporal lobe epilepsy, with increasing frequency of discharges with sleep depth (Malow et al., 1998). A complete one-night sleep recording not only increases the likelihood of the patient falling asleep and recording interictal activity, but also increases the chance of recording seizures.

Routine EEG has important limitations. The short duration of recordings often does not allow the identification of interictal epileptiform activity (sampling effect). Approximately one-half of patients with epilepsy will have a normal first EEG and close to 10% will always have a normal interictal EEG (Salinsky et al., 1987). In addition, the routine EEG is an indirect assessment of epilepsy, with rare opportunity to record seizures, which are the events that require treatment. In some patients who have both epileptic and nonepileptic seizures, or both partial and generalized epilepsy, interictal epileptiform EEG abnormalities may be unreliable for diagnosis and classification of the most clinically relevant seizures (Goodin and Aminoff, 1984). Finally, normal electrographic patterns are sometimes difficult to differentiate from epileptiform activity, and spikes or sharp waves may be present in patients without epilepsy; in these cases routine EEG can lead to a wrong diagnosis of seizures in patients with nonepileptic events, such as syncope and psychogenic seizures (Benbadis and Tatum, 2003; Krauss et al., 2005). For all these reasons, prolonged EEG combined with video is often used earlier in the diagnosis of epilepsy. The longer EEG samples obtained with such studies help to improve the diagnostic yield and specificity of EEG.

The duration of prolonged V-EEG studies should be decided depending upon the need to record the episodes studied, the episode frequency, and the possibility of inducing them with antiepileptic drug withdrawal, activation procedures, or induction protocols. In a study of 248 adult patients admitted to a V-EEG unit for diagnosis or presurgical evaluation, 167 (67%) had episodes during admission, including 119 with epileptic seizures and 48 with nonepileptic events (Friedman and Hirsch, 2009). The median time to first diagnostic event (epileptic and nonepileptic) was 2 days; mean time to epileptic seizure was 3.1 days, whereas the mean time for nonepileptic events was shorter at 1 day. Among patients with recorded epileptic seizures, 88% had a seizure within 5 days. Some 12% of patients with a definite diagnosis of epilepsy never had interictal epileptiform discharges; all of these patients had focal epilepsy. Interictal epileptiform activity was recorded in 17% of patients with nonepileptic events. Although self-reported seizure frequency is often used to determine the chance of recording seizures, at least one study has demonstrated that this parameter has a poor predictive value. According to this study, the mean time to first episode during V-EEG ranged between 2.1 and 2.8 days, and was independent of self-reported seizure frequency (Eisenman et al., 2005). This is in part explained by the fact that patients and their families are often unaware of seizures (Blum et al., 1996). Thus, a low self-reported outpatient seizure frequency should not preclude referral for V-EEG monitoring. In children, the duration of studies tends to be shorter than in adults, because of the presence of more abundant epileptiform activity and often higher seizure frequency. Different studies have reported an average length of recording of 1.2–1.5 days in children (Mizrahi, 1999; Nordli, 2006).

Activation procedures

Hyperventilation should be performed for a minimum of 3 minutes, unless there are medical contraindications. Adequate photic stimulation must include flash frequencies ranging from 1 to 60 Hz, with the lamp positioned at 30 cm from the eyes, and including the eyes-open then eyes-closed condition for each 10-second photic stimulation train (Kasteleijn-Nolst Trenite et al., 1999). During the procedure the technologist should monitor changes in the EEG and abort the light stimulus if definite epileptiform activity appears in the tracing. Other activating procedures that can induce epileptiform activity or seizures in specific reflex epilepsies should be used either routinely during V-EEG monitoring or in specific clinical situations. Praxis induces interictal epileptiform activity and seizures in nearly one-quarter of patients with juvenile myoclonic epilepsy (Guaranha et al., 2009). Other precipitating factors that can be analyzed during V-EEG in specific patients are mental calculation (Matsuoka et al., 2000), visual patterns (Zifkin and Inoue, 2004), video games and other games (Chuang et al., 2006), specific pieces of music and startle (Garcia-Morales et al., 2009). As for interictal epileptiform activity, recording of EEG during awakening, especially after sleep deprivation, increases the likelihood of recording myoclonic seizures in juvenile myoclonic epilepsy. Sleep deprivation has also been shown to increase the probability of recording seizures, especially in generalized epilepsies; however, there is no evidence that acute sleep deprivation is effective in inducing seizures and thus in decreasing the duration of V-EEG recording in focal epilepsies during surgical evaluation (Malow et al., 2002).

Additional electrodes

Different approaches are available to improve the yield of surface EEG and V-EEG by increasing the number of exploring electrodes. In most cases this includes the addition of additional temporal electrodes, for example, inferior–anterior temporal electrodes such as T1–T2 (Bromfield et al., 1989), cheek electrodes (Krauss et al., 1992), zygomatic electrodes, or sphenoidal electrodes. In a study comparing anterior temporal and sphenoidal electrodes (Kanner et al., 2002), it was identified that sphenoidals allowed earlier identification of ictal onset in temporal lobe epilepsy. The authors guided electrode placement with fluoroscopy, thus confirming their accurate position at the level of the foramen ovale. Both inferior–anterior temporal and sphenoidal electrodes may improve the diagnosis of temporal lobe epilepsy, but are not adequate to identify extratemporal seizure onset. Dense-array electrodes (10/10 System; see Fig. 20.1C) increase the possibility of identifying and localizing epileptiform activity throughout the scalp. The whole system can be placed, or selected electrodes positioned in areas of interest bilaterally, to improve localization over the suspicious area of seizure onset and compare with the contralateral hemisphere. In the past, nasopharyngeal electrodes were used to improve coverage of inferior temporal regions; however, these are uncomfortable and therefore not suited to prolonged studies. In addition, they are easily dislodged with movement, as may occur during a seizure, and they are susceptible to artifacts caused by swallowing and other pharyngeal movements, making the recordings difficult to read.

Intracranial electrodes are used for direct recording from the epidural surface (epidural electrodes), from the subdural surface (subdural and foramen ovale electrodes), and from within the cerebral cortex (depth electrodes). Intracranial electrodes are more sensitive to small field potentials than scalp electrodes, although their area of recording is restricted to potentials localized within a few millimeters (Gloor, 1985). Their placement is associated with potential morbidity and complications; therefore, their use is restricted to patients with refractory focal epilepsy not adequately localized with noninvasive procedures, and to patients requiring cortical mapping of functional cortex with electrical stimulation (usually speech, motor, sensory, and visual systems). Epidural electrodes are not used frequently, because the number that can be placed is limited due to the lower compliance of the epidural space, and because their use for functional mapping with electrical cortical stimulation is limited. Foramen ovale electrodes provide information of activity only in mesial temporal structures; therefore, their use is restricted to analysis of side of ictal onset in patients with bilateral mesial temporal lobe epilepsy. In addition, when foramen ovale electrodes show initial activation of posterior mesial temporal lobe, they highly suggest an extratemporal onset, similarly to when surface posterior temporal electrodes are activated first during focal seizures of apparent temporal lobe origin. Subdural electrodes can be placed in grids and strips of sizes from 4 to 64 contact points. They allow coverage of relatively large areas of the cortex, and can be used for electrical stimulation mapping. The number of subdural electrodes that can be placed is limited by the risks of increased intracranial pressure, midline shift, and by bridging veins in the subdural space. Subdural electrodes provide accurate information about interictal and ictal activity originating directly in the underlying cerebral cortex, but not from the depth of sulci, the amygdala or hippocampus, the sylvian fissure, or the insula. Depth electrodes are placed stereotactically in the depth of sulci and can reach deep cortical structures such as the hippocampal formation or the insula. They can also be used for functional mapping with electrical stimulation, although subdural electrodes are better suited to that function.

Physiological monitoring during V-EEG

Physiological phenomena may accompany seizures or may produce electrical activity that needs to be distinguished from seizures. They need to be monitored with specific electrodes or techniques. The electrocardiogram (ECG) must be recorded during both short-term and prolonged EEG studies. This is because identification of abnormalities of cardiac rhythm is relevant in all patients undergoing EEG, and is important in the differential diagnosis of paroxysmal events and in the identification of patients at risk of sudden death associated with epilepsy. In some cases, eye movement artifact can be difficult to differentiate from frontal slow activity. Infraorbital electrodes can help distinguish eye movement artifact by showing opposite polarity from that of frontopolar electrodes. A specific montage using additional electrodes placed above and below the epicanthal folds can also be used to assist in this differentiation (Picton et al., 2000). The time relationship of electromyographic (EMG) with paroxysmal EEG activity may be important in the diagnosis of myoclonic seizures, epileptic spasms, and subtle tonic seizures. EMG electrodes can also help measure the extent of muscle involvement. This can be achieved by placing EMG electrodes in selected muscles, usually deltoids and quadriceps muscles. Other physiological parameters that might require monitoring are oxygen saturation, breathing, skin resistance, and movements (using accelerometry). In the differential diagnosis of seizures and sleep disorders, the use of complete EEG in addition to polysomnography can be necessary.

Choice of montages and filters in the review and analysis of EEGs

Analysis of background and epileptiform activity requires the use of appropriate montages. Different montages are necessary in order to assess the nature and localization of particular patterns. Optimal EEG analysis requires the use of both bipolar and referential montages. It is recommended that routine EEG should include the use of a longitudinal bipolar, transverse bipolar, as well as referential montages (most commonly average reference and ipsilateral ear or linked ear reference). Digital EEG allows the evaluation of any EEG finding with a variety of montages to clarify its nature. In referential montages the ideal reference should be neutral with respect to the activity of interest. Thus the ear reference is not well suited for the analysis of temporal lobe sharp waves, because the ear electrode on the side of the sharp waves is likely to be contaminated. On the other hand, the ear electrodes are excellent for analysis of generalized epileptiform discharges and other generalized activity, because the ears tend to be the least involved in such situations. The average reference is well suited to analysis of focal EEG discharges, particularly when the electrodes involved in these discharges are removed from the average. However, the average reference is expected to be contaminated by discharges with a wide field. Recommendations of each montage can be reviewed in selected articles and specific EEG books. In general, EEG evaluation is optimized by the analysis of multiple episodes and the selection of different montages in order to enhance the rhythms of interest.

After reviewing the EEG with the recommended filter setting (0.3 Hz LFF and 70 Hz HFF), change of filter setting may be necessary to enhance the representation of rhythms and patterns of interest. Slow activity due to movement artifact is reduced by use of a LFF of 1–5 Hz, although this may mask relevant slow frequencies of cortical origin. Similarly, muscle artifact can be decreased by use of 15–35 HFF, but this has the risk of causing muscle artifact to appear like spikes, polyspikes, or beta activity. To avoid errors due to signal filtering, EEG activity should first be viewed without filtering.

EEG IN THE DIAGNOSIS OF EPILEPSY

Description and recording of epileptiform discharges

In patients suspected of having epilepsy, the interictal EEG often demonstrates epileptiform activity and nonspecific abnormalities. Interictal epileptiform activity includes spikes, sharp waves, and paroxysmal fast activity, and their combinations with slow waves, such as spike-and-wave complexes (spike followed by a slow wave) and polyspike-and-wave complexes (multiple spikes followed by a slow wave). Spikes are predominantly negative potentials with characteristic steep ascending and descending phases, with a duration of 20–80 milliseconds (ms). Sharp waves are longer in duration, lasting 80–200 ms. Sharp waves and spikes are distinguished from sharp nonepileptiform potentials by a number of features, not all of which may be present at the same time. However, the more epileptiform features that are present, the greater the confidence in the epileptiform nature of these discharges. The features include asymmetrical morphology, typically with shorter and smaller initial phase and longer and larger second phase (Gotman, 1980), high voltage, aftergoing slow wave, and an appearance that is different from background activity. A biphasic or polyphasic morphology also favors an epileptiform nature. The epileptiform potential should also have a field and should be different from physiological activity that could be seen in that field. The number of interictal epileptiform discharges per unit of time is not a good predictor of seizure recurrence and does not indicate the severity of epilepsy. Interictal epileptiform activity reveals the "irritative zone" (Rosenow and Luders, 2001), and its morphology and localization is usually closely related to seizure-type classification (partial versus generalized), epileptic syndrome, and localization of the epileptogenic zone.

In patients with documented epilepsy, interictal epileptiform activity can be identified in the first routine EEG in up to 50%, by the third EEG in 84%, and by the fourth in 92% of those in whom interictal epileptiform activity was eventually recorded in subsequent studies (Salinsky et al., 1987). The yield of an EEG can be increased and new abnormalities found if the EEG includes sleep recordings (Binnie and Stefan, 1999), if the recording is performed within 48 hours of a seizure (Schreiner and Pohlmann-Eden, 2003), and with prolonged studies (Gotman and Koffler, 1989). Patients with seizures beginning in childhood present a higher incidence of interictal epileptiform activity, whereas interictal epileptiform activity is less likely to be seen when epilepsy starts in old age (Drury and Beydoun, 1998). Approximately 10% of patients will not show epileptiform activity during wakefulness or sleep after repeated recordings (Adachi et al., 1998; Salinsky et al., 1987). Drug treatment with the classical antiepileptic drugs carbamazepine and phenytoin does not mask interictal epileptiform activity in patients with partial epilepsy. However, some studies suggest that this may not be the case in patients with idiopathic generalized epilepsy treated with valproic acid (Bruni et al., 1980). Some of the newer drugs, particularly levetiracetam and lamotrigine, also seem to suppress epileptiform activity, in both partial and generalized epilepsy (Marciani et al., 1996; Stodieck et al., 2001).

Nonspecific patterns include generalized and focal slow activity, and amplitude asymmetries, which indicate the presence of diffuse or focal pathology. These can be seen frequently in the absence of epilepsy. However, one type of slow activity, temporal intermittent rhythmic delta activity (TIRDA), may be specific for epilepsy, whereas irregular delta activity is nonspecific (Geyer et al., 1999).

The overall yield of diagnostic V-EEG is high, with most series reporting that 73–85% of studies demonstrated clinical events or epileptiform activity on the EEG that allowed the diagnosis of the episodes motivating the study (Mohan et al., 1996; Benbadis et al., 2004). The results of these studies may change the initially suspected diagnosis (epilepsy or nonepileptic) in approximately 25% of patients (Alsaadi et al., 2004), with similar results among children, adults, and the elderly (McBride et al., 2002; Reuber et al., 2002).

Specificity of epileptiform activity

Patients with interictal epileptiform activity have a higher risk of having seizures than patients with a normal EEG. However, about 0.5–1% of the normal population (Bennett, 1967; Gregory et al., 1993; Walczak and Jayakar, 1997) and up to 12% of patients with brain pathology (Sam and So, 2001) may have interictal epileptiform activity despite a negative history of seizures. Epileptiform activity without clinical epilepsy is more common in children with centrotemporal spikes (Verrotti et al., 1999), occipital spikes (Lerman and Kivity-Ephraim, 1981; Okubo et al., 1994), and a photoparoxysmal response (Verrotti et al., 2002). Therefore, an EEG showing interictal epileptiform activity indicates an increased risk of having seizures compared with the general population, and may support a diagnosis of epilepsy when the clinical information is not definitive, but it is *not diagnostic* of epilepsy. Because of the increasing yield of serial EEGs it is recommended to obtain three or four recordings in patients with suspected epilepsy, with one of the recordings including sleep with sleep deprivation; there is relatively little yield to serial EEGs beyond this point. However, with the widespread availability of prolonged inpatient and outpatient V-EEG monitoring, the use of early prolonged studies is rapidly gaining support and may substitute for repeated short EEGs in many situations (Falip et al., 2007).

A definite diagnosis of epilepsy can be reached only when a seizure is recorded. However, this is not usually required for the management of patients with suspected epileptic seizures; in most cases an accurate clinical diagnosis can be reached with interview of the patient and witnesses. In cases where the diagnosis is questionable, prolonged V-EEG is mandatory. These studies are usually more efficient in patients with frequent episodes, but patients with seizures often have unrecognized subtle episodes that can be captured during 24-hour V-EEG recordings. In addition, prolonged studies increase the chance of recording infrequent interictal epileptiform activity, which can be necessary in the diagnosis of some types of epilepsy, such as frontal lobe epilepsies and late-onset epilepsies, epilepsies that often present a difficult differential diagnosis. It is considered that a normal EEG recording during a seizure with impairment of consciousness does exclude a diagnosis of epilepsy. However, simple partial seizures and brief frontal lobe seizures are often associated with a normal ictal EEG even in the presence of bilateral motor activity (Devinsky et al., 1988; Bautista et al., 1998). This is the case because the synchronous activation of a minimum of 6 cm^2 is necessary in order to record an electrical potential with surface electrodes (Tao et al., 2005). An even larger surface area, as well as sufficient synchrony, is necessary for ictal activity to appear on the scalp (Hashiguchi et al., 2007; Tao et al., 2007). In addition, epileptic foci located in the mesial and inferior aspects of the hemispheres often fail to show surface epileptiform discharges.

EEG IN FOCAL EPILEPSIES

In partial epilepsies, focal epileptiform activity is distinguished from normal background activity and artifacts because of some characteristics of spikes and sharp waves. Epileptiform potentials interrupt the background activity, and have different morphology from the ongoing background. These potentials often occur in an area of focal slow activity and display a physiological cerebral field involving several electrodes, which differentiates them from artifacts. Focal interictal epileptiform activity can be activated with hyperventilation and sleep deprivation, but very rarely with photic stimulation. It is frequently, but not always, in the region of the epileptogenic zone and the epileptogenic lesion. Seizure onset is often marked by substitution of normal background by diffuse, regional, or localized attenuation of background activity, or by suppression of ongoing focal slow or interictal epileptiform activity (Geiger and Harner, 1978; Blume et al., 1984). After this, a distinct pattern of EEG activity appears that is different from the baseline background activity. Multiple rhythmic patterns can occur, including fast rhythms in the beta or alpha range, rhythmic theta or delta activity, and runs of sharp waves or spikes. These electrographic changes often have an evolution characterized by progressive slowing of frequency and propagation to adjacent and contralateral channels, or secondary generalization as the seizure evolves. Although there are no specific patterns for seizure localization, certain EEG features may support a specific area of focal onset or early involvement in focal epilepsies.

Benign focal epilepsies of childhood and related syndromes

Centrotemporal spikes are recorded in a majority of patients with *benign rolandic epilepsy* (*benign childhood epilepsy with centrotemporal spikes*) and may be present despite clinical remission of the syndrome. These are negative sharp waves typically with aftergoing slow waves with maximal amplitude midway between central and midtemporal regions (Legarda et al., 1994), and a horizontal dipole with bifrontal positivity. Although sometimes unilateral, centrotemporal spikes are often bilateral independent. They are activated during stages I–IV of sleep, where they are usually abundant, easily recorded, and frequently occur in clusters. Somatosensory stimulation of fingers or toes may activate the spikes (Tassinari et al., 1988). The background activity is normal, although transient focal slow activity can be observed during epochs of increased interictal activity. It should be noted that patients with benign rolandic epilepsy may have focal sharp waves outside the centrotemporal region, and may also have associated generalized spike-and-wave discharges (Drury and Beydoun, 1991; Beydoun et al., 1992).

Although occipital spikes predominate in *Panayiotopoulos syndrome*, EEGs show more variability (Panayiotopoulos, 2007b). Recordings are often normal, or show spikes of diverse location, multifocal discharges, brief generalized slow waves mixed with spikes, and positive spikes. Epileptiform activity is accentuated by sleep and can be abolished by fixation. In *idiopathic childhood occipital epilepsy of Gastaut*, the main EEG characteristic is occipital paroxysms with fixation-off sensitivity. Occipital photosensitivity may be seen (Gastaut, 1982). Other rare benign epilepsies of childhood with different focality have been described, and are characterized by different seizure semiology and interictal spikes localized in different regions.

Temporal lobe epilepsy

Temporal intermittent irregular delta activity is a common, but nonspecific, finding in temporal lobe epilepsy. However, temporal intermittent rhythmic delta activity (TIRDA) appears to be more specific (Reiher et al., 1989; Blume et al., 1993). TIRDA was found to have a strong correlation with mesial temporal sclerosis (Gambardella et al., 1995) (Fig. 20.2A). Temporal interictal epileptiform activity is the most specific abnormal feature in temporal lobe epilepsy, found in more than 90% of patients in some epilepsy surgery series (Fig. 20.3A). However, in nonsurgical series this abnormality was found in a smaller number of patients, ranging from 75% in a series of medically treated patients with temporal lobe epilepsy (Currie et al., 1971) to

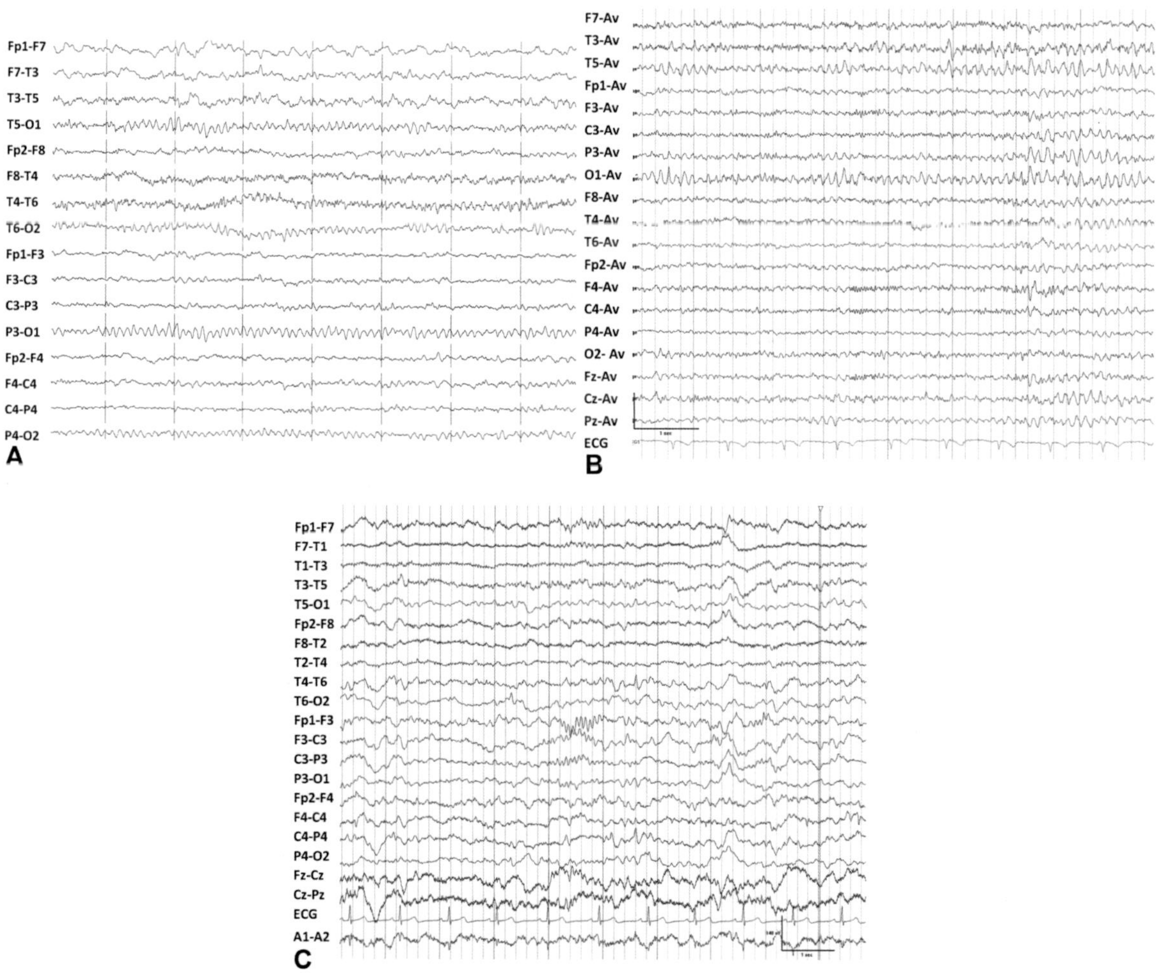

Fig. 20.2. Nonepileptiform abnormalities in focal epilepsies. (**A**) Left temporal intermittent rhythmic delta activity in a patient with left mesial temporal sclerosis. (**B**) Absence of dominant occipital rhythm on the right in occipital lobe epilepsy secondary to head trauma. (**C**) Absence of sleep spindles in the right hemisphere in congenital middle cerebral artery infarct.

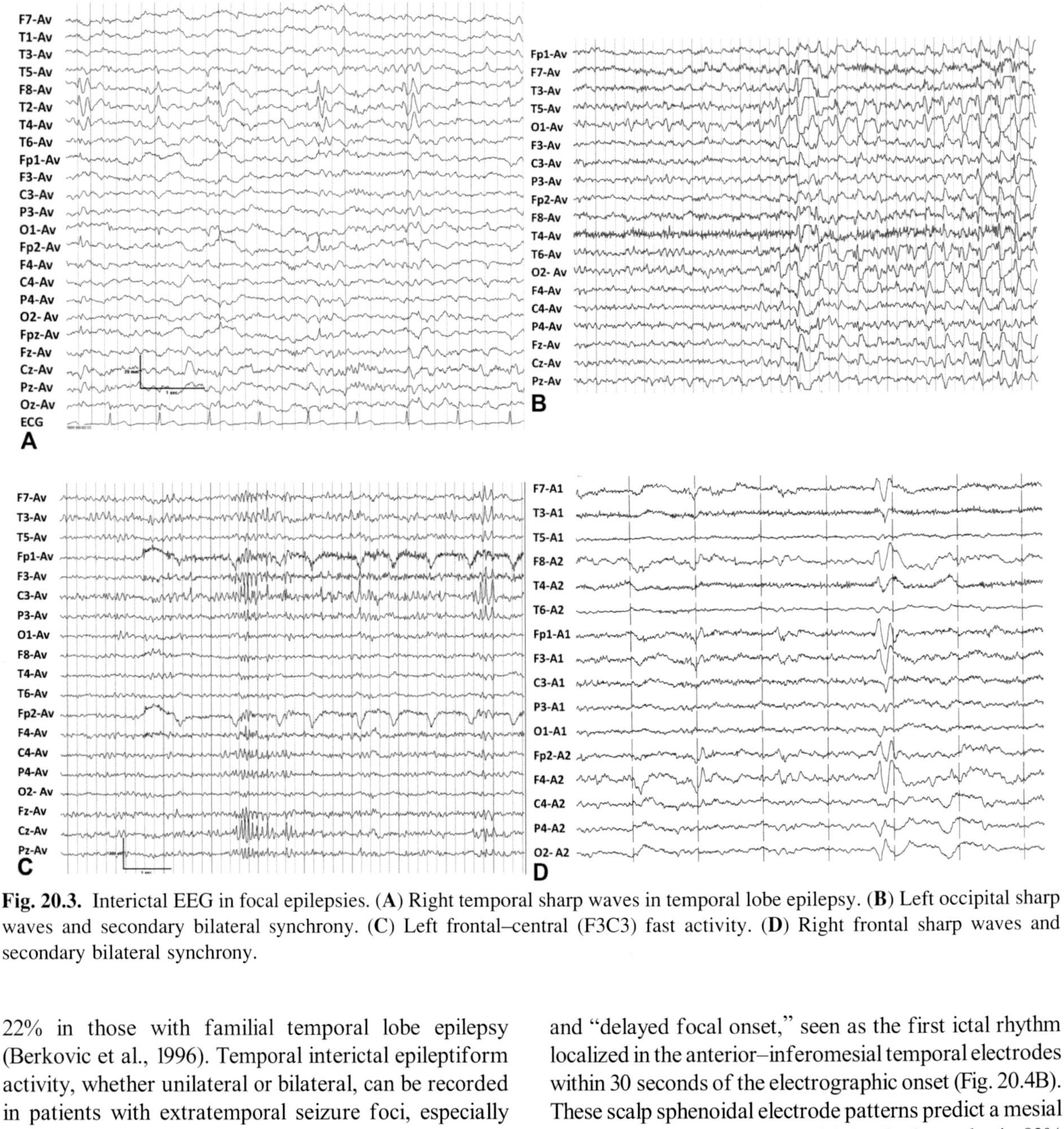

Fig. 20.3. Interictal EEG in focal epilepsies. (**A**) Right temporal sharp waves in temporal lobe epilepsy. (**B**) Left occipital sharp waves and secondary bilateral synchrony. (**C**) Left frontal–central (F3C3) fast activity. (**D**) Right frontal sharp waves and secondary bilateral synchrony.

22% in those with familial temporal lobe epilepsy (Berkovic et al., 1996). Temporal interictal epileptiform activity, whether unilateral or bilateral, can be recorded in patients with extratemporal seizure foci, especially those with occipital, orbitofrontal, and cingulate cortex epileptogenic zones. Bilateral independent temporal epileptiform discharges are common in temporal lobe epilepsy. Even though bilateral independent temporal epileptiform activity does not necessarily indicate bilateral seizure onsets, it reduces the probability of postoperative seizure control. However, this finding should not be considered alone in the decision about surgical candidacy.

In anterior–mesial temporal lobe seizures two different ictal patterns can be recorded in the majority of patients: "early focal onset" (Fig. 20.4A), characterized by localized anterior–inferomesial temporal rhythmic sharp theta activity (5–7 Hz) as the first electrographic change; and "delayed focal onset," seen as the first ictal rhythm localized in the anterior–inferomesial temporal electrodes within 30 seconds of the electrographic onset (Fig. 20.4B). These scalp sphenoidal electrode patterns predict a mesial temporal onset with intracranial depth electrodes in 82% of cases (Risinger et al., 1989).

Although most commonly seen in temporal lobe seizures, where it rarely falsely lateralizes, these patterns of ictal onset can also appear in extratemporal seizures. A slow initial pattern (<5 Hz) with maximal potential over the posterior temporal electrodes has a higher likelihood of neocortical and extratemporal onset and is associated with a less favorable surgical outcome (Ebersole and Pacia, 1996; Vossler et al., 1998; Assaf and Ebersole, 1999). Ictal activity may appear to start, then stop and reappear again; the initial onset of this "start–stop–start phenomenon" is more reliable for localization than the subsequent restart phase

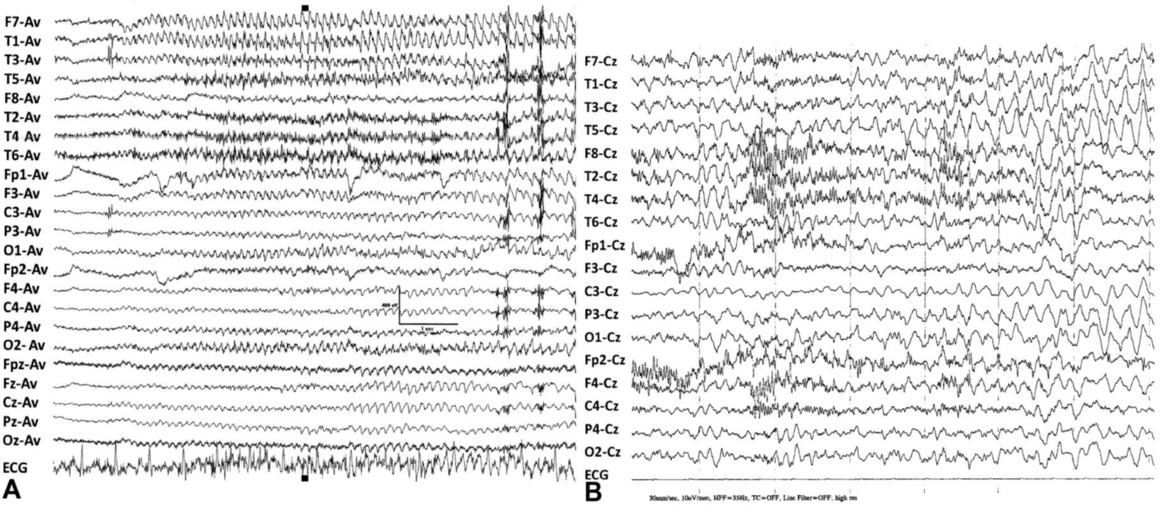

Fig. 20.4. Ictal EEG in temporal lobe epilepsy. Patterns commonly associated with mesial temporal lobe seizures: (**A**) left temporal early focal and (**B**) delayed focal patterns. (**B**) Right temporal initial fast activity in neocortical epilepsy.

(Blume and Kaibara, 1993; Atalla et al., 1996). The specificity of these patterns has not been validated, but their widespread application reveals that they are reliable for localization when consistent with other clinical findings. Common ictal manifestations of temporal lobe seizures include epigastric aura, tachycardia, arrest of ongoing activity, oral and manual automatisms, and vocalization. Ictal speech and early postictal recovery of speech reliably lateralizes to the nondominant temporal lobe (Gabr et al., 1989; Privitera et al., 1991). Dystonic posturing of an upper extremity lateralizes to the contralateral hemisphere (Kotagal et al., 1989). Oral automatisms tend to occur earlier in mesial temporal lobe epilepsy compared with neocortical epilepsy (Gil-Nagel and Risinger, 1997).

Extratemporal epilepsy

Changes and distortion in normal EEG patterns are often helpful and should be looked for in extratemporal epilepsy. Unilateral absence or slowing of the alpha rhythm (see Fig. 20.2B), with a difference exceeding 1.5 Hz, should raise the suspicion of an occipital lobe abnormality on the slower side. Beta activity can be decreased on the side of a lesion involving the frontal cortex. A persistent asymmetry of sleep spindles, exceeding 50% of the recording time, should also suggest a lesion in the hemisphere with the lower voltage, usually involving a large area of the frontal or parietal lobes (see Fig. 20.2C). Focal slow activity, either theta or delta, rhythmic or irregular, indicates the possibility of focal pathology in the involved area, but can also be caused by transient neurological pathology, such as head trauma, migraine, or transient ischemic attack. Localized spikes, sharp waves, or fast activity indicate the localization of the irritative zone (see Fig. 20.3B–D). Multifocal epileptiform activity is present in multifocal or symptomatic generalized epilepsies (see Fig. 20.7D), and in the presence of widespread pathology. Multifocal epileptiform activity can also appear in focal epilepsies with a single localized epileptogenic area, especially those localized in occipital and parietal lobes or in the mesial cortex. Interictal epileptiform activity in extratemporal epilepsy frequently involves the temporal lobes, with either unilateral or bilateral temporal lobe epileptiform activity. Closely spaced electrodes (10/10 System) over the area of suspected origin can assist in the localization of extratemporal seizure onset.

The localizing value of ictal EEG patterns in seizures of extratemporal origin is inferior to that in temporal lobe seizures. Frontal lobe seizures tend to be of shorter duration and often occur in clusters, and ictal semiology is often characterized by marked movement, dystonic posturing, and complex automatisms. Prominent motor activity often results in excessive artifact obscuring the EEG (Fig. 20.5E). Even in the absence of movement, the EEG may show poorly localized or diffuse patterns, or even no EEG changes, indicating a deep origin of abnormal electrographic activity. A focal ictal onset involving three or fewer contiguous electrodes is less common than in temporal lobe seizures. When present, it can consist of rhythmic fast (beta or alpha) (Fig. 20.5A) or theta activity, or runs of repetitive spikes (Fig. 20.5C,D), localized in frontal electrodes (Morris et al., 1988; Quesney, 1991; Laskowitz et al., 1995; Bautista et al., 1998). These focal patterns are more often observed in seizures of dorsolateral onset. Focal beta activity at ictal onset is predictive of favorable outcome after epilepsy surgery (Worrell et al., 2002).

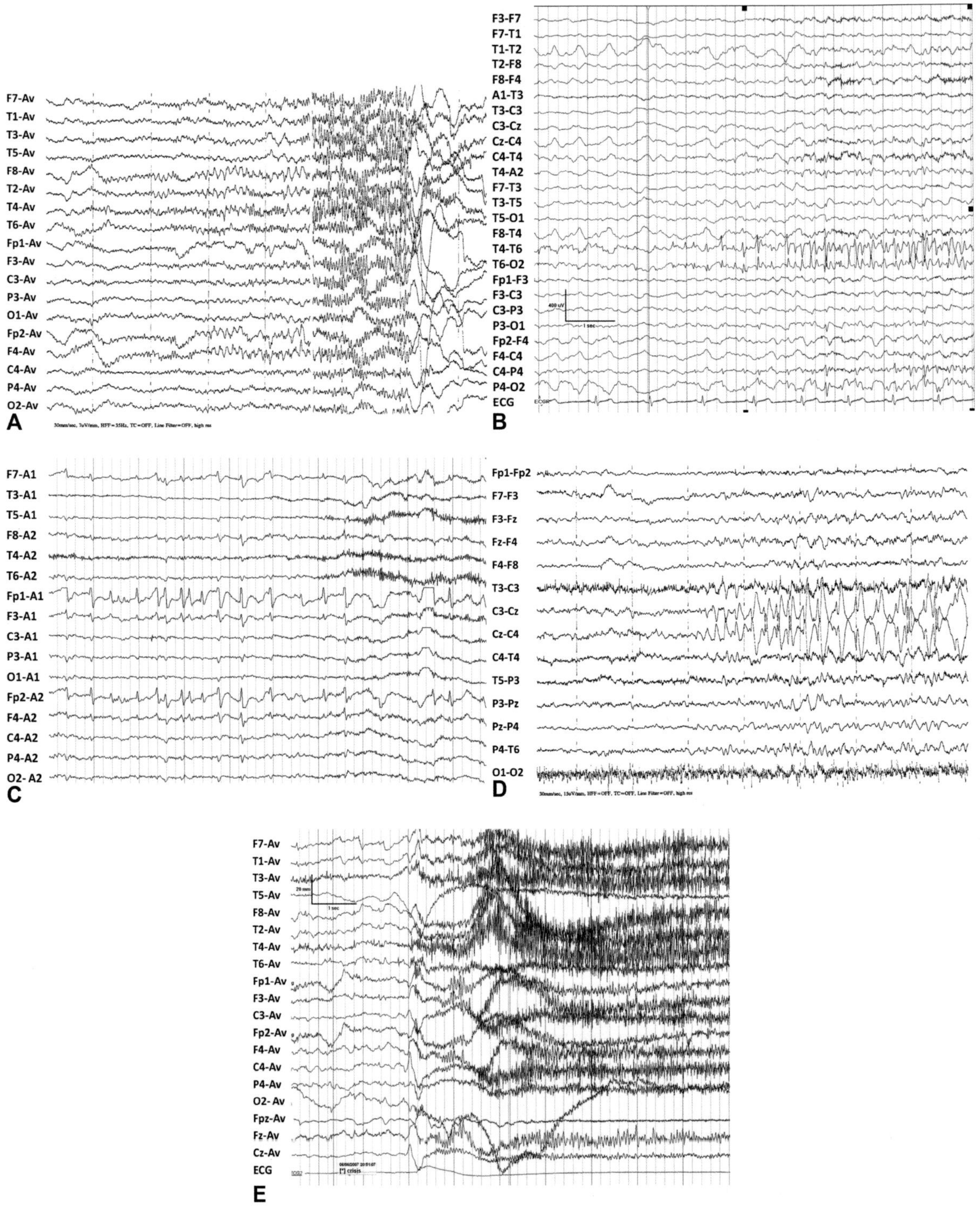

Fig. 20.5. Ictal EEG in extratemporal epilepsy. (**A**) Fast right frontal alpha activity evolving to bilateral fast frequencies in a dorsolateral frontal lobe seizure. (**B**) Right occipital–posterior temporal rapid spikes during an occipital lobe seizure. (**C**) Bilateral frontal (left predominance) repetitive spikes in a frontal lobe seizure. (**D**) Central repetitive spikes during a mesial frontal lobe seizure. (**E**) Nonlocalizing fast activity associated with prominent muscle and movement artifact during a mesial frontal lobe seizure.

Parietal lobe seizures may present with lateralized elementary sensory phenomena. As an extensive area of the parietal lobes are constituted by association cortex, parietal lobe seizures often lack specific ictal symptoms and ictal semiology is related to propagation to temporal or frontal lobes. As in frontal seizures, ictal EEG changes in parietal seizures are often obscured by movement artifact (Williamson et al., 1992a). In many cases ictal changes are better observed when the seizure propagates to temporal (usually posterior) or frontal lobes but not during initial activation of the parietal cortex. Because of this propagation, parietal seizures can be difficult to distinguish from temporal or frontal seizures (Cascino et al., 1993; Salanova et al., 1995). A similar situation occurs with occipital lobe seizures (Fig. 20.5B). Ictal onset may be heralded by specific occipital auras (hemianopsia, elementary visual illusions, blurred vision, and tunnel vision) or abnormalities in eye movements (nystagmus, eye version, and unilateral or bilateral eye blinking). However, visual manifestations are often absent (Jobst et al., 2010). Infrasylvian propagation may cause temporal lobe ictal manifestations, whereas suprasylvian propagation will cause frontal or parietal clinical characteristics, with both types of seizure occasionally present in the same patient. Ictal patterns localized to posterior electrodes and ictal semiology allow the diagnosis of occipital lobe seizures in approximately 50% of patients (Salanova et al., 1992; Williamson et al., 1992b).

EEG IN GENERALIZED EPILEPSIES

Idiopathic generalized epilepsies

Generalized spike-and-wave complexes represent the EEG hallmark in generalized seizures and epilepsies (Fig. 20.6A,B). In idiopathic generalized epilepsies, spike-and-wave complexes occur over a normal EEG background, and the frequency of the complexes is above 2.5 Hz in waking (in sleep, spike-and-wave discharges may be slower, as well as more irregular). Depending

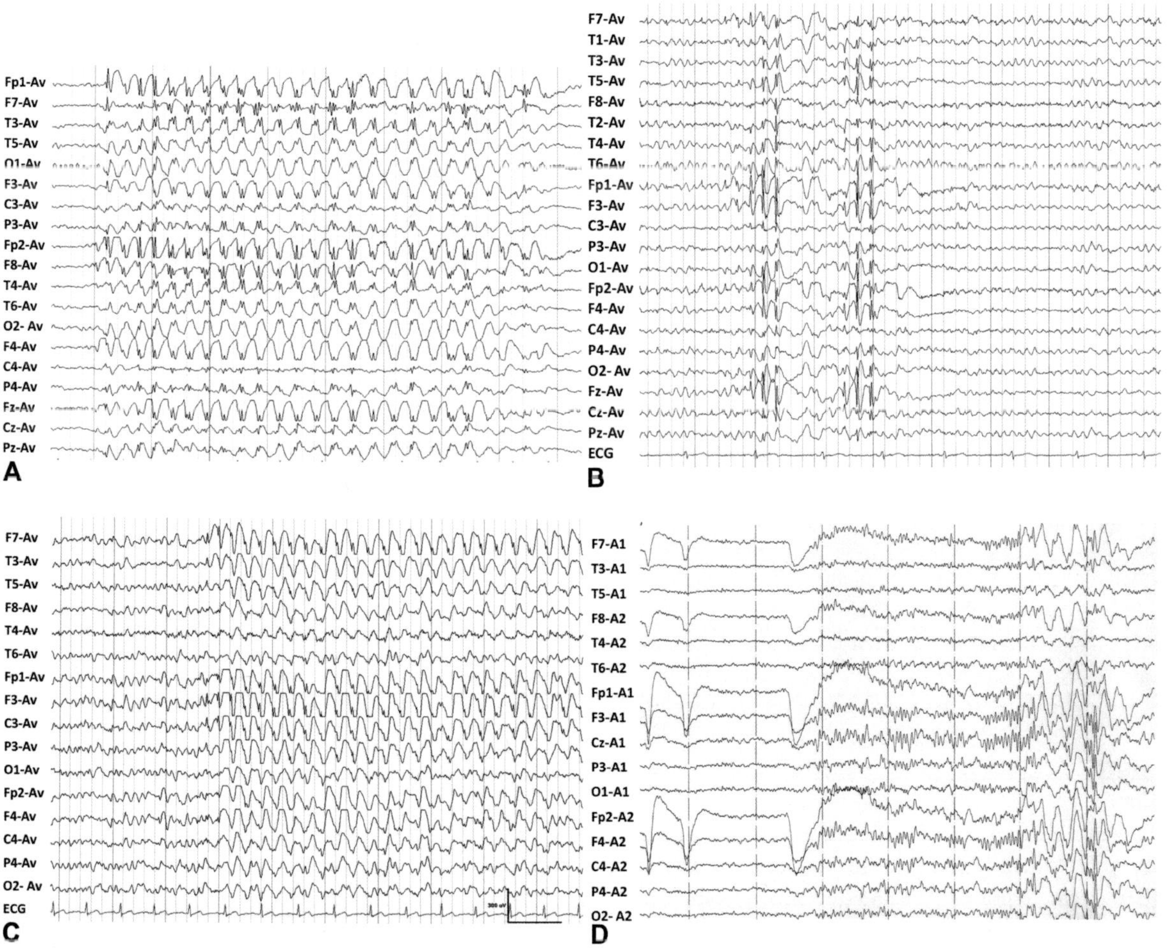

Fig. 20.6. EEG in idiopathic generalized epilepsies. (**A**) 3-Hz spike–wave during a typical absence. (**B**) Interictal 5-Hz spike-and-wave in juvenile myoclonic epilepsy. (**C**) Asymmetrical (left side predominant) 3-Hz spike-and-wave in a patient with typical absence seizures. (**D**) Eye closure artifact followed by mixed slow waves and multiple spikes in Jeavons syndrome.

on the specific syndrome, they may be activated during sleep and on awakening, and their occurrence and duration is incremented with hyperventilation, and at times during intermittent photic stimulation (photoparoxysmal response) and praxis. Although these are the general rules of EEG activity in idiopathic generalized epilepsies, exceptions are not rare, with abnormalities of background activity (focal or generalized slowing) also present in cases with concomitant focal pathology, diffuse toxic or metabolic encephalopathies, or for unknown reasons. In addition, spike-and-wave discharges may have predominance or appear over only one hemisphere (Fig. 20.6C). These asymmetries, which have been described extensively in juvenile myoclonic epilepsy (Asconape and Penry, 1984; Aliberti et al., 1994; Lombroso, 1997; Usui et al., 2005), are often a cause of diagnostic error and the selection of inappropriate antiepileptic drug treatment.

Myoclonic seizures (in *idiopathic myoclonic epilepsy of infancy* and *juvenile myoclonic epilepsy*) are always associated with spike-and-wave discharges (Fig. 20.6B), but not all spike-and-wave discharges are associated with myoclonus, especially in the juvenile form. Myoclonic seizures usually involve upper extremities and are occasionally aggregated in arrhythmic bursts. In juvenile myoclonic epilepsy they are more often recorded in the first hour after awakening. In myoclonic epilepsy of infancy, seizures tend to occur at any time of the day and more often involve axial and cephalic muscles. Intermittent photic stimulation often elicits spike-and-wave discharges and myoclonic seizures (photoparoxysmal response).

Typical absence seizures are also always associated with generalized rhythmic 2.5–4-Hz spike-and-wave complexes (Fig. 20.6A). Clinical manifestations are most likely to be observed when the duration of the discharge exceeds 3 seconds, especially in children. The main clinical features of typical absence seizures are impairment of consciousness and arrest of ongoing activity, returning immediately to normal behavior when the discharge ends. Impairment of consciousness is more evident in *childhood absence epilepsy*, and in this syndrome automatisms may also occur during long episodes. Nevertheless automatisms are less pronounced than in complex partial seizures, and usually involve mild oral movements, hand automatisms, or wandering, and also, unlike complex partial seizures, may not be stereotypical in every patient. Other subtle motor or autonomic manifestations may also be seen (Penry et al., 1975). In adults, typical absence seizures may less conspicuous. Instead of clear impairment of consciousness, patients may appear slow and have erratic responses to commands. Other types of absence seizures are described in specific syndromes. In *absence epilepsy of early childhood*, which is often associated with a less favorable prognosis than typical childhood absence epilepsy, spike-and-wave complexes are more irregular, with a 2–3-Hz frequency, and may be associated with myoclonic–astatic seizures. *Eyelid myoclonia with absence* (Jeavons syndrome) is characterized by the occurrence of generalized multiple spikes associated with slow waves lasting for 3–6 seconds (Fig. 20.6D) and mainly occurring at eye closure, and often associated with upward deviation of the eyeballs and retropulsion of the head. In *perioral myoclonia with absence*, spike–wave discharges are associated with downward rhythmic movement of perioral muscles, often with jaw anteropulsion.

Interictal abnormalities in idiopathic generalized epilepsies can be abolished by valproic acid and other antiepileptic drugs; in this case, the yield of EEG may increase when performed on awakening after partial sleep deprivation. Epilepsy with *myoclonic astatic seizures* (*Doose syndrome*) is characterized by axial and limb myoclonus followed by brief loss of postural tone with atonia. Frequent clusters of 2–3-Hz generalized polyspike discharges, followed by a high-voltage slow wave, characterize ictal and interictal EEG. During seizures the myoclonic phase is associated with the polyspike component, whereas the atonic phase corresponds to the subsequent high-voltage slow-wave component (Oguni et al., 1991).

Symptomatic/cryptogenic generalized epilepsies and epileptic encephalopathies

In symptomatic and cryptogenic generalized epilepsies there is usually diffuse or focal slowing of background activity, of different degree and persistence, more often involving the frontal regions. In more severe cases normal background activity during wakefulness and the normal architecture of sleep are absent or evident for only short epochs. Most of these syndromes were placed among the "epileptic encephalopathies" in a recent proposal of classification (Engel, 2001). In early childhood and infancy, *early myoclonic encephalopathy* and *Otahara syndrome* represent two forms of symptomatic generalized epilepsy. Early myoclonic encephalopathy is characterized by complete absence of normal background during wakefulness and sleep, a burst suppression pattern, with bilateral synchronous and asynchronous paroxysms of slow waves mixed with bursts of spikes and sharp waves, in epochs of 1–5 seconds in duration alternating with epochs of EEG silence. The burst suppression pattern is especially evident during sleep and less pronounced during wakefulness. Erratic limb and axial myoclonus occurs, and may or may not correlate with epileptiform discharges on the EEG (Otani et al., 1989). Similar EEG findings characterize the Ohtahara syndrome; however, in this syndrome the burst suppression pattern remains unchanged during wakefulness and sleep, and clinically the condition is characterized by brief tonic spasms instead of myoclonic seizures (Kobayashi et al., 2007). The occurrence of spasms in the first year of life associated with developmental regression and hypsarrhythmia is typical of *West syndrome*. Asymmetrical or symmetrical high-amplitude, continuous and asynchronous slow waves and spikes characterize hypsarrhythmia (Fig. 20.7A). This activity is usually associated with short epochs of electrodecrement, mostly during sleep (Hrachovy and Frost, 2003). *Severe myoclonic epilepsy of infancy* (*Dravet syndrome*), a syndrome classified among "epilepsies and syndromes undetermined as to whether they are focal or generalized" shows both generalized and focal epileptiform abnormalities. The EEG shows a similar progression to that of the clinical severity, from normal in the initial stages to very frequent epileptiform activity in the more severe phases. Seizures may have generalized (myoclonic and absence) or focal onset, and the corresponding EEG can show generalized or focal patterns. Photoparoxysmal response is common. With increasing age, the EEG may become remarkably free of epileptiform activity despite the presence of refractory epilepsy and developmental delay (Arzimanoglou et al., 2004; Dravet and Bureau, 2005). In *myoclonic absence epilepsy*, interictal and ictal EEG findings are similar to those of typical childhood absence epilepsy, demonstrating normal background and generalized 3-Hz spike–wave discharges (Tassinari et al., 1995). In this syndrome, however, each spike component of the discharge is associated with a prominent myoclonic jerk, typically involving shoulders, perioral muscles, or limbs, but usually not the eyelids. In some cases there is progressive clinical deterioration that may correlate with the appearance of generalized slowing of background activity and more irregular spike-and-wave discharges.

Although there is no consensus for the seizure and EEG diagnostic criteria of *Lennox–Gastaut syndrome*,

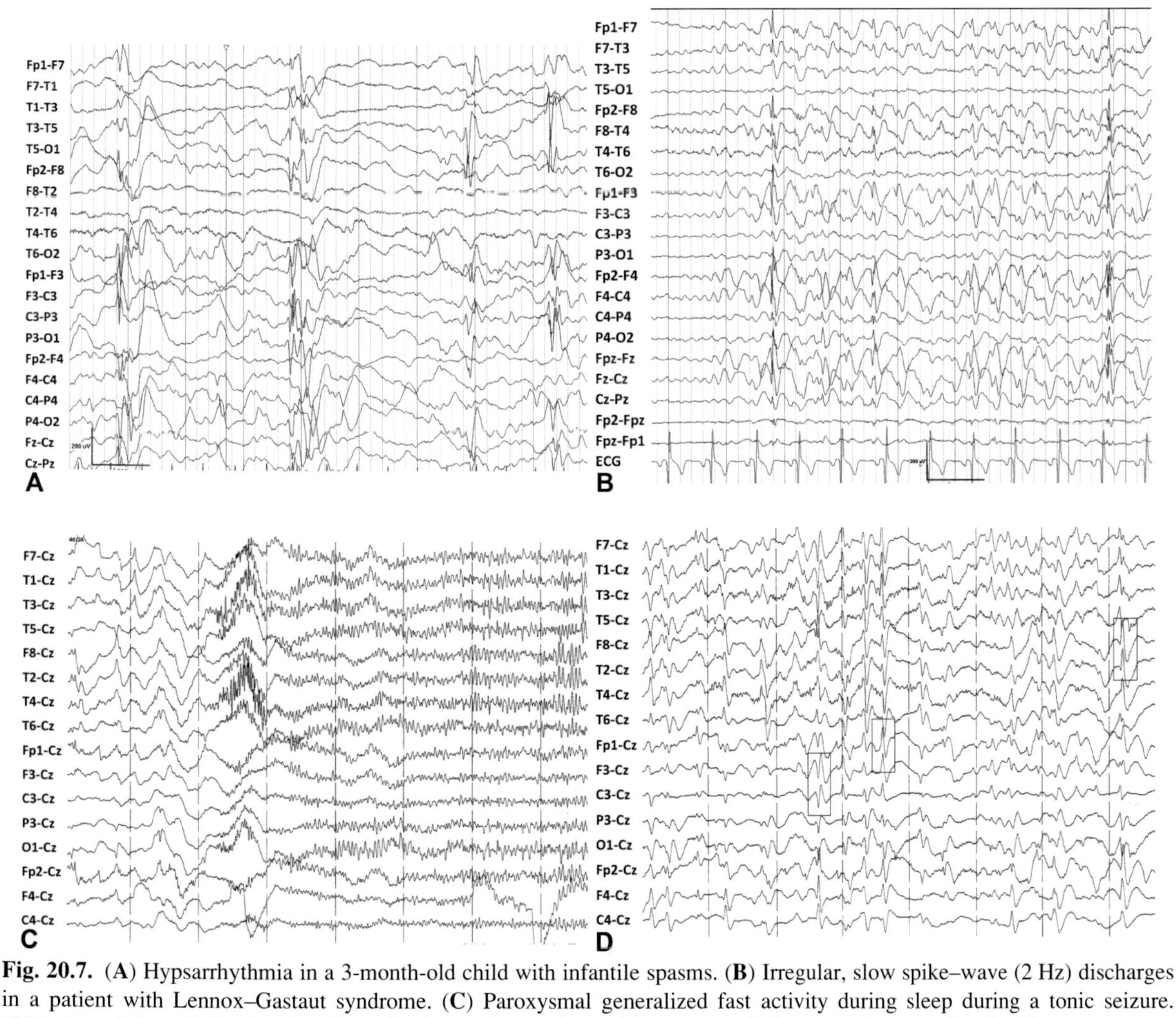

Fig. 20.7. (**A**) Hypsarrhythmia in a 3-month-old child with infantile spasms. (**B**) Irregular, slow spike–wave (2 Hz) discharges in a patient with Lennox–Gastaut syndrome. (**C**) Paroxysmal generalized fast activity during sleep during a tonic seizure. (**D**) Independent multifocal epileptiform discharges in a patient with symptomatic/cryptogenic generalized epilepsy.

all authors agree on a minimum of generalized slow spike-and-wave discharge (< 2.5 Hz) (Fig. 20.7B) and at least two seizure types among atypical absences, tonic and atonic (Panayiotopoulos, 2007a). When V-EEG recordings are of adequate duration and include wakefulness throughout the different periods of the day and all stages of sleep, additional components of the syndrome are often detected (Bare et al., 1998). These include generalized slowing of the background activity, independent multifocal epileptiform activity (Fig. 20.7D), and fast paroxysms (Fig. 20.7C), which are more pronounced or observed only during sleep. Fast paroxysms are sometimes associated with *tonic or atonic seizures*, which may be obvious or subtle (brief rigidity, turning of the head, or slight tonic eyelid opening; slight decrease in tone).

In *Landau–Kleffner syndrome* and *epilepsy with continuous spikes and waves during slow-wave sleep*, EEG at the time of the first seizures may be normal or show unilateral or bilateral centrotemporal, posterior temporal, or multifocal epileptiform activity (Tassinari et al., 2005). At some stage of the disease, continuous spike-and-wave activity during NREM sleep appears. Some patients may not show this sleep pattern, but this may be related to failure to record all stages of sleep. Because of this, repetition of a full night's recording is recommended in order to increase the diagnostic yield.

In *progressive myoclonus epilepsies*, myoclonic seizures are the first manifestation in more than 50% of patients. Myoclonic seizures are focal and multifocal, involving the face, trunk, and distal limbs. Generalized tonic–clonic seizures are usually infrequent and are not present in all patients. Although initial EEG recordings may be normal, different degrees of generalized slowing develop as the disease evolves. At the same time, generalized spike- and polyspike-and-wave discharges become more abundant. During V-EEG monitoring, spontaneous and action triggered jerks may or may not be associated with spike- or polyspike-and-wave discharges (Berkovic et al., 1991). Occipital focal epileptiform discharges and focal seizures are present in *Lafora disease* (Tinuper et al., 1983). Photic activation is present in some syndromes, may be prominent, and includes photoparoxysmal response at low frequencies. Myoclonic status is common, especially at advanced stage of the disease.

EEG IN THE DIAGNOSIS OF STATUS EPILEPTICUS

One of the most important applications of EEG is in the detection of nonconvulsive or subtle convulsive status epilepticus. The EEG for this indication is most often recorded in the ICU. Because of the number of devices that can produce electrical interference, performing EEGs in the ICU can be a technical challenge. In order to avoid electrical artifacts, several actions should be considered: unplugging electrical equipment whenever this is safe for the patient; keeping electrode wires parallel to each other and away from other cables; simultaneous video recording and careful annotations to help identify artifacts. In the presence of scalp wounds, electrodes should be placed on healthy skin around the lesion. Continuous EEG recording in patients with acute changes in mental status or other neurological symptoms in the emergency room and the ICU can reveal epileptiform activity and electrical seizures, even in situations when these are not expected. In a series of 100 patients with acute stroke studied systematically with prolonged EEG monitoring (1–36 hours in duration), abundant epileptiform activity was present in 17 patients and electrical seizures in 2 (Carrera et al., 2006). Another study of 201 patients admitted to the ICU without known neurological pathology revealed electrical seizures in 21 (10%), periodic epileptiform discharges in 34 (17%), and both in 10 (5%) (Oddo et al., 2009). Seizures were purely electrographic, with no detectable clinical correlate, in the majority of patients, and patients with sepsis had a higher rate of epileptiform abnormality.

Overt generalized convulsive status epilepticus is usually easily diagnosed on clinical grounds and EEG confirmation is rarely needed. However, when overt convulsive status epilepticus is left untreated, or when status occurs in a severely injured brain (for example, after hypoxic injury, massive stroke, or severe head trauma), subtle generalized nonconvulsive status epilepticus may be seen. The diagnostic criteria for subtle generalized convulsive status epilepticus are coma with ictal discharges on the EEG, with or without subtle clinical activity such as rhythmic twitching of extremities, trunk, face, or eyes, or tonic eye deviation (Treiman et al., 1998). This form of status epilepticus has a worse prognosis than overt generalized convulsive status epilepticus. In status epilepticus the EEG shows a progressive sequence of EEG changes (Treiman et al., 1990). The initial pattern in the sequence, discrete recurrent seizure discharges, is followed by a pattern merging seizures with waxing and waning amplitude and frequency of EEG rhythms, then continuous ictal activity, continuous ictal activity punctuated by low voltage "flat periods," and finally periodic epileptiform discharges on a "flat" background (Treiman et al., 1990).

The clinical features noted with nonconvulsive status epilepticus are variable and include impairment or loss of responsiveness with eyes open, head or eye deviation to one side, impairment of cognition, alteration of behavior, or subtle twitching of face or limb. Because these manifestations may be nonspecific, the diagnosis of nonconvulsive status epilepticus requires EEG confirmation. Criteria for the EEG diagnosis of nonconvulsive status epilepticus have been suggested (Chong and Hirsch, 2005). Nonconvulsive status epilepticus includes generalized absence status and focal nonconvulsive status epilepticus. Generalized absence status is the less common variety, but often the easier one to recognize. There may be continuous or extremely frequent generalized spike-and-wave and polyspike-and-wave activity. However, the activity is often irregular or characterized by generalized frontally predominant mixed sharp alpha, theta, and delta activity with some recognizable spike-and-wave and polyspike-and-wave activity (Fig. 20.8A).

Complex partial nonconvulsive status epilepticus is often harder to recognize. A progressive sequence of EEG changes described during generalized convulsive status epilepticus (Treiman et al., 1990) can also be seen in with more focal patterns (Fig. 20.8B–F). The initial pattern in the sequence, discrete recurrent seizure discharges, may be the easiest to diagnose. The subsequent patterns in the sequence (merging seizures, continuous ictal activity, continuous ictal activity with periods of attenuation, and periodic epileptiform discharges) can be very challenging to diagnose (Uthman and Bearden, 2008). The definitive identification of nonconvulsive status often requires clinical features consistent with nonconvulsive status as well as convincing clinical and EEG response to short-acting therapy (e.g., benzodiazepines). The patterns of generalized or lateralized periodic “epileptiform discharges” are not specific for electrographic status epilepticus and may be shared with some forms of toxic–metabolic encephalopathy, anoxic encephalopathy, and Creutzfeld–Jakob disease. When associated with clinical seizure activity at other times, these periodic patterns may be considered intermediate along the interictal–ictal continuum (Chong and Hirsch, 2005).

EEG in simple partial status may demonstrate rhythmic or repetitive spikes or focal or generalized rhythmic slow activity. EEG changes may be mild or even absent when the focus is too small and localized in deeper cortical structures. Continuous clonic activity of the affected parts of the body is the best recognized clinical manifestation, although involvement of sensory, visual, and auditory cortex causes the corresponding sensory illusion, involvement of speech areas is associated with aphasia, and involvement of association cortex with different types of cognitive impairment. *Epilepsia partialis continua*, a form of refractory simple partial status, is most frequently associated with Rasmussen syndrome, although other etiologies (cortical dysplasia, gliomas, head trauma, stroke) can also manifest this pattern. EEG is characterized by repetitive spikes or rhythmic focal slowing. *Nonconvulsive status* usually is associated with different patterns and clinical manifestations. *Complex partial status* is characterized by continuous or repetitive complex partial seizures. Long runs of generalized 3-Hz spike–wave discharges are characteristic of *absence status* and *myoclonic status*. *Subtle status* is characterized by subtle clinical manifestations (such as mild clonic activity, eye deviation, or nystagmus) associated with focal spikes or slowing.

EEG IN PRESURGICAL EVALUATION OF EPILEPSY

Epilepsy is resistant to antiepileptic drug treatment in approximately 35% of patients (Kwan and Brodie, 2000). In these patients, epilepsy surgery must be considered through proper presurgical evaluation. During this evaluation, prolonged V-EEG allows the recording of seizures; this is relevant in order to provide demonstration of epilepsy and is primordial in the localization of the epileptogenic zone, the zone that has to be removed or disconnected to achieve seizure freedom. As discussed above, there are different ictal EEG patterns, which are related to the localization of the area of seizure onset, extent of cortex involved, and distance from electrodes, among other factors. EEG recordings must be interpreted in the context of the clinical information and other tests (neuropsychological evaluation, brain imaging). When ictal onset is concordant with a well localized epileptogenic structural abnormality on brain magnetic resonance imaging (MRI) (i.e., mesial temporal sclerosis, cavernous angioma, tumor), further testing to confirm the epileptogenic zone may not be necessary. In patients with a known epileptogenic lesion on brain MRI, ictal EEG may demonstrate a different ictal onset in approximately 20% of patients undergoing presurgical evaluation, and the epileptogenic zone may be more closely related to the ictal EEG zone or to the abnormality observed on brain imaging (Fish et al., 1991; Clarke et al., 1996; Holmes et al., 1999). On the other hand, analysis of ictal EEG and seizure semiology may provide important clues for the identification of focal or widespread neuronal migration disorders in postprocessing brain imaging (Von Oertzen et al., 2002). The localization yield of ictal EEG varies with seizure type and location of the epileptogenic zone. In a review of 486 seizures from 72 patients, ictal EEG provided correct localization in 93% of mesial temporal seizures, 74% of neocortical temporal, 65% of lateral frontal, 46% of parietal, 41% of occipital, and only 24% of mesial frontal foci (Foldvary et al., 2001). When ictal semiology is also considered, the localizing yield increases and may be helpful in establishing a hypothesis that will direct the implantation of intracranial electrodes.

MISDIAGNOSIS OF EPILEPSY

Misdiagnosis of epilepsy is common (Chowdhury et al., 2008). In one retrospective study, the most common causes of misdiagnosis were an incomplete clinical

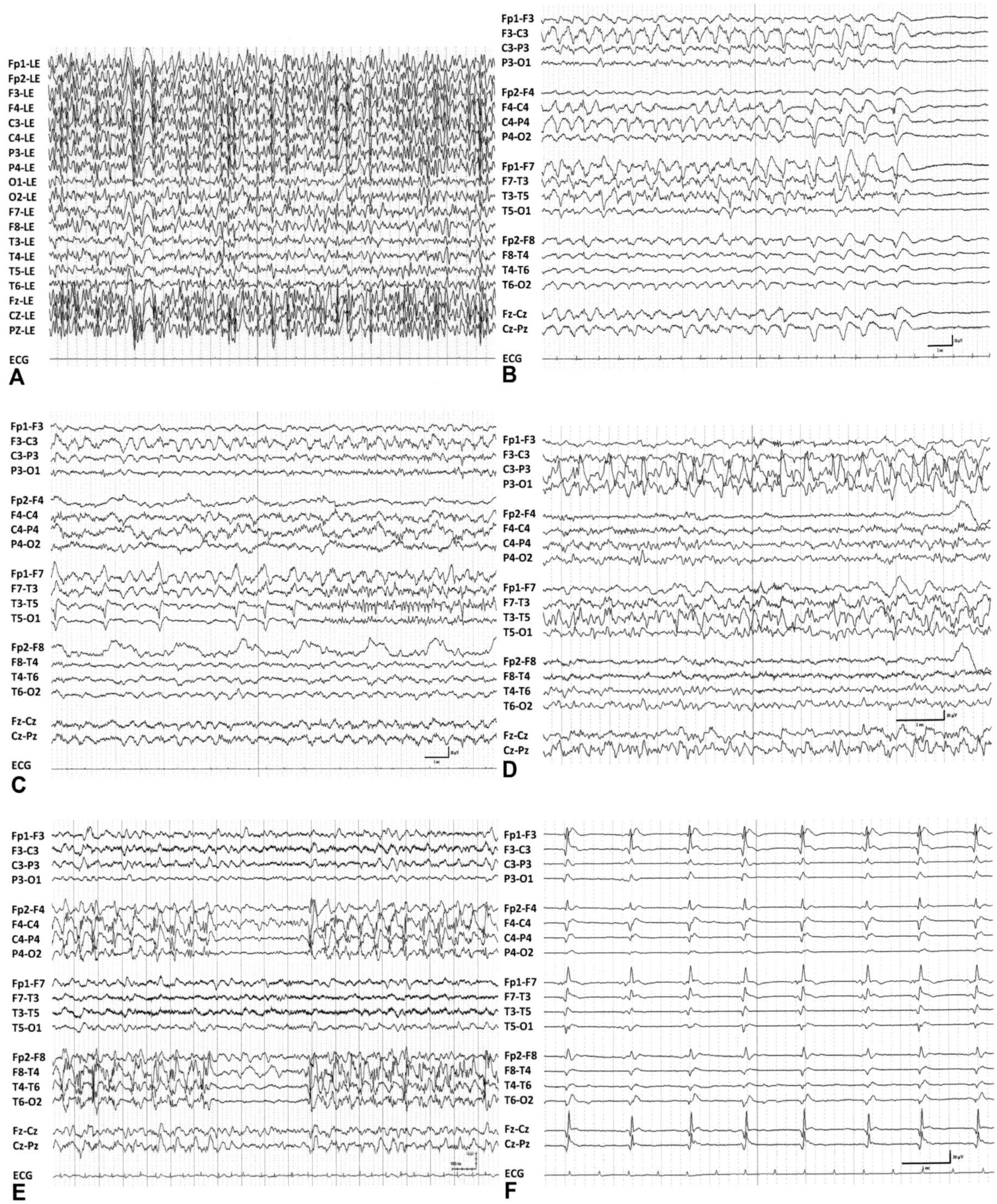

Fig. 20.8. The EEG shows status epilepticus. Generalized absence status with atypical EEG pattern (**A**). Nonconvulsive partial status epilepticus sequence of EEG changes: (**B**) discrete seizures; (**C**) merging seizures; (**D**) continuous seizure activity; (**E**) continuous seizure activity with periods of attenuation; (**F**) periodic epileptiform discharges with a flat background.

history and misinterpretation of EEG (Smith et al., 1999). Overinterpretation of EEGs can lead to erroneous diagnosis of epilepsy and the unnecessary use of antiepileptic drugs (Smith et al., 1999; Fowle and Binnie, 2000). In reviews of previous EEGs performed on patients wrongly diagnosed as epileptic and eventually diagnosed with psychogenic nonepileptic events, the over-read patterns were often simple variations of normal background activity (fragmentation or sharp configuration) (Benbadis and Tatum, 2003), as well as normal variants, particularly wicket patterns (Krauss et al., 2005). Because of this, electroencephalographers should be familiar with certain normal variants (Cobb et al., 1979; Klass and Westmoreland, 1985) and be able to identify artifacts. A number of normal sharp or rhythmic nonepileptiform patterns have been described. The majority can be identified based on their morphology, pattern, and topography. Some of the benign rhythmic variants such as midline theta and rhythmic theta bursts of drowsiness can have a waxing and waning amplitude, but with no significant change in frequency. The normal variants most likely to be overdiagnosed as epileptiform are commonly encountered in the setting of drowsiness and tend to disappear in deeper sleep (Westmoreland, 1996).

Psychogenic seizures are the most common nonepileptic events that may be misdiagnosed as epileptic seizures, and occur in 20–40% of patients referred to epilepsy centers (Benbadis and Hauser, 2000). Their occurrence can be suspected from certain clinical characteristics, some of which can be obtained from the medical history. However, witness descriptions are often unreliable (Mannan and Wieshmann, 2003) and misleading, whereas V-EEG monitoring provides reliable information that can be reviewed as many times as necessary and presented to the witness for confirmation. Nonepileptic events should be considered in all patients with difficult-to-control epilepsy, and should be strongly suspected in patients with prolonged episodes, seizures of fluctuating intensity, seizure worsening with increased dosage and number of antiepileptic drugs, and in the presence of significant psychiatric conditions or the precedent of a stressful traumatic event (Duncan and Oto, 2008). V-EEG diagnosis of psychogenic nonepileptic events is based on EEG and video review of semiology. First, there should be absence of ictal abnormalities before, during, and immediately after the episode. As EEG is often obscured by movement artifact, attention should be directed to epochs during which the patient is relatively quiet and the background EEG can be interpreted. Analysis of these epochs usually demonstrates normal rhythms, including the occipital dominant rhythm, while the patient is still unresponsive. Second, analysis of semiology usually demonstrates atypical motor activity or behavior during the episodes, such as preparation for the event, weeping, eye closure, absence of facial involvement despite apparent bilateral tonic or clonic activity, asynchronous limb movements, side-to-side head movements, crescendo–decrescendo evolution of the event, tremor or shaking, and pelvic thrusting. Caution should be exerted as some of these features have also been described in frontal epilepsies (i.e., side-to-side head motions, alternating pedaling movements of lower extremities, pelvic thrusting) (Kanner et al., 1990; Saygi et al., 1992). Of help in the differentiation among psychogenic events and frontal lobe seizures are the shorter duration and stereotypical nature of the latter compared with prolonged duration (often minutes) and marked variability over time and among multiple events recorded during a monitoring session in psychogenic events. It has to be remembered that ictal EEG is often normal during simple partial seizures and during seizures of mesial frontal lobe origin, despite the presence of marked bilateral motor activity. In these cases definitive diagnosis based on V-EEG may not be possible, unless the seizures evolve to secondary generalization with medication withdrawal. Other diagnostic methods have to be considered (brain imaging, psychiatric interview, evolution over time, response to medication) (Gates, 2000). To complicate matters further, approximately 10–20% of patients with nonepileptic psychogenic seizures also have epilepsy, so that a diagnosis of nonepileptic seizures does not necessarily exclude epileptic seizures (Lesser et al., 1983; Devinsky and Thacker, 1995; Benbadis et al., 2001). Therefore, recorded episodes should be reviewed with the family or witness and an attempt made to determine whether these are the only spells or there are other types. Occasionally patients with documented psychogenic nonepileptic events may have interictal epileptiform activity or a previous history of clear epileptic seizures; in these patients reduction in the dose or number of drugs is usually acceptable, but maintaining at least monotherapy with one drug is usually recommended.

Although there is no agreement among centers on the use of induction protocols, multiple techniques have been used to induce psychogenic nonepileptic events (Krumholz, 1999; McGonigal et al., 2004). In order to avoid deceiving the patient, the use of simultaneous hyperventilation and photic stimulation is recommended by some authors, as both can induce epileptic seizures (Parra et al., 1998; McGonigal et al., 2004). Most studies report high efficacy of induction protocols, although one study demonstrated that the majority of patients with nonepileptic events will have them spontaneously early during V-EEG monitoring (Pierelli et al., 1989; Parra et al., 1998). Patients with nonepileptic events may fail to have them during induction procedures, and, more worryingly, patients with epileptic seizures may present a nonepileptic spell during induction protocols; although rare, a true epileptic seizure may also be caused by induction procedure using the intravenous administration of placebo (Walczak et al., 1994).

Syncope is the second most common cause that may lead to a wrong diagnosis of seizure. Patients with syncope may have preliminary symptoms that may be confused with auras. During syncope, bilateral motor activity (brief clonic movements and tonic rigidity), focal signs (eye or head deviation), and incontinence are not unusual (Schuele et al., 2007). In one study of normal volunteers, multifocal myoclonus was recorded in 90% of individuals (Lempert et al., 1994). This multifocal myoclonus had a mean duration of 6.6 seconds, with a maximal duration of 15.9 seconds, which should help to distinguish it from the typically longer duration of synchronous clonic activity of generalized tonic–clonic seizures. For proper diagnosis of cardiogenic syncope in the V-EEG unit, appropriate ECG recording is mandatory in all patients. Loss of consciousness due to cardiogenic syncope should be differentiated from ictal asystole and arrhythmia in patients with epilepsy (Strzelczyk et al., 2008; Winesett et al., 2009).

QUANTIFICATION OF EPILEPTIC SEIZURES

Patient reports of seizure frequency are often inaccurate. The patients and witnesses frequently miss seizures with impairment of consciousness. Several authors, using prolonged V-EEG monitoring, have evaluated the extent of the problem of unrecognized seizures. In a series of 134 consecutive patients who had seizures during inpatient V-EEG, Heo et al. (2006) found that 31 (23%) were unable to identify that they had an episode. Patients with a higher risk of not recognizing their seizures were older, and had bilateral temporal epileptiform activity or bilateral brain pathology. However, the predictive value of these findings was low. Other authors have reported higher rates of seizure unawareness, ranging from 35% to 61% (Blum et al., 1996; Tatum et al., 2001; Kerling et al., 2006; Hoppe et al., 2007), and some studies also demonstrate that caretakers and family members may be unaware of the patient's seizure. Missed seizures include generalized tonic–clonic, complex partial, and absence seizures. Seizures occurring during sleep are more often missed, especially, but not only, in patients sleeping alone. The lack of awareness of seizures calls for the need to have adequate supervision during V-EEG monitoring studies.

LIMITATIONS OF SURFACE ELECTROENCEPHALOGRAPHY

Not all cortical activity is visible on scalp EEG. A 6-cm^2 area of synchronous discharge is required for epileptiform activity to be identified by scalp electrodes (Cooper, 1965); more recent studies suggest that an even larger area of at least 10 cm^2 of activated cortex is necessary to generate scalp ictal activity (Tao et al., 2005). This explains why most simple partial seizures do not have a surface EEG correlate (Devinsky et al., 1988). Other factors also influence how electrical currents are recorded; the EEG signal is filtered differently by the intervening brain tissue, cerebrospinal fluid, meninges, skull, and scalp, with fast frequencies having more attenuation than slow frequencies; signals recorded from scalp include variable degrees of volume conduction; activity from perpendicularly oriented superficial cortex predominate over horizontal currents; and orthogonally oriented dipoles are better recorded (Gloor, 1985). Also, electrical activity arising from midline cortex, deep structures, and depth of sulci may be too distant from scalp electrodes to be recorded. All of these modifications of electrical currents alter the recording and reduce the possibility of their localization by scalp EEG. It is possible to predict how an electrical potential will display on surface EEG, what is known as the *direct question*. However, of more clinical relevance is the *inverse question*: what is the exact location of a potential recorded on surface EEG. The inverse question can be answered with only a limited degree of certainty; however, with appropriate technique and training, the number of possible sources for a given EEG potential can be limited, and when clinical information is also considered the possibilities are often reduced to a number that can be adequate for localization, surgical resection, or intracranial electrode placing. Finally, movement and electromyogram artifacts can obscure important portions of the EEG, and make them noninterpretable; this can be partially compensated by the use of filters and longer sampling of EEG, and the recording of multiple clinical episodes.

References

Adachi N, Alarcon G, Binnie CD et al. (1998). Predictive value of interictal epileptiform discharges during non-REM sleep on scalp EEG recordings for the lateralization of epileptogenesis. Epilepsia 39: 628–632.

Aliberti V, Grunewald RA, Panayiotopoulos CP et al. (1994). Focal electroencephalographic abnormalities in juvenile myoclonic epilepsy. Epilepsia 35: 297–301.

Alsaadi TM, Thieman C, Shatzel A et al. (2004). Video-EEG telemetry can be a crucial tool for neurologists experienced in epilepsy when diagnosing seizure disorders. Seizure 13: 32–34.

American Clinical Neurophysiology Society (2006a). Guideline 1: Minimum technical requirements for performing clinical electroencephalography. J Clin Neurophysiol 23: 86–91.

American Clinical Neurophysiology Society (2006b). Guideline 5: Guidelines for standard electrode position nomenclature. J Clin Neurophysiol 23: 107–110.

American Electroencephalographic Society (1994). Guideline one: minimum technical requirements for performing clinical electroencephalography. J Clin Neurophysiol 11: 2–5.

Arzimanoglou A, Guerrini R, Aicardi J (2004). Dravet syndrome: severe myoclonic epilepsy or severe polymorphic epilepsy of infants. In: Epilepsy in Children. 3rd edn. Lippincott Williams and Wilkins, Philadelphia.

Asconape J, Penry JK (1984). Some clinical and EEG aspects of benign juvenile myoclonic epilepsy. Epilepsia 25: 108–114.

Assaf BA, Ebersole JS (1999). Visual and quantitative ictal EEG predictors of outcome after temporal lobectomy. Epilepsia 40: 52–61.

Atalla N, Abou-Khalil B, Fakhoury T (1996). The start-stop-start phenomenon in scalp-sphenoidal ictal recordings. Electroencephalogr Clin Neurophysiol 98: 9–13.

Bare MA, Glauser TA, Strawsburg RH (1998). Need for electroencephalogram video confirmation of atypical absence seizures in children with Lennox–Gastaut syndrome. J Child Neurol 13: 498–500.

Bautista RE, Spencer DD, Spencer SS (1998). EEG findings in frontal lobe epilepsies. Neurology 50: 1765–1771.

Benbadis SR, Allen Hauser W (2000). An estimate of the prevalence of psychogenic non-epileptic seizures. Seizure 9: 280–281.

Benbadis SR, Tatum WO (2003). Overinterpretation of EEGs and misdiagnosis of epilepsy. J Clin Neurophysiol 20: 42–44.

Benbadis SR, Agrawal V, Tatum WO (2001). How many patients with psychogenic nonepileptic seizures also have epilepsy? Neurology 57: 915–917.

Benbadis SR, O'Neill E, Tatum WO et al. (2004). Outcome of prolonged video-EEG monitoring at a typical referral epilepsy center. Epilepsia 45: 1150–1153.

Bennett DR (1967). Spike-wave complexes in "normal" flying personnel. Aerosp Med 38: 1276–1282.

Berkovic SF, So NK, Andermann F (1991). Progressive myoclonus epilepsies: clinical and neurophysiological diagnosis. J Clin Neurophysiol 8: 261–274.

Berkovic SF, McIntosh A, Howell RA et al. (1996). Familial temporal lobe epilepsy: a common disorder identified in twins. Ann Neurol 40: 227–235.

Beydoun A, Garofalo EA, Drury I (1992). Generalized spike-waves, multiple loci, and clinical course in children with EEG features of benign epilepsy of childhood with centrotemporal spikes. Epilepsia 33: 1091–1096.

Binnie CD, Stefan H (1999). Modern electroencephalography: its role in epilepsy management. Clin Neurophysiol 110: 1671–1697.

Blum DE, Eskola J, Bortz JJ et al. (1996). Patient awareness of seizures. Neurology 47: 260–264.

Blume WT, Kaibara M (1993). The start-stop-start phenomenon of subdurally recorded seizures. Electroencephalogr Clin Neurophysiol 86: 94–99.

Blume WT, Young GB, Lemieux JF (1984). EEG morphology of partial epileptic seizures. Electroencephalogr Clin Neurophysiol 57: 295–302.

Blume WT, Borghesi JL, Lemieux JF (1993). Interictal indices of temporal seizure origin. Ann Neurol 34: 703–709.

Bromfield E, Sato S, McBurney J et al. (1989). Anterior temporal (T1/T2) electrodes in the evaluation of patients with seizure disorders. Clin Electroencephalogr 20: VII–VIII.

Bruni J, Wilder BJ, Bauman AW et al. (1980). Clinical efficacy and long-term effects of valproic acid therapy on spike-and-wave discharges. Neurology 30: 42–46.

Carrera E, Michel P, Despland PA et al. (2006). Continuous assessment of electrical epileptic activity in acute stroke. Neurology 67: 99–104.

Cascino GD, Hulihan JF, Sharbrough FW et al. (1993). Parietal lobe lesional epilepsy: electroclinical correlation and operative outcome. Epilepsia 34: 522–527.

Chong DJ, Hirsch LJ (2005). Which EEG patterns warrant treatment in the critically ill? Reviewing the evidence for treatment of periodic epileptiform discharges and related patterns. J Clin Neurophysiol 22: 79–91.

Chowdhury FA, Nashef L, Elwes RD (2008). Misdiagnosis in epilepsy: a review and recognition of diagnostic uncertainty. Eur J Neurol 15: 1034–1042.

Chuang YC, Chang WN, Lin TK et al. (2006). Game-related seizures presenting with two types of clinical features. Seizure 15: 98–105.

Clarke DB, Olivier A, Andermann F et al. (1996). Surgical treatment of epilepsy: the problem of lesion/focus incongruence. Surg Neurol 46: 579–585.

Cobb WA, Guiloff RJ, Cast J (1979). Breach rhythm: the EEG related to skull defects. Electroencephalogr Clin Neurophysiol 47: 251–271.

Cooper R (1965). Development of a technique for recording the cerebral activity of conscious animals during complex accelerations. Med Electron Biol Eng 3: 447.

Currie S, Heathfield KW, Henson RA et al. (1971). Clinical course and prognosis of temporal lobe epilepsy. A survey of 666 patients. Brain 94: 173–190.

Devinsky O, Thacker K (1995). Nonepileptic seizures. Neurol Clin 13: 299–319.

Devinsky O, Kelley K, Porter RJ et al. (1988). Clinical and electroencephalographic features of simple partial seizures. Neurology 38: 1347–1352.

Dravet C, Bureau M (2005). Benign myoclonic epilepsy in infancy. In: J Roger, M Bureau, C Dravet et al. (Eds.), Epileptic Syndromes in Infancy, Childhood and Adolescence. 4th edn. John Libbey, London, pp. 77–88.

Drury I, Beydoun A (1991). Benign partial epilepsy of childhood with monomorphic sharp waves incentrotemporal and other locations. Epilepsia 32: 662–667.

Drury I, Beydoun A (1998). Interictal epileptiform activity in elderly patients with epilepsy. Electroencephalogr Clin Neurophysiol 106: 369–373.

Duncan R, Oto M (2008). Predictors of antecedent factors in psychogenic nonepileptic attacks: multivariate analysis. Neurology 71: 1000–1005.

Ebersole JS, Pacia SV (1996). Localization of temporal lobe foci by ictal EEG patterns. Epilepsia 37: 386–399.

Eisenman LN, Attarian H, Fessler AJ et al. (2005). Self-reported seizure frequency and time to first event in the seizure monitoring unit. Epilepsia 46: 664–668.

Engel J Jr (2001). A proposed diagnostic scheme for people with epileptic seizures and with epilepsy: report of the ILAE Task Force on Classification and Terminology. Epilepsia 42: 796–803.

Falip M, Gil-Nagel A, Viteri Torres C et al. (2007). Diagnostic problems in the initial assessment of epilepsy. Neurologist 13: S2–S10.

Fish D, Andermann F, Olivier A (1991). Complex partial seizures and small posterior temporal or extratemporal structural lesions: surgical management. Neurology 41: 1781–1784.

Foldvary N, Klem G, Hammel J et al. (2001). The localizing value of ictal EEG in focal epilepsy. Neurology 57: 2022–2028.

Fowle AJ, Binnie CD (2000). Uses and abuses of the EEG in epilepsy. Epilepsia 41: S10–S18.

Friedman DE, Hirsch LJ (2009). How long does it take to make an accurate diagnosis in an epilepsy monitoring unit? J Clin Neurophysiol 26: 213–217.

Gabr M, Luders H, Dinner D et al. (1989). Speech manifestations in lateralization of temporal lobe seizures. Ann Neurol 25: 82–87.

Gambardella A, Gotman J, Cendes F et al. (1995). Focal intermittent delta activity in patients with mesiotemporal atrophy: a reliable marker of the epileptogenic focus. Epilepsia 36: 122–129.

Garcia-Morales I, Maestu F, Perez-Jimenez MA et al. (2009). A clinical and magnetoencephalography study of MRI-negative startle epilepsy. Epilepsy Behav 16: 166–171.

Gastaut H (1982). A new type of epilepsy: benign partial epilepsy of childhood with occipital spike-waves. Clin Electroencephalogr 13: 13–22.

Gates J (2000). Epidemiology and classification of non-epileptic events. In: J Gates, A Rowan (Eds.), Non-Epileptic Seizures. Butterworth-Heinemann, Boston, pp. 3–14.

Geiger LR, Harner RN (1978). EEG patterns at the time of focal seizure onset. Arch Neurol 35: 276–286.

Geyer JD, Bilir E, Faught RE et al. (1999). Significance of interictal temporal lobe delta activity for localization of the primary epileptogenic region. Neurology 52: 202–205.

Gil-Nagel A, Risinger MW (1997). Ictal semiology in hippocampal versus extrahippocampal temporal lobe epilepsy. Brain 120: 183–192.

Gloor P (1985). Neuronal generators and the problem of localization in electroencephalography: application of volume conductor theory to electroencephalography. J Clin Neurophysiol 2: 327–354.

Goodin DS, Aminoff MJ (1984). Does the interictal EEG have a role in the diagnosis of epilepsy? Lancet 1: 837–839.

Gotman J (1980). Quantitative measurements of epileptic spike morphology in the human EEG. Electroencephalogr Clin Neurophysiol 48: 551–557.

Gotman J, Koffler DJ (1989). Interictal spiking increases after seizures but does not after decrease in medication. Electroencephalogr Clin Neurophysiol 72: 7–15.

Gregory RP, Oates T, Merry RT (1993). Electroencephalogram epileptiform abnormalities in candidates for aircrew training. Electroencephalogr Clin Neurophysiol 86: 75–77.

Guaranha MS, da Silva Sousa P, de Araujo-Filho GM et al. (2009). Provocative and inhibitory effects of a video-EEG neuropsychologic protocol in juvenile myoclonic epilepsy. Epilepsia 50: 2446–2455.

Hashiguchi K, Morioka T, Yoshida F et al. (2007). Correlation between scalp-recorded electroencephalographic and electrocorticographic activities during ictal period. Seizure 16: 238–247.

Heo K, Han SD, Lim SR et al. (2006). Patient awareness of complex partial seizures. Epilepsia 47: 1931–1935.

Holmes MD, Wilensky AJ, Ojemann GA et al. (1999). Hippocampal or neocortical lesions on magnetic resonance imaging do not necessarily indicate site of ictal onsets in partial epilepsy. Ann Neurol 45: 461–465.

Hoppe C, Poepel A, Elger CE (2007). Epilepsy: accuracy of patient seizure counts. Arch Neurol 64: 1595–1599.

Hrachovy RA, Frost JD Jr (2003). Infantile epileptic encephalopathy with hypsarrhythmia (infantile spasms/West syndrome). J Clin Neurophysiol 20: 408–425.

Jasper HH (1983). The ten-twenty electrode system of the International Federation. In: International Federation of Societies for Electroencephalography and Clinical Neurophysiology: Recommendations for the Practice of clinical electroencephalography. Elsevier, Amsterdam, pp. 3–9.

Jobst BC, Williamson PD, Thadani VM et al. (2010). Intractable occipital lobe epilepsy: clinical characteristics and surgical treatment. Epilepsia 51: 2334–2337.

Kanner AM, Morris HH, Luders H et al. (1990). Supplementary motor seizures mimicking pseudoseizures: some clinical differences. Neurology 40: 1404–1407.

Kanner AM, Parra J, Gil-Nagel A et al. (2002). The localizing yield of sphenoidal and anterior temporal electrodes in ictal recordings: a comparison study. Epilepsia 43: 1189–1196.

Kasteleijn-Nolst Trenite DG, Binnie CD, Harding GF et al. (1999). Photic stimulation: standardization of screening methods. Epilepsia 40: 75–79.

Kerling F, Mueller S, Pauli E et al. (2006). When do patients forget their seizures? An electroclinical study. Epilepsy Behav 9: 281–285.

King MA, Newton MR, Jackson GD et al. (1998). Epileptology of the first-seizure presentation: a clinical, electroencephalographic, and magnetic resonance imaging study of 300 consecutive patients. Lancet 352. 1007–1011.

Klass DW, Westmoreland BF (1985). Nonepileptogenic epileptiform electroencephalographic activity. Ann Neurol 18: 627–635.

Kobayashi K, Inoue T, Kikumoto K et al. (2007). Relation of spasms and myoclonus to suppression-burst on EEG in epileptic encephalopathy in early infancy. Neuropediatrics 38: 244–250.

Kotagal P, Luders H, Morris HH et al. (1989). Dystonic posturing in complex partial seizures of temporal lobe onset: a new lateralizing sign. Neurology 39: 196–201.

Krauss GL, Lesser RP, Fisher RS et al. (1992). Anterior "cheek" electrodes are comparable to sphenoidal electrodes for the identification of ictal activity. Electroencephalogr Clin Neurophysiol 83: 333–338.

Krauss GL, Abdallah A, Lesser R et al. (2005). Clinical and EEG features of patients with EEG wicket rhythms misdiagnosed with epilepsy. Neurology 64: 1879–1883.

Krumholz A (1999). Nonepileptic seizures: diagnosis and management. Neurology 53: S76–S83.

Kwan P, Brodie MJ (2000). Early identification of refractory epilepsy. N Engl J Med 342: 314–319.

Labate A, Ambrosio R, Gambardella A et al. (2007). Usefulness of a morning routine EEG recording in patients with juvenile myoclonic epilepsy. Epilepsy Res 77: 17–21.

Laskowitz DT, Sperling MR, French JA et al. (1995). The syndrome of frontal lobe epilepsy: characteristics and surgical management. Neurology 45: 780–787.

Leach JP, Stephen LJ, Salveta C et al. (2006). Which electroencephalography (EEG) for epilepsy? The relative usefulness of different EEG protocols in patients with possible epilepsy. J Neurol Neurosurg Psychiatry 77: 1040–1042.

Legarda S, Jayakar P, Duchowny M et al. (1994). Benign rolandic epilepsy: high central and low central subgroups. Epilepsia 35: 1125–1129.

Lempert T, Bauer M, Schmidt D (1994). Syncope: a videometric analysis of 56 episodes of transient cerebral hypoxia. Ann Neurol 36: 233–237.

Lerman P, Kivity-Ephraim S (1981). Focal epileptic EEG discharges in children not suffering from clinical epilepsy: etiology, clinical significance, and management. Epilepsia 22: 551–558.

Lesser RP, Lueders H, Dinner DS (1983). Evidence for epilepsy is rare in patients with psychogenic seizures. Neurology 33: 502–504.

Lombroso CT (1997). Consistent EEG focalities detected in subjects with primary generalized epilepsies monitored for two decades. Epilepsia 38: 797–812.

Malow BA, Lin X, Kushwaha R et al. (1998). Interictal spiking increases with sleep depth in temporal lobe epilepsy. Epilepsia 39: 1309–1316.

Malow BA, Passaro E, Milling C et al. (2002). Sleep deprivation does not affect seizure frequency during inpatient video-EEG monitoring. Neurology 59: 1371–1374.

Mannan JB, Wieshmann UC (2003). How accurate are witness descriptions of epileptic seizures? Seizure 12: 444–447.

Marciani MG, Spanedda F, Bassetti MA et al. (1996). Effect of lamotrigine on EEG paroxysmal abnormalities and background activity: a computerized analysis. Br J Clin Pharmacol 42: 621–627.

Marsan CA, Zivin LS (1970). Factors related to the occurrence of typical paroxysmal abnormalities in the EEG records of epileptic patients. Epilepsia 11: 361–381.

Matsuoka H, Takahashi T, Sasaki M et al. (2000). Neuropsychological EEG activation in patients with epilepsy. Brain 123: 318–330.

McBride AE, Shih TT, Hirsch LJ (2002). Video-EEG monitoring in the elderly: a review of 94 patients. Epilepsia 43: 165–169.

McGonigal A, Russell AJ, Mallik AK et al. (2004). Use of short term video EEG in the diagnosis of attack disorders. J Neurol Neurosurg Psychiatry 75: 771–772.

Mizrahi EM (1999). Pediatric electroencephalographic video monitoring. J Clin Neurophysiol 16: 100–110.

Mohan KK, Markand ON, Salanova V (1996). Diagnostic utility of video EEG monitoring in paroxysmal events. Acta Neurol Scand 94: 320–325.

Morris HH 3rd, Dinner DS, Luders H et al. (1988). Supplementary motor seizures: clinical and electroencephalographic findings. Neurology 38: 1075–1082.

Nordli DR Jr (2006). Usefulness of video-EEG monitoring. Epilepsia 47: 26–30.

Oddo M, Carrera E, Claassen J et al. (2009). Continuous electroencephalography in the medical intensive care unit. Crit Care Med 37: 2051–2056.

Oguni H, Imaizumi Y, Uehara T et al. (1991). A video-EEG study of astatic seizures observed in patients with myoclonic astatic epilepsy of early childhood (Doose syndrome). Jpn J Psychiatry Neurol 45: 380–382.

Okubo Y, Matsuura M, Asai T et al. (1994). Epileptiform EEG discharges in healthy children: prevalence, emotional and behavioral correlates, and genetic influences. Epilepsia 35: 832–841.

Oostenveld R, Praamstra P (2001). The five percent electrode system for high-resolution EEG and ERP measurements. Clin Neurophysiol 112: 713–719.

Otani K, Abe J, Futagi Y et al. (1989). Clinical and electroencephalographical follow-up study of early myoclonic encephalopathy. Brain Dev 11: 332–337.

Panayiotopoulos CP (2007a). Epileptic encephalopathies in infancy and early childhood. In: A Clinical Guide to Epileptic Syndromes and their Treatment. 2nd edn. Springer, London, pp. 275–326.

Panayiotopoulos CP (2007b). Benign childhood focal seizures and related epileptic syndromes. In: A Clinical Guide to Epileptic Syndromes and their Treatment. 2nd edn. Springer, London, pp. 339–376.

Parra J, Kanner AM, Iriarte J et al. (1998). When should induction protocols be used in the diagnostic evaluation of patients with paroxysmal events? Epilepsia 39: 863–867.

Patel VM, Maulsby RL (1987). How hyperventilation alters the electroencephalogram: a review of controversial viewpoints emphasizing neurophysiological mechanisms. J Clin Neurophysiol 4: 101–120.

Penry JK, Porter RJ, Dreifuss RE (1975). Simultaneous recording of absence seizures with video tape and electroencephalography. A study of 374 seizures in 48 patients. Brain 98: 427–440.

Picton TW, van Roon P, Armilio ML et al. (2000). The correction of ocular artifacts: a topographic perspective. Clin Neurophysiol 111: 53–65.

Pierelli F, Chatrian GE, Erdly WW et al. (1989). Long-term EEG-video-audio monitoring: detection of partial epileptic seizures and psychogenic episodes by 24-hour EEG record review. Epilepsia 30: 513–523.

Privitera MD, Morris GL, Gilliam F (1991). Postictal language assessment and lateralization of complex partial seizures. Ann Neurol 30: 391–396.

Quesney LF (1991). Preoperative electroencephalographic investigation in frontal lobe epilepsy: electroencephalographic and electrocorticographic recordings. Can J Neurol Sci 18: 559–563.

Reiher J, Beaudry M, Leduc CP (1989). Temporal intermittent rhythmic delta activity (TIRDA) in the diagnosis of complex partial epilepsy: sensitivity, specificity and predictive value. Can J Neurol Sci 16: 398–401.

Reuber M, Fernandez G, Bauer J et al. (2002). Diagnostic delay in psychogenic nonepileptic seizures. Neurology 58: 493–495.

Risinger MW, Engel J Jr, Van Ness PC et al. (1989). Ictal localization of temporal lobe seizures with scalp/sphenoidal recordings. Neurology 39: 1288–1293.

Rosenow F, Luders H (2001). Presurgical evaluation of epilepsy. Brain 124: 1683–1700.

Salanova V, Andermann F, Olivier A et al. (1992). Occipital lobe epilepsy: electroclinical manifestations, electrocorticography, cortical stimulation and outcome in 42 patients treated between 1930 and 1991. Surgery of occipital lobe epilepsy. Brain 115: 1655–1680.

Salanova V, Andermann F, Rasmussen T et al. (1995). Parietal lobe epilepsy. Clinical manifestations and outcome in 82 patients treated surgically between 1929 and 1988. Brain 118: 607–627.

Salinsky M, Kanter R, Dasheiff RM (1987). Effectiveness of multiple EEGs in supporting the diagnosis of epilepsy: an operational curve. Epilepsia 28: 331–334.

Sam MC, So EL (2001). Significance of epileptiform discharges in patients without epilepsy in the community. Epilepsia 42: 1273–1278.

Saygi S, Katz A, Marks DA et al. (1992). Frontal lobe partial seizures and psychogenic seizures: comparison of clinical and ictal characteristics. Neurology 42: 1274–1277.

Schalk G, Mellinger J (2010). A Practical Guide to Brain–Computer Interfacing with BCI2000: General-Purpose Software for Brain–Computer Interface Research, Data Acquisition. (Human–Computer Interaction Series). Springer Science and Business Media, London.

Schreiner A, Pohlmann-Eden B (2003). Value of the early electroencephalogram after a first unprovoked seizure. Clin Electroencephalogr 34: 140–144.

Schuele SU, Bermeo AC, Alexopoulos AV et al. (2007). Video-electrographic and clinical features in patients with ictal asystole. Neurology 69: 434–441.

Smith D, Defalla BA, Chadwick DW (1999). The misdiagnosis of epilepsy and the management of refractory epilepsy in a specialist clinic. Q J Med 92: 15–23.

Stodieck S, Steinhoff BJ, Kolmsee S et al. (2001). Effect of levetiracetam in patients with epilepsy and interictal epileptiform discharges. Seizure 10: 583–587.

Strzelczyk A, Bauer S, Knake S et al. (2008). Ictal asystole in temporal lobe epilepsy before and after pacemaker implantation. Epileptic Disord 10: 39–44.

Tao JX, Ray A, Hawes-Ebersole S et al. (2005). Intracranial EEG substrates of scalp EEG interictal spikes. Epilepsia 46: 669–676.

Tao JX, Baldwin M, Ray A et al. (2007). The impact of cerebral source area and synchrony on recording scalp electroencephalography ictal patterns. Epilepsia 48: 2167–2176.

Tassinari CA, De Marco P, Plasmati R et al. (1988). Extreme somatosensory evoked potentials (ESEPs) elicited by tapping of hands or feet in children: a somatosensory cerebral evoked potentials study. Neurophysiol Clin 18: 123–128.

Tassinari CA, Michelucci R, Rubboli G et al. (1995). Myoclonic absence epilepsy. In: JS Duncan, CP Panayiotopoulos (Eds.), Typical Absences and Related Epileptic Syndromes. Churchill Livingstone, London, pp. 187–195.

Tassinari CA, Rubboli G, Volpi I et al. (2005). Electrical status epilepticus during slow sleep (ESES or CSWS) including acquired epileptic aphasia (Landau–Kleffner syndrome). In: J Roger, M Bureau, C Dravet et al. (Eds.), Epileptic Syndromes in Infancy, Childhood and Adolescence. 4th edn. John Libbey, London, pp. 295–314.

Tatum WO, Winters L, Gieron M et al. (2001). Outpatient seizure identification: results of 502 patients using computer-assisted ambulatory EEG. J Clin Neurophysiol 18: 14–19.

Tinuper P, Aguglia U, Pellissier JF et al. (1983). Visual ictal phenomena in a case of Lafora disease proven by skin biopsy. Epilepsia 24: 214–218.

Treiman DM, Walton NY, Kendrick C (1990). A progressive sequence of electroencephalographic changes during generalized convulsive status epilepticus. Epilepsy Res 5: 49–60.

Treiman DM, Meyers PD, Walton NY et al. (1998). A comparison of four treatments for generalized convulsive status epilepticus. Veterans Affairs Status Epilepticus Cooperative Study Group. N Engl J Med 339: 792–798.

Usui N, Kotagal P, Matsumoto R et al. (2005). Focal semiologic and electroencephalographic features in patients with juvenile myoclonic epilepsy. Epilepsia 46: 1668–1676.

Uthman B, Bearden S (2008). Rhythmic diffuse delta frequency activity presenting as an unusual EEG correlate of nonconvulsive status epilepticus: three case studies. Epilepsy Behav 12: 191–199.

Verrotti A, Greco R, Altobelli E et al. (1999). Centro-temporal spikes in non-epileptic children: a long-term follow up. J Paediatr Child Health 35: 60–62.

Verrotti A, Basciani F, Trotta D et al. (2002). Photoparoxysmal responses in non-epileptic children in long-term follow-up. Acta Neurol Scand 105: 400–402.

Von Oertzen J, Urbach H, Jungbluth S et al. (2002). Standard magnetic resonance imaging is inadequate for patients with refractory focal epilepsy. J Neurol Neurosurg Psychiatry 73: 643–647.

Vossler DG, Kraemer DL, Knowlton RC et al. (1998). Temporal ictal electroencephalographic frequency correlates with hippocampal atrophy and sclerosis. Ann Neurol 43: 756–762.

Walczak TS, Jayakar P (1997). Interictal EEG. In: J Engel, Jr, TA Pedley (Eds.), Epilepsy: A Comprehensive Textbook. Vol. 1. Lippincott-Raven, Philadelphia, pp. 831–848.

Walczak TS, Williams DT, Berten W (1994). Utility and reliability of placebo infusion in the evaluation of patients with seizures. Neurology 44: 394–399.

Westmoreland BF (1996). Epileptiform electroencephalographic patterns. Mayo Clin Proc 71: 501–511.

Williamson PD, Boon PA, Thadani VM et al. (1992a). Parietal lobe epilepsy: diagnostic considerations and results of surgery. Ann Neurol 31: 193–201.

Williamson PD, Thadani VM, Darcey TM et al. (1992b). Occipital lobe epilepsy: clinical characteristics, seizure spread patterns, and results of surgery. Ann Neurol 31: 3–13.

Winesett P, Feliciano CA, Tatum WO (2009). Temporal lobe seizures triggering recurrent syncope by ictal asystole. Epilepsy Behav 14: 258–260.

Worrell GA, So EL, Kazemi J et al. (2002). Focal ictal beta discharge on scalp EEG predicts excellent outcome of frontal lobe epilepsy surgery. Epilepsia 43: 277–282.

Zifkin BG, Inoue Y (2004). Visual reflex seizures induced by complex stimuli. Epilepsia 45: 27–29.

Handbook of Clinical Neurology, Vol. 107 (3rd series)
Epilepsy, Part I
H. Stefan and W.H. Theodore, Editors

Chapter 21

Magnetoencephalography

HERMANN STEFAN[1]*, NOBUKAZU NAKASATO[2], AND ANDREW C. PAPANICOLAOU[3]
[1]*Epilepsy Center, Neurology Clinic, Erlangen University Hospital, Erlangen, Germany*
[2]*Department of Neurosurgery, Kohnan Hospital and Tohoku University, Sendai, Japan*
[3]*Department of Pediatrics, University of Tennessee, Memphis, TN, USA*

INTRODUCTION

Optimal treatment of patients with epilepsy requires accurate determination of the type of seizure and syndrome. Thus, it has been standard practice to use the patient's case history, electroencephalography (EEG) and structural magnetic resonance imaging (MRI) findings for diagnosis. In cases where the initial or subsequent antiepileptic drug treatments prove ineffective, the application of additional, newly developed, methods for localizing the epileptogenic zones has shown promise in improving treatment options and planning surgical interventions. These methods include sophisticated electrophysiological and magnetoencephalographic (MEG) recordings and source localization techniques applicable even in "MRI-negative" cases in which the epileptogenic lesions are too subtle to be detected with conventional neuroimaging.

Focal epileptic activity can be generated in both the superficial cortex and deeper brain regions, a fact that influences the detectability of the generators (Shigeto et al., 2002). However, the feasibility of localizing these generators must be explored for both types of focal epilepsy, neocortical and limbic. In either case, a certain amount of tissue must be involved in epileptic discharges in order to be localized noninvasively using electrophysiological methods (EEG) (Sutherling et al., 1988; Alarcon et al., 1994; Oishi et al., 2002; Tao et al., 2005). Therefore, presurgical evaluation requires extensive experience to decide whether noninvasive interictal or ictal recordings are sufficient for the localization of focal epileptic activity in any individual patient, or whether invasive recordings have to be carried out in order to improve the accuracy of the noninvasive results.

If the seizure generator is located in the hippocampus, for instance, noninvasive detection of focal epileptic activity may be difficult or impossible using EEG. The distribution of interictal spikes in deep hippocampal electrodes and surface electrodes was analyzed by Alarcon et al. (1994). The results of this study indicated that single hippocampal discharges could not always be detected by scalp EEG. In contrast, excision of "leading regions of spike activity" in the temporal lobe yielded a good surgical outcome.

According to experience with simultaneous invasive recording from several neocortical surface and deep temporal lobe structures in many patients with cryptogenic temporal lobe epilepsy, it appears that hippocampal parahippocampal, basal temporal areas, and the inferior temporal gyrus are involved in the development of epileptic seizures. Spike onset was often observed in the entorhinal or parahippocampal–basal cortex, and it was sometimes observed in the lateral neocortex (Stefan et al., 2008). Invasive ictal recordings have also revealed that the entorhinal cortex of the basal temporal cortex itself can be the region of ictal onset (Spencer and Spencer, 1994). In some cases, the hippocampus is involved only secondarily in the epileptic excitation process. The epileptic network in such cases involves temporomesiobasal areas in addition to the hippocampus. Depending on the spike amplitude and the characteristics of the MEG recording (gradiometer or magnetometer), the detection probability of mesial temporal spikes varies from 25% to 60%. It remains unclear

*Correspondence to: Professor Hermann Stefan, Universitätsklinikum Erlangen (FAU), Neurologische Klinik – Biomagnetismus, 10, Schwabachanlage, 91054 Erlangen, Germany. Tel: +49 (0)9131 8536989, Fax: +49 (0)9131 8534226, E-mail: hermann.stefan@uk-erlangen.de

how frequently mesial temporal spikes can be detected (Santuiste et al., 2008; Agirre-Arrizubieta et al., 2009).

As only discharges that involve several thousand neurons can be assessed through noninvasive means, only approximate localization of seizure-related circuitry within the neuronal network of the brain is possible. If MEG is able to define "critical hotspots" in the neuronal network, it is important to determine which regions are necessary and sufficient for seizure generation and control. This chapter discusses the procedures and applications of magnetic source imaging (MSI) for the detection of focal epileptic interictal and ictal activity and functionally important areas in epileptic patients.

TECHNICAL CONSIDERATIONS

Excited neuronal populations in the brain produce not only electrical potentials that can be recorded by surface or depth EEG electrodes, but also magnetic fields that are detectable on the head surface in the range of 50–1000 fT (extremely low intensity). The brain's magnetic field is weak and is considerably smaller then the ambient magnetic noise in an urban environment; therefore, the development of extremely sensitive measurement tools, such as superconducting quantum interference devices (SQUIDs), has allowed for major breakthroughs in the investigation of both abnormal and normal cerebral activation. MEG recordings are usually performed in a magnetically shielded chamber that attenuates the influence of external magnetic noise.

The technical details concerning recording and instrumentation have been provided elsewhere (e.g., Hämäläinen et al., 1993; Baumgartner et al., 1995; Mäkelä et al., 2006; Rampp and Stefan, 2007; Papanicolaou, 2009). The first MEG recordings in humans were performed using single-channel MEG systems. Currently, multichannel MEG systems with as many as 300 sensors are commercially available, enabling simultaneous whole-head recordings with improved sensors (gradiometers or magnetometers) arranged inside a helmet-shaped dewar. MEG is a noninvasive method that provides temporal resolution in the millisecond range and, unlike EEG, requires no "referencing" or physical contact between the sensors and the patient's head. The new whole-head systems have also significantly improved spatial resolution.

Interpretation of the recorded magnetic field signals requires the solution of the so-called "inverse problem," the estimation of an unknown source within the brain from magnetic field data recorded outside the head. The solution is attempted using alternative assumptions concerning the type of underlying sources that produce the recorded magnetic fields and the shape and structure of the head as a volume conductor. For the determination of the location, orientation and strength of focal activity, the source is modeled after a single "equivalent current dipole." However, when sources overlap both spatially and temporally, as in the case of multiple sources, the alternative approach of a multidipole model may be more appropriate (Hämäläinen, 1992; Mosher et al., 1992; Scherg et al., 1999). Furthermore, different current density (e.g., minimum norm, weighted minimum norm, and low-resolution electromagnetic tomography, LORETA) (Pascual Marqui et al., 1994; Ebersole, 1999) and beamformer methods (Robinson et al., 2004) may also be used for the localization of more extended sources, as well as spike-related frequency power concerning the modeling (Guggisberg et al., 2007). Correlates of epileptic high gamma oscillations in invasive EEG and MEG were reported by Rampp et al. (2010). Aside from the most frequently used spherical model, more realistically shaped models are also available (e.g. boundary element method, BEM). In the case of BEM, the head model consists of the three different compartments, brain, skull, and scalp, with the assumption that each compartment has homogeneous and isotropic conductivity (Fuchs et al., 1998a). The BEM model is based on the segmentation of structural MRI data sets, thus accounting for the individual patient's anatomy. This concept was further developed by finite element models (FEM), which also take conductivity anisotropies into account (Wolters et al., 2006). For further descriptions of MEG and EEG analysis, see De Munck and van Dijk (1999). Clinical aspects of MEG methodology have been presented by Stefan and Hummel (1999).

APPLICATIONS OF MEG/MSI IN EPILEPSY

Evoked activity

In cases in which neurosurgery remains the only therapeutic option for epileptic patients, it is essential both to know the site of the epileptogenic region (see below), and to determine whether removal of the tissue in question may cause functional deficits.

Recently, functional validation of the results of the inverse problem solution, called magnetic source imaging (MSI), has been obtained with various sensory modalities. These results are based on recording-evoked magnetic responses to repeated stimulation, in accordance with the well-established technique also used for evoked potentials, averaged over a number of stimulus-related EEG epochs.

Evoked magnetic responses to acoustic (AEF) (Hari et al., 1980; Paetau et al., 1995), visual (VEF) (Drasdo and Thompson, 1992; Aine et al., 1995; Seki et al., 1996; Grover et al., 2006), somatosensory (SEF) (Baumgartner, 1993; Kawamura et al., 1996), gustatory (GEF) (Murayama et al., 1996), and olfactory (OEF) (Kettenmann et al., 1996) field stimulation can be obtained. Magnetic fields that represent motor activity (motor evoked fields, MEF) generated by voluntary finger, limb, and tongue movements have also been recorded (Deecke et al., 1985; Cheyne et al., 1991; Ganslandt et al., 1999; Nakasato et al., 2001), and their sources were estimated using MSI. Thus, localization of cortical generators estimated from magnetic evoked activity has become an established source of information about functionally significant brain areas. This is particularly true when MSI and neurosurgery use compatible systems of spatial coordinates. Operation theaters already use neuronavigation systems in which the structural MRI of the patient with coregistered activation sources (indicative of both epileptogenic and eloquent brain) is used in conjunction with the surgical instruments online (Fig. 21.1). Using a variety of stimulating sites, SEF localizations illustrate the "somatosensory homunculus" and its variations in the organization of the somatosensory cortex of particular patients (Yang et al., 1993; Ganslandt et al., 1997; Stefan and Hummel, 1999). In a similar manner, the localization of functional brain regions subserving language are established and used for epilepsy surgery (Papanicolaou et al., 1998, 2004; Bowyer et al., 2005; Kamada et al., 2007).

Spontaneous activity

An increasing number of publications that discuss the application of MEG/MSI in presurgical evaluation evidence its capability to localize spontaneous epileptic activity (Fig. 21.2).

Validation of epileptogenic source localizations provided by MEG/MSI is necessary. MEG findings on epileptogenic foci need to be compared with the results of other diagnostic techniques considered to provide more accurate detection of the epileptogenic brain tissue. One of these techniques is ictal video-EEG, which is generally regarded as the "gold standard" (Engel, 1993). Invasive EEG monitoring and intraoperative electrocorticography (ECoG) are also options, and such comparisons have shown that MEG/MSI yields fairly good localization accuracy, even though the activity investigated is mostly interictal (Sutherling et al., 1987; Nakasato et al., 1994; Smith et al., 1994; Stefan et al.,

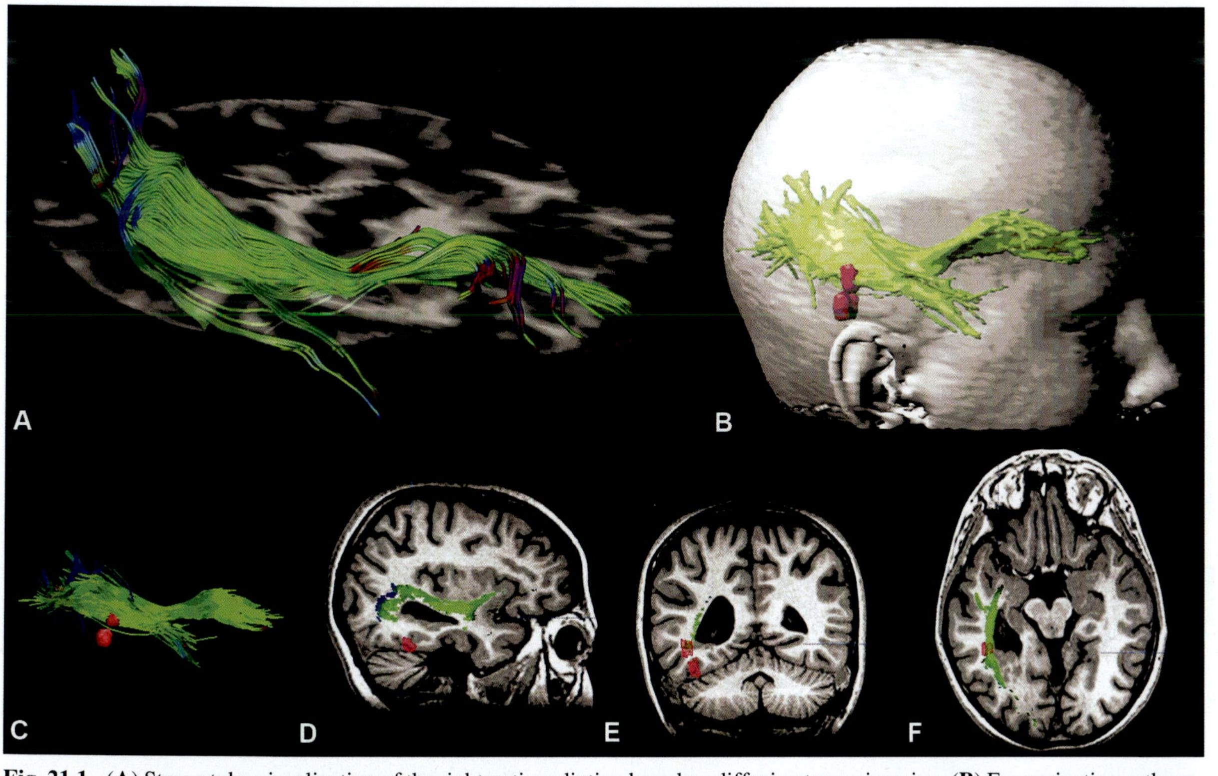

Fig. 21.1. (**A**) Streamtube visualization of the right optic radiation based on diffusion tensor imaging. (**B**) For navigation, a three-dimensional object representing the optic radiation (wrapping the individual fibers) and two distinct MSI foci (red) are generated. (**C**) Relation of optic radiation (visualized as streamlines) to MSI foci. (**D–F**) Sagittal/coronal/axial view of T1-weighted images with registered diffusion tensor imaging (DTI) and MSI data. Localization of focal epileptic activity is below the optic tract. (Reproduced from Stefan et al. (2007). © Elsevier.)

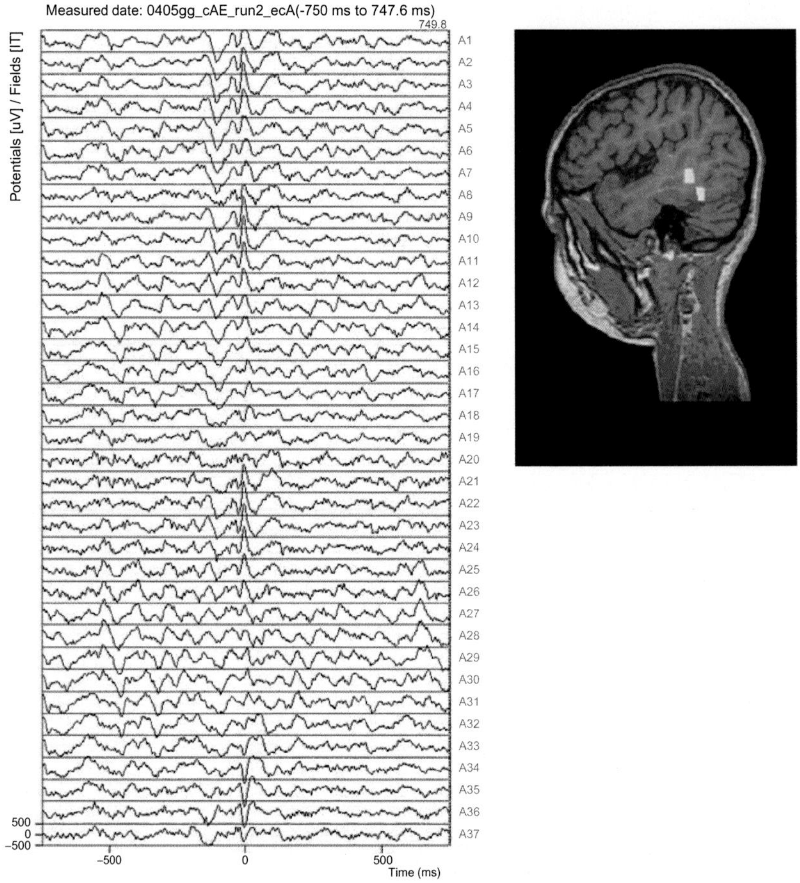

Fig. 21.2. A typical MEG spike of the patient in Figure 21.1. Two distinct MSI foci are shown in a sagittal view. (Stefan et al., 2007.)

1994, 2003; Ebersole et al., 1995; Papanicolaou et al., 2005; Paulini et al., 2007).

Eliashiv et al. (1998) reported congruency between MEG localizations and other findings from presurgical evaluations in 70–80% of cases studied. A similar percentage (72%) of patients after successful temporal lobe epilepsy surgery were found to have good spatial correlation between predominant focal epileptic activity in MEG and other localization results from presurgical evaluation and intraoperative ECoG (Stefan et al., 1993). In another study, a comparison of MEG localizations with MRI and various video-EEG findings in 58 patients with pharmacologically intractable epilepsy showed that in patients who, after surgery, were seizure-free (class 1, according to Engel's classification) or had infrequent seizures, MEG was inferior only to subdural video-EEG recordings in predicting the epileptogenic zone. MEG was superior to MRI, interictal and ictal noninvasive video-EEG (Wheless et al., 1999), and equal in efficacy to both ictal and interictal invasive EEG (Papanicolaou et al., 2005). These data suggest that in neocortical temporal and extratemporal lobe epilepsies MEG is at least as effective as the established methods for localizing the epileptogenic region. In a study that compared MEG with positron emission tomography (PET) and stereo-EEG (SEEG), MEG localizations agreed with PET and SEEG results in 7 of 9 patients, and in cases in which PET and MEG findings agreed, the surgical outcome after surgery was favorable (Lamusuo et al., 1999).

King et al. (2000) reported outcome data (according to Engel's classification) for 19 patients after resection of the primary MEG spike region. Fourteen patients were grouped in class 1, 4 in class 2, 1 in class 3, and none in class 4. However, of 17 patients who underwent resection of tissue with marginal or no relationship to MEG spike localization, only 3 were in the best or second-best outcome categories. In 4 patients the outcome ranked in class 3 and most of the cases (7) were placed in the worst outcome class.

These results indicate that resection of the primary MEG spike focus strongly correlates with excellent outcome. In this context, it seems important to note that MEG/MSI dipole localizations are thought neither to represent point-sources with millimeter accuracy nor to yield an outline of the epileptogenic tissue, but rather to indicate centers of epileptic activity and to reveal compartmental information on a sublobar level. In many patients with pharmacoresistant focal epilepsies, circumscribed clusters of interictal spike sources indicating centers of predominant focal epileptic activity can be found (Stefan et al., 1991). If spike source localizations in temporal lobe epilepsy show more than one spatially distinct cluster, the pattern might be interpreted as an indication of multifocal temporal lobe epilepsy. Similar results have been reported for neocortical extratemporal epilepsies (Oishi et al., 2006).

In many cases, brain MRI scans of epileptic patients show abnormal morphology, varying from subtle alterations to extensive mass lesions. However, abnormal MRI findings are not necessarily epileptogenic, and, even if they are, it may be important to clarify the relationship between anatomical and functional pathology. Furthermore, if there is more than one MRI-visible lesion, the specific lesions crucial to epileptogenicity must be discerned. In a considerable number of patients with neocortical temporal or extratemporal epilepsies, MEG/MSI allows the localization of epileptiform activity proximal to epileptogenic structural lesions (Stefan et al., 1994, 2004; Knowlton et al., 1997; Jin et al., 2007).

In contrast, there is sometimes no evidence of a structural lesion associated with epilepsy prior to surgery (Swartz et al., 1989; Cascino et al., 1992). With the availability of powerful new imaging systems and more sophisticated software to identify discrete alterations, the number of patients with "cryptogenic" etiology is decreasing. However, it is not yet possible to identify a structural abnormality that would account for any epileptic focus. The lack of morphological clues renders functional diagnostic methods such as MEG more significant because they may facilitate the detection of subtle morphological changes in MRI re-evaluation (Moore et al., 2002). MSI has been found to offer useful epileptogenic source locations of cryptogenic epileptic activity in concordance with other noninvasive results, thus facilitating the detailed planning of invasive procedures that include surgical rejection. In a study by Knowlton et al. (1997), in 11 out of 12 patients without focal abnormality (as determined by MRI) the sources of MEG-recorded discharges were localized in the epileptogenic zone as determined by standard preoperative evaluation.

King et al. (2000) published a review of numerous studies showing that MEG can detect interictal epileptiform discharges in patients with intractable epilepsy. There are, however, cases in which MEG spike source localization does not result in finding the focal source.

A major problem in using MEG for localization of the epileptogenic focus arises from the fact that sources of spontaneous epileptic activity are often located less superficially than, for example, the comparatively easily accessible cortical generators of evoked responses. With increasing source depth, the amplitude of the signals recorded at the head surface declines drastically; consequently, deep sources are more difficult to locate than superficial ones. A crucial question in the management of drug-resistant epilepsy is the capacity of magnetic field recordings of spontaneous brain activity to assess deep sources in the mesial structures of the temporal lobe. Initial attempts have been made to address this issue. Recent results show some success in the use of MSI localizations for presumed deep epileptic foci. However, the circular arrangement of cell layers, such as in the amygdala, may cause the cancellation of magnetic fields, thus jeopardizing signal detection. In addition, an unfavorable sensor configuration may also impair sensitivity. Comparing MEG localization with standard localizations (based upon MRI, noninvasive and invasive EEG), a correlation was found by Smith et al. (1995) in about two-thirds of the cases studied, with spontaneous spikes available in approximately half of patients with mesial temporal lobe epilepsy (MTLE). Knowlton et al. (1997) confirmed that the yield of MEG is higher in patients with neocortical epilepsy than in those with MTLE.

Averaging of similar specific patterns is frequently used to increase the signal-to-noise ratio when dealing with small amplitudes of epileptic discharges in patients with foci in deeper brain regions. The resulting signals, subjected to spatiotemporal analysis, are more likely to produce a valid estimate of focal epileptic activity compared with the unaveraged data (Sutherling and Barth, 1989; Stefan et al., 1990).

Based primarily on single dipole analyses of EEG spikes, Ebersole et al. (1995) stressed the usefulness of interpreting dipole orientation in order to obtain additional information about sublobar attribution of localizations in the temporal lobe. This was also described by Pataraia et al. (2005).

Owing to the distribution of focal origins of seizure disorders, early clinical MSI studies in epileptic patients were restricted mostly to temporal lobe cases (Rose et al., 1987; Ebersole et al., 1993; Stefan et al., 1994; Ebersole et al., 1995; Pataraia et al., 2005). Nevertheless, presurgical evaluation of patients with extratemporal epilepsy has also been reported to benefit from MSI (Hari et al., 1993; Stefan et al., 1995; Mamelak et al., 2002; Genow et al., 2004; Ossenblok et al., 2007). In frontal and other extratemporal epilepsies, intralobar localizations (predominantly lateral and frontobasal) have been confirmed by invasive recordings, but few cases have been investigated to date. Figure 21.1 shows an example of localization results in a patient with frontal lobe epilepsy. Propagation analysis is a special challenge in frontal lobe cases (Ossenblok et al., 1999).

The newer generations of biomagnetic systems allow for simultaneous examination of a broader spectrum of interest. Whole-head systems are particularly suited to the investigation of epileptic spikes (Paetau et al., 1992), as they offer the opportunity to investigate temporal relationships of events, such as mirror foci, with extended spatial distribution (Hari et al., 1993; Jin et al., 2007).

MEG can detect spikes even without concurrent activity in conventional scalp EEG (Knowlton et al., 1997; Zijlmans et al., 2002; Lin et al., 2003; Park et al., 2004; Iwasaki et al., 2005). There is no significant difference in equivalent current dipole (ECD) location between the unique MEG spikes and the concurrent EEG–MEG spikes, whereas the ECD moment of the unique MEG spikes tends to be smaller than that of the concurrent EEG–MEG spikes (Park et al., 2004). The higher spatial resolution of MEG compared with scalp EEG helps to separate small spikes from background brain noise, providing a higher yield of spike detection in typical clinical settings.

Higher spatial resolution of MEG, with the aid of the whole-head recording, may distinguish primary and secondary bilateral synchrony (Yu et al., 2004; Salayev et al., 2006). Such an application remains challenging because of the limited power of the source estimation algorithm to analyze extended and multiple sources in MEG. However, MEG may provide sufficient information to indicate callosotomy and/or focal cortical resection (Yu et al., 2004; Salayev et al., 2006).

Owing to relatively short MEG recording times compared with long-term EEG monitoring, spikes are not detected in all patients with focal epilepsy. The rate of MEG spike detection in focal epilepsies varies between 70% and 90% of spontaneous spikes. In order to induce more frequent spiking, activation using methohexital and/or clonidine or etomidate (Stefan et al., 2010) can be used (Kirchberger et al., 1998b; Kettenmann et al., 2005).

Furthermore, with limited recording duration, most MEG recordings miss ictal activity, even in patients whose antiepileptic medication is reduced for presurgical evaluation purposes. The restricted access to ictal recording presents one of the basic problems of MSI. Even if ictal activity is obtained, it is known from EEG recordings that motor artifacts are likely to disturb the brain signals. Yet, MEG data recorded during auras or seizure onset (Sutherling et al., 1987; Stefan et al., 1992; Ebersole et al., 1995; Watanabe et al., 1996; Assaf et al., 2003) may yield dipole localizations reflecting focal activity. According to investigations by Ebersole et al. (1995) and Tilz et al. (2002), ictal recordings permitted the detection of epileptiform signals in the MEG in 40–50% of patients. Prolonged MEG recordings, split into repeated sessions and interspersed with breaks to allow the patient to stretch, may provide ictal data during spontaneous seizures. Another way to obtain seizure-related MEG measurements is to take advantage of procedures that provoke the attacks. Sleep deprivation and antiepileptic drug withdrawal can be used to precipitate seizures.

The correlation between ictal and interictal localizations is one of the most important issues that should be assessed systematically by future studies of different types of epilepsy.

In small children, limited cooperation and small head size may impose limitations on recording and analysis. Even under such conditions, MEG has proven to be advantageous. Using a whole-head system to study childhood epilepsy connected with Landau–Kleffner syndrome, Paetau et al. (1999) showed that in all investigated patients the earliest spike activity originated in the intrasylvian cortex. In one subject, activity spread to the contralateral sylvian cortex within 20 ms. Secondary spikes occurred within 10–60 ms in the ipsilateral perisylvian temporo-occipital and parietal–occipital areas. In these cases, MEG provided useful presurgical information regarding cortical spike dynamics.

Studies that include simultaneous recording and analysis of MEG and EEG data (Ebersole et al., 1993; Stefan et al., 2000; Scheler et al., 2007) are of particular interest. They enable clinicians to take full advantage of the merits of both methods and to overcome their respective drawbacks. Combining EEG and MEG has produced the best accuracy, both in computer simulation studies (Liu et al., 2002) and in clinical applications (Fuchs et al., 1998b; Baillet et al., 2002; Verrotti et al., 2003).

MEG correlation to ictal signs showed association of mediotemporohorizontal dipole clusters with autonomic seizures, whereas superotemporovertical clusters correlated with auditory and psychic signs (Fukao et al., 2010).

Etiologies and syndromes

In cases of epilepsy associated with brain tumors, Patt et al. (2000) found a correlation between histological changes and the distance between localizations of focal epileptic activity on the tumor boundaries. In patients with glioma, compared with those with mixed glioneural tumors or metastases, the focal epileptic activity was closer to the tumor boundary. In temporal lobe epilepsies, Stefan et al. (1994) found a close correlation between astrocytoma, ganglioglioma, and the source of leading spike activity (distance 10–20 mm). In patients with neurocytoma focal epileptic activity, sources were localized in the cortex around the tumor (Morioka et al., 2000b).

Cortical malformations

To date, limited clinical experience has been gained with the heterogeneous group of cortical malformations.

High epileptogenic activity has been assessed by MEG in focal cortical dysplasia (FCD) with balloon cells (Bast et al., 2004). Moreover, MEG was used to detect the location in cases of FCD in the presence of normal structural MRI (Ishibashi et al., 2002) or in subcortical alterations (Widjaja et al., 2009). In other cases, MEG localized epileptic activity sources outside the border of the MRI-visible cortical malformation that had to be resected to obtain seizure control (Morioka et al., 1999; Otsubo et al., 2001b; Bast et al., 2004). In patients with double cortex, epileptic activity in both heterotopic and normal cortex was reported by Toulouse et al. (2003), with the primary focal epileptic activity localized in the normocortex and propagated into the heterotopic cortex. In a case of periventricular heterotopia, MEG was used to guide subdural and depth electrode placement for intraoperative confirmation of noninvasive finding for resective surgery (Figs 21.1 & 21.2) (Stefan et al., 2004, 2007). Despite bilateral EEG changes, Tanaka et al. (2000) found MEG-recorded epileptic activity restricted to one hemisphere in perisylvian syndrome. In patients with tuberous sclerosis, the epileptogenic focal activity was correlated with certain tubers (Peresson et al., 1998).

Vascular malformation

The correlation of vascular malformation and focal epileptic activity was investigated by Morioka et al. (2000a). The localization of high-frequency magnetic activity was closely correlated with spike source localization on intraoperative ECoG. In patients with cavernoma, the correlation between localization of focal epileptic activity and surgical outcome showed that the outcome was good if the distance was less than 30 mm (Stefan and Buchfelder, 2007). In additional studies, bilateral focal epileptic activity was detected in patients with cavernomas.

To date, for patients with symptomatic epilepsies after stroke, only sporadic observations of focal encephalitis have been reported (Ishibashi et al., 2002; Assenza et al., 2009).

Temporal plus epilepsies

Temporal plus epilepsies are a special challenge for presurgical evaluation. Whereas MTLE can often be easily diagnosed with the methods of presurgical evaluation previously described, the evaluation of temporal plus epilepsies is much more difficult. Clinical ictal signs may resemble those of epilepsies originating in the temporal lobe, but in the case of temporal lobe plus epilepsies initial focal epileptic activity can be generated in the temporal–occipital, temporal–parietal, temporal–frontal, or insular regions (Kahane and Landré, 2008). In these cases, noninvasive source localization can provide important information to improve the assessment of the epileptogenic regions and provide useful information for optimal placement of invasive electrodes (Stefan and Buchfelder, 2007).

West syndrome

Diffuse or focal MEG source localizations have been reported, and they impact the planning of epilepsy surgery (Hattori et al., 2001).

Epileptic spasms in older patients

Epileptic spasms in older patients were investigated by RamachandranNair et al. (2008), who found that, whereas ictal spasms were generalized and ictal EEG/MEG showed unilateral focal epileptic overlapping with invasive ictal onset zones (including high-frequency oscillations), patients were seizure-free postoperatively.

Landau–Kleffner syndrome

MEG has been found to be especially useful in patients with Landau–Kleffner syndrome (Paetau et al., 1999; Sobel et al., 2000; Rodin et al., 2004). Paetau et al. (1999) used MEG-derived information to decide whether patients qualified for multiple subpial transections. In patients with malignant rolandic–sylvian epilepsy syndrome, the interictal irritative brain area and eloquent cortex were identified through MEG/MSI and confirmed by ECoG, whereas scalp EEG was not informative (Otsubo et al., 2001a).

Idiopathic generalized epilepsies

Systematic neurophysiological research of epileptic networks has been stimulated by recent electrophysiological high-resolution MEG analysis indicating onset and propagation of spike and slow-wave discharges in human absence epilepsy (Westmijse et al., 2009). Focal cortical activation of epileptic activity was demonstrated in idiopathic generalized epilepsies with predominant involvement of frontal perinsular and subcortical thalamic areas. In all patients, a unilateral frontal accentuation of activity could be observed. Patients with juvenile myoclonic and myoclonic absence epilepsy presented with localizations mainly in the central and premotor regions, compared with prefrontal accentuation in patients with other absences (Stefan et al., 2009). The findings indicate in "generalized" epilepsies a subgroup with regional activity in bilateral homologous regions. Dynamic statistical parametric mapping (dSPM) was performed to estimate the cortical source distribution of generalized spike–wave activity. In addition to medial prefrontal activation in all patients, posterior cingulate and precuneus activity was also found in three of five patients after medial prefrontal activation. Cortical regions constituting a default mode network are strongly involved in the generalized spike–wave process (Sakurai et al., 2010).

MEG-guided re-evaluation in patients with normal or nonlocalizing MRI

The detection of lesions is of great importance for presurgical evaluation with regard to epileptic surgery. Studies by Funke et al. (2002) and Moore et al. (2002) showed that previously undetected lesions were identified via MEG in up to 17.5% of cases, and MEG-guided review of previously normal MRI scans led to the detection of subtle abnormalities consistent with histological examination after successful epilepsy surgery (Morioka et al., 1999; Zhang et al., 2003; Bast et al., 2004). MEG predicted outcome following surgery for intractable epilepsy in children with normal or nonfocal MRI findings. Some 77% of patients in whom MEG detected focal epileptic activity had a good postsurgical outcome (RamachandranNair et al., 2007).

Persistent seizures after surgery

It is difficult to evaluate patients after lesionectomy or unsuccessful epilepsy surgery because the placement of subdural electrodes may be difficult with regard to subdural scarring and arachnoidal adhesions. In addition, the shifting of normal brain into the resection cavities may cause distortions of anatomy in these patients. Because the magnetic fields are not distorted by skull and dura defects that may produce incorrect localizations on scalp EEG, MEG has clear advantages compared with EEG, especially in these patients (Kirchberger et al., 1998a; Pataraia et al., 2002).

Controlled prospective studies comparing MSI localizations with intracranial EEG showed that MSI had a positive predictive value for seizure onset localization in more than 80% (Knowlton et al., 2006) and that MSI indicated in 23% additional invasive electrode coverage, increasing the chance that seizure-onset region could be localized (Knowlton et al., 2009). MSI provided nonredundant information in 33% of patients, and benefited 21% who underwent surgery (Sutherling et al., 2008). These prospective studies showed the clinical usefulness of presurgical diagnostics for patient management.

There are specific limitations to the MSI technique. MEG can detect only tangential components of sources because of the comparatively short MEG recording periods that render spontaneous ictal recordings unlikely. However, the advantages of MEG/MSI are undeniable: it is noninvasive, it has high spatial and temporal resolution, it provides superior accuracy because the magnetic fields are nearly independent of conductivity, and it merges functional and anatomical information. These characteristics give MEG/MSI a prominent role among the diagnostic methods that contribute to the localization of epileptic foci (Colon et al., 2009). Because MEG/MSI is not invasive, it can be used to screen outpatients and is not restricted to inpatients or presurgical evaluation. Patients carrying a vagus nerve stimulator can also be investigated (Carrette et al., 2011). It may be particularly useful in postoperative patients in whom seizures have decreased but not altogether ceased, and where, due to asymmetrical conductivities, the defect of the cranial vault and the cavity resulting after resection impedes EEG but not MEG analysis. Strengths and limitations of MEG with regard to basic methodological and clinical aspects have been summarized by Stefan and colleagues (2011); the two methods, MEG and EEG, are complementary.

The applications of MEG/MSI in presurgical epilepsy evaluation can be summarized as follows.

1. Delineation of functionally significant areas that must be spared during surgery by means of evoked or event-related normal activity.
2. Localization of focal epileptic activity sources to guide invasive electrophysiological procedures.
3. Localization of focal epileptic activity sources to guide detailed planning of neurosurgical procedures, for example with neuronavigation, with the goal of minimal tissue removal.
4. Elucidation of spatial relationships of epileptic spike generation and subtle anatomical lesions.
5. Postoperative follow-up and, in cases where the first neurosurgical treatment has failed to render the patient seizure-free, facilitation of the decision concerning the possibility of a second operation.
6. Screening of patients who are possible candidates for epilepsy surgery.

Source localization using MEG/EEG is still a clinical work in progress, but there is significant evidence that important clinical findings can be obtained and that these complementary approaches in early diagnosis and in noninvasive presurgical evaluation can improve a patient's clinical condition.

References

Agirre-Arrizubieta Z, Huiskamp GJM, Ferrier CH et al. (2009). Interictal magnetoencephalography and the irritative zone in the electrocorticogram. Brain 132: 3060–3071.

Aine CJ, Supek S, George JS (1995). Temporal dynamics of visual-evoked neuromagnetic sources: effects of stimulus parameters and selective attention. Int J Neurosci 80: 79–104.

Alarcon G, Guy CN, Binnie CD et al. (1994). Intracerebral propagation of interictal activity in partial epilepsy: implications for source localisation. J Neurol Neurosurg Psychiatry 57: 435–449.

Assaf BA, Karkar KM, Laxer KD et al. (2003). Ictal magnetoencephalography in temporal and extratemporal lobe epilepsy. Epilepsia 44: 1320–1327.

Assenza G, Zappasodi F, Squitti R et al. (2009). Neuronal functionality assessed by magnetoencephalography is related to oxidative stress system in acute ischemic stroke. Neuroimage 44: 1267–1273.

Baillet S, Adam C, Schwartz D et al. (2002). Combined MEG and EEG source imaging of interictal activity in partial epilepsy. In: H Nowak, J Haueisen, F Giessler et al., (Eds.), BIOMAG: Proceedings of the 13th International Conference on Biomagnetism. VDE, Berlin, pp. 223–225.

Bast T, Oezkan O, Rona S et al. (2004). EEG and MEG source analysis of single and averaged interictal spikes reveals intrinsic epileptogenicity in focal cortical dysplasia. Epilepsia 45: 621–631.

Baumgartner C (1993). Clinical Electrophysiology of the Somatosensory Cortex. Springer, Vienna.

Baumgartner C, Deecke L, Stroink G et al. (Eds) (1995). Biomagnetism: Fundamental Research and Clinical Applications. Elsevier, Vienna.

Bowyer SM, Fleming T, Greenwald ML et al. (2005). Magnetoencephalographic localization of basal temporal language area. Epilepsy Behav 6: 229–234.

Carrette E, De Tiege X, Op De Beeck M et al. (2011). Magnetencephalography in epilepsy patients carrying a vagus nerve stimulator. Epilepsy Res 93: 44–52.

Cascino GD, Jack CR, Jr, Parisi JE (1992). Magnetic resonance imaging in intractable frontal lobe epilepsy. Pathologic correlation and prognostic significance. Epilepsy Res 11: 171–178.

Cheyne D, Kristeva R, Deecke L (1991). Homuncular organization of human motor cortex as indicated by neuromagnetic recordings. Neurosci Lett 122: 17–20.

Colon AJ, Ossenblok P, Nieuwenhuis L et al. (2009). Use of routine MEG in the primary diagnostic process of epilepsy. J Clin Neurophysiol 26: 326–332.

Deecke L, Kornhuber HH, Lang W et al. (1985). Timing function of the frontal cortex in sequential motor and learning tasks. Hum Neurobiol 4: 143–154.

De Munck JC, van Dijk BW (1999). The spatial distribution of spontaneous EEG and MEG. In: C Uhl (Ed.), Analysis of Neurophysiological Brain Functioning. Springer, Berlin, pp. 202–228.

Drasdo N, Thompson DA (1992). An optical stimulator for studying the topography of electrical and magnetic visual evoked responses. Doc Ophthalmol 81: 219–225.

Ebersole JS (1999). EEG source modeling. The last word (editorial). J Clin Neurophysiol 16: 297–302.

Ebersole JS, Squires K, Gamelin J et al. (1993). Simultaneous MEG and EEG provide complementary dipole maps of temporal lobe spikes. Epilepsia 34: 143.

Ebersole JS, Squires KC, Eliashiv SD et al. (1995). Applications of magnetic source imaging in evaluation of candidates for epilepsy surgery. Neuroimaging Clin N Am 5: 267–288.

Eliashiv SD, Squires K, Fried I et al. (1998). Magnetic source imaging as a localization tool in patients with surgically remediable epilepsies. Epilepsia 39: 80–90.

Engel J (1993). Surgical Treatment of the Epilepsies. Raven Press, New York.

Fuchs M, Drenckhahn R, Wischmann HA et al. (1998a). An improved boundary element method for realistic volume-conductor modeling. IEEE Trans Biomed Eng 45: 980–997.

Fuchs M, Wagner M, Wischmann HA et al. (1998b). Improving source reconstructions by combining bioelectric and biomagnetic data. Electroencephalogr Clin Neurophysiol 107: 93–111.

Fukao K, Inoue Y, Yagi K (2010). Magnetoencephalographic correlates of different types of aura in temporal lobe epilepsy. Epilepsia 51: 1846–1851.

Funke ME, Lewine JD, Orrison WW et al. (2002). MEG-guided identification of structural brain lesions in patients with neocortical epilepsy. In: H Nowak, J Haueisen, F Giessler et al., (Eds.) BIOMAG: Proceedings of the 13th International Conference on Biomagnetism. VDE, Berlin, pp. 212–215.

Ganslandt O, Steinmeier R, Kober H et al. (1997). Magnetic source imaging combined with image-guided frameless stereotaxy: a new method in surgery around the motor strip. Neurosurgery 41: 621–628.

Ganslandt O, Fahlbusch R, Nimsky C et al. (1999). Functional neuronavigation with magnetoencephalography outcome in 50 patients with lesions around the motor cortex. Neurosurg Focus 6: e3.

Genow A, Hummel C, Scheler G et al. (2004). Epilepsy surgery, resection volume and MSI localization in lesional frontal lobe epilepsy. Neuroimage 21: 444–449.

Grover KM, Bowyer SM, Rock J et al. (2006). Retrospective review of MEG visual evoked hemifield responses prior to resection of temporo-parieto-occipital lesions. J Neurooncol 77: 161–166.

Guggisberg AG, Dalal SS, Findlay AM et al. (2007). High-frequency oscillations in distributed neural networks reveal the dynamics of human decision making. Front Hum Neurosci 1: 14–28.

Hämäläinen MS (1992). Magnetoencephalography: a tool for functional brain imaging. Brain Topogr 5: 95–102.

Hämäläinen M, Hari R, Ilmoniemi LJ et al. (1993). Magnetoencephalography – theory, instrumentation, and applications to noninvasive studies of the working human brain. Rev Modern Phys 65: 413–497.

Hari R, Aittoniemi K, Jarvinen ML et al. (1980). Auditory evoked transient and sustained magnetic fields of the human brain. Localization of neural generators. Exp Brain Res 40: 237–240.

Hari R, Ahonen A, Forss N et al. (1993). Parietal epileptic mirror focus detected with a whole-head neuromagnetometer. Neuroreport 5: 45–48.

Hattori H, Yamano T, Tsutada T et al. (2001). Magnetoencephalography in the detection of focal lesions in West syndrome. Brain Dev 23: 528–532.

Ishibashi H, Simos PG, Wheless JW et al. (2002). Localization of ictal and interictal bursting epileptogenic activity in focal cortical dysplasia: agreement of magnetoencephalography and electrocorticography. Neurol Res 24: 525–530.

Iwasaki M, Pestana E, Burgess RC et al. (2005). Detection of epileptiform activity by human interpreters: blinded comparison between electroencephalography and magnetoencephalography. Epilepsia 46: 59–68.

Jin K, Nakasato N, Shamoto H et al. (2007). Neuromagnetic localization of spike sources in perilesional, contralateral mirror, and ipsilateral remote areas in patients with cavernoma. Epilepsia 48: 2160–2166.

Kahane P, Landré E (2008). The epileptic zone. Neurochirurgie 54: 265–271.

Kamada K, Toto T, Masutani Y et al. (2007). Visualization of the frontotemporal language fibers by tractography combined with functional magnetic resonance imaging and magnetoencephalography. J Neurosurg 106: 90–98.

Kawamura T, Nakasato N, Seki K et al. (1996). Neuromagnetic evidence of pre- and post-central cortical sources of somatosensory evoked responses. Electroencephalogr Clin Neurophysiol 100: 44–50.

Kettenmann B, Jousmäki V, Portin K et al. (1996). Odourants activate the human superior temporal sulcus. Neurosci Lett 203: 1–3.

Kettenmann B, Feichtinger M, Tilz C et al. (2005). Comparison of clonidine to sleep deprivation in the potential to induce spike or sharp-wave activity. Clin Neurophysiol 116: 905–912.

King DW, Park YD, Smith JR et al. (2000). Magnetoencephalography in neocortical epilepsy. Adv Neurol 84: 23.

Kirchberger K, Hummel C, Stefan H (1998a). Postoperative multichannel magnetoencephalography in patients with recurrent seizures after epilepsy surgery. Acta Neurol Scand 98: 1–7.

Kirchberger KG, Schmitt H, Hummel C et al. (1998b). Clonidine and methohexital induced epileptic MEG discharges in patients with focal epilepsies. Epilepsia 39: 1104–1112.

Knowlton RC, Laxer KD, Aminoff MJ et al. (1997). Magnetoencephalography in partial epilepsy: clinical yield and localization accuracy. Ann Neurol 42: 622–631.

Knowlton RC, Elgavish R, Howell J et al. (2006). Magnetic source imaging versus intracranial electroencephalogram in epilepsy surgery: a prospective study. Ann Neurol 59: 835–842.

Knowlton RC, Razdan SN, Limdi N et al. (2009). Effect of epilepsy magnetic source imaging of intracranial electrode placement. Ann Neurol 65: 716–723.

Lamusuo S, Forss N, Ruottinen HM et al. (1999). [^{18} F]FDG-PET and whole-scalp MEG localization of epileptogenic cortex. Epilepsia 40: 921–930.

Lin YY, Shih YH, Hsieh JC et al. (2003). Magnetoencephalographic yield of interictal spikes in temporal lobe epilepsy. Comparison with scalp EEG recordings. Neuroimage 19: 1115–1126.

Liu AK, Dale AM, Belliveau JW (2002). Monte Carlo simulation studies of EEG and MEG localization accuracy. Hum Brain Mapp 16: 47–62.

Mäkelä JP, Forss N, Jääskelöinen J et al. (2006). Magnetoencephalography in neurosurgery. Neurosurgery 59: 493–510.

Mamelak AN, Lopez N, Akhtari M et al. (2002). Magnetoencephalography-directed surgery in patients with neocortical epilepsy. J Neurosurg 97: 865–873.

Moore KR, Funke ME, Constantino T et al. (2002). Magnetoencephalographically directed review of high-spatial-resolution surface-coil MR images improves lesion detection in patients with extratemporal epilepsy. Radiology 225: 880–887.

Morioka T, Nishio S, Ishibashi H et al. (1999). Intrinsic epileptogenicity of focal cortical dysplasia as revealed by magnetoencephalography and electrocorticography. Epilepsy Res 33: 177–187.

Morioka T, Nishio S, Hisada K et al. (2000a). Neuromagnetic assessment of epileptogenicity in cerebral arteriovenous malformation. Neurosurg Rev 23: 206–212.

Morioka T, Nishio S, Shigeto H et al. (2000b). Surgical management of intractable epilepsy associated with cerebral neurocytoma. Neurol Res 22: 449–456.

Mosher JC, Lewis PS, Leahy RM (1992). Multiple dipole modeling and localization from spatio-temporal MEG data. IEEE Trans Biomed Eng 39: 541–557.

Murayama N, Nakasato N, Hatanaka K et al. (1996). Gustatory evoked magnetic fields in humans. Neurosci Lett 210: 121–123.

Nakasato N, Levesque MF, Barth DS et al. (1994). Comparisons of MEG, EEG, and ECoG source localization in neocortical partial epilepsy in humans. Electroencephalogr Clin Neurophysiol 91: 171–178.

Nakasato N, Itoh H, Hatanaka K et al. (2001). Movement-related magnetic fields to tongue protrusion. Neuroimage 14: 924–935.

Oishi M, Otsubo H, Kameyama S et al. (2002). Epileptic spikes: magnetoencephalography versus simultaneous electrocorticography. Epilepsia 43: 1390–1395.

Oishi M, Kameyama S, Masuda H et al. (2006). Single and multiple clusters of magnetoencephalographic dipoles in neocortical epilepsy: significance in characterizing the epileptogenic zone. Epilepsia 47: 355–364.

Ossenblok P, Fuchs M, Velis DN et al. (1999). Source analysis of lesional frontal-lobe epilepsy. IEEE Eng Med Biol Mag 18: 67–77.

Ossenblok P, de Munck JC, Colon A et al. (2007). Magnetoencephalography is more successful for screening and localizing frontal lobe epilepsy than electroencephalography. Epilepsia 48: 2139–2249.

Otsubo H, Chitoku S, Ochi A et al. (2001a). Malignant rolandic-sylvian epilepsy in children: diagnosis, treatment, and outcomes. Neurology 57: 590–596.

Otsubo H, Ochi A, Elliott I et al. (2001b). MEG predicts epileptic zone in lesional extrahippocampal epilepsy: 12 pediatric surgery cases. Epilepsia 42: 1523–1530.

Paetau R, Kajola M, Karhu J et al. (1992). Magnetoencephalographic localization of epileptic cortex – impact on surgical treatment. Ann Neurol 32: 106–109.

Paetau R, Ahonen A, Salonen O et al. (1995). Auditory evoked magnetic fields to tones and pseudowords in healthy children and adults. J Clin Neurophysiol 12: 177–185.

Paetau R, Granstrom ML, Blomstedt G et al. (1999). Magnetoencephalography in presurgical evaluation of children with the Landau–Kleffner syndrome. Epilepsia 40: 326–335.

Papanicolaou A (2009). Clinical Magnetoencephalography and Magnetic Source Imaging. Cambridge University Press, Cambridge.

Papanicolaou AC, Breier JI, Gormley W et al. (1998). Comparison of language mapping using extra and intraoperative electrocortical stimulation and magnetoencephalography. Epilepsia 39: 107.

Papanicolaou AC, Simos PG, Castillo EM et al. (2004). Magnetocephalography: a noninvasive alternative to the Wada procedure. J Neurosurg 100: 867–876.

Papanicolaou AC, Pataraia E, Billingsley-Marshall R et al. (2005). Toward the substitution of invasive electroencephalography in epilepsy surgery. J Clin Neurophysiol 22: 231–237.

Park HM, Nakasato N, Iwasaki M et al. (2004). Comparison of magnetoencephalographic spikes with and without concurrent electroencephalographic spikes in extratemporal epilepsy. Tohoku J Exp Med 203: 165–174.

Pascual Marqui RD, Michel CM, Lehmann D (1994). Low resolution electromagnetic tomography: a new method for localizing electrical activity in the brain. Int J Psychophysiol 18: 49–65.

Pataraia E, Baumgartner C, Lindinger G et al. (2002). Magnetoencephalography in presurgical epilepsy evaluation. Neurosurg Rev 25: 141–159.

Pataraia E, Lindinger G, Deecke L et al. (2005). Combined MEG/EEG analysis of the interictal spike complex in mesial temporal lobe epilepsy. Neuroimage 24: 607–614.

Patt S, Steenbeck J, Hochstetter A et al. (2000). Source localization and possible causes of interictal epileptic activity in tumor-associated epilepsy. Neurobiol Dis 7: 260–269.

Paulini A, Fischer M, Rampp S et al. (2007). Lobar localization information in epilepsy patients: MEG – a useful tool in routine presurgical diagnosis. Epilepsy Res 76: 123–130.

Peresson M, Lopez L, Narici L et al. (1998). Magnetic source imaging and reactivity to rhythmical stimulation in tuberous sclerosis. Brain Dev 20: 512–518.

RamachandranNair R, Otsubo H, Shroff MM et al. (2007). MEG predicts outcome following surgery for intractable epilepsy in children with normal or nonfocal MRI findings. Epilepsia 48: 149–157.

RamachandranNair R, Ochi A, Imai K et al. (2008). Epileptic spasms in older pediatric patients: MEG and ictal high-frequency oscillations suggest focal-onset seizures in a subset of epileptic spasms. Epilepsy Res 78: 216–224.

Rampp S, Stefan H (2007). Magnetoencephalography in presurgical epilepsy diagnosis. Expert Rev Med Devices 4: 335–347.

Rampp S, Kaltnehäuser M, Weigel D et al. (2010). MEG correlates of epileptic high gamma oscillations in invasive EEG. Epilepsia 51: 1638–1642.

Robinson SE, Nagarajan SS, Mantle M et al. (2004). Localization of interictal spikes using SAM(g2) and dipole fit. Neurol Clin Neurophysiol 2004: 74.

Rodin E, Funke M, Berg P et al. (2004). Magnetoencephalographic spikes not detected by conventional electroencephalography. Clin Neurophysiol 115: 2041–2047.

Rose DF, Sato S, Smith PD et al. (1987). Localization of magnetic interictal discharges in temporal lobe epilepsy. Ann Neurol 22: 348–354.

Sakurai K, Takeda Y, Tanaka N et al. (2010). Generalized spike-wave discharges involve a default mode network in patients with juvenile absence epilepsy: a MEG study. Epilepsy Res 89: 176–184.

Salayev KA, Nakasato N, Ishitobi M et al. (2006). Evaluation of interhemispheric time difference by magnetoencephalography before and after total callosotomy: report of two cases. Neurol Med Chir 46: 136–142.

Santuiste M, Nowak R, Russi A et al. (2008). Simultaneous magnetoencephalography and intracranial EEG registration: technical and clinical aspects. J Clin Neurophysiol 25: 331–339.

Scheler G, Fischer MJ, Genow A et al. (2007). Spatial relationship of source localizations in patients with focal epilepsy: comparison of MEG and EEG with a three spherical shells and a boundary element volume conductor model. Hum Brain Map 28: 315–322.

Scherg M, Bast T, Berg P (1999). Multiple source analysis of interictal spikes: goals, requirements, and clinical value. J Clin Neurophysiol 16: 214–224.

Seki K, Nakasato N, Fujita S et al. (1996). Neuromagnetic evidence that the P100 component of pattern reversal visual evoked response originates in the bottom of calcarine fissure. Electroencephalogr Clin Neurophysiol 100: 436–442.

Shigeto H, Morioka T, Hisada K et al. (2002). Feasibility and limitations of magnetoencephalographic detection of epileptic discharges: simultaneous recording of magnetic fields and electrocorticography. Neurol Res 24: 531–536.

Smith JR, Gallen C, Orrison W et al. (1994). Role of multichannel magnetoencephalography in the evaluation of ablative seizure surgery candidates. Stereotact Funct Neurosurg 62: 238–244.

Smith JR, Schwartz BJ, Gallen C et al. (1995). Utilization of multichannel magnetoencephalography in the guidance of ablative seizure surgery. J Epilepsy 8: 119–130.

Sobel DF, Aung M, Otsubo H et al. (2000). Magnetoencephalography in children with Landau–Kleffner syndrome and acquired epileptic aphasia. AJNR Am J Neuroradiol 21: 301–307.

Spencer SS, Spencer DD (1994). Entorhinal–hippocampal interactions in medial temporal lobe epilepsy. Epilepsia 35: 721–727.

Stefan H, Buchfelder M (2007). Diagnosis of sylvian and perisylvian epilepsies. Excitation symptoms of the insula reilii. Nervenarzt 78: 1175–1181.

Stefan H, Hummel C (1999). Magnetoencephalography. In: A Meinardi (Ed.), Handbook of Clinical Neurology. Elsevier, Amsterdam, pp. 319–336.

Stefan H, Schneider S, Abraham Fuchs K et al. (1990). Magnetic source localization in focal epilepsy. Multichannel magnetoencephalography correlated with magnetic resonance brain imaging. Brain 113: 1347–1359.

Stefan H, Schneider S, Abraham Fuchs K et al. (1991). The neocortico to mesio-basal limbic propagation of focal epileptic activity during the spike-wave complex. Electroencephalogr Clin Neurophysiol 79: 1–10.

Stefan H, Schneider S, Feistel H et al. (1992). Ictal and interictal activity in partial epilepsy recorded with multichannel magnetoelectroencephalography: correlation of electroencephalography/electrocorticography, magnetic resonance imaging, single photon emission computed tomography, and positron emission tomography findings. Epilepsia 33: 874–887.

Stefan H, Abraham-Fuchs K, Schneider S et al. (1993). Multichannel magneto-electroencephalography recordings of interictal and ictal activity. Physiol Meas 14: A109–A111.

Stefan H, Schüler P, Abraham-Fuchs K et al. (1994). Magnetic source localization and morphological changes in temporal lobe epilepsy: comparison of MEG/EEG, ECoG and volumetric MRI in presurgical evaluation of operated patients. Acta Neurol Scand Suppl 152: 83–88.

Stefan H, Quesney LF, Feistel HK et al. (1995). Presurgical evaluation in frontal lobe epilepsy. A multimethodological approach. Adv Neurol 66: 213–220.

Stefan H, Hummel C, Hopfengärtner R et al. (2000). Magnetoencephalography in extratemporal epilepsy. J Clin Neurophysiol 17: 190–200.

Stefan H, Hummel C, Scheler G et al. (2003). Magnetic brain source imaging of focal epileptic activity: a synopsis of 455 cases. Brain 126: 2396–2405.

Stefan H, Scheler G, Hummel C et al. (2004). Magnetoencephalography (MEG) predicts focal epileptogenicity in cavernomas. J Neurol Neurosurg Psychiatry 75: 1309–1313.

Stefan H, Nimsky C, Scheler G et al. (2007). Periventricular nodular heterotopia: a challenge for epilepsy surgery. Seizure 16: 81–86.

Stefan H, Hopfengärtner R, Kreiselmeyer G et al. (2008). Interictal triple ECoG characteristics of temporal lobe epilepsies: an intraoperative ECoG analysis correlated with surgical outcome. Clin Neurophysiol 119: 642–652.

Stefan H, Paulini-Ruf A, Hopfengärtner R et al. (2009). Network characteristics of idiopathic generalized epilepsies in combined MEG/EEG. Epilepsy Res 85: 187–198.

Stefan H, Heers M, Schmitt HJ et al. (2010). Increased spike frequency during general anesthesia with etomidate for magnetoencephalography in patients with focal epilepsies. Clin Neurophysiol 121: 1220–1226.

Stefan H, Rampp S, Knowlton RC (2011). Magnetoencephalography adds to the surgical evaluation process. Epilepsy Behav 20: 172–177.

Sutherling WW, Barth DS (1989). Neocortical propagation in temporal lobe spike foci on magnetoencephalography and electroencephalography. Ann Neurol 25: 373–381.

Sutherling WW, Crandall PH, Engel J, Jr et al. (1987). The magnetic field of complex partial seizures agrees with intracranial localizations. Ann Neurol 21: 548–558.

Sutherling WW, Crandall PH, Darcey TM et al. (1988). The magnetic and electric fields agree with intracranial localizations of somatosensory cortex. Neurology 38: 1705–1714.

Sutherling WW, Mamelak AN, Thyerlei D et al. (2008). Influence of magnetic source imaging for planning intracranial EEG in epilepsy. Neurology 71: 990–996.

Swartz B, Halgren E, Delgado-Escuetta AV et al. (1989). Neuroimaging in patients with seizures of probable frontal lobe origin. Epilepsia 30: 547–558.

Tanaka M, Yamada K, Watanabe Y et al. (2000). Electroclinical and magnetoencephalographic analysis of epilepsy in patients with congenital bilateral perisylvian syndrome. Epilepsia 41: 1584–1591.

Tao JX, Ray A, Hawes-Ebersole S et al. (2005). Intracranial EEG substrates of scalp EEG interictal spikes. Epilepsia 46: 669–676.

Tilz C, Hummel C, Hopfengärtner R et al. (2002). Ictal onset localization of epileptic seizures by magnetoencephalography. Acta Neurol Scand 106: 190–195.

Toulouse P, Agulhon C, Taussig D et al. (2003). Magnetoencephalographic studies of two cases of diffuse subcortical laminar heterotopia or so-called double cortex. Neuroimage 19: 1251–1259.

Verrotti A, Pizzella V, Madonna L et al. (2003). Magnetoencephalographic and electroencephalographic evaluation in patients with cryptogenetic partial epilepsy. Neurophysiol Clin 33: 174–179.

Watanabe Y, Fukao K, Watanabe M et al. (1996). Epileptic events observed by multichannel MEG. Electroencephalogr Clin Neurophysiol Suppl (Ireland) 47: 383–391.

Westmijse I, Ossenblock P, Gunnin B et al. (2009). Onset and propagation of spikes and slow wave discharges in human absence epilepsy: a MEG study. Epilepsia 50: 2538–2548.

Wheless JW, Willmore LJ, Breier JI et al. (1999). A comparison of magnetoencephalography, MRI, and V-EEG in patients evaluated for epilepsy surgery. Epilepsia 40: 931–941.

Widjaja E, Zarei Mahmoodabadi S, Otsubo H et al. (2009). Subcortical alterations in tissue microstructure adjacent to focal cortical dysplasia: detection at diffusion-tensor MR imaging by using magnetoencephalographic dipole cluster localization. Radiology 251: 206–215.

Wolters CH, Anwander A, Tricoche X et al. (2006). Influence of tissue conductivity anisotropy on EEG/MEG field and return current computation in a realistic head model: a simulation and visualization study using high-resolution finite element modeling. Neuroimage 30: 813–826.

Yang TT, Gallen CC, Schwartz BJ et al. (1993). Noninvasive somatosensory homunculus mapping in humans by using a large-array biomagnetometer. Proc Natl Acad Sci U S A 90: 3098–3102.

Yu HY, Nakasato N, Iwasaki M et al. (2004). Neuromagnetic separation of secondarily bilateral synchronized spike foci: report of three cases. J Clin Neurosci 11: 644–648.

Zhang W, Simos PG, Ishibashi H et al. (2003). Multimodality neuroimaging evaluation improves the detection of subtle cortical dysplasia in seizure patients. Neurol Res 25: 53–57.

Zijlmans M, Huiskamp GM, Leijten FS et al. (2002). Modality-specific spike identification in simultaneous magnetoencephalography/electroencephalography: a methodological approach. J Clin Neurophysiol 19: 183–191.

Handbook of Clinical Neurology, Vol. 107 (3rd series)
Epilepsy, Part I
H. Stefan and W.H. Theodore, Editors

Chapter 22

Structural brain imaging

REETTA KÄLVIÄINEN[1]* AND ARND DÖRFLER[2]
[1]*Kuopio Epilepsy Center, Kuopio University Hospital, Kuopio, Finland*
[2]*Department of Neuroradiology, University Hospital of Erlangen, Friedrich Alexander University Erlangen-Nürnberg, Erlangen, Germany*

INTRODUCTION

Magnetic resonance imaging (MRI) has become part of the basic assessment of patients with epilepsy. It has been suggested that all patients with epileptic seizure and/or epilepsy should, in the ideal situation, have high-quality MRI (Commission on Neuroimaging of the International League Against Epilepsy, 1997). MRI assessment requires knowledge of the clinical semiology of the seizures and abnormality shown in the EEG, and excellent interaction between the neurologist and the radiologist. Lesions are detected in 13–14% of unselected patients with first seizure or newly diagnosed epilepsy (King et al., 1998; Berg et al., 2000) and in up to 26% when 3-Tesla (T) MRI is applied in an epileptic patient population with localization-related epilepsies (Griffiths et al., 2005). The highest yield (up to 83%) in the detection of epileptogenic lesions is observed in patient groups with intractable temporal lobe epilepsy who are considered candidates for epilepsy surgery (Urbach et al., 2004).

The success of medical treatment in epilepsy is predetermined greatly by the syndrome and etiology of the epilepsy (Table 22.1, Semah et al., 1998). Complete resection of a clearly defined and imaged epileptogenic lesion can lead to total seizure freedom in up to 70–90% of cases, whereas patients who have negative findings on imaging have a less successful outcome (Immonen et al., 2010).

METHODOLOGY

The imaging sequences used, slice positioning, and experience of the radiologist play an important role in the sensitivity of the MRI technique. Standard MRI protocols fail to detect up to 50% fail to detect the majority of lesions in patients with refractory epilepsy (von Oertzen et al., 2002). Therefore, a specific, preplanned epilepsy protocol should be used. Transaxial T2-weighted fast spin-echo imaging with 3–5-mm thick sections covers the whole brain and is used for efficient screening of any space-occupying lesion. Coronal T2-weighted fast spin-echo images are necessary for precise anatomical localization within the temporal lobe and are mandatory for adequate evaluation of mesial temporal sclerosis (MTS). A coronal or sagittal three-dimensional (3D) T1-weighted gradient echo volume acquisition with isotropic voxels covers the whole brain with 1.2–2-mm partitions, allows reformatting in any orientation, and enables hippocampal volumetry. Fluid-attenuated inversion recovery (FLAIR) sequences are also induced in the protocol, usually in both transaxial and coronal orientations and preferably with a thin slice thickness. Inversion recovery (IR) sequences provide superior contrast between the gray and white matter, and double inversion recovery (DIR) sequencing has been reported to increase detection of subtle gray matter alterations (Rugg-Gunn et al., 2006). T2*-weighted or susceptibility-weighted sequences may be used to detect traces of hemosiderin in, for example, cavernomas or after trauma. The coronal sequences are best oriented at a right angle to the long axis of the hippocampus. The studies are monitored by a neuroradiologist, and contrast agent is administered for further characterization only if a space-occupying lesion (tumor or cavernoma) is identified.

MAJOR FINDINGS IN MRI IN PATIENTS WITH EPILEPSY

Hippocampal sclerosis (HS)

HS is the most frequently encountered cause of refractory temporal lobe epilepsy, and unilateral temporal lobe epilepsy due to HS is a surgically remediable focal

*Correspondence to: Professor Reetta Kälviäinen, Kuopio Epilepsy Center, Kuopio University Hospital, POB 1777, 70211 Kuopio, Finland. Tel: 358-17-173311, Fax: 358-17-173031, E-mail: reetta.kalviainen@kuh.fi

Table 22.1

Response to medical treatment as a function of syndrome and lesion in chronic focal epilepsy (Semah et al., 1998)

Syndrome and etiology	Seizure control (> 1 year seizure-free) (%)
Cryptogenic focal epilepsy	45
Symptomatic focal epilepsy	35
TLE	20
With HS	11
Without HS	31
Dual pathology (with HS)	3
Extratemporal focal epilepsy	36
Cerebral dysgenesis	24

HS, hippocampal sclerosis; TLE, temporal lobe epilepsy.

epilepsy syndrome. The diagnosis of HS on MRI has a positive predictive value on seizure outcome after surgery (Berkovic et al., 1995; Jack et al., 1996; Gilliam et al., 2000). Patients are less likely to be operated on when no hippocampal anomalies are detected on MRI, which further underlines the impact of MRI on patient management and stresses the importance of adequate imaging.

Typical imaging features of a sclerotic hippocampus are a high signal on FLAIR and T2-weighted images (Fig. 22.1), a low signal on T1-weighted images, and atrophy (volume loss) (Jackson et al., 1993). The high signal on T2-weighted and FLAIR images is due to dentate gliosis (Briellmann et al., 2002). Other related findings suggestive of HS are loss of internal structure of the hippocampus, atrophy of extrahippocampal temporal lobe structures (ipsilateral temporal pole, fornix, parahippocampal gyrus), and decreased signal intensity on T1-weighted images.

Bilateral HS is difficult to detect visually, but probably occurs more commonly than it is diagnosed. Measurement of hippocampal T2 time (T2 relaxometry) may help to identify bilateral disease (Okujava et al., 2004). HS may occur also in association with other lesions. This is called dual pathology. Most commonly these lesions include low-grade tumors, cortical malformations, vascular malformations, or ischemic lesions (Cendes et al., 1995).

In the differential diagnosis of hippocampal T2 hyperintensities on FLAIR of T2 images, especially in acute setting, limbic encephalitis and edema following continuous seizure activity (status epilepticus) should be borne in mind (Kavuk et al., 2005). The appearance of the hippocampus is not atrophic, but more swollen in these acute situations. In follow-up, however, after increased signal intensity in the acute stage, gradual atrophy of the hippocampus with increased T2 signal may develop (Bien et al., 2007; Provenzale et al., 2008). Bilateral MRI features of hippocampal atrophy with or without hippocampal T2 hyperintensity can also be the consequence of a hypoxic injury or atrophy related to dementia or depression. However, the severity of hippocampal atrophy correlates with the elongation of T2 relaxation time in temporal lobe epilepsy but not in Alzheimer's disease (Pitkänen et al., 1996).

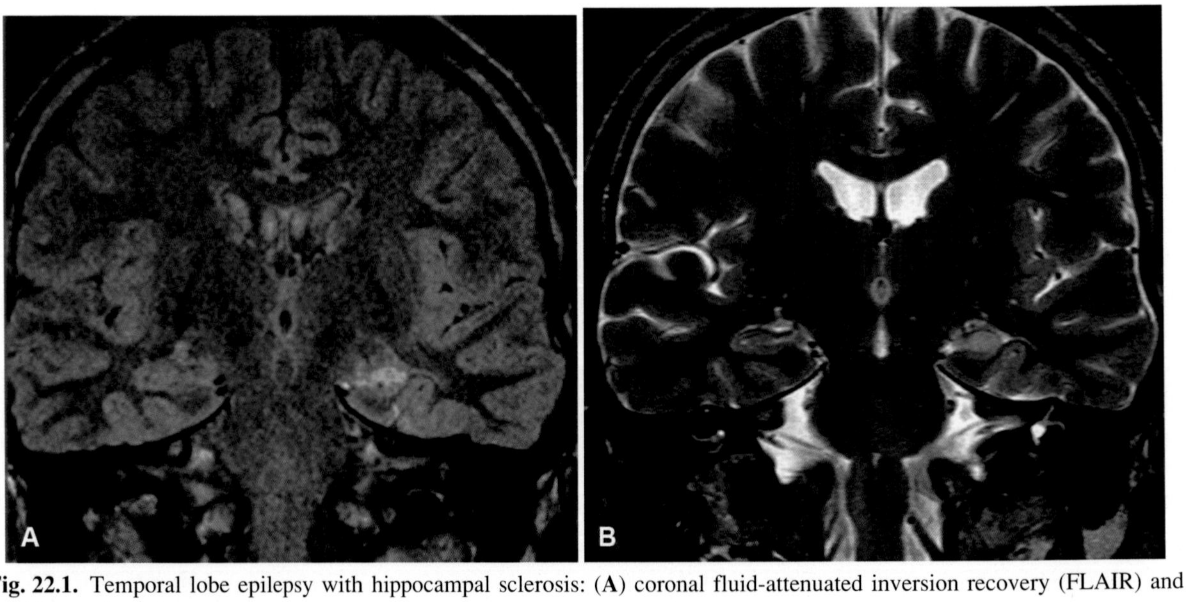

Fig. 22.1. Temporal lobe epilepsy with hippocampal sclerosis: (**A**) coronal fluid-attenuated inversion recovery (FLAIR) and (**B**) T2-weighted images.

Malformations of cortical development (MCD)

MCD are generally qualified according to the stage in which cortical development was disrupted. To date, the most comprehensive classification has been proposed by Barkovich et al. (2001). MRI for MCD should be performed using high-resolution T1-weighted gradient echo volume acquisitions: magnetization-prepared rapid gradient echo (MP-RAGE) and spoiled gradient recalled acquisition in steady state (SPGR). The inversion recovery-like contrast of the 3D T1-weighted images provides a strong contrast between gray and white matter. Additional FLAIR/T2-weighted images are necessary. In the neonate and infant, FLAIR images have little contrast between gray and white matter, but are useful in children older than 24 months in whom myelination is accomplished. If the study is obtained before the age of 6–8 months, T2-weighted images should be used (Barkovich and Raybaud, 2004). In the classification scheme of Barkovich et al. (2001), the existence of focal cortical dysplasias (FCDs) was not emphasized, and therefore an expert panel has suggested that these be divided into mild MCDs and FCDs, which are further divided into types I and II (Palmini et al., 2004).

Focal cortical dysplasia

FCD is probably the most common cause of refractory extratemporal focal epilepsy. Isolated architectural without dysplastic neurons are called FCD type I. FCD type II additionally show dysmorphic neurons, some with balloon cells – dysmorphic neurons without (Taylor type IIA) or with (Taylor type IIB) balloon cells (Palmini et al., 2004). Identifying the lesion on MRI remains one of the most important factors in determining the surgical outcome (Krsek et al., 2009; Lerner et al., 2009).

Imaging findings of FCDs include thickening of the cortex, blurring of the gray–white matter junction, abnormal cortical signal, and increased T_2/FLAIR and/or T_1 hypointense signal extending from the ependymal surface to the cortical surface (transmantle sign) (Barkovich et al., 1997) (Fig. 22.2). Additional imaging features that have been described include

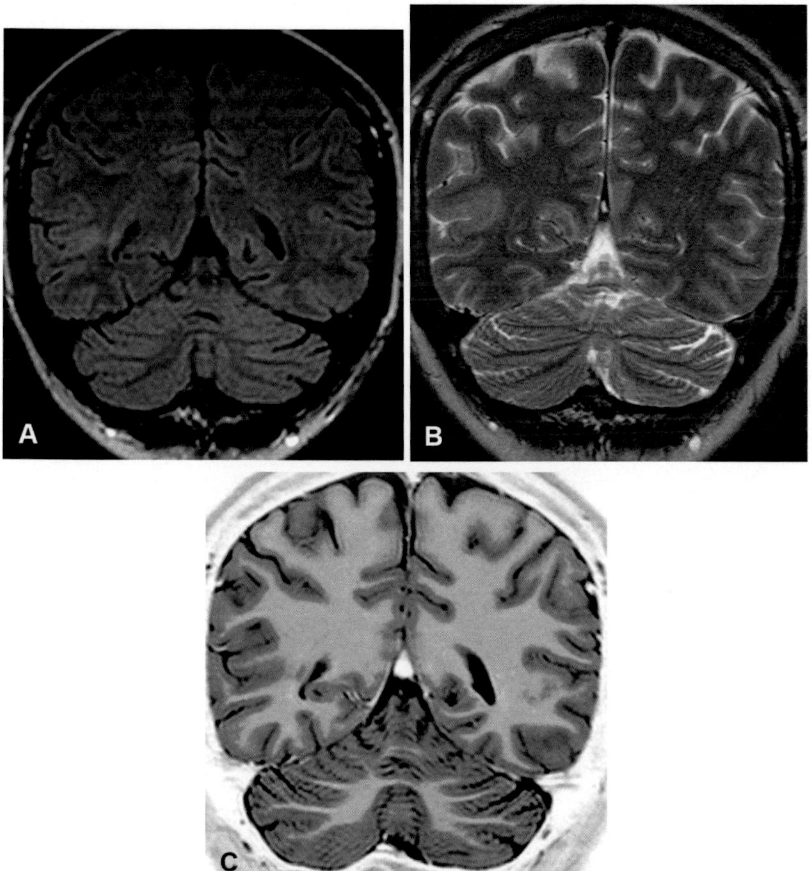

Fig. 22.2. Type II focal cortical dysplasia: (**A**) fluid-attenuated inversion recovery (FLAIR), (**B**) T2-weighted and (**C**) inversion recovery images, showing lesion and transmantle sign.

focal hypoplasia, a deep sulcus with malformations at the depths of the sulci, broadening of the gyri, and white matter atrophy. Previously it was thought that mild MCDs and type I FCDs could not be seen on MRI, but recently MRI abnormalities have been described in these pathologies (Krsek et al., 2008). Type II or Taylor-type FCDs are the most frequently identified FCDs on MRI; however, MRI findings can still be normal (Bronen et al., 1997; Chan et al., 1998; Lee et al., 1998).

HETEROTOPIA

Heterotopia is defined as a cluster of normal neurons in abnormal locations, and is divided into three main groups: periventricular nodular heterotopia, subcortical heterotopia, and band or laminar heterotopia. Subependymal or periventricular heterotopia (Fig. 22.3) consists of round or ovoid nodules of gray matter that reside in the wall of the lateral ventricles or that lie directly lateral to the ventricular wall. Nodules remain isointense to gray matter on all sequences, which differentiates these lesions from the periventricular lesions found in tuberous sclerosis. Subependymal or periventricular heterotopias do not calcify and do not enhance after contrast administration. Approximately 90% of patients with periventricular heterotopia have epilepsy (Dubeau et al., 1995), which can begin at any age.

Subcortical heterotopias are a heterogeneous group and affected patients most frequently present with seizures. Large bilateral subcortical heterotopia may be associated with impaired cognitive development (Barkovich and Kjos, 1992a). Imaging characteristics of these heterotopias are the same as those of subependymal heterotopia, and the distribution of these nodules may vary from localized groups to long subcortical curvilinear bands of gray matter nodules (band heterotopia) (Fig. 22.4).

POLYMICROGYRIA AND SCHIZENCEPHALY

Polymicrogyria is characterized by an excessive number of small and prominent convolutions spaced out by shallow and enlarged sulci. Cortical infolding and secondary, irregular thickening due to packing of microgyri are visible on MRI, although mild forms are difficult to recognize on neuroimaging (Guerrini et al., 1992). The distribution can be very variable, and theoretically all parts of the brain can be affected, although the most frequently affected part is the perisylvian region. Typical distribution patterns can be observed; one of the best known bilateral, symmetrical syndromes is bilateral perisylvian polymicrogyria, also known as congenital bilateral perisylvian syndrome (Kuzniecky et al., 1993).

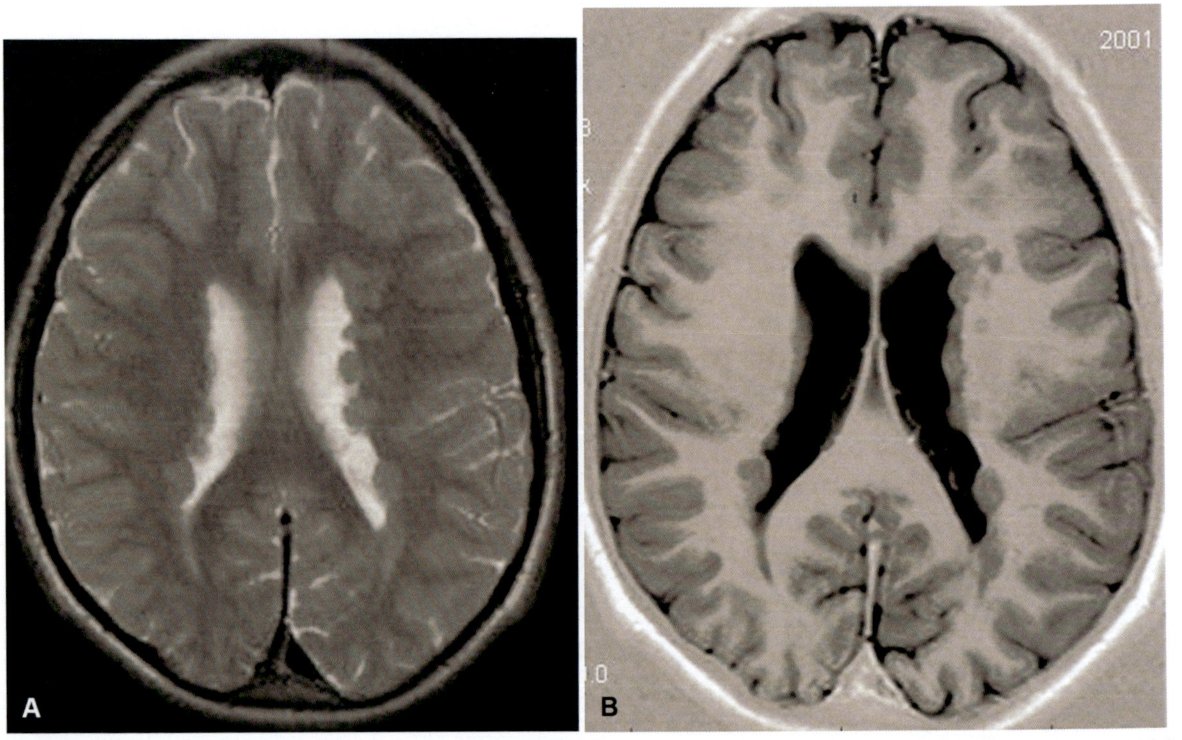

Fig. 22.3. Subependymal heterotopia: (**A**) T2-weighted and (**B**) inversion recovery images. (From Dörfler et al. (2006). © Thieme.)

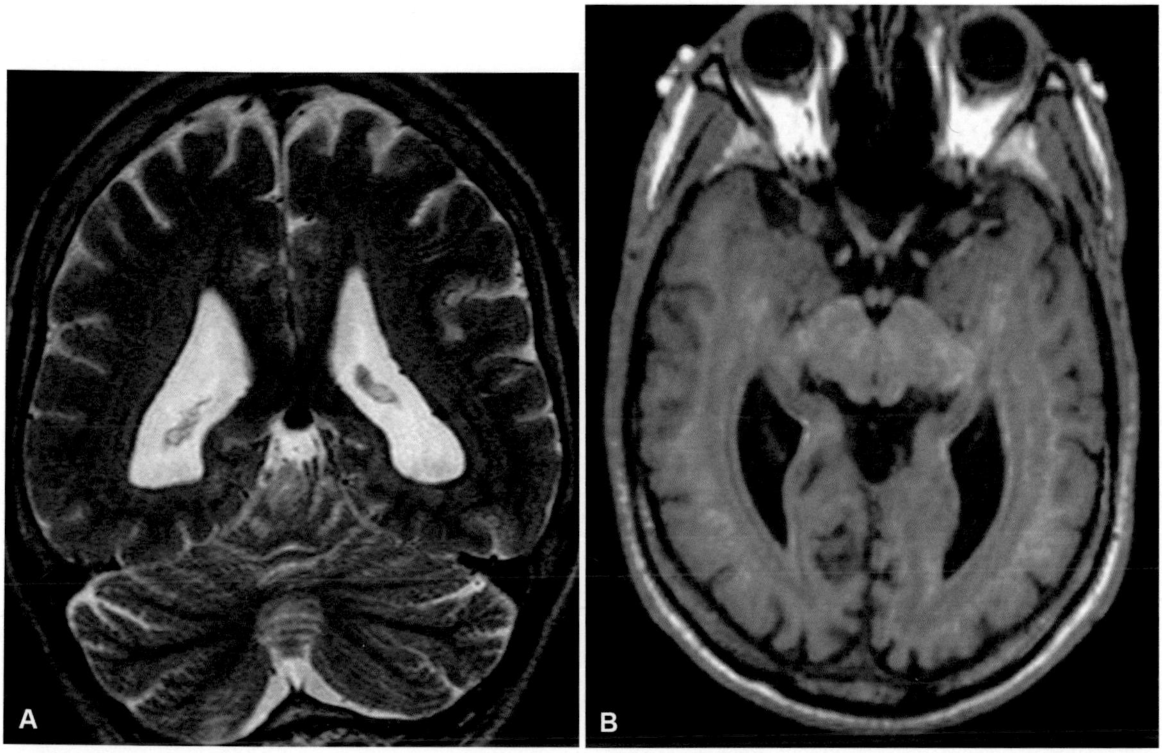

Fig. 22.4. Band heterotopia: (**A**) T2-weighted and (**B**) inversion recovery images.

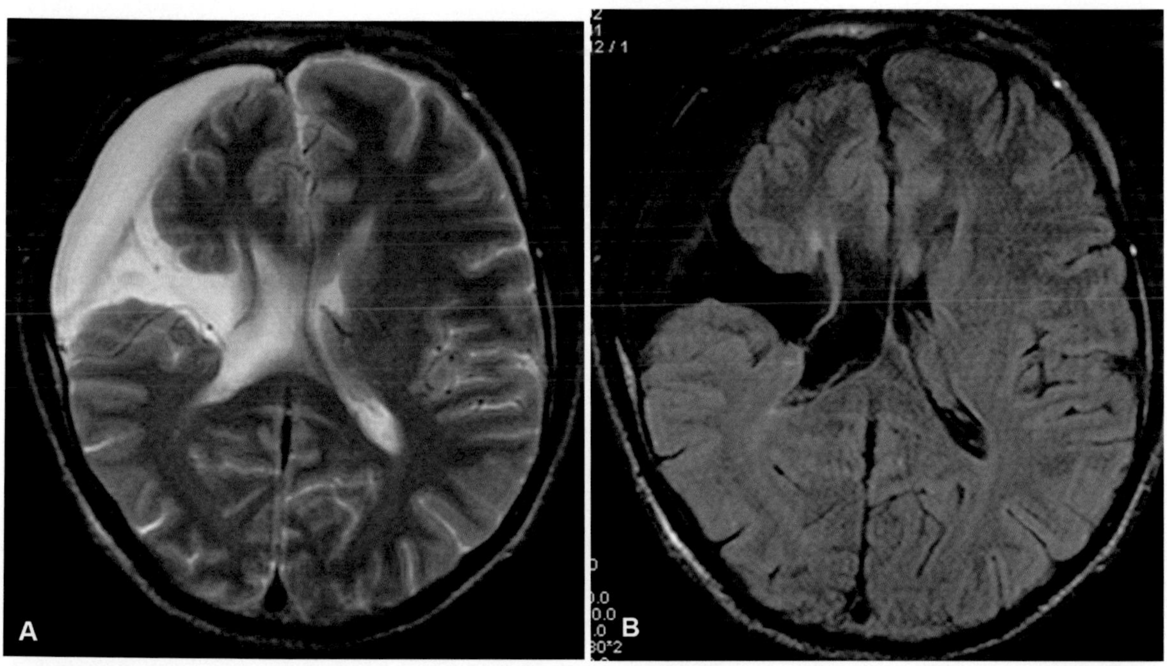

Fig. 22.5. Open-lip perisylvian schizencephaly: (**A**) T2-weighted and (**B**) fluid-attenuated inversion recovery (FLAIR) images. (From Dörfler et al. (2006). © Thieme.)

Schizencephaly (cleft brain) consists of a unilateral or bilateral full-thickness cleft of the cerebral hemispheres with communication between the ventricle and extra-axial subarachnoid spaces. The clefts are found most often in the perisylvian area. The walls of the clefts may be widely separated (open-lip; Fig. 22.5) or closely adjacent (closed-lip). Bilateral clefts are usually symmetrical. The cleft is lined by dysmorphic appearing gray matter, which is usually polymicrogyric (Fig. 22.6) (Barkovich and Kjos, 1992b).

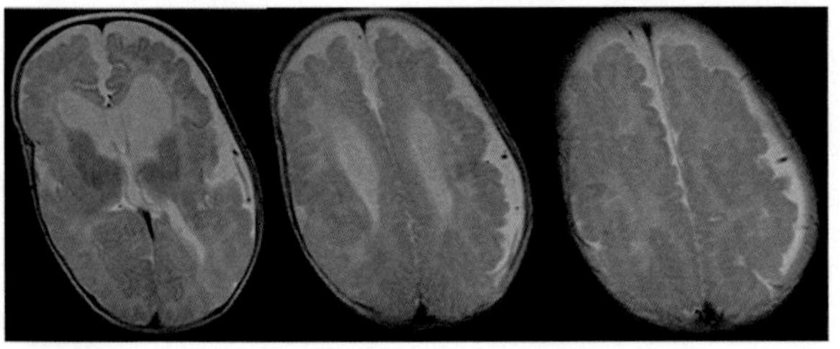

Fig. 22.6. Extensive holocephalic polymicrogyria: T2-weighted image.

Dysplastic tumors

Dysembryoplastic neuroepitheliomas (DNETs) and gangliogliomas are tumoral lesions frequently associated with refractory epilepsy. These lesions may be surrounded by cortical regions displaying abnormal cytoarchitecture and large (dysmorphic) neurons. Both lesions have a good prognosis after surgery.

MRI of patients with DNETs shows a cortical and well-delineated lesion exceeding the thickness of the normal cortex and involving the white matter. DNETs can be found anywhere in the brain, but most frequently involve the temporal lobe. Lesions are usually intracortical and exhibit low signal on T1-weighted images and high signal on T2-weighted images (Fig. 22.7), with occasional contrast enhancement (Koeller and Dillon, 1992; Fernandez et al., 2003). Calcifications may be present in up to 30% of cases.

Gangliogliomas are usually benign intra-axial neoplasms that are composed of dysplastic neurons and neoplastic glial cells. They can occur at any age, but are found most commonly in children and young adults, with a predilection for the temporal lobe. The classical imaging features are a combination of intracortical cysts, a circumscribed area of cortical and subcortical signal increase on FLAIR and T2-weighted images (Fig. 22.8), and a contrast-enhancing nodule (Zentner et al., 1994). Calcifications are present in 30% of cases. If contrast enhancement is absent (which happens in 50% of cases), gangliogliomas may be difficult to distinguish from cortical dysplasias. In these patients it is important to pay special attention to intracortical cysts.

Other tumors

In 20–30% of patients with long-term drug-resistant epilepsy, epilepsy-associated tumors are to be found (Luyken et al., 2003). There are two clinically different groups (Urbach, 2008). The first contains typical epilepsy-associated tumors such as gangliogliomas, DNETs, pleomorphic astrocytomas, and supratentorial pilocytic astrocytomas (World Health Organization (WHO) grade I), usually with benign behavior. The second group consists of diffuse astrocytomas (WHO grade II), oligodendrogliomas (WHO grade II), with a 5-year survival rate of 50–65%, and a few anaplastic cases, classified as WHO grade III, with a median survival time of 2–3 years. It is recommended that the low-grade tumors should also be recognized and removed early because of the high chance of seizure freedom and the rare but possible risk of malignant degeneration (Luyken et al., 2003).

Vascular lesions

The two most frequently encountered vascular lesions associated with epilepsy are arteriovenous malformations (AVMs) and cavernomas. In particular,

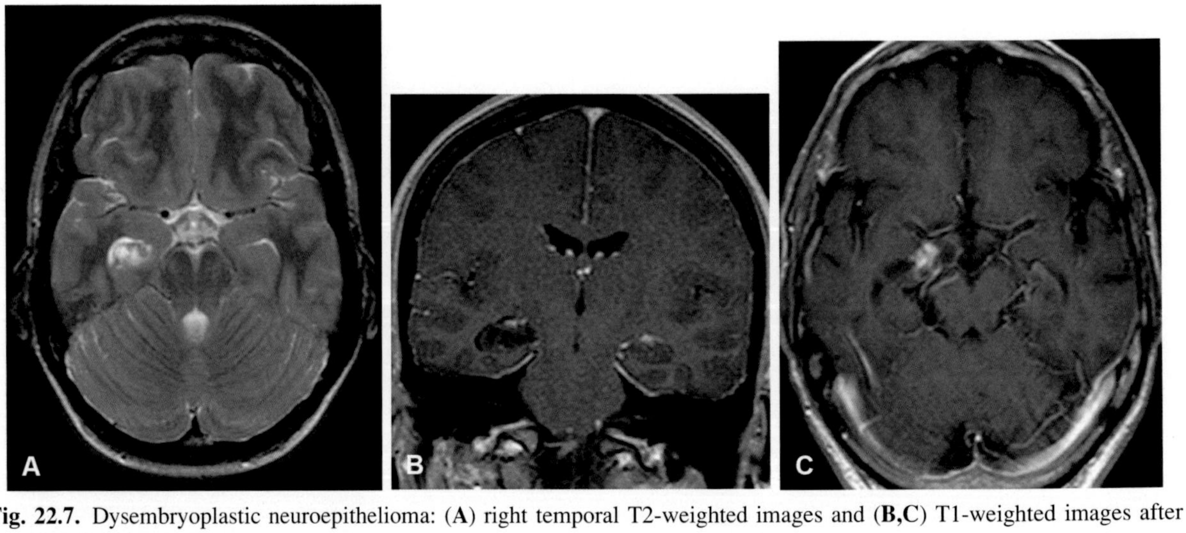

Fig. 22.7. Dysembryoplastic neuroepithelioma: (**A**) right temporal T2-weighted images and (**B,C**) T1-weighted images after contrast administration.

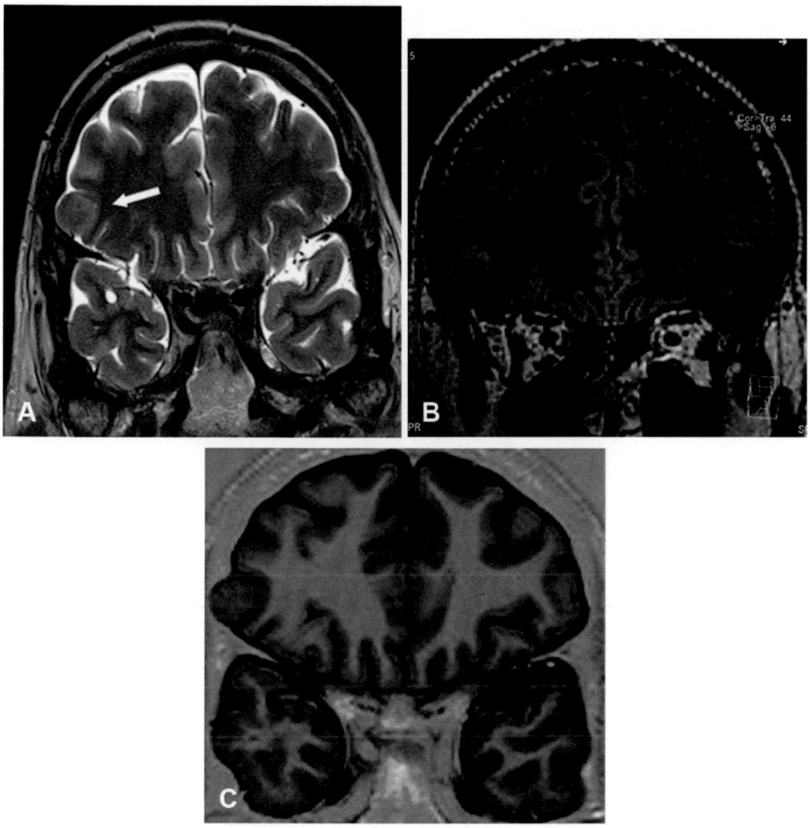

Fig. 22.8. Ganglioglioma: (**A**) right frontal T2-weighted, (**B**) fluid-attenuated inversion recovery (FLAIR), and (**C**) inversion recovery images.

supratentorial cavernomas are frequently associated with seizures and epilepsy (Awad and Jabbour, 2006). Cavernomas have a mixed signal core, due to the locules filled with blood in different stages of degradation. There is a hypointense fringe surrounding the lesions on T2*-weighted images due to hemosiderin (Fig. 22.9). Complete resection of hemosiderin fringe surrounding the cavernoma has been shown to correlate to a lower postoperative seizure frequency than that following incomplete resection of the hemosiderin fringe (Hammen et al., 2007). Gradient echo T2-weighted images (T2*) are extremely useful in identifying small cavernomas.

RECENT IMPROVEMENTS IN IMAGING

Although MRI in epileptic patients with optimal scanning protocols at 1.5-T machines yields a large number of positive studies, some small or subtle lesions remain undetected. The evolution of 3-T MRI techniques can improve the presurgical evaluation of patients with focal epilepsy, who were previously considered MRI negative with 1.5-T MRI (Knake et al., 2005). Strandberg et al. (2008) showed that MRI at 3 T could identify abnormalities in 20% of patients with previously unremarkable pathology, above all those with MCD. Recently, encouraging results have been reported for statistical methods such as statistical parametric mapping, which allows comparison of individual 3D imaging data with a group of healthy control individuals, and may increase the sensitivity of interpretation (Rugg-Gunn et al., 2006).

Diffusion tensor imaging (DTI) is a relatively new technique that provides 3D information regarding tissue water diffusion. It is sensitive to the molecular movement of water, which indicates cellular integrity and pathology. Some reports have shown that DTI could help to localize the epileptogenic areas in patients with refractory epilepsy showing normal findings on conventional MRI (Rugg-Gunn et al., 2001; Chen et al., 2008) (Fig. 22.10).

CONCLUSION

Patients who could be candidates for surgical treatment, and who have had previously unremarkable findings on MRI, should be rescanned when more advanced equipment and methods become available. As MRI techniques continue to evolve, more and more lesions will be detected.

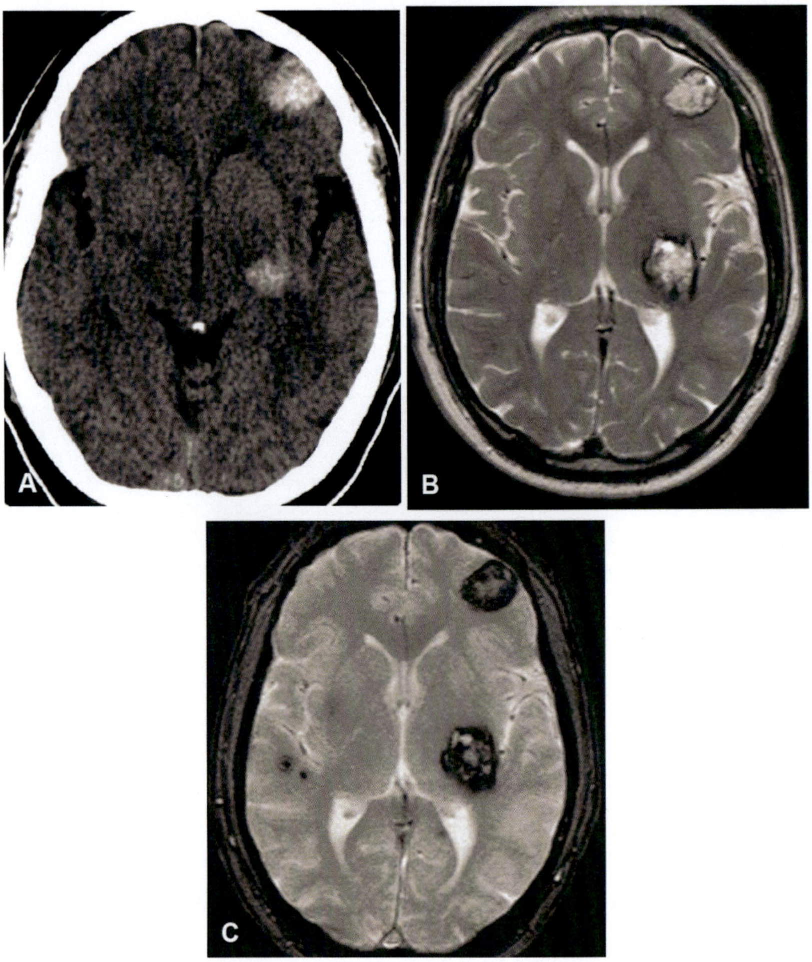

Fig. 22.9. Multiple cavernomas: (**A**) computed tomogram; (**B**) T2-weighted image showing hemosiderin fringe and "popcorn" pattern; and (**C**) sensitive T2*-weighted gradient-echo image revealing additional right temporal cavernomas and in the splenium, respectively. (From Dörfler et al. (2006). © Thieme.)

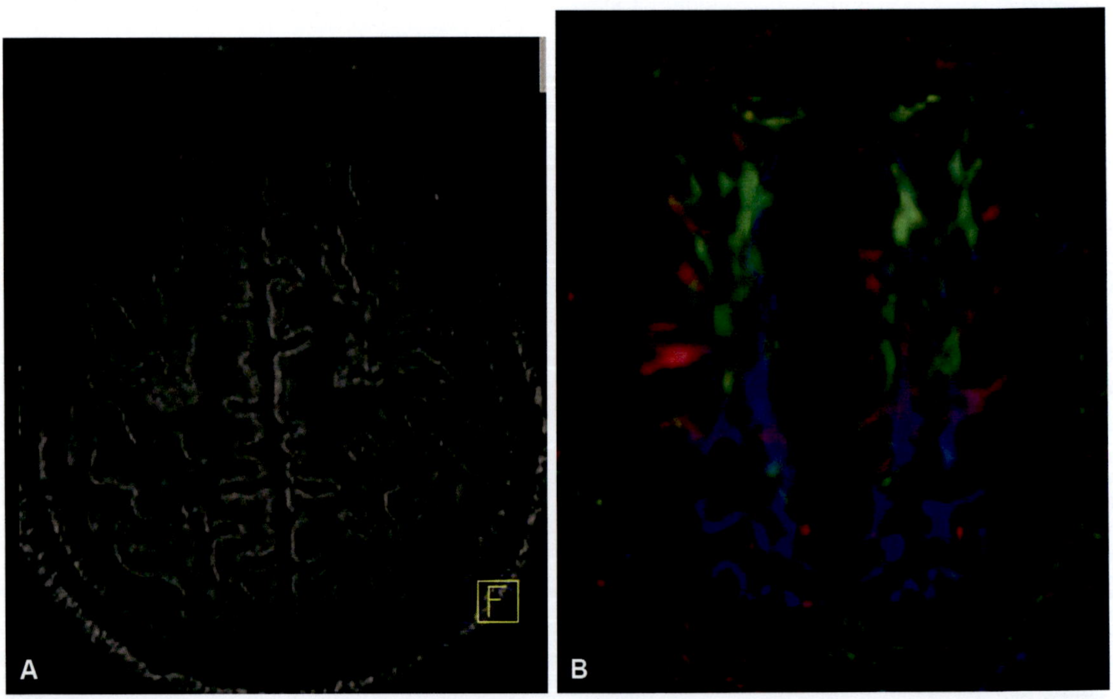

Fig. 22.10. Focal cortical dysplasia: (**A**) fluid-attenuated inversion recovery (FLAIR) image, and (**B**) with fractional anisotropy in diffusion tensor imaging (DTI).

Whether these lesions are the cause of the epilepsy will become one of the most important questions. Thus, a multidisciplinary approach with neurologists, other imaging modalities, and electrophysiologists is essential in the investigation of patients with epilepsy.

References

Awad I, Jabbour P (2006). Cerebral cavernous malformations and epilepsy. Neurosurg Focus 21: e7.

Barkovich AJ, Kjos BO (1992a). Gray matter heterotopias: MR characteristics and correlation with developmental and neurologic manifestations. Radiology 182: 493–499.

Barkovich AJ, Kjos BO (1992b). Schizencephaly: correlation of clinical findings with MR characteristics. AJNR Am J Neuroradiol 13: 85–94.

Barkovich AJ, Raybaud CA (2004). Malformations of cortical development. Neuroimaging Clin N Am 14: 401–423.

Barkovich AJ, Kuzniecky RI, Bollen AW et al. (1997). Focal transmantle dysplasia: a specific malformation of cortical development. Neurology 49: 1148–1152.

Barkovich AJ, Kuzniecky RI, Jackson GD et al. (2001). Classification system for malformations of cortical development: update 2001. Neurology 57: 2168–2178.

Berg AT, Testa FM, Levy SR et al. (2000). Neuroimaging in children with newly diagnosed epilepsy: a community-based study. Pediatrics 106: 527–532.

Berkovic SF, McIntosh AM, Kalnins RM et al. (1995). Preoperative MRI predicts outcome of temporal lobectomy: an actuarial analysis. Neurology 45: 1358–1363.

Bien CG, Urbach H, Schramm J et al. (2007). Limbic encephalitis as a precipitating event in adult-onset temporal lobe epilepsy. Neurology 69: 1236–1244.

Briellmann RS, Kalnins RM, Berkovic SF et al. (2002). Hippocampal pathology in refractory temporal lobe epilepsy: T2-weighted signal change reflects dentate gliosis. Neurology 58: 265 271.

Bronen RA, Vives KP, Kim JH et al. (1997). Focal cortical dysplasia of Taylor, balloon cell subtype: MR differentiation from low-grade tumors. AJNR Am J Neuroradiol 18: 1141–1151.

Cendes F, Cook MJ, Watson C et al. (1995). Frequency and characteristics of dual pathology in patients with lesional epilepsy. Neurology 45: 2058–2064.

Chan S, Chin SS, Nordli DR et al. (1998). Prospective magnetic resonance imaging identification of focal cortical dysplasia, including the non-balloon cell subtype. Ann Neurol 44: 749–757.

Chen Q, Lui S, Li CX et al. (2008). MRI-negative refractory partial epilepsy: role for diffusion tensor imaging in high field MRI. Epilepsy Res 80: 83–89.

Commission on Neuroimaging of the International League Against Epilepsy (1997). Recommendations for neuroimaging of patients with epilepsy. Epilepsia 38: 1255–1256.

Dörfler A, Hammen T, Doelken M et al. (2006). MRT- und CT-Diagnostik bei Epilepsiepatienten mit chronischem Verlauf. Akt Neurol 33: 458–466.

Dubeau F, Tampieri D, Lee N et al. (1995). Periventricular and subcortical nodular heterotopia: a study of 33 patients. Brain 118: 1273–1287.

Fernandez C, Girard N, Paz Paredes A et al. (2003). The usefulness of MR imaging in the diagnosis of dysembryoplastic neuroepithelial tumor in children: a study of 14 cases. AJNR Am J Neuroradiol 24: 829–834.

Gilliam F, Faught E, Martin R et al. (2000). Predictive value of MRI identified mesial temporal sclerosis for surgical outcome in temporal lobe epilepsy: an intent-to-treat analysis. Epilepsia 41: 963–966.

Griffiths PD, Coley SC, Connolly DJA et al. (2005). MR imaging of patients with localisation-related seizures: initial experience at 3.0 T and relevance to the NICE guidelines. Clin Radiol 60: 1090–1099.

Guerrini R, Dravet C, Raybaud C et al. (1992). Epilepsy and focal gyral anomalies detected by magnetic resonance imaging: electroclinicomorphological correlations and follow-up. Dev Med Child Neurol 34: 706–718.

Hammen T, Romstöck J, Dörfler A et al. (2007). Prediction of postoperative outcome with special respect to removal of hemosiderin fringe: a study in patients with cavernous haemangiomas associated with symptomatic epilepsy. Seizure 16: 248–253.

Immonen A, Jutila L, Muraja-Murro A et al. (2010). Long-term epilepsy surgery outcomes in patients with MRI-negative temporal lobe epilepsy. Epilepsia 51: 2260–2269.

Jack CR, Jr, Rydberg CH, Krecke KN et al. (1996). Mesial temporal sclerosis: diagnosis with fluid-attenuated inversion-recovery versus spin-echo MR imaging. Radiology 199: 367–373.

Jackson GD, Berkovic SF, Duncan JS et al. (1993). Optimizing the diagnosis of hippocampal sclerosis using MR imaging. AJNR Am J Neuroradiol 14: 753–762.

Kavuk I, Hufnagel A, Agelink MW et al. (2005). MRI changes associated with partial status epilepticus. Eur J Med Res 10: 243–246.

King MA, Newton MR, Jackson GD et al. (1998). Epileptology of the first seizure presentation: a clinical, electroencephalographic, and magnetic resonance imaging study of 300 consecutive patients. Lancet 352: 1007–1011.

Koeller KK, Dillon WP (1992). Dysembryoplastic neuroepithelial tumors: MR appearance. AJNR Am J Neuroradiol 13: 1319–1325.

Knake S, Triantafyllou C, Wald LL et al. (2005). 3T phased array MRI improves the presurgical evaluation in focal epilepsies: a prospective study. Neurology 65: 1026–1031.

Krsek P, Maton B, Korman B et al. (2008). Different features of histopathological subtypes of pediatric focal cortical dysplasia. Ann Neurol 63: 758–769.

Krsek P, Maton B, Jayakar P et al. (2009). Incomplete resection of focal cortical dysplasia is the main predictor of poor postsurgical outcome. Neurology 72: 217–223.

Kuzniecky R, Andermann F, Guerrini R (1993). Congenital bilateral perisylvian syndrome: study of 31 patients. The CBPS Multicenter Collaborative Study. Lancet 341: 608–612.

Lee BC, Schmidt RE, Hatfield GA et al. (1998). MRI of focal cortical dysplasia. Neuroradiology 40: 675–683.

Lerner JT, Salamon N, Hauptman JS et al. (2009). Assessment and surgical outcomes for mild type I and severe type II cortical dysplasia: a critical review and the UCLA experience. Epilepsia 50: 1310–1335.

Luyken C, Blumcke I, Fimmers R et al. (2003). The spectrum of long-term epilepsy-associated tumors: long-term seizure and tumor outcome and neurosurgical aspects. Epilepsia 44: 822–830.

Okujava M, Schulz R, Hoppe M et al. (2004). Bilateral mesial temporal lobe epilepsy: comparison of scalp EEG and hippocampal MRI-T2 relaxometry. Acta Neural Scand 110: 148–153.

Palmini A, Najm I, Avanzini G et al. (2004). Terminology and classification of the cortical dysplasias. Neurology 62: S2–S8.

Pitkänen A, Laakso M, Kälviäinen R et al. (1996). Severity of hippocampal atrophy correlates with the elongation of T2 relaxation time in temporal lobe epilepsy but not in Alzheimer's disease. Neurology 46: 1724–1730.

Provenzale JM, Barboriak DP, Van Landingham K et al. (2008). Hippocampal MRI signal hyperintensity after febrile status epilepticus is predictive of subsequent mesial temporal lobe sclerosis. AJR Am J Roentgenol 190: 976–983.

Rugg-Gunn FJ, Eriksson SH, Symms MR et al. (2001). Diffusion tensor imaging of cryptogenic and acquired partial epilepsies. Brain 124: 627–636.

Rugg-Gunn FJ, Boulby PA, Symms MR et al. (2006). Imaging the neocortex in epilepsy with double inversion recovery imaging. Neuroimage 31: 39–50.

Semah F, Picot MC, Adam C et al. (1998). Is the underlying cause of epilepsy a major prognostic factor for recurrence? Neurology 51: 1256.

Strandberg M, Larsson EM, Backman S et al. (2008). Presurgical epilepsy evaluation using 3T MRI. Do surface coils provide additional information? Epileptic Disord 10: 83–92.

Urbach H (2008). MRI of long-term epilepsy-associated tumors. Semin Ultrasound CT MR 29: 40–46.

Urbach H, Hattingen J, Von Oertzen J et al. (2004). MR imaging in the presurgical workup of patients with drug-resistant epilepsy. AJNR Am J Neuroradiol 25: 919–926.

Von Oertzen J, Urbach H, Jungbluth S et al. (2002). Standard magnetic resonance imaging is inadequate for patients with refractory focal epilepsy. J Neurol Neurosurg Psychiatry 73: 643.

Zentner J, Wolf HK, Ostertun B et al. (1994). Gangliogliomas: clinical, radiological and histopathological findings in 51 patients. J Neurol Neurosurg Psychiatry 57: 1497–1502.

Handbook of Clinical Neurology, Vol. 107 (3rd series)
Epilepsy, Part I
H. Stefan and W.H. Theodore, Editors

Chapter 23

Functional magnetic resonance imaging: focus localization

GRAEME D. JACKSON[1,2,3]*, RADWA BADAWY[1,2,3], AND JEAN GOTMAN[4]

[1]*Department of Neurology, Austin Health, Heidelberg, Victoria, Australia*

[2]*Department of Medicine, University of Melbourne, Melbourne, Victoria, Australia*

[3]*Brain Research Institute, Florey Neuroscience Institutes, Heidelberg West, Victoria, Australia*

[4]*Brain Imaging Center, Montreal Neurological Institute, McGill University, Montreal, Quebec, Canada*

INTRODUCTION

Functional magnetic resonance imaging (fMRI) allows the exploration of the local vascular response, and indirectly the coupled neural response to particular stimuli. It utilizes differences in the paramagnetic properties of oxyhemoglobin and deoxyhemoglobin, known as blood oxygen level-dependent (BOLD) contrast, to generate images of cerebral activity (Ogawa and Lee, 1990). Oxyhemoglobin is diamagnetic (nonmagnetic), whereas deoxyhemoglobin is paramagnetic, creating minor distortions in the local magnetic field that reduce the MR signal from the vessel and immediately adjacent tissues. When an area of the brain is activated, there is a regional increase in neuronal activity that results in an increase in cerebral blood flow and cerebral blood volume which exceeds the rate of oxygen extraction from the blood, resulting in a decrease in the local deoxyhemoglobin concentration. These events reduce local magnetic field inhomogeneities, and ultimately increase MR image voxel (a three-dimensional volume element) intensity when the brain is imaged using specific MR sequences (e.g., gradient echo imaging). Currently, it is believed that the magnitude of the BOLD signal reflects more the synaptic input and intracortical processing of a given volume (i.e., its total/overall synaptic activity) than the spiking output of the neurons in that area (Logothetis et al., 2001), and hence the increase in synaptic activity accompanying epileptiform activity is believed to give rise to a BOLD signal. The temporal evolution of BOLD signal changes is in the form of a characteristic curve called the hemodynamic response function (HRF) (Fig. 23.1) (Menon, 2001; Logothetis, 2003). An HRF models the typical change in BOLD signal over time following a stimulus or an epileptiform discharge measured with electroencephalography (EEG). Immediately following a stimulus, the BOLD signal and the oxyhemoglobin concentration have been shown in some studies to decrease briefly, often called the "initial dip," which is thought to reflect an increase in oxygen metabolism and oxygen extraction before blood flow increases to the area (Malonek and Grinvald, 1996; Yacoub and Hu, 2001). Following the initial dip is the characteristic increase in cerebral blood flow and cerebral blood volume that gives rise to an increase in BOLD signal, which returns slowly to baseline over several seconds, potentially dipping temporarily below baseline (called the poststimulus undershoot) (Malonek and Grinvald, 1996; Yacoub et al., 2006).

In a typical experimental setting, fMRI is used to detect changes in neuronal activity in response to tasks (e.g., cognitive and motor) or stimuli (e.g., visual and sensory). In the context of epilepsy, one can consider the control condition to occur when the EEG is at baseline and the experimental condition to correspond to the presence of an epileptic discharge. To be able to perform such an experiment, it is necessary to record EEG while the subject is in the scanner.

EEG–fMRI

fMRI has the advantage both of high spatial resolution and the ability to sample brain function with relatively good temporal resolution, albeit less than that of EEG. EEG delivers excellent information on the timing of the spikes but is not always capable of precisely locating the source of the discharge. Intracranial EEG gives more precise temporal and spatial information but is invasive, expensive, and limited to the implanted area.

*Correspondence to: Professor Graeme Jackson, M.D., F.R.A.C.P., Brain Research Institute, Florey Neuroscience Institutes, Austin Repatriation Hospital, Heidelberg West, Victoria 3081, Australia. E-mail: g.jackson@brain.org.au

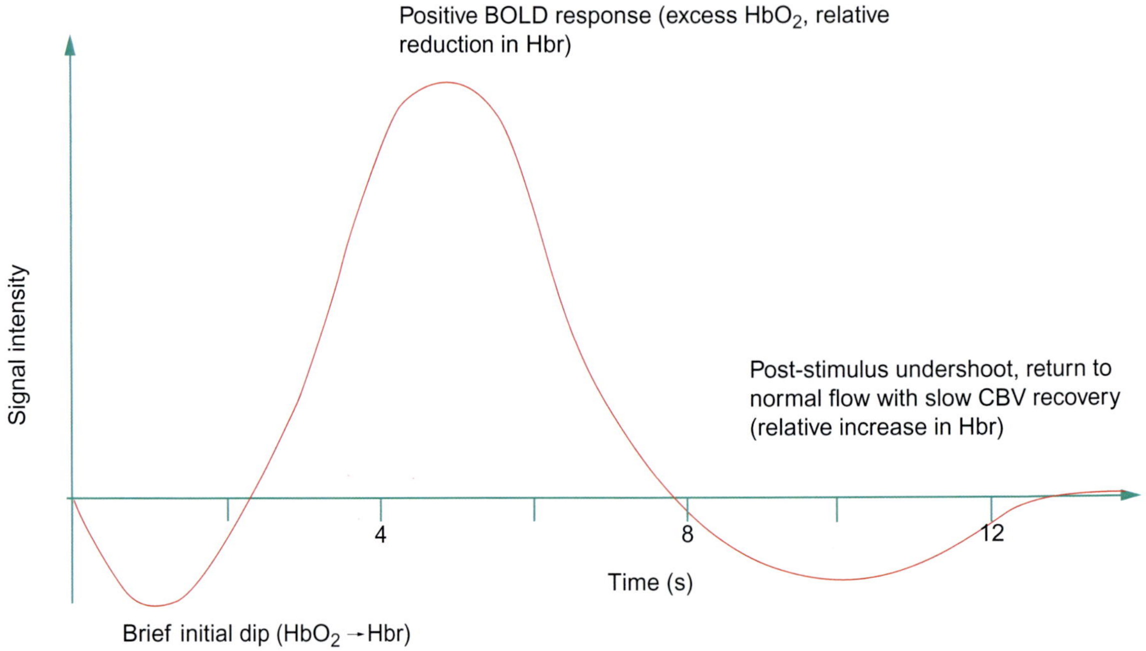

Fig. 23.1. Hemodynamic response function (HRF) showing an increase in blood oxygen level-dependent (BOLD) signal following a measured event, as well as an "initial dip" in BOLD signal immediately after the event and a "poststimulus undershoot" after the response peak. CBV, cerebral blood volume; HbO_2, oxyhemoglobin; Hbr, deoxyhemoglobin.

Combined EEG–fMRI is thus a very promising technique that allows combination of the spatial localization of fMRI and the temporal precision of EEG to map hemodynamic changes associated with epileptic activity noninvasively (Hamandi et al., 2004; Gotman et al., 2006). The possibility of recording the EEG inside an MR scanner was first reported by Ives et al. (1993), and later by the groups of Hill (Hill et al., 1995) and Lemieux (Lemieux et al., 1997). These reports established the safety of recording a good-quality EEG inside the scanner, as well as the possibility of obtaining high-quality MR images despite the presence of EEG electrodes and equipment, opening the way to fMRI studies of spontaneous EEG events such as α activity or epileptic spikes.

Patient safety and data quality

The MR scanner is a very difficult environment in which to record EEG. While EEG recording assemblies typically have high impedances and current-limiting resistors to prevent induced current, care must be taken to prevent the formation of low-impedance loops through bridging of leads or contact of wires with the subject (Lemieux et al., 1997). Heating at the contact points between the electrodes and scalp is a potential hazard, which could lead to a localized burn to the patient's scalp. It has, however, been shown that using nonferrous electrodes and leads, perhaps with current-limiting resistors (Lemieux et al., 1997), and avoiding current loops involving the patient (Lazeyras et al., 2001), result in safe recordings.

The quality of the EEG within the scanner is reduced compared with that of the EEG outside, because of the presence of conducting electrodes and wires within the static magnetic field. Any movement of the electrode wires inside the large static magnetic field, or any variation of the field around the wires, will induce currents that manifest as an artifact in the EEG. This problem can be avoided by a careful EEG setup, involving immobilization of the wires between the head and the amplifier with sand bags, of the head with a vacuum cushion, and of the wires by a head bandage (Benar et al., 2003).

During scanning the situation is different. Although the currents induced in the electrodes and leads by the rapidly changing magnetic fields may be sufficiently small to be safe for the patient, they result in EEG artifacts that can be of the order of 50 times the background ("gradient artifacts"). In order to remove such large artifacts, they must be recorded with an amplifier having a dynamic range sufficiently large to prevent saturation. Several commercial amplifiers are now available that can be placed in the scanner room and allow short cables from the electrodes to the amplifier (minimizing noise pick-up), and are connected to a recording computer outside the scanner room via fiberoptic cable. The optic cable ensures the absence of an electrically conductive bridge between the outside and inside of the scanner room, which would break the magnetic shielding and deteriorate the quality of MR images. In general, good-quality MR images can be achieved despite the EEG apparatus (Krakow et al., 2000).

Gradient and pulse artifact removal

Gradient artifact is an example of a field variation artifact caused by gradient switching during fMRI image acquisition, which renders the EEG apparently noninterpretable. The most widely used method to remove gradient artifact was originally proposed by Allen et al. (2000), and consists of estimating the artifact and subtracting it from each frame, followed by adaptive noise cancellation. This approach assumes that the recorded signal consists of artifact plus EEG, which is reasonable assuming that the amplifier remains within the linear range (i.e., does not saturate). Moreover, the artifact must have been recorded faithfully, which requires a sampling rate of several kilohertz. Several variations on the subtraction scheme have been proposed (Goldman et al., 2000; Anami et al., 2003; Benar et al., 2003; Garreffa et al., 2003; Negishi et al., 2004). Another artifact often observed on EEG recorded within the scanner is pulse or ballistocardiogram artifact. This consists of deviations following each heartbeat and possibly originates from small movements of the head or the electrodes following each pulsation because of fast movement of blood in the arteries. It can be removed by averaging and subtraction (Allen et al., 1998), the application of adaptive filtering (Bonmassar et al., 2002), wavelet filtering (Kim et al., 2004), or independent component analysis (ICA) (Benar et al., 2003; Srivastava et al., 2005). The most elegant of all these has been recently proposed by Masterton et al. (2007), and involves measurement of the artifact by coils placed on the head but not electrically coupled to the scalp.

Data acquisition and analysis

Spike-triggered fMRI

This paradigm was developed to avoid the problems associated with gradient artifacts and relies on reading the undistorted EEG between image acquisitions. The spike-triggered fMRI paradigm takes advantage of the lagging nature of the BOLD hemodynamic response. In this technique, one whole-head echo-planar imaging (EPI) frame is acquired 3–4 seconds after each epileptic spike when the hemodynamic response is thought to be close to its maximum (Warach et al., 1996; Seeck et al., 1998; Krakow et al., 1999). An equivalent number of baseline frames also has to be acquired to allow statistical comparison of the postevent and baseline periods. This method is relatively simple, but it has the disadvantage that only a small time window after a discharge can be assessed and no EEG information can be obtained during scanning. In addition, low-frequency drifts cannot be taken into account, and an experienced observer needs to be actively monitoring the EEG during the whole recording session.

Continuous scanning

While technically more challenging, it is now possible to remove the gradient artifact after the recording or in real time, and see the EEG during an EPI sequence, thus allowing a continuous fMRI recording with visualization of the EEG. This makes it possible to plot the actual BOLD response to epileptic events (Lemieux et al., 2001b; Benar et al., 2002; Masterton et al., 2007). The continuous fMRI recording allows assessment of the entire hemodynamic response after a discharge. Continuous imaging and EEG recording allows investigation of changes before, during, and after interictal discharges. The collection of several images for each spike also increases statistical power. However, continuous recording does require correct recording and removal of artifacts, as discussed above. Studies typically last 30–90 minutes, requiring the patient to remain still in the scanner.

Most recent studies from major centers have focused on continuous, simultaneously acquired, fMRI and EEG (Fig. 23.2). Analysis of these data uses a method known as spike-related fMRI–EEG (Lemieux et al., 2001a; Benar et al., 2002; Iannetti et al., 2002). This approach follows simultaneous acquisition of fMRI and EEG with postscan EEG analysis. The EEG is first processed to minimize the pulse and gradient artifacts mentioned above, and then read by an epileptologist to classify all EEG changes. Those considered to be interictal epileptiform discharges (IEDs) are then treated as events of interest in an event-related analysis of the fMRI data. This involves creating a model time course that is switched on during the IED and convolving this function with an appropriate HRF to model the delay caused by the vascular origin of the BOLD contrast in fMRI. This is the so-called general linear model. This basis function is included in the analysis, and variance correlated to this model is compared with residual variance. Voxels are considered to be activated during the IEDs when the modeled variance is significant compared with the residual variance. The main benefit of the spike-related approach is the increased amount of data acquired, so that shorter studies can lead to a significant result. Further, continuous acquisition of data allows the measurement of the actual HRF of a region (Benar et al., 2002; Waites et al., 2005).

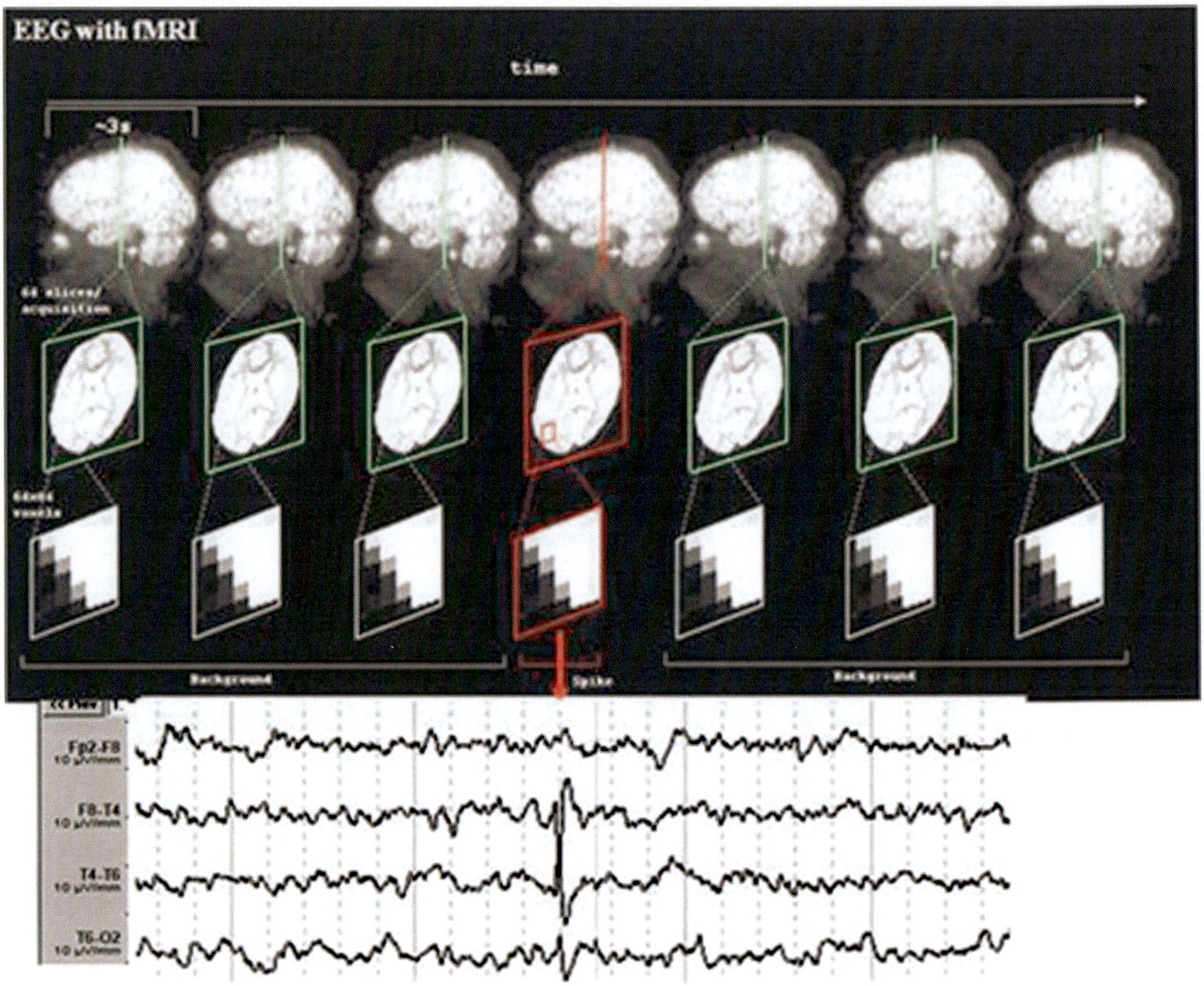

Fig. 23.2. Summary of a continuous EEG–fMRI design. The actual MR signal acquired continuously throughout a study is compared to an epileptiform discharge on a voxel by voxel basis. The EEG trace shows a focal left central epileptiform discharge recorded on a bipolar montage.

Investigators vary in their analysis approach, including acquisition method (spike-triggered or continuous, spike-related), HRF model (canonical HRF, or a set of cosine or gaussian basis functions), as well as the statistical threshold reported as significant. The most common approach is to fit a canonical HRF derived from cognitive studies to the data (Friston et al., 1995; Josephs and Henson, 1999). It is simple to implement but inflexible, because it expects the BOLD response to follow the form of the canonical HRF, which may not be valid for IEDs. Fitting the BOLD response is also possible using a set of basis functions such as cosine or gamma functions. This approach is more flexible, and can model many different forms of the HRF. The advantage of this approach is that it will detect nonstandard BOLD responses, but it is also more likely to detect false-positives, such as non-BOLD-related variance possibly due to artifacts (Waites et al., 2005).

Using a basis function approach, the HRF in a subject with epilepsy was found to have a similar form to the canonical HRF but reached its peak at a later time (10 s versus 5 s for the canonical model) (Lemieux et al., 2001a, b). In another approach, the HRF was modeled by a set of gamma functions with peak latencies varying from 3 to 9 s, in an attempt to account specifically for the variable nature of the response latency (Bagshaw et al., 2004). It is also possible to model the HRF by a set of sine and cosine basis functions (Josephs et al., 1997).

Another strategy is to try directly to measure the (average) BOLD time course following an IED (Benar et al., 2002; Kang et al., 2003). The problem with this approach is that a time course must be measured from a specific region. The choice of region has been based on the position of activations using an initial analysis that selects for regions with a response similar in form to the canonical HRF, and thus preselects for similar responses. Despite this limitation, distinct differences were seen between subjects in the observed BOLD time course (Waites et al., 2005). A localization analysis using the group-average response provided increased sensitivity and specificity compared with the canonical HRF in a group of patients with benign rolandic epilepsy with centrotemporal spikes (Masterton et al., 2010). This suggests that all of these approaches are likely to be statistically valid but may detect different aspects of the BOLD response, with regard to both spatial distribution and time course (Waites et al., 2005). A recent study compared several approaches and evaluated the influence of the number of spikes on the likelihood of positive results (van Houdt et al., 2010). It has also been shown that incorporating some characteristics of the EEG event in the analysis may improve the specificity of the BOLD response (LeVan et al., 2010).

Other analysis methods make minimal assumptions regarding the shape of the HRF. This is the class of data-driven methods which do not require building a model of the expected response. This may be useful because it is known that the shape of the response and its latency are quite variable in epilepsy (Benar et al., 2002; Bagshaw et al., 2004). In this approach, the analysis method knows only the time at which events (typically the EEG spikes) occur, but makes weak assumption regarding its shape (for instance that it must be over within 30 s). Such a method is deconvolution, which attempts to find a voxel-specific response with the only constraint that the response is constant within every voxel (Lu et al., 2006, 2007). This approach appeared better than the modeled HRF approach at detecting activations related to spikes. Finally, some methods analyze all the voxels together rather than each individually, looking for regions that act in concert (multivariate methods). The most common of these methods, ICA, was first applied in epilepsy by Rodionov et al. (2007) and then shown to be robust to variability in fluctuations of the HRF (Jacobs et al., 2008).

APPLICATIONS IN EPILEPSY

Ictal and preictal fMRI

Early fMRI studies of epilepsy focused on the ictal state, because, in the absence of EEG information, this state was easiest to identify, typically using prior anatomical information and searching for focal variance changes (Jackson et al., 1994; Detre et al., 1995, 1996; Krings et al., 2000). The first report appeared in 1994 (Jackson et al., 1994), and was of a 4-year-old boy with Rasmussen's encephalitis and recurrent simple partial seizures of the face. Single-slice fMRI was taken through the area of maximum anatomical abnormality, with one slice being taken every 10 s for 10 min. The time of clinical seizure onset was noted, and images analyzed by subtracting baseline images from those obtained during clinical seizures. In addition, the time course of signal change from specific regions of interest was analyzed. The study demonstrated that seizures were associated with a regional increase in BOLD contrast in specific gyri in the left hemisphere, but also that the rise in BOLD signal commenced 60 s prior to clinical seizure onset. Unfortunately techniques of EEG recording in the magnet were not available, so electrographic seizure onset was not known. In addition, due to the single-slice technique it is not known what activation may have been occurring outside the imaging plane.

Detre et al. (1995) reported a case study that suggested fMRI could localize the epileptiform focus during subclinical seizure activity. The subject was a 25-year-old with multiple daily simple partial seizures of the right face. Analysis was based on subtracting the mean pixel intensity found over the 11-min epoch from each slice. There were marked fluctuations in signal intensity from the presumed epileptogenic zone, despite there being no clinical seizures. Confirmation that this was the epileptogenic zone was later provided by placement of intracranial electrodes prior to resective surgery. The fMRI study defined the area of final electrocorticography-guided surgical resection more precisely than did ictal single-photon emission computed tomography (SPECT), positron emission tomography (PET), or EEG. Although analysis was limited by the absence of EEG monitoring during the fMRI study, prohibiting correlation between electrical discharges and blood flow changes, it is interesting to note that the rise in blood flow from the epileptogenic zone occurred gradually over 30 s, suggesting a gradual buildup of activity over this time.

A case study of a patient with simple partial seizures characterized by psychomotor arrest without falls demonstrated BOLD signal increase at the seizure focus, and decrease in surrounding areas, before a gradual return to baseline (Salek-Haddadi et al., 2002a). The authors speculated that BOLD increases might have occurred several seconds prior to distinguishable EEG changes, perhaps indicating preictal changes in BOLD signal. Animal models have confirmed both that ictal BOLD signal changes occur in the seizure focus (as determined by intracranial EEG) (Opdam et al., 2002) and that BOLD signal changes can occur before appreciable EEG changes in response to epileptiform activity (Makiranta et al., 2005). Another case study of a patient with late-onset Rasmussen's encephalitis was performed in which 15 electroclinical events were recorded (Di Bonaventura et al., 2006). In this patient, no deactivations were evident and activations were measured in the ipsilateral thalamus and right perisylvian structures (especially in the temporal lobe), which was highly concordant with the EEG findings (Di Bonaventura et al., 2006). A recent study of 25 brief electrographic seizures in a patient with temporoparietal gray matter nodular heterotopia found BOLD signal changes lasting up to 30 s after each 3–4-s event (Kobayashi et al., 2006c). BOLD signal increases were seen in the malformation and surrounding cortex. The site of maximum BOLD signal change was in the angular gyrus (i.e., outside the visible malformation), and distant from the site of maximal EEG discharge amplitude, thus raising questions about the precise location of the ictal focus in this patient. In a study of eight patients with malformations of cortical development, in whom short seizures and spikes were recorded in the scanner, Tyvaert et al. (2008) demonstrated that ictal and interictal activations sometimes involve the same structures (see Fig. 23.4) and sometimes different structures, thus shedding some light on the variability of their relationships. In subsequent studies of BOLD changes during brief seizures in a similar group of patients, Tyvaert et al. (2009) and LeVan et al. (2010) demonstrated the ability of dynamic analysis of the BOLD signal to follow the propagation of seizure activity within one seizure, sometimes revealing the onset in an unexpected region.

Preictal studies

Two case reports have shown that BOLD signal increases occur 1–2 min before clinical or electrographic onset in a patient with Rasmussen's encephalitis (Jackson et al., 1994) and in a patient with a malignant glioma (Krings et al., 2000). In the only multisubject study examining preictal BOLD changes to date, changes in BOLD signal were found up to 20 min prior to onset of the seizure (Federico et al., 2005a) (Fig. 23.3). These observations may be related to recent studies of interictal discharges showing that hemodynamic changes may occur prior to the occurrence of interictal discharges measured using scalp EEG (Hawco et al., 2007; Jacobs et al., 2009). The authors concluded that the results suggest the potential to investigate where and when preictal brain activation changes occur with promising seizure focus localization and therapeutic gains.

Although ictal and preictal studies showed that epileptic seizures may be associated with and preceded by dramatic rises in BOLD signal, the widespread use of fMRI for seizure localization is unlikely. First, most seizures cause some head motion, causing significant degradation of the fMR image. Second, in the majority of patients seizures are infrequent and unpredictable. It is impractical to scan a patient for several hours while waiting for an event to occur. On the other hand, short electrographic seizures, lasting only a few seconds, may provide very useful localizing information (Tyvaert et al., 2008, 2009). In patients in whom these are not infrequent, they are valuable to analyze. Nevertheless, most studies rely mainly on the analysis of interictal epileptiform abnormalities.

Interictal fMRI

Focal epilepsy

The spikes of focal epilepsies are not easily detected in the MRI environment because they are most prominent in only one or a few EEG channels, making them hard to distinguish from artifact. Despite this difficulty, a number of studies have attempted to study focal epilepsy with EEG–fMRI and found that BOLD activation changes were frequently concordant with the localization of epileptiform discharges using EEG and other modalities (Warach et al., 1996; Seeck et al., 1998; Krakow et al., 2001; Lemieux et al., 2001b; Benar et al., 2002; Salek-Haddadi et al., 2002b, 2006; Al-Asmi et al., 2003; Bagshaw et al., 2004; Federico et al., 2005b; Tyvaert et al., 2008). The first attempt to study the localization of interictal discharges using spike-triggered fMRI involved multiple investigations of 10 patients (Krakow et al., 1999). The authors recorded between 21 and 50 interictal discharges per experiment. Reproducible focal BOLD signal changes that were largely concordant with EEG spike localization were seen in 6 patients; 3 patients showed no significant BOLD activation, and 1 patient failed to show reproducible activation in a subsequent investigation. Another spike-triggered fMRI study published the same year demonstrated spike-associated BOLD signal changes that were correlated with EEG discharge localization in 9 of 10 subjects (Patel et al., 1999). A study of 11 patients examined the spatial correlation between spike-associated BOLD signals and a variety of presurgical investigations including scalp and intracranial video-EEG monitoring, structural MRI, PET, and SPECT, and neuropsychological testing (Lazeyras et al., 2000). Overall, the BOLD response showed good spatial concordance with clinical findings in 8 of the 11 patients in total, and in 5 of 6 patients who had subsequent intracranial EEG recordings. Using spike-triggered fMRI, BOLD signal changes have been found in areas that are consistent with clinical presentation of specific epilepsy syndromes (Archer et al., 2003b, c).

The first report of continuous EEG of diagnostic quality during fMRI was in a group of 10 patients with focal epilepsy (Jager et al., 2002). After exclusion of 5 patients owing to lack of discharges, high discharge rate (resulting in inadequate baseline), and motion, the remaining 5 subjects all showed BOLD signal increases that were temporally correlated to spikes detected with

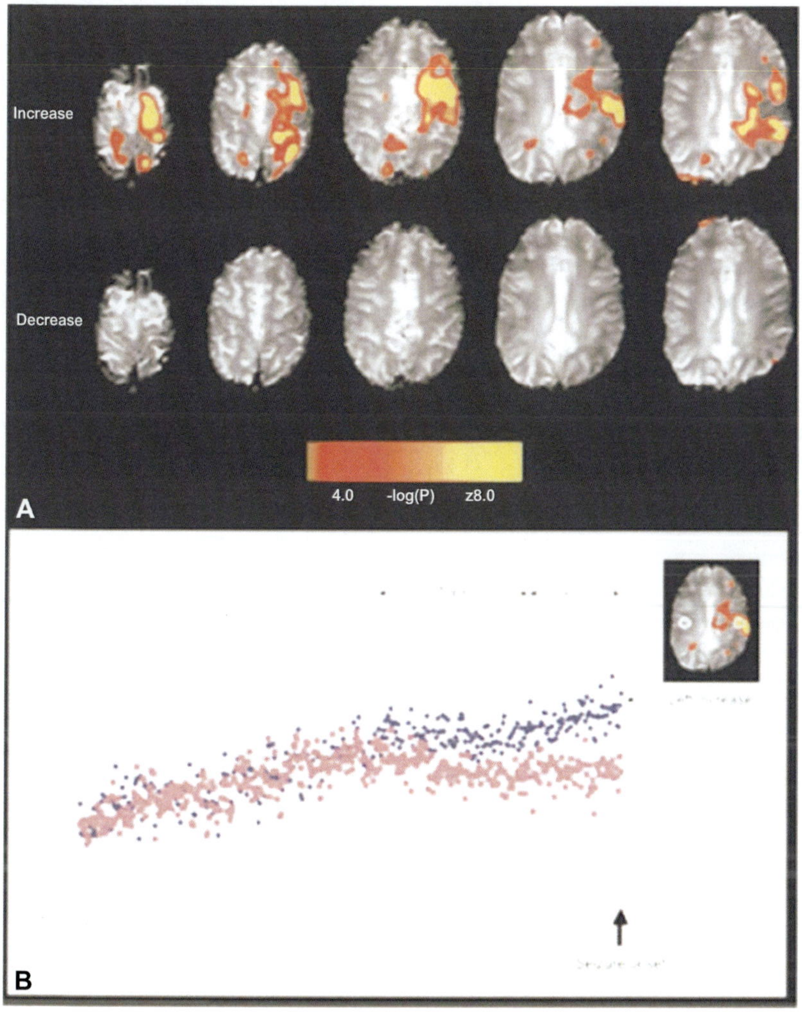

Fig. 23.3. Preictal blood oxygen level-dependent (BOLD) signal changes in a patient with refractory seizures. (**A**) *Top row:* BOLD signal increases were seen in the left frontal lobe and postcentral gyrus. *Bottom row:* No significant BOLD signal decreases were seen. (**B**) The time course of the BOLD signal for 25 min prior to seizure. This was measured in a 25-voxel region of interest (ROI) in the area of maximal BOLD signal (*small image*). This ROI corresponded to the patient's seizure focus. Increase is shown as diamonds and the BOLD signal in the homologous contralateral region is shown as squares. Image intensity in both regions was normalized to 1 in the first volume (y-axis) and plotted as a function of volume number (1 volume every 3.6 s, x-axis). Note that the signal fluctuates in a similar way in both regions for the first few minutes, followed by a divergence of BOLD signal 11 min before the seizure event, with relatively increased signal in the ROI ipsilateral to the seizure focus. This increase is biphasic, with an initial change maintained for about 4 min, followed by a progressive increase until the seizure (vertical lines). (Reproduced with permission from Federico et al. (2005a). © Oxford University Press.)

EEG. In this study, the authors found peak signal intensity 6–7 s after spike detection (Jager et al., 2002). A larger report of 48 fMRI studies performed on 38 patients with partial epilepsy using either spike-triggered or continuous EEG–fMRI showed significant BOLD activations in 22% (2 of 9) and 45% (10 of 22) of the experiments, respectively, after removal of studies with no EEG discharges or with complicating issues such as subject movement (Al-Asmi et al., 2003). The yield over all studies was 39% (12 of 31 studies) (Al-Asmi et al., 2003). Based on these and other results, continuous EEG–fMRI has been deemed more sensitive to the detection of discharges than spike-triggered fMRI. This study also showed that BOLD activation was more likely for subjects with bursts of discharges, rather than isolated discharges. In the 12 patients with BOLD signal changes, a total of 38 different regions showed increases in signal. The 29 sites of largest activation volume were concordant with EEG localization in all but one case. Subsequent intracranial EEG recordings in 4 patients further validated the EEG–fMRI results (Al-Asmi et al., 2003).

In addition to BOLD signal increases, BOLD signal decreases or deactivations have also been reported in relation to focal epileptiform discharges. A large review of EEG–fMRI studies of focal epilepsy reported deactivations in 26 of 34 experiments that demonstrated robust BOLD responses to focal discharges, and noted deactivations were often found with concomitant activations (Kobayashi et al., 2006b). There was spatial concordance of deactivations and EEG localization in 16 patients, which is less than the typical concordance between activations and EEG localization. The underlying neurophysiological mechanisms for this BOLD deactivation, particularly when correlated to epileptiform discharges, remains unclear but may reflect decreases in neuronal activity and blood flow (Stefanovic et al., 2005; Kobayashi et al., 2006; Shmuel et al., 2006; Northoff et al., 2007). It was noted that isolated spikes were more likely to produce activations or deactivations individually, whereas bursts of spikes were more likely to produce activations and deactivations together. Similar results were reported in a group of 6 children with lesional and nonlesional pharmacoresistant focal epilepsy, where significant activations were found in 4 children, activation and deactivation in 1 child, and widespread deactivation in another. In 4 of the children activations colocalized with the presumed seizure focus, one of which was confirmed by intracranial EEG (De Tiege et al., 2007). A recent study indicated that the deactivation can be sometimes caused by an earlier activation, although not in the majority of cases (Rathakrishnan et al., 2010).

Focal epileptic networks

Another phenomenon repeatedly observed is that BOLD signal changes can occur at sites distant to the presumed seizure focus in focal epilepsies. In one study, 35 EEG–fMRI studies derived from 27 patients with temporal lobe epilepsy with a variety of underlying structural abnormalities were analyzed (Kobayashi et al., 2006a). BOLD responses occurred in 83% of studies, predominantly in the spiking temporal lobe, and manifested as activation or deactivation. Responses were sometimes very focal, but often involved also the contralateral homologous cortex as well as extratemporal regions, suggesting a widespread effect of temporal lobe epileptic spikes. The authors postulated that the contralateral response may be due to projected neuronal activity that is not sufficiently synchronized to be visible in the EEG, a hypothesis that was subsequently confirmed (Yu et al., 2009). The same group also evaluated a series of patients with gray matter heterotopia (Kobayashi et al., 2006c) and malformations of cortical development (Tyvaert et al., 2008) (Fig. 23.4). These patients, as the temporal lobe group, showed a broad spectrum of results, including activations and deactivations, sometimes located in or very close to the lesion, and sometimes in a region unrelated to the lesion. Several patients also showed BOLD signal changes in subcortical structures such as the brainstem reticular formation, basal ganglia, or thalamus. These findings are consistent with human and animal evidence that support thalamic involvement in temporal lobe epilepsy (Blumenfeld et al., 2007; Keller and Roberts, 2008), as well as animal studies that show subcortical involvement in cortical epileptiform discharges (Silva-Barrat et al., 1986; Zilles et al., 1998; Holmes et al., 1999). Furthermore, in a feline model of epilepsy, epileptiform discharges were detected in subcortical structures prior to cortical detection of the discharges (Morillo et al., 1982). Another study of two patients with reading epilepsy using spike-triggered fMRI found fMRI activation of bilateral cortical and subcortical areas associated with reading-induced epileptiform discharges in one subject, but no fMRI activation in the other, likely due to the fact that only four spikes were recorded in this patient (Archer et al., 2003b). Based on these studies and others, it is likely that distant cortical and subcortical circuits are involved in the generation of "focal" discharges.

In children with benign epilepsy with centrotemporal spikes (BECTS, rolandic epilepsy), spike-related BOLD signal increased in the face area of the sensorimotor cortex, restricted to the postcentral gyrus (Archer et al., 2003b). On the other hand, Lengler and colleagues (2007) reported decreased BOLD signal in the postcentral gyrus. These opposing hemodynamic changes may reflect a difference in EEG–fMRI analysis methodology used in these studies. The overall findings are consistent with the facial sensorimotor involvement in BECTS seizures.

Source localization

Most studies use EEG data primarily to identify the time points of interictal discharges for subsequent event-related fMRI analysis. However, EEG data can be used further to provide information about the area producing interictal discharges by source localization techniques (Bagshaw et al., 2006). Many EEG localization techniques use a boundary element method, which attempts to model the electrical conductance of the human head based on the properties of various tissue layers. A fine cubic grid is then projected onto an image of the brain, creating points representing potential electrical sources at each intersection of the three-dimensional grids (Benar et al., 2006). Electrical source imaging (ESI) analysis calculates possible sources of electrical activity in the brain as it changes over time (moving dipole), or averaged over a certain time period (stationary dipole). From a number of discrete calculated dipoles, a current density reconstruction can be created that maps the dipole moment per unit volume and is overlaid onto the

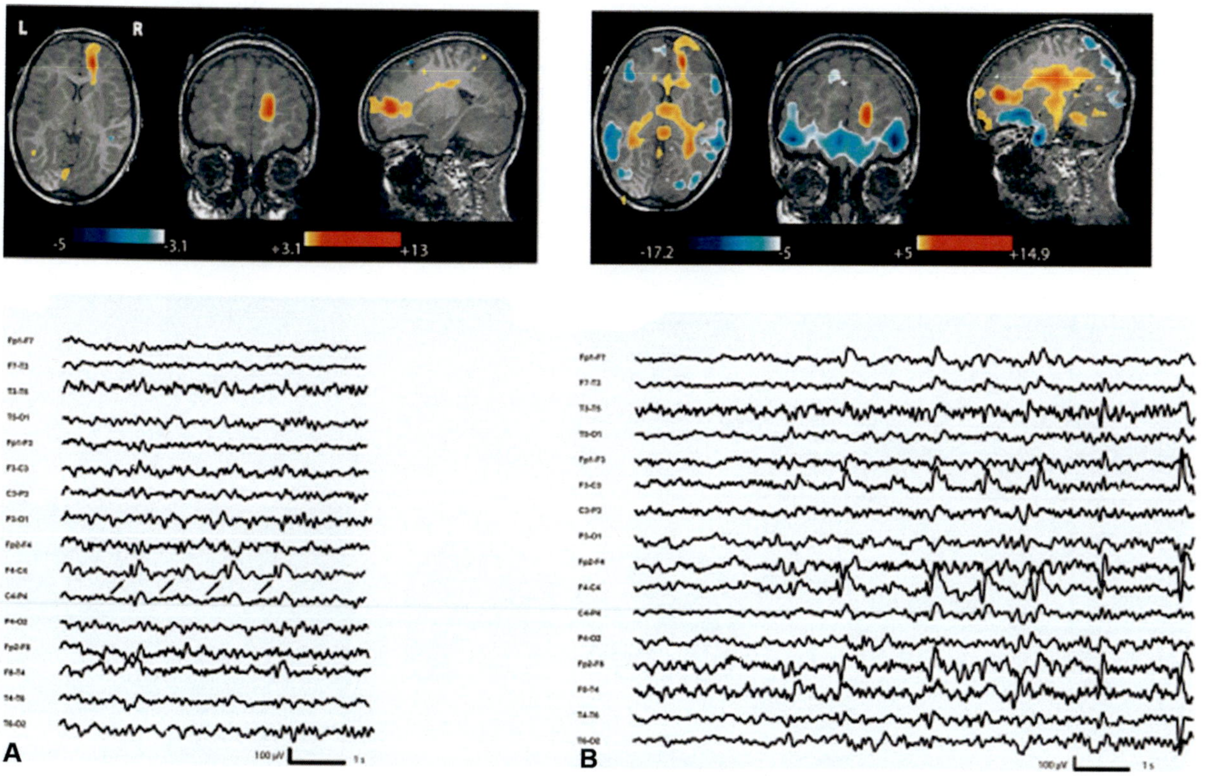

Fig. 23.4. Blood oxygen level-dependent (BOLD) changes in a patient with focal cortical dysplasia. (**A**) Activation in the dysplasia during interictal right frontal spike and waves. (**B**) BOLD signal changes observed during clinical seizures with prolonged rhythmic discharge of right frontal spike and waves with synchronous contralateral activity. Maximum activation is again in the lesion with propagation over the right frontopolar area, thalami, and midbrain. The seizure discharge also leads to deactivations in areas distant from the focus. (Reproduced with permission from Tyvaert et al. (2008). © Oxford University Press.)

surface of a model of the cerebral cortex. Good concordance between ESI, EEG–fMRI data, and intracranial EEG recording performed on separate settings has been reported in several studies (Benar et al., 2006; Grova et al., 2008). A single study performed ESI analysis on 13 interictal discharge types recorded inside the scanner from 8 patients (Vulliemoz et al., 2010a). ESI at discharge onset was anatomically closest to the positive BOLD cluster in 4 cases, and closest to negative BOLD responses in another 4. ESI at a later time frame showed propagation to remote source colocalized with other BOLD clusters in half the cases. In concordant cases, the distance between the maximum ESI and the closest EEG–fMRI cluster was less than 33 mm. The authors concluded that simultaneous ESI and EEG–fMRI analysis may thus be useful to distinguish areas of BOLD response related to initiation of epileptiform discharges from propagation areas (Fig. 23.5).

Intracranial EEG–fMRI

To increase the yield of EEG–fMRI studies, combining intracranial EEG with fMRI has recently been applied successfully in patients with epilepsy (Vulliemoz et al., 2010b).

Use of this technique allows the detection of much smaller interictal epileptiform discharges than could be recorded using scalp EEG–fMRI, and demonstrates BOLD increases and decreases in different cortical and subcortical areas as well as activation near the epileptogenic zone. This has the potential to provide a means by which the different circuits involved in generation can be investigated and possibly more precise seizure focus localization.

Clinical utility

The clinical role of EEG–fMRI is expanding. Recently, 29 patients were studied who were previously rejected for epilepsy surgery because of an unclear seizure focus or presumed multifocality (Zijlmans et al., 2007). These patients underwent EEG–fMRI studies and 8 were reevaluated for surgery because of the results of the studies. In addition, EEG–fMRI was used to confirm that some patients were not suitable for surgery due to multifocal pathology or extensive subcortical involvement. The authors proposed EEG–fMRI should play a role in seizure focus localization when results from other investigations are inconclusive, as well as to confirm

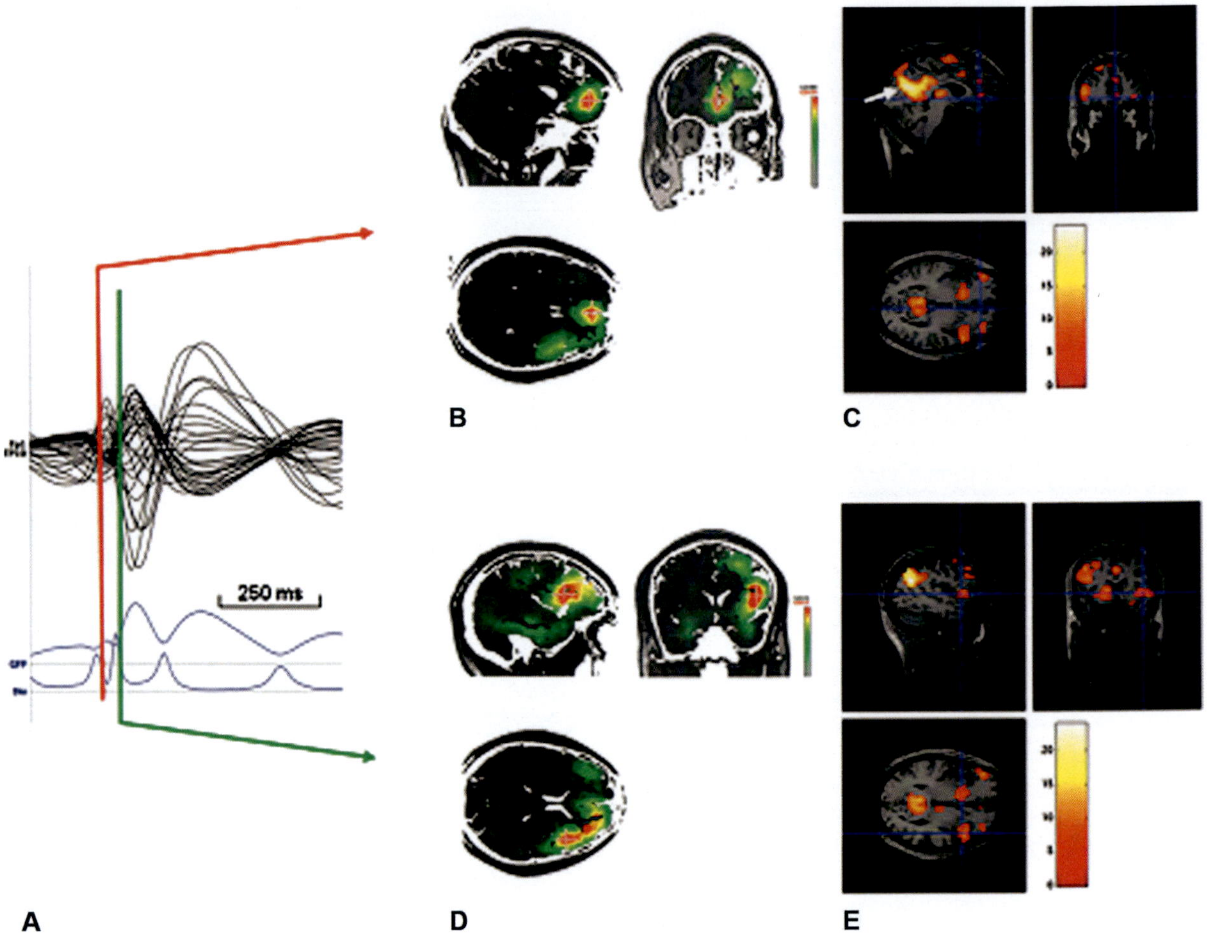

Fig. 23.5. Example of mesial frontal onset with lateral propagation. Electrical source imaging (ESI) and EEG–fMRI map overlaid on coregistered T1-weighted image. (**A**) Averaged intra-MR interictal epileptic discharges (IEDs). The first rising phase of the averaged IED and global field power (GFP) is used for IED onset (ESIo, red line) and a later time frame for IED propagation (ESIp, +88 ms, second rising phase of the averaged IED, green line). Dis, dissimilarity is a measure inversely related to the spatial correlation between two scalp voltage map topographies (not shown): a minimum of Dis therefore reflects a period of map stability (Lantz et al., 2003; Michel et al., 2004). (**B**) EEG source imaging at IED onset (ESIo) in orbitofrontal cortex (bilateral but maximum in left hemisphere). (**C**) Right orbitofrontal blood oxygen level-dependent (BOLD) cluster concordant with ESIo (positive BOLD response, cross-line at maximum). The highly significant BOLD response in the mesial parietal cortex corresponds to negative BOLD response in the "default mode" network (arrow). (**D**) EEG source imaging just after second maximum of the averaged IED showing a shift of maximal source activity to frontal–opercular region (ESIp). (**E**) Right lateral frontal BOLD cluster closest to ESIp (positive BOLD response, cross-line at maximum). (Reproduced from Vulliemoz et al. (2010a) © Wiley.)

multifocal epilepsy in order to prevent operations that may have a minimal chance of success (Zijlmans et al., 2007). Recent results in patients with nonlesional frontal epilepsy are also encouraging (Moeller et al., 2009). Furthermore, the confidence with which clinical studies can be considered is increased by a recent study showing good reproducibility (Gholipour et al., 2011).

Generalized epilepsy

The first EEG–fMRI study of patients with generalized spike-and-wave (GSW) discharges was performed by Hill et al. (1999). They studied patients with generalized discharges induced by photic stimulation and observed BOLD signal increases in the occipital lobe of patients compared with controls during photic stimulation, regardless of whether epileptiform discharges were present or not. BOLD signal changes were not observed elsewhere, most notably the thalamus. Archer et al. (2003a), first showed consistent areas of deactivation and activation associated with GSW discharges in a group of 5 patients using spike-triggered EEG–fMRI at 3 Tesla. Deactivation was seen in 4 patients, consistently located in posterior cingulate gyrus. Variable BOLD activation was detected in the same 4 patients in precentral sulci bilaterally.

Continuous EEG–fMRI was first applied to generalized epilepsy in a single patient with frequent absence seizures associated with 3-Hz GSW activity (Salek-Haddadi et al., 2003). The thalamus exhibited focal activation during runs of generalized discharges, in addition to widespread cortical deactivation that was maximal frontally. These changes underscore the role of the thalamus in generation of GSW activity suggested by animal studies (McCormick and Contreras, 2001). A more recent report in a group of 15 patients with GSW activity was performed for better characterization of spike-associated thalamic and cortical BOLD signal changes (Aghakhani et al., 2004). The BOLD signal changes were seen in 14 patients (93%), with bilateral thalamic changes in 12 (80%), and activation predominating over deactivation. In subjects with measurable cortical BOLD changes, deactivation predominated in 9 patients and activation in 5 (Aghakhani et al., 2004). The cortical BOLD changes were seen to the same extent both in frontal and posterior head regions, which was not consistent with the typical anterior to posterior predominance of the GSW discharges seen in these patients using EEG. A group analysis was later performed using the same patient data sets (Gotman et al., 2005). From this analysis, activations were seen bilaterally in the thalamus as well as bilaterally in insulae, mesial mid-frontal regions, and cerebellum. The focal cortical activation seen in these studies suggest that "generalized" discharges are perhaps not as generalized over the entire brain as once thought.

Deactivations were seen bilaterally in the posterior cingulate gyrus, as discussed earlier (Archer et al., 2003a), as well as in anterior frontal and parietal lobes. The location of the frontal and parietal deactivations in this study corresponded closely to sites of activation seen in the "default or resting state" (Raichle et al., 2001; Gotman et al., 2005). The default or resting state refers to a pattern of activation associated with a wakeful resting state, which is suspended temporarily once a task is presented to a subject (Raichle et al., 2001). It is believed that thalamic activation (and therefore frontal and parietal BOLD deactivation) associated with GSW discharges may cause the momentary interruption of the resting state of the brain. This, in turn, may explain transient reductions of responsiveness seen in some patients during GSW discharges (Archer et al., 2003a; Gotman et al., 2005). These findings were later confirmed in a number of studies showing BOLD signal change in the thalamus, parietal cortex, and caudate nuclei during spike-and-wave (Hamandi et al., 2006) and absence (Labate et al., 2005; Laufs et al., 2006; Moeller et al., 2008) seizures, and recently negative BOLD signal change was found in the posterior brainstem, which includes the brainstem reticular formation (Carney et al., 2010) (Fig. 23.6). Recent studies have evaluated the time course of BOLD signal changes before, during, and after absence seizures, showing that there can be focal changes before the EEG onset and that some regions show continued increased BOLD after the end of the EEG discharge (Bai et al., 2010; Moeller et al., 2010).

Symptomatic generalized epilepsy

Generalized paroxysmal fast activity (PFA) and 2–2.5-Hz slow spike–wave (SSW) discharges are the two cardinal features found in the EEG recordings of patients with Lennox–Gastaut syndrome. These two epileptiform discharge types were recently studied in 8 patients with Lennox–Gastaut syndrome. PFA showed intense positive diffuse cortical BOLD signal in the cortex and subcortical structures, whereas SSW discharges showed diffuse cortical involvement with both positive and negative BOLD responses. The cortical regions showing BOLD deactivation during SSW discharges were different from those showing BOLD activation during PFA. Whereas activation was present mainly in association cortex in PFA, deactivation was seen predominantly in primary visual, auditory, and sensorimotor cortex in SSW discharges, suggesting involvement of different networks in the generation of the two discharge types (N. Pillay et al., unpublished results).

BRAIN CONNECTIVITY

Functional and effective connectivity are descriptions of the relationships between patterns of neural activity and therefore involve measurements of neural function. Functional connectivity is a descriptive measure of spatiotemporal correlations between spatially distinct regions of cerebral cortex (Friston et al., 1993), whereas effective connectivity is defined as the influence that one neural system exerts over another (Friston et al., 1993). Functional connectivity is a statistical description of the degree to which two brain regions demonstrate similar behavior and cooperate at a network level. It does not reflect a causal relationship between cortical regions and does not assume an underlying anatomical model for the connections. On the other hand, effective connectivity makes assumptions about the structure and directionality of the interactions based on prior knowledge of brain regions involved in the system, and the possible anatomical connections between those brain regions (Friston, 1997). However, the two concepts of functional and effective connectivity are not mutually exclusive, as the description of the connecting brain regions through functional connectivity can also be used to propose a theory that specifies the causal links between correlating regions. Various methodologies have been used to measure functional connectivity, such as

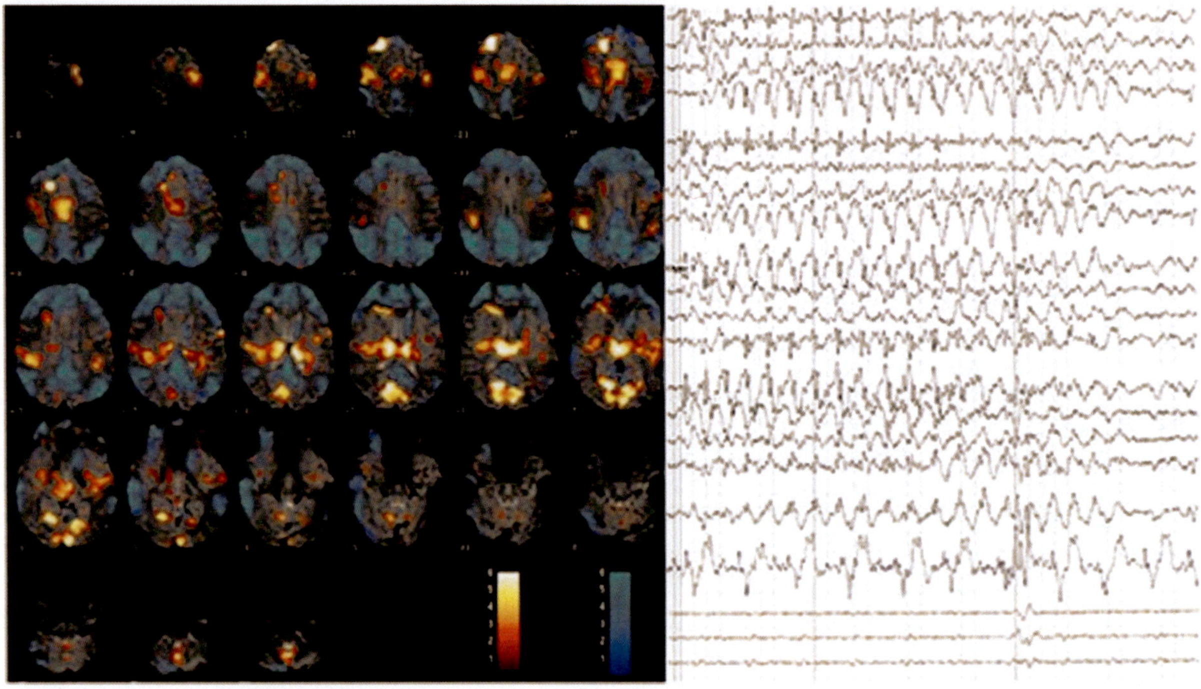

Fig. 23.6. Blood oxygen level-dependent (BOLD) signal changes associated with generalized 3-Hz spike–wave interictal discharges in a subject with idiopathic generalized epilepsy (IGE). The maps of BOLD signal changes are overlaid onto the corresponding T1 axial image (5 mm between slices). Highest scores are seen in the thalamus (positive; yellow) and posterior midline structures (negative; blue). The deactivations largely cover the "default mode" network. The images on the right show the corresponding epileptiform discharges recorded inside the scanner.

scalp EEG synchrony (Astolfi et al., 2004; Babiloni et al., 2005), corticocortical evoked potentials (Matsumoto et al., 2004), and activity correlation in PET (Grady et al., 2001). These studies measured brain networks involved in specific task states and documented network changes in patients with various diseases (Grady et al., 2001; Irwin et al., 2004; Saini et al., 2004). Although these methods measure variations in neuronal activity with high temporal resolution, they produce *very* low spatial resolution, and EEG-based methods cannot investigate the whole brain. fMRI, on the other hand, gives better spatial resolution and can investigate the whole brain, but provides lower temporal resolution. It has become a method of choice in investigating brain functional connectivity.

BOLD functional connectivity mapping is an fMRI approach that seeks to identify the interrelationship between different regions of the brain that are activated during the resting state. The BOLD signal of fMRI reflects neural activity (Logothetis et al., 2001). The implicit assumption is that BOLD signal functional connectivity maps represent correlated neural activity of spatially segregated brain regions (Leopold and Logothetis, 2003).

Synchronous low-frequency fluctuation (< 0.08 Hz) in the MR time course is temporally correlated between functionally related regions of resting brain (Biswal et al., 1995; Lowe et al., 1998; Xiong et al., 1999; Cordes et al., 2000; Hampson et al., 2002). The biological basis of these low-frequency correlations may be related to low-frequency oscillations in cerebral hemodynamics (Biswal et al., 1997). This low-frequency MR signal is used in a functional connectivity analysis that employs the seed voxel approach to assess connectivity maps for a specific region of interest (ROI). First, a single or a cluster of seed voxels is selected based on anatomical (e.g., gyral or sulcal landmarks) or functional knowledge (e.g., center of mass of clusters on task activation statistical maps). Second, a ROI is drawn around the seed voxel. Finally, the average referenced time course of the ROI is then cross-correlated with all the remaining brain voxels, producing a functional connectivity map. This map is a three-dimensional representation of a functional network that shows regions of the brain with time courses similar to the ROI. This technique can be applied to investigate structures involved in different epileptic networks. By performing an initial spike-related analysis using spikes identified using EEG, one can identify a focal region involved in the spike generation network, and probably associated with generation of those spikes detectable by scalp electrodes (Fig. 23.7). These regions are presumably a subset

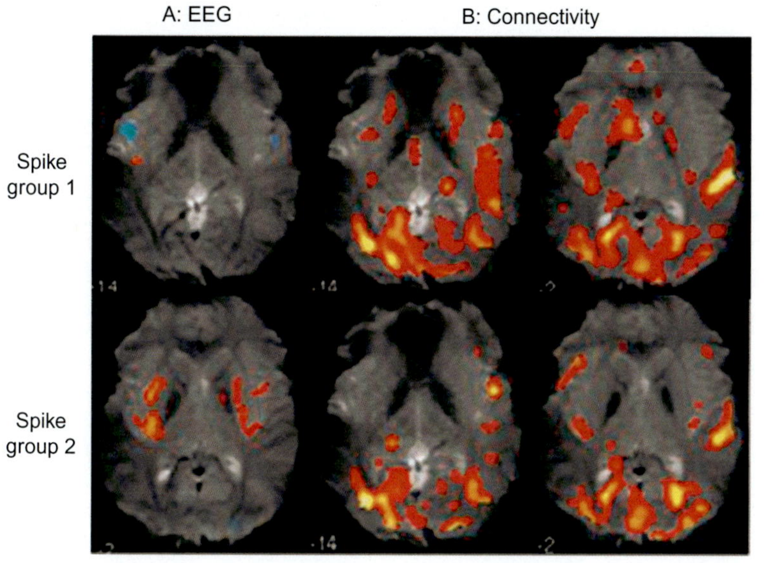

Fig. 23.7. Combined EEG–fMRI and functional connectivity analysis of a patient with idiopathic generalized epilepsy (IGE). (**A**) Event-related analysis of spikes with two morphologies (group 1, 12 spikes; group 2, 2 spikes) show different patterns of activation (red) and deactivation (blue). (**B**) Connectivity analysis shows greater sensitivity, yielding a widespread network that is consistent for the two spike groups, indicating that functional connectivity is more sensitive to the underlying seizure network. (Reproduced from Waites et al. (2005). © Elsevier.)

of all regions involved in the epileptogenic circuit that is sought after. By using the signal time course of this region, a wider network is identified including subcortical regions (Waites et al., 2005). Recent studies have shown evidence for abnormal connectivity in the temporal lobe (Pereira et al., 2010).

It is also possible to study functional connectivity with methods other than the seed-based approach described above. ICA applied to whole-brain fMRI data can identify sets of voxels that are fluctuating together. This has been applied to identify multiple resting state networks (van de Ven et al., 2008), but has not yet been applied in epilepsy.

CONCLUSION

Precise seizure focus localization and unraveling different structures involved in the genesis of the epileptic process is a major challenge that faces epilepsy research. The combination of EEG and fMRI is a well-established method that offers the unique advantage of measuring noninvasively specific hemodynamic changes related to epileptic discharges, providing unique localizing information on seizure foci and different cortical and subcortical structures that may be involved in this process. In addition, functional connectivity studies are emerging as a promising tool that can be used to interrogate epileptic networks and possible changes within physiological networks in epileptic brain. fMRI is thus an excellent tool that provides novel and unique insights into the genesis of epileptiform activity and how this differs in various epileptic syndromes. With the improved sensitivity as more sophisticated data analysis and EEG event localization and artifact elimination paradigms evolve, there is no doubt that fMRI will continue to help our understanding of the genesis of epilepsy and contribute to clinical evaluations.

ACKNOWLEDGMENTS

The authors gratefully thank Dr. Danny Flanagan for his help with the figures and text review.

REFERENCES

Aghakhani Y, Bagshaw AP, Benar CG et al. (2004). fMRI activation during spike and wave discharges in idiopathic generalized epilepsy. Brain 127: 1127–1144.

Al-Asmi A, Benar CG, Gross DW et al. (2003). fMRI activation in continuous and spike-triggered EEG-fMRI studies of epileptic spikes. Epilepsia 44: 1328–1339.

Allen PJ, Polizzi G, Krakow K et al. (1998). Identification of EEG events in the MR scanner: the problem of pulse artifact and a method for its subtraction. Neuroimage 8: 229–239.

Allen PJ, Josephs O, Turner R (2000). A method for removing imaging artifact from continuous EEG recorded during functional MRI. Neuroimage 12: 230–239.

Anami K, Mori T, Tanaka F et al. (2003). Stepping stone sampling for retrieving artifact-free electroencephalogram during functional magnetic resonance imaging. Neuroimage 19: 281–295.

Archer JS, Abbott DF, Waites AB et al. (2003a). fMRI "deactivation" of the posterior cingulate during generalized spike and wave. Neuroimage 20: 1915–1922.

Archer JS, Briellman RS, Abbott DF et al. (2003b). Benign epilepsy with centro-temporal spikes: spike triggered fMRI shows somato-sensory cortex activity. Epilepsia 44: 200–204.

Archer JS, Briellmann RS, Syngeniotis A et al. (2003c). Spike-triggered fMRI in reading epilepsy: involvement of left frontal cortex working memory area. Neurology 60: 415–421.

Astolfi L, Cincotti F, Mattia D et al. (2004). Estimation of the effective and functional human cortical connectivity with structural equation modeling and directed transfer function applied to high-resolution EEG. Magn Reson Imaging 22: 1457–1470.

Babiloni F, Cincotti F, Babiloni C et al. (2005). Estimation of the cortical functional connectivity with the multimodal integration of high-resolution EEG and fMRI data by directed transfer function. Neuroimage 24: 118–131.

Bagshaw AP, Aghakhani Y, Benar CG et al. (2004). EEG-fMRI of focal epileptic spikes: analysis with multiple haemodynamic functions and comparison with gadolinium-enhanced MR angiograms. Hum Brain Mapp 22: 179–192.

Bagshaw AP, Kobayashi E, Dubeau F et al. (2006). Correspondence between EEG-fMRI and EEG dipole localisation of interictal discharges in focal epilepsy. Neuroimage 30: 417–425.

Bai X, Vestal M, Berman R et al. (2010). Dynamic time course of typical childhood absence seizures: EEG, behavior, and functional magnetic resonance imaging. J Neurosci 30: 5884–5893.

Benar CG, Gross DW, Wang Y et al. (2002). The BOLD response to interictal epileptiform discharges. Neuroimage 17: 1182–1192.

Benar C, Aghakhani Y, Wang Y et al. (2003). Quality of EEG in simultaneous EEG-fMRI for epilepsy. Clin Neurophysiol 114: 569–580.

Benar CG, Grova C, Kobayashi E et al. (2006). EEG-fMRI of epileptic spikes: concordance with EEG source localization and intracranial EEG. Neuroimage 30: 1161–1170.

Biswal B, Yetkin FZ, Haughton VM et al. (1995). Functional connectivity in the motor cortex of resting human brain using echo-planar MRI. Magn Reson Med 34: 537–541.

Biswal BB, Van Kylen J, Hyde JS (1997). Simultaneous assessment of flow and BOLD signals in resting-state functional connectivity maps. NMR Biomed 10: 165–170.

Blumenfeld H, Rivera M, Vasquez JG et al. (2007). Neocortical and thalamic spread of amygdala kindled seizures. Epilepsia 48: 254–262.

Bonmassar G, Purdon PL, Jaaskelainen IP et al. (2002). Motion and ballistocardiogram artifact removal for interleaved recording of EEG and EPs during MRI. Neuroimage 16: 1127–1141.

Carney PW, Masterton RAJ, Harvey AS et al. (2010). The core network in absence epilepsy: differences in cortical and thalamic BOLD response. Neurology 75: 904–911.

Cordes D, Haughton VM, Arfanakis K et al. (2000). Mapping functionally related regions of brain with functional connectivity MR imaging. AJNR Am J Neuroradiol 21: 1636–1644.

De Tiege X, Laufs H, Boyd SG et al. (2007). EEG-fMRI in children with pharmacoresistant focal epilepsy. Epilepsia 48: 385–389.

Detre JA, Sirven JI, Alsop DC et al. (1995). Localization of subclinical ictal activity by functional magnetic resonance imaging: correlation with invasive monitoring. Ann Neurol 38: 618–624.

Detre JA, Alsop DC, Aguirre GK et al. (1996). Coupling of cortical and thalamic ictal activity in human partial epilepsy: demonstration by functional magnetic resonance imaging. Epilepsia 37: 657–661.

Di Bonaventura C, Carnfi M, Vaudano AE et al. (2006). Ictal hemodynamic changes in late-onset Rasmussen encephalitis. Ann Neurol 59: 432–433.

Federico P, Abbott DF, Briellmann RS et al. (2005a). Functional MRI of the pre-ictal state. Brain 128: 1811–1817.

Federico P, Archer JS, Abbott DF et al. (2005b). Cortical/subcortical BOLD changes associated with epileptic discharges: an EEG-fMRI study at 3 T. Neurology 64: 1125–1130.

Friston KJ (1997). Testing for anatomically specified regional effects. Hum Brain Mapp 5: 133–136.

Friston KJ, Frith CD, Liddle PF et al. (1993). Functional connectivity: the principal-component analysis of large (PET) data sets. J Cereb Blood Flow Metab 13: 5–14.

Friston KJ, Holmes AP, Poline JB et al. (1995). Analysis of fMRI time-series revisited. Neuroimage 2: 45–53.

Garreffa G, Carni M, Gualniera G et al. (2003). Real-time MR artifacts filtering during continuous EEG/fMRI acquisition. Magn Reson Imaging 21: 1175–1189.

Gholipour T, Moeller F, Pittau F et al. (2011). Reproducibility of interictal EEG-fMRI results in patients with epilepsy. Epilepsia 52: 433–442.

Goldman RI, Stern JM, Engel J Jr et al. (2000). Acquiring simultaneous EEG and functional MRI. Clin Neurophysiol 111: 1974–1980.

Gotman J, Grova C, Bagshaw A et al. (2005). Generalized epileptic discharges show thalamocortical activation and suspension of the default state of the brain. Proc Natl Acad Sci U S A 102: 15236–15240.

Gotman J, Kobayashi E, Bagshaw AP et al. (2006). Combining EEG and fMRI: a multimodal tool for epilepsy research. J Magn Reson Imaging 23: 906–920.

Grady CL, Furey ML, Pietrini P et al. (2001). Altered brain functional connectivity and impaired short-term memory in Alzheimer's disease. Brain 124: 739–756.

Grova C, Daunizeau J, Kobayashi E et al. (2008). Concordance between distributed EEG source localization and simultaneous EEG-fMRI studies of epileptic spikes. Neuroimage 39: 755–774.

Hamandi K, Salek-Haddadi A, Fish DR et al. (2004). EEG/functional MRI in epilepsy: the Queen Square Experience. J Clin Neurophysiol 21: 241–248.

Hamandi K, Salek-Haddadi A, Laufs H et al. (2006). EEG-fMRI of idiopathic and secondarily generalized epilepsies. Neuroimage 31: 1700–1710.

Hampson M, Peterson BS, Skudlarski P et al. (2002). Detection of functional connectivity using temporal correlations in MR images. Hum Brain Mapp 15: 247–262.

Hawco CS, Bagshaw AP, Lu Y et al. (2007). BOLD changes occur prior to epileptic spikes seen on scalp EEG. Neuroimage 35: 1450–1458.

Hill RA, Chiappa KH, Huang-Hellinger F et al. (1995). EEG during MR imaging: differentiation of movement artifact from paroxysmal cortical activity. Neurology 45: 1942–1943.

Hill RA, Chiappa KH, Huang-Hellinger F et al. (1999). Hemodynamic and metabolic aspects of photosensitive epilepsy revealed by functional magnetic resonance imaging and magnetic resonance spectroscopy. Epilepsia 40: 912–920.

Holmes GL, Sarkisian M, Ben-Ari Y et al. (1999). Consequences of cortical dysplasia during development in rats. Epilepsia 40: 537–544.

Iannetti GD, Di Bonaventura C, Pantano P et al. (2002). fMRI/EEG in paroxysmal activity elicited by elimination of central vision and fixation. Neurology 58: 976–979.

Irwin W, Anderle MJ, Abercrombie HC et al. (2004). Amygdalar interhemispheric functional connectivity differs between the non-depressed and depressed human brain. Neuroimage 21: 674–686.

Ives JR, Warach S, Schmitt F et al. (1993). Monitoring the patient's EEG during echo planar MRI. Electroencephalogr Clin Neurophysiol 87: 417–420.

Jackson GD, Connelly A, Cross JH et al. (1994). Functional magnetic resonance imaging of focal seizures. Neurology 44: 850–856.

Jacobs J, Hawco C, Kobayashi E et al. (2008). Variability of the hemodynamic response as a function of age and frequency of epileptic discharge in children with epilepsy. Neuroimage 40: 601–614.

Jacobs J, LeVan P, Moeller F et al. (2009). Hemodynamic changes preceding the interictal EEG spike in patients with focal epilepsy investigated using simultaneous EEG-fMRI. Neuroimage 45: 1220–1231.

Jager L, Werhahn KJ, Hoffmann A et al. (2002). Focal epileptiform activity in the brain: detection with spike-related functional MR imaging – preliminary results. Radiology 223: 860–869.

Josephs O, Henson RN (1999). Event-related functional magnetic resonance imaging: modelling, inference and optimization. Philos Trans R Soc Lond B Biol Sci 354: 1215–1228.

Josephs O, Turner R, Friston K (1997). Event-related fMRI. Hum Brain Mapp 5: 243–248.

Kang JK, Benar C, Al-Asmi A et al. (2003). Using patient-specific hemodynamic response functions in combined EEG-fMRI studies in epilepsy. Neuroimage 20: 1162–1170.

Keller SS, Roberts N (2008). Voxel-based morphometry of temporal lobe epilepsy: an introduction and review of the literature. Epilepsia 49: 741–757.

Kim KH, Yoon HW, Park HW (2004). Improved ballistocardiac artifact removal from the electroencephalogram recorded in fMRI. J Neurosci Methods 135: 193–203.

Kobayashi E, Bagshaw AP, Benar CG et al. (2006a). Temporal and extratemporal BOLD responses to temporal lobe interictal spikes. Epilepsia 47: 343–354.

Kobayashi E, Bagshaw AP, Grova C et al. (2006b). Negative BOLD responses to epileptic spikes. Hum Brain Mapp 27: 488–497.

Kobayashi E, Bagshaw AP, Grova C et al. (2006c). Grey matter heterotopia: what EEG-fMRI can tell us about epileptogenicity of neuronal migration disorders. Brain 129: 366–374.

Krakow K, Woermann FG, Symms MR et al. (1999). EEG-triggered functional MRI of interictal epileptiform activity in patients with partial seizures. Brain 122: 1679–1688.

Krakow K, Allen PJ, Symms MR et al. (2000). EEG recording during fMRI experiments: image quality. Hum Brain Mapp 10: 10–15.

Krakow K, Lemieux L, Messina D et al. (2001). Spatio-temporal imaging of focal interictal epileptiform activity using EEG-triggered functional MRI. Epileptic Disord 3: 67–74.

Krings T, Topper R, Reinges MH et al. (2000). Hemodynamic changes in simple partial epilepsy: a functional MRI study. Neurology 54: 524–527.

Labate A, Briellmann RS, Abbott DF et al. (2005). Typical childhood absence seizures are associated with thalamic activation. Epileptic Disord 7: 373–377.

Lantz G, Spinelli L, Seeck M et al. (2003). Propagation of interictal epileptiform activity can lead to erroneous source localizations: a 128-channel EEG mapping study. J Clin Neurophysiol 20: 311–319.

Laufs H, Lengler U, Hamandi K et al. (2006). Linking generalized spike-and-wave discharges and resting state brain activity by using EEG/fMRI in a patient with absence seizures. Epilepsia 47: 444–448.

Lazeyras F, Blanke O, Perrig S et al. (2000). EEG-triggered functional MRI in patients with pharmacoresistant epilepsy. J Magn Reson Imaging 12: 177–185.

Lazeyras F, Zimine I, Blanke O et al. (2001). Functional MRI with simultaneous EEG recording: feasibility and application to motor and visual activation. J Magn Reson Imaging 13: 943–948.

Lemieux L, Allen PJ, Franconi F et al. (1997). Recording of EEG during fMRI experiments: patient safety. Magn Reson Med 38: 943–952.

Lemieux L, Krakow K, Fish DR (2001a). Comparison of spike-triggered functional MRI BOLD activation and EEG dipole model localization. Neuroimage 14: 1097–1104.

Lemieux L, Salek-Haddadi A, Josephs O et al. (2001b). Event-related fMRI with simultaneous and continuous EEG: description of the method and initial case report. Neuroimage 14: 780–787.

Lengler U, Kafadar I, Neubauer BA et al. (2007). fMRI correlates of interictal epileptic activity in patients with idiopathic benign focal epilepsy of childhood. A simultaneous EEG-functional MRI study. Epilepsy Res 75: 29–38.

Leopold DA, Logothetis NK (2003). Spatial patterns of spontaneous local field activity in the monkey visual cortex. Rev Neurosci 14: 195–205.

LeVan P, Tyvaert L, Moeller F et al. (2010). Independent component analysis reveals dynamic ictal BOLD responses in EEG-fMRI data from focal epilepsy patients. Neuroimage 49: 366–378.

Logothetis NK (2003). The underpinnings of the BOLD functional magnetic resonance imaging signal. J Neurosci 23: 3963–3971.

Logothetis NK, Pauls J, Augath M et al. (2001). Neurophysiological investigation of the basis of the fMRI signal. Nature 412: 150–157.

Lowe MJ, Mock BJ, Sorenson JA (1998). Functional connectivity in single and multislice echoplanar imaging using resting-state fluctuations. Neuroimage 7: 119–132.

Lu Y, Bagshaw AP, Grova C et al. (2006). Using voxel-specific hemodynamic response function in EEG-fMRI data analysis. Neuroimage 32: 238–247.

Lu Y, Grova C, Kobayashi E et al. (2007). Using voxel-specific hemodynamic response function in EEG-fMRI data analysis: an estimation and detection model. Neuroimage 34: 195–203.

Makiranta M, Ruohonen J, Suominen K et al. (2005). BOLD signal increase precedes EEG spike activity – a dynamic penicillin induced focal epilepsy in deep anesthesia. Neuroimage 27: 715–724.

Malonek D, Grinvald A (1996). Interactions between electrical activity and cortical microcirculation revealed by imaging spectroscopy: implications for functional brain mapping. Science 272: 551–554.

Masterton RA, Abbott DF, Fleming SW et al. (2007). Measurement and reduction of motion and ballistocardiogram artefacts from simultaneous EEG and fMRI recordings. Neuroimage 37: 202–211.

Masterton RA, Harvey AS, Archer JS et al. (2010). Focal epileptiform spikes do not show a canonical BOLD response in patients with benign rolandic epilepsy (BECTS). Neuroimage 51: 252–260.

Matsumoto R, Nair DR, LaPresto E et al. (2004). Functional connectivity in the human language system: a cortico-cortical evoked potential study. Brain 127: 2316–2330.

McCormick DA, Contreras D (2001). On the cellular and network bases of epileptic seizures. Annu Rev Physiol 63: 815–846.

Menon RS (2001). Imaging function in the working brain with fMRI. Curr Opin Neurobiol 11: 630–636.

Michel CM, Murray MM, Lantz G et al. (2004). EEG source imaging. Clin Neurophysiol 115: 2195–2222.

Moeller F, Siebner HR, Wolff S et al. (2008). Simultaneous EEG-fMRI in drug-naive children with newly diagnosed absence epilepsy. Epilepsia 49: 1510–1519.

Moeller F, Tyvaert L, Nguyen DK et al. (2009). EEG-fMRI: adding to standard evaluations of patients with nonlesional frontal lobe epilepsy. Neurology 73: 2023–2030.

Moeller F, Levan P, Muhle H et al. (2010). Absence seizures: Individual patterns revealed by EEG-fMRI. Epilepsia 51: 2000–2010.

Morillo LE, Ebner TJ, Bloedel JR (1982). The early involvement of subcortical structures during the development of a cortical seizure focus. Epilepsia 23: 571–585.

Negishi M, Abildgaard M, Nixon T et al. (2004). Removal of time-varying gradient artifacts from EEG data acquired during continuous fMRI. Clin Neurophysiol 115: 2181–2192.

Northoff G, Walter M, Schulte RF et al. (2007). GABA concentrations in the human anterior cingulate cortex predict negative BOLD responses in fMRI. Nat Neurosci 10: 1515–1517.

Ogawa S, Lee TM (1990). Magnetic resonance imaging of blood vessels at high fields: in vivo and in vitro measurements and image simulation. Magn Reson Med 16: 9–18.

Opdam HI, Federico P, Jackson GD et al. (2002). A sheep model for the study of focal epilepsy with concurrent intracranial EEG and functional MRI. Epilepsia 43: 779–787.

Patel MR, Blum A, Pearlman JD et al. (1999). Echo-planar functional MR imaging of epilepsy with concurrent EEG monitoring. AJNR Am J Neuroradiol 20: 1916–1919.

Pereira FR, Alessio A, Sercheli MS et al. (2010). Asymmetrical hippocampal connectivity in mesial temporal lobe epilepsy: evidence from resting state fMRI. BMC Neurosci 11: 66.

Raichle ME, MacLeod AM, Snyder AZ et al. (2001). A default mode of brain function. Proc Natl Acad Sci U S A 98: 676–682.

Rathakrishnan R, Moeller F, Levan P et al. (2010). BOLD signal changes preceding negative responses in EEG-fMRI in patients with focal epilepsy. Epilepsia 51: 1837–1845.

Rodionov R, De Martino F, Laufs H et al. (2007). Independent component analysis of interictal fMRI in focal epilepsy: comparison with general linear model-based EEG-correlated fMRI. Neuroimage 38: 488–500.

Saini S, DeStefano N, Smith S et al. (2004). Altered cerebellar functional connectivity mediates potential adaptive plasticity in patients with multiple sclerosis. J Neurol Neurosurg Psychiatry 75: 840–846.

Salek-Haddadi A, Lemieux L, Fish DR (2002a). Role of functional magnetic resonance imaging in the evaluation of patients with malformations caused by cortical development. Neurosurg Clin N Am 13: 63–69, viii.

Salek-Haddadi A, Merschhemke M, Lemieux L et al. (2002b). Simultaneous EEG-Correlated Ictal fMRI. Neuroimage 16: 32–40.

Salek-Haddadi A, Lemieux L, Merschhemke M et al. (2003). Functional magnetic resonance imaging of human absence seizures. Ann Neurol 53: 663–667.

Salek-Haddadi A, Diehl B, Hamandi K et al. (2006). Hemodynamic correlates of epileptiform discharges: an EEG-fMRI study of 63 patients with focal epilepsy. Brain Res 1088: 148–166.

Seeck M, Lazeyras F, Michel CM et al. (1998). Non-invasive epileptic focus localization using EEG-triggered functional MRI and electromagnetic tomography. Electroencephalogr Clin Neurophysiol 106: 508–512.

Shmuel A, Augath M, Oeltermann A et al. (2006). Negative functional MRI response correlates with decreases in neuronal activity in monkey visual area V1. Nat Neurosci 9: 569–577.

Silva-Barrat C, Menini C, Bryere P et al. (1986). Multiunitary activity analysis of cortical and subcortical structures in paroxysmal discharges and grand mal seizures in photosensitive baboons. Electroencephalogr Clin Neurophysiol 64: 455–468.

Srivastava G, Crottaz-Herbette S, Lau KM et al. (2005). ICA-based procedures for removing ballistocardiogram artifacts from EEG data acquired in the MRI scanner. Neuroimage 24: 50–60.

Stefanovic B, Warnking JM, Kobayashi E et al. (2005). Hemodynamic and metabolic responses to activation, deactivation and epileptic discharges. Neuroimage 28: 205–215.

Tyvaert L, Hawco C, Kobayashi E et al. (2008). Different structures involved during ictal and interictal epileptic activity in malformations of cortical development: an EEG-fMRI study. Brain 131: 2042–2060.

Tyvaert L, LeVan P, Dubeau F et al. (2009). Noninvasive dynamic imaging of seizures in epileptic patients. Hum Brain Mapp 30: 3993–4011.

van de Ven V, Bledowski C, Prvulovic D et al. (2008). Visual target modulation of functional connectivity networks revealed by self-organizing group ICA. Hum Brain Mapp 29: 1450–1461.

van Houdt PJ, de Munck JC, Zijlmans M et al. (2010). Comparison of analytical strategies for EEG-correlated fMRI data in patients with epilepsy. Magn Reson Imaging 28: 1078–1086.

Vulliemoz S, Carmichael DW, Rosenkranz K et al. (2010a). Simultaneous intracranial EEG and fMRI of interictal epileptic discharges in humans. Neuroimage 54: 182–190.

Vulliemoz S, Lemieux L, Daunizeau J et al. (2010b). The combination of EEG source imaging and EEG-correlated functional MRI to map epileptic networks. Epilepsia 51: 491–505.

Waites A, Abbott D, Fleming S et al. (2005). Magnetic resonance neurophysiology: simultaneous EEG and fMRI. In: R Kuzniecky, G Jackson, (Eds.), Magnetic Resonance in Epilepsy. 2nd edn. Elsevier Academic Press, London, pp. 299–314.

Warach S, Ives JR, Schlaug G et al. (1996). EEG-triggered echo-planar functional MRI in epilepsy. Neurology 47: 89–93.

Xiong J, Parsons LM, Gao JH et al. (1999). Interregional connectivity to primary motor cortex revealed using MRI resting state images. Hum Brain Mapp 8: 151–156.

Yacoub E, Hu X (2001). Detection of the early decrease in fMRI signal in the motor area. Magn Reson Med 45: 184–190.

Yacoub E, Ugurbil K, Harel N (2006). The spatial dependence of the poststimulus undershoot as revealed by high-resolution BOLD- and CBV-weighted fMRI. J Cereb Blood Flow Metab 26: 634–644.

Yu JM, Tyvaert L, Levan P et al. (2009). EEG spectral changes underlying BOLD responses contralateral to spikes in patients with focal epilepsy. Epilepsia 50: 1804–1809.

Zijlmans M, Huiskamp G, Hersevoort M et al. (2007). EEG-fMRI in the preoperative work-up for epilepsy surgery. Brain 130: 2343–2353.

Zilles K, Qu M, Schleicher A et al. (1998). Characterization of neuronal migration disorders in neocortical structures: quantitative receptor autoradiography of ionotropic glutamate, GABA(A) and GABA(B) receptors. Eur J Neurosci 10: 3095–3106.

Handbook of Clinical Neurology, Vol. 107 (3rd series)
Epilepsy, Part I
H. Stefan and W.H. Theodore, Editors

Chapter 24

Functional magnetic resonance imaging: functional mapping

WILLIAM D. GAILLARD [1,2]* AND MADISON M. BERL [1]

[1] *Center for Neuroscience, Children's National Medical Center, Washington, DC, USA*

[2] *Clinical Epilepsy Section, National Institute of Neurological Disease and Stroke, National Institutes of Health, Bethesda, MD, USA*

INTRODUCTION

Functional magnetic resonance imaging (fMRI) has assumed an increasing role for mapping eloquent cortex during epilepsy surgery planning. This chapter reviews principles and methods for acquisition of fMRI data, then considers applications for motor, sensory, language, and memory systems mapping. fMRI may also be used to identify the source of interictal EEG spikes and, rarely, to capture seizures and hence map the seizure focus. Limitations of fMRI methods are also discussed. This review does not consider the use of these methods to explore the neurobiology of epilepsy and effects of brain function, nor does it consider in detail more recent applications of functional connectivity and diffusion tensor imaging (DTI).

Conventional fMRI is based on the blood oxygen level-dependent (BOLD) response, an indirect and surrogate measure of brain activity that derives from synaptic activity (Logothetis, 2003). Increased neuronal activity elicits a regionally specific increase in blood flow, a concomitant increase in blood volume, and an increase in the ratio of oxyhemoglobin to deoxyhemoglobin (Fox and Raichle, 1986). These changes, principally in the hemoglobin moieties, results in a change in T2* signal assessed by fast MRI gradients (Moonen and Bandettini, 2000). The anatomical resolution possible is 1 mm^3, although in practice it is closer to 3 mm^3, and after conventional image processing with smoothing it is 6–10 mm^3. The peak in hemodynamic response occurs 4–6 seconds after the neuronal activity; thus distributed networks are captured. Serial processing requires real time techniques such as magnetoencephalography (MEG) and electroencephalography (EEG).

fMRI data are collected by imaging the brain while a subject performs a selected task. As fMRI is a relative measure there must be at least two conditions. Analysis compares MRI signal in each voxel that composes brain tissue between images acquired during the control and experimental condition. The most common presentation is to present task in alternating blocks of 20–40 seconds for 3–5 repetitions (4 is usually sufficient). However, data can also be obtained with single items or events (e.g. single words, pictures); 30 items and 30 control points are generally considered necessary for reliable data analysis. Clinical motor, sensory, and language paradigms are usually obtained with block designs; memory paradigms work better with event-related designs. Block designs yield superior signal to noise, but event-related designs allow data to be analyzed based on correct or incorrect response. Thus, memory data may be analyzed based on BOLD response to those items correctly encoded or recalled (see below). Items not properly encoded generally do not elicit a BOLD response; incorporation of these data would diminish capacity to image the functional anatomy for task.

For clinical application it is important that tasks can be performed by the patient; thus, material may need to be adapted to match task difficulty with patient ability. It is also helpful to have a stark contrast in task and experimental conditions. Simple paradigms that yield a robust response on an individual basis are best for clinical purposes. Effort may also be as important as performance. From a cognitive perspective it is preferred that responses in the scanner may be monitored to assure compliance with task and to help interpret results when atypical or unexpected. In practice, some unmonitored

*Correspondence to: William Davis Gaillard, M.D., Center for Neuroscience, Children's National Medical Center, 111 Michigan Ave NW, Washington, DC 20010, USA. Tel: 202-476-2120, E-mail: wgaillar@childrensnational.org

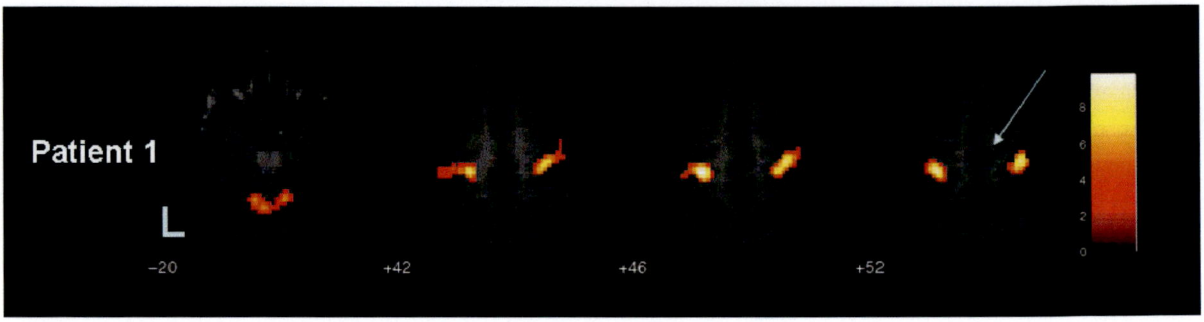

Fig. 24.1. Images from a 9-year-old child with left frontal lobe epilepsy. Motor tapping of hands identifies the primary motor cortex, posterior to a cavernous angioma (arrow) that has bled and is now the focus for the child's focal motor seizures. Left image is left brain.

paradigms (see verbal fluency below) have consistently yielded reliable and reproducible results. Furthermore, demand for a response often changes the cognitive nature of the task (e.g., from one of generation to decision) and brain areas engaged in task.

Data can be analyzed in either native (individual) space – typically superimposed on a high resolution image – or in the normalized space of a standard anatomical atlas, commonly that of either Talairach and Tournoux (1988) or the Montreal Neurological Institute (MNI). Normative data are presented as group data in normalized space mostly because random-effects analysis may be performed that allows extrapolation of results to a broad population. Whether individual or group data, the processed data are set to mark voxels that exceed set statistical criteria for signal difference between conditions by a color-based code; these voxels are then deemed "activated" for the task. Data can be displayed as t or z maps. A variety of programs exist for these purposes, SPM, AFNI, FSL, and MEDX being the more common. Some patient data are also presented in group space, but these studies are often flawed as patient populations are heterogeneous and important variability or atypical patterns are lost. None the less, group maps provide a sense of what the typical pattern for task should be and allow statistical extrapolation of experimental findings to the broad population when random-effects analytical tools are used. For surgical planning, individual or native space needs to be used. These data can be coregistered to higher resolution images in addition to those used for intraoperative navigation.

MOTOR AND SENSORY MAPPING

Motor and sensory paradigms readily elicit the most robust of MR signal – 3–4% at 1.5 T compared with cognitive tasks of 0.5–1% signal. Correlation with electrocortical stimulation (ECS) and evoked response finds agreement within 1 cm and usually within 5 mm (Lehericy et al., 2000b). Finger tapping paradigms (versus rest as control) identify primary motor cortex, in addition to contralateral motor cortex, and often basal ganglia and cerebellar networks and supplementary motor area (SMA) (Kim et al., 1993; Rao et al., 1993; Jack et al., 1994) (Fig. 24.1). More complex movements and planned movements are more likely to recruit SMA (Nelson et al., 2002). Foot tapping and tongue wiggling can also be used but are more likely to be accompanied by movement artifact. Sensory cortex can be identified by brushing the face, arm, hand, leg, or foot (Kwong et al., 1992; Hammeke et al., 1994). Primary auditory cortex can be identified by presenting a series of tones (Binder et al., 1994) and occipital cortex by alternating grid patterns as used in evoked response or flashing light. When used as a seed point for DTI-based tractography, the occipital radiations that link the lateral geniculate bodies with the calcarine cortex can be identified. These methods have been advocated as a way to avoid disruption of Meyer's loop in temporal lobe surgery and thus limit visual field cuts (Powell et al., 2008a; Yogarajah et al., 2009). Motor and sensory mapping is used when planning surgery in frontal and parietal lobe (and occipital lobe for visual cortex), and is usually obtained for resection of focal lesions, typically tumor and malformations of cortical development. As with visual systems, motor fMRI may be used as a seed region to identify sensorimotor tracts (Guye et al., 2003).

LANGUAGE MAPPING

The most widespread use of fMRI is to map language networks. fMRI has in large part replaced the intracarotid amobarbital procedure (IAT or Wada test). fMRI findings alter surgical planning (Medina et al., 2005). In over 290 reports, including meta-analysis, there is excellent agreement with the IAT for the determination of hemispheric language dominance (Desmond et al., 1995; Binder et al., 1996; Bahn et al., 1997; Hertz-Pannier et al., 1997; Worthington et al., 1997; Yetkin et al., 1998; Gaillard et al., 2002; Spreer et al., 2002; Lehericy et al.,

2000a; Rutten et al., 2002a; Adcock et al., 2003; Sabbah et al., 2003; Woermann et al., 2003; Benke et al., 2006; Medina et al., 2007; Arora et al., 2009). Complete agreement between the two methods occurs in 84–92% of patients; the remainder exhibit partial concordance – where one modality is lateralized and the other bilateral. Reports of complete discordance are rare and in these circumstances either modality has proved to yield the correct answer (Pardo and Fox, 1993; Hunter et al., 1999; Kho et al., 2005; Lanzenberger et al., 2005). fMRI can be viewed as a means of excluding the need for IAT in approximately 80% of patients when language issues are clinically important, or as a complement to IAT. In contrast to IAT, fMRI can also provide localization as well as lateralization of language functions. It is easier to repeat fMRI studies when results are inconclusive or uncertain. Unlike IAT or ECS, normal data are also available for interpretation of fMRI. There are a few studies that compare fMRI to direct intraoperative or subdural mapping with ECS (FitzGerald et al., 1997; Pouratian et al., 2002; Rutten et al., 2002b; Roux et al., 2003). These studies are limited as they do not use the same stimuli for their comparisons (the exception is an ^{15}O water positron emission tomography (PET) study; Bookheimer et al., 1997); they show 90% sensitivity and 65% specificity. The principal implication of these studies is that fMRI-negative areas are safe to resect; some fMRI-positive areas may not be essential for task.

Several paradigms have been used to identify brain areas that sustain language functions. Although anterior and posterior language networks reside mostly in the same hemisphere, they may occur in opposite hemispheres (crossed dominance) (Baciu et al., 2003; Gaillard, 2004; Ries et al., 2004; Lee et al., 2008); thus, it is important to select a task that targets the region to be operated on. While an oversimplification, it is helpful to consider tasks targeted at identifying "receptive" language in posterior or temporal neocortex (Wernicke's region) and "expressive" speech in anterior or inferior frontal cortex (Broca's region) (Geschwind and Levitsky, 1968). Of course, both regions are also involved in a complex interplay that underlies both aspects of receptive and expressive speech. Verbal fluency tasks activate dominant inferior frontal gyrus (Broca) and dorsolateral prefrontal cortex (mostly BA46/9, implicated in verbal working memory). Some paradigms place an emphasis on phonological processing – generating words that begin with letters (C, L, F for children; F, A, S for adults) or words that rhyme with target words; others place a emphasis on semantic processing – generating words that belong to a particular category (animals, food) or noun–verb generation (present: ball; answer: throw, pitch, bounce) (Hertz-Pannier et al., 1997; Yetkin et al., 1998; Pujol et al., 1999; Lehericy et al., 2000a; Gaillard et al., 2001; Woermann et al., 2003). As a rule, these paradigms yield little or less in the way of temporal activation. The noun–verb task does a better job of eliciting temporal activation as there are more stimuli that increase receptive comprehension burden (Wood et al., 2001, 2004; Anderson et al., 2006). All fluency tasks also identify anterior cingulate and mesial SMA, areas not critical to language dominance. These tasks are generally covert and unmonitored; they may be adapted to provide for a semantic or phonological decision. Rather than generate words that fall within the category "animal," the task is modified to ask whether the given words fall into the presented category "animal" (Binder et al., 1995, 1996; Springer et al., 1999). This task also elicits activation in BA47. Tasks that identify temporal receptive cortex (Schlosser et al., 1999; Lehericy et al., 2000a; Carpentier et al., 2001; Ahmad et al., 2003; Holland et al., 2007) use phrases or sentences, such as reading stories or listening to stories. However, the more complex the syntax and complicated the story the greater the recruitment of right homologs (Just et al., 1996; Gaillard et al., 2001). Simple phrases or sentences are best; those that require a semantic decision or response combine aspects of both and are the better tasks for identifying temporal and frontal cortex at the same time. The lingual gyrus, or basal temporal cortex (especially BA20/37), is identified when patients imagine or must recall specific items named or imagined (Balsamo et al., 2006). Ironically, the object naming tasks used for ECS have not proved useful in fMRI for mapping temporal neocortical language-processing regions. Object naming paradigms can elicit the same frontal activation as observed in verbal fluency/decision paradigms when some form of expressive language output or decision is required based on the presented picture.

Paradigm presentation can be visual or auditory. For auditory tasks, several methods have been used to control for first- and second-order auditory processing, which is bilateral, in order to isolate linguistic aspect of the task: (1) series of tones (Binder et al., 1996); speech in an unfamiliar language (Schlosser et al., 1998); or reverse speech of items from experimental condition (Gaillard et al., 2007).

Language laterality can be rated visually (Fernandez et al., 2001; Gaillard et al., 2004) or by quantitative methods using region of interest (ROI) approaches. ROI methods either rely on counting voxels that exceed a given threshold in each region or calculate the mean t score of voxels. The ROI may be hemispheric (Binder et al., 1996), smaller anatomical regions (e.g., Broca's or Wernicke's; Gaillard et al., 2002; Spreer et al., 2002), or regions defined by group activation maps and then applied to patients (Holland et al., 2001; Weber et al., 2006; Wellmer et al., 2009). The smaller region approach is generally preferred as it is targeted at language-specific regions; the anatomical region approach has theoretical advantages in circumstances where patient activation lies outside or margins of typical activation.

There are strategies that can be used to increase assurance of fMRI findings. One strategy is to use several similar paradigms that target same areas, such as employing different forms of verbal fluency (letter, categories, noun–verb) that all yield IFG activation (Ramsey et al., 2001). The other is to use paradigms that target different areas within the distributed network for language, such as employing a verbal fluency task that targets IFG and a comprehension task that targets temporal receptive cortex (Gaillard et al., 2004; Thivard et al., 2005). Other studies find that the area of conjunction across studies is helpful in increasing concordance between fMRI and IAT (Ramsey et al., 2001; Arora et al., 2009). The use of multiple paradigms increases interrater agreement (Gaillard et al., 2002, 2004) (Figs 24.2 & 24.3). There may be a less strong correlation with invasive methods when language is atypical and if MRI is normal (Woermann et al., 2003; Brazdil et al., 2005; Benke et al., 2006), but many of these studies rely on verbal fluency paradigms directed at frontal language areas.

In addition to determining language dominance, semantic decision fMRI tasks are also predict postoperative naming deficits identified on the Boston Naming Task (Sabsevitz et al., 2003). There are no other

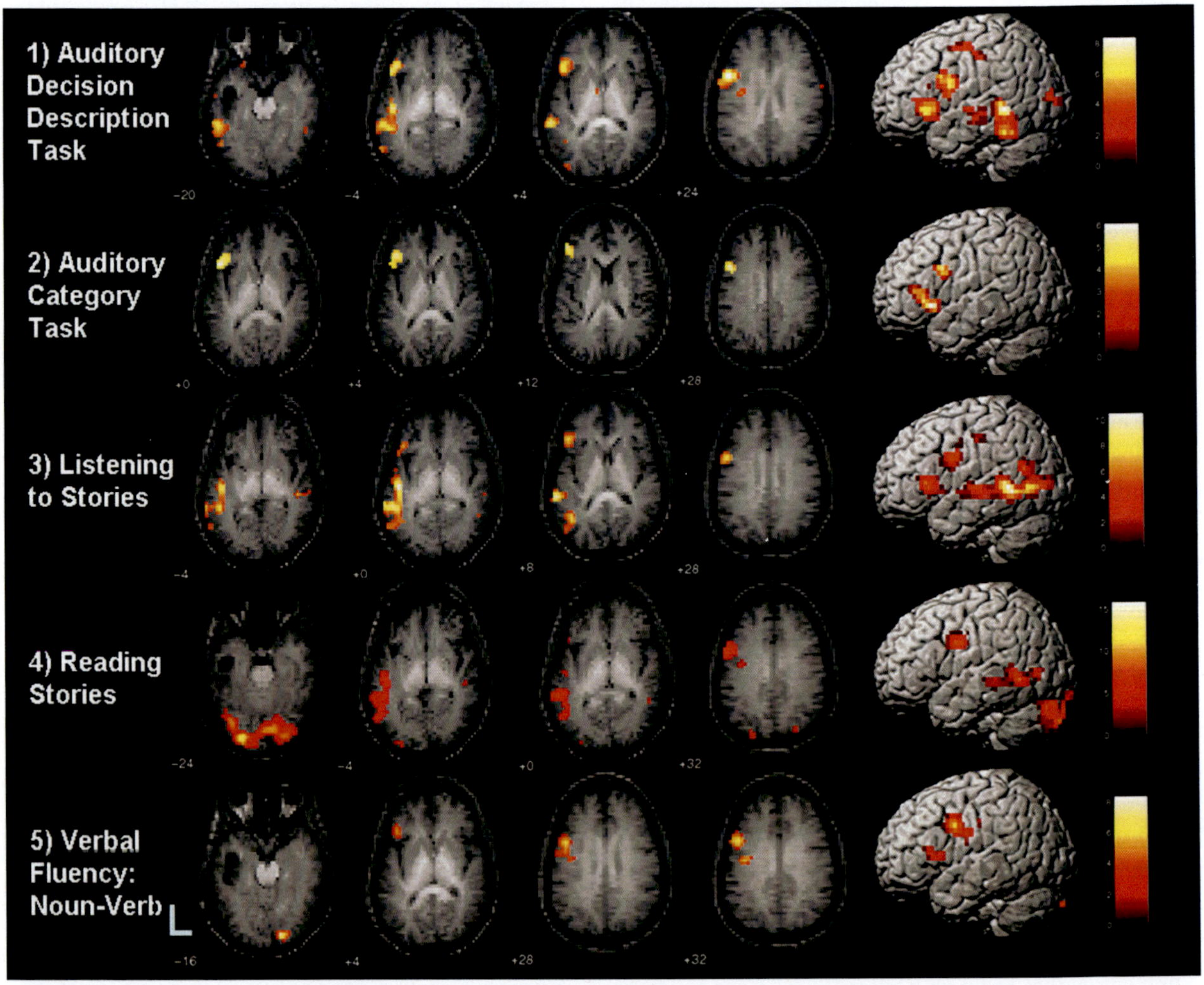

Fig. 24.2. Images from a 19-year-old man with a 5-year history of focal seizures and mass lesion in the anterior left temporal lobe. Five tasks are performed, verbal fluency (visual noun–verb generation) compared with rest; auditorily based category (semantic) decision (whether a presented item matched a specified category); auditory-based word definition decision (e.g., a large gray animal is an elephant); listening to stories; reading stories (control viewing open or filled circles). The auditory tasks use a reverse speech control task. The panel of tasks demonstrates typical left hemisphere activation, hence left dominance for language. The tasks are targeted at anterior and posterior language-processing regions, and the panel also provides redundancy to assure findings. Left image is left brain.

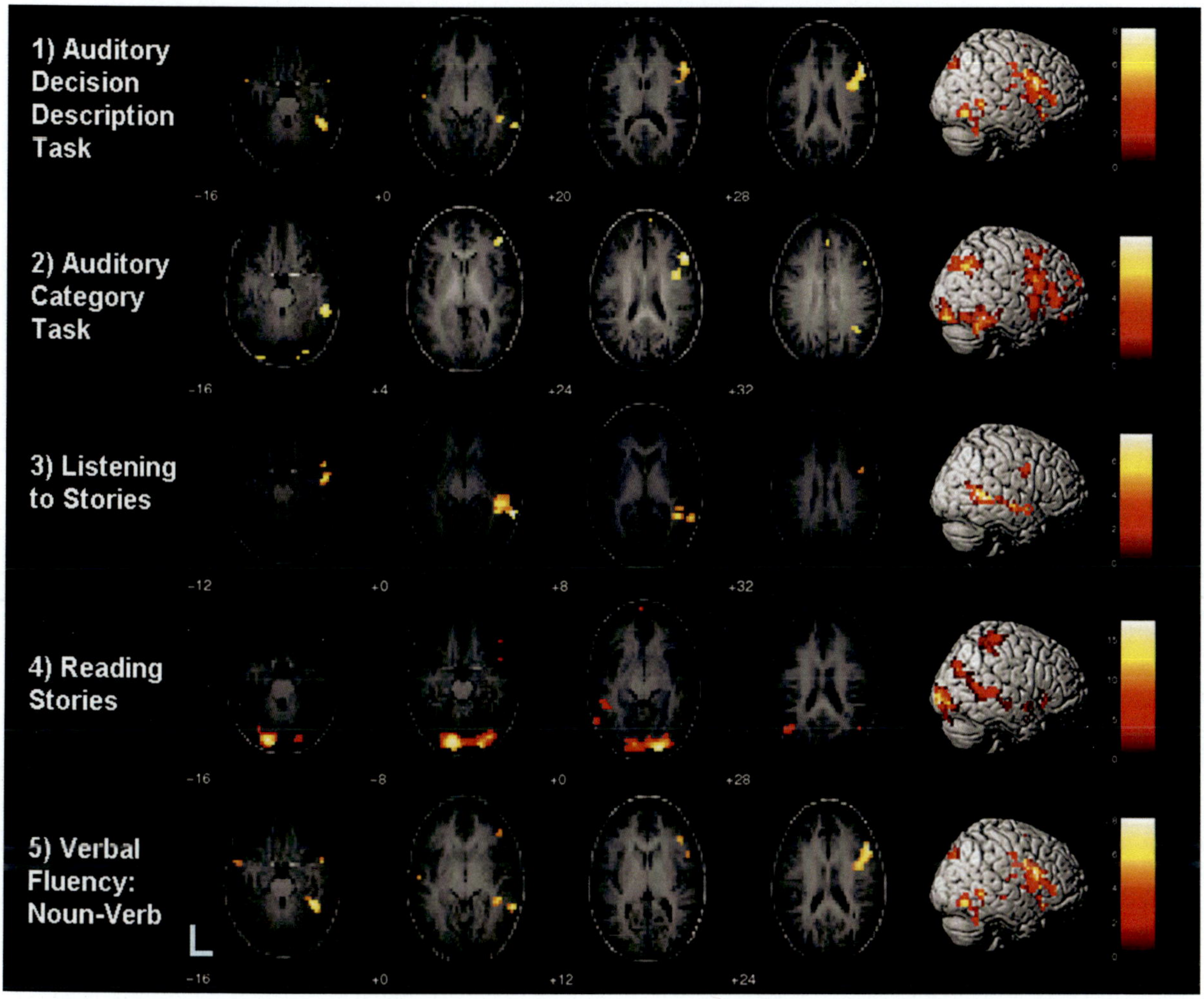

Fig. 24.3. Images from an 11-year-old left-handed child with recent-onset epilepsy and left mid frontal mass and seizure focus. Tasks include verbal fluency, category decision, word definition, and listening to stories (see Fig. 24.2). The patient demonstrates activation in right homologs of Broca's and Wernicke's regions and in the right hemisphere, dominant for language. Left image is left brain.

postoperative outcome studies based on fMRI language measures, only comparisons with invasive methods.

There are circumstances in which fMRI may provide false information. In these circumstances the physiological basis of the BOLD response is perturbed, activation in true language cortex is not elicited, but a modest amount of activation commonly seen in homologous regions is falsely interpreted as primary activation. There are four circumstances to note: (1) when there is critical carotid stenosis; (2) large tumors (e.g., glioma blastoma multiforme) with edema and mass effect; (3) arteriovascular malformations with vascular steal; and (4) postictal state (Jayakar et al., 2002; Lehericy et al., 2002; Rother et al., 2002; Wellmer et al., 2009). The fourth category is of particular concern for epilepsy populations; care should be made to note the nature, extent, and severity of ictal activity preceding fMRI. There are some concerns that smaller lesions may have a measurable effect on local BOLD response and calculated asymmetry indices by these methods (Wellmer et al., 2009). There are also case reports where language asymmetry index has normalized following successful surgery (Helmstaedter et al., 2006). Some medications, such as topiramate, may influence the BOLD response or interfere with cognitive capacity and hence effort or performance, and have indirect effects on activation maps (Jansen et al., 2006).

fMRI language studies find that 20–30% of patients exhibit atypical language and that atypical language may take many forms (Thivard et al., 2005; Gaillard et al., 2007) (Figs 24.3 & 24.4). One-fifth of patients with atypical language are right hemisphere dominant; the other 80% are bilateral (Gaillard, 2004). Bilateral expression can be truly bilateral, or a crossed dominance between frontal and temporal areas, or task dependent. A fair

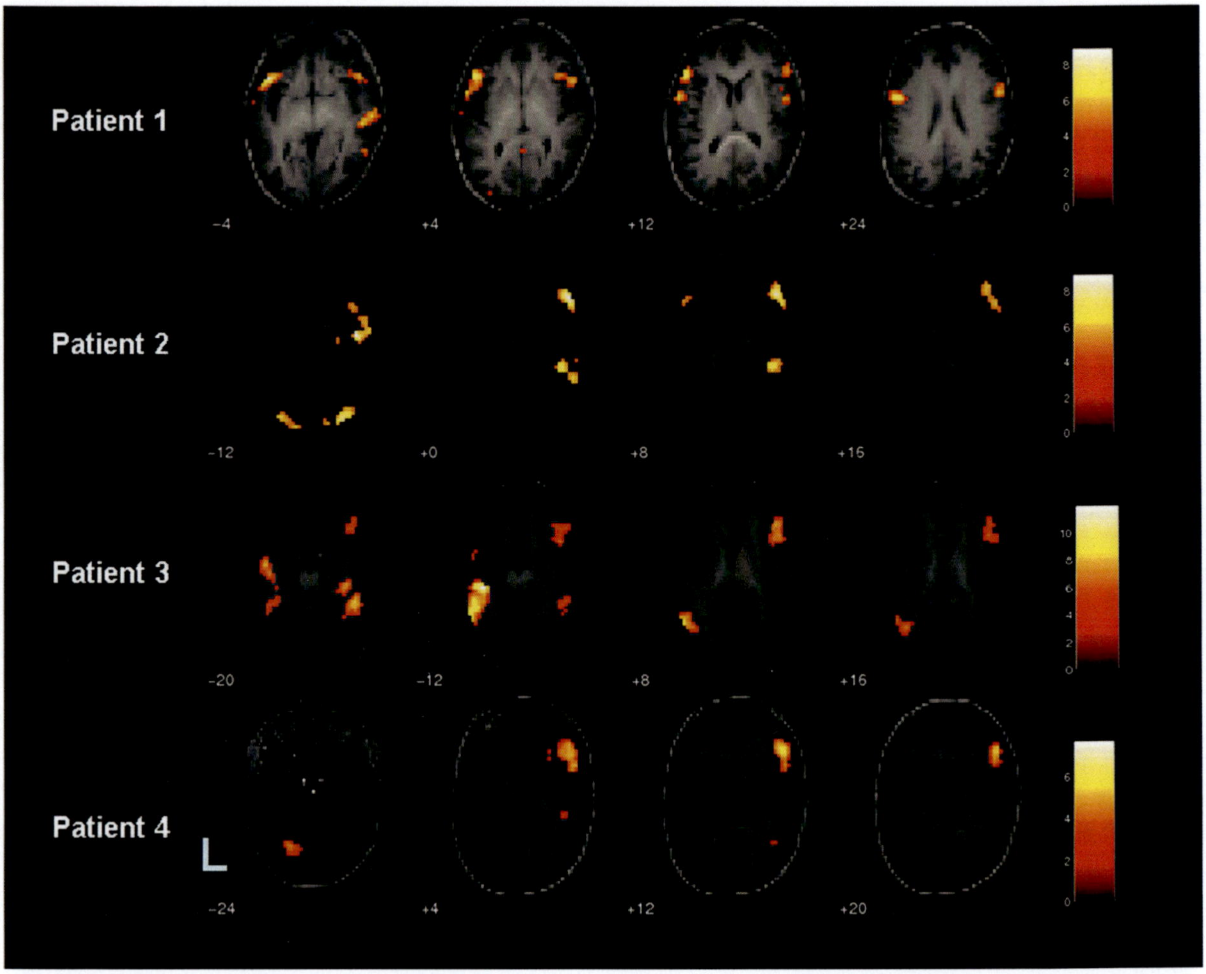

Fig. 24.4. Different atypical language patterns seen with the auditory-based word definition decision task. Patient 1, bilateral frontal, right temporal activation; Patient 2, right frontal and temporal activation; Patient 3, crossed dominance, right frontal, and left temporal activation; Patient 4, right frontal activation. Left image is left brain.

proportion of patients will be bilateral in one region (mostly frontal) and unilateral in the other (usually posterior). In one recent study atypical language representation occurred in 25–30% of right-handed patients (where population norms for right-handers is about 5%) and in 60% of left-handed patients (population norms about 24%). When activation is bilateral it is not possible with fMRI to determine whether one, both, or neither hemisphere areas are critical to sustaining speech processing. Right hemisphere language processing – intrahemispheric reorganization – occurs in homologs of Wernicke's and Broca's areas (Staudt et al., 2001, 2002; Liegeois et al., 2008; Mbwana et al., 2009; Rosenberger et al., 2009). There is slight evidence for intrahemispheric reorganization or compensation, typically along the margins of typically activated area in the left hemisphere (Mbwana et al., 2009; Rosenberger et al., 2009).

Nearly one-third of patients with normal MRI have atypical language. Not surprisingly, all patients with a history of left hemispheric stroke have atypical language. Approximately 15% of patients with small developmental tumors or focal cortical dysplasia also have atypical language representation; this percentage is higher if the dysplasia occupies a large portion of language cortex (Liegeois et al., 2004; Smith et al., 2004; Briellmann et al., 2006; Gaillard et al., 2007; Hadac et al., 2007; Wellmer et al., 2009). One-fifth to one-quarter of patients with left mesial temporal sclerosis (MTS) exhibit atypical language dominance. The effect of MTS on language representation is interesting as this area is remote from primary receptive or expressive cortex; its role in verbal working memory may be involved in this instance (Thivard et al., 2005; Weber et al., 2006; Gaillard et al., 2007). It is uncommon to find atypical language if onset of epilepsy or its symptomatic cause occurred after age 6 years beyond that expected as a normal variant (Springer et al., 1999; Woermann et al., 2003; Gaillard et al., 2007).

fMRI findings in children are comparable to those in adults (Balsamo et al., 2002; Liegeois et al., 2002; Ahmad et al., 2003; Gaillard et al., 2000, 2003; Wood et al., 2004; Balsamo et al., 2006). It may be helpful to adapt paradigms for children's abilities. Children as young as 4 years of age may be readily studied (Byars et al., 2002; Yerys et al., 2009). Younger children with developmental delays, attention-deficit/hyperactivity disorder (ADHD), or anxiety disorders are more difficult to scan; older children with learning, cognitive, and behavioral disabilities do quite well in scanners (Byars et al., 2002; Yerys et al., 2009). For the youngest children, decreasing time in scanner and length of paradigms increases success rates. Passive studies for motor control, sensation, and auditory comprehension can elicit typical activation patterns (Souweidane et al., 1999; Altman and Bernal, 2001). Success with sedation depends on type and depth of sedation/anesthesia (B. Bernal, personal communication).

As with motor control and vision, functional imaging may also be used to determine seed points for DTI-based tractography. The identification of short and long tract fibers that provide structural connectivity for language may help to direct surgical approaches (Catani et al., 2005, 2007; Frey et al., 2008; Powell et al., 2008a; Yogarajah et al., 2008).

MEMORY MAPPING

Memory studies are more problematic than language fMRI. The mesial temporal structures are technically more challenging to image, particularly at the higher magnetic fields used to improve signal to noise. As the monitoring, maintenance, and laying down of memory is constant, it is more difficult to achieve contrast between experimental and control conditions. Event-related paradigms analyzed on the basis of items correctly encoded or recalled are superior to block design studies and yield more robust finding in individual subjects (Stern et al., 1996; Brewer et al., 1998). Unlike language fMRI, there is only a fair correlation with memory paradigms and with IAT (Detre et al., 1998). The basis for IAT as a means of evaluating memory is less firmly established than for language, but IAT may be able to predict patients at risk of some forms of troubling memory loss following temporal lobectomy (Rabin et al., 2004; Richardson et al., 2004; Janszky et al., 2005; Powell et al., 2008b; Bonelli et al., 2010). Part of the difficulty lies in the complexities of the various types of memory. Most efforts are directed at declarative (explicit) memory, in particular encoding. There has been less attention paid to imaging retrieval of encoded information. There is evidence of material specificity for fMRI paradigms (Golby et al., 2001, 2002; Richardson et al., 2004; Powell et al., 2005; Bonelli et al., 2010); those that are primarily verbal provide more activation in the left, language-dominant, hippocampal formation (HF) and other mesial temporal structures; those that are purely visuospatial preferentially activate the right HF; tasks that require both (e.g., picture or scene encoding, and imaginary navigation) provide more greater bilateral activation (Detre et al., 1998; Rabin et al., 2004; Binder et al., 2008). The components of material specificity may be tempered by novelty (Kennepohl et al., 2007). Furthermore, there may be a gradient in anterior and posterior HF based on retrieval or encoding (Binder et al., 2005). The control condition is particularly important to minimize HF activation in order to optimize contrast, as the hippocampus is virtually constantly engaged in memory function.

The most successful tasks are picture-encoding paradigms compared with scrambled pictures for control. These paradigms yield bilateral hippocampal and parahippocampal activation. There is a correlation with activation in resected (left) HF and postoperative deficits on the Boston Naming Task (Rabin et al., 2004) (less activation, better postoperative naming); this correlation is superior to IAT but does not apply to other memory measures. The Roland Hometown Navigation Task (where patients image a walk through their town) also results in bilateral activation, and may be useful for visuospatial outcomes following resection of right mesial structures (Jokeit et al., 2001; Janszky et al., 2005). The primary goal of imaging, however, is to anticipate large insults to verbal memory. Some small-scale studies have examined verbal encoding as part of a panel of memory tasks (Golby et al., 2001, 2002). There is mounting evidence that activation in resected cortex predicts postoperative outcome for that task – for picture encoding, verbal encoding, and face encoding – that is, hippocampal adequacy (activation in resected HF) rather than hippocampal reserve (activation in remaining HF) is important for outcomes (Rabin et al., 2004; Richardson et al., 2004; Powell et al., 2008b; Bonelli et al., 2010). Postoperative verbal deficits appear to follow language dominance (Binder et al., 2008). In the absence of reorganization of language there is little evidence for memory compensation (Richardson et al., 2003; Powell et al., 2007). It may be that determination of temporal lobe language dominance and a determination hippocampal volume integrity may be all that is necessary to determine risk of postoperative verbal memory loss (i.e., highest risk for removing intact hippocampus in language-dominant temporal lobe). As with language paradigms, use of a panel of memory paradigms targeted at material specificity, encoding, and retrieval is likely to provide the most valuable information (Golby et al., 2002; Powell et al., 2005; Powell et al., 2008b; Bonelli et al., 2010). Large-scale studies powered to link these paradigms to outcome are forthcoming.

ICTAL AND INTERICTAL MAPPING

fMRI may also be used to help identify the epileptogenic zone. Capturing ictal events in the scanner is uncommon, but may be achieved following weaning medications, as is commonly performed for video-EEG monitoring and ictal single-photon emission computed tomography (SPECT) acquisition (E. Kobayashi, personal communication). They are also problematic as movement usually ensues and motion impedes quality image acquisition. However, the same principles apply and the time course can be modeled to identify areas that exhibit increased blood flow and mark seizure propagation (Jackson et al., 1994; Detre et al., 1995; Schwartz et al., 1998; Krings et al., 2000). There is also evidence that a preictal state may be identified that precedes the ictus by a substantial interval (Federico et al., 2005). More common, however, is the use of EEG spike-triggered event-related fMRI (Gotman, 2008). Event-related methods may be harnessed to model a hemodynamic response function that typically peaks 5 seconds after the event, here an interictal spike (Krakow et al., 1999; Symms et al., 1999; Bagshaw et al., 2004). Older studies imaged the brain after identification of an EEG spike or sharp wave compared with data acquired when the EEG was quiescent. Current software and filters enable continuous acquisition of MRI data simultaneously with EEG. The EEG signal may be recovered, and segments with and without spikes then identified for BOLD signal analysis (Al-Asmi et al., 2003; Lemieux, 2004). In this manner the "source" of the spike may be identified by its BOLD signal (Krakow et al., 2001; Benar et al., 2006). Propagation effects may also be identified (Kobayashi et al., 2006). The method usually requires 5–30 spikes; multifocal spikes are more problematic to model. The utility of this method, like MEG, is based on the supposition that the interictal source is concordant with the ictal zone. Rather than interrogation of data by individual spike, it may be possible to identify the epileptogenic zone by disruptions and alteration of background signal and noise (Morgan et al., 2004).

Finally, arterial spin methods, which provide for direct measure of cerebral blood flow (CBF), allow the determination of regional decreases in perfusion, analogous to interictal SPECT and ^{15}O water PET (Wolf et al., 2001; Lim et al., 2008), although interictal CBF abnormalities may not be reliable identifiers of the epileptogenic zone (Gaillard et al., 1995).

CONCLUSION

fMRI provides a reliable, replicable, and noninvasive means of identifying the functional anatomy of essential cerebral functions including motor control, sensory systems, language-processing networks, and the different forms of memory. Language mapping is best performed with a panel of tasks that have redundant features and target the area of planned surgical resection. It is also important to remember the limitations to functional mapping. In many instances, fMRI may replace or at least complement IAT. When the findings are unusual, not replicable, or null then confirmation by invasive methods is necessary. Memory paradigms are becoming established; the extent of activation in targeted hippocampus likely predicts deficits in some forms of memory. Event-related fMRI of interictal spikes may provide source localization of interictal epileptic activity.

References

Adcock JE, Wise RG, Oxbury JM et al. (2003). Quantitative fMRI assessment of the differences in lateralization of language-related brain activation in patients with temporal lobe epilepsy. Neuroimage 18: 423–438.

Ahmad Z, Balsamo LM, Sachs BC et al. (2003). Auditory comprehension of language in young children: neural networks identified with fMRI. Neurology 60: 1598–1605.

Al-Asmi A, Benar CG, Gross DW et al. (2003). fMRI activation in continuous and spike-triggered EEG-fMRI studies of epileptic spikes. Epilepsia 44: 1328–1339.

Altman NR, Bernal B (2001). Brain activation in sedated children: auditory and visual functional MR imaging. Radiology 221: 56–63.

Anderson DP, Harvey AS, Saling MM et al. (2006). fMRI lateralization of expressive language in children with cerebral lesions. Epilepsia 47: 998–1008.

Arora J, Pugh K, Westerveld M et al. (2009). Language lateralization in epilepsy patients: fMRI validated with the Wada procedure. Epilepsia 50: 2225–2241.

Baciu MV, Watson JM, McDermott KB et al. (2003). Functional MRI reveals an interhemispheric dissociation of frontal and temporal language regions in a patient with focal epilepsy. Epilepsy Behav 4: 776–780.

Bagshaw AP, Aghakhani Y, Benar CG et al. (2004). EEG-fMRI of focal epileptic spikes: analysis with multiple haemodynamic functions and comparison with gadolinium-enhanced MR angiograms. Hum Brain Mapp 22: 179–192.

Bahn MM, Lin W, Silbergeld DL et al. (1997). Localization of language cortices by functional MR imaging compared with intracarotid amobarbital hemispheric sedation. AJR Am J Roentgenol 169: 575–579.

Balsamo LM, Xu B, Grandin CB et al. (2002). A functional magnetic resonance imaging study of left hemisphere language dominance in children. Arch Neurol 59: 1168–1174.

Balsamo LM, Xu B, Gaillard WD (2006). Language lateralization and the role of the fusiform gyrus in semantic processing in young children. Neuroimage 31: 1306–1314.

Benar CG, Grova C, Kobayashi E et al. (2006). EEG-fMRI of epileptic spikes: concordance with EEG source localization and intracranial EEG. Neuroimage 30: 1161–1170.

Benke T, Koylu B, Visani P et al. (2006). Language lateralization in temporal lobe epilepsy: a comparison between fMRI and the Wada test. Epilepsia 47: 1308–1319.

Binder JR, Rao SM, Hammeke TA et al. (1994). Functional magnetic resonance imaging of human auditory cortex. Ann Neurol 35: 662–672.

Binder J, Rao S, Hammeke T et al. (1995). Lateralized human brain language systems demonstrated by task subtraction functional magnetic resonance imaging. Arch Neurol 52: 593–601.

Binder JR, Swanson SJ, Hammeke TA et al. (1996). Determination of language dominance using functional MRI: a comparison with the Wada test. Neurology 46: 978–984.

Binder JR, Bellgowan PS, Hammeke TA et al. (2005). A comparison of two fMRI protocols for eliciting hippocampal activation. Epilepsia 46: 1061–1070.

Binder JR, Sabsevitz DS, Swanson SJ et al. (2008). Use of preoperative functional MRI to predict verbal memory decline after temporal lobe epilepsy surgery. Epilepsia 49: 1377–1394.

Bonelli SB, Powell RH, Yogarajah M et al. (2010). Imaging memory in temporal lobe epilepsy: predicting the effects of temporal lobe resection. Brain 133: 1186–1199.

Bookheimer SY, Zeffiro TA, Blaxton T et al. (1997). A direct comparison of PET activation and electrocortical stimulation mapping for language localization. Neurology 48: 1056–1065.

Brazdil M, Chlebus P, Mikl M et al. (2005). Reorganization of language-related neuronal networks in patients with left temporal lobe epilepsy – an fMRI study. Eur J Neurol 12: 268–275.

Brewer JB, Zhao Z, Desmond JE et al. (1998). Making memories: brain activity that predicts how well visual experience will be remembered. Science 281: 1185–1187.

Briellmann RS, Labate A, Harvey AS et al. (2006). Is language lateralization in temporal lobe epilepsy patients related to the nature of the epileptogenic lesion? Epilepsia 47: 916–920.

Byars AW, Holland SK, Strawsburg RH et al. (2002). Practical aspects of conducting large-scale functional magnetic resonance imaging studies in children. J Child Neurol 17: 885–890.

Carpentier A, Pugh KR, Westerveld M et al. (2001). Functional MRI of language processing: dependence on input modality and temporal lobe epilepsy. Epilepsia 42: 1241–1254.

Catani M, Jones DK, Ffytche DH (2005). Perisylvian language networks of the human brain. Ann Neurol 57: 8–16.

Catani M, Allin MP, Husain M et al. (2007). Symmetries in human brain language pathways correlate with verbal recall. Proc Natl Acad Sci U S A 104: 163–168.

Desmond JE, Sum JM, Wagner AD et al. (1995). Functional MRI measurement of language lateralization in Wada-tested patients. Brain 118: 1411–1419.

Detre JA, Sirven JI, Alsop DC et al. (1995). Localization of subclinical ictal activity by functional magnetic resonance imaging: correlation with invasive monitoring. Ann Neurol 38: 618–624.

Detre JA, Maccotta L, King D et al. (1998). Functional MRI lateralization of memory in temporal lobe epilepsy. Neurology 50: 926–932.

Federico P, Abbott DF, Briellmann RF et al. (2005). Functional MRI of the pre-ictal state. Brain 128: 1811–1817.

Fernandez G, de Greiff A, von Oertzen J et al. (2001). Language mapping in less than 15 minutes: real-time functional MRI during routine clinical investigation. Neuroimage 14: 585–594.

FitzGerald DB, Cosgrove GR, Ronner S et al. (1997). Location of language in the cortex: a comparison between functional MR imaging and electrocortical stimulation. AJNR Am J Neuroradiol 18: 1529–1539.

Fox PT, Raichle ME (1986). Focal physiological uncoupling of cerebral blood flow and oxidative metabolism during somatosensory stimulation of human subjects. Proc Natl Acad Sci U S A 323: 806–809.

Frey S, Campbell JSW, Pike GB et al. (2008). Dissociating the human language pathways with high angular resolution diffusion fiber tractography. J Neurosci 28: 11435.

Gaillard WD (2004). Functional MR imaging of language, memory, and sensorimotor cortex. Neuroimaging Clin N Am 14: 471–485.

Gaillard WD, Fazilat S, White S et al. (1995). Interictal metabolism and blood flow are uncoupled in temporal lobe cortex of patients with complex partial epilepsy. Neurology 45: 1841–1847.

Gaillard WD, Hertz-Pannier L, Mott SH et al. (2000). Functional anatomy of cognitive development: fMRI of verbal fluency in children and adults. Neurology 54: 180–185.

Gaillard WD, Pugliese M, Grandin CB et al. (2001). Cortical localization of reading in normal children: an fMRI language study. Neurology 57: 47–54.

Gaillard WD, Balsamo L, Xu B et al. (2002). Language dominance in partial epilepsy patients identified with an fMRI reading task. Neurology 59: 256–265.

Gaillard WD, Balsamo LM, Ibrahim Z et al. (2003). fMRI identifies regional specialization of neural networks for reading in young children. Neurology 60: 94–100.

Gaillard WD, Balsamo L, Xu B et al. (2004). fMRI language task panel improves determination of language dominance. Neurology 63: 1403–1408.

Gaillard WD, Berl MM, Moore EN et al. (2007). Atypical language in lesional and nonlesional complex partial epilepsy. Neurology 69: 1761–1771.

Geschwind N, Levitsky W (1968). Human brain: left–right asymmetries in temporal speech region. Science 161: 186–187.

Golby AJ, Poldrack RA, Brewer JB et al. (2001). Material-specific lateralization in the medial temporal lobe and prefrontal cortex during memory encoding. Brain 124: 1841–1854.

Golby AJ, Poldrack RA, Illes J et al. (2002). Memory lateralization in medial temporal lobe epilepsy assessed by functional MRI. Epilepsia 43: 855–863.

Gotman J (2008). Epileptic networks studied with EEG-fMRI. Epilepsia 49: 42–51.

Guye M, Parker GJ, Symms M et al. (2003). Combined functional MRI and tractography to demonstrate the connectivity of the human primary motor cortex in vivo. Neuroimage 19: 1349–1360.

Hadac J, Brozová K, Tintera J et al. (2007). Language lateralization in children with pre- and postnatal epileptogenic lesions of the left hemisphere: an fMRI study. Epileptic Disord 9: S19–S27.

Hammeke TA, Yetkin FZ, Mueller WM et al. (1994). Functional magnetic resonance imaging of somatosensory stimulation. Neurosurgery 35: 677–681.

Helmstaedter C, Fritz NE, Gonzalez Perez PA et al. (2006). Shift-back of right into left hemisphere language dominance after control of epileptic seizures: evidence for epilepsy driven functional cerebral organization. Epilepsy Res 70: 257–262.

Hertz-Pannier L, Gaillard WD, Mott SH et al. (1997). Noninvasive assessment of language dominance in children and adolescents with functional MRI: a preliminary study. Neurology 48: 1003–1012.

Holland SK, Plante E, Byars A et al. (2001). Normal fMRI brain activation patterns in children performing a verb generation task. Neuroimage 14: 837–843.

Holland SK, Vannest J, Mecoli M et al. (2007). Functional MRI of language lateralization during development in children. Int J Audiol 46: 533–551.

Hunter KE, Blaxton TA, Bookheimer SY et al. (1999). (15)O water positron emission tomography in language localization: a study comparing positron emission tomography visual and computerized region of interest analysis with the Wada test. Ann Neurol 45: 662–665.

Jack CR, Thompson RM, Butts RK et al. (1994). Sensory motor cortex: correlation of presurgical mapping with functional MR imaging and invasive cortical mapping. Radiology 190: 85–92.

Jackson GD, Connelly A, Cross JH et al. (1994). Functional magnetic resonance imaging of focal seizures. Neurology 44: 850–856.

Jansen JF, Aldenkamp AP, Marian Majoie HJ et al. (2006). Functional MRI reveals declined prefrontal cortex activation in patients with epilepsy on topiramate therapy. Epilepsy Behav 9: 181–185.

Janszky J, Jokeit H, Kontopoulou K et al. (2005). Functional MRI predicts memory performance after right mesiotemporal epilepsy surgery. Epilepsia 46: 244–250.

Jayakar P, Bernal B, Santiago Medina L et al. (2002). False lateralization of language cortex on functional MRI after a cluster of focal seizures. Neurology 58: 490–492.

Jokeit H, Okujava M, Woermann FG (2001). Memory fMRI lateralizes temporal lobe epilepsy. Neurology 57: 1786–1793.

Just MA, Carpenter PA, Keller TA et al. (1996). Brain activation modulated by sentence comprehension. Science 274: 114–116.

Kennepohl S, Sziklas V, Garver KE et al. (2007). Memory and the medial temporal lobe: hemispheric specialization reconsidered. Neuroimage 36: 969–978.

Kho KH, Leijten FS, Rutten GJ et al. (2005). Discrepant findings for Wada test and functional magnetic resonance imaging with regard to language function: use of electrocortical stimulation mapping to confirm results. Case report. J Neurosurg 102: 169–173.

Kim SG, Ashe J, Georgopoulos AP et al. (1993). Functional imaging of human motor cortex at high magnetic field. J Neurophysiol 69: 297–302.

Kobayashi E, Bagshaw AP, Benar CG et al. (2006). Temporal and extratemporal BOLD responses to temporal lobe interictal spikes. Epilepsia 47: 343–354.

Krakow K, Woermann FG, Symms MR et al. (1999). EEG-triggered functional MRI of interictal epileptiform activity in patients with partial seizures. Brain 122: 1679–1688.

Krakow K, Lemieux L, Messina D et al. (2001). Spatio-temporal imaging of focal interictal epileptiform activity using EEG-triggered functional MRI. Epileptic Disord 3: 67–74.

Krings T, Topper R, Reinges MH et al. (2000). Hemodynamic changes in simple partial epilepsy: a functional MRI study. Neurology 54: 524–527.

Kwong KK, Belliveau JW, Chesler DA et al. (1992). Dynamic magnetic resonance imaging of human brain activity during primary sensory stimulation. Proc Natl Acad Sci U S A 89: 5675–5679.

Lanzenberger R, Wiest G, Geissler A et al. (2005). fMRI reveals functional cortex in a case of inconclusive Wada testing. Clin Neurol Neurosurg 107: 147–151.

Lee D, Swanson SJ, Sabsevitz DS et al. (2008). Functional MRI and Wada studies in patients with interhemispheric dissociation of language functions. Epilepsy Behav 13: 350–356.

Lehericy S, Cohen L, Bazin B et al. (2000a). Functional MR evaluation of temporal and frontal language dominance compared with the Wada test. Neurology 54: 1625–1633.

Lehericy S, Duffau H, Cornu P et al. (2000b). Correspondence between functional magnetic resonance imaging somatotopy and individual brain anatomy of the central region: comparison with intraoperative stimulation in patients with brain tumors. J Neurosurg 92: 589–598.

Lehericy S, Biondi A, Sourour N et al. (2002). Arteriovenous brain malformations: is functional MR imaging reliable for studying language reorganization in patients? Initial observations. Radiology 223: 672–682.

Lemieux L (2004). Electroencephalography-correlated functional MR imaging studies of epileptic activity. Neuroimaging Clin N Am 14: 487–506.

Liegeois F, Connelly A, Salmond CH et al. (2002). A direct test for lateralization of language activation using fMRI: comparison with invasive assessments in children with epilepsy. Neuroimage 17: 1861–1867.

Liegeois F, Connelly A, Cross JH et al. (2004). Language reorganization in children with early-onset lesions of the left hemisphere: an fMRI study. Brain 127: 1229–1236.

Liegeois F, Connelly A, Baldeweg T et al. (2008). Speaking with a single cerebral hemisphere: fMRI language organization after hemispherectomy in childhood. Brain Lang 106: 195–203.

Lim YM, Cho YW, Shamim S et al. (2008). Usefulness of pulsed arterial spin labeling MR imaging in mesial temporal lobe epilepsy. Epilepsy Res 82: 183–189.

Logothetis NK (2003). The underpinnings of the BOLD functional magnetic resonance imaging signal. J Neurosci 23: 3963–3971.

Mbwana J, Berl MM, Ritzl EK et al. (2009). Limitations to plasticity of language network reorganization in localization related epilepsy. Brain 132: 347–356.

Medina LS, Bernal B, Dunoyer C et al. (2005). Seizure disorders: functional MR imaging for diagnostic evaluation and surgical treatment – prospective study. Radiology 236: 247–253.

Medina LS, Bernal B, Ruiz J (2007). Role of functional MR in determining language dominance in epilepsy and nonepilepsy populations: a Bayesian analysis. Radiology 242: 94–100.

Moonen CTW, Bandettini PA (Eds.), (2000). Functional MRI. Springer, Heidelberg.

Morgan VL, Price RR, Arain A et al. (2004). Resting functional MRI with temporal clustering analysis for localization of epileptic activity without EEG. Neuroimage 21: 473–481.

Nelson L, Lapsiwala S, Haughton VM et al. (2002). Preoperative mapping of the supplementary motor area in patients harboring tumors in the medial frontal lobe. J Neurosurg 97: 1108–1114.

Pardo JV, Fox PT (1993). Preoperative assessment of the cerebral hemispheric dominance for language with CBF PET. Hum Brain Mapp 1: 57–68.

Pouratian N, Bookheimer SY, Rex DE et al. (2002). Utility of preoperative functional magnetic resonance imaging for identifying language cortices in patients with vascular malformations. J Neurosurg 97: 21–32.

Powell HW, Koepp MJ, Symms MR et al. (2005). Material-specific lateralization of memory encoding in the medial temporal lobe: blocked versus event-related design. Neuroimage 27: 231–239.

Powell HW, Richardson MP, Symms MR et al. (2007). Reorganization of verbal and nonverbal memory in temporal lobe epilepsy due to unilateral hippocampal sclerosis. Epilepsia 48: 1512–1525.

Powell HW, Parker GJ, Alexander DC et al. (2008a). Imaging language pathways predicts postoperative naming deficits. J Neurol Neurosurg Psychiatry 79: 327–330.

Powell HW, Richardson MP, Symms MR et al. (2008b). Preoperative fMRI predicts memory decline following anterior temporal lobe resection. J Neurol Neurosurg Psychiatry 79: 686–693.

Pujol J, Deus J, Losilla JM et al. (1999). Cerebral lateralization of language in normal left-handed people studied by functional MRI. Neurology 52: 1038–1043.

Rabin ML, Narayan VM, Kimberg DY et al. (2004). Functional MRI predicts post-surgical memory following temporal lobectomy. Brain 127: 2286–2298.

Ramsey NF, Sommer I, Rutten GJ et al. (2001). Combined analysis of language tasks in fMRI improves assessment of hemispheric dominance for language functions in individual subjects. Neuroimage 13: 719–733.

Rao SM, Binder JR, Bandettini PA et al. (1993). Functional magnetic resonance imaging of complex human movements. Neurology 43: 2311–2318.

Richardson MP, Strange BA, Duncan JS et al. (2003). Preserved verbal memory function in left medial temporal pathology involves reorganisation of function to right medial temporal lobe. Neuroimage 20: S112–S119.

Richardson MP, Strange BA, Thompson PJ et al. (2004). Preoperative verbal memory fMRI predicts post-operative memory decline after left temporal lobe resection. Brain 127: 2419–2426.

Ries ML, Boop FA, Griebel ML et al. (2004). Functional MRI and Wada determination of language lateralization: a case of crossed dominance. Epilepsia 45: 85–89.

Rosenberger LR, Zeck J, Berl MM et al. (2009). Interhemispheric and intrahemispheric language reorganization in complex partial epilepsy. Neurology 72: 1830–1836.

Rother J, Knab R, Hamzei F et al. (2002). Negative dip in BOLD fMRI is caused by blood flow–oxygen consumption uncoupling in humans. Neuroimage 15: 98–102.

Roux FE, Boulanouar K, Lotterie JA et al. (2003). Language functional magnetic resonance imaging in preoperative assessment of language areas: correlation with direct cortical stimulation. Neurosurgery 52: 1335–1345.

Rutten GJ, Ramsey NF, van Rijen PC et al. (2002a). fMRI-determined language lateralization in patients with unilateral or mixed language dominance according to the Wada test. Neuroimage 17: 447–460.

Rutten GJ, Ramsey NF, van Rijen PC et al. (2002b). Development of a functional magnetic resonance imaging protocol for intraoperative localization of critical temporoparietal language areas. Ann Neurol 51: 350–360.

Sabbah P, Chassoux F, Leveque C et al. (2003). Functional MR imaging in assessment of language dominance in epileptic patients. Neuroimage 18: 460–467.

Sabsevitz DS, Swanson SJ, Hammeke TA et al. (2003). Use of preoperative functional neuroimaging to predict language deficits from epilepsy surgery. Neurology 60: 1788–1792.

Schlosser MJ, Aoyagi N, Fulbright RK et al. (1998). Functional MRI studies of auditory comprehension. Hum Brain Mapp 6: 1–13.

Schlosser MJ, Luby M, Spencer DD et al. (1999). Comparative localization of auditory comprehension by using functional magnetic resonance imaging and cortical stimulation. J Neurosurg 91: 626–635.

Schwartz TH, Resor SR Jr De La Paz R et al. (1998). Functional magnetic resonance imaging localization of ictal onset to a dysplastic cleft with simultaneous sensorimotor mapping: intraoperative electrophysiological confirmation and postoperative follow-up: technical note. Neurosurgery 43: 639–644.

Smith ML, Bernal B, Duchowny M et al. (2004). Severity of focal cortical dysplasia and functional organization of the brain. Epilepsia 45: 357.

Souweidane MM, Kim KH, McDowall R et al. (1999). Brain mapping in sedated infants and young children with passive-functional magnetic resonance imaging. Pediatr Neurosurg 30: 86–92.

Spreer J, Arnold S, Quiske A et al. (2002). Determination of hemisphere dominance for language: comparison of frontal and temporal fMRI activation with intracarotid amytal testing. Neuroradiology 44: 467–474.

Springer JA, Binder JR, Hammeke TA et al. (1999). Language dominance in neurologically normal and epilepsy subjects: a functional MRI study. Brain 122: 2033–2046.

Staudt M, Grodd W, Niemann G et al. (2001). Early left periventricular brain lesions induce right hemispheric organization of speech. Neurology 57: 122–125.

Staudt M, Lidzba K, Grodd W et al. (2002). Right-hemispheric organization of language following early left-sided brain lesions: functional MRI topography. Neuroimage 16: 954–967.

Stern CE, Corkin S, Gonzalez RG et al. (1996). The hippocampal formation participates in novel picture encoding: evidence from functional magnetic resonance imaging. Proc Natl Acad Sci U S A 93: 8660–8665.

Symms MR, Allen PJ, Woermann FG et al. (1999). Reproducible localization of interictal epileptiform discharges using EEG-triggered fMRI. Phys Med Biol 44: N161–N168.

Talairach J, Tournoux P (1988). Co-planar Stereotaxic Atlas of the Human Brain: 3-Dimensional Proportional System – an Approach to Cerebral Imaging. Thieme Medical Publishers, New York.

Thivard L, Hombrouck J, du Montcel ST et al. (2005). Productive and perceptive language reorganization in temporal lobe epilepsy. Neuroimage 24: 841–851.

Weber B, Wellmer J, Reuber M et al. (2006). Left hippocampal pathology is associated with atypical language lateralization in patients with focal epilepsy. Brain 129: 346–351.

Wellmer J, Weber B, Urbach H et al. (2009). Cerebral lesions can impair fMRI-based language lateralization. Epilepsia 50: 2213–2224.

Woermann FG, Jokeit H, Luerding R et al. (2003). Language lateralization by Wada test and fMRI in 100 patients with epilepsy. Neurology 61: 699–701.

Wolf RL, Alsop DC, Levy-Reis I et al. (2001). Detection of mesial temporal lobe hypoperfusion in patients with temporal lobe epilepsy by use of arterial spin labeled perfusion MR imaging. AJNR Am J Neuroradiol 22: 1334–1341.

Wood AG, Saling MM, Abbott DF et al. (2001). A neurocognitive account of frontal lobe involvement in orthographic lexical retrieval: an fMRI study. Neuroimage 14: 162–169.

Wood AG, Harvey AS, Wellard RM et al. (2004). Language cortex activation in normal children. Neurology 63: 1035–1044.

Worthington C, Vincent DJ, Bryant AE et al. (1997). Comparison of functional magnetic resonance imaging for language localization and intracarotid speech amytal testing in presurgical evaluation for intractable epilepsy. Preliminary results. Stereotact Funct Neurosurg 69: 197–201.

Yerys BE, Jankowski KF, Shook D et al. (2009). The fMRI success rate of children and adolescents: typical development, epilepsy, attention deficit/hyperactivity disorder, and autism spectrum disorders. Hum Brain Mapp 30: 3426–3435.

Yetkin FZ, Swanson S, Fischer M et al. (1998). Functional MR of frontal lobe activation: comparison with Wada language results. AJNR Am J Neuroradiol 19: 1095–1098.

Yogarajah M, Powell HW, Parker GJ et al. (2008). Tractography of the parahippocampal gyrus and material specific memory impairment in unilateral temporal lobe epilepsy. Neuroimage 40: 1755–1764.

Yogarajah M, Focke NK, Bonelli S et al. (2009). Defining Meyer's loop–temporal lobe resections, visual field deficits and diffusion tensor tractography. Brain 132: 1656–1668.

Handbook of Clinical Neurology, Vol. 107 (3rd series)
Epilepsy, Part I
H. Stefan and W.H. Theodore, Editors

Chapter 25

Magnetic resonance spectroscopy in epilepsy

THILO HAMMEN[1]* AND RUBEN KUZNIECKY[2]

[1]*Neurological Clinic, University Hospital, Erlangen, Germany*

[2]*NYU Epilepsy Center, Department of Neurology, New York University School of Medicine, New York, NY, USA*

INTRODUCTION

Nuclear magnetic resonance spectroscopy (MRS) is a noninvasive method for detecting brain metabolites. MRS has been applied to the study of human disease for several decades. It has advanced the study of neurological disorders by providing a metabolic biopsy of the living brain. Although a large number of metabolites and enzymatic pathways can be studied with MRS, two main techniques have been applied to study epilepsy. The most common one is ^{1}H-MRS, in which compounds such as *N*-acetylaspartate (NAA), choline (Cho), creatine (Cr), myoinositol, γ-aminobutyric acid (GABA), and glutamate are detected. The second technique employs phosphorus (^{31}P), which provides information about the energetics of human tissue. Today, clinical ^{1}H-MRS can be carried out in routine MR scanners and at high field in research settings. This chapter reviews our current knowledge of MRS as applied to epilepsy.

BASICS OF MAGNETIC RESONANCE SPECTROSCOPY

MRS, like magnetic resonance imaging (MRI), uses the spin of the nuclei rotating in the presence of a magnetic field with the Larmor frequency $f = \gamma B_0$ parallel or antiparallel to the direction of B_0. The thermal excess spins can be excited with radiofrequency (RF) – pulses to induce an echo or free induction decay (FID) into a receiver coil. The FID contains information about the tissue obtained via the mathematical operation called Fourier transformation. Magnetic field gradients are used to encode spatial positions. The slice selection gradient is applied during the RF pulse and results in only a narrow region for which the frequency from the RF pulse is resonant. The phase-encoding gradient is applied between the RF pulse and the echo. The MR information is obtained by repeating the slice excitation and signal detection multiple times, each with a different amplitude of the phase-encoding gradient.

In contrast to MRI, MRS signals are detected without gradients for frequency encoding, because the information in frequency variation is needed for identification of the metabolites, as described below.

The local environment alters the effect of the applied magnetic field at the location of the nucleus. The effective magnetic field felt at the nucleus is the difference between the applied magnetic field B_0 and the field generated by the electrons in its neighborhood. The resonance frequency of the nucleus is then proportional to the effective magnetic field. The frequency difference is known as "chemical shift." The chemical shift is the most important parameter in MRS because it is unique with regard to the chemical environment, except for overlap and signal broadening, and is used to characterize the various metabolites.

The strength of the signal depends on the concentration of the metabolite; thus, signals from metabolites such as NAA are about 1/10 000 the intensity of the water signal in the proton spectra. The presence of this large water signal is essential for brain imaging but a problem for proton spectroscopy, because it complicates the detection of the smaller spectroscopic signals. Therefore, one needs to reduce the intensity of the water signal by special techniques ("water suppression"); a chemical shift selective (CHESS) presaturation pulse is used most commonly. Similarly, the signals from the relatively concentrated extracranial fat component are usually eliminated with one of the various methods of "spectral editing." Unlike MRI, in which the voxel size is usually $1 \times 1 \times 3$ mm^3 or less, MRS voxel sizes are typically $10 \times 10 \times 10$ mm^3 or larger, but can be smaller at higher field. Based on the number of measured voxels, MRS is divided into single-voxel spectroscopy (SVS) (Fig. 25.1) and chemical shift imaging (CSI) (Fig. 25.2).

*Correspondence to: Thilo Hammen, M.D., Epilepsiezentrum – Neurolgoische Klinik, Universitätsklinikum Erlangen, Schwabachanlage 6, 91054 Erlangen, Germany. E-mail: thilo.hammen@uk-erlangen.de

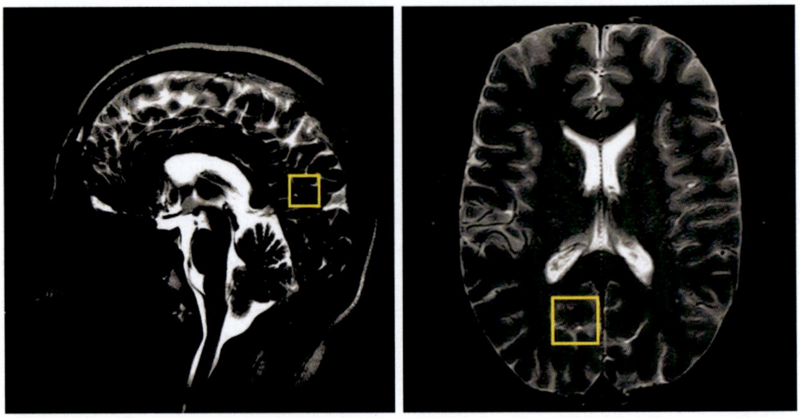

Fig. 25.1. Single-voxel spectroscopy.

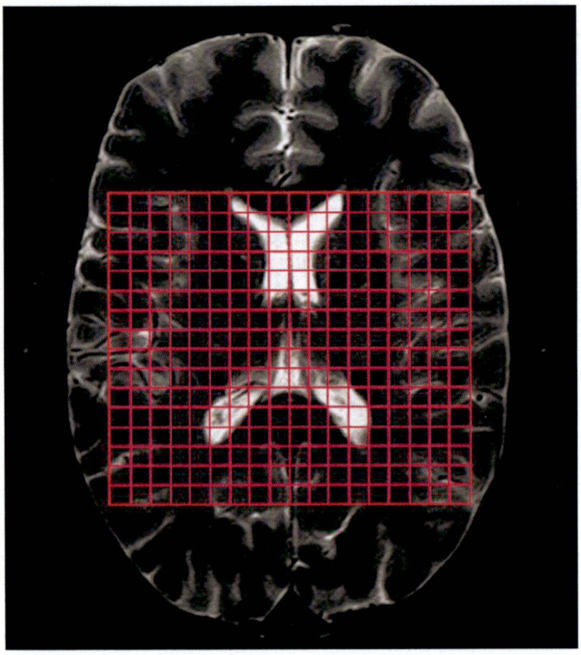

Fig. 25.2. Chemical shift imaging (multivoxel spectroscopy).

INTRACEREBRAL METABOLITES DETECTED BY CLINICAL ^{1}H-MRS AND THEIR CLINICAL SIGNIFICANCE

N-acetylaspartate compounds

NAA is the dominant peak in normal adult brain spectra. The *N*-acetylmethyl (CH_3) group of NAA provides the NAA peak at 2.02 parts per million (p.p.m.) (Fig. 25.3). NAA is thought to be a marker of neuronal/axonal density and viability. NAA, which is a cerebral amino acid, is specific for the central and peripheral nervous systems. Today, NAA is accepted as an objective marker for neuronal loss or dysfunction.

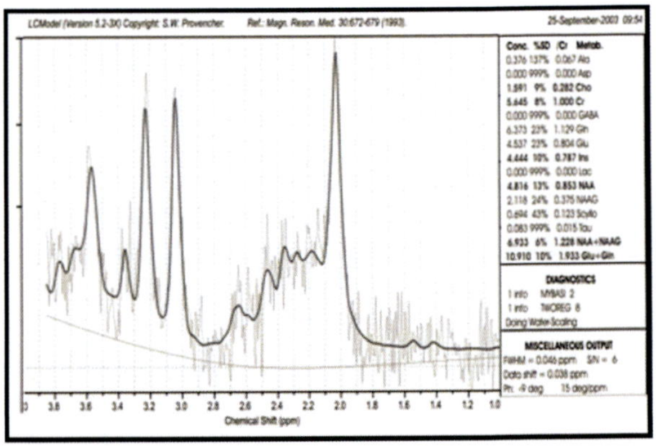

Fig. 25.3. Spectra of the hippocampus analyzed by LCModel. (Courtesy of S. Provencher.)

Creatine + phosphocreatine (Cr + PCr)

Cr and PCr are referred to as total Cr, which is used as an internal reference in ^{1}H-MRS. Concentrations of other brain metabolites are related to Cr because it is considered a relatively stable compound. The major peak of total Cr occurs at 3.02 p.p.m. (Fig. 25.3). The Cr peak is a marker for brain cell density in glial and neuronal cells, and is also correlated with brain energetics. This compound is found mainly in skeletal muscle, brain, and heart. Cr plays an important role in energy metabolism. Although found in all types of neuronal cell, Cr concentrations are greater in glial cells. Increased Cr parameters correlate with histopathologically diagnosed astrocytes and oligodendrocytes (glial cells), in which increased Cho and Cr levels are found.

Choline

Phosphorylcholine and glycerophosphorylcholine are the main metabolites that contribute to the choline resonance peak, located at 3.2 p.p.m. (Fig. 25.3). Cho is mainly bound to cell membranes and myelin. Cho, which is involved in the synthesis and decomposition of cell membranes, is a marker for membrane damage and gliosis. In adults, increased Cho levels reflect diseases that affect membrane turnover. Increased Cho is correlated to astrocytes and oligodendrocytes in which increased Cho and Cr levels are found. Increased Cho may reflect myelin breakdown, increased cell density, or gliosis. Increased Cho levels may indicate Alzheimer's disease, epilepsy and tumors (gliomas I–IV).

Myoinositol

The myoinositol peak is located at 3.6 p.p.m. in the ^{1}H-MRS spectrum (Fig. 25.3). Myoinositol is a sugar-like molecule, detected in brain and kidney. It is located in astrocytes, in which the molecule is an important osmolyte and cell volume generator. Myoinositol is a glial marker. Increased levels represent glial changes and osmolarity disturbances such as hypernatremia and/or dehydration.

Glutamate and glutamine (Glx)

Because of a large overlap of the peaks of glutamate and glutamine, these metabolites cannot be measured unequivocally at 1.5 Tesla (T). To distinguish glutamate from glutamine, higher field strengths (3–7 T) and special editing sequences are necessary. The Glx peaks are defined between 2.15 and 2.45 p.p.m. Glx is needed for neurotransmission. Increased levels of Glx have neurotoxic potential. Glx is an epileptogenic excitatory neurotransmitter.

γ-Aminobutyric acid

To detect GABA, high field strengths (3 T or above) are necessary. The small coupled spectral peaks of GABA are located at 3.02 p.p.m., which is overlapped by intense resonances of NAA, Cr, and Glx. Unfortunately, the use of *in vivo* ^{1}H-MRS to study GABA is complicated by the proton resonances of GABA being overlapped by the larger resonances of Cr, Glx, and NAA, as well as resonances from macromolecules. Over the past decade special sequences have been developed to avoid signal overlap, although technical implementation remains difficult. The concentration of GABA in cortical gray matter is extremely low (approximately 1 mmol/L *in vivo*), making reliable quantification of GABA extremely difficult. To assess the GABA peak properly, these surrounding signals have to be edited out by special editing sequences and the use of multiple quantum filters. GABA is an inhibitory neurotransmitter which prevents and terminates epileptic seizures. GABA and Glx probably define the epileptic focus in biochemical terms.

CLINICAL APPLICATION OF ^{1}H-MRS IN EPILEPSY

^{1}H-MRS in extratemporal epilepsy

^{1}H-MRS plays an increasing role in the clinical diagnosis and evaluation of therapeutic strategies in patients with epilepsy (Cendes et al., 1997; Vermathen et al., 1997; Achten, 1998; Hajek et al., 1998; Kuzniecky et al., 1998; Hammen et al., 2003). Most studies were carried out in patients with temporal lobe epilepsy (TLE), because TLE is the most common focal epilepsy. The ^{1}H-MRS abnormalities found in temporal lobes of patients with mesial temporal sclerosis led investigators to examine patients with epilepsy of extratemporal origin, particularly nonlesional frontal lobe epilepsy (Garcia et al., 1995; Stanley et al., 1998; Lundbom et al., 2001). A few of these studies showed reduced NAA/Cr or NAA/Cho ratios in the affected frontal lobe compared with the homologous nonepileptic contralateral region. Compared with normal controls, reduced NAA ratios can be detected in both frontal lobes, also including the homologous region of the contralateral frontal lobe. Reduction is most distinct in the hemisphere in which the seizure focus is localized. The results demonstrate that ^{1}H-MRS in general is able to lateralize the frontoparietal epileptogenic focus in patients with no pathological findings on MRI. Furthermore, the results of these studies provide evidence that epileptogenic seizures are based on a widespread neuronal dysfunction that exceeds the epileptogenic foci detected by EEG and spreads to the nonepileptic frontal lobe, which also demonstrated altered metabolite ratios compared with controls. Unfortunately, owing to limited brain coverage and large voxel size, the localization power of ^{1}H-MRS in extratemporal lobe epilepsy is very restricted.

^{1}H-MRS in temporal lobe epilepsies

The first studies performed more than a decade ago established the ability of ^{1}H-MRS to lateralize the seizure focus in temporal lobes and to test the validity of the method with already established methods of focus localization, employing video-EEG as the "gold standard" as well as MRI volumetry (MRIV), fluorodeoxyglucose-positron emission tomography (FDG-PET), and single-photon emission computed tomography (SPECT). Hugg et al. (1993) demonstrated a significant asymmetry of NAA left/right metabolite ratios. In all patients with TLE, lower NAA signals were observed in the affected hippocampal formation (Hugg et al., 1993). The reduced NAA signals were consistent with histopathological findings of mesial temporal sclerosis with selective neuronal loss and gliosis. Further studies demonstrated similar results. These studies demonstrated a decrease in NAA in the affected temporal lobe of patients with TLE.

In general, the results can be distinguished into three groups. Most authors found a decrease in NAA/Cr or NAA/Cho + Cr ratio ipsilateral to the EEG focus (Cendes et al., 1994; Gadian et al., 1994; Cross et al., 1996). The second group reported reduced concentrations of NAA with no significant changes in the levels of Cr or Cho (Hugg et al., 1993; Knowlton et al., 1997). Finally, single increases of Cho and Cr ipsilateral to the focus have been reported in few cases as well (Cendes et al., 1994; Connelly et al., 1998). The different results are probably based on different measurements, field strength, postprocessing techniques, and heterogeneous patient groups. Kuzniecky et al. (1998) investigated the validity of ^{1}H-MRS in lateralizing the pathological area before surgery in 30 consecutive patients with TLE with mesial temporal lobe sclerosis on MRI. Volumetry correctly lateralized 93% of patients, compared with 97% for ^{1}H-MRS. Incorrect lateralization compared with EEG was found by volumetry in two patients, and by ^{1}H-MRS in one patient. Concordance between the described MRI modalities was 73%. No correlation was found between the degree of hippocampal volume loss and the degree of metabolic disturbance in ^{1}H-MRS. Comparable results were described by Cendes et al. (1997), who investigated 100 consecutive patients with intractable mesial TLE. An asymmetry index for NAA/Cr values of temporal lobes was calculated. This study likewise found that the EEG, MRIV findings, and ^{1}H-MRS were highly concordant. ^{1}H-MRS was abnormal in 99 of 100 patients, demonstrating bilateral changes in 54%. Correct lateralization was obtained in 86% of patients with single-proton spectroscopy. MRIV was abnormal in 86 of 98 patients, with bilateral changes in 28%. Correct lateralization was obtained in 83% using MRIV alone and in 90% using combined MRIV and ^{1}H-MRS (versus 93% lateralization by EEG). In addition to lateralization of the affected hemisphere, ^{1}H-MRS proved to be a sensible method for detecting bilateral dysfunction. In some patients, NAA/Cr values in the contralateral temporal lobe were also reduced compared with homologous regions of controls. In general, the reduction of NAA/Cr ratio was less pronounced in the contralateral lobe. The degree of asymmetry of NAA/Cr ratios correlated with the degree of one-sidedness of EEG abnormalities. The asymmetry ratios were less pronounced in patients with more frequent bilateral (ictal and interictal) EEG abnormalities. These results support the fact that ^{1}H-MRS is a valid method even in bilateral focus detection, giving high concordance with the degree of bilateral EEG findings in patients with TLE.

In another correlative study, Knowlton et al. (1997) compared results of FDG-PET with those of ^{1}H-MRS at 1.5 T in focus localization in 23 patients with TLE and no lesional findings on MRI. PET had a concordance of 87% with no discordant results; MRV showed a 65% and ^{1}H-MRS a 61% concordance. In patients with hippocampal atrophy, PET was sensitive in 75% and ^{1}H-MRS in 50%. The combination of ^{1}H-MRS and MRIV demonstrated comparable lateralization sensitivity to FDG-PET. Bilateral abnormalities were detected in 17% with volumetric studies and in 33% with ^{1}H-MRS. Doelken et al. (2007) compared video-EEG monitoring in 49 patients with TLE with high-resolution MRI, ^{1}H-MRS, and SPECT. Some 25 patients had evidence of hippocampal sclerosis in MRI (MRI-positive) and 24 demonstrated no pathological findings on MRI (MRI-negative). Twenty-two of 25 patients with TLE and evidence of hippocampal sclerosis were graded as unilateral by EEG findings, whereas 3 were classified as bilateral. Of 24 MRI-negative patients, 14 were graded as unilateral by EEG and 10 as bitemporal. ^{1}H-MRS indicated concordant lateralization compared with EEG in 82% of MRI-positive patients and in 71% of MRI-negative patients. ^{1}H-MRS indicated concordance with SPECT in 84% of MRI-positive patients and 67% of MRI-negative patients with TLE. In unilateral TLE, the concordance rate for both modalities was 74% for MRI-positive patients and 67% for MRI-negative patients. Contralateral findings to EEG focus were found in 28% by ^{1}H-MRS and in 27% by SPECT. The data demonstrate that multimodal imaging in patients with TLE improves lateralization of affected hemispheres, especially in patients without pathological findings on MRI also indicating bilateral dysfunction.

^{1}H-MRS in assessment of MRI-negative TLE

Up to 30% of patients with intractable TLE have normal findings on MRI. Lateralization of the affected temporal lobe in this group remains a challenge. Multimodal focus localization in which clinical features are added to imaging techniques seems to be a promising approach in this patient group. The results of multiple studies investigating the role of ^{1}H-MRS in MRI-negative patients have shown a reduction of NAA in the affected hemisphere (Achten et al., 1997; Connelly et al., 1998; Woermann et al., 1999; Simister et al., 2002). NAA reduction is most likely based on neuronal dysfunction rather than tissue lesions, because high-resolution MRI shows no evidence of hippocampal atrophy or lesional alterations in temporomesial structures. Hammen et al. (2006) reported a study in which 22 consecutive patients diagnosed with TLE were investigated by high-resolution MRI and ^{1}H-MRS. The results of metabolite alterations were correlated with scalp EEG. Reduction of NAA in the affected hemisphere was found in 66% of patients with unilateral TLE. Group comparison revealed a significant reduction of NAA in the involved temporal lobe compared with controls. Cho levels were significantly increased in the affected hemisphere compared with levels in healthy controls. The results of this study and others indicate that ^{1}H-MRS can provide valuable information for assessing the affected hemisphere in MRI-negative TLE. Although there is evidence for a clear tendency of reduced NAA in the involved hemisphere, it should be noted that ^{1}H-MRS demonstrates only moderate sensitivity in hemispheric lateralization in this patient group. ^{1}H-MRS should therefore be used only as an additional tool in combination with clinical features, high-resolution MRI, intensive EEG monitoring, and, if possible, SPECT and PET in terms of multimodal focus localization, especially if surgery is being considered.

Distinguishing subgroups of TLE by ^{1}H-MRS

The Commission on Classification and Terminology of the International Classification of Epilepsy Syndromes (1989) distinguishes between mesiobasal temporal lobe epilepsy (MBTLE) and lateral (neocortical) temporal lobe epilepsy (NCTLE). Differentiation of the various subgroups by clinical features, EEG, MRI, SPECT, or FDG-PET is still difficult. Vermathen et al. (1997) investigated NAA changes in the hippocampal formation in neocortical and mesial TLE. The authors compared NAA levels in patients with unilateral mesial TLE with levels in patients with neocortical epilepsy. They found that alterations of hippocampal NAA were able to differentiate mesiobasal TLE from neocortical TLE. The patients with mesial TLE showed a significantly marked reduction of NAA in the hippocampal formation. In the neocortical epilepsy group, NAA was reduced in neither the ipsilateral nor the contralateral hippocampus. These results are similar to those of others (Hammen et al., 2003; Riederer et al., 2006). In these studies, hippocampal metabolite alterations were greater in patients with a mesiobasal focus compared with those in the lateral neocortical TLE group. This suggests that the absence of spectroscopic abnormalities in the hippocampus of temporal neocortical epilepsies may help to distinguish them from mesiotemporal lobe epilepsies. The fact that neither the ipsilateral nor the contralateral hippocampus of patients with neocortical TLE showed significant metabolic alterations supports the notion that neocortical TLE is neither caused by nor does it lead to hippocampal alterations. The findings of ^{1}H-MRS underline the utility of the classification system of TLE mentioned above.

Predictors of surgical outcome using ^{1}H-MRS in intractable TLE

Although the significance of bilateral, diffuse metabolite alterations is poorly understood, they may have important influence on therapeutic strategies. A number of investigators (Kuzniecky et al., 1999; Eberhardt et al., 2000; Stefan et al., 2000) have demonstrated that bilateral metabolite alterations in patients with TLE with hippocampal sclerosis have a predictive value for postoperative outcome. Patients demonstrating severe bilateral or even metabolic changes contralateral to the planned hippocampectomy had a poorer postoperative seizure outcome than those demonstrating unilateral metabolite alterations ipsilateral to the hemisphere in which surgery was performed. Kuzniecky et al. (1999) investigated the spectral metabolite alterations in 40 consecutive patients who underwent temporal lobe surgery for mesial TLE. The postoperative outcome was analyzed after 24 months and was classified as seizure-free or not seizure-free. A poor postoperative outcome was associated with contralateral or bitemporal abnormalities of ^{1}H-MRS spectra. Comparable results were reported by Eberhardt et al. (2000), who evaluated the significance of preoperative bilateral spectral changes for the prognosis of postoperative seizure outcome. ^{1}H-MRS was performed in 26 consecutive patients with TLE prior to epilepsy surgery. Discriminant analysis of ipsilateral and contralateral CSI was performed. The NAA/Cho ratios were determined from the hippocampal regions of both hemispheres and were correlated to results in healthy controls. The results indicated that contralateral changes in ^{1}H-MRS are a good predictor of poor seizure outcome, whereby 92% of patients who became seizure-free had no severe bilateral metabolic deviations and were classified correctly by means of this method.

Focal unilateral metabolite abnormalities that are in agreement with the EEG focus indicate a good prognostic outcome, whereas contralateral or widespread, bilateral abnormal metabolite spectra are associated with a poor postoperative outcome. Nevertheless, in some cases of bilateral disease, one hemisphere is still the leader in the initiation of most seizures. It is important to be aware that the hemisphere with the greatest MRS abnormality is not always the side of seizure origin. The rate of false localization by spectroscopy alone may be as high as 10–15%. For this reason, a multimodal imaging approach including EEG, MRIV, PET, SPECT, and, if possible, myeloencephalography (MEG) should be undertaken. If these methods provide concordant information concerning focus localization, a seizure-free outcome after surgery is likely. In cases of discrepancy and bilateral findings of seizure origin with these methods, the likelihood of a favorable outcome is reduced.

Correlation between metabolite alterations in ^{1}H-MRS and histopathology

Several studies correlated spectral metabolite alterations with histopathological alterations. This is an important topic because it helps us to understand the role of spectral metabolites and what metabolite alterations in ^{1}H-MRS indicate. There are only a few studies that have correlated spectral alterations with histopathological findings of hippocampal sclerosis, which is the most common lesion in patients with mesial TLE (Hugg et al., 1993; Duc et al., 1998; Stefan et al., 2001; Cohen-Gadol et al., 2004). Hugg et al. (1993) found that focal NAA reductions were based on findings of mesial temporal sclerosis in surgically resected epileptogenic foci. NAA reductions correlated with selective neuron loss and gliosis. Similar findings were reported by Duc et al. (1998). A reduction in NAA before surgery showed a high correlation with the degree of hippocampal sclerosis, reflecting neuronal loss. However, these studies were qualitative in nature, making a correlation difficult. Another study gave similar results (Hammen et al., 2008). Spectral metabolite alterations in hippocampal sclerosis correlated with the degree of segmental neuronal cell loss and amount of astrogliosis, as indicated by astroglial fibrillary acidic protein (GFAP) expression. A positive correlation was found between the reduction in NAA and the reduction of neuronal density in hippocampal CA1, CA3, and CA4 subfields and in the dentate gyrus. Neuronal cell loss in CA1 was found to be the most predictive. A positive association was found between myoinositol increase and hippocampal gliosis, as determined by GFAP expression. Significantly increased myoinositol levels were associated with diffuse hippocampal astrogliosis. However, another quantitative study by Kuzniecky et al. (2001) found a strong correlation between MRI hippocampal volumes and neuronal/glial ratios but no correlation between NAA and neuronal/glial abnormalities. Thus, current data is conflicting and further studies are needed to resolve the divergent results.

Monitoring of intracerebral GABA by ^{1}H-MRS for assessment of conservative treatment schedules

Increasing cerebral GABA is one of multiple mechanisms of action of anticonvulsant drugs. Recent *in vivo* ^{1}H-MRS studies have demonstrated that increased GABA occurs following the administration of certain anticonvulsants in humans. Determination of intracerebral GABA by ^{1}H-MRS contributes to the understanding of epileptogenesis and mechanisms of action of antiepileptic drugs. GABA is an inhibitory transmitter. Up to now, spectral *in vivo* GABA measurements have been undertaken to monitor GABA levels following antiepileptic drug administration. Petroff et al. (1996, 1998) carried out several studies that investigated human brain GABA levels under the influence of vigabatrin therapy. Vigabatrin increases the level of brain GABA by irreversibly inhibiting GABA transaminase. In one study, patients were treated with vigabatrin 50 mg per kg per day. Single-voxel spectroscopy was carried out in the occipital lobe before, 2 hours after vigabatrin intake, and 1, 5, and 8 days after the initial titration. Some 2 hours after vigabatrin administration the GABA peak increased by more than 40%. A further moderate increase of intracerebral GABA was detected on the day after the first titration. In the course of titration, levels of GABA declined gradually from day 5 to day 8. This study supports the notion that vigabatrin offers prompt protection against further seizures by raising GABA levels. In a second study the authors also investigated an increase in the levels of homocarnosine (a dipeptide of GABA), which is also thought to be an inhibitory neuromodulator. Daily low-dose administration of vigabatrin (2 g) increased both metabolites, GABA and homocarnosine, whereas larger doses of vigabatrin (4 g) further increased homocarnosine but changed GABA levels only minimally. In general, seizure control improved with increasing homocarnosine and GABA concentrations. The authors found that improved seizure control with vigabatrin therapy was associated with higher mean homocarnosine levels in responders than in the nonresponder group. Responders and nonresponders did not differ in terms of the mean GABA level.

Mueller et al. (2003) investigated responder profiles in patients who were treated with vigabatrin by analyzing GABA+ (including homocarnosine and macromolecules) to a Cr ratio (GABA+/Cr). Spectral measurements were performed before and after a titration period of 1 and 3 months. The authors correlated clinical responder groups depending on the therapeutic efficacy of vigabatrin with changes in the GABA+/Cr signal. The nonresponders (patients who showed no increase in seizure reduction with vigabatrin) demonstrated no significant increase in the GABA+/Cr signal compared with baseline during the whole treatment. The full responders demonstrated a significant increase in the GABA+/Cr signal during the whole treatment phase in month 1 and month 3 after the start of vigabatrin titration. Compared with non or partial responders, the GABA level was lower at baseline before antiepileptic medication. The partial responders also showed lower ipsilateral GABA+/Cr signals before antiepileptic drug treatment. The GABA+/Cr ratio increased at the beginning of the treatment (1 month after titration) and decreased when seizures under antiepileptic medication started again after 3 months.

More recent studies have investigated other antiepileptic drugs and their influence on GABA metabolites. Kuzniecky et al. (2002) investigated the modulation of cerebral GABA by topiramate, lamotrigine, and gabapentin in 17 healthy adults. Spectral GABA was measured from a 13.5-mL volume over the occipital lobe using a 4.1-T magnet. GABA measurements were undertaken 3 and 6 hours after administration of an acute single drug dose. Drugs were titrated to target doses within a time period of 4 weeks. Additional GABA measurements were performed at 2 and 4 weeks for each antiepileptic drug. Compared with baseline in the acute phase, cerebral GABA concentrations rose by 70% for topiramate and by 48% for gabapentin at 6 hours after drug administration. Lamotrigine did not result in an increase of intracerebral GABA in the acute titration period. In long-term dosing, after 4 weeks, there was a significant increase in GABA compared with baseline for all three drugs (topiramate, 46%; gabapentin, 25%; lamotrigine, 25%). The study showed that topiramate and gabapentin increased cerebral GABA within 6 hours after drug administration, whereas GABA levels achieved at 4 weeks of drug titration resulted in a spectral cerebral GABA increase for all three drugs. More recently, another study using similar methods showed no changes in brain GABA concentrations after the addition of levetiracetam (Kuzniecky et al., 2008).

^{31}P SPECTROSCOPY

Unlike ^{1}H spectra where the abundance of the ^{1}H resonance provides a vast array of resonances, the ^{31}P spectrum is limited in its content reflecting five primary groups of resonances: phosphocreatine (PCr), inorganic phosphate (Pi), adenosine triphosphate (ATP), and phosphomonoesters (PME) and phosphodiesters (PDE) (Fig. 25.4). Thus, although limited in the types of resonance that can be measured, the ^{31}P spectrum provides great detail with regard to the bioenergetic status of the tissue (PCr, ATP, and Pi). This has proven to be useful in studies of TLE, where marked energetic impairment, decreased PCr/Pi, and PCr/ATP are present in both the ipsilateral and contralateral hippocampi. Additionally, due to the chemical exchange characteristics of the Pi resonance, pH can be determined from its chemical shift. Similarly, although less used, the free magnesium content can be determined from the chemical shift of the β-ATP resonance. The PDE and PME resonances give information about lipid head groups.

Owing to the relatively large chemical shift range and the relatively low number of major resonances, the ^{31}P spectrum is relatively free of spectral overlap such that advanced methods of spectral editing are not required. Thus, methodologically, ^{31}P spectra are relatively easy to acquire and analyze. However, due to its decreased gyromagnetic ratio, and the relatively low brain concentrations (<4 mmol/L), the available signal to noise ratio (SNR) in the ^{31}P spectrum is limited. Thus, the primary challenges for ^{31}P spectroscopy in the brain are: (1) to achieve an adequate SNR in localized spectra; and (2) to compensate for the effects of tissue heterogeneity.

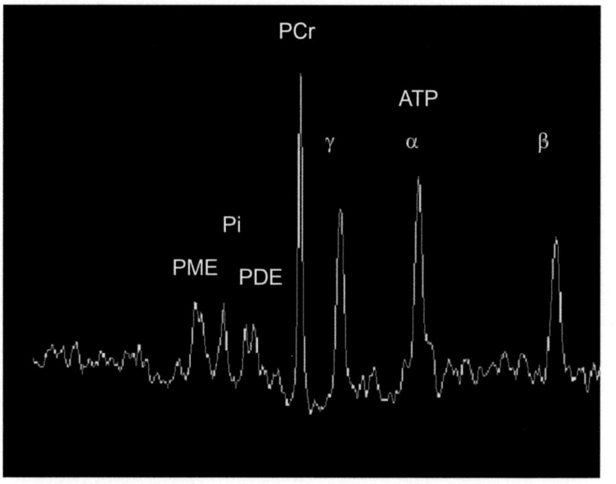

Fig. 25.4. Example of a ^{31}P spectrum acquired from the human brain using a 3.4-mL nominal voxel. ATP, adenosine triphosphate; PCr, phosphocreatine; PDE, phosphodiesters; Pi, inorganic phosphate; PME, phosphomonoesters.

Spectroscopic imaging

A major advantage of ^{31}P spectroscopy is the ability to image the entire brain. At 4 T and above, nominal volume sizes of 10–12 mL are possible with volume head coils with acquisition times of less than 1 hour. Figure 25.4 gives an example of a ^{31}P spectrum acquired from the human brain using a 3.4-mL nominal voxel. In this spectrum the resonances of PCr, ATP, Pi, PDE and PME are all well resolved and easily quantifiable. Despite the spectral quality, three additional factors can limit the interpretability of the ^{31}P data: (1) the spatial distribution of tissue contributing to the acquired voxel; (2) natural tissue heterogeneity in the ^{31}P spectrum; and (3) the coarseness of the spectroscopic imaging grid. However, there are methods to deal with these technical issues.

^{31}P-magnetic resonance spectroscopy in epilepsy

^{31}P-MRS allows evaluation of the energetic state of the brain, by providing a measure of nucleoside triphosphates (predominantly ATP), PCr, PME, PDE, and Pi in brain tissue (Buchli et al., 1994). Information about the levels of high-energy phosphate metabolites is derived from ATP and PCr. Typically the PCr/ATP ratio is quoted as an indicator of the tissue energy status. Although cerebral ATP is depleted only under severe metabolic conditions, changes in PCr have been observed with ^{31}P-MRS following neuronal activity (Sappey-Marinier et al., 1992). The PME peak predominantly comprises phosphatidylethanolamine, phosphatidylcholine (precursors of cell membranes; Bretscher, 1972). The PDE resonance includes glycerophosphatidylcholine (GPCh), glycerophosphatidylethanolamine (GPEth), and mobile phospholipids. The GPCh and GPEth represent membrane breakdown products (Bretscher, 1972), but the majority of the signal (> 80%) probably originates from intracellular mobile phospholipids. Additionally, the chemical shift of the Pi resonance provides an excellent measure of intracellular pH (pHi) (Gadian et al., 1982). Changes in the relative PME and PDE concentrations have been associated with membrane turnover (Bluml et al., 1999). Figure 25.5 shows phosphorus and proton spectra obtained at very high field strengths of 7 T and above. These studies were performed on excised epileptogenic tissue.

Phosphoesters are of considerable interest because they represent precursors of membrane synthesis and breakdown products. However, these metabolites contain both protons and phosphorus in close proximity, and the components absorb energy from each other, making their MR detection, differentiation, and quantification difficult. It is possible to increase the sensitivity and improve the differentiation of phosphoesters by simultaneously transmitting two RF signals, one of which is tuned to the proton nuclei to disrupt the interaction between proton and phosphorus nuclei (known as decoupling). The increase in signal is greater than 50%, which is sufficient to allow quantitation of the different phosphoester components in the tissue. An added advantage of this technique is the reduction in time taken for data acquisition, reducing potential patient discomfort.

In ^{31}P-MRS studies of patients with epilepsy, changes in PCr can be expected. During and shortly after a seizure in animals, changes in pHi and high-energy phosphates may be found (Petroff et al., 1984). Interestingly, these metabolites have been reported to be abnormal in relatively seizure-free patients (Chu et al., 1998). ^{31}P-MRS also provides information on mobile PME and PDE associated with membranes (Gadian, 1995). ^{31}P-MRS has shown potential for lateralizing metabolic dysfunction (Chu et al., 1998). Decreased PCr/Pi was observed in 65–75% of patients with TLE (Laxer et al., 1992). This may relate to the timing of measurements relative to recent seizure activity. Altered ^{31}P metabolites and pHi have been reported in the postictal period. An important feature of the findings reported to date is that abnormalities are present in regions that are normal to a range of other measurements, including MRI.

Temporal lobe epilepsy and ^{31}P-MRS

Several groups have investigated a potential reduction in PCR/Pi in patients with TLE (Hugg et al., 1992; Kuzniecky et al., 1992; Laxer et al., 1992; van der Grond et al., 1998). In one study (Kuzniecky et al., 1992) there were significant differences between patients and

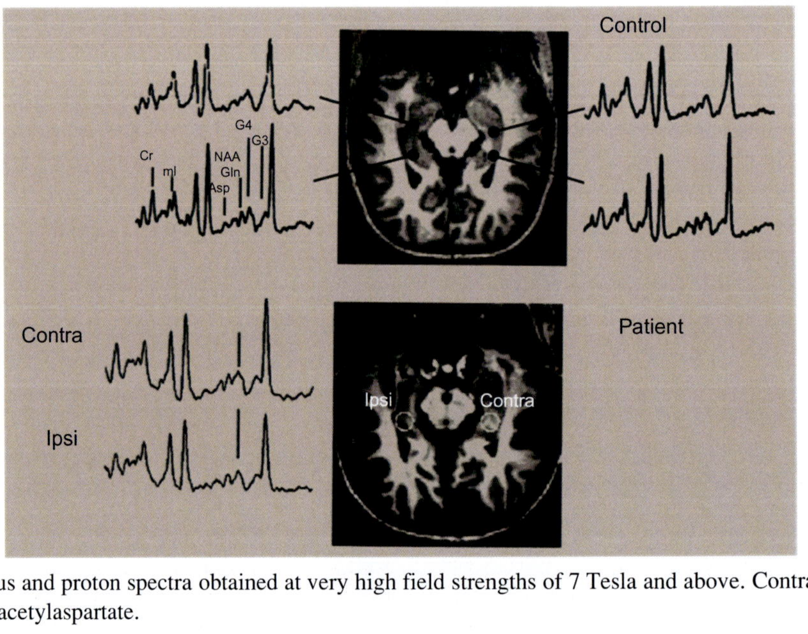

Fig. 25.5. Phosphorus and proton spectra obtained at very high field strengths of 7 Tesla and above. Contra, contralateral; Ipsi, ipsilateral; NAA, *N*-acetylaspartate.

controls with respect to the PCr/Pi ratio. However, no significant differences were found between patients and controls with respect to pH. In contrast, others have found an increase in pH, along with increased Pi and reduced PME in the ipsilateral temporal lobe (Hugg et al., 1992; van der Grond et al., 1998). Reduced ATP/Pi and PCr/Pi ratios in the temporal lobe were predictive for the side of the seizure focus in more than 70% of patients studied (Chu et al., 1998). More recently, high field studies (4.1 T) with excellent spectral resolution have indicated that pH is indeed normal in the interictal state.

References

Achten E (1998). Aspects of proton MR spectroscopy in the seizure patient. Neuroimaging Clin N Am 8: 849–862.

Achten E, Boon P, Van De Kerckhove T et al. (1997). Value of single-voxel proton MR spectroscopy in temporal lobe epilepsy. AJNR Am J Neuroradiol 18: 1131–1139.

Bluml S, Tan J, Harris K et al. (1999). Quantitative proton-decoupled ^{31}P MRS of the schizophrenic brain in vivo. J Comput Assist Tomogr 23: 272–275.

Bretscher MS (1972). Asymmetrical lipid bilayer structure for biological membranes. Nat New Biol 236: 11–12.

Buchli R, Duc CO, Martin E et al. (1994). Assessment of absolute metabolite concentrations in human tissue by 31P MRS in vivo. Part I: Cerebrum, cerebellum, cerebral gray and white matter. Magn Reson Med 32: 447–452.

Cendes F, Andermann F, Preul MC et al. (1994). Lateralization of temporal lobe epilepsy based on regional metabolic abnormalities in proton magnetic resonance spectroscopic images. Ann Neurol 35: 211–216.

Cendes F, Caramanos Z, Andermann F et al. (1997). Proton magnetic resonance spectroscopic imaging and magnetic resonance imaging volumetry in the lateralization of temporal lobe epilepsy: a series of 100 patients. Ann Neurol 42: 737–746.

Chu WJ, Hetherington HP, Kuzniecky RI et al. (1998). Lateralization of human temporal lobe epilepsy by ^{31}P NMR spectroscopic imaging at 4.1 T. Neurology 51: 472–479.

Cohen-Gadol AA, Pan JW, Jim JH et al. (2004). Mesial temporal lobe epilepsy: a proton magnetic resonance spectroscopy study and a histopathological analysis. J Neurosurg 101: 613–620.

Connelly A, Van Paesschen W, Porter DA et al. (1998). Proton magnetic resonance spectroscopy in MRI-negative temporal lobe epilepsy. Neurology 51: 61–66.

Cross JH, Connelly A, Jackson GD et al. (1996). Proton magnetic resonance spectroscopy in children with temporal lobe epilepsy. Ann Neurol 39: 107–113.

Doelken MT, Richter G, Stefan H et al. (2007). Multimodal coregistration in patients with temporal lobe epilepsy – results of different imaging modalities in lateralization of the affected hemisphere in MR imaging positive and negative subgroups. AJNR Am J Neuroradiol 28: 449–454.

Duc CO, Trabesinger AH, Weber OM et al. (1998). Quantitative ^{1}H MRS in the evaluation of mesial temporal lobe epilepsy in vivo. Magn Reson Imaging 16: 969–979.

Eberhardt KE, Stefan H, Buchfelder M et al. (2000). The significance of bilateral CSI changes for the postoperative outcome in temporal lobe epilepsy. J Comput Assist Tomogr 24: 919–926.

Gadian DG (1995). NMR and its Application to Living Systems. Oxford University Press, New York.

Gadian DG, Radda GK, Dawson MJ et al. (1982). pH Measurements of Cardiac and Skeletal Muscle Using ^{31}P NMR. Liss, New York.

Gadian DG, Connelly A, Duncan JS et al. (1994). ^{1}H magnetic resonance spectroscopy in the investigation of intractable epilepsy. Acta Neurol Scand Suppl 152: 116–121.

Garcia PA, Laxer KD, van der Grond J et al. (1995). Proton magnetic resonance spectroscopic imaging in patients with frontal lobe epilepsy. Ann Neurol 37: 279–281.

Hajek M, Dezortova M, Komárek V et al. (1998). ^{1}H MR spectroscopy in patients with mesial temporal epilepsy. MAGMA 7: 95–114.

Hammen T, Stefan H, Pauli E et al. (2003). ^{1}H-MR spectroscopy: a promising method in distinguishing subgroups in temporal lobe epilepsy? J Neurol Sci 215: 21–25.

Hammen T, Kerling F, Schwarz M et al. (2006). Identifying the affected hemisphere by (1)H-MR spectroscopy in patients with temporal lobe epilepsy and no pathological findings in high resolution MRI. Eur J Neurol 13: 482–490.

Hammen T, Hildebrandt M, Stadlbauer A et al. (2008). Non-invasive detection of hippocampal sclerosis: correlation between metabolite alterations detected by (1)H-MRS and neuropathology. NMR Biomed 21: 545–552.

Hugg JW, Matson GB, Twieg DB et al. (1992). Phosphorus-31 MR spectroscopic imaging (MRSI) of normal and pathological human brains. Magn Reson Imaging 10: 227–243.

Hugg JW, Laxer KD, Matson GB et al. (1993). Neuron loss localizes human temporal lobe epilepsy by in vivo proton magnetic resonance spectroscopic imaging. Ann Neurol 34: 788–794.

Knowlton RC, Laxer KD, Ende G et al. (1997). Presurgical multimodality neuroimaging in electroencephalographic lateralized temporal lobe epilepsy. Ann Neurol 42: 829–837.

Kuzniecky R, Elgavish GA, Hetherington HP et al. (1992). In vivo ^{31}P nuclear magnetic resonance spectroscopy of human temporal lobe epilepsy. Neurology 42: 1586–1590.

Kuzniecky R, Hugg JW, Hetherington H et al. (1998). Relative utility of ^{1}H spectroscopic imaging and hippocampal volumetry in the lateralization of mesial temporal lobe epilepsy. Neurology 51: 66–71.

Kuzniecky R, Hugg J, Hetherington H et al. (1999). Predictive value of ^{1}H MRSI for outcome in temporal lobectomy. Neurology 53: 694–698.

Kuzniecky R, Palmer C, Hugg J et al. (2001). Magnetic resonance spectroscopic imaging in temporal lobe epilepsy: neuronal dysfunction or cell loss? Arch Neurol 58: 2048–2053.

Kuzniecky R, Ho S, Pan J et al. (2002). Modulation of cerebral GABA by topiramate, lamotrigine, and gabapentin in healthy adults. Neurology 58: 368–372.

Kuzniecky R, Pan J, Burns A et al. (2008). Levetiracetam has no acute effects on brain GABA. Epilepsy Behav 12: 242–244.

Laxer KD, Hubesch B, Sappey-Marinier D et al. (1992). Increased pH and inorganic phosphate in temporal seizure foci demonstrated by [^{31}P]MRS. Epilepsia 33: 618–623.

Lundbom N, Gaily E, Vuori K et al. (2001). Proton spectroscopic imaging shows abnormalities in glial and neuronal cell pools in frontal lobe epilepsy. Epilepsia 42: 1507–1514.

Mueller SG, Weber OM, Duc CO et al. (2003). Effects of vigabatrin on brain GABA+/Cr signals in focus-distant and focus-near brain regions monitored by ^{1}H-NMR spectroscopy. Eur J Neurol 10: 45–52.

Petroff OA, Prichard JW, Behar KL et al. (1984). In vivo phosphorus nuclear magnetic resonance spectroscopy in status epilepticus. Ann Neurol 16: 169–177.

Petroff OA, Rothman DL, Behar KL et al. (1996). Human brain GABA levels rise rapidly after initiation of vigabatrin therapy. Neurology 47: 1567–1571.

Petroff OA, Mattson RH, Behar KL et al. (1998). Vigabatrin increases human brain homocarnosine and improves seizure control. Ann Neurol 44: 948–952.

Riederer F, Bittsansky M, Schmidt C et al. (2006). 1 H magnetic resonance spectroscopy at 3 T in cryptogenic and mesial temporal lobe epilepsy. NMR Biomed 19: 544–553.

Sappey-Marinier D, Calabrese G, Fein G et al. (1992). Effect of photic stimulation on human visual cortex lactate and phosphates using 1 H and 31P magnetic resonance spectroscopy. J Cereb Blood Flow Metab 12: 584–592.

Simister RJ, Woermann FG, McLean MA et al. (2002). A short-echo-time proton magnetic resonance spectroscopic imaging study of temporal lobe epilepsy. Epilepsia 43: 1021–1031.

Stanley JA, Cendes F, Dubeau F et al. (1998). Proton magnetic resonance spectroscopic imaging in patients with extratemporal epilepsy. Epilepsia 39: 267–273.

Stefan H, Pauli E, Eberhardt KE et al. (2000). MRI spectroscopy, T2 relaxometry, and postoperative prognosis in cryptogenic temporal lobe epilepsy. Nervenarzt 71: 282–287.

Stefan H, Feichtinger M, Pauli E et al. (2001). Magnetic resonance spectroscopy and histopathological findings in temporal lobe epilepsy. Epilepsia 42: 41–46.

van der Grond J, Gerson JR, Laxer KD et al. (1998). Regional distribution of interictal ^{31}P metabolic changes in patients with temporal lobe epilepsy. Epilepsia 39: 527–536.

Vermathen P, Ende G, Laxer KD et al. (1997). Hippocampal N-acetylaspartate in neocortical epilepsy and mesial temporal lobe epilepsy. Ann Neurol 42: 194–199.

Woermann FG, McLean MA, Bartlett PA et al. (1999). Short echo time single-voxel ^{1}H magnetic resonance spectroscopy in magnetic resonance imaging-negative temporal lobe epilepsy: different biochemical profile compared with hippocampal sclerosis. Ann Neurol 45: 369–376.

Handbook of Clinical Neurology, Vol. 107 (3rd series)
Epilepsy, Part I
H. Stefan and W.H. Theodore, Editors

Chapter 26

Epilepsy diagnosis: positron emission tomography

AJAY KUMAR [1], FRANCK SEMAH [2], HARRY T. CHUGANI [1]*, AND WILLIAM H. THEODORE [3]

[1] *Departments of Pediatrics & Neurology, School of Medicine, Wayne State University, Children's Hospital of Michigan, Detroit, MI, USA*

[2] *Department of Nuclear Medicine, University Hospital of Lille, Lille, France*

[3] *Clinical Epilepsy Section, National Institute of Neurological Disease and Stroke, National Institutes of Health, Bethesda, MD, USA*

INTRODUCTION

Positron emission tomography (PET) can play a very important role in the evaluation of epilepsy, particularly when surgery is considered. The most commonly used PET tracer in epilepsy is [^{18}F]2-fluoro-2-deoxy-D-glucose ([^{18}F]FDG), used to measure the cerebral metabolic rate of glucose consumption (CMRglc). Other PET tracers with potential for detecting epileptic foci include: [^{11}C]α-methyl-L-tryptophan (AMT), which measures tryptophan metabolism; [^{11}C]flumazenil ([^{11}C]FMZ), which binds to α subunits of the γ-aminobutyric acid type A ($GABA_A$) benzodiazepine receptor, and most recently 5-hydroxytryptamine type 1A ($5HT_{1A}$) receptor ligands. Other radioligands that bind to opioid, histamine, *N*-methyl-D-aspartate (NMDA), "peripheral benzodiazepine," or acetylcholine receptors have been explored; their clinical role in epilepsy is not established, but they have very important research applications.

LOCALIZATION-RELATED EPILEPSY

Temporal lobe epilepsy

[^{18}F]FDG-PET

In the early 1980s Engel and collaborators showed the value of [^{18}F]FDG-PET in the investigation of epilepsy (Kuhl et al., 1978; Engel et al., 1982a, b, c). Their work was based on the autoradiographic methods developed by Louis Sokoloff, extended to human PET imaging by Reivich, Huang, Phelps, and others. The role of [^{18}F]FDG-PET in the presurgical evaluation of patients with intractable epilepsy is to lateralize and, if possible, localize epileptic foci. The overall sensitivity of [^{18}F]FDG-PET for detection of temporal lobe epilepsy (TLE) foci has been as high as 80%, and seems to be increasing as scanner design and resolution improve (Swartz et al., 1989; Gaillard et al., 1995a; Knowlton et al., 1997; Ryvlin et al., 1998; O'Brien et al., 2001). Several studies have suggested that [^{18}F]FDG-PET can impact on surgical decision-making in 50–70%, sometimes changing initial decisions based on magnetic resonance imaging (MRI) and video-EEG (Ollenberger et al., 2005; Uijl et al., 2007). [^{18}F]FDG-PET was found to be most useful in cases of negative MRI or when ictal EEG was discordant with MRI or videotaped seizure semiology (Uijl et al., 2007).

Temporal lobe interictal hypometabolic regions often extend beyond the presumed epileptogenic zone. Involvement of temporal neocortex probably occurs in the majority of patients, and it is difficult to distinguish medial from lateral TLE based on CMRglc patterns (Hajek et al., 1993; Kim et al., 2003) (Figs 26.1–26.4). Patients may have ipsilateral parietal and frontal cortex as well as thalamus and even occasionally contralateral temporal lobe hypometabolism (Swartz et al., 1989; Henry et al., 1993a, b; Gaillard et al., 1995a; Van Bogaert et al., 2000). This may represent the epileptic network involved in seizure propagation (Chassoux et al., 2004) and be related to behavioral and neuropsychological changes of chronic epilepsy. [^{18}F]FDG-PET, in conjunction with other imaging, clinical, and neurophysiological data, can be used to guide electrode placement in such instances.

[^{18}F]FDG-PET has been reported to be useful in predicting surgery outcome in some but not all studies. Ipsilateral PET hypometabolism appears to have a high

*Correspondence to: Harry T. Chugani, M.D., Children's Hospital of Michigan, Department of Neurology, 3901 Beaubien Blvd., Detroit, MI 48201, USA. E-mail: hchugani@pet.wayne.edu

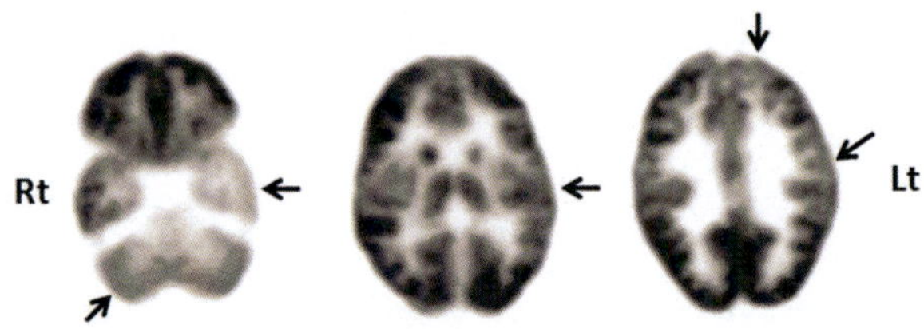

Fig. 26.1. Interictal [18F]FDG-PET scan in a child with intractable temporal lobe epilepsy, showing hypometabolism involving left temporal lobe and extending up to the left parietal and left frontal lobe (arrows). Also noted is right cerebellar diaschisis (arrow).

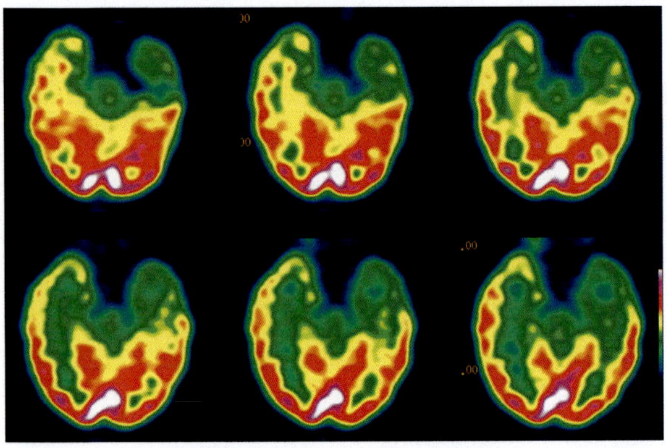

Fig. 26.2. Interictal [18F]FDG-PET scan in a patient with temporal lobe epilepsy, showing hypometabolism involving the left temporal lobe. The hypometabolism is more pronounced in the temporopolar region but involves the mesial part of the temporal lobe and extends to the lateral part (axial image in the hippocampal plane).

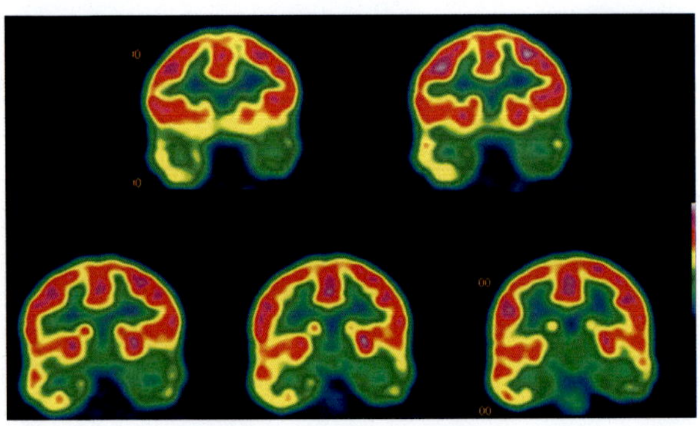

Fig. 26.3. Interictal [18F]FDG-PET scan in the same patient with temporal lobe epilepsy, showing hypometabolism involving the left temporal lobe (coronal in the hippocampal plane).

predictive value (86%) for good surgical outcome, even in patients with normal findings on MRI (80%) or those with nonlocalized ictal scalp EEG (72%) (Willmann et al., 2007). Patients with more severe temporal lobe hypometabolism appear to have better postsurgical seizure control (Theodore et al., 1983, 1992b). The temporal pole appears to be a significant predictor of

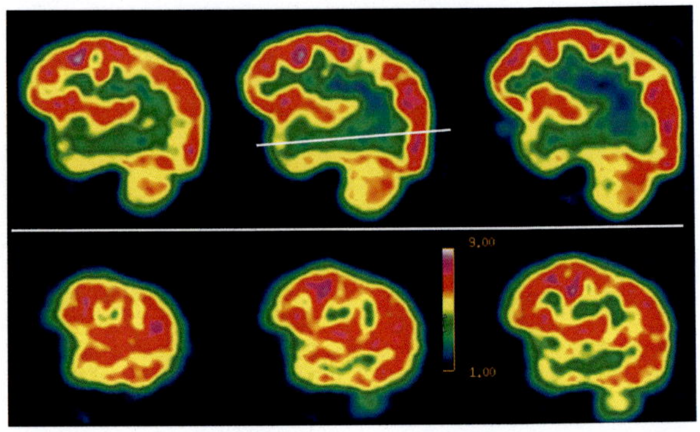

Fig. 26.4. Interictal [18F]FDG-PET scan showing the axial hippocampal plane that could be delineated on the [18F]FDG-PET scan (white line).

postoperative outcome (Dupont et al., 2000). In nonlesional TLE, completeness of hypometabolic cortex resection may predict surgical outcome (Vinton et al., 2007). An odds ratio of 7.1 has been reported for [18F]FDG-PET in predicting seizure-free outcome following epilepsy surgery (Knowlton et al., 2008). However, it is difficult to predict who will not become seizure-free after surgery (Uijl et al., 2008). A recent study found that incomplete resection, mild neuropathological findings, or the presence of secondary generalized tonic–clonic seizures was associated with a greater chance of surgical failure in patients with intractable epilepsy related to focal cortical dysplasia (Kim et al., 2009). Interestingly, none of the findings from [18F]FDG-PET, MRI, EEG, or ictal single-photon emission computed tomography (SPECT) was associated with surgical outcome. Medial temporal compared with lateral temporal hypometabolism (Delbeke et al., 1996), restricted temporal hypometabolism (Manno et al., 1994; Salanova et al., 1998), and greater inferior lateral temporal hypometabolism (Theodore et al., 1997) appear to be independent predictors for seizure control in TLE. Contralateral hypometabolism is a negative prognostic factor (Wong et al., 2010). Several studies have suggested that CMRglc could improve after surgery in some anatomically connected regions, suggesting a relationship with postoperative cognitive improvement (Dupont et al., 2001; Takaya et al., 2009).

Unilateral temporal lobe hypometabolism can be "falsely lateralized" in 1–2% (Sperling et al., 1995). Rarely, [18F]FDG-PET may show lateral or medial temporal lobe *hyper*metabolism, related to subclinical seizures or interictal spiking, which may or may not be detected by scalp EEG (Theodore et al., 1983; Chugani et al., 1993a). Increased metabolism has been reported in large cortical malformations (Poduri et al., 2007). [18F]FDG-PET shows hypometabolism in almost 20% of children (Gaillard et al., 1995b, 2002), and in up to 50% of adults with new-onset seizure (Weitemeyer et al., 2005).

PET hypometabolism is related to underlying pathology, neuronal loss, seizure evolution, and specific seizure characteristics (Semah et al., 1995). In children with new partial seizure onset, a shorter time since last seizure and higher seizure frequency predicted abnormal [18F]FDG-PET findings, which was significantly associated with seizure outcome; those with normal initial PET scan had good seizure control (Gaillard et al., 2007). Interestingly, no evidence was found for progression of hypometabolism. Other studies found that children with persistent or increased seizure frequency showed increased hypometabolic cortex (Benedek et al., 2006). Increased CMRglc may persist for up to 48 hours after a seizure (Leiderman et al., 1994). Wider spread of discharges during the most recent seizure before [18F]FDG-PET may lead to more extensive hypometabolism (Savic et al., 1997).

[18F]FDG-PET becomes most valuable when MRI is normal or equivocal (Lamusuo et al., 2001). Detection of hypometabolism in MRI-negative TLE varies from 50% to 85%, depending on both MRI and PET technique; it may be more common in mesial than neocortical TLE (Semah et al., 1995; Theodore et al., 1997; Lamusuo et al., 2000, 2001; Swartz et al., 2002; Carne et al., 2004). Surgical outcome can be excellent in [18F]FDG-PET-positive MRI-negative mesial TLE (Carne et al., 2004). In MRI-negative neocortical TLE, agreement of any two modalities among interictal or ictal surface EEG, [18F]FDG-PET, and subtraction ictal SPECT predicted good surgical outcome; results did not appear to be improved by implanted electrodes (Lee et al., 2005). As many as 30–50% of patients with cortical dysplasia, particularly children, have nonlocalized scalp EEG and normal MRI scans; [18F]FDG-PET is positive in 75–90% (Lerner et al., 2009). However, based on a few studies, [11C]methionine-PET may be superior to [18F]FDG-PET for distinguishing focal cortical dysplasia from mixed glial–neuronal tumors (Phi et al., 2010). PET can play a role in cases of dual pathology (coexistence of medial temporal and neocortical seizure foci) or "secondary" epileptic foci.

$GABA_A$ RECEPTOR IMAGING

[11C]FMZ is the neuroreceptor tracer used most widely in epilepsy. [11C]FMZ-PET shows decreased $GABA_A$ receptor binding in temporal and extratemporal epileptic foci; the extent of decreased binding is usually less than the area of hypometabolism on [18F]FDG-PET (Henry et al., 1993a; Savic et al., 1993; Szelies et al., 1996; Ryvlin et al., 1998) (Fig. 26.5). [11C]FMZ-PET is highly sensitive in TLE (Ryvlin et al., 1998), particularly in patients with a sclerotic hippocampus (Henry et al., 1993a; Koepp et al., 1996). The reduction in [11C]FMZ binding appears to be greater than that due to the loss of hippocampal volume alone (Koepp et al., 1997). Although GABA receptor density is increased in cortical layers V–VI of epileptogenic cortex, there is decreased [11C]FMZ affinity for these receptors, leading to an overall decrease in the distribution volume, shown as an area of decreased [11C]FMZ uptake on PET (Juhasz et al., 1999; Nagy et al., 1999).

The sensitivity of [11C]FMZ-PET in detection of unilateral hippocampal sclerosis has been reported to be up to 100%, although specificity may be lower; contralateral abnormalities appear in as many as one-third of patients with apparently unilateral hippocampal sclerosis, and false lateralization has been reported (Henry et al., 1993a; Koepp et al., 1996; Ryvlin et al., 1998, 1999). In patients with MRI-negative TLE, [11C]FMZ-PET may be abnormal in up to 85% (Koepp et al., 2000; Lamusuo et al., 2000; Koepp and Woermann, 2005). Some authors have suggested that [11C]FMZ-PET is associated with better surgical outcome than [18F]FDG-PET, even when MRI is normal (Ryvlin et al., 1998). A shorter interval between the last seizure and [11C]FMZ-PET may lead to lower [11C] FMZ binding in the epileptogenic region (Bouvard et al., 2005).

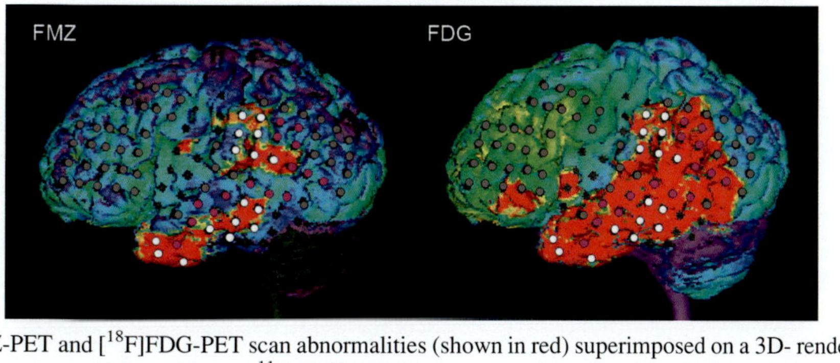

Fig. 26.5. [11C]FMZ-PET and [18F]FDG-PET scan abnormalities (shown in red) superimposed on a 3D- rendered brain MRI in a child with intractable temporal lobe epilepsy. [11C]FMZ-PET shows a much smaller area of abnormality compared with [18F] FDG-PET. (White circles, electrodes showing seizure onset; pink circles, electrodes showing rapid seizure propagation.)

Statistical parametric mapping (SPM) can increase [^{11}C]FMZ-PET accuracy, with detection of subtle changes in [^{11}C]FMZ binding, which may be difficult to appreciate visually (Koepp et al., 1996; Bouilleret et al., 2002). These SPM studies have sometimes also found *increased* [^{11}C]-FMZ binding (Koepp et al., 1996, 1997; Richardson et al., 1998; Hammers et al., 2001), which, in some cases, suggested cortical developmental malformations (Koepp et al., 1997). Use of SPM occasionally revealed increased [^{11}C]FMZ binding in normal-appearing temporal white matter, found to harbor microdysgenesis on histopathological examination (Hammers et al., 2002). As ectopic neuronal clusters may lead to epileptogenesis via aberrant circuitry, [^{11}C]FMZ-PET may provide information complementary to MRI and [^{18}F]FDG-PET.

Serotonin receptors

Serotonin influences a wide range of neurophysiological processes and behavioral functions; there are at least 16 different receptor subtypes. Three $5HT_{1A}$ receptor ligands, piperazine compounds [^{18}F]FCWAY100635 (Toczek et al., 2003; Giovacchini et al., 2005), [^{11}C]WAY100635 (Savic et al., 2004), and [^{18}F]MPPF (Merlet et al., 2004a, b), have been used to study patients with epilepsy. The ^{18}F ligands have the advantage of a higher signal to noise ratio, but FCWAY has a fluorinated metabolite that can accumulate in bone leading to partial volume effects that need to be corrected. MPPF has lower specific activity, and is sensitive to endogenous 5HT levels, but can be studied with a reference region approach. It is also a *p*-glycoprotein transporter substrate (la Fougère et al., 2010).

Studies with all three ligands showed reduced binding in mesial temporal regions, including hippocampus, amygdala, parahippocampal, and fusiform gyrus ipsilateral to the epileptic focus in patients with TLE; reduced binding was most prominent in the region of ictal onset (Merlet et al., 2004a). The abnormalities were not dependent on MRI lesions; the reduction in binding ipsilateral to the epileptic focus was reduced by only about 20% when partial volume correction for structural atrophy was performed (Giovacchini et al., 2005) (Fig. 26.6). Decreased [^{18}F]MPPF binding potential localized the epileptogenic zone in 40%, and lateralized it in about 80% of patients with mesial TLE and 33% with other TLE subtypes (Didelot et al., 2008). A comparison of [^{18}F]FCWAY-PET and [^{18}F]FDG-PET in a series of patients with MRI-negative TLE suggested that [^{18}F]FCWAY-PET was less sensitive, but more specific, for localization of epileptic foci (Liew et al., 2009).

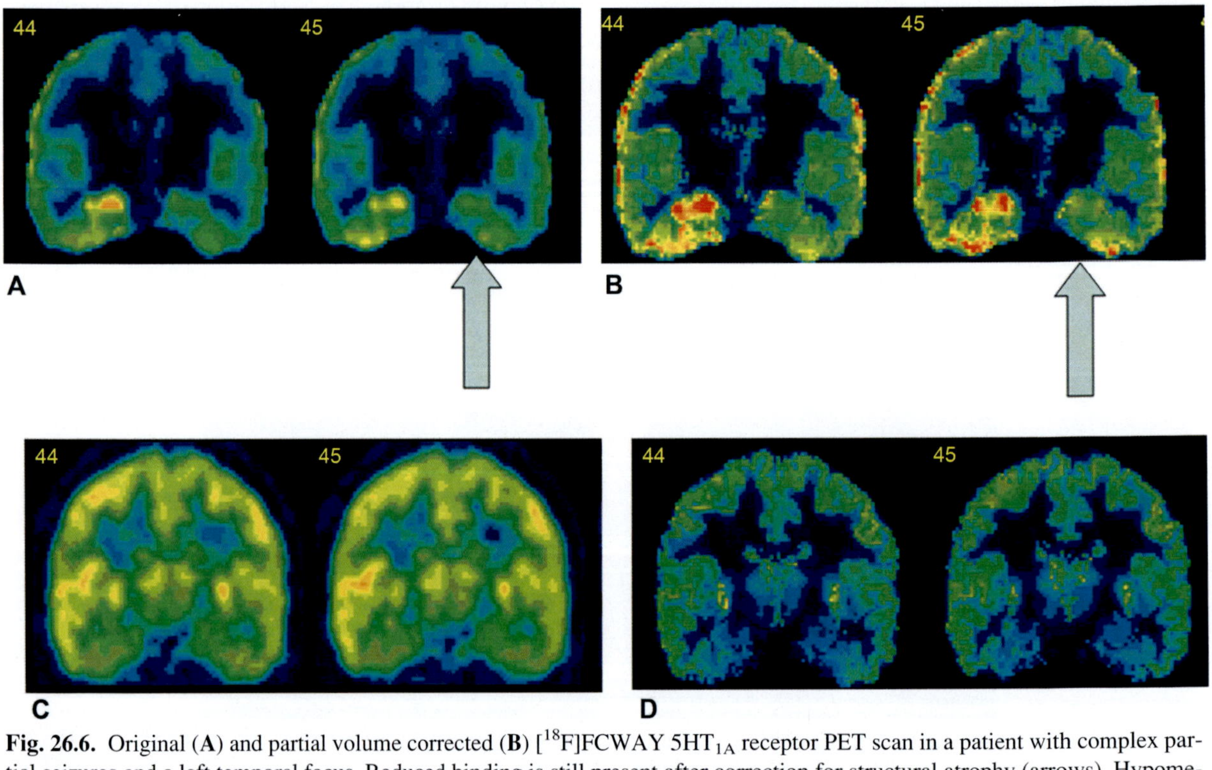

Fig. 26.6. Original (**A**) and partial volume corrected (**B**) [^{18}F]FCWAY $5HT_{1A}$ receptor PET scan in a patient with complex partial seizures and a left temporal focus. Reduced binding is still present after correction for structural atrophy (arrows). Hypometabolism is less prominent on original (**C**) and partial volume corrected (**D**) [^{18}F]FDG-PET.

Depression, epilepsy, and $5HT_{1A}$ receptor binding

Reduced [^{11}C]WAY binding in anterior cingulate in TLE had a significant correlation with the Montgomery–Asberg mood rating scale, and reduced [^{18}F]FCWAY hippocampal binding ipsilateral to the epileptic focus with the Beck Depression Inventory (BDI) (Savic et al., 2004; Theodore et al., 2007). Patients with TLE and a diagnosis of major depressive disorder based on the Structured Clinical Interview for the Diagnostic and Statistical Manual for Mental Disorders, 4th edition (DSM-IV), had greater reductions in FCWAY binding than either controls or patients with epilepsy alone in limbic regions and cingulate gyrus, independent of focus side and mesial temporal sclerosis (Hasler et al., 2007). In contrast, BDI correlated positively with [^{18}F]MPPF binding potential in raphe and in the insula contralateral to seizure onset, and somatic symptoms with binding potential in the hippocampal/parahippocampal region ipsilateral to seizure onset (Lothe et al., 2008). MPPF has much higher sensitivity to synaptic 5HT levels than FCWAY or CWAY (Zimmer et al., 2002). Lower levels of endogenous serotonin in depressed than in nondepressed patients with epilepsy would lead to relatively increased MPPF but not WAY binding, explaining the contrast with previous results. Patients with major depressive disorder have reductions of $5HT_{1A}$ receptor binding in limbic regions and cingulate cortex (Drevets et al., 2007). No effects of antiepileptic drugs on [^{18}F]FCWAY receptor binding were found (Theodore et al., 2006).

Experience with another PET tracer, [^{11}C]AMT is limited. AMT is an analog of tryptophan, the precursor for serotonin synthesis but, unlike tryptophan, AMT is not incorporated into protein in significant amounts. After transport of AMT across the blood–brain barrier, it is converted to α-methylserotonin (AM-5HT) by tryptophan hydroxylase, and accumulates in neurons and nerve terminals along with the releasable pool of serotonin, as, unlike serotonin, AM-5HT is not a substrate for the degradative enzyme monoamine oxidase. Although one study found it to be useful in identifying the epileptic foci in patients with TLE and normal hippocampal volume (Natsume et al., 2003), AMT does not seem to be very useful in patients with mesial TLE, particularly with hippocampal sclerosis.

Extratemporal lobe epilepsy

PET can also be very helpful in presurgical evaluation of extratemporal lobe epilepsy (ETLE). MRI is negative in a large number of cases (Wyllie et al., 1998). For example, incomplete myelination in infants may limit MRI detection of focal cortical dysplasia, (Depositario-Cabacar et al., 2008). This is probably reflected in suboptimal surgical outcome (seizure freedom in only 50–60% of patients) in ETLE compared with that in TLE. Outcome is worse if MRI is normal (Engel et al., 1993; Duchowny et al., 1998), because the placement of intracranial electrodes would be guided only by seizure semiology and scalp EEG findings, subject to significant sampling error. [^{18}F]FDG-PET can provide important lateralizing and localizing information to guide intracranial electrode placement (Fig. 26.7).

Frontal lobe epilepsy is usually associated with subtle structural changes, such as cortical dysplasia or heterotopias, which may not appear on MRI, but show hypometabolism on [^{18}F]FDG-PET. [^{18}F]FDG-PET may distinguish frontal and temporal seizure foci in cases of lateralized but not localized scalp ictal video-EEG (Theodore et al., 1997). In lesional cases, PET may show hypometabolism extending beyond the lesion or very restricted areas of hypometabolism. These areas should be sampled with intracranial EEG during surgery, as perilesional cortex may also be epileptogenic and lesionectomy alone may lead to surgical failure (Fig. 26.8). When hypometabolism is

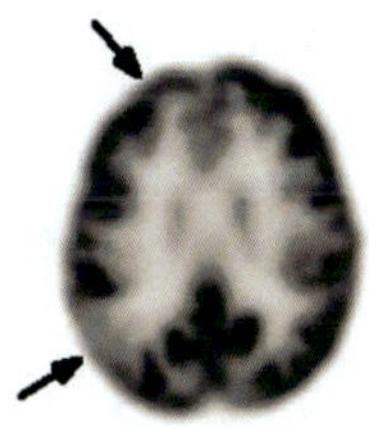

Fig. 26.7. [^{18}F]FDG-PET showing frontal–parietal hypometabolism (arrows) in an epileptic child with nonlateralizing scalp EEG and normal MRI.

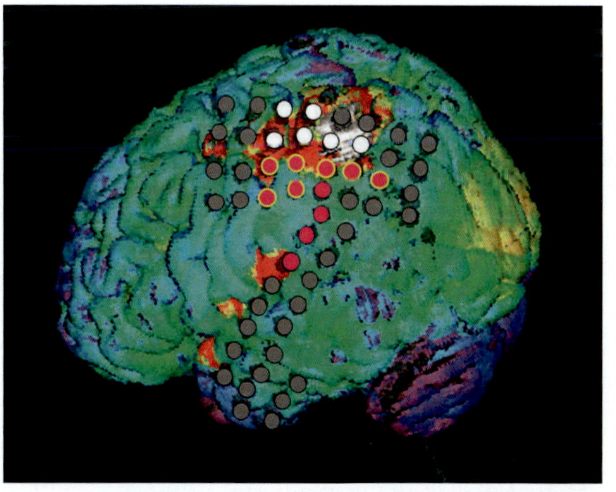

Fig. 26.8. Coregistration of [^{18}F]FDG-PET and intracranial electrodes on a 3D-rendered brain MRI showing an MRI-visible brain lesion (white), PET hypometabolic region (red), and intracranial electrodes (white circles, seizure onset; pink circles with yellow border, spike with rapid seizure spread; pink circles, rapid seizure spread; gray circles, no seizure activity). Note that the hypometabolic region is larger and extends beyond the MRI lesion, and contains some of the epileptogenic areas.

found on $[^{18}F]$FDG-PET in patients with normal MRI, a subtle lesion may have been missed.

In frontal lobe epilepsy, the sensitivity of $[^{18}F]$FDG-PET in localizing the epileptogenic zone is in the range of 45–73% (Henry et al., 1991; Swartz et al., 1995; da Silva et al., 1997; Kim et al., 2002; Honbolygo et al., 2006). Using high-resolution $[^{18}F]$FDG-PET and semiautomated analysis, sensitivity was 92% and specificity 62.5% in detection of frontal lobe epileptic foci in children (da Silva et al., 1997). In occipital lobe epilepsy, lower sensitivity has been reported (Patil et al., 2007). Localized hypometabolism on $[^{18}F]$FDG-PET was significantly associated with seizure-free surgery outcome in patients with neocortical epilepsy (Yun et al., 2006), but other investigators did not find a relation (Lee et al., 2008).

Flumazenil

$[^{11}C]$FMZ-PET may have higher sensitivity than $[^{18}F]$FDG-PET for detecting epileptogenic cortex in neocortical epilepsy (Savic et al., 1995; Ryvlin et al., 1998; Muzik et al., 2000). Although $[^{11}C]$FMZ-PET abnormalities also typically extend beyond MRI-visible structural lesions, they are usually smaller than the large hypometabolism seen with $[^{18}F]$FDG-PET and show better correlation with intracranial EEG findings (Arnold et al., 2000; Juhasz et al., 2000; Szelies et al., 2002). Sometimes $[^{11}C]$FMZ-PET may show a neocortical abnormality without any MRI correlate, and if there is concordance with scalp EEG data, further investigation with intracranial EEG is warranted. In MRI-negative patients with ETLE, $[^{11}C]$FMZ-PET has been reported to be abnormal in up to 70% of patients (Koepp and Woermann, 2005). Complete resection of the $[^{11}C]$FMZ-PET abnormality is associated with better surgical outcome, even in MRI-negative cases (Muzik et al., 2000; Juhasz et al., 2001). Use of SPM can further enhance the utility of $[^{11}C]$FMZ-PET, including those with normal MRI findings (Richardson et al., 1998; Hammers et al., 2001).

AMT may play an important role in ETLE, particularly in children. Histologically verified (macroscopic or microscopic) cortical dysplasia is associated with more frequent increased AMT uptake compared with that in patients with nonspecific gliosis (Juhasz et al., 2003). The area of increased AMT uptake is significantly less than reduced CMRglc, corresponding more to the epileptic *focus* rather than *epileptogenic areas*. In some instances, AMT-PET can identify the epileptogenic cortex even when $[^{18}F]$FDG-PET and $[^{11}C]$FMZ-PET scans are normal. In 73 children with intractable neocortical epilepsy with and without malformations of cortical development, sensitivity and specificity of focally increased AMT uptake, using intracranial EEG localization of seizure onset as the standard, specificity of AMT-PET for detecting the lobe of seizure onset was equally high in lesional (97%) and nonlesional (100%) groups, whereas sensitivity was higher in the lesional than in the nonlesional group (47% versus 29% respectively) (Wakamoto et al., 2008). AMT-PET showed the epileptic focus in 25% of patients with nonlocalizing MRI.

Other ligands in localization-related epilepsy

Mu-opiate receptor binding imaged with $[^{11}C]$carfentanil was increased in temporal neocortex, but not in amygdala or hippocampus ipsilateral to temporal lobe seizure foci compared with the contralateral side (Frost et al., 1988). $[^{11}C]$diprenorphine (a ligand with comparable affinity for mu, delta, and kappa receptors) binding was not significantly different between temporal regions ipsilateral and contralateral to the focus, suggesting that an increase in mu-receptor binding might be offset by a decrease in delta- and/or kappa-receptor binding. (Mayberg et al., 1991). However, increased binding of the delta-receptor-selective antagonist was present in mid-inferior and anterior aspects of the middle and superior temporal cortex (Madar et al., 1997). $[^{18}F]$cyclofoxy, a mu- and kappa-receptor antagonist, showed no group asymmetry (Theodore et al., 1992a). Kappa-receptor downregulation might offset mu-receptor upregulation.

Patients with reading epilepsy had lower left parieto-temporo-occipital $[^{11}C]$diprenorphine binding while reading than during a control task, whereas healthy volunteers had increased binding suggesting ictal release of an endogenous opioid-like substance (Koepp et al., 1998). Patients scanned within hours of spontaneous temporal lobe seizures had increased temporal pole and fusiform gyrus $[^{11}C]$diprenorphine binding ipsilateral to the seizure focus (Bartenstein et al., 1994; Hammers et al., 2007). The data suggest initial endogenous ictal opioid release, followed by an overshoot to below basal levels, and increased receptor availability for the exogenous tracer for up to 8 hours after seizures. After selective amygdalohippocampectomy, two patients had greater reduction of $[^{11}C]$diprenorphine binding, possibly reflecting reduced receptor availability, after successful surgery. Could upregulation of opiate receptors be an endogenous antiepileptic response? Naloxone infusion reduced both overall cerebral blood flow (CBF) and the degree of temporal asymmetry in TLE, suggesting that increased opiate levels might be related to CBF abnormalities (Theodore et al., 1993).

The irreversible monoamine oxidase B (MAO-B, which has high levels in astrocytes and sclerotic hippocampi in surgical specimens) inhibitor ligand $[^{11}C]$

deuterium-deprenyl had increased uptake in the temporal lobe ipsilateral to EEG foci (Kumlien et al., 1992, 1995; Bergström et al., 1998). A subsequent study, however, did not confirm these results, showing lower initial ipsilateral temporal lobe tracer distribution volume, probably reflecting reduced CBF, but no difference at equilibrium (Kumlien et al., 2001).

Subcortical structures may play a regulatory role in both partial and generalized epilepsy syndromes. [^{18}F]FDG-PET showed decreased CMRglc in caudate and/or thalamus (Henry et al., 1993b; Arnold et al., 1996; Khan et al., 1997). Similar findings in drug-resistant generalized seizures, and in patients with mesial temporal lobe partial seizures, suggest that the decrease is not dependent on epilepsy type (Bouilleret et al., 2005). Reduced dopamine receptor binding was not due to striatal volume loss (Bouilleret et al., 2008).

Compared with controls, [^{18}F]fallypride, a dopamine D2/D3-receptor ligand, showed significantly decreased binding potential in epileptogenic temporal lobe in TLE (Werhahn et al., 2006). There was a small reduction of D_1-receptor ligand [^{11}C]SCH23390 binding in the right putamen of patients with autosomal dominant nocturnal frontal lobe epilepsy (ADNFLE) (Fedi et al., 2008). However, potential effects of structural atrophy were not excluded in these studies.

Patients with TLE had reduced NMDA-receptor binding on [^{11}C](*S*)-[*N*-methyl]ketamine-PET ipsilateral to the side of seizure onset, matching [^{18}F]FDG-PET hypometabolism (Kumlien et al., 1999). Patients with ADNFLE had increased midbrain, pons, and cerebellar, and decreased dorsolateral prefrontal cortex binding, with [^{18}F]F-A-85380, a high-affinity $\alpha_4\beta_2$ nicotinic acetylcholine receptor agonist (Picard et al., 2006). [^{11}C]doxepin activity was 10–50% higher in temporal neocortex ipsilateral to the seizure focus, inversely correlated with CMRglc (Iinuma et al., 1993).

A study with PET and [^{11}C]verapamil, a *p*-glycoprotein substrate, showed no statistically significant binding alterations in patients with refractory TLE (Langer et al., 2007).

SECONDARY GENERALIZED EPILEPTIC SYNDROMES

Infantile spasms or West syndrome

[^{18}F]FDG-PET findings not only help in understanding the pathogenesis of the infantile spasms, but may have significant prognostic and therapeutic implications. In a study of 140 children with cryptogenic infantile spasms, 95% had one or more cortical abnormalities on [^{18}F]FDG-PET scan (Chugani and Conti, 1996).

[^{18}F]FDG-PET often shows unifocal or multifocal areas of cortical hypometabolism that correspond well with the EEG localization of focal ictal or interictal abnormalities (Chugani et al., 1990, 1993b). These hypometabolic areas may change with time, with persistence of hypometabolism indicating continuation of spasms and worse developmental prognosis (Maeda et al., 1994; Itomi et al., 2002). Reduced CMRglc was associated with delayed myelination (Natsume et al., 1996). Rarely, [^{18}F]FDG-PET may show areas of hypermetabolism, which have lower [^{11}C]FMZ binding on [^{11}C]FMZ-PET scan, usually related to cortical dysplasia (Chugani et al., 1990, 1993b; Juhasz et al., 2001; Kumada et al., 2006). [^{18}F]FDG-PET may show hypermetabolism in lenticular nuclei and brainstem in infants with infantile spasms (Fig. 26.9) (Chugani et al., 1992). A nonlesional etiology, such as neurometabolic or neurodegenerative disorders, should be suspected if [^{18}F]FDG-PET shows symmetrical, diffuse hypometabolism (Depositario-Cabacar et al., 2008). Asymmetrical and asynchronous spasms may show abnormalities in the primary sensorimotor area (Gaily et al., 1995). Bitemporal hypometabolism may be suggestive of autistic features and poor seizure control (Chugani et al., 1996). AMT-PET can be very useful in tuberous sclerosis complex with infantile spasms, showing increased AMT uptake in epileptic and decreases in non-epileptic tubers (Curatolo et al., 2001).

Children with a distinct unifocal cortical lesion, concordant with EEG, may be considered for epilepsy surgery (Chugani et al., 1990, 1993b; Kramer et al., 1997). Spasms may be associated with a "leading" spike followed by fast-wave bursts, starting within 2 cm of a hypometabolic region; failure to resect this region resulted in poor surgical outcome (Asano et al., 2005).

Landau–Kleffner syndrome (LKS)

LKS is a disorder of unknown etiology characterized by acquired aphasia and epilepsy occurring between 4 and 8 years in a child developing typically until that time.

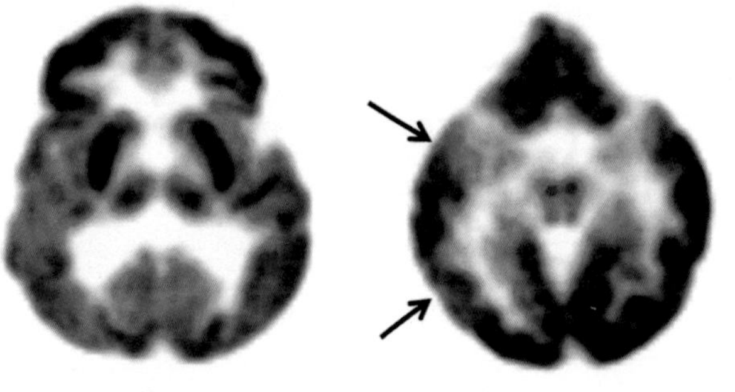

Fig. 26.9. [^{18}F]FDG-PET scan in a child with infantile spasms, showing increased glucose metabolism in bilateral lentiform nuclei and hypometabolism in right temporal lobe (arrows), probably representing the complex cortical–subcortical interactions thought to be important in the secondary generalization of focal cortical discharges resulting in spasms.

[^{18}F]FDG-PET shows bitemporal hypometabolism, particularly in superior and medial regions (da Silva et al., 1997; Honbolygo et al., 2006; Shiraishi et al., 2007). [^{11}C]FMZ-PET shows reduced [^{11}C]FMZ binding at the tip of the temporal lobe (Shiraishi et al., 2007). Children may have additional areas of neocortical hypometabolism, including those in the occipital cortex, indicating extensive brain functional disturbances (Rintahaka et al., 1995; da Silva et al., 1997). During continuous spike–waves in slow-wave sleep, bitemporal *hyper*metabolism is seen, suggesting possible involvement of the temporal lobes in the generation of continuous spike–waves (Maquet et al., 1990; Rintahaka et al., 1995). Specific cognitive impairment may be related to increased CMRglc in cortical association areas with spike–wave discharges (Metz-Lutz and Filippini, 2006). [^{18}F]FDG-PET can be used to monitor dynamic changes in temporal lobe CMRglc during episodes of aphasia and remission (Luat et al., 2006) (Fig. 26.10).

Tuberous sclerosis complex (TSC)

Approximately 70–90% of patients with TSC present with seizures. [^{18}F]FDG-PET shows hypometabolism in and around tubers, believed to be due to decreased neuronal number and simplified dendritic pattern (Szelies et al., 1983; Rintahaka and Chugani, 1997). Delta-slowing and frequent spike activity were independently and additively associated with reduced CMRglc in children with focal epilepsy associated with TSC (Nishida et al., 2008).

CMRglc in bilateral, lateral temporal cortex was associated with severity of communication disturbance, and hypermetabolism in deep cerebellar nuclei and increased caudate AMT uptake with stereotyped behavior and impaired social interaction, as well as communication disturbance (Asano et al., 2001; Luat et al., 2007; Depositario-Cabacar et al., 2008). Decreased glucose metabolism and increased AMT uptake occurs in cerebellar tubers (Eluvathingal et al., 2006). Children with right cerebellar lesions had higher social isolation and communicative and developmental disturbance than children with left cerebellar lesions.

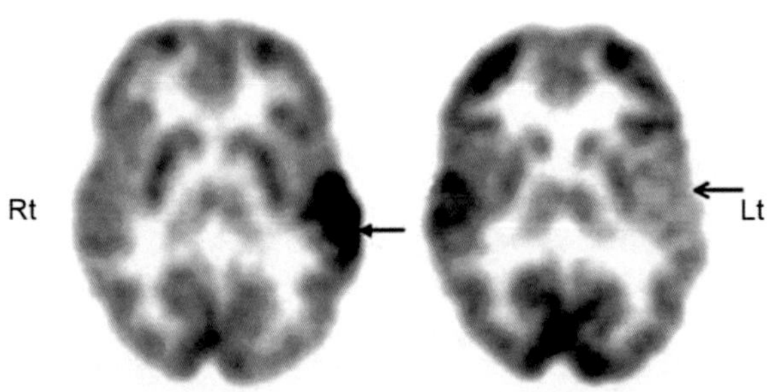

Fig. 26.10. [^{18}F]FDG-PET images from a child with Landau–Kleffner syndrome showing (*left*) marked hypermetabolism in the left temporal cortex (arrow) during the peak of his aphasic episode. EEG during the PET tracer uptake period showed frequent and repetitive spike-and-wave activities from this area. *Right:* A repeat [^{18}F]FDG-PET scan during remission showed hypometabolism in the same region (arrow).

Although [^{18}F]FDG-PET can detect small cortical tubers not visualized on T2-weighted MRI, hypometabolism often extends beyond structural lesions (Asano et al., 2000). However, both epileptic and nonepileptic tubers show reduced CMRglc on interictal [^{18}F]FDG-PET scans. AMT-PET shows increased AMT uptake interictally in epileptic but not quiescent tubers in almost two-thirds of children with tuberous sclerosis and intractable epilepsy, perhaps due to activation of the kynurenine pathway; all tubers with at least 10% AMT increase were found to be epileptogenic. (Chugani et al., 1998; Asano et al., 2000; Fedi et al., 2003; Kagawa et al., 2005) (Fig. 26.11). Although the specificity of AMT-PET is very high, sensitivity is modest. However, MRI-based quantitative analysis can double its sensitivity, from 44.4% to 79% with visual assessment (Juhász et al., 2002). AMT-PET can provide independent complementary information regarding localization of epileptogenic regions in TSC and assist patient selection for epilepsy surgery (Ohta et al., 2001; Kagawa et al., 2005).

Sturge–Weber syndrome (SWS)

SWS is a neurocutaneous disorder characterized by facial port-wine stain, glaucoma, and pial angiomatosis involving one cerebral hemisphere in 85% of the patients, and both hemispheres in the remainder. [^{18}F]FDG-PET often demonstrates cortical hypometabolism, ipsilateral to the facial nevus, and extending beyond structural abnormalities on MRI (Chugani et al., 1989; Juhasz et al., 2007a). However, early in the course, [^{18}F]FDG-PET may show transient interictal hypermetabolism (not associated with ongoing seizures or interictal spiking) that becomes hypometabolic with time (Chugani et al., 1989). In some children, serial [^{18}F]FDG-PET scans show rapidly progressing hypometabolism of affected cortex, probably related to its destruction; these patients usually show decreased seizures and, if progression occurs at a young age, improvement in neurocognitive function (Behen et al., 2006; Juhasz et al., 2007a) (Fig. 26.12). Early and rapid progression of the brain tissue beneath the unilateral lesion leads to early and more efficient reorganization in contralateral cortex (Batista et al., 2007). High CMRglc in contralateral visual cortex suggests cortical reorganization and transfer of some functions to the contralateral healthy side.

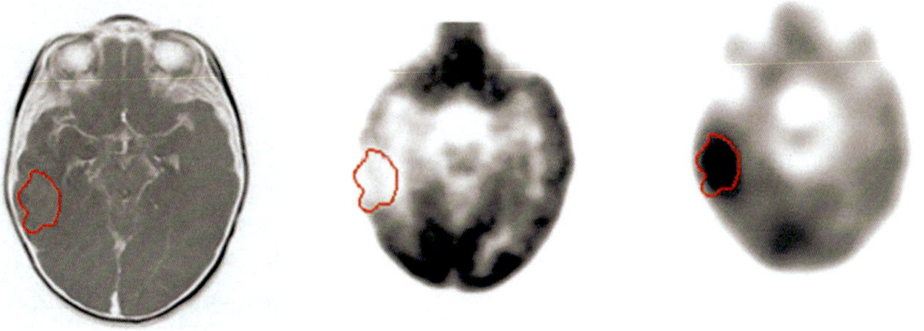

Fig. 26.11. MRI and PET images from a child with tuberous sclerosis and intractable seizures being evaluated for epilepsy surgery. Whereas [^{18}F]FDG-PET (*middle*) showed glucose hypometabolism in the right temporal tuber (inverted FLAIR, *left*), AMT-PET (*right*) showed intense uptake (red circle), corresponding to the EEG focus.

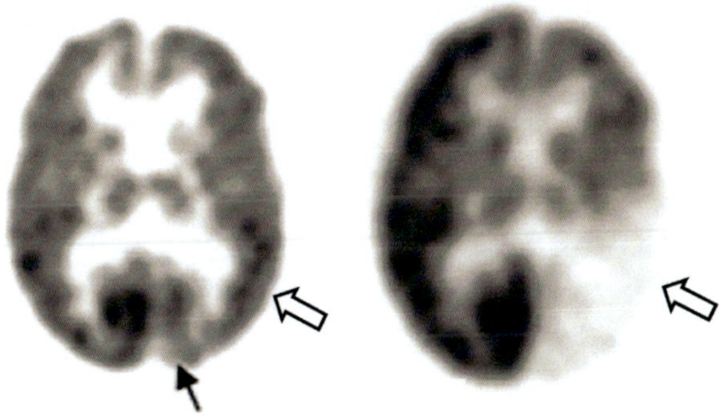

Fig. 26.12. Serial [^{18}F]FDG-PET scans showing progression of the cortical hypometabolism (closed arrow), indicating degenerative changes in the brain tissue associated with the angioma in a child with Sturge–Weber syndrome and meningeal hemangioma of the left posterior quadrant. Also noted is the severe hypometabolism in the adjacent parieto-occipital region (open arrow), initially showing preserved metabolism. With this rapid progression, the child showed improvement in seizure status and cognitive function.

Persistence of mild hypometabolism in underlying cortex indicates ongoing functional worsening, usually associated with persistent seizures and developmental delay (Lee et al., 2001a). These children should undergo early surgical intervention to control seizures and improve development. Earlier surgical resection enhances the chance of cortical reorganization, while brain plasticity is still at its maximum. In SWS, maximum metabolic changes and cortical damage occur in the first few years of life (Juhasz et al., 2007a), coinciding with sustained increase in cerebral metabolic demand (Chugani et al., 1987). Metabolic abnormalities may remain stable or partially recover later in some children with well controlled seizures (Müller et al., 1997). Both structural and functional abnormalities were found to extend well beyond the angioma, indicating widespread abnormalities of growth and development of the affected hemisphere (Pfund et al., 2003). Increased white-matter volume underlying the angioma was seen in infants, but ipsilateral white-matter regions outside the angioma showed volume loss in both infants and older patients. Extensive gray- and white-matter volume loss and hypometabolism ipsilateral to the angioma likely contributes to progressive cognitive dysfunctions, regardless of the extent of angioma (Juhasz et al., 2007b).

Lennox–Gastaut syndrome

Lennox–Gastaut syndrome is a generalized epilepsy often refractory to antiepileptic treatment. [^{18}F]FDG-PET may show unifocal or multifocal metabolic abnormalities (Fig. 26.13), even when MRI is normal or EEG nonlocalizing. [^{18}F]FDG-PET can reveal cortical abnormalities in cryptogenic cases, with classification into four subtypes: unilateral focal, unilateral diffuse, or bilateral diffuse hypometabolism, and normal CMRglc (Chugani et al., 1987; Theodore et al., 1987). [^{18}F]FDG-PET may help in understanding the etiopathogenesis of this disorder and may reveal the neurosubstrates of various functional abnormalities seen in this condition (Gur et al., 1982; Chugani et al., 1987; Iinuma et al., 1987; Theodore et al., 1987; Yanai et al., 1987; Miyauchi et al., 1988; Ferrie et al., 1996). Occasionally, [^{18}F]FDG-PET can also help in surgical treatment by showing a focal lesion and normal functioning in the rest of the cortex. Resective surgery

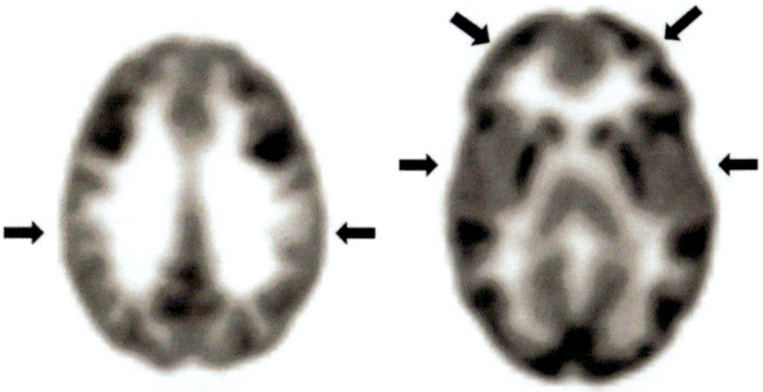

Fig. 26.13. [^{18}F]FDG-PET scan showing bilateral cortical hypometabolism affecting frontal, parietal, and temporal cortex (arrows) in a child with Lennox–Gastaut syndrome and multiple seizure types.

may be considered if the lesion is concordant with neurophysiological data, and may result in seizure freedom and normal development (You et al., 2007).

Hemimegalencephaly (HME)

HME is a congenital hypertrophy of one cerebral hemisphere associated with epilepsy, hemianopsia, and varying degrees of developmental delay. [^{18}F]FDG-PET usually shows hypometabolism in the affected hemisphere (Rintahaka et al., 1993). Occasionally hypermetabolism is associated with frequent spiking. Children with intractable epilepsy should undergo hemispherectomy in the first year of life to allow maximal brain plasticity to take place. Preoperative evaluation should include an assessment of integrity of the apparently normal non-HME hemisphere. Metabolic abnormalities, sometimes subtle, in the apparently normal hemisphere on [^{18}F]FDG-PET indicates some degree of functional impairment (Fig. 26.14). These children are still surgical candidates but outcome may be less favorable (Rintahaka et al., 1993).

Rasmussen's encephalitis and epilepsy of inflammatory origin

Rasmussen's syndrome is a chronic encephalitis characterized by intractable focal epilepsy and progressive neurological deterioration with lateralized brain destruction. In the early stages, the diagnosis can be difficult to make, as structural brain imaging is usually normal and brain biopsy often is needed. In children with Rasmussen's syndrome evaluated within 1 year of seizure onset, [^{18}F]FDG-PET showed areas of hypermetabolism or hypometabolism restricted mostly to frontal and temporal regions; posterior cortex was preserved (Lee et al., 2001b). Pathological changes seen in resected cortex were more pronounced in regions of abnormal than normal CMRglc. In children evaluated more than 1 year after seizure onset, PET showed more diffuse hemispheric abnormalities including occipital cortex, but still highly lateralized. These CMRglc patterns in early and late disease stages may facilitate Rasmussen's diagnosis and assist biopsy guidance when structural neuroimaging is still normal. Focal CMRglc abnormalities indicate earlier disease stages and depict extent better than concomitant MRI (Fogarasi et al., 2003).

PET studies with [^{11}C]PK11195, a ligand for the "peripheral benzodiazepine receptor" more recently known as the "translocator protein 18 kD," found on astrocyte mitochondrial membranes and activated microglia, showed diffusely increased binding in the affected hemisphere in Rasmussen's encephalitis (Banati et al., 1999; Kumar et al., 2008). Neuroinflammation, mediated by activated microglia, plays an important role in Rasmussen's pathogenesis and may be the underlying cause in other cases of intractable epilepsy of unknown etiology (Fig. 26.15). Several patients with epilepsy attributed to encephalitis of unknown origin studied with [^{11}C]PK11195-PET had increased binding in regions of possible seizure onset or neuronal injury (Goerres et al., 2001; Kumar et al., 2008).

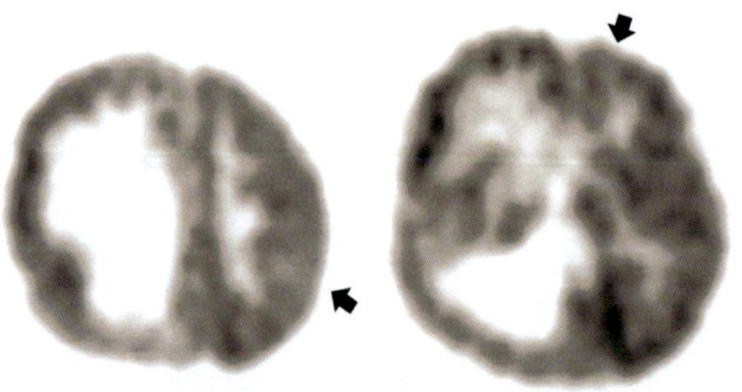

Fig. 26.14. [^{18}F]FDG-PET scan in a child with right hemimegalencephaly and intractable seizures. [^{18}F]FDG-PET revealed subtle hypometabolism (arrows) in the apparently normal hemisphere, indicating some degree of functional impairment.

PET IN PRIMARY GENERALIZED EPILEPSY

[^{18}F]FDG-PET generally has shown normal interictal patterns with diffusely increased CMRglc and CBF during seizures (Theodore et al., 1985; Prevett et al., 1995a; de Jong et al., 2008). Some data suggest thalamic activation and cortical deactivation (Duncan, 2005). Binding of the dopamine transporter ligand [^{11}C]PE2I was reduced in the midbrain in juvenile myoclonic epilepsy (JME) and in the putamen in patients with primary generalized tonic–clonic seizures (Ciumas et al., 2010). Using the high-affinity dopamine D2/D3 receptor PET ligand [^{18}F]fallypride, patients with JME showed a reduction in D2/3 receptor binding restricted to the bilateral posterior putamen (Landvogt et al., 2010). PET studies with [^{18}F]L-dopa (a presynaptic dopaminergic marker) in patients with ring chromosome 20-type epilepsy, characterized

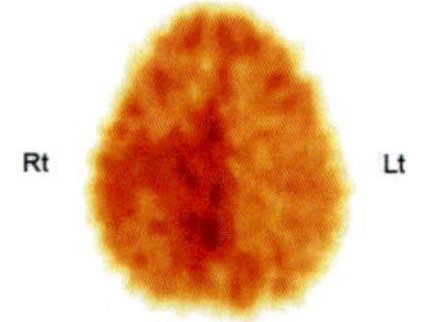

Fig. 26.15. [^{11}C]PK11195-PET scan showing an area of increased tracer binding in the right frontoparietal cortex in a child with intractable epilepsy and normal MRI, indicating neuroinflammation, which was confirmed on postsurgical histopathology.

by drug-resistant and very longlasting seizures, showed decreased uptake (Biraben et al., 2004).

There were no interictal or ictal differences from controls in [^{11}C]FMZ-PET in absence seizures in one study (Prevett et al., 1995b). Another found that patients with generalized seizures had increased benzodiazepine receptor density in cerebellar nuclei and decreased density in the thalamus (Savic et al., 1994). Differences in the patient population may explain the disparate results.

Reduced [^{11}C]FMZ binding was found in two genetic epilepsy syndromes, familial generalized epilepsy with the *GABRG2* (R43Q) mutation and succinic semialdehyde dehydrogenase deficiency (Fedi et al., 2006; Pearl et al., 2009). These two studies illustrate the value of receptor PET in showing how specific mutations lead to physiological effects.

Increased [^{11}C]diprenorphine opiate-receptor ligand elimination from association cortex during serial absences suggested endogenous opioid release and increased receptor occupancy (Bartenstein et al., 1993). [^{11}C]WAY 5HT$_{1A}$ receptor binding was reported to be reduced in bilateral dorsolateral prefrontal cortex, raphe nuclei, and hippocampus in JME (Meschaks et al., 2005).

There is little clinical role for PET in primary generalized epilepsy. It should not be used for seizure classification or distinction from localization-related epilepsy.

CONCLUSION: THE FUTURE OF PET IN EPILEPSY

The only current clinical role for PET in epilepsy is presurgical evaluation. [^{18}F]FDG will remain the most important tracer in this role, although [^{11}C]FMZ may be useful in limited circumstances. Advances in MRI may gradually reduce its value, as there will be fewer patients with negative structural imaging studies. An alternative view suggests that even when MRI is localizing, PET may reveal additional regions of cortical dysfunction that may have prognostic value for epilepsy surgery. Additional studies will be needed to address this possibility. Another hypothesis worthy of testing is that a combination of imaging procedures, which might include at least [^{18}F]FDG-PET in concert with surface interictal EEG, might obviate the need for ictal video-EEG monitoring.

Receptor PET, in contrast, should continue to be important for elucidating the pathophysiology of epilepsy, as well as comorbidities such as depression. One particularly important aspect of receptor PET is its role in translating experimental animal and *ex vivo* tissue studies to human imaging.

References

Arnold S, Schlaug G, Niemann H et al. (1996). Topography of interictal glucose hypometabolism in unilateral mesiotemporal epilepsy. Neurology 46: 1422–1430.

Arnold S, Berthele A, Drzezga A et al. (2000). Reduction of benzodiazepine receptor binding is related to the seizure onset zone in extratemporal focal cortical dysplasia. Epilepsia 41: 818–824.

Asano E, Chugani DC, Muzik O et al. (2000). Multimodality imaging for improved detection of epileptogenic foci in tuberous sclerosis complex. Neurology 54: 1976–1984.

Asano E, Chugani DC, Muzik O et al. (2001). Autism in tuberous sclerosis complex is related to both cortical and subcortical dysfunction. Neurology 57: 1269–1277.

Asano E, Juhasz C, Shah A et al. (2005). Origin and propagation of epileptic spasms delineated on electrocorticography. Epilepsia 46: 1086–1097.

Banati RB, Goerres GW, Myers R et al. (1999). [^{11}C](R)-PK11195 positron emission tomography imaging of activated microglia in vivo in Rasmussen's encephalitis. Neurology 53: 2199–2203.

Bartenstein PA, Duncan JS, Prevett MC et al. (1993). Investigation of the opioid system in absence seizures with positron emission tomography. J Neurol Neurosurg Psychiatry 56: 1295–1302.

Bartenstein PA, Prevett MC, Duncan JS et al. (1994). Quantification of opiate receptors in two patients with mesiobasal temporal lobe epilepsy, before and after selective amygdalohippocampectomy, using positron emission tomography. Epilepsy Res 18: 119–125.

Batista CE, Juhasz C, Muzik O et al. (2007). Increased visual cortex glucose metabolism contralateral to angioma in children with Sturge–Weber syndrome. Dev Med Child Neurol 49: 567–573.

Behen ME, Juhász C, Helder E et al. (2006). Cognitive function in Sturge–Weber syndrome: effect of side and extent of severe hypometabolism on PET scanning. Ann Neurol 60: S122. (Abstract).

Benedek K, Juhasz C, Chugani DC et al. (2006). Longitudinal changes in cortical glucose hypometabolism in children with intractable epilepsy. J Child Neurol 21: 26–31.

Bergström M, Kumlien E, Lilja A et al. (1998). Temporal lobe epilepsy visualized with PET with ^{11}C-L-deuterium-deprenyl – analysis of kinetic data. Acta Neurol Scand 98: 224–231.

Biraben A, Semah F, Ribeiro MJ et al. (2004). PET evidence for a role of the basal ganglia in patients with ring chromosome 20 epilepsy. Neurology 63: 73–77.

Bouilleret V, Dupont S, Spelle L et al. (2002). Insular cortex involvement in mesiotemporal lobe epilepsy: a positron emission tomography study. Ann Neurol 51: 202–208.

Bouilleret V, Semah F, Biraben A et al. (2005). Involvement of the basal ganglia in refractory epilepsy: an ^{18}F-fluoro-L-DOPA PET study using 2 methods of analysis. J Nucl Med 46: 540–547.

Bouilleret V, Semah F, Chassoux F et al. (2008). Basal ganglia involvement in temporal lobe epilepsy: a functional and morphologic study. Neurology 70: 177–184.

Bouvard S, Costes N, Bonnefoi F et al. (2005). Seizure-related short-term plasticity of benzodiazepine receptors in partial epilepsy: a [11 C]flumazenil-PET study. Brain 128: 1330–1343.

Carne RP, O'Brien TJ, Kilpatrick CJ et al. (2004). MRI-negative PET-positive temporal lobe epilepsy: a distinct surgically remediable syndrome. Brain 127: 2276–2285.

Chassoux F, Semah F, Bouilleret V et al. (2004). Metabolic changes and electro-clinical patterns in mesio-temporal lobe epilepsy: a correlative study. Brain 127: 164–174.

Chugani HT, Conti JR (1996). Etiologic classification of infantile spasms in 140 cases: role of positron emission tomography. J Child Neurol 11: 44–48.

Chugani HT, Mazziotta JC, Engel J, Jr et al. (1987). The Lennox–Gastaut syndrome: metabolic subtypes determined by 2-deoxy-2[^{18}F]fluoro-D-glucose positron emission tomography. Ann Neurol 21: 4–13.

Chugani HT, Mazziotta JC, Phelps ME (1989). Sturge–Weber syndrome: a study of cerebral glucose utilization with positron emission tomography. J Pediatr 114: 244–253.

Chugani HT, Shields WD, Shewmon DA et al. (1990). Infantile spasms: I. PET identifies focal cortical dysgenesis in cryptogenic cases for surgical treatment. Ann Neurol 27: 406–413.

Chugani HT, Shewmon DA, Sankar R et al. (1992). Infantile spasms: II. Lenticular nuclei and brain stem activation on positron emission tomography. Ann Neurol 31: 212–219.

Chugani HT, Shewmon DA, Khanna S et al. (1993a). Interictal and postictal focal hypermetabolism on positron emission tomography. Pediatr Neurol 9: 10–15.

Chugani HT, Shewmon DA, Shields WD et al. (1993b). Surgery for intractable infantile spasms: neuroimaging perspectives. Epilepsia 34: 764–771.

Chugani HT, Da Silva E, Chugani DC (1996). Infantile spasms: III. Prognostic implications of bitemporal hypometabolism on positron emission tomography. Ann Neurol 39: 643–649.

Chugani DC, Muzik O, Chakraborty P et al. (1998). Human brain serotonin synthesis capacity measured in vivo with alpha-[C-11]methyl-L-tryptophan. Synapse 28: 33–43.

Ciumas C, Wahlin TB, Espino C et al. (2010). The dopamine system in idiopathic generalized epilepsies: identification of syndrome-related changes. Neuroimage 51: 606–615.

Curatolo P, Seri S, Verdecchia M et al. (2001). Infantile spasms in tuberous sclerosis complex. Brain Dev 23: 502–507.

da Silva EA, Chugani DC, Muzik O et al. (1997). Identification of frontal lobe epileptic foci in children using positron emission tomography. Epilepsia 38: 1198–1208.

de Jong BM, van de Hoeven JH, Pruim J et al. (2008). Cortico-thalamic activation in generalized status epilepticus, a PET study. Clin Neurol Neurosurg 110: 182–185.

Delbeke D, Lawrence SK, Abou-Khalil BW et al. (1996). Postsurgical outcome of patients with uncontrolled complex partial seizures and temporal lobe hypometabolism on 18FDG-positron emission tomography. Invest Radiol 31: 261–266.

Depositario-Cabacar DT, Riviello JJ et al. (2008). Present status of surgical intervention for children with intractable seizures. Curr Neurol Neurosci Rep 8: 123–129.

Didelot A, Ryvlin P, Lothe A et al. (2008). PET imaging of brain 5-HT1A receptors in the preoperative evaluation of temporal lobe epilepsy. Brain 131: 2751–2764.

Drevets WC, Thase ME, Moses-Kolko EL et al. (2007). Serotonin-1A receptor imaging in recurrent depression: replication and literature review. Nucl Med Biol 34: 865–877.

Duchowny M, Jayakar P, Resnick T et al. (1998). Epilepsy surgery in the first three years of life. Epilepsia 39: 737–743.

Duncan JS (2005). Brain imaging in idiopathic generalized epilepsies. Epilepsia 46: 108–111.

Dupont S, Semah F, Clemenceau S et al. (2000). Accurate prediction of postoperative outcome in mesial temporal lobe epilepsy: a study using positron emission tomography with 18fluorodeoxyglucose. Arch Neurol 57: 1331–1336.

Dupont S, Croize AC, Semah F et al. (2001). Is amygdalohippocampectomy really selective in medial temporal lobe epilepsy? A study using positron emission tomography with (18)fluorodeoxyglucose. Epilepsia 42: 731–740.

Eluvathingal TJ, Behen ME, Chugani HT et al. (2006). Cerebellar lesions in tuberous sclerosis complex: neurobehavioral and neuroimaging correlates. J Child Neurol 21: 846–851.

Engel J, Jr, Kuhl DE, Phelps ME et al. (1982a). Comparative localization of epileptic foci in partial epilepsy by PCT and EEG. Ann Neurol 12: 529–537.

Engel J, Jr, Kuhl DE, Phelps ME et al. (1982b). Interictal cerebral glucose metabolism in partial epilepsy and its relation to EEG changes. Ann Neurol 12: 510–517.

Engel J, Jr, Kuhl DE, Phelps ME (1982c). Patterns of human local cerebral glucose metabolism during epileptic seizures. Science 218: 64–66.

Engel JJ, Van Ness PC, Rasmussen TB et al. (1993). Outcome with respect to epileptic seizures. In: JJ Engel (Ed.), Surgical Treatment of the Epilepsies. 2nd edn. Raven, New York, pp. 609–622.

Fedi M, Reutens DC, Andermann F et al. (2003). α-[^{11}C]-methyl-L-tryptophan PET identifies the epileptogenic tuber and correlates with interictal spike frequency. Epilepsy Res 52: 203–213.

Fedi M, Berkovic SF, Marini C et al. (2006). A $GABA_A$ receptor mutation causing generalized epilepsy reduces benzodiazepine receptor binding. Neuroimage 32: 995–1000.

Fedi M, Berkovic SF, Scheffer IE et al. (2008). Reduced striatal D1 receptor binding in autosomal dominant nocturnal frontal lobe epilepsy. Neurology 71: 795–798.

Ferrie CD, Maisey M, Cox T et al. (1996). Focal abnormalities detected by 18FDG PET in epileptic encephalopathies. Arch Dis Child 75: 102–107.

Fogarasi A, Hegyi M, Neuwirth M et al. (2003). Comparative evaluation of concomitant structural and functional neuroimages in Rasmussen's encephalitis. J Neuroimaging 13: 339–345.

Frost JJ, Mayberg HS, Fisher RS et al. (1988). Mu-opiate receptors measured by positron emission tomography are increased in temporal lobe epilepsy. Ann Neurol 23: 231–237.

Gaillard WD, Bhatia S, Bookheimer SY et al. (1995a). [^{18}F]-FDG-PET and volumetric MRI in the evaluation of patients with partial epilepsy. Neurology 45: 123–126.

Gaillard WD, White S, Malow B et al. (1995b). [^{18}F]-FDG-PET in children and adolescents with partial seizures: role in epilepsy surgery evaluation. Epilepsy Res 20: 77–84.

Gaillard WD, Kopylev L, Weinstein S et al. (2002). Low incidence of abnormal (18)FDG-PET in children with new-onset partial epilepsy: a prospective study. Neurology 58: 717–722.

Gaillard WD, Weinstein S, Conry J et al. (2007). Prognosis of children with partial epilepsy: MRI and serial 18FDG-PET. Neurology 68: 655–659.

Gaily EK, Shewmon DA, Chugani HT et al. (1995). Asymmetric and asynchronous infantile spasms. Epilepsia 36: 873–882.

Giovacchini G, Toczek MT, Bonwetsch R et al. (2005). 5-HT 1A receptors are reduced in temporal lobe epilepsy after partial-volume correction. J Nucl Med 46: 1128–1135.

Goerres GW, Revesz T, Duncan J et al. (2001). Imaging cerebral vasculitis in refractory epilepsy using [^{11}C](R)-PK11195 positron emission tomography. AJR Am J Roentgenol 176: 1016–1018.

Gur RC, Sussman NM, Alavi A et al. (1982). Positron emission tomography in two cases of childhood epileptic encephalopathy (Lennox–Gastaut syndrome). Neurology 32: 1191–1194.

Hajek M, Antonini A, Leenders KL et al. (1993). Mesiobasal versus lateral temporal lobe epilepsy: metabolic differences in the temporal lobe shown by interictal 18 F-FDG positron emission tomography. Neurology 43: 79–86.

Hammers A, Koepp MJ, Labbe C et al. (2001). Neocortical abnormalities of [^{11}C]-flumazenil PET in mesial temporal lobe epilepsy. Neurology 56: 897–906.

Hammers A, Koepp MJ, Hurlemann R et al. (2002). Abnormalities of grey and white matter [^{11}C]flumazenil binding in temporal lobe epilepsy with normal MRI. Brain 125: 2257–2271.

Hammers A, Asselin MC, Hinz R et al. (2007). Upregulation of opioid receptor binding following spontaneous epileptic seizures. Brain 130: 1009–1016.

Hasler G, Bonwetsch R, Giovacchini G et al. (2007). 5-HT_{1A} receptor binding in temporal lobe epilepsy patients with and without major depression. Biol Psychiatry 62: 1258–1264.

Henry TR, Sutherling WW, Engel J, Jr et al. (1991). Interictal cerebral metabolism in partial epilepsies of neocortical origin. Epilepsy Res 10: 174–182.

Henry TR, Frey KA, Sackellares JC et al. (1993a). In vivo cerebral metabolism and central benzodiazepine-receptor binding in temporal lobe epilepsy. Neurology 43: 1998–2006.

Henry TR, Mazziotta JC, Engel J, Jr (1993b). Interictal metabolic anatomy of mesial temporal lobe epilepsy. Arch Neurol 50: 582–589.

Honbolygo F, Csepe V, Fekeshazy A et al. (2006). Converging evidences on language impairment in Landau–Kleffner syndrome revealed by behavioral and brain activity measures: a case study. Clin Neurophysiol 117: 295–305.

Iinuma K, Yanai K, Yanagisawa T et al. (1987). Cerebral glucose metabolism in five patients with Lennox–Gastaut syndrome. Pediatr Neurol 3: 12–18.

Iinuma K, Yokoyama H, Otsuki T et al. (1993). Histamine H1 receptors in complex partial seizures. Lancet 341: 238.

Itomi K, Okumura A, Negoro T et al. (2002). Prognostic value of positron emission tomography in cryptogenic West syndrome. Dev Med Child Neurol 44: 107–111.

Juhasz C, Nagy F, Muzik O et al. (1999). [^{11}C]Flumazenil PET in patients with epilepsy with dual pathology. Epilepsia 40: 566–574.

Juhasz C, Chugani DC, Muzik O et al. (2000). Electroclinical correlates of flumazenil and fluorodeoxyglucose PET abnormalities in lesional epilepsy. Neurology 55: 825–835.

Juhasz C, Chugani DC, Muzik O et al. (2001). Relationship of flumazenil and glucose PET abnormalities to neocortical epilepsy surgery outcome. Neurology 56: 1650–1658.

Juhász C, Chugani DC, Asano E et al. (2002). Alpha[^{11}C] methyl-L-tryptophan positron emission tomography scanning in 176 patients with intractable epilepsy. Ann Neurol S118. (Abstract).

Juhasz C, Chugani DC, Muzik O et al. (2003). Alpha-methyl-L-tryptophan PET detects epileptogenic cortex in children with intractable epilepsy. Neurology 60: 960–968.

Juhasz C, Batista CE, Chugani DC et al. (2007a). Evolution of cortical metabolic abnormalities and their clinical correlates in Sturge–Weber syndrome. Eur J Paediatr Neurol 11: 277–284.

Juhasz C, Lai C, Behen ME et al. (2007b). White matter volume as a major predictor of cognitive function in Sturge–Weber syndrome. Arch Neurol 64: 1169–1174.

Kagawa K, Chugani DC, Asano E et al. (2005). Epilepsy surgery outcome in children with tuberous sclerosis complex evaluated with alpha-[^{11}C]methyl-L-tryptophan positron emission tomography (PET). J Child Neurol 20: 429–438.

Khan N, Leenders KL, Hajek M et al. (1997). Thalamic glucose metabolism in temporal lobe epilepsy measured with 18 F-FDG positron emission tomography (PET). Epilepsy Res 28: 233–243.

Kim YK, Lee DS, Lee SK et al. (2002). (18)F-FDG PET in localization of frontal lobe epilepsy: comparison of visual and SPM analysis. J Nucl Med 43: 1167–1174.

Kim YK, Lee DS, Lee SK et al. (2003). Differential features of metabolic abnormalities between medial and lateral temporal lobe epilepsy: quantitative analysis of (18)F-FDG PET using SPM. J Nucl Med 44: 1006–1012.

Kim DW, Lee SK, Chu K et al. (2009). Predictors of surgical outcome and pathologic considerations in focal cortical dysplasia. Neurology 72: 211–216.

Knowlton RC, Laxer KD, Ende G et al. (1997). Presurgical multimodality neuroimaging in electroencephalographic lateralized temporal lobe epilepsy. Ann Neurol 42: 829–837.

Knowlton RC, Elgavish RA, Bartolucci A et al. (2008). Functional imaging: II. Prediction of epilepsy surgery outcome. Ann Neurol 64: 35–41.

Koepp MJ, Woermann FG (2005). Imaging structure and function in refractory focal epilepsy. Lancet Neurol 4: 42–53.

Koepp MJ, Richardson MP, Brooks DJ et al. (1996). Cerebral benzodiazepine receptors in hippocampal sclerosis. An objective in vivo analysis. Brain 119: 1677–1687.

Koepp MJ, Labbe C, Richardson MP et al. (1997). Regional hippocampal [^{11}C]flumazenil PET in temporal lobe epilepsy with unilateral and bilateral hippocampal sclerosis. Brain 120: 1865–1876.

Koepp MJ, Richardson MP, Brooks DJ et al. (1998). Focal cortical release of endogenous opioids during reading-induced seizures. Lancet 352: 952–955.

Koepp MJ, Hammers A, Labbe C et al. (2000). ^{11}C-flumazenil PET in patients with refractory temporal lobe epilepsy and normal MRI. Neurology 54: 332–339.

Kramer U, Sue WC, Mikati MA (1997). Focal features in West syndrome indicating candidacy for surgery. Pediatr Neurol 16: 213–217.

Kuhl DE, Engel J, Jr, Phelps ME et al. (1978). Epileptic patterns of local cerebral metabolism and perfusion in humans determined by emission computed tomography of ^{18}FDG and $^{13}NH_3$. Ann Neurol 8: 348–360.

Kumada T, Okazawa H, Yamauchi H et al. (2006). Focal glucose hypermetabolism in interictal state of West syndrome. Pediatr Neurol 34: 47–50.

Kumar A, Chugani HT, Luat A et al. (2008). Epilepsy surgery in a case of encephalitis: use of ^{11}C-PK11195 positron emission tomography. Pediatr Neurol 38: 439–442.

Kumlien E, Hilton-Brown P, Spannere B et al. (1992). In vitro quantitative autoradiography of (^{3}H)-L-deprenyl and (^{3}H)-PK 11195 binding sites in human epileptic hippocampus. Epilepsia 33: 610–617.

Kumlien E, Hartvig P, Valind S et al. (1999). NMDA-receptor activity visualized with (S)-[N-methyl-^{11}C]ketamine and positron emission tomography in patients with medial temporal lobe epilepsy. Epilepsia 40: 30–37.

Kumlien E, Nilsson A, Hagberg G et al. (2001). PET with ^{11}C-deuterium-deprenyl and ^{18}F-FDG in focal epilepsy. Acta Neurol Scand 103: 360–366.

la Fougère C, Böning G, Bartmann H et al. (2010). Uptake and binding of the serotonin 5-HT1A antagonist [18 F]-MPPF in brain of rats: effects of the novel P-glycoprotein inhibitor tariquidar. Neuroimage 49: 1406–1415.

Lamusuo S, Pitkanen A, Jutila L et al. (2000). [^{11}C]Flumazenil binding in the medial temporal lobe in patients with temporal lobe epilepsy: correlation with hippocampal MR volumetry, T2 relaxometry, and neuropathology. Neurology 54: 2252–2260.

Lamusuo S, Jutila L, Ylinen A et al. (2001). [^{18}F]FDG-PET reveals temporal hypometabolism in patients with temporal lobe epilepsy even when quantitative MRI and histopathological analysis show only mild hippocampal damage. Arch Neurol 58: 933–939.

Landvogt C, Buchholz HG, Bernedo V et al. (2010). Alteration of dopamine D2/D3 receptor binding in patients with juvenile myoclonic epilepsy. Epilepsia 51: 1699–1706.

Langer O, Bauer B, Hammers A et al. (2007). Pharmacoresistance in epilepsy: a pilot PET study with the p-glycoprotein substrate R-[^{11}C]verapamil. Epilepsia 48: 1774–1784.

Lee JS, Asano E, Muzik O et al. (2001a). Sturge–Weber syndrome: correlation between clinical course and [^{18}F]-FDG PET findings. Neurology 57: 189–195.

Lee JS, Juhasz C, Kaddurah AK et al. (2001b). Patterns of cerebral glucose metabolism in early and late stages of Rasmussen's syndrome. J Child Neurol 16: 798–805.

Lee SK, Lee SY, Kim KK et al. (2005). Surgical outcome and prognostic factors of cryptogenic neocortical epilepsy. Ann Neurol 58: 525–532.

Lee JJ, Lee SK, Lee SY et al. (2008). Frontal lobe epilepsy: clinical characteristics, surgical outcomes and diagnostic modalities. Seizure 17: 514–523.

Leiderman DB, Albert P, Balish M et al. (1994). The dynamics of metabolic change following seizures as measured by positron emission tomography with fludeoxyglucose F18. Arch Neurol 51: 932–936.

Lerner JT, Salamon N, Hauptman JS et al. (2009). Assessment and surgical outcomes for mild type I and severe type II cortical dysplasia: a critical review and the UCLA experience. Epilepsia 50: 1310–1335.

Liew CJ, Lim YM, Bonwetsch R et al. (2009). ^{18}F-FCWAY and ^{18}F-FDG PET in MRI-negative temporal lobe epilepsy. Epilepsia 50: 234–239.

Lothe A, Didelot A, Hammers A et al. (2008). Comorbidity between temporal lobe epilepsy and depression: a [^{18}F] MPPF PET study. Brain 131: 2765–2782.

Luat AF, Chugani HT, Asano E et al. (2006). Episodic receptive aphasia in a child with Landau–Kleffner syndrome: PET correlates. Brain Dev 28: 592–596.

Luat AF, Makki M, Chugani HT (2007). Neuroimaging in tuberous sclerosis complex. Curr Opin Neurol 20: 142–150.

Madar I, Lesser RP, Krauss G et al. (1997). Imaging of delta- and mu-opioid receptors in temporal lobe epilepsy by positron emission tomography. Ann Neurol 41: 358–367.

Maeda N, Watanabe K, Negoro T et al. (1994). Evolutional changes of cortical hypometabolism in West's syndrome. Lancet 343: 1620–1623.

Manno EM, Sperling MR, Ding X et al. (1994). Predictors of outcome after anterior temporal lobectomy: positron emission tomography. Neurology 44: 2331–2336.

Maquet P, Hirsch E, Dive D et al. (1990). Cerebral glucose utilization during sleep in Landau–Kleffner syndrome: a PET study. Epilepsia 31: 778–783.

Mayberg HS, Sadzot B, Meltzer CC et al. (1991). Quantification of mu and non-mu opiate receptors in temporal lobe epilepsy using positron emission tomography. Ann Neurol 30: 3–11.

Merlet I, Ostrowsky K, Costes N et al. (2004a). 5-HT1A receptor binding and intracerebral activity in temporal lobe epilepsy: an [^{18}F]MPPF-PET study. Brain 127: 900–913.

Merlet I, Ryvlin P, Costes N et al. (2004b). Statistical parametric mapping of 5-HT1A receptor binding in temporal lobe epilepsy with hippocampal ictal onset on intracranial EEG. Neuroimage 22: 886–896.

Meschaks A, Lindstrom P, Halldin C et al. (2005). Regional reductions in serotonin 1A receptor binding in juvenile myoclonic epilepsy. Arch Neurol 62: 946–950.

Metz-Lutz MN, Filippini M (2006). Neuropsychological findings in Rolandic epilepsy and Landau–Kleffner syndrome. Epilepsia 47: 71–75.

Miyauchi T, Nomura Y, Ohno S et al. (1988). Positron emission tomography in three cases of Lennox–Gastaut syndrome. Jpn J Psychiatry Neurol 42: 795–804.

Müller RA, Chugani HT, Muzik O et al. (1997). Language and motor functions activate calcified hemisphere in patients with Sturge–Weber syndrome: a positron emission tomography study. J Child Neurol 12: 431–437.

Muzik O, da Silva EA, Juhasz C et al. (2000). Intracranial EEG versus flumazenil and glucose PET in children with extratemporal lobe epilepsy. Neurology 54: 171–179.

Nagy F, Chugani DC, Juhasz C et al. (1999). Altered in vitro and in vivo flumazenil binding in human epileptogenic neocortex. J Cereb Blood Flow Metab 19: 939–947.

Natsume J, Watanabe K, Maeda N et al. (1996). Cortical hypometabolism and delayed myelination in West syndrome. Epilepsia 37: 1180–1184.

Natsume J, Kumakura Y, Bernasconi N et al. (2003). Alpha-[^{11}C] methyl-L-tryptophan and glucose metabolism in patients with temporal lobe epilepsy. Neurology 60: 756–761.

Nishida M, Asano E, Juhasz C et al. (2008). Cortical glucose metabolism correlates negatively with delta-slowing and spike-frequency in epilepsy associated with tuberous sclerosis. Hum Brain Mapp 29: 1255–1264.

O'Brien TJ, Hicks RJ, Ware R et al. (2001). The utility of a 3-dimensional, large-field-of-view, sodium iodide crystal-based PET scanner in the presurgical evaluation of partial epilepsy. J Nucl Med 42: 1158–1165.

Ohta Y, Nariai T, Akimoto H et al. (2001). Tuberous sclerosis: epileptogenicity and multimodal presurgical evaluations. Childs Nerv Syst 17: 313–319.

Ollenberger GP, Byrne AJ, Berlangieri SU et al. (2005). Assessment of the role of [^{18}F]-FDG PET in the diagnosis and management of children with refractory epilepsy. Eur J Nucl Med Mol Imaging 32: 1311–1316.

Patil S, Biassoni L, Borgwardt L (2007). Nuclear medicine in pediatric neurology and neurosurgery: epilepsy and brain tumors. Semin Nucl Med 37: 357–381.

Pearl PL, Gibson KM, Quezado Z et al. (2009). Decreased GABA-A binding on [^{11}C]-FMZ-PET in succinic semialdehyde dehydrogenase (SSADH) deficiency. Neurology 73: 423–429.

Pfund Z, Kagawa K, Juhász C et al. (2003). Quantitative analysis of gray- and white-matter volumes and glucose metabolism in Sturge–Weber syndrome. J Child Neurol 18: 119–126.

Phi JH, Paeng JC, Lee HS et al. (2010). Evaluation of focal cortical dysplasia and mixed neuronal and glial tumors in pediatric epilepsy patients using ^{18}F-FDG and ^{11}C-methionine pet. J Nucl Med 51: 728–734.

Picard F, Bruel D, Servent D et al. (2006). Alteration of the in vivo nicotinic receptor density in ADNFLE patients: a PET study. Brain 129: 2047–2060.

Poduri A, Golja A, Takeoka M et al. (2007). Focal cortical malformations can show asymmetrically higher uptake on interictal fluorine-18 fluorodeoxyglucose positron emission tomography (PET). J Child Neurol 22: 232–237.

Prevett MC, Duncan JS, Jones T et al. (1995a). Demonstration of thalamic activation during typical absence seizures using $H_2(^{15})O$ and PET. Neurology 45: 1396–1402.

Prevett MC, Lammertsma AA, Brooks DJ et al. (1995b). Benzodiazepine-$GABA_A$ receptor binding during absence seizures. Epilepsia 36: 592–599.

Richardson MP, Koepp MJ, Brooks DJ et al. (1998). ^{11}C-flumazenil PET in neocortical epilepsy. Neurology 51: 485–492.

Rintahaka PJ, Chugani HT (1997). Clinical role of positron emission tomography in children with tuberous sclerosis complex. J Child Neurol 12: 42–52.

Rintahaka PJ, Chugani HT, Messa C et al. (1993). Hemimegalencephaly: evaluation with positron emission tomography. Pediatr Neurol 9: 21–28.

Rintahaka PJ, Chugani HT, Sankar R (1995). Landau–Kleffner syndrome with continuous spikes and waves during slow-wave sleep. J Child Neurol 10: 127–133.

Ryvlin P, Bouvard S, Le Bars D et al. (1998). Clinical utility of flumazenil-PET versus [^{18}F]fluorodeoxyglucose-PET and MRI in refractory partial epilepsy. A prospective study in 100 patients. Brain 121: 2067–2081.

Ryvlin P, Bouvard S, Le Bars D et al. (1999). Transient and falsely lateralizing flumazenil-PET asymmetries in temporal lobe epilepsy. Neurology 53: 1882–1885.

Salanova V, Markand O, Worth R et al. (1998). [^{18}F]-FDG-PET and MRI in temporal lobe epilepsy: relationship to febrile seizures, hippocampal sclerosis and outcome. Acta Neurol Scand 97: 146–153.

Savic I, Ingvar M, Stone-Elander S (1993). Comparison of [^{11}C]flumazenil and [^{18}F]FDG as PET markers of epileptic foci. J Neurol Neurosurg Psychiatry 56: 615–621.

Savic I, Pauli S, Thorell JO et al. (1994). In vivo demonstration of altered benzodiazepine receptor density in patients with generalised epilepsy. J Neurol Neurosurg Psychiatry 57: 797–804.

Savic I, Thorell JO, Roland P (1995). [^{11}C]flumazenil positron emission tomography visualizes frontal epileptogenic regions. Epilepsia 36: 1225–1232.

Savic I, Altshuler L, Baxter L, Jr (1997). Pattern of interictal hypometabolism in PET scans with fludeoxyglucose F18 reflects prior seizure types in patients with mesial temporal lobe seizures. Arch Neurol 54: 129–136.

Savic I, Lindstrom P, Gulyas B et al. (2004). Limbic reductions of 5-HT1A receptor binding in human temporal lobe epilepsy. Neurology 62: 1343–1351.

Semah F, Baulac M, Hasboun D et al. (1995). Is interictal temporal hypometabolism related to mesial temporal sclerosis? A positron emission tomography/magnetic resonance imaging confrontation. Epilepsia 36: 447–456.

Shiraishi H, Takano K, Shiga T et al. (2007). Possible involvement of the tip of temporal lobe in Landau–Kleffner syndrome. Brain Dev 29: 529–533.

Sperling MR, Alavi A, Reivich M et al. (1995). False lateralization of temporal lobe epilepsy with [^{18}F]-FDG positron emission tomography. Epilepsia 36: 722–727.

Swartz BE, Halgren E, Delgado-Escueta AV et al. (1989). Neuroimaging in patients with seizures of probable frontal lobe origin. Epilepsia 30: 547–558.

Swartz BW, Khonsari A, Vrown C et al. (1995). Improved sensitivity of 18FDG-positron emission tomography scans in frontal and “frontal plus” epilepsy. Epilepsia 36: 388–395.

Swartz BE, Brown C, Mandelkern MA et al. (2002). The use of 2-deoxy-2-[18 F]fluoro-D-glucose (FDG-PET) positron emission tomography in the routine diagnosis of epilepsy. Mol Imaging Biol 4: 245–252.

Szelies B, Herholz K, Heiss WD et al. (1983). Hypometabolic cortical lesions in tuberous sclerosis with epilepsy: demonstration by positron emission tomography. J Comput Assist Tomogr 7: 946–953.

Szelies B, Weber-Luxenburger G, Pawlik G et al. (1996). MRI-guided flumazenil- and [^{18}F]-FDG-PET in temporal lobe epilepsy. Neuroimage 3: 109–118.

Szelies B, Sobesky J, Pawlik G et al. (2002). Impaired benzodiazepine receptor binding in peri-lesional cortex of patients with symptomatic epilepsies studied by [(11)C]-flumazenil PET. Eur J Neurol 9: 137–142.

Takaya S, Mikuni N, Mitsueda T et al. (2009). Improved cerebral function in mesial temporal lobe epilepsy after subtemporal amygdalohippocampectomy. Brain 132: 185–194.

Theodore WH, Newmark ME, Sato S et al. (1983). [^{18}F]fluorodeoxyglucose positron emission tomography in refractory complex partial seizures. Ann Neurol 14: 429–437.

Theodore WH, Brooks R, Margolin R et al. (1985). Positron emission tomography in generalized seizures. Neurology 35: 684–690.

Theodore WH, Rose D, Patronas N et al. (1987). Cerebral glucose metabolism in the Lennox–Gastaut syndrome. Ann Neurol 21: 14–21.

Theodore WH, Carson RE, Andreasen P et al. (1992a). PET imaging of opiate receptor binding in human epilepsy using [^{18}F]cyclofoxy. Epilepsy Res 13: 129–139.

Theodore WH, Sato S, Kufta C et al. (1992b). Temporal lobectomy for uncontrolled seizures: the role of positron emission tomography. Ann Neurol 32: 789–794.

Theodore WH, Leiderman D, Gaillard WD et al. (1993). The effect of naloxone on cerebral blood flow and glucose metabolism in patients with complex partial seizures. Epilepsy Res 16: 51–54.

Theodore WH, Sato S, Kufta CV et al. (1997). [^{18}F]-FDG-positron emission tomography and invasive EEG: seizure focus detection and surgical outcome. Epilepsia 38: 81–86.

Theodore WH, Giovacchini G, Bonwetsch R et al. (2006). The effect of antiepileptic drugs on 5-HT1A receptor binding measured by positron emission tomography. Epilepsia 47: 499–503.

Theodore WH, Hasler G, Giovacchini G et al. (2007). Reduced hippocampal 5HT1A PET receptor binding and depression in temporal lobe epilepsy. Epilepsia 48: 1526–1530.

Toczek MT, Carson RE, Lang L et al. (2003). PET imaging of 5-HT1A receptor binding in patients with temporal lobe epilepsy. Neurology 60: 749–756.

Uijl SG, Leijten FS, Arends JB et al. (2007). The added value of [^{18}F]-fluoro-D-deoxyglucose positron emission tomography in screening for temporal lobe epilepsy surgery. Epilepsia 48: 2121–2129.

Uijl SG, Leijten FS, Arends JB et al. (2008). Prognosis after temporal lobe epilepsy surgery: the value of combining predictors. Epilepsia 49: 1317–1323.

Van Bogaert P, Massager N, Tugendhaft P et al. (2000). Statistical parametric mapping of regional glucose metabolism in mesial temporal lobe epilepsy. Neuroimage 12: 129–138.

Vinton AB, Carne R, Hicks RJ et al. (2007). The extent of resection of [^{18}F]-FDG-PET hypometabolism relates to outcome of temporal lobectomy. Brain 130: 548–560.

Wakamoto H, Chugani DC, Juhasz C et al. (2008). Alpha-methyl-L-tryptophan positron emission tomography in epilepsy with cortical developmental malformations. Pediatr Neurol 39: 181–188.

Weitemeyer L, Kellinghaus C, Weckesser M et al. (2005). The prognostic value of [F]FDG-PET in nonrefractory partial epilepsy. Epilepsia 46: 1654–1660.

Werhahn KJ, Landvogt C, Klimpe S et al. (2006). Decreased dopamine D2/D3-receptor binding in temporal lobe epilepsy: an [^{18}F]fallypride PET study. Epilepsia 47: 1392–1396.

Willmann O, Wennberg R, May T et al. (2007). The contribution of 18 F-FDG PET in preoperative epilepsy surgery evaluation for patients with temporal lobe epilepsy: a meta-analysis. Seizure 16: 509–520.

Wong CH, Bleasel A, Wen L et al. (2010). The topography and significance of extratemporal hypometabolism in refractory mesial temporal lobe epilepsy examined by FDG-PET. Epilepsia 51: 1365–1373.

Wyllie E, Comair YG, Kotagal P et al. (1998). Seizure outcome after epilepsy surgery in children and adolescents. Ann Neurol 44: 740–748.

Yanai K, Iinuma K, Matsuzawa T et al. (1987). Cerebral glucose utilization in pediatric neurological disorders determined by positron emission tomography. Eur J Nucl Med 13: 292–296.

You SJ, Lee JK, Ko TS (2007). Epilepsy surgery in a patient with Lennox–Gastaut syndrome and cortical dysplasia. Brain Dev 29: 167–170.

Yun CH, Lee SK, Lee SY et al. (2006). Prognostic factors in neocortical epilepsy surgery: multivariate analysis. Epilepsia 47: 574–579.

Zimmer L, Mauger G, Le Bars D et al. (2002). Effect of endogenous serotonin on the binding of the 5-HT1A PET ligand 18 F-MPPF in the rat hippocampus: kinetic beta measurements combined with microdialysis. J Neurochem 80: 278–286.

Handbook of Clinical Neurology, Vol. 107 (3rd series)
Epilepsy, Part I
H. Stefan and W.H. Theodore, Editors

Chapter 27

Peri-ictal single-photon emission computed tomography: principles and applications in epilepsy evaluation

ELSON L. SO [1]* AND TERRENCE J. O'BRIEN [2]
[1] *Department of Neurology, Mayo Clinic, Rochester, MN, USA*
[2] *Department of Medicine, University of Melbourne, Melbourne, Victoria, Australia*

INTRODUCTION

Localization of seizure activity in the brain is a *sine qua non* for surgery to control seizures. Seizures are localized by integration, by an experienced clinician, of information from the clinical history, seizure description, magnetic resonance imaging (MRI), interictal electroencephalography (EEG), ictal video-EEG recording, and functional imaging, for example [^{18}F] fluorodeoxyglucose positron emission tomography (FDG-PET), single-photon emission computed tomography (SPECT), magnetic resonance spectroscopy (MRS), and magnetic source imaging (MSI). High concordance of the evidence from these diagnostic modalities is necessary for confident localization of seizures before resective epilepsy surgery. This principle is especially important when localizing seizures in patients with nonlesional epilepsy, i.e. when MRI shows no potentially epileptogenic lesion.

The main objective of this chapter is to discuss the usefulness of different types of peri-ictal SPECT study to aid localization of the seizure focus. Peri-ictal SPECT studies refer to studies obtained by ictal or postictal injection of the radiotracer. Different radiotracers have also been used in SPECT. The development and application of digital subtraction and statistical analysis of SPECT data will also be discussed.

Positron emission tomography (PET) was formally evaluated 30 years ago as a functional imaging modality to assess both regional cerebral metabolism and perfusion in epilepsy (Kuhl et al., 1980). SPECT ensued as a method for measuring regional cerebral blood flow (rCBF) in epilepsy (Kuhl et al., 1982; Bonte et al., 1983; Uren et al., 1983; Biersack et al., 1986; Matsuda et al., 1986; Stefan et al., 1987a, b, 1990). The development of technetium-99 m (^{99m}Tc)-linked radiotracers soon led to the study of SPECT in evaluating rCBF during the interictal and the peri-ictal periods (Sharp et al., 1986; Lee et al., 1987, 1988).

In a study that evaluated nonlesional epilepsy with interictal EEG, ictal scalp EEG, FDG-PET, and subtraction ictal SPECT coregistered to MRI (SISCOM), 80% of patients became seizure-free when all four modalities were concordant; in contrast, only about 45% became seizure-free when fewer than two modalities were concordant (Lee et al., 2005).

Overall, nonlesional epilepsy surgery is associated with a lower chance of excellent outcome than lesional epilepsy surgery. The probability of excellent seizure control following temporal lobe lesional surgery is as high as 90%, but the probability is approximately 65% in nonlesional temporal lobe surgery (Radhakrishnan et al., 1998). A discrepancy in outcomes is also observed between lesional and nonlesional frontal lobe epilepsy surgery (72% versus 41% probability for excellent postsurgical outcome; i.e., seizure-free, or only aura or nondisabling nocturnal seizures) (Mosewich et al., 2000). Therefore, the absence of a structural lesion on MRI in nonlesional epilepsy requires the use of functional imaging to detect surrogate evidence of a focus of potential epileptogenicity. Functional imaging may also be valuable in epilepsy surgery evaluation when MRI shows an ambiguous lesion or multiple lesions or when diagnostic modalities are not concordant.

*Correspondence to: Elson L. So, M.D., Department of Neurology, Director, Section of Electroencephalography, Mayo Clinic Rochester, MN 55905, USA. E-mail: eso@mayo.edu

UNIQUE ROLE OF PERFUSION SPECT IN EPILEPSY

SPECT dynamics and radiotracer characteristics

Several modalities are available for imaging the regional cerebral dysfunction that potentially corresponds to the epileptogenic zone (i.e., the focus that has to be resected for optimal seizure control). Of all functional imaging modalities, SPECT is the only one that is feasible for imaging interictal, ictal, and postictal alterations in brain function. The radiotracer FDG used in metabolism PET has a cerebral uptake duration of about 40 minutes, which greatly exceeds the typical duration of seizure activity of 1–3 minutes. On the other hand, perfusion PET is not feasible as an ictal test because its radiotracer, ^{15}O-labeled water, has a very short half-life of about 2 minutes, which would require that the patient be in the scanner and experiencing a seizure at the time of the scan. Functional MRI, MRS, and magnetoencephalography (MEG) also require the patient to be in the scanning machine at the time of the occurrence of the event of interest. Because the precise time of seizure occurrence is unpredictable, the application of these modalities is practically limited to the interictal period. Moreover, the high susceptibility of these procedures to movement artifacts requires the patient to be very still and cooperative. In addition, MEG and functional MRI equipment and technology are the least widely available diagnostic modalities for seizure localization.

SPECT images are acquired by camera detection of gamma energy rays emitted by a radiotracer that had been administered to the patient. Multiple planar imaging data are obtained at different angles, and computer-aided reconstruction of the data results in axial, coronal, and sagittal series of images of the organ of interest. Perfusion brain SPECT was initially evaluated as a clinical imaging procedure by using the radiotracer *N*-isopropyl-(iodine 123)-*p*-iodoamphetamine ([^{123}I]IMP) (Matsuda et al., 1986). Although [^{123}I]IMP kinetics are favorable for peri-ictal SPECT use, this agent has not been readily available on a commercial basis, and ^{99m}Tc-linked radiotracers have been in use for peri-ictal SPECT studies for at least two decades. The first-pass brain extraction rate of ^{99m}Tc-linked radiotracers used in SPECT is very high, so that fixation of the radiotracer to brain receptors is sufficiently prompt after intravenous injection of the radiotracer during a seizure. This characteristic permits snapshot imaging of perfusion changes associated with epileptic seizure activity. Moreover, radioactivity decay of ^{99m}Tc-linked radiotracers is sufficiently slow, and the fixation of the radiotracers to brain receptors is sufficiently long, to allow the brain SPECT images to be scanned for up to 3–4 hours after radiotracer injection (Neirinckx et al., 1988; Jacquier-Sarlin et al., 1996). This interval allows enough time for administering antiseizure or sedative medications to enhance patient safety and reduce movement artifacts, and for arranging the availability of staff and equipment to conduct SPECT. Furthermore, SPECT is more readily available in medical centers worldwide than most other diagnostic modalities mentioned in the preceding paragraphs.

Early studies of peri-ictal SPECT in epilepsy used the radiotracer hexamethyl propylene amine oxime (^{99m}Tc-HMPAO), which had to be constituted immediately before its injection (Harvey et al., 1993a, b; Newton et al., 1993). This prevented prompt injection of ^{99m}Tc-HMPAO during the ictal period and has resulted in most injections being conducted during the postictal period. ^{99m}Tc-labeled ethyl cysteinate diethylester (^{99m}Tc-ECD) was later developed as a preconstituted stable radiotracer, ready for immediate injection when a seizure occurs (Walovitch et al., 1991). Thus, ^{99m}Tc-ECD can be injected more quickly after seizure onset than ^{99m}Tc-HMPAO (O'Brien et al., 1999a). A stabilized form of ^{99m}Tc-HMPAO that does not require preparation immediately before injection is now available for peri-ictal SPECT use in some countries.

Although the peak uptake of ^{99m}Tc-ECD is only about 5% of the dose injected, ^{99m}Tc-ECD has a much longer washout period than ^{99m}Tc-HMPAO. The regional distribution of ^{99m}Tc-ECD reflects the rCBF in a more linear fashion than that of ^{99m}Tc-HMPAO (Devous et al., 1993). The back-diffusion of ^{99m}Tc-ECD is higher in extracerebral tissues than in cerebral tissues, which offers better image definition of cerebral tissue perfusion at lower radioisotope doses. Compared with ^{99m}Tc-HMPAO, ^{99m}Tc-ECD uptake is relatively less in extracerebral and subcortical white-matter regions (Leveille et al., 1992; Patterson et al., 1997; O'Brien et al., 1999a). However, it is not known whether these pharmacokinetic advantages increase the sensitivity of ^{99m}Tc-ECD over that of stabilized ^{99m}Tc-HMPAO in identifying the epileptogenic zone (Asenbaum et al., 1998; O'Brien et al., 1999a; Lee et al., 2002).

Neurophysiological basis of peri-ictal SPECT

The development of localized hyperemia during focal seizure activity was observed many years ago by direct visualization of the cerebral cortex during brain surgery (Horsley, 1892). The phenomenon was also observed in animal models of focal epilepsy (Penfield et al., 1939). Subsequent development of technology for measuring rCBF has permitted the characterization and measurement of the phenomenon.

The state of ictal hyperperfusion is brief, lasting only a few minutes at most. With temporal lobe seizures, the hyperperfusion typically involves the mesial and

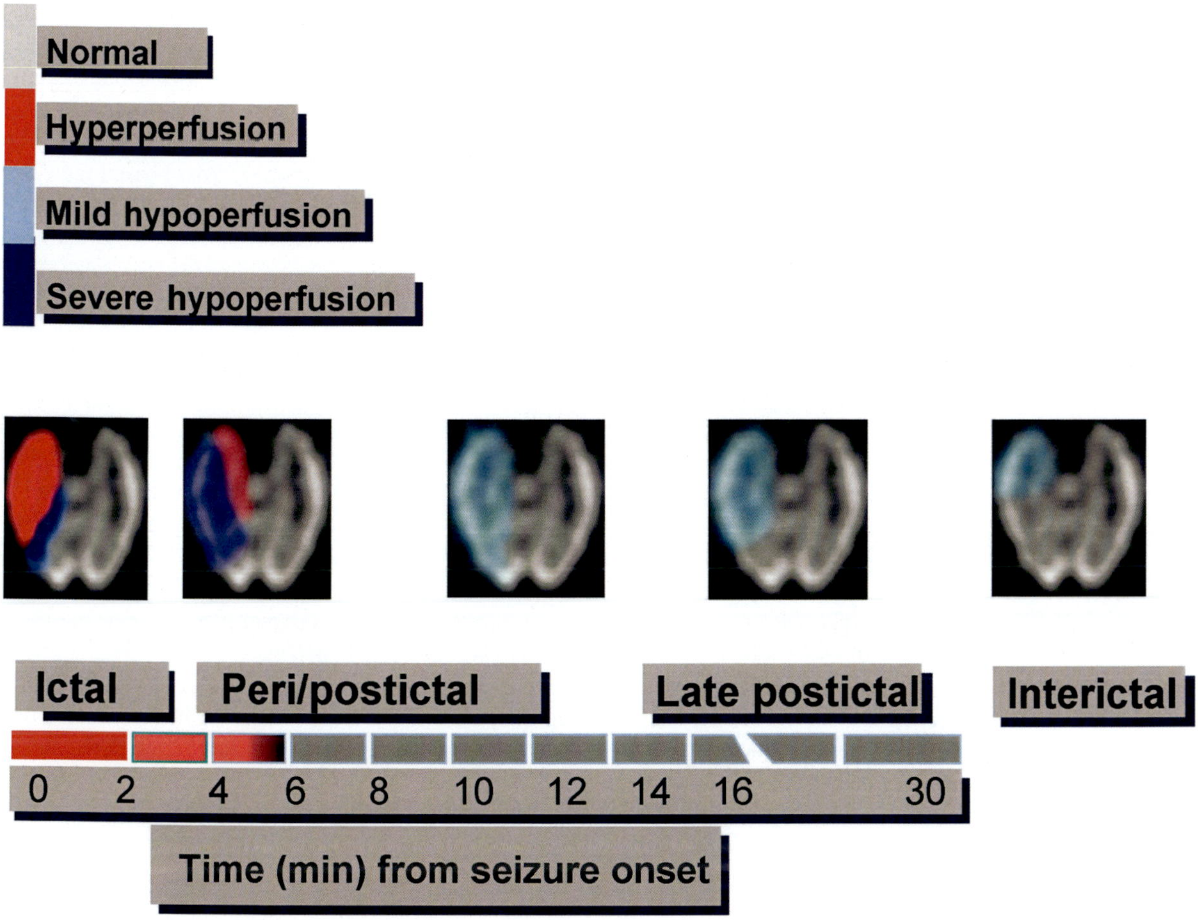

Fig. 27.1. Depiction (not actual) of peri-ictal perfusion changes in relation to epileptic seizure activity detected by SPECT. (Adapted from Rowe et al. [1991], with permission.)

anterolateral regions of the temporal lobe (Fig. 27.1). Within 30 seconds after the end of the seizure, there is often a switch from hyperperfusion to marked hypoperfusion at the lateral temporal neocortical region, while the mesial temporal region remains hyperperfused (Rowe et al., 1991; Newton et al., 1992). This pattern then evolves over the next few minutes to hypoperfusion involving both the lateral and mesial temporal regions, followed by gradual return to the baseline interictal state of mild focal hyperperfusion. This pattern of interictal, ictal, and postictal rCBF alterations at the seizure focus is the basis for using peri-ictal SPECT to help identify the seizure focus. The rate of focal cerebral uptake of SPECT radiotracers such as ^{99m}Tc-ECD has satisfactory linear correlation with rCBF dynamics at the focus (Devous et al., 1993; Friberg et al., 1994). With extratemporal seizures, the pattern of rCBF changes associated with the stage of seizure activity is less well defined. The postictal switch in the state of perfusion typically occurs earlier in extratemporal seizures than in temporal lobe seizures (O'Brien et al., 2000). Even when extratemporal seizures are brief, early injection of the radiotracer can still demonstrate focal hyperperfusion at the epileptogenic zone (O'Brien et al., 1999b).

PREREQUISITES FOR CONDUCTING PERI-ICTAL SPECT IMAGING

As will be discussed later in this chapter, imaging ictal perfusion abnormalities is clinically more useful than imaging either interictal or postictal abnormalities. Therefore, the primary goal of SPECT imaging in epilepsy has been the prompt intravenous injection of the radiotracer as soon as possible after seizure activity has begun. Peri-ictal SPECT has to be conducted simultaneously with video-EEG recording of seizures so that the timing of the radiotracer injection can be related to the stage of electrographic seizure activity. Experienced staff must be available for prompt recognition of both clinical and EEG onset of seizures. Personnel who handle the radiotracer must have training in radiation safety. Female patients with childbearing potential should be tested routinely for pregnancy before the SPECT injection is arranged.

SPECT findings in epilepsy should be interpreted with the knowledge of the relationship between the time of injection and the stage of the seizure activity, as detected by video-EEG recording (Rowe et al., 1991; Avery et al., 1999). Ictal injection of SPECT radiotracer is not always possible. The duration of some seizures, especially frontal lobe seizures, is short. Seizures could also have subtle manifestations unrecognized by the patient, especially when there is no aura, and observers may not be aware of their onset or occurrence. Therefore, the ability to interpret postictal hypoperfusion is also important. Because the timing of the switch from focal hyperperfusion to hypoperfusion is not predictable in each patient, every peri-ictal study must be assessed for both hyperperfusion and hypoperfusion abnormalities (O'Brien et al., 1999b; H.W. Lee et al., 2000).

Display of the SPECT abnormality on three-dimensional MRI studies makes it possible to relate the abnormality to locations of other normal or abnormal brain anatomy and function (Fig. 27.2). This capability is particularly helpful for assessing the concordance of the SPECT focus with MRI lesions, the eloquent cortical structure, other functional imaging abnormalities, or the intracranial electrode contacts at which interictal and ictal EEG discharges occur (So, 2000). This three-dimensional map is important in presurgical planning and assessment of the surgical benefits and risks to the patient.

Precision in the alignment and registration of images between studies is crucial for accurate identification of the abnormal SPECT focus and its relation to other normal or abnormal brain structures or function (Sychra et al., 1994; O'Brien et al., 1998a). When digitally subtracting ictal or postictal SPECT from the interictal SPECT, alignment of the images for subtraction must be precise; otherwise, artifactual perfusion differences may be derived at pixels that do not correspond anatomically between studies. Imprecise alignment can also mask true perfusion differences, thus reducing the sensitivity of the SPECT procedure. Voxel-based matching has been demonstrated to improve SPECT-to-SPECT registration for ictal image subtraction (Brinkmann et al., 1999).

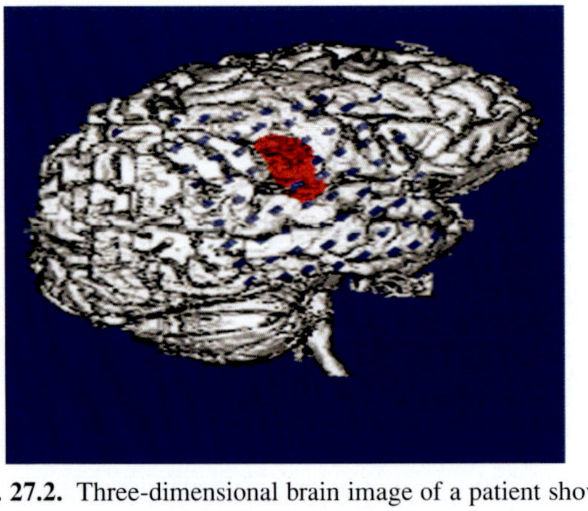

Fig. 27.2. Three-dimensional brain image of a patient showing SISCOM hyperperfusion focus (red) and contacts (blue) of subdural grid electrodes. The four contacts (black) that recorded EEG onset of seizures are concordant with the SISCOM hyperperfusion focus.

CLINICAL INTERPRETATION OF SPECT IMAGES

SPECT images should be reconstructed in the three standard orthogonal views (axial, coronal, and sagittal). Oblique transaxial slices oriented along the long axis of the temporal lobe should also be obtained because they improve visualization of blood flow changes in the temporal lobe (Mullan et al., 1995). Peri-ictal images should always be compared with interictal images in the same patient to detect focal patterns in perfusion changes. This is important because the interictal SPECT images in patients with epilepsy often show baseline focal asymmetries that may be misinterpreted as focal peri-ictal hyperperfusion or hypoperfusion abnormalities.

The images are best reviewed on a high-resolution computer monitor where the corresponding slices from the peri-ictal and interictal scans can be viewed side by side and "normalized" if necessary to account for differences in overall image intensity. Ideally, 255 gray-scale images should be used for the interpretation, but in practice multicolor lookup tables are often used to emphasize visually changes in gray-scale values within the image. These color lookup tables should be used with caution because the finite number of intensities that are displayed can create artificial contours, and they are usually skewed so that small changes in intensity at one part of the scale may result in a dramatic color change. If color tables are used, they should be relatively linear without dramatic color switches, such as the "hot iron" table that is used most commonly in our programs. Furthermore, both hyperfusion and hypoperfusion subtraction images or data must be reviewed in each patient, regardless of the timing of radiotracer injection. SISCOM interpretation, which is based on combined reviews of both hyperperfusion and hypoperfusion images, is superior to review of only hyperperfusion or only hypoperfusion images (O'Brien et al., 1999b; H.W. Lee et al., 2000).

For the interpretation of peri-ictal SPECT studies to be accurate, peri-ictal SPECT images must be compared carefully with interictal images. This comparison, whether by direct visual observation or by digital subtraction of the SPECT data, is the basis for deriving difference images that are attributable to seizure activity. Without interictal SPECT images for comparison, ictal hyperperfusion at a seizure focus may not be obvious if the focus is markedly hypoperfused in the interictal state. Degrees of perfusion at different brain regions may also vary between individuals during the baseline nonictal state.

SISCOM

Rationale for subtraction SPECT

Interictal SPECT is now rarely used by itself to localize the seizure focus for epilepsy surgery. Its sensitivity and specificity are quite low for detecting the phenomenon of hypoperfusion at the seizure focus that is sometimes observable during the interictal period. Only 48% of patients with unilateral temporal lobe seizures and 28% of those with extratemporal lobe epilepsy have correctly localizing abnormalities (Newton et al., 1995). The false localization rate of interictal SPECT is as high as 10%. However, interictal SPECT continues to serve as the basis for comparison of peri-ictal (ictal and postictal) SPECT studies for deducing signal changes that are attributable to the ictal activity or the postictal state. The comparison is conventionally made by side-by-side visual inspection of the peri-ictal SPECT images and the interictal images.

Conventional side-by-side visual comparison of peri-ictal and interictal images can be difficult because the intensity of the images usually varies, depending on the injected dose of radioisotope and the time from injection to scanning. The image slice level and orientation, which depend on the position of the patient's head in the scanner, may also vary between the peri-ictal and the interictal studies. In addition, the precise anatomical location of abnormal perfusion may be difficult to determine because of poor spatial resolution and structural detail of SPECT images compared with those of MRI images.

Advances in computer-aided image analysis and coregistration techniques have helped overcome many of the limitations associated with the traditional side-by-side visual inspection of images. Methods have been described by our group (O'Brien et al., 1998a) and others (Zubal et al., 1995; Vera et al., 1999; Lee et al., 2003) for the normalization, coregistration, and subtraction of interictal from ictal SPECT data to create a "difference image" of the location, extent, and degree of peri-ictal change in perfusion. This difference image is then coregistered to the brain MRI to aid accurate anatomical localization within the patient's brain image (Fig. 27.3). We have termed our method SISCOM – subtraction ictal SPECT coregistered to MRI (O'Brien et al., 1998a).

The potential advantages of these methods over traditional visual inspection are numerous. First, subtraction SPECT should be more objective and specific because subjective decisions are not required about changes in relative regional blood flow between two scans that differ in overall intensity and head position. Second, subtraction SPECT has the potential to improve the sensitivity of ictal SPECT by bringing out regions with a marked peri-ictal alteration in blood flow that are otherwise difficult to detect by visual inspection. Third, MRI coregistration improves the anatomical localization of the regions of peri-ictal blood flow change and allows a closer correlation with other underlying structural abnormalities. The abnormal subtraction SPECT focus can be targeted with stereotactic MRI and surgical navigational systems for intracranial electrode implantation or surgical resection (So, 2000; Ackerly et al., 2004; Thadani et al., 2004).

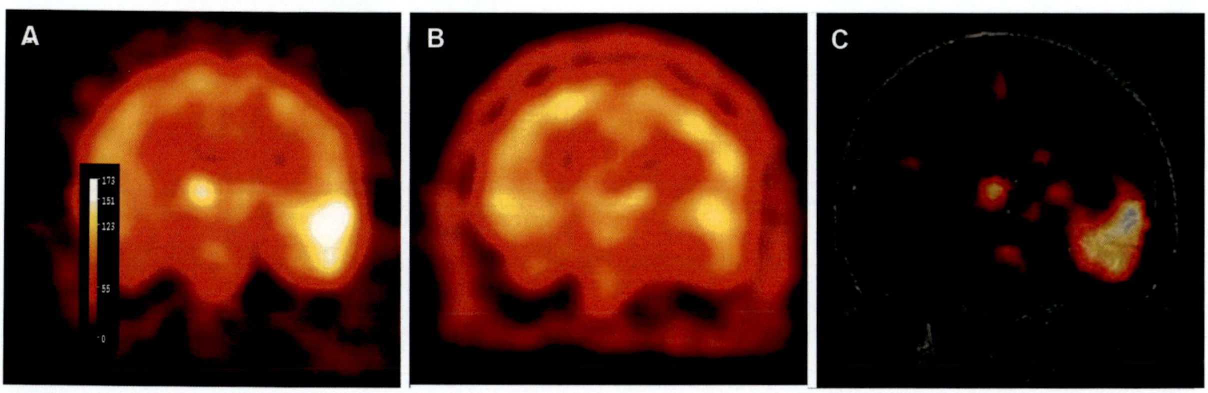

Fig. 27.3. Ictal (**A**), interictal (**B**), and hyperperfusion (**C**) SISCOM images in a patient with medically refractory left temporal onset seizures.

Technical basis of SISCOM

The SISCOM method consists of four major steps, as outlined in Figure 27.4 and described previously (O'Brien et al., 1998a). The SISCOM method uses Analyze software (Mayo Foundation, Rochester, MN, USA), but other image analysis software can also be used to achieve the same purpose. However, any method should undergo technical and clinical validations before clinical application for seizure localization. The SISCOM method is objective, reproducible, and semiautomated, and can be performed in less than 10 minutes with minimal user intervention.

Usefulness of SISCOM versus traditional SPECT interpretation

Computer-aided subtraction of ictal-interictal SPECT has been demonstrated at different institutions to advance the detection of the seizure focus (Zubal et al., 1995; O'Brien et al., 1998b; Vera et al., 1999). The SISCOM method was validated in 51 patients whose seizure focus could not be localized adequately after diagnostic evaluations with clinical history and examination, epilepsy-protocol MRI, interictal EEG, ictal video-EEG monitoring, and PET in some cases (O'Brien et al., 1998b). We found SISCOM to be superior to conventional side-by-side visual inspection of peri-ictal and interictal images. SISCOM detected an abnormal focus in 88% of the patients, whereas the conventional method of SPECT review detected a focus in only 39%. The interobserver rate was also better with SISCOM than with the conventional method. The interrater agreement rate between two blinded reviewers was 84% ($\kappa = 0.83$) for SISCOM versus 41% ($\kappa = 0.26$) for the conventional method. Patients whose SISCOM localization was concordant with the site of surgical resection were more likely to have excellent postsurgical outcomes than those who did not (63% versus 20%). In contrast, seizure localization by the conventional method of visual inspection was not associated with excellent postsurgical seizure control. The usefulness of SISCOM in epilepsy surgery evaluation has also been reported by others (Lee et al., 2006; Ahnlide et al., 2007).

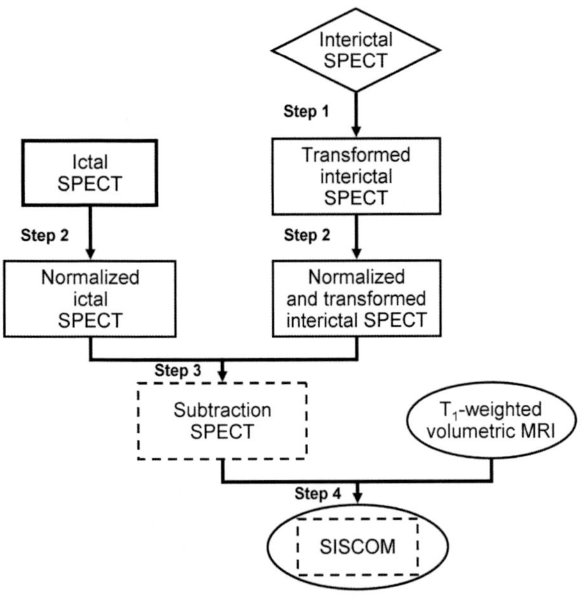

Fig. 27.4. Flow diagram outlining the four primary steps of the SISCOM method. Step 1: Coregister and transform the interictal SPECT into the three-dimensional space of the ictal SPECT by either surface matching or a voxel-based method. Step 2: Normalize the intensity of both images to a standard value (most commonly the mean cerebral intensity). Step 3: Subtract the normalized and coregistered images to derive a difference (activation) image in cerebral blood flow related to the partial seizure. This subtraction image is thresholded to display only the pixels with intensities greater than 2 standard deviations above (hyperperfusion image) or below (hypoperfusion image) zero. Step 4: Coregister the subtracted and thresholded image onto the structural MRI to produce the SISCOM image.

Although ictal injection of the SPECT radioligand should always be attempted, SISCOM analysis of postictal SPECT is still useful in the event that the radiotracer is injected after the seizure has ended (O'Brien et al., 1999b; Oommen et al., 2004). With SISCOM analysis, two-thirds of the positive postictal SPECT studies showed a hypoperfusion focus (Fig. 27.5), and the remaining third showed a hyperperfusion focus. It should be noted that ictal SPECT injection can also be associated with focal hypoperfusion, rather than focal hyperperfusion changes (H.W. Lee et al., 2000). This is more apt to occur in extratemporal lobe seizures than in temporal lobe seizures. Therefore, SISCOM interpretation based on combined reviews of both hypoperfusion and hyperperfusion images is superior to review of only hypoperfusion or only hyperperfusion images, regardless of the timing of the radiotracer injection (O'Brien et al., 1999b; H.W. Lee et al., 2000). In our experience, combined review of postictal SPECT images was localizing in 83% of the patients versus 74% for hypoperfusion images alone and 66% for hyperperfusion images alone (O'Brien et al., 1999b). All three types of review compare favorably with the localization rate of 31% for the conventional method of image review. Logistic regression analysis showed that surgical resection of the combined SISCOM localization focus is predictive of excellent postsurgical seizure control.

Medically intractable epilepsy of extratemporal origin presents several challenges to seizure localization for epilepsy surgery (Quesney et al., 1992; Williamson, 1992; Mosewich et al., 2000). Extratemporal seizures are often very brief and without obvious scalp EEG

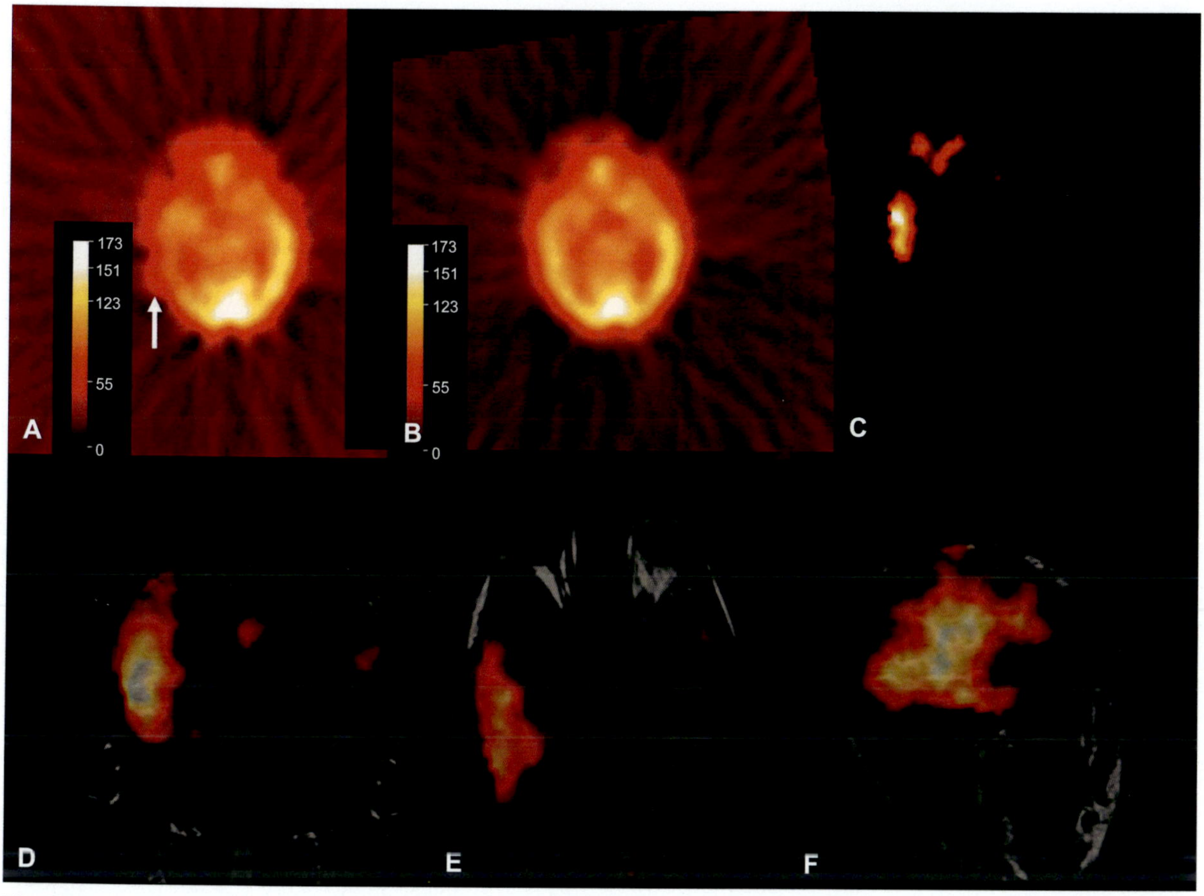

Fig. 27.5. Postictal (**A**), interictal (**B**), and hypoperfusion (**C**) subtraction images thresholded to 1 standard deviation in a patient with right temporal lobe epilepsy. The SISCOM images demonstrate an extensive region of hypoperfusion at the right lateral temporal region (**D–F**).

discharges. SISCOM has been shown to be effective in localizing the epileptogenic zone in patients with medically refractory extratemporal epilepsy (O'Brien et al., 2000). SISCOM revealed an abnormally perfused focus in 67% of the patients whose seizures could not otherwise be localized with noninvasive tests. Moreover, SISCOM revealed an abnormal focus in 77% of the patients with nonlesional MRI. Excellent postsurgical seizure control was achieved in 58% when surgical resection involved the SISCOM focus (Fig. 27.6) versus 17% when the resection did not. Logistic regression also showed that SISCOM results were predictive of postsurgical outcome, independent of MRI or scalp EEG findings. In fact, the extent of resection of the cortical region of the SISCOM focus was associated with excellent postsurgical outcome. All of the patients whose SISCOM focus was completely resected had excellent outcomes, compared with 60% of those with partial resection and 20% of those with no resection of the focus.

SISCOM has also been shown to be useful for localizing the seizure focus in patients with focal malformations of cortical development (O'Brien et al., 2004). In these patients, SISCOM images were localizing in 86%, including 80% of patients with nonlocalizing MRI. SISCOM localization was concordant with 91% of MRI localization, with 93% of scalp ictal EEG localization, and with 100% of intracranial EEG localization. Concordance between SISCOM localization and the surgical resection site was associated with greater postsurgical improvement in seizure frequency. On multiple regression analysis, a model combining SISCOM concordance with the surgical resection site and the extent of MRI lesion resection was predictive of lower postoperative seizure frequency. Kim and colleagues (2009) also found their method of subtraction SPECT with MRI coregistration to be useful for epilepsy surgery evaluation in patients with cortical dysplasia. In their series, incomplete lesion resection and a milder degree of pathology were independent predictors of poor surgical outcome.

The role of SISCOM in the investigation of patients for repeat epilepsy surgery has also been evaluated (Wetjen et al., 2006). SISCOM showed a focus of abnormal perfusion in 79% of 58 patients who had prior

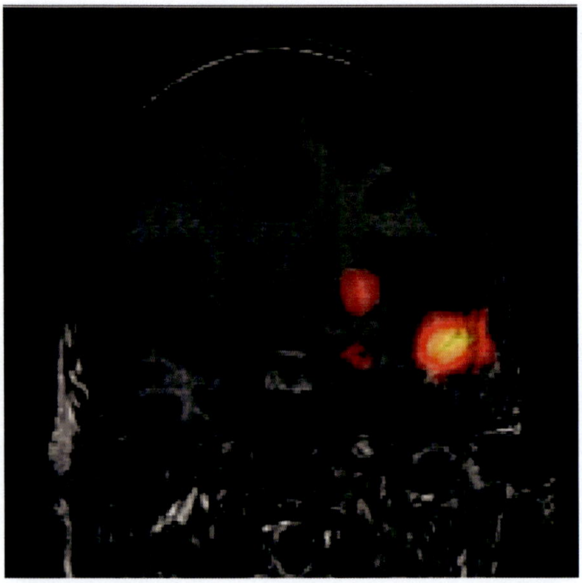

Fig. 27.6. SISCOM showing the hyperperfusion focus superior to the site of previous partial temporal lobectomy. Repeat surgery with resection that included the SISCOM focus resulted in excellent seizure control.

temporal or extratemporal epilepsy surgery. About 72% of SISCOM localization was in the immediate vicinity of the site of previous resection (see Fig. 27.6). Although SISCOM localization was concordant with scalp ictal EEG localization in 70% of the patients, SISCOM concordance was only 47% with the intracranial EEG onset zone in a subgroup of 15 patients who underwent intracranial electrode implantation. The number of patients who eventually had repeat surgery was too small to permit association with outcome of the surgery. For now, SISCOM localization in repeat surgery evaluation should best be used as a guide for careful correlation with other diagnostic tests and for guiding intracranial electrode implantation. Although more than half the SISCOM localizations did not totally concur with the intracranial EEG onset, many were close to the EEG onset zone.

Prospective blinded evaluations of diagnostic modalities for epilepsy surgery are lacking in the literature. However, the influence of SISCOM on epilepsy surgery decision-making and planning was assessed prospectively in patients whose noninvasive evaluations showed nonlocalizing findings (Tan et al., 2008). During an epilepsy surgery conference where each patient was discussed, the consensus decision was documented after presentation of standard noninvasive test results. A consensus decision was documented again after presentation of the SISCOM finding. The consensus decision changed after the SISCOM result was known in 31% when SISCOM was localizing, and in only 6% when it was nonlocalizing. Changes in consensus decisions for the whole group included: (1) obviating intracranial electrode implantation before epilepsy surgery; (2) offering resective surgery, intracranial electrode implantation, or further diagnostic tests in patients judged initially to be nonsurgical candidates; (3) increasing the extent of intracranial electrode coverage; and (4) recommending an antiepileptic drug trial or vagal nerve stimulation instead of intracranial electrode implantation.

It is uncommon for all major functional imaging modalities to be available in a single institution (Knowlton, 2006). However, Knowlton and colleagues (2008) conducted a prospective observational study that compared SISCOM, MEG, and PET, and found that SISCOM localization had the best sensitivity for excellent postsurgical outcome. The sensitivity was 62% for SISCOM, 31% for MEG, and 54% for PET. Both SISCOM and PET localizations have high specificity for excellent postsurgical outcome. The specificity of either SISCOM or PET was 86%, compared with 79% for MEG.

PERI-ICTAL SPECT ANALYSIS WITH STATISTICAL PARAMETRIC MAPPING

As explained in the foregoing section, the distinction of SPECT from other functional imaging modalities is its capability to depict both seizure and nonseizure states of brain function and compare the two states by subtraction to derive changes attributable to seizure activity. Although subtraction with the SISCOM technique has been shown to be substantially superior to conventional visual comparison of ictal and interictal images (O'Brien et al., 1998b), SISCOM images of peak hyperperfusion changes are generated by arbitrary, not statistical, thresholding at the 95th percentile of global cerebral perfusion (O'Brien et al., 1998a). This threshold level is assumed to be sufficiently stringent to permit only clinically meaningful degrees of perfusion differences to be displayed for interpretation. Also, because multiple pixels with peak perfusion changes have to be adjacent to one another to result in an obvious focus of altered perfusion, it has been assumed the focus is unlikely to have become observable by chance alone. Despite SISCOM's superiority to other functional imaging modalities for association with postsurgical seizure freedom (Knowlton et al., 2008), the assumptions made about the SISCOM technique lack the vigor of statistical analysis for determining perfusion changes that are significant.

Statistical parametric mapping (SPM) compares the patient's SPECT data statistically with those of control data (Knowlton et al., 2004). Control data may consist of interictal SPECT from a group of patients with epilepsy or SPECT from nonepilepsy subjects (Friston et al., 1991). SPM can be further applied to subtraction SPECT to ascertain that the difference between ictal and interictal studies in a patient is unlikely to have occurred by chance. Our group developed a method of statistically comparing the patient's ictal–interictal difference SPECT data with the difference data derived from pairs of sequential SPECT studies in each normal volunteer (Brinkmann et al., 2000). The statistical atlas formed by data from the normal volunteers represents the extent of random variations between any two SPECT studies in the resting or nonseizure state. Our updated method, statistical ictal SPECT coregistered to MRI (STATISCOM), was compared with SISCOM in 87 patients. Preliminary results showed that STATISCOM was superior to SISCOM in detecting a hyperperfusion focus (84% versus 66%; $p < 0.05$) (unpublished data, December 2008). Moreover, the probability of seizure-free outcome was higher when STATISCOM correctly localized the temporal lobe epilepsy subtype than when the STATISCOM result was indeterminate (81% versus 53%; $p < 0.05$). McNally and colleagues (2005) had used a similar method of ictal–interictal subtraction SPECT analyzed by SPM (ISAS) to assess patients with seizures that had previously been well localized by other diagnostic modalities. Their ISAS results agreed with the previous localizations in 5 of 7 patients with mesial temporal lobe epilepsy and in 5 of 6 patients with neocortical epilepsy. However, they found no correlation between ISAS results and surgical outcome.

SPM analysis had also been applied to ictal SPECT data instead of ictal–interictal subtraction data. The method has the theoretical advantage of obviating the need for interictal SPECT study (J.D. Lee et al., 2000). However, analysis of ictal SPECT alone against control data could result in the phenomenon of pseudonormalization. This phenomenon occurs when the degree of increased perfusion at the seizure focus becomes insignificant and undetectable, because ictal perfusion at the focus was compared directly with control data. The level to which the ictal perfusion increased from an interictally hypoperfused state at the seizure focus may fail to exceed to a notable extent the level of perfusion in the corresponding area of control subjects.

PERI-ICTAL SPECT: ADVANTAGES, LIMITATIONS, AND PRECAUTIONS

Unlike EEG, peri-ictal SPECT is unable to display seizure activity and sites of its involvement over the time course of the seizure episode. A peri-ictal SPECT image provides a snapshot of cerebral perfusion corresponding to a particular time related to the seizure activity. Achieving true ictal injection and imaging may be difficult in many instances. Some seizures are not heralded by auras. Others have subtle clinical manifestations, especially at the beginning of the seizures. It takes time for the medical staff to detect and confirm seizure activity and to rush to the patient's room to inject the radiotracer. Injection of the radiotracer at a time when the seizure has already secondarily generalized increases the chance of indeterminate or false localizing findings. Moreover, the ictal and postictal duration of some epileptic seizures can be very short (Noe et al., 2004). Extratemporal seizures often last no longer than 30 seconds. Staff responsible for ictal SPECT injection must be experienced in the prompt identification of clinical or EEG seizure onset.

A few measures can improve the chance of true ictal injection of the radiotracer. We have preferentially situated SPECT candidates in rooms closest to our seizure monitoring station, where the radiotracer is kept ready for injection. A patient's family or friends who are familiar with the appearance of the habitual seizure are invited to stay in the room with the patient. Intravenous access to the patient is kept patent by a short indwelling catheter and heparin lock. Patency of the access is checked every few hours. When the patient or guest triggers the seizure alarm, a light by the door to the patient's room also flashes to identify the location of the patient. Traffic in the hallway outside the rooms is restricted to staff and the patient's visitors. Radiation safety procedures require that gloves be worn by personnel when they inject the radiotracer. Therefore, our personnel wear gloves while awaiting seizure occurrence. We have also developed a system that allows personnel quickly to slip on their gloves before grabbing the syringe of radiotracer material (Budde et al., 1995). If habitual seizures are short but frequent, or have a predictable time of occurrence, personnel may sit by the patient's bedside with the radiotracer ready for injection. If habitual seizures typically occur during sleep, the patient is asked to avoid sleep at night and to sleep instead in the daytime when staff are available to conduct SPECT injection and imaging. The use of an automated injection system has been described, but it has not gained widespread use (Sepkuty et al., 1998; Feichtinger et al., 2007). The reliability and safety of the injection system and process need to be fully evaluated, because keeping radioactive materials near a patient for many hours while awaiting seizure occurrence has implications as a potential breach of radiation safety for patient, visitors, and staff.

As described above, the logistics for ictal SPECT injection are quite complex. As a result, peri-ictal SPECT is conducted only in selected institutions that have the availability of personnel during most hours of the day to perform prompt ictal SPECT injection and imaging (Burneo et al., 2007). Most medical centers are able to perform the procedures for only 8 hours a day, and a few have extended that window to 16 hours a day. Additional drawbacks of peri-ictal imaging are that hospitalization for video-EEG monitoring is required and the radiotracers used in the study are expensive. Because of the decay in radioactivity, radiotracer agents have to be replaced every 4–6 hours with newly prepared agents. We usually do not arrange for an ictal SPECT procedure until the patient has had at least one seizure recorded by video-EEG. The initial seizure occurrence in the setting of antiepileptic drug withdrawal during monitoring signals that more seizures are likely to follow soon. Besides, information gained from assessing the initial seizures may guide the staff and family in the prompt detection of the next seizure occurrence.

Interpretation of SISCOM studies must be made in the context of the patient's history and MRI, EEG, and video-EEG localization of seizures. SISCOM localization that contradicts findings with these modalities must be assessed carefully for possible false localization due to seizure spread or technical problems. In situations where few or none of the other modalities provide seizure-localizing information, the SISCOM focus should be further confirmed with intracranial electrode recording. In addition, the focus of abnormal perfusion is not always precisely the seizure onset location (Hogan et al., 1997). For example, abnormal SPECT may primarily involve the lateral temporal neocortex even when seizure onset is at the mesial temporal region. Compared with the SISCOM hyperperfusion focus, the SISCOM hypoperfusion focus is usually larger and less precise, because it is best detected at perfusion difference threshold of 1 standard deviation (see Fig. 27.5). Although the entire SISCOM focus should ideally be resected, the extent of the resection should be guided by intracranial seizure recording and cortical function mapping to optimize safety and seizure outcome. However, intracranial recording may be obviated when SISCOM localization agrees with MRI epileptogenic lesion that could be safely resected and when there is no contradictory EEG finding (Tan et al., 2008).

Finally, peri-ictal SPECT data are derived from a single seizure during or after which the radiotracer was injected. The relevance of the peri-ictal SPECT study to the patient's epilepsy can be reliably inferred only when that seizure is identical to the patient's habitual seizures. This should be verified with the patient and with persons familiar with the habitual seizures. Video-recording of the seizure may have to be reviewed with them if necessary. Care should be taken when evaluating a patient with multifocal epilepsy. Several seizures may have to be recorded and assessed to ensure that the patient does not have multiple types of seizure, especially when there are clues to the presence of multifocal epilepsy in the patient's history, EEG, or MRI.

References

Ackerly T, Geso M, O'Keefe G et al. (2004). Stereotactic radiosurgery planning with ictal SPECT images. Australas Phys Eng Sci Med 27: 136–147.

Ahnlide JA, Rosen I, Linden-Mickelsson Tech P et al. (2007). Does SISCOM contribute to favorable seizure outcome after epilepsy surgery? Epilepsia 48: 579–588.

Asenbaum S, Brucke T, Pirker W et al. (1998). Imaging of cerebral blood flow with technetium-99 m-HMPAO and technetium-99 m-ECD: a comparison. J Nucl Med 39: 613–618.

Avery RA, Spencer SS, Spanaki MV et al. (1999). Effect of injection time on postictal SPET perfusion changes in medically refractory epilepsy. Eur J Nucl Med 26: 830–836.

Biersack HJ, Stefan H, Reichmann K et al. (1986). Brain imaging with ^{99m}Tc-HMPAO SPECT, CT, and NMR-results in epilepsy [abstract]. J Nucl Med 27: 1028.

Bonte FJ, Devous MD, Sr, Stokely EM et al. (1983). Single-photon tomographic determination of regional cerebral blood flow in epilepsy. AJNR Am J Neuroradiol 4: 544–546.

Brinkmann BH, O'Brien TJ, Aharon S et al. (1999). Quantitative and clinical analysis of SPECT image registration for epilepsy studies. J Nucl Med 40: 1098–1105.

Brinkmann BH, O'Brien TJ, Webster DB et al. (2000). Voxel significance mapping using local image variances in subtraction ictal SPET. Nucl Med Commun 21: 545–551.

Budde PA, Hung JC, Mahoney DW et al. (1995). Rapid quality control procedure for technetium-99 m-bicisate. J Nucl Med Technol 23: 190–194.

Burneo JG, Vezina W, Romsa J et al. (2007). Evaluating the development of a SPECT protocol in a Canadian epilepsy unit. Can J Neurol Sci 34: 225–229.

Devous MD, Sr, Payne JK, Lowe JL et al. (1993). Comparison of technetium-99 m-ECD to xenon-133 SPECT in normal controls and in patients with mild to moderate regional cerebral blood flow abnormalities. J Nucl Med 34: 754–761.

Feichtinger M, Eder H, Holl A et al. (2007). Automatic and remote controlled ictal SPECT injection for seizure focus localization by use of a commercial contrast agent application pump. Epilepsia 48: 1409–1413.

Friberg L, Andersen AR, Lassen NA et al. (1994). Retention of ^{99m}Tc-bicisate in the human brain after intracarotid injection. J Cereb Blood Flow Metab 14: S19–S27.

Friston KJ, Frith CD, Liddle PF et al. (1991). Comparing functional (PET) images: the assessment of significant change. J Cereb Blood Flow Metab 11: 690–699.

Harvey AS, Bowe JM, Hopkins IJ et al. (1993a). Ictal ^{99m}Tc-HMPAO single photon emission computed tomography in children with temporal lobe epilepsy. Epilepsia 34: 869–877.

Harvey AS, Hopkins IJ, Bowe JM et al. (1993b). Frontal lobe epilepsy: clinical seizure characteristics and localization with ictal ^{99m}Tc-HMPAO SPECT. Neurology 43: 1966–1980.

Hogan RE, Cook MJ, Binns DW et al. (1997). Perfusion patterns in postictal ^{99m}Tc-HMPAO SPECT after coregistration with MRI in patients with mesial temporal lobe epilepsy. J Neurol Neurosurg Psychiatry 63: 235–239.

Horsley V (1892). An address on the origin and seat of epileptic disturbance: delivered before the Cardiff Medical Society. Br Med J 1: 693–696.

Jacquier-Sarlin MR, Polla BS, Slosman DO (1996). Cellular basis of ECD brain retention. J Nucl Med 37: 1694–1697.

Kim DW, Lee SK, Chu K et al. (2009). Predictors of surgical outcome and pathologic considerations in focal cortical dysplasia. Neurology 72: 211–216.

Knowlton RC (2006). The role of FDG-PET, ictal SPECT, and MEG in the epilepsy surgery evaluation. Epilepsy Behav 8: 91–101.

Knowlton RC, Lawn ND, Mountz JM et al. (2004). Ictal SPECT analysis in epilepsy: subtraction and statistical parametric mapping techniques. Neurology 63: 10–15.

Knowlton RC, Elgavish RA, Bartolucci A et al. (2008). Functional imaging: II. Prediction of epilepsy surgery outcome. Ann Neurol 64: 35–41.

Kuhl DE, Engel J, Jr, Phelps ME et al. (1980). Epileptic patterns of local cerebral metabolism and perfusion in humans determined by emission computed tomography of 18FDG and 13NH3. Ann Neurol 8: 348–360.

Kuhl DE, Barrio JR, Huang SC et al. (1982). Quantifying local cerebral blood flow by N-isopropyl-p-[123I] iodoamphetamine (IMP) tomography. J Nucl Med 23: 196–203.

Lee BI, Markand ON, Wellman HN et al. (1987). HIPDM single photon emission computed tomography brain imaging in partial onset secondarily generalized tonic–clonic seizures. Epilepsia 28: 305–311.

Lee BI, Markand ON, Wellman HN et al. (1988). HIPDM-SPECT in patients with medically intractable complex partial seizures: ictal study. Arch Neurol 45: 397–402.

Lee HW, Hong SB, Tae WS (2000). Opposite ictal perfusion patterns of subtracted SPECT: hyperperfusion and hypoperfusion. Brain 123: 2150–2159.

Lee JD, Kim HJ, Lee BI et al. (2000). Evaluation of ictal brain SPET using statistical parametric mapping in temporal lobe epilepsy. Eur J Nucl Med 27: 1658–1665.

Lee DS, Lee SK, Kim YK et al. (2002). Superiority of HMPAO ictal SPECT to ECD ictal SPECT in localizing the epileptogenic zone. Epilepsia 43: 263–269.

Lee SK, Yun CH, Oh JB et al. (2003). Intracranial ictal onset zone in nonlesional lateral temporal lobe epilepsy on scalp ictal EEG. Neurology 61: 757–764.

Lee SK, Lee SY, Kim KK et al. (2005). Surgical outcome and prognostic factors of cryptogenic neocortical epilepsy. Ann Neurol 58: 525–532.

Lee SK, Lee SY, Yun CH et al. (2006). Ictal SPECT in neocortical epilepsies: clinical usefulness and factors affecting the pattern of hyperperfusion. Neuroradiology 48: 678–684.

Leveille J, Demonceau G, Walovitch RC (1992). Intrasubject comparison between technetium-99 m-ECD and technetium-99 m-HMPAO in healthy human subjects. J Nucl Med 33: 480–484.

Matsuda H, Seki H, Sumiya H et al. (1986). Quantitative cerebral blood flow measurements using N-isopropyl-(iodine 123) p-iodoamphetamine and single photon emission computed tomography with rotating gamma camera. Am J Physiol Imaging 1: 186–194.

McNally KA, Paige AL, Varghese G et al. (2005). Localizing value of ictal-interictal SPECT analyzed by SPM (ISAS). Epilepsia 46: 1450–1464.

Mosewich RK, So EL, O'Brien TJ et al. (2000). Factors predictive of the outcome of frontal lobe epilepsy surgery. Epilepsia 41: 843–849.

Mullan BP, O'Connor MK, Hung JC (1995). Single photon emission computed tomography. Neuroimaging Clin N Am 5: 647–673.

Neirinckx RD, Burke JF, Harrison RC et al. (1988). The retention mechanism of technetium-99 m-HM-PAO: intracellular reaction with glutathione. J Cereb Blood Flow Metab 8: S4–S12.

Newton MR, Berkovic SF, Austin MC et al. (1992). Postictal switch in blood flow distribution and temporal lobe seizures. J Neurol Neurosurg Psychiatry 55: 891–894.

Newton MR, Austin MC, Chan JG et al. (1993). Ictal SPECT using technetium-99 m-HMPAO: methods for rapid preparation and optimal deployment of tracer during spontaneous seizures. J Nucl Med 34: 666–670.

Newton MR, Berkovic SF, Austin MC et al. (1995). SPECT in the localisation of extratemporal and temporal seizure foci. J Neurol Neurosurg Psychiatry 59: 26–30.

Noe KH, Rathke KM, So EL et al. (2004). Factors influencing SISCOM yield in extratemporal epilepsy surgery candidates [abstract]. Epilepsia 45: 303–304.

O'Brien TJ, O'Connor MK, Mullan BP et al. (1998a). Subtraction ictal SPET co-registered to MRI in partial epilepsy: description and technical validation of the method with phantom and patient studies. Nucl Med Commun 19: 31–45.

O'Brien TJ, So EL, Mullan BP et al. (1998b). Subtraction ictal SPECT co-registered to MRI improves clinical usefulness of SPECT in localizing the surgical seizure focus. Neurology 50: 445–454.

O'Brien TJ, Brinkmann BH, Mullan BP et al. (1999a). Comparative study of ^{99m}Tc-ECD and ^{99m}Tc-HMPAO for peri-ictal SPECT: qualitative and quantitative analysis. J Neurol Neurosurg Psychiatry 66: 331–339.

O'Brien TJ, So EL, Mullan BP et al. (1999b). Subtraction SPECT co-registered to MRI improves postictal SPECT localization of seizure foci. Neurology 52: 137–146.

O'Brien TJ, So EL, Mullan BP et al. (2000). Subtraction peri-ictal SPECT is predictive of extratemporal epilepsy surgery outcome. Neurology 55: 1668–1677.

O'Brien TJ, So EL, Cascino GD et al. (2004). Subtraction SPECT coregistered to MRI in focal malformations of cortical development: localization of the epileptogenic zone in epilepsy surgery candidates. Epilepsia 45: 367–376.

Oommen KJ, Saba S, Oommen JA et al. (2004). The relative localizing value of interictal and immediate postictal SPECT in seizures of temporal lobe origin. J Nucl Med 45: 2021–2025.

Patterson JC, Early TS, Martin A et al. (1997). SPECT image analysis using statistical parametric mapping: comparison of technetium-99 m-HMPAO and technetium-99 m-ECD. J Nucl Med 38: 1721–1725.

Penfield W, von Santha K, Cipriani A (1939). Cerebral blood flow during induced epileptiform seizures in animal and man. J Neurophysiol 2: 257–267.

Quesney LF, Constain M, Rasmussen T et al. (1992). Presurgical EEG investigation in frontal lobe epilepsy. Epilepsy Res Suppl 5: 55–69.

Radhakrishnan K, So EL, Silbert PL et al. (1998). Predictors of outcome of anterior temporal lobectomy for intractable epilepsy: a multivariate study. Neurology 51: 465–471.

Rowe CC, Berkovic SF, Austin MC et al. (1991). Patterns of postictal cerebral blood flow in temporal lobe epilepsy: qualitative and quantitative analysis. Neurology 41: 1096–1103.

Sepkuty JP, Lesser RP, Civelek CA et al. (1998). An automated injection system (with patient selection) for SPECT imaging in seizure localization. Epilepsia 39: 1350–1356.

Sharp PF, Smith FW, Gemmell HG et al. (1986). Technetium-99 m HM-PAO stereoisomers as potential agents for imaging regional cerebral blood flow: human volunteer studies. J Nucl Med 27: 171–177.

So EL (2000). Integration of EEG, MRI, and SPECT in localizing the seizure focus for epilepsy surgery. Epilepsia 41: S48–S54.

Stefan H, Kuhnen C, Biersack HJ et al. (1987a). Initial experience with ^{99m}Tc-hexamethyl-propylene amine oxime (HM-PAO) single photon emission computed tomography (SPECT) in patients with focal epilepsy. Epilepsy Res 1: 134–138.

Stefan H, Pawlik G, Bocher-Schwarz HG et al. (1987b). Functional and morphological abnormalities in temporal lobe epilepsy: a comparison of interictal and ictal EEG, CT, MRI, SPECT and PET. J Neurol 234: 377–384.

Stefan H, Bauer J, Feistel H et al. (1990). Regional cerebral blood flow during focal seizures of temporal and frontocentral onset. Ann Neurol 27: 162–166.

Sychra JJ, Pavel DG, Chen Y et al. (1994). The accuracy of SPECT brain activation images: propagation of registration errors. Med Phys 21: 1927–1932.

Tan KM, Britton JW, Buchhalter JR et al. (2008). Influence of subtraction ictal SPECT on surgical management in focal epilepsy of indeterminate localization: a prospective study. Epilepsy Res 82: 190–193.

Thadani VM, Siegel A, Lewis P et al. (2004). Validation of ictal single photon emission computed tomography with depth encephalography and epilepsy surgery. Neurosurg Rev 27: 27–33.

Uren RF, Magistretti PL, Royal HD et al. (1983). Single-photon emission computed tomography: a method of measuring cerebral blood flow in three dimensions (preliminary results of studies in patients with epilepsy and stroke). Med J Aust 1: 411–413.

Vera P, Kaminska A, Cieuta C et al. (1999). Use of subtraction ictal SPECT co-registered to MRI for optimizing the localization of seizure foci in children. J Nucl Med 40: 786–792.

Walovitch RC, Franceschi M, Picard M et al. (1991). Metabolism of 99mTc-L, L-ethyl cysteinate dimer in healthy volunteers. Neuropharmacology 30: 283–292.

Wetjen NM, Cascino GD, Fessler AJ et al. (2006). Subtraction ictal single-photon emission computed tomography coregistered to magnetic resonance imaging in evaluating the need for repeated epilepsy surgery. J Neurosurg 105: 71–76.

Williamson PD (1992). Frontal lobe seizures: problems of diagnosis and classification. Adv Neurol 57: 289–309.

Zubal IG, Spencer SS, Imam K et al. (1995). Difference images calculated from ictal and interictal technetium-99 m-HMPAO SPECT scans of epilepsy. J Nucl Med 36: 684–689.

Handbook of Clinical Neurology, Vol. 107 (3rd series)
Epilepsy, Part I
H. Stefan and W.H. Theodore, Editors

Chapter 28

Clinical neuropsychology in epilepsy: theoretical and practical issues

CHRISTOPH HELMSTAEDTER* AND JURI-ALEXANDER WITT
Department of Epileptology, University Clinic of Epileptology, Bonn, Germany

INTRODUCTION

Neuropsychology in epilepsy is characterized by its close connection to neurophysiology, neuropathology and neuroradiology, and neuropharmacology. The synergy of these faculties has been stimulated decisively by epilepsy surgery. Neuropsychology traditionally is synonymous with the detection, lateralization, and localization of brain dysfunctions and associated behaviors. However, today, in the presence of powerful high-resolution brain imaging techniques and sophisticated electroencephalographic (EEG) evaluation tools, the role of neuropsychology is changing (Baxendale and Thompson, 2010). Apart from revealing cerebral dysfunctions related to epilepsy, neuropsychology is increasingly becoming a tool for the monitoring of epilepsy outcome and for quality control of the treatment of epilepsy (Elger et al., 2004; Helmstaedter, 2009a). Standardized neuropsychological evaluation has become an integrated and essential tool in the diagnostic and clinical evaluation of surgical patients with epilepsy, and it will be extended to play a critical role in the routine care of patients with epilepsy on a more general level. This change of the diagnostic focus, however, does not supersede the examination of specific brain dysfunctions. On the contrary, if the cognitive effects of epilepsies and underlying pathologies are to be detected, or if the cognitive consequences of pharmacological or surgical treatment are the focus of interest, then it is essential to have sensitive and specific measures that respond to the etiological factors involved and that reflect focal and systemic changes in affected brain regions and functional networks (Hoppe and Helmstaedter, 2010). There is a diverse range of different test instruments available, leaving the examiner spoilt for choice (Jones-Gotman et al., 2010). After 20–30 years of intensive research on the neuropsychology of epilepsy, PubMed (http://www.ncbi.nlm.nih.gov/sites/entrez) lists over 3000 publications when the terms "epilepsy and cognition" are searched. Based on this knowledge, test selection should be evidence-based and oriented to predefined criteria and clinically relevant questions. Concommitant with diagnostic and therapeutic improvements in epilepsy, neuropsychological instruments themselves should become the subject of ongoing quality control. The specific role of neuropsychology in epilepsy and the diagnostic options for clinicians are best illustrated on the basis of the following etiological model of cognitive impairments in epilepsy.

ETIOLOGY OF COGNITIVE IMPAIRMENTS IN EPILEPSY

Epilepsies are classified according to their etiology, topography, and seizure characteristics. The traditional classification system differentiates idiopathic, symptomatic, and cryptogenic epilepsies, the major differential criteria being the presence, suggestion, or absence of a cerebral lesion and the degree of genetic determination. Classifications of the epilepsies change with the number of etiological factors revealed (Berg et al., 2010). For the neuropsychology of the epilepsy, however, all factors are of interest that may affect cognition along with the course of the disease and its treatment.

For cognitive impairments in epilepsy an etiological model can be suggested, according to which dysfunctions may result from more stable and irreversible structural morphological cerebral changes on the one hand and from more dynamic and principally reversible epilepsy and treatment-related dysfunctions on the other hand (Fig. 28.1). The relative contribution of these

*Correspondence to: Professor Christoph Helmstaedter, Dipl. Psych., University Clinic of Epileptology, Sigmund-Freud-Str. 25, 53105 Bonn, Germany. Tel: +49-(0)228-287-16108, Fax: +49-(0)228-287-14486, E-mail: C.Helmstaedter@uni-bonn.de

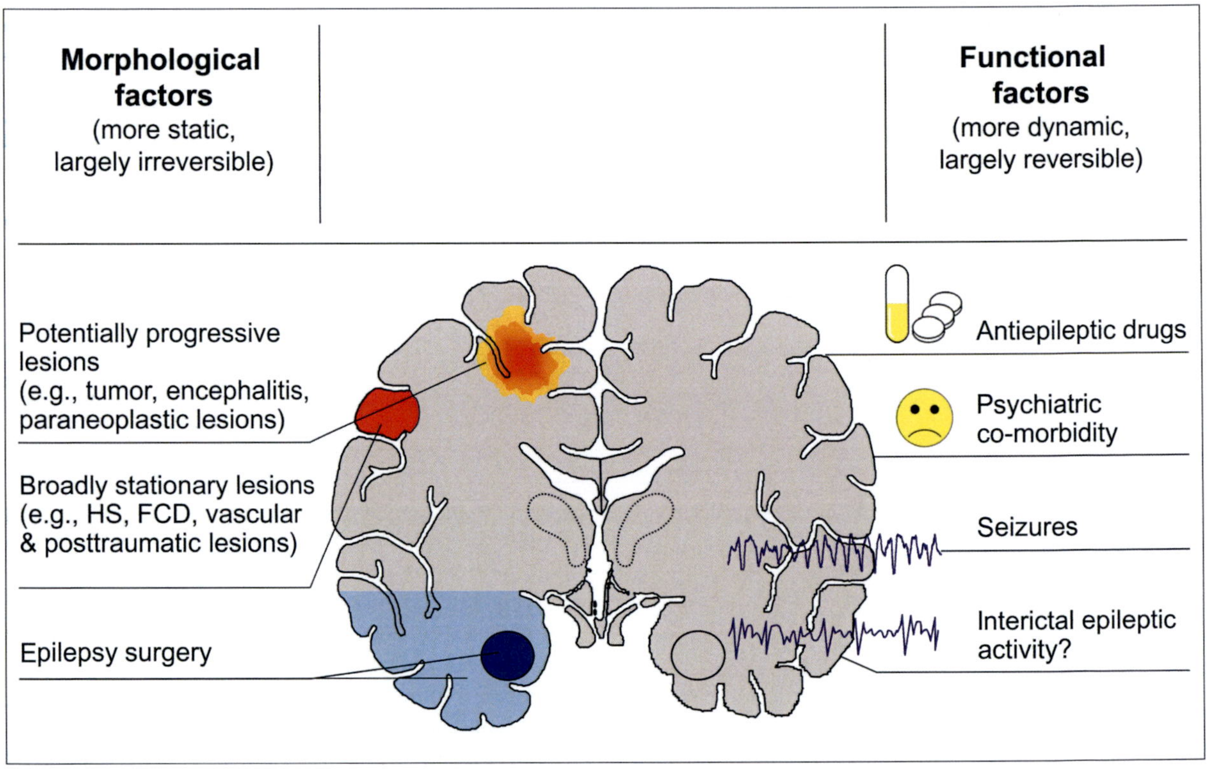

Fig. 28.1. Etiological model of cognitive dysfunction in epilepsy. FCD, focal cortical dysplasia; HS, hippocampal sclerosis. (From Elger et al. (2004). © Elsevier.)

factors may differ depending on subject variables, the localization and lateralization of the epilepsy, and variables such as age, age at onset, and the duration of epilepsy, which place the impairments within a neurodevelopmental framework (Elger et al., 2004). In addition to lesions, epilepsy, and treatment-related factors, the influence of psychiatric comorbidity on cognition needs to be taken into consideration.

Taking this model as a basis, the practical clinical questions to be asked regarding neuropsychology are shown in Table 28.1.

NEUROPSYCHOLOGICAL ASSESSMENT

Mental status examination and evaluation of change

With regard to the neuropsychological examination of patients with epilepsy, a principal distinction to be made is whether the neuropsychological status is to be evaluated or whether the evaluation aims at performance change resulting from changes arising from epilepsy or its treatment. Cognitive status evaluations should at best be performed following an adequate interval from

Table 28.1

Neuropsychology: questions to be asked

Questions to neuropsychology
General practice

- Can cognitive impairments be discerned (global vs. partial)?
- Can these impairments be related in a plausible way to the epilepsy and the underpinning pathology?
- What do the impairments tell us about neurodevelopment (mental retardation vs. loss of acquired functions)
- In case of repeated measures, what do the impairments tell us about the course of the disease (accelerated decline, recovery/release, developmental hindrance or catch-up)?
- Which impairments can be observed in the context of seizures, i.e. ictal (during the seizures), postictal (after the seizure)? How long do these impairments persist, is permanent damage the result?
- Is there a behavioural correlate of epileptic activity as indicated by EEG during waking states and sleep (paroxysmal or continuous activity, spike-wave complexes etc.)?
- Does the antiepileptic medication taken alone or via its impact on seizures or mood have a positive/negative impact on cognition?

Epilepsy surgery

- Are the impairments consistent with known lesions, the type of lesion (AHS, tumor, developmental, dysplasia) and the localization of the lesion/epilepsy?
- Is there evidence for impairments exceeding what would be expected from MRI and type of epilepsy?
- Is there evidence for cerebral plasticity (dominance patterns, hemispheric reorganization)?
- What are the direct and longer-term consequences of invasive treatments (surgery, radiotherapy, deep brain stimulation, vagal nerve stimulation)?
- What are the patient's resources to compensate for additional damage (plasticity, reserve capacity, compensation)?

Superordinate

- What are the consequences for everyday life, school, occupational achievement, interpersonal relations, quality of life?
- Suggestions for interventions (ergotherapy, logopedics, neuropsychological rehabilitation, etc.)?

AHS, Ammon's horn sclerosis; MRI, magnetic resonance imaging.

the last seizure, when the seizure situation is stable and when the patient is on an antiepileptic medication that can be rated as harmless for cognition. This must be taken into account in advance in order to prevent hours of invalid testing. This is particularly relevant when the test routine considers application of comprehensive standard batteries. Because of the dynamic impairments that are characteristic of epilepsy and because neuropsychology in epilepsy also means outcome and quality control, assessment of cognitive change is an essential part of patient care. Evaluation of change along with the course of epilepsy or treatment requires knowledge about the reliability (stability) of the applied instruments: are parallel versions available, is the same test repeated, which practice effects can be expected, does the instrument provide reliable change indices (RCI)? Many tests are not standardized for repeated application and this needs to be considered when interpreting changes in cognitive measures (Hermann et al., 1996).

Individual versus standardized evaluations

A second important differentiation is whether to approach the patient individually by eclectic test selection or by use of a standard test battery. Individual diagnostics reveal more information about a given patient, but, particularly in research-oriented epilepsy centers, a standard diagnostic approach might be preferable in order to learn across patients and to modify the approach depending on diagnostic outcomes. Most epilepsy centers use test batteries and, although there is some agreement on which domains need to be assessed, there appears to be great heterogeneity regarding individual test selection. This is indicated by the international overview of tests commonly used in 1993 (Jones-Gotman et al., 1993), and also by a recent evaluation that assessed the question of evidence-based diagnosis in 14 epilepsy centers in German-speaking countries (Witt and Helmstaedter, 2009, 2011). This evaluation counted more than 200 different test instruments in use; only 25% of the tests selected were evidence-based, about 30% were selected for subjective and pragmatic reasons, and for the rest no explicit rationale for selection was provided. Different tests provide different outcomes, and in order to overcome this babylonian diversity some pediatric and adult epilepsy centers in Germany now use the same core test battery (Helmstaedter, 2009a; Witt and Helmstaedter, 2009). In the USA, the same issue is followed by the National Institute of Neurological Disorders and Stroke (NINDS) Common Data Elements Project, which provides detailed recommendations for neuropsychology in patients with epilepsy (http://www.commondataelements.ninds.nih.gov/Epilepsy.aspx). Such agreements are required to facilitate communication of neuropsychological results (on scientific issues as well as on individual patients) across different centers.

Most centers assess intelligence (IQ). Testing of IQ is very time-consuming and is only partly aimed at basic neuropsychological functions. It can, however, be indicative of mental retardation and developmental hindrance, particularly when compared with the performance levels of parents and siblings. In children, IQ is still the best predictor of school performance. However, because the majority of epilepsies start early, and because this often results in lower IQ, the intelligence level as assessed by full-scale IQ tests should not be considered as a reference or correction to identify partial impairments in specific cognitive domains. This would lead to an underestimation of the patient's impairments. Interpretation of neuropsychological results in consideration of the IQ should be applied only in patients with epilepsy/lesions acquired later.

For the diagnosis of partial impairments in the different cognitive domains, for instance in order to lateralize or localize impairments, or to isolate the major reason for dysfunctional behavior, specific and well-validated measures should be chosen according to evidence in the epilepsy literature. This information, however, is not necessarily provided by common compendia of neuropsychological test instruments for adults or children (Baron, 2004; Lezak et al., 2004; Strauss et al., 2006).

The experience and agreement on which tests to use for the diagnosis of partial impairments covary with the prevalence of the different epilepsies. For temporal lobe epilepsy verbal and figural memory list learning tests are preferred; for frontal lobe epilepsy tests on motor coordination, attention, planning, mental flexibility, and response inhibition are preferred. Posterior parietal or occipital epilepsies have not been evaluated systematically, although tests on sensory tactile discrimination appear to be valid.

In general, the same tests may be used for localization diagnostics that have been shown to be valid in regard to progressive, traumatic, or vascular lesions in the respective brain regions. Syndrome-oriented tests such as aphasia examinations, however, may prove to be insensitive with regard to the often mild to moderate impairments in epilepsy. A very important issue is that tests claiming to assess the same cognitive domain (e.g., for memory the Auditory Verbal Learning Test, California Verbal Learning Test, Wechsler Memory Scale) may have different sensitivity and specificity to localized lesions and dysfunctions in epilepsy. The use of different tests results in different outcomes, which cannot be directly compared (Loring et al., 2008; Helmstaedter et al., 2009).

Neurodevelopmental aspects

In younger children, developmental aspects of motor and language development need to be considered and it should be remembered that, depending on the time of injury/epilepsy onset, there is potential for reorganization, and that with progressive brain maturation symptoms may change and children may develop impairments not seen previously (Gleissner and Helmstaedter, 2008). Tests and structured developmental interviews that are commonly used for the presurgical evaluation of children and intellectually impaired adults with epilepsy have been listed by Gleissner and Helmstaedter (2008). As developing children represent a "moving target" and because, depending on age, different tests must often be used, a standardized evaluation of children across ages and mental capabilities can be difficult. For orientation, normalized and standardized questionnaires for parents of children with epilepsy may provide information about cognitive and behavioral dysfunction (Gleissner et al., 2006). In children, the direct monitoring of adaptive behaviors is essential because motivational and attentional problems may lead to an underestimation of the child's performance (performance–competence discrepancy).

Hemispheric organization, plasticity, reserve capacity

Questions regarding the localization and hemispheric lateralization of an impairment, postoperative outcomes, and reserve capacities require knowledge of the hemispheric dominance for the performance in question. This information is needed mainly in the context of epilepsy surgery, and it is important in the prevention of aphasia or amnesia. In hemispherectomy and callosotomy, information on motor and visual organization is of additional interest.

Left-handedness or ambidexterity are good markers of atypical language dominance, particularly in early-onset left-hemisphere epilepsies. In addition, neuropsychological test profiles with comparably well-preserved language and unexpectedly affected nonlanguage functions can be indicative of atypical language dominance in left-hemisphere epilepsies. Traditional neuropsychological techniques such as dichotic listening or tachistoscopy, which assess ear or visual field dominance, may serve as a gross orientation, but for clinical decision-making such tests do not suffice.

The most reliable tool for determining hemispheric dominance is still the intracarotid application of amobarbital for anesthesia of the individual hemispheres, which was first described by Juhn Atsushi Wada and is therefore also known as the Wada test. The intracarotid amobarbital test (IAT) is invasive and its indication is limited to brain surgery. It was initially introduced to prevent postoperative aphasia, and later also used for the prevention of global amnesia resulting from temporal lobe surgery. The IAT provides the unique possibility for assessing the functions of an isolated hemisphere by temporarily deactivating the contralateral hemisphere, thereby disclosing deficits and compensatory capabilities of the isolated hemispheres. For a long time the IAT was obligatory before epilepsy surgery, but it is now rarely indicated (Baxendale et al., 2008; Helmstaedter, 2008c), mainly because of the availability of more selective surgical procedures and alternative noninvasive tools for the assessment of cerebral dominance. Alternatives to the IAT that provide determination of language dominance in the individual patient include functional magnetic resonance imaging (fMRI), magnetoencephalography (MEG), positron emission tomography (PET), single-photon emission computed tomography (SPECT), near-infrared spectroscopy (NIRS), and functional transcranial Doppler sonography (fTCD) (Abou-Khalil, 2007). The majority of these noninvasive techniques register hemodynamic responses to language paradigms. A problem with nearly all of these approaches is the lack of normative data and the use of different protocols/paradigms in different centers (Dodrill and Ojemann, 1997; Haag et al., 2008). Additionally, almost all alternatives to the Wada test carry the risk of false-positive and -negative findings. If resection in or close to probable eloquent cortex is planned, electrocorticographic functional mapping via implanted electrodes or during awake surgery is used to delineate the exact resection borders (Baxendale, 2002; Helmstaedter and Kurthen, 2002; Gaillard, 2004; Baxendale et al., 2008; Haag et al., 2008; Helmstaedter, 2008c).

Modular testing

Taking the time constraints for neuropsychologists and the need for evidence-based neuropsychological evaluation in epilepsy into account, a modular neuropsychological assessment can be proposed that is directly

Table 28.2

Question-guided modular evaluations

- Evaluation and screening of major impairments is performed using computerized testing (Hoppe et al., 2009), which includes attention, reaction times, memory, and executive functions, and which can be applied repeatedly if required (approximately 25 minutes)
- The question of developmental hindrance, delay, retardation, and catch-up is assessed via IQ tests and/or application of standardized neurodevelopmental interviews (Gleissner et al., 2008) (about 1–1½ hours)
- Aura, seizure semiology, ictal and/or postictal testing provide information about which cognitive functions are positively (semiology) or negatively (testing) affected in the context of seizures (Helmstaedter et al., 1994a; Lux et al., 2002; Jordan, 2007) (up to 5 minutes)*
- Before performing extended testing, patients are screened for cognitive antiepileptic side-effects (Lutz and Helmstaedter, 2005; Helmstaedter, 2008b, 2010). If the drug regimen is critical and if this test indicates serious impairment of executive functions, further testing is postponed until AEDs have been changed (about 10–15 minutes)
- For presurgical evaluation or differential diagnosis, when a localization or lateralization diagnosis is required, a battery of frontal executive and of verbal and figural memory functions is applied (Muller et al., 1997; Gleissner et al., 1998; Helmstaedter and Durwen, 1990; Helmstaedter et al., 1991, 1996b, 1998, 2001b) (about 1–1½ hours)
- For a decision regarding surgery, this is extended by assessing IQ (WAIS short version based on 5 subtests), motor, language, visuoconstructive, visuospatial, and semantic memory functions (total test battery including the tests mentioned above: approximately 3½ hours). The overall information is assumed to have greater external validity than single tests and the results, for example, may be given to therapeutic training or rehabilitation services if this is indicated
- Language/memory lateralization is noninvasively assessed via fMRI, (language in younger children by fTCD)
- In selected cases language dominance is determined invasively by means of the Wada test. If surgery in eloquent cortex is planned, cognitive mapping by electrocortical stimulation is performed in addition (Kurthen et al., 1994; Fernandez et al., 2003; Deppe et al., 2004; Weber et al., 2006; Wellmer et al., 2009)
- Cognitive evaluation is accompanied by assessment of depression (Beck Depression Inventory), anxiety (Zung Self-Rating Anxiety Scale), personality (Fragebogen zur Persönlichkeit bei zerebralen Erkrankungen; FPZ), and a measure on Quality of Life in Epilepsy Inventory 10 (QOLIE-10) (Helmstaedter and Witt, 2011)

*EEG-locked continuous performance testing in order to assess the impact of epileptic activity is not included because in this regard no standards are yet available.

AED, antiepileptic drug; fMRI, functional magnetic resonance imaging; fTCD, functional transcranial Doppler sonography.

concerned with the questions to neuropsychology posed in Table 28.1. Table 28.2 provides the schedule and rationale for this modular diagnostic approach, which is simply an example of what can be done for and around patients with epilepsy.

NEUROPSYCHOLOGICAL FINDINGS IN EPILEPSIES

This section reviews the neuropsychological features of different types of epilepsy that are listed in Table 28.3, including information about the age at manifestation, precipitating conditions, and the suggested course of cognitive development.

Idiopathic epilepsies

Idiopathic epilepsies are traditionally defined as having a genetic predisposition in the absence of brain lesions. Whereas idiopathic generalized epilepsies (IGEs) are characterized by generalized EEG patterns that involve the whole cortex, idiopathic partial epilepsies show epileptic activity limited to particular brain regions.

Idiopathic epilepsies generally appear to be more easy to treat and, because of the lack of lesions, they are reported to be associated with less severe cognitive impairments than focal symptomatic epilepsies. This, however, must not hide the fact that there are cognitive and behavioral problems in idiopathic epilepsies. In idiopathic epilepsies there is a stronger relationship between epileptic activity and cognition than in symptomatic focal epilepsy. It is difficult to separate the degree to which epileptic activity in these epilepsies marks dysfunctional brain development, which is associated with cognitive impairment, from the degree to which it directly affects cognition. Different from what would be expected from the term "generalized epilepsy," a wide range of partial rather than generalized impairments can be discerned in generalized and partial idiopathic epilepsy. EEG, histological findings, and findings from structural and functional imaging studies support an involvement of the frontal lobes, the thalamus, and thalamocortical loops in IGE (Meencke and Janz, 1985; Woermann et al., 1999; Salek-Haddadi et al., 2003; Aghakhani et al., 2004). The cognitive impairments in the idiopathic epilepsies differ, depending on whether the epilepsy interferes with critical periods or so-called spurts of cognitive development, for example before, at, or after language acquisition, or at the time

Table 28.3

Cognitive function in different types of epilepsy

Type of epilepsy	Manifestation	Precipitating condition	Course of cognitive development
Idiopathic epilepsies			
Early childhood epilepsy with GTCS and hemi grand mal	Age 5–15 years	Normal	Unfavorable/mental decline
Benign myoclonic epilepsy	Until age 3 years	Normal	Positive/retardation possible
Severe myoclonic epilepsy (mitochondrial defects)	Age 1 year	Normal	Unfavorable/mental decline
Myoclonic–astatic epilepsy	Until age 5 years	Mostly normal	Ranges from partial deficits to dementia
Absence epilepsy			
Early onset	Age 1–4 years	Normal	Partial deficits possible
Pyknolepsia	Age 5–8 years	Normal	Partial deficits possible
Juvenile	Age 9-12 years	Normal	Partial deficits possible
Juvenile myoclonic epilepsy	Age 12–18 years	Normal	Frontal lobe partial deficits
Juvenile epilepsy with GTCS	Age 12–18 years	Normal	Partial deficits (frontal?)
Symptomatic or cryptogenic epilepsies			
Focal epilepsies	All ages	Normal or impaired	Dependent on onset and localization; partial deficits and low IQ
Frontal lobe	All ages	Normal or impaired	Predominant impairment of executive functions
Temporal lobe	All ages; often early	Normal or impaired	Predominant episodic memory impairment (material-specific)
Parieto-occipital	All ages; often early	Normal or impaired	Frontal or temporal rather than classical parietal dysfunctions
Epilepsia partialis continua	All ages	Mostly impaired	Often one hemisphere affected
Rasmussen encephalitis			The course and outcome is unfavorable and mental decline is common
Encephalopathy/catastrophic epilepsies			
West syndrome	Age 1 year	Mostly impaired	Unfavorable/retardation
Lennox–Gastaut syndrome	Age 2–7 years	Mostly impaired	Unfavorable/retardation
Benign partial epilepsies and related syndromes			
Rolando Epilepsy (benign epilepsy with centrotemporal spikes)	Age 3–13 years	Maturation disorder (hereditary)	Partial deficits
Benign epilepsy with centrotemporal spikes			
Pseudo-Lennox development syndrome	Age 2–7 years	Maturation disorder (hereditary)	Impaired language and other partial deficits
CSWS/ESES (continuous spike–wave)	Age 2–10 years	Maturation disorder (hereditary)	Onset and course-dependent retardation and mental decline
Landau–Kleffner syndrome	Age 4–10 years	Maturation disorder (hereditary)	Auditory agnosia and aphasia predominant/ retardation and mental decline

CSWS, continuous spike–wave during sleep; ESES, electrical status epilepticus during sleep; GTCS, generalized tonic–clonic seizures.

before or during development of frontal executive functions. Frontal executive dysfunctions are seen in both partial and generalized idiopathic epilepsies, and appear to mark the common endpoint of a neurodevelopmental interference. Despite the mostly good prognosis, long-term residual deficits cannot be excluded.

Patients with IGE comprise about 6–12% of children with epilepsy. IGE appears to have peaks in early childhood, at 5–8 years, and at 9–12 years of age (Table 28.3). Patients with IGE show only minor problems with respect to global intelligence, but they experience problems in attention, psychomotor speed, visuospatial skills, and nonverbal memory. Language and verbal memory appear unaffected (Mirsky et al., 2001; Pavone et al., 2001; Hommet et al., 2006). In IGE, impairments become evident as a function of epileptic activity, but cognitive processes can also induce epileptic discharges and seizures (Matsuoka et al., 2000). It may be of interest that such a relationship can sometimes also be seen in focal symptomatic epilepsies (Helmstaedter et al., 1992). Epileptic spike–wave activity in IGE specifically affects sensory and executive functions, and tests requiring sustained attention in continuous visual and auditory tasks seem to be suited for the identification of epilepsy-related dysfunction in this group of patients (Jambaque et al., 2001). Continuing epileptic activity experienced over a long period of time interferes with brain development. Consequently, patients with early-onset absence epilepsies starting in early childhood or at school age are at greater risk of a poor outcome than those with juvenile absence epilepsy.

Benign partial epilepsies and related syndromes. Benign childhood epilepsy with centrotemporal spikes (BECTS) is a common form of epilepsy (10–15% of epileptic children), with onset between ages 3 and 13 (most between 5 and 10 years). BECTS has a good prognosis as most patients become seizure-free after puberty. It should be noted that rolandic discharges, which are typically seen in this type of epilepsy, are also frequently seen in healthy children as well as in nonepileptic children with cognitive or behavioral disorders, with headaches and some genetic disorders (Stephani and Carlsson, 2006). Language problems are a major characteristic of BECTS (Papavasiliou et al., 2005; Liasis et al., 2006). In this context it may be of interest that rolandic discharges were reported in 10% of 300 dyslexic children (Stephani and Carlsson, 2006). In the active phase of BECTS, neuropsychological deficits comprise attention, motor functions, short-term memory, visual and perceptive abilities. Despite normal IQ, most patients have neuropsychological and language problems suggestive of a developmental learning disability, and problems appear more severe in those with complex partial seizures (Vinayan et al., 2005; Giordani et al., 2006; Stephani and Carlsson, 2006). With seizure remission children can catch up with normal development, although minor persisting problems may be found in executive functions and verbal comprehension (Lindgren et al., 2004; Monjauze et al., 2005). Thus, absence of seizures and complete remission of epileptic activity appear to be essential for a good cognitive outcome.

According to its localization, benign partial epilepsy with occipital discharges appears to affect visual information processing (Wolff et al., 2005), but patients also score worse than normal controls in intellectual functions, memory, and attention (Gulgonen et al., 2000).

The particular conditions of Landau–Kleffner syndrome (LKS), continuous spike–wave during sleep (CSWS), and electrical status epilepticus during sleep (ESES) (Van Hirtum-Das et al., 2006) are also associated with language problems. Strong parallels and transitions from LKS to ESES, as well as from partial generalized epilepsy to ESES, have been discussed (Rossi et al., 1999; Saltik et al., 2005; Van Hirtum-Das et al., 2006). Compared with BECTS, however, patients with LKS, CSWS, and ESES experience a progressive loss and decline of already acquired functions, which can result in severe mental retardation (Debiais et al., 2007). An early age at onset and a longer duration of these conditions appear essential for poorer mental outcome. As with BECTS, more frequent epileptic discharges and generalized epileptic activity seem to be related to greater cognitive problems (Van Hirtum-Das et al., 2006).

Juvenile myoclonic epilepsy (JME) starts predominantly between 12 and 18 years of age, and is characterized by neuropsychological and behavioral features of a frontal dysexecutive syndrome (Janz, 2002). This is indicated by neuropsychological findings of problems in reasoning, concept formation, mental speed, and cognitive flexibility, or in visual working memory as assessed in an experimental [^{18}F]fluorodeoxyglucose (FDG)-PET study (Swartz et al., 1996; Devinsky et al., 1997; Sonmez et al., 2004). According to Trinka et al. (2006), 35% of 43 patients with JME showed one or more Axis I or II behavioral disorders. Some 23% of this sample had a personality disorder, which would be supportive for the suggestion by Janz (2002) that frontal lobe cognitive dysfunction together with personality change (e.g., limited self-control, suggestibility, indifference, rapid mood changes) form a syndrome characteristic of JME.

Focal symptomatic epilepsies

Epileptic encephalopathies (West and Lennox–Gastaut syndrome, Dravet syndrome)

Having already considered LKS in the context of BECTS, the other so called severe epilepsy syndromes, West syndrome (catastrophic epilepsy with infantile spasms) and Lennox–Gastaut syndrome with predominant atypical absences and tonic seizures, are characterized by diffuse and multifocal epileptic activity due to diverse, diffuse, and multifocal lesions (Crumrine, 2002; Shields, 2002). The West syndrome is often accompanied by mental deterioration, behavioral regression with visual unresponsiveness, and reduction of social interaction with autistic features. The majority of patients will not achieve normal intelligence in adulthood (Jambaque et al., 2001). In about 40% of patients, Lennox–Gastaut syndrome evolves from West Syndrome, and this group also shows rapid progressive intellectual decline (Jambaque et al., 2001). As with most other epilepsies, cognitive outcome is worse with an earlier onset that interferes with brain maturation and hinders cognitive development. Standardized neuropsychological testing can hardly be performed because the IQ ranges below 50 in most patients. Behaviorally, impairment of motor speed, apraxia, autistic or psychotic traits, hyperkinesia, spatial disorientation, and perseveration can be observed and the long-term outcome is generally poor (Besag, 2004). Although Wet and Lennox–Gastaut syndromes are etiologically and clinically very heterogeneous, 35% of patients with Dravet syndrome (severe myoclonic epilepsy of infancy) have in common a dominantly inherited sodium channel-related gene defect (*SCN1A*) (Oguni et al., 2005). This syndrome is characterized by myoclonic seizures, absence, and focal seizures. Developmental hindrance ranges from mild to severe, and most children suffer from behavioral problems in terms of hyperactivity and autistic traits. According to a recent longitudinal study, mental retardation, psychotic or autistic traits, and hyperactivity are very common between the ages of 1 and 4 years, stabilizing thereafter on a level that remains subnormal (Jambaque et al., 2001; Caraballo and Fejerman, 2006; Wolff et al., 2006).

Localization-related epilepsies

Temporal lobe epilepsies (TLEs) represent about 70–80% of the chronic symptomatic epilepsies, about half of them associated with hippocampal sclerosis and/or atrophy. Because of the high prevalence and because the temporal lobe structures represent morphologically distinct and well-defined brain structures, the functional correlates of TLEs are the best evaluated. Whether mesial TLE represents a nosological entity or a syndrome is a matter of debate (Wieser, 2004). The temporal lobe structures are involved in memory processing, and impairment of declarative episodic memory (knowledge fixed in space and time) represents the major cognitive impairment in this group of epilepsies. Semantic memory (context-free world knowledge) is also found to be impaired in TLE, but this appears more related to temporolateral neocortical dysfunction than episodic memory, which appears to be related directly to hippocampal pathology and dysfunction (Helmstaedter, 2002). Correlations between test performance and mesial structures in TLE have, for example, been demonstrated for hippocampal volume (Sawrie et al., 2001), hippocampal cell loss in distinct subfields (Pauli et al., 2006), event-related potentials (Fernandez et al., 2002; Vannucci et al., 2008), rhinal–hippocampal gamma-band coupling (Fell et al., 2001), long-term potentiation (Beck et al., 2000), and fMRI (Bonelli et al., 2010). In clinical practice this means that memory assessment in TLE can be taken as a good marker of temporomesial pathology/dysfunction.

Episodic memory impairment in TLE tends to be material specific (verbal/nonverbal) according to whether the left (language-dominant) or right hemisphere is affected. Whereas the relationship between verbal memory and the left temporal lobe is a fairly consistent feature of left TLE, the relationship between the right temporal lobe and figural visuospatial memory appears inconsistent. Major reasons for erroneous lateralization of material-specific memory impairment are age (material specificity develops with brain maturation), sex differences (females show advantages in verbal and disadvantages in figural memory), atypical language dominance (verbal memory is often preserved at the cost of figural memory, and this is also related to sex), verbalization strategies (these account for figural memory), and test materials (figural: abstractness, allocentric versus egocentric; verbal load on working memory, semantic processing, organization, IQ). Hermann et al. (1997), in their definition of the neuropsychological characteristics of mesial TLE, stated that these patients often suffer from low IQ. In this respect, some authors suggest mental decline with a longer duration of epilepsy (Jokeit and Ebner, 2002). However, such studies rarely take educational levels into account. Poor intelligence in chronic TLE is related mostly to poorer educational levels, and poor education can hardly be interpreted in terms of a loss of previously acquired functions due to longer duration of epilepsy (Kaaden and Helmstaedter, 2009).

As discussed above, the impairments seen in TLE appear to be present from the commencement of the disease, and active epilepsy does not necessarily add to this. Secondarily acquired trauma or progressive pathologies (e.g., tumors, encephalitis) are an exception (Malter et al., 2010). As for other epilepsies, early-onset TLE interferes with cognitive and brain development, and patients fail to develop an adequate performance in comparison to healthy subjects. Early-onset TLE impairs functions of directly affected structures (temporal) but also interferes with the development of structures (mainly frontal) that mature later (Weber et al., 2007; Helmstaedter and Elger, 2009; Kaaden et al., 2009). Apart from memory problems, patients with TLE also show impairments in frontal lobe-associated executive functions. This can be explained partly neurodevelopmentally, as just discussed, and also in part by reversible effects of irradiating epileptic dysfunction or diaschisis phenomena on distant brain areas (Hermann et al., 1988; Jokeit et al., 1997).

Temporomesial pathology affects not only memory but also emotion processing and reward learning. Accordingly patients with TLE often show comorbid depression, impaired social cognition, and preference learning (Frisch et al., 2009a; Johnsrude et al., 2000; Schacher et al., 2006). An extreme may be seen in autism, which appears to be a special characteristic of patients with tuberous sclerosis with temporal lobe tubers (Bolton et al., 2002). In comparison to frontal lobe epilepsies, in patients with TLE introversion, neuroticism, cognitive (memory) impairment, and social limitations are the prominent behavioral features (Helmstaedter and Witt, 2011). In this context, the old literature referred to the so-called "temporal lobe personality," which comprised a mixture of behaviors that from today's point of view would be better explained psychiatrically or neuropsychologically (Blumer et al., 2004; Devinsky and Schachter, 2009).

Frontal lobe epilepsies (FLE) represent the second most common group of symptomatic epilepsies. In contrast to TLE, in which hippocampal sclerosis is a predominant and quite homogeneous morphological feature, very heterogeneous etiological factors are involved in FLE. Frontal lobe executive functions are involved in most other cognitive domains, resulting in diffuse and comparably nonspecific impairments. However, the cognitive and behavioral impairments characteristic of FLE largely resemble those described in the lesion-related literature. On a superordinate level they can best be described as a dysexecutive syndrome with impairment of response selection, initiation, execution, and inhibition. In particular, patients have been shown to have attention problems, problems with short-term or working memory, mental flexibility, response selection, response inhibition, planning, and motor coordination (Helmstaedter et al., 1996b; Upton and Thompson, 1996; Exner et al., 2002). FLEs also affect memory performance, but in a different manner than TLE (Centeno et al., 2010). In keeping with the frontal dysexecutive functions, discriminative elements in verbal learning and memory as assessed with the Auditory Verbal Learning Test are, for example: irregular learning curves across subsequent learning trials (ups and downs instead of steady increase), perseverations due to monitoring problems, interference phenomena in terms of proactive interference, problems with source memory as two lists had to be learned, distractibility in recognition memory, and comparatively well-preserved long-term retention of what had been learned (Helmstaedter et al., 2001b). As with TLE, the neuropsychology of FLE can hardly be appreciated without taking behavioral changes into consideration. The frontal lobe is traditionally referred to as the "social brain" and, as with TLE, dysfunctional behaviors can be discerned in FLE that characteristically correspond to the affected brain region. Compared with patients with TLE, FLE is more likely to be associated with hyperactivity, impulsivity, conscientiousness, obsession, and behaviors, which might traditionally have been termed "organic psycho-syndrome" (Helmstaedter and Witt, 2011).

Posterior, parietal, and occipital epilepsies (PLEs) represent a very small proportion of symptomatic epilepsies. Consequently, studies focusing on cognition in patients with parietal or occipital lesions are rare. Compared with patients with cerebrovascular or traumatic lesions, in posterior epilepsies symptoms such as aphasia, apraxia, neglect, or anopsia are a rare phenomenon (Busch, 2011). These typically posterior symptoms are, if seen at all, a correlate of late and acquired brain lesions or in the context of ictal and postictal seizure semiology. Instead the impairments seen in PLE rather resemble those seen in temporal or frontal lobe epilepsy. Neuropsychological data of pediatric patients with PLE indicate subaverage intelligence and domain overspanning impairments in memory, attention, and executive functions (Gleissner et al., 2008). Similarly, a corresponding evaluation in adult patients with PLE demonstrated deficits in almost all cognitive domains (Witt et al., 2008a), including frontal and temporal lobe functions. Comparison of the cognitive profiles of TLE, FLE, and PLE in a large series of surgical patients revealed the generally poorest performance levels in PLE (Helmstaedter et al., 2007). Two explanations may account for this observation. First, developmental hindrance can be suggested as in most other early-onset epilepsies and an impaired input system can be suggested to have greater negative effects on downstream functions than an impaired memory or executive system. Second, a negative impact of epileptic dysfunction irradiating along the axis of dorsolateral and frontomedian long-fiber tracts may serve as an explanation for the impairment pattern. This would at least mirror the conditions seen with the spread of seizures in posterior epilepsies, which often mimic temporal or frontal lobe seizures (Akimura et al., 2003).

DIFFERENTIAL DIAGNOSTICS OF NEUROPSYCHOLOGICAL IMPAIRMENT IN EPILEPSY

As already mentioned above, cognitive impairments in epilepsy result from the epilepsy, its medical treatment, and the underpinning morphological structural change or damage. Whilst the impact of each of these factors can well be proven, the way in which these factors interact is largely unknown. In the individual patient, repeated testing along with changes in therapy or the seizure situation is the only way to disentangle the relative contribution of these factors. Neuropsychological monitoring of the treatment of patients with limbic encephalitis may serve as an example (Malter et al., 2010).

Epileptic dysfunction and seizures

With regard to the factor "epilepsy," the type of epilepsy (idiopathic, symptomatic), intrahemispheric and interhemispheric localization and spread of epileptic activity, the age at onset, the duration and severity of the epilepsy (seizure type and frequency) are relevant for the cognitive outcome.

Evidence of a direct relationship between EEG epileptic potentials and cognitive impairments can be assessed only under controlled conditions, that is by running neuropsychological assessments in parallel with the EEG, or by the monitoring of cognition along with "treatment of the EEG" (Binnie, 2003). Whereas, in animal models, a relationship between epileptic activity and behavior can well be demonstrated, the establishment of such relations in humans is difficult (Zhou et al., 2007; Holmes, 2010). As already mentioned, a close relationship between epileptic activity and cognition is discussed for the idiopathic focal or generalized epilepsies. However, despite the high relevance, particularly for the developing child (Austin and Dunn, 2002), no EEG-locked standardized assessment or test procedure has yet become routine (Aldenkamp et al., 2004). In addition, it is important to note that the negative impact of epileptic activity or the positive effect of controlling epileptic activity on cognition cannot be generalized for all patients.

In focal symptomatic epilepsies a relationship between epileptic activity and cognitive impairment may exist in individual patients, but in this type of epilepsy the correlation appears different and weaker than in idiopathic focal or generalized epilepsies. Most evident, however is the relation in "subclinical" or "emotional" seizures, which proceed without the involvement of the motor system. Apart from more acute effects of epileptic activity on behavior, there are indirect indicators that can be taken as evidence that interictal epileptic dysfunction additionally affects cognition and behavior in a more chronic fashion. Positive cognitive and behavioral changes following successful epilepsy surgery, for example, indicate a slowly progressing system reset and release of functions that had been suppressed or delayed before surgery (Lendt et al., 2000; Helmstaedter et al., 2003; Witt et al., 2008b). The cognitive effects of epileptic activity during sleep and awake states in childhood epilepsies may be taken as another example (Nicolai et al., 2006). Furthermore, an impact of epilepsy on the acute and chronic functional organization of the brain has been demonstrated by correlating interictal activity with hemisphere dominance patterns (Janszky et al., 2003; Helmstaedter et al., 2006). The issue of epileptic activity and its treatment gains increasing interest independently of epilepsy, because epileptic activity without the manifestation of seizures can be observed in autistic spectrum disorders, dyslexia, attention-deficit/hyperactivity disorder (ADHD), etc. (Dunn et al., 2011).

Symptoms during, as well as after, the seizure have diagnostic relevance. Seizure semiology often provides a suggestion as to which hemisphere and which brain regions become primarily and secondarily involved (So, 2006; Jordan, 2007). Apart from seizure semiology, in terms of a *positive symptomatology* there are additional cognitive deficits in terms of a *negative symptomatology* during seizures. However, diagnosing impairment in contrast to semiology requires active testing of the patient during the seizure (Lux et al., 2002). After the seizure, the time needed to become reoriented as well as type, degree, and duration of postictal impairment are related to the seizure. Postictal aphasia, disorientation, and pareses, for example, can indicate the lateralization of the seizure origin. Seizure propagation determines the duration of the seizure, ictal consciousness, and postictal recovery. Even when patients appear completely reoriented, partial impairments in individual performance may persist for hours. Postictal impairments reflect the lateralization and localization of the seizure. Recovery is hierarchical in that cognitive functions distant from the primary focus recover earlier than functions associated with the area of the focus (Helmstaedter et al., 1994a). It may be of interest that functional release/recovery after successful epilepsy surgery shows parallels to recovery from seizures.

A highly relevant, and with regard to epileptic dysfunction essential, question is whether chronic epilepsy progressively damages the brain (Sutula and Pitkänen, 2002). In short, will chronic uncontrolled epilepsy result in dementia? According to studies in animals there is evidence for a negative effect of seizures on the brain, and on the maturing brain in particular. However, very different effects can be demonstrated depending on the animal/epilepsy model and age at damage. In humans, it is difficult to disentangle the differential influence of initial precipitating lesions, seizures, and the consequences of seizures (e.g., hypoxia). Here, seizures normally cause reversible impairment. In individual patients with severe seizure conditions (series of generalized seizures, convulsive or nonconvulsive status epilepticus) permanent damage can be the result, but even here the differential impact of the seizure/epileptic activity and the often severe underlying pathology is not self-evident (Dietl et al., 2004; Dodrill, 2004; Helmstaedter, 2007).

Cross-sectional studies indicate a very slow decline (> 30 years) with chronic uncontrolled epilepsy. Longitudinal studies indicate some impact of continuing seizure and seizure control on cognition, but hardly show continuous decline as a function of time. However, as already discussed in the context of TLEs, duration of epilepsy can hardly be separated from age in early-onset epilepsy (Jokeit et al., 2000). There now is evidence from newly diagnosed children and adults that cognitive impairments are often already present at the time of epilepsy onset (Hermann et al., 2006; Witt and Helmstaedter, 2012; Taylor et al., 2010). Between 40% and 60% of newly diagnosed patients exhibit cognitive impairments. Thus, in chronic epilepsy the factor "epilepsy" more likely hinders mental development than causes mental decline. Accordingly the onset of epilepsy and its underpinnings appear to be the decisive factors for cognition and cognitive development, and call for early and subsequent epilepsy and cognition-related interventions. Nevertheless, in older patients with chronic epilepsy an increased number of severely impaired subjects must be suggested. If patients become impaired early in the course of the disease, and if mental decline with "normal" aging runs in parallel but at a lower level compared with the course of cognition in healthy subjects, very poor levels must be reached at an earlier age (Helmstaedter and Elger, 1999).

Antiepileptic drug treatment

Pharmacological treatment of epileptic seizures carries the risk of cognitive side-effects that may affect daily functioning and quality of life. Efficacy and tolerability of the treatment are decisive for compliance and the long-term retention of the therapy (Bootsma et al., 2009). On the one hand antiepileptic drugs (AEDs) may induce or aggravate cognitive impairments in different cognitive domains. On the other hand, effective seizure control can lead to improvements in cognition and behavior. Consequently seizure control can mask adverse cognitive side-effects or falsely suggest positive side-effects of the AED in use.

The risk of cognitive side-effects increases with: (1) rapid titration, (2) higher doses, and (3) a higher overall drug load in the case of polytherapy. This at least accounts for the greater interaction potentials (e.g., enzyme induction/inhibition) of the so-called "older AEDs," compared with the "newer AEDs." Titration speed, dose, and number of AEDs also represent the points of action for the control of cognitive and behavioral side-effects. For clinical practice it might be useful to know that a recent cross-sectional evaluation in a large series of 1430 patients indicated that, independently of which drugs were used, cognitive problems were present but acceptable with monotherapy and two AEDs in comparison to controls or an off-drug condition, whereas there was significant impairment with three or more AEDs (Witt and Helmstaedter, 2010).

The individual antiepileptic agents in part differentially affect cognition. An initial crude differentiation considers that the first-generation AEDs had sedative properties and affect global (intellectual) performance, that the second generation is associated primarily with impairments in psychomotor speed and memory function, whereas the newest generation seems to have behavioral side-effects. Among the classical AEDs, bromide, benzodiazepines, and phenobarbital are more frequently associated with cognitive side-effects than phenytoin, valproic acid, or carbamazepine (Ortinski and Meador, 2004). With the exception of topiramate, and perhaps also zonisamide (Park and Kwon, 2008), the newer AEDs appear to have superior cognitive profiles than previous generations (French et al., 2004).

Table 28.4 provides an overview over the cognitive side-effects of AEDs reported in recent reviews for children (Loring and Meador, 2004) and adults (Kwan and Brodie, 2001; Aldenkamp et al., 2003; Ortinski and Meador, 2004; Park and Kwon, 2008). Preferential targets of AEDs include the attention and executive functions, but memory and language functions can also be affected. However, even when specific impacts on memory (phenytoin, carbamazepine) or language (topiramate) are assumed, attention and executive functions are almost always affected. Thus, when monitoring of cognitive side-effects in the individual patient is required, one may rely on computerized or paper–pencil screening tests that focus on these functions (Aldenkamp et al., 2005; Lutz and Helmstaedter, 2005; Hessen et al., 2006; Helmstaedter et al., 2010).

AEDs also have indications for other neurological conditions (e.g., migraine or neuralgia) and psychiatric disturbances (Spina and Perugi, 2004), and AEDs with positive psychotropic side-effects are prescribed to alleviate psychiatric comorbidity in epilepsy (Hermann et al., 2008). In this regard, Ketter's hypothesis can be taken into account, according to which AEDs that potentiate γ-aminobutyric acid (GABA) inhibitory neurotransmission (e.g., barbiturates, benzodiazepines, valproate, gabapentin, tiagabine, and vigabatrin) have a sedating effect, and those that attenuate glutamate excitatory neurotransmission (e.g., felbamate and lamotrigine) have a stimulating effect (Ketter et al., 1999). However, Ketter's assumptions are an oversimplification and do not apply equally well to all AEDs (Roberts et al., 2005).

Depending on behavioral traits, one should prevent their amplification, as has been suggested for the stimulating effect of levetiracetam in patients predisposed to be extraverted, irritable, and impulsive (Helmstaedter et al., 2008a). One should nevertheless keep in mind that

Table 28.4

Overview of the cognitive effects of common antiepileptic drugs

	Attention		Memory		Language		Psychotropic	
	Adults	Children	Adults	Children	Adults	Children	Adults	Children
Lamotrigine	0	↑	0				↑	
Levetiracetam	0	↑	0		0		↓/↑	
Tiagabine	0		0		0		0	
Vigabatrin	0		0		0			
Felbamate	(↓)							
Zonisamide	(↓)							
Oxcarbazepine	↓/↑		0					
Gabapentin	↓	↓	0		0		(↑)	
Clobazam	↓	↓	0				↓	
Valproic acid	↓		↓		0		↑	↑
Carbamazepine	↓		↓	(↓)				
Phenytoin	↓		↓	(↓)				
Phenobarbital	↓		↓			(↓)		
Topiramate	↓	↓	↓		↓	↓	(↓)	

↓, negative effect ; ↑, positive effect; ( ), possible effect; 0, no effect; blank, no evidence.

positive psychotropic effects of AEDs, whether secondarily via mood (e.g., lamotrigine) or directly via arousal (e.g., levetiracetam), can also improve cognition. Severe psychiatric conditions require treatment (Kanner, 2008), and when successful this can also have a positive effect on neuropsychological functioning.

Cognitive side-effects of AEDs are largely reversible following drug withdrawal, but there are a few important exceptions. Treatment with vigabatrin can lead to irreversible visual field defects (Gonzalez et al., 2009; Krauss, 2009) and is thus reserved mainly for severe infantile epileptic encephalopathy (West syndrome). Irreversible effects of AED treatment are of particular importance in pregnancy and lactation, and also in children with epilepsy. *In utero* as well as early childhood exposure to antiepileptic medication may chronically affect the maturing and developing brain (Holmes, 1997; Frisch et al., 2009b; Harden et al., 2009; Meador et al., 2009).

Lesions, pathology, and surgery

Cognitive capabilities in focal symptomatic epilepsies are determined by the localization, lateralization, extent, and type of lesion that underpins the epilepsy. The cognitive profile of a TLE with hippocampal sclerosis, for example, differs from that found in TLE with temporomesial or temporolateral tumors (Helmstaedter et al., 1997a). As already mentioned in the section on TLE, structural–functional relationships have also been demonstrated for different degrees of mesial pathology in terms of neuronal loss in hippocampal subregions (Pauli et al., 2006) or between other brain volumetric measures and memory (Butler et al., 2009).

Pathology is decisive for cognition because the type of pathology is correlated to the age at lesion/epilepsy onset. With early congenital, acquired, or developmental lesions (e.g., cortical dysplasia), the brain is still functionally plastic and has a greater capacity for compensation than the mature brain (e.g., traumatic, inflammatory, neoplastic lesions). Despite greater plasticity, early lesions and dysfunctions hinder mental development. Accordingly early-onset lesions/epilepsies are often characterized by nonspecific, globally reduced intellectual capabilities, whereas late-acquired lesions/late-onset epilepsies show partial impairments with largely unimpaired intelligence (see the discussion above).

Epilepsy surgery

Surgery can be a very successful treatment option for patients with focal symptomatic epilepsies. A randomized trial of surgical versus medical treatment indicated successful seizure control in 58% of surgically versus 8% of medically treated patients (Wiebe et al., 2001). Successful seizure control reduces behavioral and mood problems, and improves overall quality of life. However, apart from seizure control, brain surgery can have negative effects on cognition and behavior that quantitatively and qualitatively exceed those seen before surgery (Elger et al., 2004; Helmstaedter et al., 2007).

There are three main factors that determine the cognitive outcome of epilepsy and its treatment. The first and probably most predictive factor is the "functionality" of the affected and unaffected brain regions (Chelune, 1995; Stroup et al., 2003). Functionality of the brain even appears to be related to some degree to seizure control (Helmstaedter, 2009b). Closely connected to the question of "functionality" is the second factor, which is the patient's "mental reserve capacity" (Helmstaedter, 1999). The third factor is "seizure control" (Helmstaedter et al., 2003).

Both the functional integrity of the affected and to be resected tissues and reserve capacity are reflected by baseline performance. On the one hand, patients with a better baseline performance will also be those with the better outcomes (reserve); on the other hand, patients with a better baseline performance are at greater risk of loss after surgery (functionality). Functionality is expressed by baseline performance of directly affected brain areas. Both functionality and reserve capacity depend on the patient's age at the time of surgery. The critical phases of cerebral functional plasticity last until about puberty; the time when reserve capacities and capabilities for compensation start to decline with aging is about age 30 years (Helmstaedter, 1999). Methods to estimate functional adequacy and reserve capacity in addition to neuropsychological assessment are electroencephalographic (EEG) recordings (extracranial/intracranial, interictal/ictal) (Rosenow and Lüders, 2004), structural and functional imaging techniques (Koepp and Woermann, 2005), angiography with intracarotidal application of amobarbital, methohexital, or etomidate (Buchtel et al., 2002; Banks et al., 2010), and, last but not least, electrocortical stimulation (Wellmer et al., 2009).

Temporal lobe surgery

The logical consequences for epilepsy surgery from these findings would be to remove what is necessary to control seizures, and to leave as much functional tissue as possible in order to preserve the patient's cognitive functions. This is best illustrated by the findings regarding surgery for TLE. TLE is frequently already associated with memory impairment before surgery, and surgery can significantly add to this. In the Bonn series of 898 patients operated on and evaluated neuropsychologically between 1988 and 2003, cognitive impairments in 732 patients with TLE were clearly dominated by memory impairment (46–69%), followed by problems in language, motor functions, attention, and visuoconstruction. In addition, memory was the domain of major postoperative change (losses in 27–40%). Patients with a resected left temporal lobe are at a particularly high risk of experiencing verbal memory decline. However, at the same time cognitive improvements in mainly frontal lobe-associated functions may be observed after temporal lobe surgery (Table 28.5) (Helmstaedter et al., 2007; Helmstaedter, 2011). These changes are consistent with literature reports (Lee et al., 2002; Sherman et al., 2011).

A recent review of the quest for the most successful surgical approach in temporal lobe surgery came to the conclusion that different surgical approaches in TLE do not result in different seizure outcomes (Schramm, 2008). From a neuropsychological point of view there is, however, converging evidence that in patients with mesial TLE the cognitive outcome of more selective surgery is superior to that of standard anterior two-thirds temporal lobe resections (Renowden et al., 1995; Helmstaedter et al., 1996a, 2008c; Clusmann et al., 2002; Morino et al., 2006; Paglioli et al., 2006; Sindou

Table 28.5

Cognition before and after temporal lobe surgery

	Preoperative impairment*			Postoperative change at 12 months				
Domain	*n*	Left TLE	Right TLE	*n*	Left TLE		Right TLE	
					↓	↑	↓	↑
Verbal memory	732	69%	46%	732	40%	14%	27%	29%
Figural memory	732	49%	59%	707	31%	27%	28%	23%
Attention	717	21%	29%	709	11%	36%	11%	40%
Language	653	39%	32%	618	21%	27%	14%	32%
Motor function	717	30%	40%	449	16%	34%	16%	37%
Visuoconstruction	602	19%	21%	554	10%	35%	13%	31%
Vocabulary – IQ	591	8%	11%	NA				
Wada atypical domain	320	41%	22%	NA				

*Impairment $= x < \text{mean}_{\text{normative data}} - 1.5\text{SD}$; ↓, significant decline; ↑, significant improvement.
NA, data not available; SD, standard deviation; TLE, temporal lobe epilepsy.

et al., 2006; Alpherts et al., 2007). However, selectivity of TLE surgery has its limits in that collateral neocortical damage and dissection of fiber tracts (e.g., temporal stem) due to the surgical approach can negatively affect memory outcome (Helmstaedter et al., 2004b, 2008c). Another limitation is that preservation of function and sparing of mesial tissue conflicts with the position that the total resection of the hippocampus is essential for the achievement of seizure freedom (Olivier, 1996). A randomized trial of mesial resection length indicated superior seizure outcome but no different neuropsychological outcome following total compared with partial hippocampectomy in standard anterior temporal lobectomy (Wyler et al., 1995). The functional relevance, particularly of the more posterior parts of the hippocampus, for memory outcome has been indicated by several studies (Baxendale et al., 2000; Bonelli et al., 2010). In this regard, the question of preservation of functional tissue that can be obtained with radiosurgery may be of interest, which claims to be nondestructive and aims to change the intrinsic epileptic characteristics of the irradiated tissue (Bartolomei et al., 2008; Barbaro et al., 2009). The future cognitive outcomes of deep brain stimulation will be of comparable interest, but it still needs to be established whether stimulation does preserve function or whether it interferes with the functionality of the stimulated area (Benabid et al., 2002; Boon et al., 2007; Velasco et al., 2007). In addition, the eventual effects of chronic implantation of depth electrodes needs to be evaluated. After right-sided selective TLE surgery, for example, a lasting negative effect of bilateral depth electrode implantation on verbal memory has been described (Gleissner et al., 2002).

Extratemporal lobe surgery

What can be stated for TLE seems to be true also for the cognitive outcome of extratemporal lobe surgery. That is to say, further impairments due to surgery should be less likely if surgery is restricted to predamaged and epileptogenic tissue, and if surgery does not affect eloquent areas still involved in function. Frontal lobe resections with subpial transections (dissection of horizontal corticocortical connections) can have negative cognitive consequences on motor function, speed, response inhibition, and language, when the intervention includes the supplementary motor areas, the central region, or the motor language area. As seen after temporal lobe surgery, extrafrontal performances may improve (Helmstaedter et al., 1998; Lendt et al., 2002; Altenmuller and Schulze-Bonhage, 2007). More historical studies report only the patient's postoperative condition and do not permit conclusions regarding changes due to surgery (Elger et al., 2004). Reports on epilepsy surgery in the posterior cortex do not indicate additional cognitive deterioration (Gleissner et al., 2008; Witt et al., 2008a), but resections carry the risk of visual field defects (Luerding et al., 2004), contralateral sensory deficits (two-point discrimination, stereognosis; Salanova et al., 1995), and a transient partial Gerstmann syndrome has been described (Binder et al., 2009). As release effects due to postoperative seizure freedom are observed only in attention (Gleissner et al., 2008) and executive function (Witt et al., 2008a), most of the preoperative impairment appears to be rather static and not the result of a dynamic and reversible secondary epileptogenic involvement of temporal and frontal structures.

Callosotomy

The main objective of callosotomy – the more or less complete surgical disconnection of the hemispheres – is less a curative than a palliative treatment for the control of drop attacks and generalized tonic–clonic seizures due to rapid interhemispheric seizure spread. Patients undergoing callosotomy suffer mostly from severe epilepsies; they are often mentally retarded, and they often show atypically organized hemisphere dominance. Wada testing of these patients (see below) is essential in order to prevent disconnection syndromes. Lassonde and Sauerwein (1997) published a series of 25 pediatric patients who underwent callosotomy and who all benefited from surgery. The greatest improvements were observed in social adjustment. Younger patients showed greater gains than older patients. No negative cognitive change but positive social development has also been reported by Provinciali et al. (1990). Sass and colleagues (1990), in contrast, observed impairments after total and partial callosotomy, and raised concerns regarding motor function and language, particularly in those patients with a dissociation of hand and language dominance. One year after surgery, in a series of 15 mostly anterior callosotomies (Elger et al., 2004), there was a trend of deterioration in language functions (10 patients), significant worsening in figural memory (11 patients), but stable performance in attention, verbal memory, and visuoconstruction. Apart from mutism, which was reversible in all cases (Quattrini et al., 1997), persisting alien hand syndromes in three patients with mixed dominance were observed after anterior callosotomy. Another study did not find an increased risk of neuropsychological impairments in the presence of mixed dominance patterns (Mamelak et al., 1993).

Hemispherectomy

Hemispherectomy is the treatment of ultimate rationale in the presence of severe catastrophic epilepsies that are confined to one hemisphere (mostly Rasmussen's encephalitis, Sturge–Weber syndrome, hemimegalencephaly). In these patients the neuropsychologically most relevant question is the degree to which the contralateral nonaffected hemisphere will take over functions of the affected hemisphere. However, despite clear efficacy in controlling seizures in 65–80% of the patients, there is no place for excessive optimism with regard to plasticity. Although functional cerebral plasticity extends into puberty, Bayard and Lassonde reported in a review of studies published between 1972 and 1997 (Jambaque et al., 2001) that postoperative IQ was not related to age at surgery and that even in early surgery the right hemisphere clearly could not take over all linguistic features normally carried out by the left hemisphere. This would be in line with findings from intracarotid amobarbital testing (IAT or Wada test; see below) that atypical dominance and even complete right-hemisphere language dominance does not guarantee better language functions after surgery (Helmstaedter et al., 1997c). Motor functions seem to improve, but attention and memory generally appear to be deficient after surgery (Jambaque et al., 2001). Later studies have largely confirmed that the outcome of hemispherectomy is determined mostly by the presurgical condition and that no major positive cognitive change can be expected after surgery (Devlin et al., 2003; Pulsifer et al., 2004; Battaglia et al., 2006; Basheer et al., 2007; Lettori et al., 2008). However, parents nevertheless report significant individual improvements and positive behavioral change, as confirmed by a recent longer-term follow-up evaluation of the academic and psychosocial achievements of 57 patients (Buddewig et al., 2009). This study indicated that patients operated early (at age < 7 years) had the best seizure outcome, that patients who had surgery between ages 7 and 16 had the best preoperative to postoperative cognitive and behavioral change, and that the best overall psychosocial outcome was observed in the group operated after age 16 years. This latter group, however, also had the best baseline conditions. Overall, 23% of 57 patients successfully attended a regular school, 21% of 33 patients older than 20 years were employed on a low level, and less than half of the patients (42%) were rated as being able to lead an independent life – 15% have or had a partner (Buddewig et al., 2009).

Vagal nerve stimulation

From a neuropsychological standpoint, vagal nerve stimulation for seizure control is of particular interest because its intermittent and programmable stimulation condition allows for an experimental evaluation of the modulatory effects of peripheral vagal stimulation on central nervous system functions. Indeed, positive psychotropic effects in terms of improved attention, decision-making, or word recognition have been reported, although negative effects have also been described (Clark et al., 1999; Helmstaedter et al., 2001a; Hassert et al., 2004; Martin et al., 2004). Apart from its acute effects, no persisting changes as assessed with a neuropsychological test battery have yet been demonstrated (Hoppe et al., 2001a, b).

Weighting cognition against seizure outcome

A very important and superordinate question for surgical patients is whether they would be willing to risk additional cognitive impairment in the prospect of seizure control. In this respect, seizure outcome appears to have priority (Langfitt et al., 2007; Helmstaedter, 2008a). The respective findings call for increased attention to prevent the so-called "double loser" – the duality of not becoming seizure-free plus a postoperative additional loss of cognitive function. These patients show deterioration in quality of life in the long run. For seizure-free patients one cannot, however, exclude that additional impairments due to surgery provide the basis for later accelerated mental decline with aging (Helmstaedter et al., 2002).

Finally it should be mentioned that cognitive rehabilitation programs may be helpful to counteract losses due to surgery. Training of affected and particularly of compensatory functions can in part reverse deficits (Helmstaedter et al., 2008b). Unfortunately such interventions are often considered only in the context of epilepsy surgery, which usually means only after a long history of suffering from epilepsy and concomitant impairment. According to what has been reported so far about the negative effects of an early onset of epilepsy on cognitive development, such support would be appreciated much earlier in the course of the disease.

Hemispheric dominance and functional plasticity

Most epilepsies start early in life and the maturing and developing brain has the capacity for functional reorganization, restitution, and replacement in response to the lesion/dysfunction. This process is generally referred to as functional cerebral plasticity.

In early-onset epilepsies affecting the left hemisphere, the brain lesion and the epileptic dysfunction represent two factors that, taken alone but also in combination, may drive an intrahemispheric or interhemispheric cerebral reorganization of language functions. This compensatory plastic process promotes and supports the preservation of at least basic language-based communication skills. Intrahemispheric reorganization comprises recruitment of unaffected adjacent brain regions (Ojemann, 1993). In this case the precise topography of language function may be determined by electrical stimulation mapping (ESM) (Wellmer et al., 2009). Interhemispheric reorganization involves contralateral homologous brain structures. Here it is important to note that reorganization of language dominance does not follow an all-or-none principle. Instead it is highly economic for individual functions, e.g. dissociations of handedness, expressive and receptive language, or verbal memory are common (Kurthen et al., 1992). The transfer can, for example, be limited to expressive language functions in the presence of a left frontal lobe lesion/dysfunction, or to receptive language functions in case of a left temporoposterior lesion/dysfunction.

Whereas lesions are assumed to have a chronic and irreversible effect on cerebral hemispheric organization, epilepsy as a potentially controllable condition is assumed to have a more dynamic and eventually reversible impact on hemispheric dominance (Janszky et al., 2003, 2004; Regard et al. 1985; Helmstaedter et al., 2006).

An overview (Table 28.6) of 595 IATs performed between 1997 and 2006 in Bonn indicate atypical language dominance in 35% of presurgical patients (43% in left and 24% in right hemispheric epilepsies) (Fritz, 2009; Helmstaedter, 2010). Depending on the Wada protocol, cohort, and patient selection bias, the respective values for atypical dominance in the literature vary between 17% of 90 patients (Mateer and Dodrill, 1983) to 38% of 73 patients (Rey et al., 1988). Möddel et al. (2009) reported atypical dominance in 22% of 445 patients. The time window for plastic changes of language functions expires with the completion of language development and reaches into puberty (Helmstaedter et al., 1997c).

Table 28.6

Wada test results in presurgical patients with epilepsy

	Prevalence (%)
Presurgical patients with epilepsy (n = 595)	
Atypical language dominance	
Total	35
Left-hemisphere epilepsy	43
Right-hemisphere epilepsy	24
Presurgical patients with left-hemisphere epilepsy (n = 366)	
Atypical language dominance	
Left-handers	91
Right-handers	31
Female	46
Male	38
Early-onset epilepsy	51
Late-onset epilepsy ($\geq$ 14 years)	28
Complete right-hemisphere language dominance	
Extratemporal lobe epilepsy	29
Temporal lobe epilepsy	13

In left-hemisphere epilepsies with an onset before age 15 years, 51% were atypically dominant in contrast to 28% of those with a later onset (Helmstaedter, 2010). The degree of right-hemisphere involvement in language function correlates with the onset of the disease and the extent of structural or functional damage (i.e., the earlier the onset, the more language can be found in the right hemisphere), and the pattern of complete right dominance is seen more frequently in extratemporal lobe epilepsy directly affecting language areas (29%) than in left TLE (13%). As a trend, atypical dominance is more frequent in women, who in addition benefit more from atypical language dominance than men with regard to language related functions (Helmstaedter et al., 1999, 2004a). As already mentioned, left-handedness in combination with early onset of the disease is a good indicator for atypical language dominance (left-handed, 91%; right-handed, 31%), but not vice versa.

Atypical language dominance is often associated with a constellation of material-specific cognitive deficits that contradicts the lateralization of the epileptic focus or lesion. A patient with left-hemisphere epilepsy and atypical language dominance may show deficits in visual spatial tasks, whereas language-related functions and verbal memory are preserved. This effect is termed "crowding" or "suppression" and indicates a transfer of language to the right hemisphere at the cost of original right-hemisphere functions (Strauss et al., 1990). The findings are in keeping with a theoretical concept that suggests an incompatibility of basic aspects of verbal versus nonverbal information processing within the same (unaffected) hemisphere rather than a struggling for space (Helmstaedter et al., 1994b).

The prevalence of atypical language dominance in right-hemisphere epilepsies is greater than 20% (Helmstaedter et al., 1997c; Helmstaedter, 2010). Language within an epileptic right hemisphere seems to be genuine rather than being a consequence of the epilepsy in this hemisphere. In this regard it is remarkable that right-hemisphere language in right-hemisphere epilepsy is less likely in early-onset than in later-onset epilepsies, a finding that led to the idea of a language dominance shift from the right to left hemisphere owing to an early affected right hemisphere (Helmstaedter et al., 1997b). However, this appears to occur "silently," that is to say, with no specific effect on the patient's neuropsychological profile.

CONCLUSION

An explicit aim of this chapter was to provide the reader with an overview of what neuropsychology in epilepsy can do for the diagnosis and differential diagnosis of cognitive impairments associated with epilepsy, and the options that arise from neuropsychological diagnostics for quality and outcome control.

The main emphasis was placed on:

1. the postulation of a neuropsychology in epilepsy that is done in a modular way, that is targeted, time economical, and above all evidence-based
2. the differentiation of static and irreversible versus dynamic and reversible impairments and their determinants
3. the fact that, with the exception of epilepsies with progressive etiology, early-onset chronic epilepsy is more a developmental hindering than a progressively dementing disease
4. the finding that impairments established early in the course of epilepsy call for early interventions that take into account that outcomes depend on the functionality of the affected brain, its reserve capacities, and the control of seizures and epileptic dysfunction.

References

Abou-Khalil B (2007). An update on determination of language dominance in screening for epilepsy surgery: the Wada test and newer noninvasive alternatives. Epilepsia 48: 442–455.

Aghakhani Y, Bagshaw AP, Benar CG et al. (2004). fMRI activation during spike and wave discharges in idiopathic generalized epilepsy. Brain 127: 1127–1144.

Akimura T, Fujii M, Ideguchi M et al. (2003). Ictal onset and spreading of seizures of parietal lobe origin. Neurol Med Chir (Tokyo) 43: 534–540.

Aldenkamp AP, De Krom M, Reijs R (2003). Newer antiepileptic drugs and cognitive issues. Epilepsia 44: 21–29.

Aldenkamp AP, Arends J, Verspeek S et al. (2004). The cognitive impact of epileptiform EEG discharges; relationship with type of cognitive task. Child Neuropsychol 10: 297–305.

Aldenkamp AP, Beitler J, Arends J et al. (2005). Acute effects of subclinical epileptiform EEG discharges on cognitive activation. Funct Neurol 20: 23–28.

Alpherts WC, Vermeulen J, van Rijen PC et al. (2007). Standard versus tailored left temporal lobe resections: Differences in cognitive outcome? Neuropsychologia 46: 455–460.

Altenmuller DM, Schulze-Bonhage A (2007). Differentiating between benign and less benign: epilepsy surgery in symptomatic frontal lobe epilepsy associated with benign focal epileptiform discharges of childhood. J Child Neurol 22: 456–461.

Austin JK, Dunn DW (2002). Progressive behavioral changes in children with epilepsy. Prog Brain Res 135: 419–427.

Banks S, Sziklas V, Djordjevic J et al. (2010). Awareness of deficits during intracarotid anesthetic procedures in epilepsy: comparisons of motor, naming, and comprehension awareness under amobarbital versus under etomidate. Epilepsy Behav 19: 591–595.

Barbaro NM, Quigg M, Broshek DK et al. (2009). A multicenter, prospective pilot study of gamma knife radiosurgery for mesial temporal lobe epilepsy: seizure response, adverse events, and verbal memory. Ann Neurol 65: 167–175.

Baron IS (2004). Neuropsychological Evaluation of the Child. Oxford University Press, Oxford.

Bartolomei F, Hayashi M, Tamura M et al. (2008). Long-term efficacy of gamma knife radiosurgery in mesial temporal lobe epilepsy. Neurology 70: 1658–1663.

Basheer SN, Connolly MB, Lautzenhiser A et al. (2007). Hemispheric surgery in children with refractory epilepsy: seizure outcome, complications, and adaptive function. Epilepsia 48: 133–140.

Battaglia D, Chieffo D, Lettori D et al. (2006). Cognitive assessment in epilepsy surgery of children. Childs Nerv Syst 22: 744–759.

Baxendale S (2002). The role of functional MRI in the presurgical investigation of temporal lobe epilepsy patients: a clinical perspective and review. J Clin Exp Neuropsychol 24: 664–676.

Baxendale S, Thompson P (2010). Beyond localization: the role of traditional neuropsychological tests in an age of imaging. Epilepsia 51: 2225–2230.

Baxendale SA, Thompson PJ, Kitchen ND (2000). Postoperative hippocampal remnant shrinkage and memory decline: a dynamic process. Neurology 55: 243–249.

Baxendale S, Thompson PJ, Duncan JS (2008). The role of the Wada test in the surgical treatment of temporal lobe epilepsy: an international survey. Epilepsia 49: 715–720.

Beck H, Goussakov IV, Lie A et al. (2000). Synaptic plasticity in the human dentate gyrus. J Neurosci 20: 7080–7086.

Benabid AL, Minotti L, Koudsie A et al. (2002). Antiepileptic effect of high-frequency stimulation of the subthalamic nucleus (corpus luysi) in a case of medically intractable epilepsy caused by focal dysplasia: a 30-month follow-up: technical case report. Neurosurgery 50: 1385–1391.

Berg AT, Berkovic SF, Brodie MJ et al. (2010). Revised terminology and concepts for organization of seizures and epilepsies: report of the ILAE Commission on Classification and Terminology, 2005–2009. Epilepsia 51: 676–685.

Besag FM (2004). Behavioral aspects of pediatric epilepsy syndromes. Epilepsy Behav 5: S3–S13.

Binder DK, Podlogar M, Clusmann H et al. (2009). Surgical treatment of parietal lobe epilepsy. J Neurosurg 110: 1170–1178.

Binnie CD (2003). Cognitive impairment during epileptiform discharges: is it ever justifiable to treat the EEG? Lancet Neurol 2: 725–730.

Blumer D, Montouris G, Davies K (2004). The interictal dysphoric disorder: recognition, pathogenesis, and treatment of the major psychiatric disorder of epilepsy. Epilepsy Behav 5: 826–840.

Bolton PF, Park RJ, Higgins JN et al. (2002). Neuro-epileptic determinants of autism spectrum disorders in tuberous sclerosis complex. Brain 125: 1247–1255.

Bonelli SB, Powell RH, Yogarajah M et al. (2010). Imaging memory in temporal lobe epilepsy: predicting the effects of temporal lobe resection. Brain 133: 1186–1199.

Boon P, Vonck K, De Herdt V et al. (2007). Deep brain stimulation in patients with refractory temporal lobe epilepsy. Epilepsia 48: 1551–1560.

Bootsma HP, Ricker L, Hekster YA et al. (2009). The impact of side effects on long-term retention in three new antiepileptic drugs. Seizure 18: 327–331.

Buchtel HA, Passaro EA, Selwa LM et al. (2002). Sodium methohexital (brevital) as an anesthetic in the Wada test. Epilepsia 43: 1056–1061.

Buddewig S, Gleissner U, Elger C et al. (2009). Long term follow up of behavioral and cognitive outcome in hemispherectomized epilepsy patients. Epilepsia 50: 121.

Busch R (2011). Neuropsychological outcomes of extra temporal surgery. In: A Arzimanoglou, B Hermann, M Lasonde et al. (Eds.), Neuropsychology in the Care of People with Epilepsy. Progress in Epileptic Disorders. Vol. 11. John Libbey, Montrouge, pp. 223–238.

Butler CR, Bhaduri A, Acosta-Cabronero J et al. (2009). Transient epileptic amnesia: regional brain atrophy and its relationship to memory deficits. Brain 132: 357–368.

Caraballo RH, Fejerman N (2006). Dravet syndrome: a study of 53 patients. Epilepsy Res 70: S231–S238.

Centeno M, Thompson PJ, Koepp MJ et al. (2010). Memory in frontal lobe epilepsy. Epilepsy Res 91: 123–132.

Chelune GJ (1995). Hippocampal adequacy versus functional reserve: predicting memory functions following temporal lobectomy. Arch Clin Neuropsychol 10: 413–432.

Clark KB, Naritoku DK, Smith DC et al. (1999). Enhanced recognition memory following vagus nerve stimulation in human subjects. Nat Neurosci 2: 94–98.

Clusmann H, Schramm J, Kral T et al. (2002). Prognostic factors and outcome after different types of resection for temporal lobe epilepsy. J Neurosurg 97: 1131–1141.

Crumrine PK (2002). Lennox–Gastaut syndrome. J Child Neurol 17: S70–S75.

Debiais S, Tuller L, Barthez MA et al. (2007). Epilepsy and language development: the continuous spike–waves during slow sleep syndrome. Epilepsia 48: 1104–1110.

Deppe M, Ringelstein EB, Knecht S (2004). The investigation of functional brain lateralization by transcranial Doppler sonography. Neuroimage 21: 1124–1146.

Devinsky J, Schachter S (2009). Norman Geschwind's contribution to the understanding of behavioral changes in temporal lobe epilepsy: the February 1974 lecture. Epilepsy Behav 15: 417–424.

Devinsky O, Gershengorn J, Brown E et al. (1997). Frontal functions in juvenile myoclonic epilepsy. Neuropsychiatry Neuropsychol Behav Neurol 10: 243–246.

Devlin AM, Cross JH, Harkness W et al. (2003). Clinical outcomes of hemispherectomy for epilepsy in childhood and adolescence. Brain 126: 556–566.

Dietl T, Urbach H, Helmstaedter C et al. (2004). Persistent severe amnesia due to seizure recurrence after unilateral temporal lobectomy. Epilepsy Behav 5: 394–400.

Dodrill CB (2004). Neuropsychological effects of seizures. Epilepsy Behav 5: 21–24.

Dodrill CB, Ojemann GA (1997). An exploratory comparison of three methods of memory assessment with the intracarotid amobarbital procedure. Brain Cogn 33: 210–223.

Dunn DW, Kronenberger WG, Sherman EMS (2011). Autism spectrum disorder and attention deficit hyperactivity disorder in childhood epilepsy. In: A Arzimanoglou, B Hermann, M Lasonde et al. (Eds.), Neuropsychology in the Care of People with Epilepsy. Progress in Epileptic Disorders. Vol. 11. John Libbey, Montrouge, pp. 273–284.

Elger CE, Helmstaedter C, Kurthen M (2004). Chronic epilepsy and cognition. Lancet Neurol 3: 663–672.

Exner C, Boucsein K, Lange C et al. (2002). Neuropsychological performance in frontal lobe epilepsy. Seizure 11: 20–32.

Fell J, Klaver P, Lehnertz K et al. (2001). Human memory formation is accompanied by rhinal–hippocampal coupling and decoupling. Nat Neurosci 4: 1259–1264.

Fernandez G, Klaver P, Fell J et al. (2002). Human declarative memory formation: segregating rhinal and hippocampal contributions. Hippocampus 12: 514–519.

Fernandez G, Specht K, Weis S et al. (2003). Intrasubject reproducibility of presurgical language lateralization and mapping using fMRI. Neurology 60: 969–975.

French JA, Kanner AM, Bautista J et al. (2004). Efficacy and tolerability of the new antiepileptic drugs I: Treatment of new onset epilepsy: report of the Therapeutics and Technology Assessment Subcommittee and Quality Standards Subcommittee of the American Academy of Neurology and the American Epilepsy Society. Neurology 62: 1252–1260.

Frisch C, Hanke J, Kleineruschkamp S et al. (2009a). Positive correlation between the density of neuropeptide Y positive neurons in the amygdala and parameters of self-reported anxiety and depression in mesiotemporal lobe epilepsy patients. Biol Psychiatry 66: 433–440.

Frisch C, Husch K, Angenstein F et al. (2009b). Dose-dependent memory effects and cerebral volume changes after in utero exposure to valproate in the rat. Epilepsia 50: 1432–1441.

Fritz NE (2009). Bedingungen und Konsequenzen atypischer Sprachdominanz für Sprache bei linkshemsiphärischer Epilepsie Philosopische Fakultät. Rheinische Friedrich-Wilhelms-Universität, Bonn.

Gaillard WD (2004). Functional MR imaging of language, memory, and sensorimotor cortex. Neuroimaging Clin N Am 14: 471–485.

Giordani B, Caveney AF, Laughrin D et al. (2006). Cognition and behavior in children with benign epilepsy with centrotemporal spikes (BECTS). Epilepsy Res 70: 89–94.

Gleissner U, Helmstaedter C (2008). Presurgical work up in children and intellectually disabled adults with epilepsy. In: H Lueders (Ed.), Textbook of Epilepsy Surgery. Lippincott-Raven, Philadelphia, pp. 833–843.

Gleissner U, Helmstaedter C, Elger CE (1998). Right hippocampal contribution to visual memory: a presurgical and postsurgical study in patients with temporal lobe epilepsy. J Neurol Neurosurg Psychiatry 65: 665–669.

Gleissner U, Helmstaedter C, Schramm J et al. (2002). Memory outcome after selective amygdalohippocampectomy: a study in 140 patients with temporal lobe epilepsy. Epilepsia 43: 87–95.

Gleissner U, Lendt M, Mayer S et al. (2006). [A new questionnaire for recognizing cognitive problems in children and adolescents]. Nervenarzt 77: 449–465.

Gleissner U, Kuczaty S, Clusmann H et al. (2008). Neuropsychological results in pediatric patients with epilepsy surgery in the parietal cortex. Epilepsia 49: 700–704.

Gonzalez P, Sills GJ, Parks S et al. (2009). Binasal visual field defects are not specific to vigabatrin. Epilepsy Behav 16: 521–526.

Gulgonen S, Demirbilek V, Korkmaz B et al. (2000). Neuropsychological functions in idiopathic occipital lobe epilepsy. Epilepsia 41: 405–411.

Haag A, Knake S, Hamer HM et al. (2008). The Wada test in Austrian, Dutch, German, and Swiss epilepsy centers from 2000 to 2005: a review of 1421 procedures. Epilepsy Behav 13: 83–89.

Harden CL, Meador KJ, Pennell PB et al. (2009). Management issues for women with epilepsy – focus on pregnancy (an evidence-based review): II. Teratogenesis and perinatal outcomes: report of the Quality Standards Subcommittee and Therapeutics and Technology Subcommittee of the American Academy of Neurology and the American Epilepsy Society. Epilepsia 50: 1237–1246.

Hassert DL, Miyashita T, Williams CL (2004). The effects of peripheral vagal nerve stimulation at a memory-modulating intensity on norepinephrine output in the basolateral amygdala. Behav Neurosci 118: 79–88.

Helmstaedter CA (1999). Prediction of memory reserve capacity. Adv Neurol 81: 271–279.

Helmstaedter C (2002). Effects of chronic epilepsy on declarative memory systems. Prog Brain Res 135: 439–453.

Helmstaedter C (2007). Cognitive outcome of status epilepticus in adults. Epilepsia 48: 85–90.

Helmstaedter C (2008a). Temporal lobe resection – does the prospect of seizure freedom outweigh the cognitive risks? Nat Clin Pract Neurol 4: 66–67.

Helmstaedter C (2008b). EpiTrack Junior: Veränderungssensitives kognitives Skreening zur Qualitäts- und Erfolgskontrolle der Epilepsiebehandlung bei Kindern und Jugendlichen. UCB, Monheim.

Helmstaedter C (2008c). The role of the Wada test in the surgical treatment of temporal lobe epilepsy: an international perspective. Epilepsia 49: 720–722.

Helmstaedter C (2009a). Neurospychologie bei Epilepsie. In: W Sturm, M Herrmann, TF Münte (Eds.), Lehrbuch der klinischen Neuropsychologie. Spektrum, Heidelberg, pp. 687–700.

Helmstaedter C (2009b). Assessment of cognitive function – does it reveal the patients at risk? Epilepsia 50: 34.

Helmstaedter C (2010). WADA test: lessons on language dominance and change of indication with improvements in the diagnosis and surgical treatment of epilepsy. Epilepsy Behav 17: 585.

Helmstaedter C (2011). Neuropsychological outcomes of different surgical approaches in temporal lobe epilepsy. In: C Helmstaedter, B Hermann, M Lasonde et al. (Eds.), Neuropsychology in the Care of People with Epilepsy. Progress in Epileptic Disorders. Vol. 11. John Libbey, Montrouge, pp. 201–221.

Helmstaedter C, Durwen HF (1990). The Verbal Learning and Retention Test. A useful and differentiated tool in evaluating verbal memory performance. Schweiz Arch Neurol Psychiatr 141: 21–30.

Helmstaedter C, Elger CE (1999). The phantom of progressive dementia in epilepsy. Lancet 354: 2133–2134.

Helmstaedter C, Elger CE (2009). Chronic temporal lobe epilepsy: a neurodevelopmental or progressively dementing disease? Brain 132: 2822–2830.

Helmstaedter C, Kurthen M (2002). Validity of the WADA test. Epilepsy Behav 3: 562–563.

Helmstaedter C, Witt JA (2011). Behavioral and neuropsychological aspects of frontal and temporal lobe epilepsy. In: M Trimble, B Schmitz (Eds.), The Neuropsychiatry of Epilepsy. 2nd edn. Cambridge University Press, Cambridge, pp. 90–108.

Helmstaedter C, Pohl C, Hufnagel A et al. (1991). Visual learning deficits in nonresected patients with right temporal lobe epilepsy. Cortex 27: 547–555.

Helmstaedter C, Hufnagel A, Elger CE (1992). Seizures during cognitive testing in patients with temporal lobe epilepsy: possibility of seizure induction by cognitive activation. Epilepsia 33: 892–897.

Helmstaedter C, Elger CE, Lendt M (1994a). Postictal courses of cognitive deficits in focal epilepsies. Epilepsia 35: 1073–1078.

Helmstaedter C, Kurthen M, Linke DB et al. (1994b). Right hemisphere restitution of language and memory functions in right hemisphere language-dominant patients with left temporal lobe epilepsy. Brain 117: 729–737.

Helmstaedter C, Elger CE, Hufnagel A et al. (1996a). Different effects of left anterior temporal lobectomy, selective amygdalohippocampectomy, and temporal cortical lesionectomy on verbal learning, memory, and recognition. J Epilepsy 9: 39–45.

Helmstaedter C, Kemper B, Elger CE (1996b). Neuropsychological aspects of frontal lobe epilepsy. Neuropsychologia 34: 399–406.

Helmstaedter C, Grunwald T, Lehnertz K et al. (1997a). Differential involvement of left temporolateral and temporomesial structures in verbal declarative learning and memory: evidence from temporal lobe epilepsy. Brain Cogn 35: 110–131.

Helmstaedter C, Kurthen M, Gleissner U et al. (1997b). Natural atypical language dominance and language shifts from the right to the left hemisphere in right hemisphere pathology. Naturwissenschaften 84: 250–252.

Helmstaedter C, Kurthen M, Linke DB et al. (1997c). Patterns of language dominance in focal left and right hemisphere epilepsies: relation to MRI findings, EEG, sex, and age at onset of epilepsy. Brain Cogn 33: 135–150.

Helmstaedter C, Gleissner U, Zentner J et al. (1998). Neuropsychological consequences of epilepsy surgery in frontal lobe epilepsy. Neuropsychologia 36: 681–689.

Helmstaedter C, Kurthen M, Elger CE (1999). Sex differences in material-specific cognitive functions related to language dominance: an intracarotid amobarbital study in left temporal lobe epilepsy. Laterality 4: 51–63.

Helmstaedter C, Hoppe C, Elger CE (2001a). Memory alterations during acute high-intensity vagus nerve stimulation. Epilepsy Res 47: 37–42.

Helmstaedter C, Lendt M, Lux S (2001b). VLMT Verbaler Lern- und Merkfähigkeitstest. Beltz Test, Göttingen.

Helmstaedter C, Reuber M, Elger CC (2002). Interaction of cognitive aging and memory deficits related to epilepsy surgery. Ann Neurol 52: 89–94.

Helmstaedter C, Kurthen M, Lux S et al. (2003). Chronic epilepsy and cognition: a longitudinal study in temporal lobe epilepsy. Ann Neurol 54: 425–432.

Helmstaedter C, Brosch T, Kurthen M et al. (2004a). The impact of sex and language dominance on material-specific memory before and after left temporal lobe surgery. Brain 127: 1518–1525.

Helmstaedter C, Van Roost D, Clusmann H et al. (2004b). Collateral brain damage, a potential source of cognitive impairment after selective surgery for control of mesial temporal lobe epilepsy. J Neurol Neurosurg Psychiatry 75: 323–326.

Helmstaedter C, Fritz NE, Gonzalez Perez PA et al. (2006). Shift-back of right into left hemisphere language dominance after control of epileptic seizures: evidence for epilepsy driven functional cerebral organization. Epilepsy Res 70: 257–262.

Helmstaedter C, Schramm J, Elger CE (2007). 15 years epilepsy surgery in Bonn: cognitive and seizure outcome. Epilepsia 48: 14.

Helmstaedter C, Fritz NE, Kockelmann E et al. (2008a). Positive and negative psychotropic effects of levetiracetam. Epilepsy Behav 13: 535–541.

Helmstaedter C, Loer B, Wohlfahrt R et al. (2008b). The effects of cognitive rehabilitation on memory outcome after temporal lobe epilepsy surgery. Epilepsy Behav 12: 402–409.

Helmstaedter C, Richter S, Roske S et al. (2008c). Differential effects of temporal pole resection with amygdalohippocampectomy versus selective amygdalohippocampectomy on material-specific memory in patients with mesial temporal lobe epilepsy. Epilepsia 49: 88–97.

Helmstaedter C, Wietzke J, Lutz MT (2009). Unique and shared validity of the "Wechsler logical memory test", the "California verbal learning test", and the "verbal learning and memory test" in patients with epilepsy. Epilepsy Res 87: 203–212.

Helmstaedter C, Schoof K, Rossmann T et al. (2010). Introduction and first validation of EpiTrack-Junior, a screening tool for the assessment of cognitive side effects of antiepileptic medication on attention and executive functions in children and adolescents with epilepsy. Epilepsy Behav 19: 55–64.

Hermann BP, Wyler AR, Richey ET (1988). Wisconsin Card Sorting Test performance in patients with complex partial seizures of temporal-lobe origin. J Clin Exp Neuropsychol 10: 467–476.

Hermann BP, Seidenberg M, Schoenfeld J et al. (1996). Empirical techniques for determining the reliability, magnitude, and pattern of neuropsychological change after epilepsy surgery. Epilepsia 37: 942–950.

Hermann BP, Seidenberg M, Schoenfeld J et al. (1997). Neuropsychological characteristics of the syndrome of mesial temporal lobe epilepsy. Arch Neurol 54: 369–376.

Hermann B, Jones J, Sheth R et al. (2006). Children with new-onset epilepsy: neuropsychological status and brain structure. Brain 129: 2609–2619.

Hermann B, Seidenberg M, Jones J (2008). The neurobehavioural comorbidities of epilepsy: can a natural history be developed? Lancet Neurol 7: 151–160.

Hessen E, Lossius MI, Reinvang I et al. (2006). Influence of major antiepileptic drugs on attention, reaction time, and speed of information processing: results from a randomized, double-blind, placebo-controlled withdrawal study of seizure-free epilepsy patients receiving monotherapy. Epilepsia 47: 2038–2045.

Holmes GL (1997). Epilepsy in the developing brain: lessons from the laboratory and clinic. Epilepsia 38: 12–30.

Holmes G (2010). Is the epileptiform activity the reason for cognitive impairment or only an epiphenomenon. Epilepsia 51: 171.

Hommet C, Sauerwein HC, De Toffol B et al. (2006). Idiopathic epileptic syndromes and cognition. Neurosci Biobehav Rev 30: 85–96.

Hoppe C, Helmstaedter C (2010). Sensitive and specific neuropsychological assessments of the behavioral effects of epilepsy and its treatment is essential. Epilepsia 51: 2365–2366.

Hoppe C, Helmstaedter C, Scherrmann J et al. (2001a). Self-reported mood changes following 6 months of vagus nerve stimulation in epilepsy patients. Epilepsy Behav 2: 335–342.

Hoppe C, Helmstaedter C, Scherrmann J et al. (2001b). No evidence for cognitive side effects after 6 months of vagus nerve stimulation in epilepsy patients. Epilepsy Behav 2: 351–356.

Hoppe C, Fliessbach K, Schlegel U et al. (2009). NeuroCog FX: computerized screening of cognitive functions in patients with epilepsy. Epilepsy Behav 16: 298–310.

Jambaque I, Lassonde M, Dulac O (2001). Neuropsychology of Childhood Epilepsy. Kluwer Academic/Plenum Publishers, New York.

Janszky J, Jokeit H, Heinemann D et al. (2003). Epileptic activity influences the speech organization in medial temporal lobe epilepsy. Brain 126: 2043–2051.

Janszky J, Ollech I, Jokeit H et al. (2004). Epileptic activity influences the lateralization of mesiotemporal fMRI activity. Neurology 63: 1813–1817.

Janz D (2002). The psychiatry of idiopathic generalized epilepsy. In: MR Trimble, B Schmitz (Eds.), The Neuropsychiatry of Epilepsy. Cambridge University Press, Cambridge, pp. 41–61.

Johnsrude IS, Owen AM, White NM et al. (2000). Impaired preference conditioning after anterior temporal lobe resection in humans. J Neurosci 20: 2649–2656.

Jokeit H, Ebner A (2002). Effects of chronic epilepsy on intellectual functions. Prog Brain Res 135: 455–463.

Jokeit H, Seitz R, Markowitsch H et al. (1997). Prefrontal asymmetric interictal glucose hypometabolism and cognitive impairment in patients with temporal lobe epilepsy. Brain 120: 2283–2294.

Jokeit H, Luerding R, Ebner A (2000). Cognitive impairment in temporal-lobe epilepsy. Lancet 355: 1018–1019.

Jones-Gotman M, Smith ML, Zatorre RJ (1993). Neuropsychological testing for localizing and lateralizing the epileptogenic region. In: J Engel (Ed.), Surgical Treatment of the Epilepsies. Raven Press, New York, pp. 245–262.

Jones-Gotman M, Smith ML, Risse GL et al. (2010). The contribution of neuropsychology to diagnostic assessment in epilepsy. Epilepsy Behav 18: 3–12.

Jordan JW (2007). Semiology: witness to a seizure – what to note and how to report. Am J Electroneurodiagnostic Technol 47: 264–282.

Kaaden S, Helmstaedter C (2009). Age at onset of epilepsy as a determinant of intellectual impairment in temporal lobe epilepsy. Epilepsy Behav 15: 213–217.

Kaaden S, Quesada C, Schramm J et al. (2009). Voxel-based morphometry (VBM) supports neurodevelopmental hypothesis regarding early onset temporal lobe epilepsy (TLE). Epilepsia 50: 216.

Kanner AM (2008). The use of psychotropic drugs in epilepsy: what every neurologist should know. Semin Neurol 28: 379–388.

Ketter TA, Post RM, Theodore WH (1999). Positive and negative psychiatric effects of antiepileptic drugs in patients with seizure disorders. Neurology 53: S53–S67.

Koepp MJ, Woermann FG (2005). Imaging structure and function in refractory focal epilepsy. Lancet Neurol 4: 42–53.

Krauss GL (2009). Evaluating risks for vigabatrin treatment. Epilepsy Curr 9: 125–129.

Kurthen M, Helmstaedter C, Linke DB et al. (1992). Interhemispheric dissociation of expressive and receptive language functions in patients with complex-partial seizures: an amobarbital study. Brain Lang 43: 694–712.

Kurthen M, Helmstaedter C, Linke DB et al. (1994). Quantitative and qualitative evaluation of patterns of cerebral language dominance – an amobarbital study. Brain Lang 46: 536–564.

Kwan P, Brodie MJ (2001). Neuropsychological effects of epilepsy and antiepileptic drugs. Lancet 357: 216–222.

Langfitt JT, Westerveld M, Hamberger MJ et al. (2007). Worsening of quality of life after epilepsy surgery: effect of seizures and memory decline. Neurology 68: 1988–1994.

Lassonde M, Sauerwein C (1997). Neuropsychological outcome of corpus callosotomy in children and adolescents. J Neurosurg Sci 41: 67–73.

Lee TM, Yip JT, Jones-Gotman M (2002). Memory deficits after resection from left or right anterior temporal lobe in humans: a meta-analytic review. Epilepsia 43: 283–291.

Lendt M, Helmstaedter C, Kuczaty S et al. (2000). Behavioural disorders in children with epilepsy: early improvement after surgery. J Neurol Neurosurg Psychiatry 69: 739–744.

Lendt M, Gleissner U, Helmstaedter C et al. (2002). Neuropsychological outcome in children after frontal lobe epilepsy surgery. Epilepsy Behav 3: 51–59.

Lettori D, Battaglia D, Sacco A et al. (2008). Early hemispherectomy in catastrophic epilepsy: a neuro-cognitive and epileptic long-term follow-up. Seizure 17: 49–63.

Lezak MD, Howieson DB, Loring DW et al. (2004). Neuropsychological Assessment. Oxford University Press, Oxford.

Liasis A, Bamiou DE, Boyd S et al. (2006). Evidence for a neurophysiologic auditory deficit in children with benign epilepsy with centro-temporal spikes. J Neural Transm 113: 939–949.

Lindgren S, Kihlgren M, Melin L et al. (2004). Development of cognitive functions in children with rolandic epilepsy. Epilepsy Behav 5: 903–910.

Loring DW, Meador KJ (2004). Cognitive side effects of antiepileptic drugs in children. Neurology 62: 872–877.

Loring DW, Strauss E, Hermann BP et al. (2008). Differential neuropsychological test sensitivity to left temporal lobe epilepsy. J Int Neuropsychol Soc 14: 394–400.

Luerding R, Boesebeck F, Ebner A (2004). Cognitive changes after epilepsy surgery in the posterior cortex. J Neurol Neurosurg Psychiatry 75: 583–587.

Lutz MT, Helmstaedter C (2005). EpiTrack: tracking cognitive side effects of medication on attention and executive functions in patients with epilepsy. Epilepsy Behav 7: 708–714.

Lux S, Kurthen M, Helmstaedter C et al. (2002). The localizing value of ictal consciousness and its constituent functions: a video-EEG study in patients with focal epilepsy. Brain 125: 2691–2698.

Malter MP, Helmstaedter C, Urbach H et al. (2010). Antibodies to glutamic acid decarboxylase define a form of limbic encephalitis. Ann Neurol 67: 470–478.

Mamelak AN, Barbaro NM, Walker JA et al. (1993). Corpus callosotomy: a quantitative study of the extent of resection, seizure control, and neuropsychological outcome. J Neurosurg 79: 688–695.

Martin CO, Denburg NL, Tranel D et al. (2004). The effects of vagus nerve stimulation on decision-making. Cortex 40: 605–612.

Mateer CA, Dodrill CB (1983). Neuropsychological and linguistic correlates of atypical language lateralization: evidence from sodium amytal studies. Hum Neurobiol 2: 135–142.

Matsuoka H, Takahashi T, Sasaki M et al. (2000). Neuropsychological EEG activation in patients with epilepsy. Brain 123: 318–330.

Meador KJ, Penovich P, Baker GA et al. (2009). Antiepileptic drug use in women of childbearing age. Epilepsy Behav 15: 339–343.

Meencke HJ, Janz D (1985). The significance of microdysgenesia in primary generalized epilepsy: an answer to the considerations of Lyon and Gastaut. Epilepsia 26: 368–371.

Mirsky AF, Duncan B, Levav M (2001). Neuropsychological studies in idiopathic generalized epilepsies. In: I Jambaquet, M Lasonde, O Dulac (Eds.), Neuropsychology of Childhood Epilepsy. Plenum Press, New York, pp. 141–149.

Möddel G, Lineweaver T, Schuele SU et al. (2009). Atypical language lateralization in epilepsy patients. Epilepsia 50: 1505–1516.

Monjauze C, Tuller L, Hommet C et al. (2005). Language in benign childhood epilepsy with centro-temporal spikes abbreviated form: rolandic epilepsy and language. Brain Lang 92: 300–308.

Morino M, Uda T, Naito K et al. (2006). Comparison of neuropsychological outcomes after selective amygdalohippocampectomy versus anterior temporal lobectomy. Epilepsy Behav 9: 95–100.

Muller H, Hasse-Sander I, Horn R et al. (1997). Rey Auditory-Verbal Learning Test: structure of a modified German version. J Clin Psychol 53: 663–671.

Nicolai J, Aldenkamp AP, Arends J et al. (2006). Cognitive and behavioral effects of nocturnal epileptiform discharges in children with benign childhood epilepsy with centrotemporal spikes. Epilepsy Behav 8: 56–70.

Oguni H, Hayashi K, Osawa M et al. (2005). Severe myoclonic epilepsy in infancy: clinical analysis and relation to SCN1A mutations in a Japanese cohort. Adv Neurol 95: 103–117.

Ojemann GA (1993). Functional mapping of cortical language areas in adults. Intraoperative approaches. Adv Neurol 63: 155–163.

Olivier A (1996). Surgery of mesial temporal lobe epilepsy. In: S Shorvon, F Dreifuss, D Fish et al. (Eds.), The Treatment of Epilepsy. Blackwell Science, Oxford, pp. 689–698.

Ortinski P, Meador KJ (2004). Cognitive side effects of antiepileptic drugs. Epilepsy Behav 5: S60–S65.

Paglioli E, Palmini A, Portuguez M et al. (2006). Seizure and memory outcome following temporal lobe surgery: selective compared with nonselective approaches for hippocampal sclerosis. J Neurosurg 104: 70–78.

Papavasiliou A, Mattheou D, Bazigou H et al. (2005). Written language skills in children with benign childhood epilepsy with centrotemporal spikes. Epilepsy Behav 6: 50–58.

Park SP, Kwon SH (2008). Cognitive effects of antiepileptic drugs. J Clin Neurol 4: 99–106.

Pauli E, Hildebrandt M, Romstock J et al. (2006). Deficient memory acquisition in temporal lobe epilepsy is predicted by hippocampal granule cell loss. Neurology 67: 1383–1389.

Pavone P, Bianchini R, Trifiletti RR et al. (2001). Neuropsychological assessment in children with absence epilepsy. Neurology 56: 1047–1051.

Provinciali L, Del Pesce M, Censori B et al. (1990). Evolution of neuropsychological changes after partial callosotomy in intractable epilepsy. Epilepsy Res 6: 155–165.

Pulsifer MB, Brandt J, Salorio CF et al. (2004). The cognitive outcome of hemispherectomy in 71 children. Epilepsia 45: 243–254.

Quattrini A, Del Pesce M, Provinciali L et al. (1997). Mutism in 36 patients who underwent callosotomy for drug-resistant epilepsy. J Neurosurg Sci 41: 93–96.

Regard M, Landis T, Wieser HG et al. (1985). Functional inhibition and release: unilateral tachistoscopic performance and stereoelectroencephalographic activity in a case with left limbic status epilepticus. Neuropsychologia 23: 575–581.

Renowden SA, Matkovic Z, Adams CB et al. (1995). Selective amygdalohippocampectomy for hippocampal sclerosis: postoperative MR appearance. AJNR Am J Neuroradiol 16: 1855–1861.

Rey M, Dellatolas G, Bancaud J et al. (1988). Hemispheric lateralization of motor and speech functions after early brain lesion: study of 73 epileptic patients with intracarotid amytal test. Neuropsychologia 26: 167–172.

Roberts GM, Majoie HJ, Leenen LA et al. (2005). Ketter's hypothesis of the mood effects of antiepileptic drugs coupled to the mechanism of action of topiramate and levetiracetam. Epilepsy Behav 6: 366–372.

Rosenow F, Lüders HO (Eds.), (2004). Presurgical Assessment of the Epilepsies with Clinical Neurophysiology and Functional Imaging. Handbook of Clinical Neurophysiology Vol. 3. Elsevier, Amsterdam.

Rossi PG, Parmeggiani A, Posar A et al. (1999). Landau–Kleffner syndrome (LKS): long-term follow-up and links with electrical status epilepticus during sleep (ESES). Brain Dev 21: 90–98.

Salanova V, Andermann F, Rasmussen T et al. (1955). Parietal lobe epilepsy. Clinical manifestations and outcome in 82 patients treated surgically between 1929 and 1988. Brain 118: 607–627.

Salek-Haddadi A, Lemieux L, Merschhemke M et al. (2003). Functional magnetic resonance imaging of human absence seizures. Ann Neurol 53: 663–667.

Saltik S, Uluduz D, Cokar O et al. (2005). A clinical and EEG study on idiopathic partial epilepsies with evolution into ESES spectrum disorders. Epilepsia 46: 524–533.

Sass KJ, Novelly RA, Spencer DD et al. (1990). Postcallosotomy language impairments in patients with crossed cerebral dominance. J Neurosurg 72: 85–90.

Sawrie SM, Martin RC, Knowlton R et al. (2001). Relationships among hippocampal volumetry, proton magnetic resonance spectroscopy, and verbal memory in temporal lobe epilepsy. Epilepsia 42: 1403–1407.

Schacher M, Winkler R, Grunwald T et al. (2006). Mesial temporal lobe epilepsy impairs advanced social cognition. Epilepsia 47: 2141–2146.

Schramm J (2008). Temporal lobe epilepsy surgery and the quest for optimal extent of resection: a review. Epilepsia 49: 1296–1307.

Sherman EM, Wiebe S, Fay-McClymont TB et al. (2011). Neuropsychological outcomes after epilepsy surgery: systematic review and pooled estimates. Epilepsia 52: 857–869.

Shields WD (2002). West's syndrome. J Child Neurol 17: S76–S79.

Sindou M, Guenot M, Isnard J et al. (2006). Temporo-mesial epilepsy surgery: outcome and complications in 100 consecutive adult patients. Acta Neurochir (Wien) 148: 39–45.

So EL (2006). Value and limitations of seizure semiology in localizing seizure onset. J Clin Neurophysiol 23: 353–357.

Sonmez F, Atakli D, Sari H et al. (2004). Cognitive function in juvenile myoclonic epilepsy. Epilepsy Behav 5: 329–336.

Spina E, Perugi G (2004). Antiepileptic drugs: indications other than epilepsy. Epileptic Disord 6: 57–75.

Stephani U, Carlsson G (2006). The spectrum from BCECTS to LKS: the Rolandic EEG trait–impact on cognition. Epilepsia 47: 67–70.

Strauss E, Satz P, Wada J (1990). An examination of the crowding hypothesis in epileptic patients who have undergone the carotid amytal test. Neuropsychologia 28: 1221–1227.

Strauss E, Sherman EM, Spreen O (2006). A Compendium of Neuropsychological Tests: Administration, Norms, and Commentary. Oxford University Press, Oxford.

Stroup E, Langfitt J, Berg M et al. (2003). Predicting verbal memory decline following anterior temporal lobectomy (ATL). Neurology 60: 1266–1273.

Sutula T, Pitkänen A (Eds.), (2002). Do Seizures Damage the Brain? Progress in Brain Research, Vol. 135. Elsevier, Amsterdam.

Swartz BE, Simpkins F, Halgren E et al. (1996). Visual working memory in primary generalized epilepsy: an 18FDG-PET study. Neurology 47: 1203–1212.

Taylor J, Kolamunnage-Dona R, Marson AG et al. (2010). Patients with epilepsy: cognitively compromised before the start of antiepileptic drug treatment? Epilepsia 51: 48–56.

Trinka E, Kienpointner G, Unterberger I et al. (2006). Psychiatric comorbidity in juvenile myoclonic epilepsy. Epilepsia 47: 2086–2091.

Upton D, Thompson PJ (1996). General neuropsychological characteristics of frontal lobe epilepsy. Epilepsy Res 23: 169–177.

Van Hirtum-Das M, Licht EA, Koh S et al. (2006). Children with ESES: variability in the syndrome. Epilepsy Res 70: S248–S258.

Vannucci M, Pezer N, Helmstaedter C et al. (2008). Hippocampal response to visual objects is related to visual memory functioning. NeuroReport 19: 965–968.

Velasco AL, Velasco F, Velasco M et al. (2007). Electrical stimulation of the hippocampal epileptic foci for seizure control: a double-blind, long-term follow-up study. Epilepsia 48: 1895–1903.

Vinayan KP, Biji V, Thomas SV (2005). Educational problems with underlying neuropsychological impairment are common in children with benign epilepsy of childhood with centrotemporal spikes (BECTS). Seizure 14: 207–212.

Weber B, Wellmer J, Schur S et al. (2006). Presurgical language fMRI in patients with drug-resistant epilepsy: effects of task performance. Epilepsia 47: 880–886.

Weber B, Luders E, Faber J et al. (2007). Distinct regional atrophy in the corpus callosum of patients with temporal lobe epilepsy. Brain 130: 3149–3154.

Wellmer J, Weber C, Mende M et al. (2009). Multitask electrical stimulation for cortical language mapping: hints for necessity and economic mode of application. Epilepsia 50: 2267–2275.

Wiebe S, Blume WT, Girvin JP et al. (2001). A randomized, controlled trial of surgery for temporal-lobe epilepsy. N Engl J Med 345: 311–318.

Wieser HG (2004). Mesial temporal lobe epilepsy with hippocampal sclerosis. Epilepsia 45: 695–714.

Witt JA, Helmstaedter C (2009). [Neuropsychology in epilepsy]. Fortschr Neurol Psychiatr 77: 691–698.

Witt JA, Helmstaedter C (2010). The impact of antiepileptic drug treatment on attention and executive functions. Epilepsia 51: 20.

Witt JA, Helmstaedter C (2012). Cognitive outcome of antiepileptic treatment with levetiracetam versus carbamazepine monotherapy: a non-interventional surveillance trial. Epilepsy Behav 18: 74–80.

Witt JA, Elger CE, Helmstaedter C (2008a). Preoperative cognitive profile and postoperative change in patients with epilepsy surgery in the parietal cortex. Epilepsia 49: 143.

Witt JA, Hollmann K, Helmstaedter C (2008b). The impact of lesions and epilepsy on personality and mood in patients with symptomatic epilepsy: a pre- to postoperative follow-up study. Epilepsy Res 82: 139–146.

Woermann FG, Free SL, Koepp MJ et al. (1999). Abnormal cerebral structure in juvenile myoclonic epilepsy demonstrated with voxel-based analysis of MRI. Brain 122: 2101–2108.

Wolff M, Weiskopf N, Serra E et al. (2005). Benign partial epilepsy in childhood: selective cognitive deficits are related to the location of focal spikes determined by combined EEG/MEG. Epilepsia 46: 1661–1667.

Wolff M, Casse-Perrot C, Dravet C (2006). Severe myoclonic epilepsy of infants (Dravet syndrome): natural history and neuropsychological findings. Epilepsia 47: 45–48.

Wyler AR, Hermann BP, Somes G (1995). Extent of medial temporal resection on outcome from anterior temporal lobectomy: a randomized prospective study. Neurosurgery 37: 982–990.

Zhou JL, Lenck-Santini PP, Zhao Q et al. (2007). Effect of interictal spikes on single-cell firing patterns in the hippocampus. Epilepsia 48: 720–731.

Handbook of Clinical Neurology, Vol. 107 (3rd series)
Epilepsy, Part I
H. Stefan and W.H. Theodore, Editors

Chapter 29

Neuropsychiatric complications of epilepsy

ANDRES M. KANNER [1]* AND DALE C. HESDORFFER [2]

[1]*Department of Neurological Sciences, Rush Medical College at Rush University, Chicago, IL, USA*

[2]*Gertrude H. Sergievsky Center and Department of Epidemiology, Columbia University, New York, NY, USA*

INTRODUCTION

Psychiatric comorbidities have long been recognized in people with epilepsy, yet a significant proportion of patients with psychiatric comorbidities remain undiagnosed and untreated. Historically, psychiatric comorbidities were conceptualized as "complications" of the epileptic seizure disorder; recent longitudinal epidemiological studies have established a more complex relation between psychiatric disorders and epilepsy.

Psychiatric comorbidities impact negatively the quality of life of people with epilepsy and are associated with a worse response to pharmacological and surgical treatment. This chapter reviews the epidemiological, clinical, pathogenic, and therapeutic aspects of psychiatric comorbidities in epilepsy.

EPIDEMIOLOGICAL ASPECTS OF PSYCHIATRIC DISORDERS IN EPILEPSY

A number of studies have evaluated the frequency of current psychiatric disorders and disturbances in people with prevalent epilepsy. These reports are generally cross-sectional, from referral centers, fail to take into account the time order of the two conditions, and lack a comparison group.

The question arises: why are psychiatric disorders more prevalent than expected in patients with epilepsy? This question is impossible to answer in cross-sectional studies of prevalent populations with epilepsy or with psychiatric disorder; instead other study designs are needed. One possibility is that epilepsy or its correlates may cause psychiatric disorders. Answering this question requires a study of people with new-onset (incident) epilepsy who have never had the psychiatric disorder of interest and who are followed over time to examine the risk for a first episode of the psychiatric disorder. It is also possible that the prevalent psychiatric disorder represents a recurrent episode of a disorder that first occurred before the onset of epilepsy. Such recurrent psychiatric disorder could be independent of or dependent upon factors associated with epilepsy (e.g., temporal lobe pathology) that could influence vulnerability both to recurrence of the psychiatric disorder and to the continued seizures that would define prevalent epilepsy. Answering this question requires a follow-up study of incident epilepsy with and without a history of the psychiatric disorder of interest before epilepsy onset to examine the risk for recurrent and new-onset disorder. Understanding the reasons for the occurrence of psychiatric disorders in prevalent epilepsy by addressing these questions could guide treatment and the prevention of psychosocial morbidity in epilepsy.

Mood disorders

DEPRESSION

Depression is the most common psychiatric comorbidity in epilepsy. In cross-sectional studies of people with prevalent epilepsy, 10–24% have a moderate to severe number of symptoms of depression (Dominian et al., 1963; Jacoby et al., 1996; O'Donoghue et al., 1999; Beghi et al., 2002; Boylan et al., 2004; Cramer et al., 2004; Tellez-Zenteno et al., 2007). The prevalence of depressive symptoms has been shown to increase with increasing seizure frequency in two community surveys from the British general practice system (Jacoby et al., 1996; O'Donoghue et al., 1999). In these studies, a moderate to severe number of depressive symptoms occurred in 4–20% of patients in remission, 10–39% of those with less than one seizure per month, and 21–55% of those with one or more seizures per month. In a cross-sectional study of less severe epilepsy (Beghi et al., 2002),

*Correspondence to: Andres M. Kanner, M.D., Department of Neurological Sciences, Rush University Medical Center, 1653 West Congress Parkway, Chicago, IL 60612, USA. Tel: +1-312-942-2238, Fax: +1-312-942-2238, E-mail: akanner@rush.edu

in which 60% of patients had generalized seizures and 63% were without seizures for 12 months or more, depression in epilepsy was compared to depression in blood donors. This study found that patients with epilepsy were 11.3-fold more likely to have moderate to severe depression compared with blood donors, with no difference by seizure type. Thus, associations between prevalent epilepsy and depression are not necessarily confined to individuals with frequent seizures.

Several studies have shown that a history of major depression is associated with an increased risk of *developing* unprovoked seizures, suggesting a common underlying susceptibility that may be genetic. In the earliest population-based case–control study to examine this, Forsgren and Nystrom (1990) found that a history of "depression" was associated with an increased risk of developing epilepsy, particularly "localized onset" seizures. Since then, two further studies have demonstrated that a history of depression, diagnosed according to Diagnostic and Statistical Manual of Mental Disorders (DSM) criteria, increased the risk of developing unprovoked seizures (Hesdorffer et al., 2000, 2006). The first, conducted in older adults residing in Rochester, Minnesota (Hesdorffer et al., 2000), found that a history of major depression was significantly associated with a 6-fold increased risk of developing a first idiopathic/cryptogenic unprovoked seizure. A later Icelandic population-based case–control study (Hesdorffer et al., 2006) found that a history of major depression diagnosed according to DSM-IV criteria was associated with a 1.7-fold increased risk of developing epilepsy (95% confidence interval (CI) 1.1–2.7). Similar results were reported in a hospital-based prospective study (Nilsson et al., 2003), although generalizability was limited because fewer than half of the people who meet criteria for major depression seek medical care, and even fewer are hospitalized (Kessler et al., 1999; Olfson et al., 2005).

Bipolar disorder

Bipolar disorder may be associated with prevalent epilepsy and the development of new-onset epilepsy, but methodological issues and the rarity of bipolar disorder preclude conclusions. Symptoms of bipolar disorder occur in 12.2% of adults with prevalent epilepsy, 6.6-fold greater than in the general population ($p < 0.0001$) and 1.6–2.2-fold greater than in adults with migraine ($p = 0.006$), asthma ($p < 0.0001$), or diabetes ($p < 0.0001$) (Ettinger et al., 2005). The proportion with bipolar disorder may be an overestimation as Mula et al. (2008) found that, among 11.8% of adults with prevalent epilepsy who met DSM criteria for bipolar disorder, all but 1.4% had interictal dysphoric disorder, postictal mania or hypomania and preictal dysphoria. Studies examining whether bipolar disorder is associated with an increased risk of developing epilepsy are hampered by the relative rarity of both disorders, making it difficult to assemble large enough cohorts to find statistically significant results. Nonetheless, the two studies to date suggest an association. In a study of older adults, one patient met criteria for mania prior to the onset of epilepsy; no controls were affected (Hesdorffer et al., 2000). In a population-based study from Iceland, bipolar disorder was associated with a 5-fold increased risk of developing epilepsy, which was not statistically significant (Hesdorffer et al., 2006).

Anxiety

In studies of adults with prevalent epilepsy, anxiety and depression are the most common psychiatric disorders (Mendez et al., 1986; Jacoby et al., 1996; O'Donoghue et al., 1999; Rosemarie et al., 2006; Mensah et al., 2007; Tellez-Zenteno et al., 2007), occurring in 6.5–25%. Anxiety is more common in adults with poorly controlled seizures than in those who are seizure-free (Mendez et al., 1986; Jacoby et al., 1996; O'Donoghue et al., 1999; Mensah et al., 2007) and occurs just over 2-fold more often than in people without epilepsy (Rosemarie et al., 2006; Tellez-Zenteno et al., 2007).

Studies of anxiety in children with prevalent epilepsy have reported high rates of anxiety in childhood epilepsy, ranging from 13% to 48.5% of children with prevalent epilepsy (Ettinger et al., 1998; Alwash et al., 2000; Ott et al., 2001; Oguz et al., 2002; Williams et al., 2003; Caplan et al., 2005). When comparison groups are included, anxiety with depression is more common in children with epilepsy than in normal children (Oguz et al., 2002; Caplan et al., 2005).

Attention-deficit/hyperactivity disorder (ADHD)

Clinically, there has been a perception that ADHD is more common among children with epilepsy, due to the seizure disorder or its treatment (Lindsay et al., 1984). In studies of children with prevalent epilepsy, 28.1–39% had "hyperactivity–impulsivity" (Carlton-Ford et al., 1995; McDermott et al., 1996), 42.4% had problems with attention (Holdsworth and Whitmore, 1974), and 13.9% had ADHD (Williams et al., 1998). This is in excess of the 5% prevalence of ADHD in general population samples (Kaplan and Sadock, 1991; Carlton-Ford et al., 1995). Large surveys of the general population (Carlton-Ford et al., 1995; McDermott et al., 1996) confirm associations seen in smaller studies of prevalent epilepsy, showing that hyperactivity was 5.7-fold more prevalent among 121 children with epilepsy (28.1%), aged 5–17 years, compared with 3950 controls (4.9%) in the 1988 National Health Interview study (Carlton-Ford et al., 1995), and that "highly impulsive behavior" occurred among 39% of 118 children with a history of epilepsy compared with 11% of 11 042 children without a history of epilepsy (McDermott et al., 1996).

When time order is examined, ADHD is associated with increased risk of *developing* epilepsy. This has been shown in case–control studies of children with epilepsy (Dunn et al., 1997; Austin et al., 2001; Hesdorffer et al., 2004; Jones et al., 2007) and in cohort studies of select populations of children with ADHD (Williams et al., 1998; Hughes et al., 2000; Hemmer et al., 2001; Holtmann et al., 2003). In three clinically based case–control studies of children with incident unprovoked seizure, attention problems (Dunn et al., 1997; Austin et al., 2001) and ADHD (Jones et al., 2007) were more common *before* the onset of first seizure than among controls. A population-based case–control study in Iceland (Hesdorffer et al., 2004) confirmed this association, showing that children with incident unprovoked seizure were 2.5-fold (95% CI 1.1–5.5) more likely than age- and sex-matched controls to have a history of ADHD, meeting DSM-IV criteria *prior* to seizure onset. The association was restricted to ADHD – predominantly inattentive type (odds ratio (OR) 3.7, 95% CI 1.1–13). When the occurrence of new-onset seizures was examined in selected samples of patients with ADHD (Hughes et al., 2000; Williams, 2000; Hemmer et al., 2001; Holtmann et al., 2003), the percentage of children who developed unprovoked seizures (0.2–2%) was greater than the expected rate, because the average annual incidence of seizures is about 0.047 per year in children aged 5–16 years (Hauser et al., 1993).

Psychosis

Clinical observations early in the last century suggested an inverse relationship between epilepsy and schizophrenia. It was these observations that led to the institution of convulsive therapy, initially with camphor and later with electroconvulsive therapy (ECT), as a treatment for major psychosis. Interestingly epidemiological studies have largely refuted this contention, finding instead an increased prevalence of schizophrenia in adults with epilepsy and an increased risk of developing schizophrenia after the development of epilepsy. No studies have examined whether a history of schizophrenia is associated with an increased risk of developing epilepsy.

In studies of prevalent schizophrenia from the early 1900s, epilepsy was present in 0.13–3.5% of subjects (Urstein, 1909; Glauss, 1931). When prevalent epilepsy is examined, schizophrenia is present in 0.7–1.2% (Edeh and Toone, 1987; Jalava and Sillanpaa, 1996; Stefansson et al., 1998; Gaitatzis et al., 2004), affective psychosis in 0.7% (Jalava and Sillanpaa, 1996), and psychosis not otherwise specified in 0.6–9% (Edeh and Toone, 1987; Jalava and Sillanpaa, 1996; Stefansson et al., 1998; Gaitatzis et al., 2004). If epilepsy and schizophrenia were unrelated (i.e., independent), one would expect about 0.04% of the population to have both, based upon a cumulative incidence of epilepsy to age 70 years of 3% (Hauser et al., 1993) and of schizophrenia to age 72 years of 1.17–1.59% (Thorup et al., 2007). Thus, schizophrenia is 15-fold more common than expected in prevalent epilepsy, and vice versa.

Studies examining the time order of the relationship between epilepsy and schizophrenia are restricted to those examining whether new-onset epilepsy is associated with an increased risk of schizophrenia. In a case–control study of psychiatric illness in developing countries, epilepsy in children increased the risk of schizophrenia 2-fold (Ban et al., 1979), but febrile seizures were not associated with an increased risk. Similarly, a population-based Danish registry study (Qin et al., 2005) found that epilepsy was associated with a 2.5-fold increased risk of schizophrenia in the absence of a family history of psychosis – an important exclusion because family history could explain an increased risk of schizophrenia in epilepsy. In contrast to clinic-based studies of schizophrenia and epilepsy, the risk of developing schizophrenia did not differ by seizure type. However, the risk was dependent upon age at onset of epilepsy, with an increasing risk of schizophrenia observed with increasing age at onset ($p < 0.001$), suggesting that the median age at onset of schizophrenia after epilepsy is greater than the onset of 22 years reported in the general population (Thorup et al., 2007). The risk of developing schizophrenia is also increased in the presence of febrile seizures, but only when febrile seizures are followed by the development of epilepsy (Vestergaard et al., 2005) (relative risk (RR) 1.4 for schizophrenia after febrile seizures only; RR 3.04 for schizophrenia after febrile seizures plus epilepsy). Febrile seizure type was unknown in this study, but it is possible that the association was due to hippocampal damage associated with prolonged febrile seizure.

Conclusion

Psychiatric disorders are more common than expected in prevalent epilepsy. Mood disorders and ADHD are associated with an increased risk of developing epilepsy. Epilepsy is associated with an increased risk of developing schizophrenia. However, it is unknown whether a bidirectional relationship exists between epilepsy and these disorders, and further studies are needed to address this question.

PSYCHIATRIC COMORBIDITY AS AN EXPRESSION OF EPILEPSY-RELATED ACTIVITY

Peri-ictal psychiatric disturbances in epilepsy may precede (preictal), follow (postictal), or be concurrent with (ictal) epileptic activity. Some epilepsy-related psychiatric phenomena occur as paraictal disorders, epileptic disorders associated with significant cognitive and psychiatric disturbances at the onset of the seizure disorder that remit or improve markedly following clinical or electrographic seizure freedom.

Peri-ictal psychiatric disturbances may present as isolated symptoms of depression, anxiety, psychosis, behavioral problems, or clusters of symptoms of one or more of these psychiatric conditions. Often, they may mimic full-blown depressive, anxiety, or psychotic episodes. Recognized for more than 100 years, their clinical manifestations, course, and response to treatment are still not well characterized. With the exception of ictal disturbances, pathogenic mechanisms operant remain poorly understood.

Preictal disturbances

Preictal psychiatric symptoms can herald a seizure and most involve changes in mood with symptoms of anxiety and irritability, short attention span, and impulsive behavior (Blanchet and Frommer, 1986). In the Blanchet and Frommer (1986) study, changes in dysphoric symptoms were rated daily over 56 days in 27 patients with epilepsy and were associated with seizures in the next 3 days in 81.5%.

Postictal disturbances

The prevalence of postictal psychiatric episodes in the general population of prevalent epilepsy is unknown. In selected samples with partial epilepsy, the yearly incidence of postictal episodes, mostly postictal psychotic episodes (PIPE) during video-encephalography (V-EEG) is 7.9% (Kanner et al., 1996).

Postictal psychiatric symptoms

The prevalence and clustering of postictal psychiatric symptoms has been ascertained in 100 patients with pharmacoresistant partial epilepsy (Kanner et al., 2004). A median of five *postictal psychiatric* symptoms (PPS) were identified and 74 patients experienced at least one type of PPS. These included anxiety, depression, and neurovegetative symptoms, which overlapped in 81% of patients with other psychiatric symptoms. Most symptoms lasted for 24 hours or more. More than half of the patients with epilepsy and PPS had a history of mood disorders and a quarter had a history of anxiety, suggesting a predisposition to PPS. Though none acted on their symptoms, 13 patients reported habitual *postictal suicidal ideation*; eight experienced passive and active suicidal thoughts, whereas five reported only passive suicidal ideation. A history of major depression or bipolar disorder occurred in three-quarters of patients with postictal suicidal ideation and was significantly associated with previous psychiatric hospitalization.

Postictal anxiety occurred in 60.8% of patients with PPS, with most having one or more symptoms lasting for more than 24 hours. Again, prior history of anxiety disorder occurred in one-third of patients. Far rarer were postictal psychotic symptoms, occurring in 9.5% of patients with PPS. Most lasted for more than 24 hours and included referential thinking (people are staring and talking about me), auditory hallucinations, paranoid delusions, religious delusions, and visual hallucinations. Comorbidity with postictal anxiety and depression were common. A history of anxiety disorder was associated with a greater number of postictal psychotic symptoms.

Postictal hypomanic symptoms, including excessive energy and racing thoughts, occurred in 29.7% of patients with PPS. There was no significant association between a psychiatric history and the development of hypomanic symptoms.

Postictal psychotic episodes (PIPE)

Case series of PIPE reveal the following clinical characteristics: (1) a 12–120-hour delay between the onset of psychiatric symptoms and the last seizure; (2) relatively short duration; (3) affect-laden psychotic symptomatology, often with a religious delusional content; (4) high frequency of secondarily generalized tonic–clonic seizures preceding PIPE; (5) onset of PIPE in a seizure disorder lasting for more than 10 years.

Unusual presentations of postictal psychotic episodes include cases of Capgras syndrome (Drake, 1987) and a case mimicking Kluver–Bucey syndrome reported in a patient with persistent seizures following a left temporal lobectomy (Anson and Kuhlman, 1993). In children, PIPE have been reported *only* following status epilepticus (SE) in which EEG recordings obtained during the psychotic episode documented the remission of seizure activity (Nissenkorn et al., 1999).

Bilateral ictal foci (Umbricht et al., 1995; Kanner and Ostrovskaya, 2008) and secondarily generalized tonic–clonic seizures (Devinsky et al., 1995; Umbricht et al., 1995; Kanner et al., 1996; Logsdail and Toone, 1988; Kanner and Ostrovskaya, 2008) are associated with PIPE, and 89% of patients with PIPE have bilateral ictal foci (Kanner and Ostrovskaya, 2008). A history of diffuse central nervous system (CNS) insults (e.g., encephalitis), poorly localized ictal onset on V-EEG, and family psychiatric history are risk factors for PIPE (Alper et al., 2001, 2007). Dysplasias in temporal lobe structures are associated with a higher risk of PIPE (Briellmann et al., 2000). PIPE have also been associated with an increased risk of postsurgical mood disorders in the first 2 years after surgery (Kanemoto et al., 2001).

In a small proportion of individuals, PIPE develop into interictal psychotic episodes (Tarulli et al., 2001; Kanner and Ostrovskaya, 2008). Among patients with both interictal psychosis and PIPE, some evolve from PIPE to interictal psychosis, whereas a smaller group evolves from interictal psychosis to PIPE (Adachi et al., 2003).

Ictal psychiatric disturbances

Ictal psychiatric phenomena occur when psychiatric symptoms are the manifestations of the actual seizure activity. The most frequent is ictal fear or panic followed by mood symptoms (Daly, 1958). In contrast, ictal psychotic episodes arise mostly with nonconvulsive SE (Kaplan, 2002).

Ictal fear is frequently misdiagnosed and treated as panic disorder, and the correct diagnosis is reached only after the patient has suffered from a generalized tonic–clonic seizure. Around 60% of auras presenting with "psychiatric" symptoms are ictal panic. A careful history can help distinguish an interictal panic disorder from ictal panic, which has the following characteristics: (1) duration <30 seconds; (2) stereotypical clinical semiology; (3) fear out of context to concurrent events; (4) panic associated with other ictal phenomena such as periods of confusion of variable duration and subtle or overt automatisms; (5) mild to moderate fear that rarely reaches the intensity of a panic attack.

Similar to other ictal psychiatric phenomenon, ictal panic is often associated with interictal panic disorder and anxiety disorder with a higher frequency than in controls (Mintzer and Lopez, 2002). Ictal panic has also been associated with a higher risk of developing postsurgical mood and anxiety disorders following a temporal lobectomy (Kohler et al., 2001).

As stated above, ictal psychotic episodes can be the clinical expression of nonconvulsive SE. In simple partial status, ictal psychosis can manifest as delusions and hallucinations (e.g., visual and, less frequently, auditory), which are usually brief and stereotyped, although the diagnosis is often difficult to document on EEG because scalp recordings may not detect ictal patterns. Unlike hallucinations occurring in psychosis, patients realize that their hallucinations reflect unreal phenomena.

Absence SE can present with bizarre behaviors that patients may be unaware of and are thus usually reported by relatives or friends. A case report (Olnes et al., 2003) described such behavior in a man whose EEG showed generalized spikes, polyspikes, and slow waves consistent with atypical absence SE. A case report of ictal catatonia as an expression of nonconvulsive status was reported (Kanemoto et al., 1999) in a man with no focal neurological signs, and no history of either epilepsy or psychiatric illness, and where the EEG showed continuous generalized spike and wave discharges (1.5–2 Hz) consistent with atypical absence SE. Thus, EEG should be considered in patients with ictal catatonia, particularly those occurring *de novo* in elderly persons.

Paraictal psychiatric disorders

Epileptic encephalopathies and the phenomenon of forced normalization illustrate the paraictal psychiatric disorders. Acquired epileptic aphasia of childhood (also known as Landau–Kleffner syndrome; LKS) is an epileptic encephalopathy that exemplifies the paraictal psychiatric disorders. This acquired epileptic aphasia or verbal auditory agnosia occurs in children who previously developed age-appropriate language function. It is thought to result from an epileptogenic lesion arising in the speech cortex during a critical period of development (Landau and Kleffner, 1957). LKS has a clearly defined set of clinical and electrographic characteristics that begin between 2 and 8 years of age. These include a receptive speech disturbance or verbal auditory agnosia, soon followed by disturbances of expressive speech, which can evolve to a state of complete mutism. Speech and behavioral disturbances are very often associated and include motor hyperactivity in up to 50% of children, impulsive and aggressive behavior, and sleep disturbances. At the height of the auditory agnosia, some autistic-like features, such as self-stimulatory behavior, may be identified. Electrographic epileptiform activity presents characteristically as spike–wave discharges with a bilateral distribution, maximal in the posterior temporal regions of each hemisphere; in 20–30% these occur without clinical seizures. This EEG pattern may occupy more than 80% of slow-wave sleep, and is known as continuous spikes and waves during slow-wave sleep (CSWS).

Children show relatively normal performance on nonverbal cognitive tasks. Often spontaneous remission of language and behavioral disturbances occur weeks or months after onset, which may explain the underrecognition of this condition. However, when symptoms persist unchanged for more than 1 year, spontaneous recovery is rare and a severe lifelong linguistic handicap is the common result.

In some of these children, however, eradication of epileptic activity fails to exert any impact on language deficits or behavioral problems, a puzzling phenomenon. In a series of 14 patients with LKS who underwent multiple subpial transection (MST) of the epileptogenic zone in the perisylvian and intrasylvian cortex, all children were mute and had lost any functional language without evidence of any recovery for more than 2 years (Morrell et al., 1995). Seven children recovered significant language functions during a mean follow-up period of 44 months, and 9 with clinical seizures became seizure-free. Findings in a second series of children supported a significant improvement of language functions after surgery (Irwin et al., 2001).

Forced normalization presents with mood and psychotic disorders in association with the cessation of epileptic seizures (Landolt, 1955; Ried and Mothersill, 1998), and has been reported in patients with temporal lobe epilepsy (TLE) and generalized epilepsies (Wolf and Trimble, 1985; Schmitz and Wolf, 1995). The terms "alternative psychosis" or "alternative depressive episodes" have also been suggested to illustrate the temporal relation of the onset of psychiatric symptomatology with the remission of seizure activity. The prevalence of alternative psychosis is about 1% of patients with epilepsy attending a tertiary care facility (Schmitz and Wolf, 1995). Both Landolt (1953) and Wolf and Trimble (1985) reported a pleomorphic clinical presentation with a paranoid psychosis without clouding of consciousness as the most frequent manifestation. Forced normalization has been associated with different antiepileptic drugs (AEDs) (phenytoin, ethosuximide, levetiracetam, vigabatrin). Whether this reflects an adverse event of the AED or results of seizure suppression is often difficult to establish.

The treatment of alternative psychotic episodes involves the reduction and/or discontinuation of the AED until overt seizure recurrence causes remission of the psychotic symptoms (Ried and Mothersill, 1998). The rapidity with which AED should be tapered is unclear. Tellenbach (1965) suggested a rapid tapering under EEG monitoring, whereas Landolt (1953) advocated the use of ECT or metrazol if necessary. Following seizure recurrence and remission of psychotic symptoms, AEDs should be reintroduced slowly (Tellenbach, 1965).

WHY ARE PSYCHIATRIC DISORDERS SO PREVALENT IN EPILEPSY?

Common pathogenic mechanisms may explain the comorbidity of epilepsy and psychiatric disorders and, when available, information on the time order of these relationships may further elucidate mechanisms.

Depression

Evidence from animal models and human studies suggests common underlying pathogenic mechanisms that may explain the comorbidity of depression and epilepsy. For example, decreased concentrations of 5-hydroxytryptamine (5HT; serotonin) in the synaptic cleft play an epileptogenic role in both animal and human studies of epilepsy (Kilian and Frey, 1973; Andrade and Nicoll, 1987; Ben-Menachem et al., 1992; Okuhara and Beck, 1994; Statnick et al., 1996; Applegate and Tecott, 1998; Okada et al., 1998; Watanabe et al., 1998; Graumlich et al., 1999; Shiah and Yatham, 2000; Murakami et al., 2001; Hernandez et al., 2002; Jakus et al., 2003; Arbatova et al., 2005), and are also associated with major depression (Delgado et al., 1994, 1999; Owens and Nemeroff, 1994; Owens et al., 1997; Placidi et al., 2001; Bhagwagar et al., 2002; Booij et al., 2002; Golden et al., 2002; Moreno et al., 2000, 2002). Positron emission tomography (PET) studies (discussed below) in major depression and epilepsy suggest dysfunction of $5HT_{1A}$ receptors.

Experimental models

Serotonin receptors are found presynaptically in the raphe nuclei, inhibiting release of 5HT into the synaptic cleft (Sotelo et al., 1990; Riad et al., 2000), and postsynaptically where they mediate effects of 5HT (Mengod et al., 1990; Jacobs and Azmitia, 1992; Aznar et al., 2003). The antiepileptic effect of $5HT_{1A}$ receptors is associated with a membrane-hyperpolarizing response linked to increased potassium conductance in hippocampal kindled seizures in cats, and in intrahippocampal kainic acid-induced seizures in freely moving rats (Beck and Choi, 1991; Jobe and Weber, 2005). In genetically epilepsy-prone rats (GEPR), the anticonvulsant effect of the selective serotonin reuptake inhibitor (SSRI) fluoxetine (Dailey et al., 1992; Watanabe et al., 1998; Hernandez et al., 2002) is enhanced through administration of $5HT_{1A}$ antagonists (Browning et al., 1997b) by enhancing the increase in extracellular 5HT produced by the SSRI. In rats, depletion of 5HT decreases seizure threshold (Kilian and Frey, 1973; Statnick et al., 1996; Trindade-Filho et al., 2008) through $5HT_{1A}$ activation (Salgado-Commissariat and Alkadhi, 1997; Lu and Gean, 1998), and administration of tryptophan, the 5HT precursor, increases seizure threshold (Kilian and Frey, 1973). As illustrated in a microdialysis study, the anticonvulsant effect has an inverted U-shaped response (Clinckers et al., 2005).

Norepinephrine (NE)

The anticonvulsant effect of NE (noradrenaline) has also been demonstrated in the GEPR animal model, as increase of this neurotransmitter in the CNS was associated with blocking of seizures whereas the administration of drugs that deplete the brain of NE resulted in worsening seizures (Jobe and Weber, 2005). The effect of vagus nerve stimulation on the locus coeruleus and raphe may be responsible for its antidepressant effects in humans (Browning et al., 1997a).

Dopamine (DA)

In the study by Clinckers et al. (2005), cited above, DA perfusions in rats were protective for limbic seizures when extracellular DA concentrations were increased by 70–400% from baseline levels. Coperfusion with the selective D_2 blocker remoxipride abolished all anticonvulsant effects. Simultaneous D_2-receptor blockade significantly aggravated pilocarpine-induced seizures at high extracellular DA concentrations (> 1000% increase relative to baseline).

Glutamate and hyperactive hypothalamic–pituitary–adrenal (HPA) axis

Hyperactive HPA axis has been identified in major depressive disorders, in TLE, and in animal models of epilepsy (Mazarati et al., 2009); high serum cortisol concentrations result from an overactive HPA axis. In studies of rats and monkeys, dendrites of pyramidal neurons in the CA3 region retract as a reaction to stress; if the stressful event is long-lasting, the changes become irreversible through a reduction of dendritic branching and loss of dendritic spines that are included in glutamatergic synaptic inputs. Stress-induced secretion of glutamate in the hippocampus has been suggested as a potential mechanism of neuronal damage (Sapolsky et al., 1990) whereby chronic exposure to high glucocorticoid concentrations results in energy depletion by blocking glucose uptake in the neuron, making it more vulnerable to excitotoxicity, such as that mediated by glutamate, which is released in excess. Furthermore, glucocorticoids increase the concentration of extracellular glutamate by preventing its reuptake into glial cells, which in turn allows a prolonged binding to *N*-methyl-D-aspartate (NMDA) receptors. Glutamate accumulation in turn yields high intracellular concentrations of calcium, further increasing the vulnerability of these cells (Sapolsky et al., 1990). This effect can be mitigated by NMDA antagonists. Interestingly, $5HT_{1A}$ agonists decrease glutamate release, but chronic exposure to glucocorticoids also decreases $5HT_{1A}$ receptor expression.

High cortisol serum levels resulting from chronic stress also have been found to interfere with the development of new granule cell neurons in the adult hippocampal dentate gyrus. This effect is thought to be mediated by a decrease in the secretion of brain-derived neurotrophic factor (BDNF) in the dentate gyrus, pyramidal cell layer of the hippocampus, amygdala, and neocortex (Smith et al., 1995). These changes can be overturned with chronic (but not acute) antidepressant therapy, because chronic administration of antidepressant drugs increases BDNF expression and prevents a stress-induced decrease in BDNF levels (Nibuya et al., 1995). There is also evidence that antidepressant drugs can increase hippocampal BDNF levels in humans (Chen et al., 2001). These data indicate that antidepressant-induced upregulation of BDNF can hypothetically repair damage to hippocampal neurons and protect vulnerable neurons from additional damage. Nonetheless, other studies have suggested that BDNF increases cell survival by inhibition of cell cascades associated with apoptosis. These data may explain the bilateral hippocampal atrophy identified in major depressive disorders in humans (Sheline, 2005).

The role of excitatory neurotransmitters and in particular the glutamate receptors, NMDA and α-amino-3-hydroxy-5-methyl-4-isoxazolepropionic acid (AMPA), has been well established in epilepsy. Likewise, NMDA antagonists have been shown to have antiepileptogenic properties in the "kindling" animal model and to display antiepileptic properties. Yet, recent data suggest their potential pathogenic role in depression as well. First, disturbances in glutamate metabolism, NMDA, and metabotropic glutamate receptor (mGluR) 1 and 5 have been implicated in depression and suicidality (Tatarczynska et al., 2001). Second, the NMDA receptor antagonists, group I mGluR (mGluR1 and mGluR5) antagonists, and positive modulators of AMPA receptors have been found to display antidepressant-like activity in a variety of preclinical models (Tatarczynska et al., 2002). Third, a single intravenous dose of an NMDA receptor antagonist has been found to be sufficient to produce sustained relief from depressive symptoms (Berman et al., 2000).

Evidence for serotonergic disturbances in humans with mood disorders and epilepsy

Studies using PET consistently demonstrate decreased 5HT receptor binding in the frontal, temporal, and limbic cortex of patients with primary depressive disorders without epilepsy (Drevets et al., 1999), in mesial temporal frontal lobe and brainstem structures in TLE (Toczek et al., 2003; Merlet et al., 2004; Savic et al., 2004; Theodore et al., 2006; Hasler et al., 2007), and in the dorsolateral prefrontal cortex, raphe nuclei, and hippocampus in juvenile myoclonic epilepsy (Meschaks et al., 2005). In TLE, reduced $5HT_{1A}$ binding is found in mesial temporal structures ipsilateral to the seizure focus (whether hippocampal atrophy was present or not), amygdala, anterior cingulate, lateral temporal neocortex ipsilateral to the seizure focus, the contralateral hippocampi, the raphe, and the ipsilateral thalamic region.

Patients with TLE and major depressive disorder show decreased $5HT_{1A}$ receptor binding in the epileptic focus and significantly more pronounced reduction in binding, extending into nonlesional limbic brain areas outside the epileptic focus compared with those with TLE and no depression (Theodore et al., 2006). An inverse correlation between increased number of symptoms of depression and $5HT_{1A}$ receptor binding at the ipsilateral hippocampus has also been observed in TLE (Hasler et al., 2007). Similar findings are found using ^{1}H magnetic resonance spectroscopy (^{1}H-MRS) (Gilliam et al., 2007).

Decreased binding potential of the $5HT_{1A}$ receptor is observed in juvenile myoclonic epilepsy in the dorsolateral prefrontal cortex, raphe nuclei, and hippocampus compared with controls (Meschaks et al., 2005). Interestingly, this epilepsy syndrome is comorbid with depression and anxiety (de Araujo Filho et al., 2006).

The anticonvulsant effect of SSRIs observed in animal models of epilepsy has also been suggested in several open trials of patients with pharmacoresistant epilepsy. For example, citalopram was found to decrease median seizure frequency by 55.6% in nondepressed patients with poorly controlled epilepsy (Favale et al., 2003). Furthermore, the tricyclic antidepressant imipramine, with reuptake inhibitory effects of NE and 5HT, was reported to suppress absence and myoclonic seizures in double-blind placebo-controlled studies (Fromm et al., 1972, 1978).

Together, these studies suggest that 5HT may have antiepileptic properties, an effect possibly mediated by $5HT_{1A}$ autoreceptors in the raphe nuclei. This impression is supported by a recent cohort study, examining seizures as adverse events in Food and Drug Administration (FDA) randomized clinical trials of SSRIs and serotonin–norepinephrine reuptake inhibitors (SNRIs) for the treatment of major depression (Alper et al., 2007). In this study, there was a 19-fold increased risk of seizures in the placebo group with major depression compared with the expected rate in the general population. However, compared with the placebo group, the group treated with antidepressants was significantly *protected* from the development of seizures.

Dopamine

Data are sparser concerning the role of DA in the comorbidity of epilepsy and depression. In major depression, the therapeutic effect of antidepressant drugs that are NE and DA reuptake inhibitors operate through increases in synaptic DA. In addition, abnormal dopaminergic function has been demonstrated in the brain of patients with primary major depressive disorders (Tremblay et al., 2005) with functional magnetic resonance imaging (MRI) blood oxygen level-dependent (BOLD) activation during a controlled task and measurement of dexamfetamine subjective effects in which patients with major depression had a 2-fold increased response to the rewarding effects of dexamfetamine in the ventrolateral prefrontal cortex, orbitofrontal cortex, caudate, and putamen compared with controls. Abnormal DA activity was also found in the brain of patients with refractory epilepsy in a PET study using [^{18}F] fluoro-DOPA in which three groups of patients were included (Bouilleret et al., 2005); one consisted of 16 patients with a ring chromosome 20 (r20); a second group included 10 patients with absence-like epilepsy, and the third included 9 patients with intractable TLE. Compared with patients with TLE, absence-like epilepsy and ring chromosome 20 each displayed a decrease of [^{18}F]fluoro-DOPA uptake, which in TLE was lateralized to the side of the seizure focus.

Structural abnormalities

Findings of studies using high-resolution MRI and volumetrics suggest that abnormalities of several neuroanatomical structures, including atrophy of the mesial temporal lobe and frontal lobe, may play a pathogenic role in epilepsy and mood and anxiety disorders, a factor that may link these disorders together. In primary major depression, the literature suggests atrophy in temporal and frontal lobe structures. Nine of 12 studies demonstrated atrophy of the hippocampi, entorhinal cortex, and amygdala, and 10 of 11 studies found atrophy of prefrontal, mesial–frontal, or orbitofrontal structures (Sheline, 2005). A significant inverse correlation was observed between duration of depression and left hippocampal volume, suggesting that patients with chronic depression were more likely to have hippocampal atrophy (Sheline, 2005).

Anxiety

Neurotransmitter abnormalities

Abnormalities in several neurotransmitters and neuropeptides are found in anxiety disorders, including γ-aminobutyric acid (GABA), NE, 5HT, and some of the hormones and neuropeptides involved in the HPA axis and with corticotropin-releasing hormone. These neurotransmitters also play a significant pathogenic role in mood disorders and epilepsy, perhaps explaining their comorbidity.

γ-Aminobutyric acid (GABA)

The neurotransmitter GABA, which promotes inhibition of neuronal excitability by its effect upon chloride ion channels, has a well-known importance in epilepsy. Several AEDs (e.g., benzodiazepines, barbiturates, and tiagabine) have anxiolytic properties through potentiation and prolongation of GABA's synaptic inhibitory actions (Stahl, 2004). The convulsant pentylenetetrazol (PTZ; a model for generalized seizures) blocks $GABA_A$ receptor function and also promotes anxiety symptoms (Jung et al., 2002). In animal models of anxiety, anxiolytic effects of valproic acid may be mediated through GABAergic processes as they are reversed by the use of $GABA_A$ receptor antagonists (Baetz and Bowen, 1998; Stahl, 2004). Anxiety disorders may result from defective neuroinhibitory processes, mediated partly through GABA (Malizia et al., 1998), whereas abnormalities in benzodiazepine receptors may play a pathogenic role in epilepsy (Chang and Lowenstein, 2003). Abnormalities in the benzodiazepine receptor system may underlie anxiety disorders, as suggested by the induction of panic symptoms in patients with panic disorder when the benzodiazepine antagonist flumazenil is administered, and by the demonstration of widespread decreased binding of flumazenil to benzodiazepine receptor in such patients (Nutt et al., 1990).

Noradrenergic abnormalities in anxiety

Fear activates neurons of the locus coeruleus, increasing NE secretion in the locus coeruleus, in limbic structures such as the amygdala, hippocampus, and hypothalamus, and in the cerebral cortex. With sustained stress in the learned helplessness animal model, NE is depleted (Harris, 1989). The NE reuptake inhibitor, reboxetine, treats panic disorders effectively (Versiani et al., 2002). Panic attacks, insomnia, startle, and autonomic hyperarousal can be alleviated by decreasing the firing of neurons in the locus coeruleus with agents such as benzodiazepines, alcohol, and opiates, whereas drugs that increase neuronal firing in the locus coeruleus (i.e., cocaine) worsen these symptoms (Davis, 1999).

Serotonergic abnormalities

The suggested role of serotonin in anxiety disorders is supported by the potent anxiolytic effects of tricyclic antidepressants (TCAs) and SSRIs (Rickels et al., 1993; Tollefson and Rosenbaum, 1998), enhancers of 5HT synaptic concentrations, which may act via inhibition of noradrenergic activation through raphe nuclei projections to the locus coeruleus, periaqueductal gray inhibition of the freeze/flight responses, hypothalamic inhibition of corticotropin-releasing hormone (CRH), and the amygdala inhibiting excitatory pathways from cortex and thalamus.

Attention-deficit/hyperactivity disorder (ADHD)

Elucidation of pathogenic mechanisms operant in epilepsy and ADHD is more problematic than in mood and anxiety disorders. Children with hyperkinetic syndromes require significantly lower doses of metrazol to elicit paroxysmal responses on EEG recordings (photometrazol threshold) than controls (Denhoff et al., 1957; Laufer and Denhoff, 1957); however, pretreatment with CNS stimulant amfetamines or D-amfetamines raised the photometrazol threshold to that of controls. DA and NE play a significant pathogenic role in ADHD and, as shown above, in epilepsy.

Genetic contributions to ADHD include the dopamine D4 receptor gene (*DRD4*), the dopamine D5 receptor gene (*DRD5*), the dopamine transporter gene (*DAT*), the dopamine β-hydroxylase gene (*DBH*), the serotonin transporter gene (*5HTT*), the serotonin receptor 1B gene (*HTR1B*), and the synaptosomal-associated protein 25 gene (*SNAP25*). DRD4 is expressed predominantly in the frontal cortex, which receives dense input from midbrain DA neurons and is associated with cognitive and emotional processes. In cortical pyramidal neurons from wild-type and DRD4-deficient mice, an increased frequency of spontaneous synaptic activity and increased frequency and duration of paroxysmal discharges is induced by epileptogenic agents, suggesting that DRD4 functions as inhibitory modulator of glutamate activity in the frontal cortex (Rubinstein et al., 2001).

Imaging studies in children with ADHD with and without epilepsy have revealed morphometric differences from controls but in different directions. Studies examining time order of the comorbidity of epilepsy and ADHD have revealed two possibly interrelated features of children with both disorders. Quantitative MRI demonstrates that ADHD in epilepsy is associated with significantly increased gray matter in regions of the frontal lobe and significantly smaller brainstem volume (Hermann et al., 2007). The earlier onset of ADHD in children with epilepsy than in controls (Hesdorffer et al., 2004) may be due to these anatomical findings. Yet in ADHD without epilepsy, imaging studies find delays in attaining normal cortical thickness throughout most of the cerebrum, particularly pronounced in prefrontal regions (Shaw et al., 2007a). The *DRD4* 7-repeat allele is associated with a thinner right orbitofrontal/inferior prefrontal and posterior parietal cortex in these children and a better clinical outcome in adolescence and a distinct trajectory of cortical development

(Shaw et al., 2007b). Explanations for these differences await further research.

Psychosis

Febrile seizures, particularly prolonged febrile seizures, may play a role in the comorbidity of epilepsy and psychosis. The risk of developing schizophrenia after febrile seizures is increased 3-fold when epilepsy is also present (Vestergaard et al., 2005); however, febrile seizure type was unknown in this study. Children with prolonged febrile seizures have the greatest risk of developing later epilepsy (Annegers et al., 1979), and imaging studies have found hippocampal pathology on MRI performed shortly after prolonged febrile seizure with subsequent volume asymmetry (VanLandingham et al., 1998; Lewis et al., 2002; Scott et al., 2002, 2003, 2006). Animal studies have shown that injury is specific to prolonged febrile seizures as it is not seen in other models of prolonged seizure in the immature brain (Dube et al., 2007). These findings are particularly interesting in the light of clinical studies of epilepsy and psychosis, in which psychosis is more common after prolonged febrile seizure (Kanemoto et al., 2001), and in TLE compared with other epilepsy types (Bartlet, 1957; Maier et al., 2000; Trimble et al., 2000; Kanemoto et al., 2001), coupled with findings of temporal lobe abnormalities in the schizophrenia literature (Seidman et al., 2003). Epidemiological data are inconsistent with these clinical data, perhaps because information on seizure type has been drawn from International Classification of Diseases (ICD) codes (Qin et al., 2005).

Role of psychosocial variables

Allostatic load is defined as the cumulative wear and tear on the body due to adapting to adverse physical or psychosocial situations (McEwen, 2000) or due to "weathering" repeated marginalization (Geronimus et al., 2006). The psychosocial impact of having epilepsy may lead to depression in vulnerable individuals (Baker et al., 2005), perhaps through allostatic load. These stressors include stigma (Hermann et al., 1990; Livneh et al., 2001), employability, and the ability to hold a driver's license. The degree to which such stressors may adversely impact a person with epilepsy and lead to depression seems to be determined by coping strategies, which mediate how life stressors are perceived. Different coping strategies have been shown to reduce or amplify perceived stress that may result from the inherent unpredictability of seizure occurrence, stigma, and the functional consequences of having epilepsy (Livneh et al., 2001; Goldstein et al., 2005). Perceived stress has been shown to increase with avoidant coping strategies and to decrease with problem-focused coping (Hermann et al., 1990), which is associated with resilience in the face of stress (Southwick et al., 2005). Similarly in the general population, mastery is inversely associated with depression (Spijker et al., 2007) and does not appear to be influenced by subthreshold depression. From an evolutionary standpoint, coping strategies reflect underlying traits (Koolhaas et al., 2007), but the extent to which coping strategies observed in people with epilepsy are stable traits over time is unknown.

Iatrogenic causes are common causes of psychiatric disturbances in epilepsy due to pharmacological and surgical therapies.

Pharmacological iatrogenic causes can result from the addition of AEDs with negative psychotropic properties or the discontinuation of AEDs with positive psychotropic properties. Most AEDs are associated with iatrogenic psychiatric disturbances of all types, particularly at toxic doses. GABAergic AEDs (e.g., barbiturates, tiagabine, vigabatrin, and occasionally benzodiazepines) facilitate the development of mood, anxiety, and behavioral disturbances, the latter mimicking ADHD. Levetiracetam, topiramate, and zonisamide, new generation AEDs, can cause depressive episodes and behavioral disturbances. For all of these iatrogenic psychiatric disturbances in response to AEDs, a prior psychiatric history or a family psychiatric history are risk factors. Of note, psychiatric adverse events associated with levetiracetam and topiramate can be prevented with concomitant lamotrigine.

Iatrogenic psychotic symptoms and episodes are reported with most AEDs including the first-generation AEDs, ethosuximide, phenytoin, phenobarbital, and primidone, as well as AEDs such as vigabatrin, topiramate, levetiracetam, and zonisamide. Clinical differentiation between alternative psychoses and a toxic reaction can be difficult if a seizure-free state followed the introduction of the AED. A toxic reaction should be considered in the presence of other toxic symptoms (e.g., ataxia, tremor) or absence of a seizure-free state.

Discontinuation of AEDs with mood-stabilizing properties can in some cases result in psychosis, and acute benzodiazepine withdrawal is well known to result in an acute psychotic episode (Ketter et al., 1994).

Postsurgical psychiatric complications

Epilepsy surgery, particularly anterotemporal lobectomy (ATL), is associated with remission of presurgical psychiatric comorbidity in about 50% of patients (Devinsky et al., 2005). Yet, postsurgical psychiatric complications presenting as depressive and anxiety disorders can occur in up to 30% of patients (Kanner and Balabanov, 2008), whereas *de novo* psychotic disorders have been reported in 3–10% of patients (Trimble, 1992) and *de novo* mood and anxiety disorders in up to 15% of patients (Kanner and Balabanov, 2008). Postsurgical psychiatric complications can present as exacerbations of presurgical conditions, particularly mood and anxiety disorders, and may require a restart or dose adjustment of psychotropic medications.

Mood lability and anxiety can be identified in the first 6 weeks after surgery, and remit by the end of the first year. Although up to 15% of patients may experience persistence of depressive disorders that fail to remit with a variety of pharmacological and other therapies, most patients with exacerbations of presurgical mood and anxiety disorders respond to pharmacotherapy with SSRIs or SNRIs. Awareness of a surgical candidate's lifetime psychiatric history, ictal fear, and PIPE is crucial as these are the patients most likely to experience postsurgical psychiatric symptomatology.

De novo postsurgical psychotic episodes can mimic schizophreniform disorders, manic episodes, or present as PIPE, and occur in 3.8–35.7% of patients with a mean occurrence of 7.6% (Taylor, 1972; Jensen and Vaernet, 1977; Stevens, 1990; Trimble, 1992; Leinonen et al., 1994; Shaw et al., 2004). In some cases, forced normalization was a possibility (Trimble, 1992). Postsurgical psychotic episodes have been associated with a right temporal seizure focus (Mace and Trimble, 1991), whereas others have associated the presence of gangliogliomas or dysembryoplastic neuroepithelial tumors (DNETs) with the development of *de novo* postsurgical psychotic disorders (Andermann et al., 1999). Larger studies are needed to explore these associations further.

CLINICAL MANIFESTATIONS OF COMMON INTERICTAL PSYCHIATRIC DISORDERS: ARE THEY UNIQUE TO EPILEPSY?

Major depression is the most commonly studied psychiatric disorder in relation to neurological disorders other than epilepsy. A bidirectional relationship between major depression and neurological disorders has been established for stroke (Jonas and Mussolino, 2000; Ohira et al., 2001; Bremmer et al., 2006; Ramasubbu et al., 2006; Salaycik et al., 2007), perhaps associated with the short arm of the serotonin transporter-linked promoter region (Ramasubbu et al., 2006), Alzheimer's disease (Ownby et al., 2006), migraine (Breslau et al., 1991, 2000), and traumatic brain injury (Fann et al., 2004). The prevalence of depression is increased in multiple sclerosis (Patten et al., 2003), but time order is not established. The prevalence of several psychiatric disorders is increased in Tourette syndrome (Robertson, 2000), including depression, anxiety, and ADHD, each of which is associated with epilepsy.

The consistency and strength of the association between prior depression and subsequent neurological diseases of the brain, including epilepsy, are compelling. It is difficult to attribute this association to a prodrome of the neurological disorder, particularly for epilepsy, because the association between depression and neurological disease remains, even when limited to depression occurring many years prior to the neurological diagnosis. Collectively, studies suggest that alterations in neurotransmitter function associated with depression or other psychiatric disorders may increase susceptibility to neurological diseases.

The clinical manifestations of the major psychiatric disorders in epilepsy can be identical to those in the absence of epilepsy. Yet, in a subset of epilepsy with mood disorders, the clinical manifestations must be classified as Depressive disorder not otherwise specified, or Atypical depression, according to DSM-III-R criteria. Kraepelin and Bleuler were the first to recognize this "unique" clinical presentation of mood disorders in patients with epilepsy consisting of recurrent episodes of "dysphoric symptoms" (Kraepelin, 1923; Bleuler, 1949); Gastaut expanded on Kraepelin's initial observations (Gastaut et al., 1953, 1955), and Blumer coined the term of interictal dysphoric disorder (Blumer and Altshuler, 1998), suggesting an atypical clinical expression of depression in epilepsy that may be frequent.

Interictal dysphoric disorder (IDD) is a chronic depression that mimics a *dysthymic* disorder with an intermittent course. Other symptoms include irritability, euphoric mood, fear, and anxiety. In patients with IDD, one-third to one-half require pharmacological treatment (Blumer and Zielinski, 1988) and 71% of patients with epilepsy and depressive symptoms requiring pharmacological treatment have a pleomorphic clinical picture consisting of anhedonia, with or without hopelessness, fatigue, anxiety, irritability, poor frustration tolerance, and mood lability with bouts of crying (Kanner et al., 2000). This is somewhat at odds with observations that depression preceding epilepsy is classifiable as major depressive disorder according to DSM criteria (Hesdorffer et al., 2000, 2006).

Psychotic disorders in epilepsy may also differ from primary schizophreniform disorders. In epilepsy, patients are older at onset, psychotic episodes are remarkable for the *absence* of negative symptoms, a better premorbid condition, and rare deterioration of personality (Slater et al., 1963).

With respect to anxiety disorders and ADHD, the clinical manifestations are identical to those of patients without epilepsy and no unique clinical characteristics have been identified.

IMPACT OF PSYCHIATRIC COMORBIDITIES

Quality of life of patients with epilepsy

Among the major psychiatric comorbidities in epilepsy, depressive and anxiety disorders have been studied most with respect to their impact on quality of life. There is consensus that mood and anxiety disorders have a negative impact in epilepsy, but these disorders are independent predictors of poor quality of life in people without epilepsy. Among patients with pharmacoresistant epilepsy, seizure frequency and severity did not predict patients' ratings of their quality of life (Perrine et al., 1995; Gilliam et al., 1997; Lehrner et al., 1999; Cramer et al., 2003; Boylan et al., 2004), but depression did.

Economic burden on family and society

Depression can also have a significant impact on healthcare costs associated with the management of the seizure disorder. When depression is untreated, more health resources are used, independent of seizure type and time since the last seizure (Cramer et al., 2004). Compared with epilepsy without depression, the frequency of medical visits was 2-fold greater with mild and moderate depression and 4-fold greater with severe depression. Presence and severity of depression was a predictor of worse disability scores independent of duration of the seizure disorder.

Suicidality risk

AED-induced depression may account for some of the depression observed in cross-sectional studies of epilepsy (Ring et al., 1993; Mula et al., 2003a, b, c, 2006). Such depression appears to occur 3.2-fold more often in association with AEDs that enhance GABA neurotransmission ($p = 0.14$, Fisher's exact test) and 5.1-fold more often with drugs that potentiate GABA-mediated neurotransmission ($p = 0.15$). Risk factors for AED-induced depression include a previous psychiatric history (Mula et al., 2003a), often previous depression (Mula et al., 2003a, c), family history of depression (Ring et al., 1993; Mula et al., 2003a), and hippocampal sclerosis (Mula et al., 2003b, 2006), which are themselves risk factors for depression in the absence of AED use (Burcusa and Iacono, 2007). It is also possible that AEDs may decrease the threshold for depression in the presence of an underlying vulnerability to depression.

Impact on response to pharmacological and surgical treatment of seizures

Recent studies have examined the impact of a psychiatric history on the risk of continued seizures, and thus for being present in a prevalent cohort with epilepsy. In an incident cohort followed for 20 years, a psychiatric history (80% depression) was associated with a 2.2-fold increased risk of having refractory epilepsy (95% CI 1.3–3.6) (Hitiris et al., 2007). Likewise, a study of 100 consecutive patients who underwent an anterotemporal lobectomy revealed that a lifetime psychiatric history, and in particular of mood disorder, was predictive of failure to achieve a seizure-free state after a mean $\pm$ SD postsurgical follow-up period of 8.1 ± 3.3 years (Kanner et al., 2009).

TREATMENT OF COMORBID PSYCHIATRIC DISORDERS

There are scant data based on randomized placebo-controlled studies (Class I and II) and no Class III trials on the treatment of comorbid psychiatric disorders. Thus, clinicians must use the same principles applied in the treatment of these psychiatric disorders in people without epilepsy.

Treatment of depressive and anxiety disorders in epilepsy

Pharmacotherapy

Depression and anxiety are considered together based on the high comorbidity of symptoms of depression or anxiety in the presence of depressive and anxiety disorders (Kanner et al., 2010). In addition, the same psychotropic agent can be used to treat both disorders (Table 29.1). The need to achieve complete symptom remission of both conditions is imperative to minimize the risk of recurrence of major depressive disorders.

Only two controlled studies have been conducted to assess the safety and efficacy of psychotropic drugs in the treatment of depressive disorders in epilepsy. The first study found no difference when comparing the efficacy of placebo, amitriptyline and mianserin (an antidepressant no longer in use in the USA) (Robertson, 1985). The second study, a double-blind randomized study of 187 patients with major depressive episodes randomized to a treatment with sertraline up to doses of 200 mg/day or cognitive behavioral therapy (CBT) (F. Gilliam et al., unpublished data), found no difference between treatments, with 60% of patients entering symptom remission.

SSRIs and SNRIs have become the first line of pharmacotherapy for primary major depressive, dysthymic,

Table 29.1

Efficacy of SSRIs and SNRIs in primary depression and anxiety disorders

Antidepressant drug	Depression	Panic disorder	Generalized anxiety	Starting dose (mg/day)	Maximum dose (mg/day)
Paroxetine*	+	+	+	10	60
Sertraline*	+	+	+	25	200
Fluoxetine*	+	+	+	10	80
Citalopram*	+	+	+	10	60
Escitalopram*	+	+	+	5	30
Venlafaxine†	+	+	+	37.5	300
Duloxetine†	+	−	+	20	120

*Selective serotonin reuptake inhibitor (SSRI).
†Serotonin–norepinephrine reuptake inhibitor (SNRI).
It should be noted, however, that there are no data on the use of duloxetine in patients with epilepsy, although the author has used it in more than 50 patients with poorly controlled epilepsy without any worsening of seizures (unpublished data).

and anxiety disorders (Stahl, 2000a) and are also recommended in patients with epilepsy. Antidepressants of the tricyclic family have been relegated to third line, because of their worse toxicity profile, particularly the greater risk of cardiotoxicity, although their efficacy is comparable to that of SSRIs and SNRIs. Monoamine oxidase inhibitors, used for selective types of pharmacoresistant depressive and anxiety disorders, should be prescribed only by psychiatrists.

Common misconceptions of a "proconvulsant" effect of antidepressants have been one of the causes of undertreatment in people with epilepsy suffering from a depressive or anxiety disorder. Antidepressants can cause seizures in patients without epilepsy and in patients with epilepsy when given in toxic doses, or in patients in whom the drug metabolism is slow, which can result in high serum concentrations at standard doses (Curran and DePauw, 1998). The only four antidepressants that have been found to be proconvulsant are bupropion, maprotiline, clomipramine, and amoxapine (Swinkels and Jonghe, 1995). One study found that sertraline, an SSRI, caused worsening seizures in 1 of 100 patients with pharmacoresistant epilepsy (Kanner et al., 2000).

Table 29.1 summarizes the SSRIs and SNRIs that have been found to be effective in the treatment of primary major depression as well as anxiety disorders. Following an unsuccessful trial with a SSRI at optimal doses, clinicians should consider using a SNRI. Patients should be referred to a psychiatrist if no symptom remission is achieved after a second trial. Although SSRIs are typically started first, patients, particularly those with retarded depression, could be started on a SNRI.

A cautionary note: the therapeutic effect of SSRIs and SNRIs may be identified 2–3 weeks after starting the drug. As SSRIs can at times cause restlessness and mild anxiety at the start of therapy, a short course of a benzodiazepine such as clonazepam (1 mg/day) should be considered.

Pharmacokinetic interactions between SSRIs, SNRIs, and AEDs

All antidepressants are metabolized in the liver via the cytochrome P450 (CP450) system. Their metabolism is accelerated in the presence of AEDs with enzyme-inducing properties, which include phenytoin, carbamazepine, phenobarbital, and primidone at any dosages, and oxcarbazepine and topiramate at doses above 900 and 400 mg respectively.

Some SSRIs are inhibitors of one or more isoenzymes of the CP450 system. These include fluoxetine, paroxetine, fluvoxamine, and, to a lesser degree, sertraline (Haselberger et al., 1997). Adjustment of some of the AED (primarily carbamazepine and phenytoin) dosages may be necessary. Citalopram and escitalopram are the SSRIs with no impact on CP450 isoenzymes. SNRIs do not have these properties.

Other treatments of anxiety disorders in epilepsy

Benzodiazepines have been used for a long time in the management of anxiety disorders but are not recommended for chronic use because of the development of tolerance. However, short trials of clonazepam can be quite effective in combination with a SSRI or SNRI, during the initial 6 weeks of therapy.

The FDA recently issued a warning that all AEDs can be associated with an increased risk of suicidal risk and behavior. This warning has been received with great skepticism by several professional epilepsy societies, which have questioned the validity of the FDA's findings because of several methodological problems

(Hesdorffer and Kanner, 2009). Nonetheless, screening for current and past history of suicidality and depressive disorders is necessary in all patients being started on an AED.

Nonpharmacological treatment

Psychotherapy, in particular CBT, has been used successfully in the treatment of major depressive episodes, as shown in a recent study of patients with major depressive disorder and epilepsy (F. Gilliam et al., unpublished data). Behavioral therapy and CBT have been used as well in the treatment of primary anxiety disorders, particularly phobic and obsessive compulsive disorders, and are expected to be useful in these conditions in patients with epilepsy.

Electroshock therapy

ECT is not contraindicated in depressed patients with epilepsy (Blackwood et al., 1980). It is a well-tolerated treatment and is worth considering in those with very severe depression that fails to respond to antidepressants (Regenold et al., 1998).

Treatment of comorbid ADHD

Pharmacotherapy

The pharmacological treatment of ADHD is identical to that for patients without seizures. It includes trials with CNS stimulants and non-CNS stimulants, including the noradrenergic agent atomoxetine and antidepressants.

First-line therapy includes the CNS stimulant families, either methylphenidate or one of the amfetamine compounds (Dunn and Kronenberger, 2005). Magnesium pemoline has been associated with rare hepatotoxicity and should be considered a third-line medication (McCurry and Cronquist, 1997).

There is a misconception among clinicians that CNS-stimulant drugs can lower the seizure threshold, based on reports included in the Physician and Desk Reference (PDR). The consensus among pediatric neurologists and epileptologists is that there is no evidence to support these concerns. In fact, several trials of methylphenidate in children with seizures have shown this agent to be safe and effective (Dunn and Kronenberger, 2005).

In general, there is no pharmacokinetic interaction between CNS stimulants and AEDs. Methylphenidate has low bioavailability (20–25%), which may account for occasional erratic responses. If a trial with methylphenidate is not effective, clinicians can switch to a dexamfetamine formulation, which has high bioavailability (75%).

In the absence of a therapeutic response with CNS stimulants, a trial with the new noradrenergic drug, atomoxetine, should be considered owing to its therapeutic effect in ADHD for both adults and children. Safety in epilepsy has not been established for this relatively new agent, although, in the authors' experience, no worsening of seizure frequency has been identified. Furthermore, regulatory trials of atomoxetine do not report an increased seizure risk. Alternative pharmacological options include the use of antidepressants, α-adrenergic agonists, and antipsychotic drugs (Green, 1995), which should be administered by an expert in ADHD pharmacotherapy.

Nonpharmacological treatment

Nonpharmacological therapy is often necessary and complementary to the therapeutic effects of pharmacotherapy. Behavioral therapy and CBT can be very efficacious in training patients to develop strategies to control their impulsivity and poor frustration tolerance.

Treatment of psychosis in epilepsy

The primary treatment for psychotic symptoms and episodes in patients with epilepsy is antipsychotic drugs (APDs) and, in refractory cases, ECT.

Antipsychotic drug use in epilepsy

Antipsychotic drugs can be separated into two classes: "conventional" (CAPDs) and "atypical" (AAPDs) APDs. Conventional APDs include 18 drugs in which the effects are mediated by blockade of DA_2 receptors at mesocortical, nigrostriatal, and tuberoinfundibular DA pathways (Stahl, 2004). In addition to their DA blockade properties, most of these CAPDs have muscarinic cholinergic, α_1, and histaminic blocking properties, responsible for anticholinergic adverse effects, weight gain, sedation, dizziness, and orthostatic hypotension.

Six AAPDs have been introduced in the USA: clozapine, risperidone, olanzapine, ziprasidone, quetiapine, and aripiprazole. AAPDs have in large part replaced CAPDs. AAPDs are dopamine–serotonin antagonists that target DA_2 and $5HT_{2A}$ receptors (Stahl, 2000b). Their main difference with CAPDs is the absence or mild occurrence of extrapyramidal adverse events and of hyperprolactinemia. A lesser blunting of affect is typical of these drugs, and several AAPDs have demonstrated mood-stabilizing properties.

Although the efficacy of CAPDs and AAPDs has been shown to be comparable, the preference for AAPDs is based on a decreased risk of CNS-mediated adverse events, in particular extrapyramidal symptoms, and the lower potential for long-term tardive dyskinesia that has typically been associated with CAPDs. Furthermore, the mood-stabilizing properties of several AAPDs makes these drugs more appealing, particularly in the management of psychotic episodes in patients with epilepsy, which are typically affectively laden.

Safety of antipsychotic drugs in epilepsy

The proconvulsant properties of CAPDs are well recognized, ranging between 0.5% and 1.2% amongst patients without epilepsy. The risk is higher with certain drugs and in the presence of: (1) a history of epilepsy; (2) abnormal EEG recordings; (3) a history of CNS disorder; (4) rapid titration of the CAPD dose; (5) high doses of APDs; and (6) the presence of other drugs that lower the seizure threshold. For example, when chlorpromazine was used at doses above 1000 mg/day, the incidence of seizures was reported to increase to 9%, in contrast to a 0.5% incidence at lower doses (Logothetis, 1967). Haloperidol, molindone, fluphenazine, perphenazine, and trifluoperazine are among the CAPDs with a lower seizure risk (Whitworth and Fleischhacker, 1995).

With the exception of clozapine, and to a lesser degree olanzapine, AAPD-related seizure incidence has not been comparable to that in the general population (Toth and Frankenburg, 1994). During premarketing studies of patients without epilepsy taking AAPDs, seizures were reported in 0.3% of those given risperidone, 0.9% for olanzapine, and 0.8% for quetiapine (versus 0.5% in those given placebo), and in 0.4% of patients treated with ziprasidone (data in PDR). In contrast, clozapine has been reported to cause seizures in 4.4% when used at doses above 600 mg/day, whereas at a dosage below 300 mg the incidence of seizures is less than 1% in patients without epilepsy.

Unfortunately, the impact of AAPDs on seizure occurrence in epilepsy has not been studied properly, with the exception of clozapine in a study of 5629 patients treated with this AAPD. In patients without epilepsy, seizures were more likely to occur at daily doses above 600 mg/day, whereas 16 patients had epilepsy before commencement of this drug and all experienced worsening of seizures while on the drug, at both high and low doses. Clearly any CAPD or AAPD should be started at a low dose with slow dose increments to minimize the risk of seizures in patients with epilepsy.

Most APDs can cause EEG changes, which include slowing of the background activity especially when used at high doses. Some of these drugs, particularly clozapine, can cause paroxysmal EEG changes in the form of interictal sharp waves and spikes. This type of epileptiform activity, however, is not predictive of seizure occurrence (Tiihonen et al., 1991).

All APDs are metabolized in the liver. Accordingly, the addition of enzyme-inducing AEDs may potentially result in recurrence of psychotic symptoms previously controlled at higher serum concentrations of APD. Conversely, discontinuation of such AEDs may result in a decrease in the clearance of APD, which in turn can lead to adverse events caused by an increase of their serum concentrations and, in particular, of extrapyramidal adverse events in the case of CAPDs. In addition, valproic acid can inhibit the glucuronidation process of AAPDs such as clozapine.

AAPDs are known to cause a metabolic syndrome associated with type 2 diabetes, hyperlipidemia, and weight gain. Their use with other AEDs that can cause weight gain (valproic acid, pregabalin, gabapentin, carbamazepine, and oxcarbazepine) can "in theory" worsen the weight gain. Furthermore, enzyme-inducing AEDs such as phenytoin and carbamazepine are also known to increase serum lipid levels, which can have an agonist effect with some of the AAPDs.

CONCLUDING REMARKS

Psychiatric comorbidities are common in prevalent epilepsy. Depression, suicide attempts, and ADHD have been shown to increase the risk of developing epilepsy, and epilepsy has been shown to increase risk of developing schizophrenia. Psychiatric disorders preceding the onset of epilepsy also predispose to preictal, postictal, and ictal psychiatric disturbances. There are several common pathogenic mechanisms that could explain the comorbidity of epilepsy and psychiatric disorders, including: disturbances in serotonin, norepinephrine, dopamine, glutamate, and GABA; a hyperactive HPA axis; structural abnormalities in several neuroanatomical structures, including atrophy of the mesial temporal lobe and frontal lobe; and febrile seizures. Psychiatric comorbidities impact upon quality of life in patients with epilepsy and are associated with a poor seizure prognosis. Psychopathology is often underrecognized in patients with epilepsy. Clinicians should assess patients with epilepsy for these comorbidities and refer them as needed for a complete psychiatric evaluation.

References

Adachi N, Kato M, Sekimoto M et al. (2003). Recurrent postictal psychosis after remission of interictal psychosis: further evidence of bimodal psychosis. Epilepsia 44: 1218–1222.

Alper K, Devinsky O, Westbrook L et al. (2001). Premorbid psychiatric risk factors for postictal psychosis. J Neuropsychiatry Clin Neurosci 13: 492–499.

Alper K, Schwartz KA, Kolts RL et al. (2007). Seizure incidence in psychopharmacological clinical trials: an analysis of Food and Drug Administration (FDA) summary basis of approval reports. Biol Psychiatry 62: 345–354.

Alwash RH, Hussein MJ, Matloub FF (2000). Symptoms of anxiety and depression among adolescents with seizures in Irbid, Northern Jordan. Seizure 9: 412–416.

Andermann LF, Savard G, Meencke HJ et al. (1999). Psychosis after resection of ganglioglioma or DNET: evidence for an association. Epilepsia 40: 83–87.

Andrade R, Nicoll RA (1987). Pharmacologically distinct actions of serotonin on single pyramidal neurones of the rat hippocampus recorded in vitro. J Physiol 394: 99–124.

Annegers JF, Hauser WA, Elveback LR et al. (1979). The risk of epilepsy following febrile convulsions. Neurology 29: 297–303.

Anson JA, Kuhlman DT (1993). Postictal Kluver–Bucy syndrome after temporal lobectomy. J Neurol Neurosurg Psychiatry 56: 311–313.

Applegate CD, Tecott LH (1998). Global increases in seizure susceptibility in mice lacking 5-HT2C receptors: a behavioral analysis. Exp Neurol 154: 522–530.

Arbatova J, D'Amato E, Vaarmann A et al. (2005). Reduced serotonin and 3-hydroxyanthranilic acid levels in serum of cystatin B-deficient mice, a model system for progressive myoclonus epilepsy. Epilepsia 46: 49–51.

Austin JK, Harezlak J, Dunn DW et al. (2001). Behavior problems in children before first recognized seizures. Pediatrics 107: 115–122.

Aznar S, Qian Z, Shah R et al. (2003). The 5-HT1A serotonin receptor is located on calbindin- and parvalbumin-containing neurons in the rat brain. Brain Res 959: 58–67.

Baetz M, Bowen RC (1998). Efficacy of divalproex sodium in patients with panic disorder and mood instability who have not responded to conventional therapy. Can J Psychiatry 43: 73–77.

Baker GA, Spector S, McGrath Y et al. (2005). Impact of epilepsy in adolescence: a UK controlled study. Epilepsy Behav 6: 556–562.

Ban TA, Vartanian FE, Sartorius N et al. (1979). Identification of high-risk criteria in the framework of W.H.O. collaborative research in the major mental disorders. Prog Neuropsychopharmacol 3: 575–578.

Bartlet JE (1957). Chronic psychosis following epilepsy. Am J Psychiatry 114: 338–343.

Beck SG, Choi KC (1991). 5-Hydroxytryptamine hyperpolarizes CA3 hippocampal pyramidal cells through an increase in potassium conductance. Neurosci Lett 133: 93–96.

Beghi E, Spagnoli P, Airoldi L et al. (2002). Emotional and affective disturbances in patients with epilepsy. Epilepsy Behav 3: 255–261.

Ben-Menachem E, Persson LI, Hedner T (1992). Selected CSF biochemistry and gabapentin concentrations in the CSF and plasma in patients with partial seizures after a single oral dose of gabapentin. Epilepsy Res 11: 45–49.

Berman RM, Cappiello A, Anand A et al. (2000). Antidepressant effects of ketamine in depressed patients. Biol Psychiatry 47: 351–354.

Bhagwagar Z, Whale R, Cowen PJ (2002). State and trait abnormalities in serotonin function in major depression. Br J Psychiatry 180: 24–28.

Blackwood DHR, Cull RE, Freeman CP et al. (1980). A study of the incidence of epilepsy following ECT. J Neurol Neurosurg Psychiatry 43: 1098–1102.

Blanchet P, Frommer GP (1986). Mood change preceding epileptic seizures. J Nerv Ment Dis 174: 471–476.

Bleuler E (1949). Lehrbuch der Psychiatrie. 8th edn. Springer, Berlin.

Blumer D, Altshuler LL (1998). Affective disorders. In: J Engel, TA Pedley (Eds.), Epilepsy: A Comprehensive Textbook. Vol. II. Lippincott-Raven, Philadelphia, pp. 2083–2099.

Blumer D, Zielinksi J (1988). Pharmacologic treatment of psychiatric disorders associated with epilepsy. J Epilepsy 1: 135–150.

Booij L, Van der Does W, Benkelfat C et al. (2002). Predictors of mood response to acute tryptophan depletion. A reanalysis. Neuropsychopharmacology 27: 852–861.

Bouilleret V, Semah F, Biraben A et al. (2005). Involvement of the basal ganglia in refractory epilepsy: an 18-F-fluoro-L-DOPA PET study using 2 methods of analysis. J Nucl Med 46: 540–547.

Boylan LS, Flint LA, Labovitz DL et al. (2004). Depression but not seizure frequency predicts quality of life in treatment-resistant epilepsy. Neurology 62: 258–261.

Bremmer MA, Hoogendijk WJ, Deeg DJ et al. (2006). Depression in older age is a risk factor for first ischemic cardiac events. Am J Geriatr Psychiatry 14: 523–530.

Breslau N, Davis GC, Andreski P (1991). Migraine, psychiatric disorders, and suicide attempts: an epidemiologic study of young adults. Psychiatry Res 37: 11–23.

Breslau N, Schultz LR, Stewart WF et al. (2000). Headache and major depression: is the association specific to migraine? Neurology 54: 308–313.

Briellmann RS, Kalnins RM, Hopwood MJ et al. (2000). TLE patients with postictal psychosis: mesial dysplasia and anterior hippocampal preservation. Neurology 55: 1027–1030.

Browning RA, Clark KB, Naritoku DK et al. (1997a). Loss of anticonvulsant effect of vagus nerve stimulation in the pentylenetetrazol seizure model following treatment with 6-hydroxydopamine or 5,7-dihydroxy-tryptamine. Soc Neurosci 23: 2424.

Browning RA, Wood AV, Merrill MA et al. (1997b). Enhancement of the anticonvulsant effect of fluoxetine following blockade of 5-HT1A receptors. Eur J Pharmacol 336: 1–6.

Burcusa SL, Iacono WG (2007). Risk for recurrence in depression. Clin Psychol Rev 27: 959–985.

Caplan R, Siddarth P, Gurbani S et al. (2005). Depression and anxiety disorders in pediatric epilepsy. Epilepsia 46: 720–730.

Carlton-Ford S, Miller R, Brown M et al. (1995). Epilepsy and children's social and psychological adjustment. J Health Soc Behav 36: 285–301.

Chang BS, Lowenstein DH (2003). Epilepsy. N Engl J Med 349: 1257–1266.

Chen B, Dowlatshahi D, MacQueen GM et al. (2001). Increased hippocampal BDNF immunoreactivity in subjects treated with antidepressant medication. Biol Psychiatry 50: 260–265.

Clinckers R, Smolders I, Meurs A et al. (2005). Hippocampal dopamine and serotonin elevations as pharmacodynamic markers for the anticonvulsant efficacy of oxcarbazepine and 10,11-dihydro-10-hydroxycarbamazepine. Neurosci Lett 390: 48–53.

Cramer JA, Blum M, Reed M et al. (2003). The influence of comorbid depression on quality of life for people with epilepsy. Epilepsy Behav 4: 515–521.

Cramer JA, Blum D, Fanning K et al. (2004). The impact of comorbid depression on health resource utilization in a community sample of people with epilepsy. Epilepsy Behav 5: 337–342.

Curran S, DePauw (1998). Selecting an antidepressant for use in a patient with epilepsy. Safety considerations. Drug Safe 18: 125–133.

Dailey JW, Yan QS, Mishra PK et al. (1992). Effects of fluoxetine on convulsions and on brain serotonin as detected by microdialysis in genetically epilepsy-prone rats. J Pharmacol Exp Ther 260: 533–540.

Daly D (1958). Ictal affect. Am J Psychiatry 115: 97–108.

Davis M (1999). Functional neuroanatomy of anxiety and fear: a focus on the amygdala. In: DS Charney, EJ Nestler, BS Bunney (Eds.), Neurobiology of Mental Illness. Oxford University Press, New York, pp. 463–474.

de Araujo Filho GM, Pascalicchio TF, Lin K et al. (2006). Neuropsychiatric profiles of patients with juvenile myoclonic epilepsy treated with valproate or topiramate. Epilepsy Behav 8: 606–609.

Delgado PL, Price LH, Miller HL et al. (1994). Serotonin and the neurobiology of depression. Effects of tryptophan depletion in drug-free depressed patients. Arch Gen Psychiatry 51: 865–874.

Delgado PL, Miller HL, Salomon RM et al. (1999). Tryptophan-depletion challenge in depressed patients treated with desipramine or fluoxetine: implications for the role of serotonin in the mechanism of antidepressant action. Biol Psychiatry 46: 212–220.

Denhoff E, Laufer MW, Solomon G (1957). Hyperkinetic impulse disorder in children's behavior problems. Psychosom Med 19: 38–49.

Devinsky O, Abrahmson H, Alper K et al. (1995). Postictal psychosis: a case control study of 20 patients and 150 controls. Epilepsy Res 20: 247–253.

Devinsky O, Barr WB, Vickrey BG et al. (2005). Changes in depression and anxiety after resective surgery for epilepsy. Neurology 65: 1744–1749.

Dominian J, Serafetinides EA, Dewhurst M (1963). A follow-up study of late-onset epilepsy. II. Psychiatric and social findings. Br Med J 1: 431–435.

Drake ME (1987). Postictal Capgras syndrome. Clin Neurol Neurosurg 89: 271–274.

Drevets WC, Frank E, Price JC et al. (1999). PET imaging of serotonin 1A receptor binding in depression. Biol Psychiatry 46: 1375–1387.

Dube CM, Brewster AL, Richichi C et al. (2007). Fever, febrile seizures and epilepsy. Trends Neurosci 30: 490–496.

Dunn DW, Kronenberger WG (2005). Childhood epilepsy, attention problems, and ADHD: review and practical considerations. Semin Pediatr Neurol 12: 222–228.

Dunn DW, Austin JK, Huster GA (1997). Behaviour problems in children with new-onset epilepsy. Seizure 6: 283–287.

Edeh J, Toone B (1987). Relationship between interictal psychopathology and the type of epilepsy. Results of a survey in general practice. Br J Psychiatry 151: 95–101.

Ettinger AB, Weisbrot DM, Nolan EE et al. (1998). Symptoms of depression and anxiety in pediatric epilepsy patients. Epilepsia 39: 595–599.

Ettinger AB, Reed ML, Goldberg JF et al. (2005). Prevalence of bipolar symptoms in epilepsy vs other chronic health disorders. Neurology 65: 535–540.

Fann JR, Burington B, Leonetti A et al. (2004). Psychiatric illness following traumatic brain injury in an adult health maintenance organization population. Arch Gen Psychiatry 61: 53–61.

Favale E, Audenino D, Cocito L et al. (2003). The anticonvulsant effect of citalopram as an indirect evidence of serotonergic impairment in human epileptogenesis. Seizure 12: 316–318.

Forsgren L, Nystrom L (1990). An incident case–referent study of epileptic seizures in adults. Epilepsy Res 6: 66–81.

Fromm GH, Amores CY, Thies W (1972). Imipramine in epilepsy. Arch Neurol 27: 198.

Fromm GH, Wessel HB, Glass JD et al. (1978). Imipramine in absence and myoclonic–astatic seizures. Neurology 28: 953.

Gaitatzis A, Trimble MR, Sander JW (2004). The psychiatric comorbidity of epilepsy. Acta Neurol Scand 110: 207–220.

Gastaut H, Roger J, Lesèvre N (1953). Différenciation psychologique des épileptiques en fonction des formes électrocliniques de leur maladie. Rev Psychol Appl 3: 237–249.

Gastaut H, Morin G, Lesèvre N (1955). Étude du comportement des épileptiques psychomoteurs dans l'intervalle de leurs crises: les troubles de l'activité globale et de la sociabilité. Ann Med Psychol (Paris) 113: 1–27.

Geronimus AT, Hicken M, Keene D et al. (2006). "Weathering" and age patterns of allostatic load scores among blacks and whites in the United States. Am J Public Health 96: 826–833.

Gilliam F, Kuzniecky R, Faught E et al. (1997). Patient-validated content of epilepsy-specific quality-of-life measurement. Epilepsia 38: 233–236.

Gilliam FG, Maton BM, Martin RC et al. (2007). Hippocampal 1 H-MRSI correlates with severity of depression symptoms in temporal lobe epilepsy. Neurology 68: 364–368.

Glauss A (1931). Ueber Kombinatiionen von Schizophrenia und Epilepsie. Z Ges Neurol Psychiatr 135: 450–500.

Golden RN, Heine AD, Ekstrom RD et al. (2002). A longitudinal study of serotonergic function in depression. Neuropsychopharmacology 26: 653–659.

Goldstein LH, Holland L, Soteriou H et al. (2005). Illness representations, coping styles and mood in adults with epilepsy. Epilepsy Res 67: 1–11.

Graumlich JF, McLaughlin RG, Birkhahn D et al. (1999). Carbamazepine pharmacokinetics–pharmacodynamics in genetically epilepsy-prone rats. Eur J Pharmacol 369: 305–311.

Green WH (1995). The treatment of attention-deficit hyperactivity disorder with nonstimulant medications. Child Adolesc Psychiatr Clin N Am 4: 169–195.

Harris JC (1989). Experimental animal modeling of depression and anxiety. Psychiatr Clin North Am 12: 815–836.

Haselberger MB, Freedman LS, Tolbert S (1997). Elevated serum phenytoin concentrations associated with coadministration of sertraline. J Clin Psychopharmacol 17: 107–109.

Hasler G, Bonwetsch R, Giovacchini G et al. (2007). 5-HT (1A) receptor binding in temporal lobe epilepsy patients with and without major depression. Biol Psychiatry 62: 1258–1264.

Hauser WA, Annegers JF, Kurland LT (1993). Incidence of epilepsy and unprovoked seizures in Rochester, Minnesota: 1935–1984. Epilepsia 34: 453–468.

Hemmer SA, Pasternak JF, Zecker SG et al. (2001). Stimulant therapy and seizure risk in children with ADHD. Pediatr Neurol 24: 99–102.

Hermann BP, Whitman S, Wyler AR et al. (1990). Psychosocial predictors of psychopathology in epilepsy. Br J Psychiatry 156: 98–105.

Hermann B, Jones J, Dabbs K et al. (2007). The frequency, complications and aetiology of ADHD in new onset paediatric epilepsy. Brain 130: 3135–3148.

Hernandez EJ, Williams PA, Dudek FE (2002). Effects of fluoxetine and TFMPP on spontaneous seizures in rats with pilocarpine-induced epilepsy. Epilepsia 43: 1337–1345.

Hesdorffer DC, Kanner AM (2009). The FDA alert on suicidality and antiepileptic drugs: Fire or false alarm? Epilepsia 50: 978–988.

Hesdorffer DC, Hauser WA, Annegers JF et al. (2000). Major depression is a risk factor for seizures in older adults. Ann Neurol 47: 246–249.

Hesdorffer DC, Ludvigsson P, Olafsson E et al. (2004). ADHD as a risk factor for incident unprovoked seizures and epilepsy in children. Arch Gen Psychiatry 61: 731–736.

Hesdorffer DC, Hauser WA, Olafsson E et al. (2006). Depression and suicide attempt as risk factors for incident unprovoked seizures. Ann Neurol 59: 35–41.

Hitiris N, Mohanraj R, Norrie J et al. (2007). Predictors of pharmacoresistant epilepsy. Epilepsy Res 75: 192–196.

Holdsworth L, Whitmore K (1974). A study of children with epilepsy attending ordinary schools. II: Information and attitudes held by their teachers. Dev Med Child Neurol 16: 759–765.

Holtmann M, Becker K, Kentner-Figura B et al. (2003). Increased frequency of rolandic spikes in ADHD children. Epilepsia 44: 1241–1244.

Hughes JR, DeLeo AJ, Melyn MA (2000). The electroencephalogram in attention deficit-hyperactivity disorder: emphasis on epileptiform discharges. Epilepsy Behav 1: 271–277.

Irwin K, Birch V, Lees J et al. (2001). Multiple subpial transaction in Landau–Kleffner syndrome. Dev Med Child Neurol 43: 248–252.

Jacobs BL, Azmitia EC (1992). Structure and function of the brain serotonin system. Physiol Rev 72: 165–229.

Jacoby A, Baker GA, Steen N et al. (1996). The clinical course of epilepsy and its psychosocial correlates: findings from a U.K. Community study. Epilepsia 37: 148–161.

Jakus R, Graf M, Juhasz G et al. (2003). 5-HT2C receptors inhibit and 5-HT1A receptors activate the generation of spike-wave discharges in a genetic rat model of absence epilepsy. Exp Neurol 184: 964–972.

Jalava M, Sillanpaa M (1996). Concurrent illnesses in adults with childhood-onset epilepsy: a population-based 35-year follow-up study. Epilepsia 37: 1155–1163.

Jensen I, Vaernet K (1977). Temporal lobe epilepsy. Follow-up investigation of 74 temporal lobe resected patients. Acta Neurochir (Wien) 37: 173–200.

Jobe PC, Weber RH (2005). Affective disorder and epilepsy comorbidity in the genetically epilepsy prone-rat (GEPR). In: F Gilliam, AM Kanner, YI Sheline (Eds.), Neurologic Dysfunction in Depression. Taylor & Francis, London, pp. 121–158.

Jonas BS, Mussolino ME (2000). Symptoms of depression as a prospective risk factor for stroke. Psychosom Med 62: 463–471.

Jones JE, Watson R, Sheth R et al. (2007). Psychiatric comorbidity in children with new onset epilepsy. Dev Med Child Neurol 49: 493–497.

Jung ME, Lal H, Gatch MB (2002). The discriminative stimulus effects of pentylenetetrazol as a model of anxiety: recent developments. Neurosci Biobehav Rev 26: 429–439.

Kanemoto K, Miyamoto T, Abe R (1999). Ictal catatonia as a manifestation of de novo absence status epilepticus following benzodiazepine withdrawal. Seizure 8: 364–366.

Kanemoto K, Tsuji T, Kawasaki J (2001). Reexamination of interictal psychoses based on DSM IV psychosis classification and international epilepsy classification. Epilepsia 42: 98–103.

Kanner AM, Balabanov AJ (2008). Psychiatric outcome of epilepsy surgery. In: HO Luders (Ed.), Textbook of Epilepsy Surgery. Informa Healthcare, London, pp. 1254–1262.

Kanner AM, Ostrovskaya A (2008). Long-term significance of postictal psychotic episodes I. Are they predictive of bilateral ictal foci? Epilepsy Behav 12: 150–153.

Kanner AM, Stagno S, Kotagal P et al. (1996). Postictal psychiatric events during prolonged video-electroencephalographic monitoring studies. Arch Neurol 53: 258–263.

Kanner AM, Kozak AM, Frey M (2000). The use of sertraline in patients with epilepsy: is it safe? Epilepsy Behav 1: 100–105.

Kanner AM, Soto A, Gross-Kanner H (2004). Prevalence and clinical characteristics of postictal psychiatric symptoms in partial epilepsy. Neurology 62: 708–713.

Kanner AM, Byrne RW, Chicharro AV et al. (2009). Is a lifetime psychiatric history predictive of a worse postsurgical seizure outcome following a temporal lobectomy? Neurology 72: 793–799.

Kanner AM, Barry JJ, Gilliam F et al. (2010). Anxiety disorders, sub-syndromic depressive episodes and major depressive episodes: do they differ on their impact on the quality of life of patients with epilepsy? Epilepsia 51: 1152–1158.

Kaplan HI, Sadock BJ (1991). Synopsis of Psychiatry: Behavioral Sciences Clinical Psychiatry. Williams and Wilkins, Baltimore.

Kaplan PW (2002). Behavioral manifestations of nonconvulsive status epilepticus. Epilepsy Behav 3: 122–139.

Kessler RC, Zhao S, Katz SJ et al. (1999). Past-year use of outpatient services for psychiatric problems in the National Comorbidity Survey. Am J Psychiatry 156: 115–123.

Ketter TA, Malow BA, Flamini R et al. (1994). Anticonvulsant withdrawal-emergent psychopathology. Neurology 44: 55–61.

Kilian M, Frey HH (1973). Central monoamines and convulsive thresholds in mice and rats. Neuropharmacology 12: 681–692.

Kohler CG, Carran MA, Bilker W et al. (2001). Association of fear auras with mood and anxiety disorders after temporal lobectomy. Epilepsia 42: 674–681.

Koolhaas JM, de Boer SF, Buwalda B et al. (2007). Individual variation in coping with stress: a multidimensional approach of ultimate and proximate mechanisms. Brain Behav Evol 70: 218–226.

Kraepelin E (1923). Psychiatrie. Vol 3. Johann Ambrosius Barth, Leipzig.

Landau WM, Kleffner F (1957). Syndrome of acquired aphasia with convulsive disorder in children. Neurology 7: 523–530.

Landolt H (1953). Some clinical electroencephalographical correlations in epileptic psychosis (twilight states). Electroencephalogr Clin Neurophysiol 5: 121.

Landolt H (1955). Über Verstimmungen, Dämmerzustände und schizophrene Zustandsbilder bei Epilepsie: Ergebnisse klinischer und elektroenzephalographischer Untersuchungen. Schweiz Arch Neurol Psychiatrie 76: 313–321.

Laufer M, Denhoff E (1957). Hyperkinetic behavior in children. J Pediatr 50: 463–474.

Lehrner J, Kalchmayr R, Serles W et al. (1999). Health-related quality of life (HRQOL), activity of daily living (ADL) and depressive mood disorder in temporal lobe epilepsy patients. Seizure 8: 88–92.

Leinonen E, Tuunainen A, Lepola U (1994). Postoperative psychoses in epileptic patients after temporal lobectomy. Acta Neurol Scand 90: 394–399.

Lewis DV, Barboriak DP, MacFall JR et al. (2002). Do prolonged febrile seizures produce medial temporal sclerosis? Hypotheses, MRI evidence and unanswered questions. Prog Brain Res 135: 263–278.

Lindsay J, Ounsted C, Richards P (1984). Long-term outcome in children with temporal lobe seizures. V: indications and contra-indications for neurosurgery. Dev Med Child Neurol 26: 25–32.

Livneh H, Wilson LM, Duchesneau A et al. (2001). Psychosocial adaptation to epilepsy: the role of coping strategies. Epilepsy Behav 2: 533–544.

Logothetis J (1967). Spontaneous epileptic seizures and EEG changes in the course of phenothiazine therapy. Neurology 17: 869–877.

Logsdail SJ, Toone BK (1988). Postictal psychosis. A clinical and phenomenological description. Br J Psychiatry 152: 246–252.

Lu KT, Gean PW (1998). Endogenous serotonin inhibits epileptiform activity in rat hippocampal CA1 neurons via 5-hydroxytryptamine1A receptor activation. Neuroscience 86: 729–737.

Mace CJ, Trimble MR (1991). Psychosis following temporal lobe surgery: a report of six cases. J Neurol Neurosurg Psychiatry 54: 639–644.

Maier M, Mellers J, Toone B et al. (2000). Schizophrenia, temporal lobe epilepsy and psychosis: an in vivo magnetic resonance spectroscopy and imaging study of the hippocampus/amygdala complex. Psychol Med 30: 571–581.

Malizia AL, Cunningham VJ, Bell CJ et al. (1998). Decreased brain GABA(A)-benzodiazepine receptor binding in panic disorder: preliminary results from a quantitative PET study. Arch Gen Psychiatry 55: 715–720.

Mazarati AM, Shin D, Kwon YS et al. (2009). Elevated plasma corticosterone level and depressive behavior in experimental temporal lobe epilepsy. Neurobiol Dis 34: 457–461.

McCurry L, Cronquist S (1997). Pemoline and hepatotoxicity. Am J Psychiatry 154: 713–714.

McDermott S, Coker AL, Mani S et al. (1996). A population-based analysis of behavior problems in children with cerebral palsy. J Pediatr Psychol 21: 447–463.

McEwen BS (2000). The neurobiology of stress: from serendipity to clinical relevance. Brain Res 886: 172–189.

Mendez MF, Cummings JL, Benson DF (1986). Depression in epilepsy. Significance and phenomenology. Arch Neurol 43: 766–770.

Mengod G, Pompeiano M, Martinez-Mir MI et al. (1990). Localization of the mRNA for the 5-HT2 receptor by in situ hybridization histochemistry. Correlation with the distribution of receptor sites. Brain Res 524: 139–143.

Mensah SA, Beavis JM, Thapar AK et al. (2007). A community study of the presence of anxiety disorder in people with epilepsy. Epilepsy Behav 11: 118–124.

Merlet I, Ostrowsky K, Costes N et al. (2004). 5-HT1A receptor binding and intracerebral activity in temporal lobe epilepsy: an [^{18}F]MPPF-PET study. Brain 127: 900–913.

Meschaks A, Lindstrom P, Halldin C et al. (2005). Regional reductions in serotonin 1A receptor binding in juvenile myoclonic epilepsy. Arch Neurol 62: 946–960.

Mintzer S, Lopez F (2002). Comorbidity of ictal fear and panic disorder. Epilepsy Behav 3: 330–337.

Moreno FA, Heninger GR, McGahuey CA et al. (2000). Tryptophan depletion and risk of depression relapse: a prospective study of tryptophan depletion as a potential predictor of depressive episodes. Biol Psychiatry 48: 327–329.

Moreno FA, Rowe DC, Kaiser B et al. (2002). Association between a serotonin transporter promoter region polymorphism and mood response during tryptophan depletion. Mol Psychiatry 7: 213–216.

Morrell F, Whisler WW, Smith MC et al. (1995). Landau–Kleffner syndrome: treatment with subpial intracortical transection. Brain 118: 1529–1546.

Mula M, Trimble MR, Lhatoo SD et al. (2003a). Topiramate and psychiatric adverse events in patients with epilepsy. Epilepsia 44: 659–663.

Mula M, Trimble MR, Sander JW (2003b). The role of hippocampal sclerosis in topiramate-related depression and cognitive deficits in people with epilepsy. Epilepsia 44: 1573–1577.

Mula M, Trimble MR, Yuen A et al. (2003c). Psychiatric adverse events during levetiracetam therapy. Neurology 61: 704–706.

Mula M, Sander JW, Trimble MR (2006). The role of hippocampal sclerosis in antiepileptic drug-related depression in patients with epilepsy: a study on levetiracetam. Seizure 15: 405–408.

Mula M, Schmitz B, Jauch R et al. (2008). On the prevalence of bipolar disorder in epilepsy. Epilepsy Behav 13: 658–661.

Murakami T, Okada M, Kawata Y et al. (2001). Determination of effects of antiepileptic drugs on SNAREs-mediated hippocampal monoamine release using in vivo microdialysis. Br J Pharmacol 134: 507–520.

Nibuya M, Morinobu S, Duman RS (1995). Regulation of BDNF and trkB mRNA in rat brain by chronic electroconvulsive seizure and antidepressant drug treatments. J Neurosci 15: 7539–7547.

Nilsson FM, Kessing LV, Bolwig TG (2003). On the increased risk of developing late-onset epilepsy for patients with major affective disorder. J Affect Disord 76: 39–48.

Nissenkorn A, Moldavsky M, Loberboym M et al. (1999). Postictal psychosis in a child. J Child Neurol 14: 818–819.

Nutt DJ, Glue P, Lawson CW et al. (1990). Flumazenil provocation of panic attacks: evidence for altered benzodiazepine receptor sensitivity in panic disorders. Arch Gen Psychiatry 47: 917–925.

O'Donoghue MF, Goodridge DM, Redhead K et al. (1999). Assessing the psychosocial consequences of epilepsy: a community-based study. Br J Gen Pract 49: 211–214.

Oguz A, Kurul S, Dirik E (2002). Relationship of epilepsy-related factors to anxiety and depression scores in epileptic children. J Child Neurol 17: 37–40.

Ohira T, Iso H, Satoh S et al. (2001). Prospective study of depressive symptoms and risk of stroke among Japanese. Stroke 32: 903–908.

Okada M, Hirano T, Mizuno K et al. (1998). Effects of carbamazepine on hippocampal serotonergic system. Epilepsy Res 31: 187–198.

Okuhara DY, Beck SG (1994). 5-HT1A receptor linked to inward-rectifying potassium current in hippocampal CA3 pyramidal cells. J Neurophysiol 71: 2161–2167.

Olfson M, Das AK, Gameroff MJ et al. (2005). Bipolar depression in a low-income primary care clinic. Am J Psychiatry 162: 2146–2151.

Olnes MJ, Golding A, Kaplan PW (2003). Nonconvulsive status epilepticus resulting from benzodiazepine withdrawal. Ann Intern Med 139: 956–958.

Ott D, Caplan R, Guthrie D et al. (2001). Measures of psychopathology in children with complex partial seizures and primary generalized epilepsy with absence. J Am Acad Child Adolesc Psychiatry 40: 907–914.

Owens MJ, Nemeroff CB (1994). Role of serotonin in the pathophysiology of depression: focus on the serotonin transporter. Clin Chem 40: 288–295.

Owens MJ, Morgan WN, Plott SJ et al. (1997). Neurotransmitter receptor and transporter binding profile of antidepressants and their metabolites. J Pharmacol Exp Ther 283: 1305–1322.

Ownby RL, Crocco E, Acevedo A et al. (2006). Depression and risk for Alzheimer disease: systematic review, meta-analysis, and metaregression analysis. Arch Gen Psychiatry 63: 530–538.

Patten SB, Beck CA, Williams JV et al. (2003). Major depression in multiple sclerosis: a population-based perspective. Neurology 61: 1524–1527.

Perrine K, Hermann BP, Meador KJ et al. (1995). The relationship of neuropsychological functioning to quality of life in epilepsy. Arch Neurol 52: 997–1003.

Placidi GP, Oquendo MA, Malone KM et al. (2001). Aggressivity, suicide attempts, and depression: relationship to cerebrospinal fluid monoamine metabolite levels. Biol Psychiatry 50: 783–791.

Qin P, Xu H, Laursen TM et al. (2005). Risk for schizophrenia and schizophrenia-like psychosis among patients with epilepsy: population based cohort study. BMJ 331: 23.

Ramasubbu R, Tobias R, Buchan AM et al. (2006). Serotonin transporter gene promoter region polymorphism associated with poststroke major depression. J Neuropsychiatry Clin Neurosci 18: 96–99.

Regenold WT, Weintraub D, Taller A (1998). Electroconvulsive therapy for epilepsy and major depression. Am J Geriatr Psychiatry 6: 180–183.

Riad M, Garcia S, Watkins KC et al. (2000). Somatodendritic localization of 5-HT1A and preterminal axonal localization of 5-HT1B serotonin receptors in adult rat brain. J Comp Neurol 417: 181–194.

Rickels K, Downing R, Schweizer E et al. (1993). Antidepressants for the treatment of generalized anxiety disorder: a placebo-controlled comparison of imipramine, trazodone and diazepam. Arch Gen Psychiatry 50: 884–895.

Ried S, Mothersill IW (1998). Forced normalization: the clinical neurologist's view. In: MR Trimble, B Schmitz (Eds.), Forced Normalization and Alternative Psychoses of Epilepsy. Wrightson Biomedical Publishing, Petersfield, pp. 77–94.

Ring HA, Crellin R, Kirker S et al. (1993). Vigabatrin and depression. J Neurol Neurosurg Psychiatry 56: 925–928.

Robertson M (1985). Depression in patients with epilepsy: an overview and clinical study. In: M Trimble (Ed.), The Psychopharmacology of Epilepsy. John Wiley, Chichester p. 65.

Robertson MM (2000). Tourette syndrome, associated conditions and the complexities of treatment. Brain 123: 425–462.

Rosemarie K, Frank G, David JT (2006). Prevalence of self-reported epilepsy or seizure disorder and its associations with self-reported depression and anxiety: results from the 2004 Healthstyles Survey. Epilepsia 47: 1915–1921.

Rubinstein M, Cepeda C, Hurst RS et al. (2001). Dopamine D4 receptor-deficient mice display cortical hyperexcitability. J Neurosci 21: 3756–3763.

Salaycik KJ, Kelly-Hayes M, Beiser A et al. (2007). Depressive symptoms and risk of stroke: the Framingham Study. Stroke 38: 16–21.

Salgado-Commissariat D, Alkadhi KA (1997). Serotonin inhibits epileptiform discharge by activation of 5-HT1A receptors in CA1 pyramidal neurons. Neuropharmacology 36: 1705–1712.

Sapolsky RM, Uno H, Rebert CS et al. (1990). Hippocampal damage associated with prolonged glucocorticoid exposure in primates. J Neurosci 10: 2897–2902.

Savic I, Lindstrom P, Gulyas B et al. (2004). Limbic reductions of 5-HT1A receptor binding in human temporal lobe epilepsy. Neurology 62: 1343–1351.

Schmitz B, Wolf P (1995). Psychosis in epilepsy: frequency and risk factors. J Epilepsy 8: 295–305.

Scott RC, Gadian DG, King MD et al. (2002). Magnetic resonance imaging findings within 5 days of status epilepticus in childhood. Brain 125: 1951–1959.

Scott RC, King MD, Gadian DG et al. (2003). Hippocampal abnormalities after prolonged febrile convulsion: a longitudinal MRI study. Brain 126: 2551–2557.

Scott RC, King MD, Gadian DG et al. (2006). Prolonged febrile seizures are associated with hippocampal vasogenic edema and developmental changes. Epilepsia 47: 1493–1498.

Seidman LJ, Pantelis C, Keshavan MS et al. (2003). A review and new report of medial temporal lobe dysfunction as a vulnerability indicator for schizophrenia: a magnetic resonance imaging morphometric family study of the parahippocampal gyrus. Schizophr Bull 29: 803–830.

Shaw P, Mellers J, Henderson M et al. (2004). Schizophrenia-like psychosis arising de novo following a temporal lobectomy: timing and risk factors. J Neurol Neurosurg Psychiatry 75: 1003–1008.

Shaw P, Eckstrand K, Sharp W et al. (2007a). Attention-deficit/hyperactivity disorder is characterized by a delay in cortical maturation. Proc Natl Acad Sci U S A 104: 19649–19654.

Shaw P, Gornick M, Lerch J et al. (2007b). Polymorphisms of the dopamine D4 receptor, clinical outcome, and cortical structure in attention-deficit/hyperactivity disorder. Arch Gen Psychiatry 64: 921–931.

Sheline YI (2005). Brain structural changes associated with depression. In: F Gilliam, AM Kanner, YI Sheline (Eds.), Depression and Brain Dysfunction. Taylor & Francis, London, pp. 85–104.

Shiah IS, Yatham LN (2000). Serotonin in mania and in the mechanism of action of mood stabilizers: a review of clinical studies. Bipolar Disord 2: 77–92.

Slater E, Beard AW, Glithero E (1963). The schizophrenia-like psychosis of epilepsy. Br J Psychiatry 109: 95–150.

Smith MA, Makino S, Kvetnansky R et al. (1995). Effects of stress on neurotrophic factor expression in the rat brain. Ann N Y Acad Sci 771: 234–239.

Sotelo C, Cholley B, El Mestikawy S et al. (1990). Direct immunohistochemical evidence of the existence of 5-HT1A autoreceptors on serotoninergic neurons in the midbrain raphe nuclei. Eur J Neurosci 2: 1144–1154.

Southwick SM, Vythilingam M, Charney DS (2005). The psychobiology of depression and resilience to stress: implications for prevention and treatment. Annu Rev Clin Psychol 1: 255–291.

Spijker J, de Graaf R, Oldehinkel AJ et al. (2007). Are the vulnerability effects of personality and psychosocial functioning on depression accounted for by subthreshold symptoms? Depress Anxiety 24: 472–478.

Stahl SM (2000a). Depression and bipolar disorders. In: SM Stahl (Ed.), Essential Pharmacology: Neuroscientific Basis and Practical Applications. 2nd edn. Cambridge University Press, New York, pp. 135–197.

Stahl SM (2000b). Antipsychotic agents. In: SM Stahl (Ed.), Essential Pharmacology: Neuroscientific Basis and Practical Applications. 2nd edn. Cambridge University Press, New York, pp. 401–458.

Stahl SM (2004). Psychopharmacology of anticonvulsants: do all anticonvulsants have the same mechanism of action? J Clin Psychiatry 65: 149–150.

Statnick MA, Maring-Smith ML, Clough RW et al. (1996). Effect of 5,7-dihydroxytryptamine on audiogenic seizures in genetically epilepsy-prone rats. Life Sci 59: 1763–1771.

Stefansson SB, Olafsson E, Hauser WA (1998). Psychiatric morbidity in epilepsy: a case controlled study of adults receiving disability benefits. J Neurol Neurosurg Psychiatry 64: 238–241.

Stevens JR (1990). Psychiatric consequences of temporal lobectomy for intractable seizures: a 20–30-year follow-up of 14 cases. Psychol Med 20: 529–545.

Swinkels J, Jonghe F (1995). Safety of antidepressants. Int Clin Psychopharmacol 9: 19–25.

Tarulli A, Devinsky O, Alper K (2001). Progression of postictal to interictal psychosis. Epilepsia 42: 1468–1471.

Tatarczynska E, Klodzinska A, Chojnacka-Wojcik E et al. (2001). Potential anxiolytic- and antidepressant-like effects of MPEP, a potent, selective and systemically active mGlu5 receptor antagonist. Br J Pharmacol 132: 1423–1430.

Tatarczynska E, Palucha A, Szewczyk B et al. (2002). Anxiolytic and antidepressant-like effects of group III metabotropic glutamate agonist (1 S,3R,4 S)-1-aminocyclopentane-1,3,4-tricarboxylic acid (ACPT-I) in rats. Pol J Pharmacol 54: 707–710.

Taylor DC (1972). Mental state and temporal lobe epilepsy. Epilepsia 13: 727–765.

Tellenbach H (1965). Epilepsie als Anfallsleiden und als Psychose: uber alternative Psychosen paranoiderpragung bei "forcierter Normalisierung" (Landolt) des Elektroencephalogramms Epilepttischer. Nervenarzt 36: 190–202.

Tellez-Zenteno JF, Patten SB, Jette N et al. (2007). Psychiatric comorbidity in epilepsy: a population-based analysis. Epilepsia 48: 2336–2344.

Theodore WH, Giovacchini G, Bonwetsch R et al. (2006). The effect of antiepileptic drugs on 5-HT-receptor binding measured by positron emission tomography. Epilepsia 47: 499–503.

Thorup A, Waltoft BL, Pedersen CB et al. (2007). Young males have a higher risk of developing schizophrenia: a Danish register study. Psychol Med 37: 479–484.

Tiihonen J, Nousiainen U, Hakola P et al. (1991). EEG abnormalities associated with clozapine treatment (letter). Am J Psychiatry 148: 1406.

Toczek MT, Carson RE, Lang L et al. (2003). PET imaging of 5-HT1A receptor binding in patients with temporal lobe epilepsy. Neurology 60: 749–756.

Tollefson GD, Rosenbaum JF (1998). Selective serotonin reuptake inhibitors. In: AF Schatzberg, CB Nemeroff (Eds.), Textbook of Psychopharmacology. 2nd edn. American Psychiatric Association Press, Washington, DC, pp. 219–237.

Toth P, Frankenburg FR (1994). Clozapine and seizures: a review. Can J Psychiatry 39: 236–238.

Tremblay LK, Naranjo CA, Graham SJ et al. (2005). Functional neuroanatomical substrates of altered reward processing in major depressive disorder revealed by a dopaminergic probe. Arch Gen Psychiatry 62: 1228–1236.

Trimble MR (1992). Behaviour changes following temporal lobectomy, with special reference to psychosis. J Neurol Neurosurg Psychiatry 55: 89–91.

Trimble MR, Rusch N, Betts T et al. (2000). Psychiatric symptoms after therapy with new antiepileptic drugs: psychopathological and seizure related variables. Seizure 9: 249–254.

Trindade-Filho EM, de Castro-Neto EF, de Carvalho RA et al. (2008). Serotonin depletion effects on the pilocarpine model of epilepsy. Epilepsy Res 82: 194–199.

Umbricht D, Degreef G, Barr WB et al. (1995). Postictal and chronic psychosis in patients with temporal lobe epilepsy. Am J Psychiatry 152: 224–231.

Urstein A (1909). Dementia praecox und ihre Stellung zum manisch-depressiven Irresein. Eine klinische Studie. Urban und Schwarzenberg, Berlin.

VanLandingham KE, Heinz ER, Cavazos JE et al. (1998). Magnetic resonance imaging evidence of hippocampal injury after prolonged focal febrile convulsions. Ann Neurol 43: 413–426.

Versiani M, Cassano G, Perugi G et al. (2002). Reboxetine, a selective norepinephrine reuptake inhibitor, is an effective and well-tolerated treatment for panic disorder. J Clin Psychiatry 63: 31–37.

Vestergaard M, Pedersen CB, Christensen J et al. (2005). Febrile seizures and risk of schizophrenia. Schizophr Res 73: 343–349.

Watanabe K, Minabe Y, Ashby CR, Jr et al. (1998). Effect of acute administration of various 5-HT receptor agonists on focal hippocampal seizures in freely moving rats. Eur J Pharmacol 350: 181–188.

Whitworth AB, Fleischhacker WW (1995). Adverse effects of antipsychotic drugs. Int Clin Psychopharmacol 9: 21–27.

Williams RL (2000). A note on robust variance estimation for cluster-correlated data. Biometrics 56: 645–646.

Williams J, Griebel ML, Dykman RA (1998). Neuropsychological patterns in pediatric epilepsy. Seizure 7: 223–228.

Williams J, Steel C, Sharp GB et al. (2003). Anxiety in children with epilepsy. Epilepsy Behav 4: 729–732.

Wolf P, Trimble MR (1985). Biological antagonism and epileptic psychosis. Br J Psychiatry 146: 272–276.

Index

NB: Page numbers in *italics* refer to boxes, figures and tables

D

F

G

M

O

Q

R

S

FSC
www.fsc.org
MIX
Papier | Fördert gute Waldnutzung
FSC® C083411

Kolibri 360 GmbH
Ferdinand-Jühlke-Straße 7
99095 Erfurt, Deutschland
produktsicherheit@kolibri360.de